Visit our website

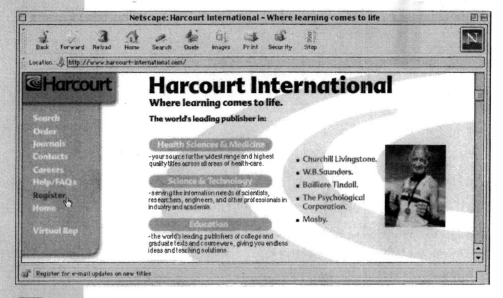
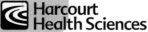

Commissioning Editor: Serena Bureau
Project Development Manager: Tim Kimber
Project Manager: Cheryl Brant/Scott Millar
Production Manager: Mark Sanderson
Designer: Ian Spick

MANUAL OF ASTHMA MANAGEMENT

is a registered trademark of Harcourt Publishers Limited

The right of Paul M. O'Byrne and Neil C. Thomson to be identified as author/s of this work has been asserted by them in accordance with the Copyright, Designs and Patents Act 1988

First edition published 1995

ISBN 0 7020 2529 1

British Library Cataloguing in Publication Data
A catalogue record for this book is available from the British Library

Library of Congress Cataloging in Publication Data
A catalog record for this book is available from the Library of Congress

Note
Medical knowledge is constantly changing. As new information becomes available, changes in treatment, procedures, equipment and the use of drugs become necessary. The editors/authors/contributors and the publishers have, as far as it is possible, taken care to ensure that the information given in this text is accurate and up to date. However, readers are strongly advised to confirm that the information, especially with regard to drug usage, complies with the latest legislation and standards of practice.

Transferred to digital printing 2005

Printed and bound by Antony Rowe Ltd, Eastbourne

MANUAL OF ASTHMA MANAGEMENT

SECOND EDITION

EDITED BY

PAUL M. O'BYRNE MB FRCPI FRCP(C)
EJ Moran Campbell Professor of Medicine
Head of Respiratory Division
McMaster University
Firestone Regional Chest and Allergy Unit
St Joseph's Hospital
Hamilton, Ontario
Canada

NEIL C. THOMSON MD FRCP
Professor of Respiratory Medicine
Department of Respiratory Medicine
Western Infirmary
Glasgow
United Kingdom

WB Saunders
London • Edinburgh • New York • Philadelphia • St Louis • Sydney • Toronto • 2001

Contents

Contributors   viii

Preface   xv

EPIDEMIOLOGY AND PATHOGENESIS OF ASTHMA

1   Definition, classification, epidemiology and risk factors   3
     AJ Woolcock, V Keena and JK Peat

2   Natural history   19
     MR Sears

3   Pathogenesis   27
     PM O'Byrne

DIAGNOSIS AND INVESTIGATIONS OF ASTHMA

4   Triggers of asthma   43
     NC Thomson

5   Diagnosis in children   53
     B Zimmerman

6   Diagnosis in adults   63
     AL Cogo, B Beghè, L Corbetta and LM Fabbri

7   Pulmonary function tests   81
     KJ Killian

8   Provocation tests   91
     DW Cockcroft

9   Investigations of allergy   101
     AB Becker

10   Examination of sputum, nasal cytology and exhaled gases   107
     PG Gibson, DH Yates and N Saltos

11   Bronchoalveolar lavage and bronchial biopsies   119
     E Ådelroth

ASSESSMENT AND TREATMENT OF ASTHMA

12   Assessment of asthma control: symptoms, drug use, PEFR   127
     JM Corne, N Chanarin and ST Holgate

13   Assessment of asthma control: quality of life   135
     EF Juniper

14   Assessment of asthma control: markers of inflammation   143
     K Parameswaran and FE Hargreave

15   Primary prevention of asthma   149
     AB Becker

16   Secondary allergen avoidance measures   157
     PL Powers, JG Wyman and TAE Platts-Mills

17   Corticosteroids   173
     PJ Barnes

18   Anti-allergic drugs   197
     A Cartier

19   Immunosuppressive agents   203
     DJ Evans and DM Geddes

20   Mediator antagonists and other new agents   223
     E Israel and JM Drazen

21   Bronchodilators   237
     J Lötvall

22   Delivery systems   261
     GK Crompton

23   Immunotherapy   273
     SM Walker and SR Durham

24   Other forms of treatment   285
     R Bhagat and DW Cockcroft

25   Patient education   295
     MR Partridge

26   Self-management plans   309
     W D'Souza, J Crane and R Beasley

27   Assessment of compliance   323
     GM Cochrane

MANAGEMENT OF ASTHMA

28 General principles 329
AP Greening

29 Management of chronic asthma in
children 339
JY Paton

30 Management of acute asthma in
children 399
S Pedersen

31 Management of chronic asthma in
adults 421
R Pauwels

32 Management of acute asthma in adults 431
BDW Harrison

33 Specific problems: occupational asthma 443
J-L Malo and M Chan-Yeung

34 Specific problems: asthma induced by
aspirin and other non-steroidal
anti-inflammatory drugs 453
B Dahlén, O Zetterström and S-E Dahlén

35 Specific problems: allergic
bronchopulmonary aspergillosis 463
RM Limbrey and PH Howarth

36 Specific problems: exercise-induced
asthma 471
SD Anderson and JD Brannan

37 Specific problems: nocturnal asthma 487
RJ Martin

38 Specific problems: asthma in pregnancy
and pre-menses 495
A Tuffaha and WW Busse

39 Specific problems: glucocorticoid-
resistant asthma 507
SJ Lane, GM Cochrane and TH Lee

40 Specific problems: psychological factors 515
RE Ruffin, AM Southcott and R Adams

41 Specific problems: gastroesophageal
reflux and asthma 521
CJ Allen and MT Newhouse

42 Specific problems: cough 525
PW Ind

43 Specific problems: chronic rhinosinusitis
and asthma 537
P Assanasen and R Naclerio

44 Specific problems: food allergy in
asthma 553
J Bousquet, D Jaffuel, P Chanez and F-B Michel

45 Specific problems: difficult, therapy-
resistant asthma 559
KF Chung

46 Specific problems: steroid-induced
side-effects 577
NC Barnes

47 Acute complications of asthma 589
B Hickey and EH Walters

48 Chronic complications of asthma 595
NHT ten Hacken, HAM Kerstjens and DS Postma

RUNNING AN ASTHMA SERVICE

49 Primary care 613
ML Levy

50 Hospital practice 631
J Garrett and J Kolbe

51 Audit in asthma 643
BDW Harrison

52 Economics of asthma 655
SD Sullivan, SD Ramsey and KB Weiss

Index 663

Contributors

Robert Adams MBBS MD FRACP
Research Fellow
Channing Laboratory
Brigham and Women's Hospital
Harvard Medical School
Boston, MA
USA

Ellinor Ädelroth MD PHD
Associate Professor
Department of Respiratory Medicine & Allergy
University Hospital
Umea, Sweden

Christopher Allen MA BM BCH MRCP (UK) FRCPC
Associate Clinical Professor of Medicine
McMaster University
Firestone Regional Chest & Allergy Unit
St Josephs Hospital
Hamilton, Ontario
Canada

Sandra Anderson PHD DSC
Principal Hospital Scientist
Department of Respiratory Medicine
Royal Prince Alfred Hospital
Camperdown, NSW
Australia

Paraya Assanasen MD
Fellow in Allergy and Rhinology
The University of Chicago
Chicago, IL
USA

Neil Barnes MD
Consultant Physician
Department of Respiratory Medicine
The London Chest Hospital
London, UK

Peter Barnes MA DM DSC FRCP
Department of Thoracic Medicine
National Heart and Lung Institute
London, UK

Richard Beasley MBCHB FRACP MD
Professor of Medicine
Department of Medicine
Wellington School of Medicine
Wellington, New Zealand

Allan Becker MD FRCPC
Professor, Section of Allergy and Clinical Immunology
Department of Pediatrics & Child Health
University of Manitoba
Winnipeg, MB
Canada

Bianca Beghé MD
Fellow, Department of Clinical and Experimental Medicine
Section of Respiratory Disease
University of Ferrara
Ferrara, Italy

Rajesh Bhagat MBBS MD
Fellow, Division of Pulmonary and Critical Care Medicine
Department of Medicine
Duke University Medical Center
Durham, NC
USA

Jean Bousquet
Service des Maladies Respiratoires
Hospital Arnaud de Villeneuve
Montpellier, France

John Brannan BSC
Research Assistant
Department of Respiratory Medicine
Royal Prince Alfred Hospital
Camperdown, NSW
Australia

William Busse MD
Professor of Medicine
Department of Medicine
University of Wisconsin Medical School
Section of Allergy/Clinical Immunology
Madison, WI
USA

André Cartier MD FRCP(C)
Clinical Professor of Medicine
Chest Department
Sacre-Coeur Hospital
Montreal, Quebec
Canada

Nicholas Chanarin MBCHB MR CP
Department of University Medicine
Southampton General Hospital
Southampton, UK

Pascal Chanez
Hospital Arnaud de Villeneuve
Service des Maladies Respiratoires
Centre Hospitalier Universitaire
Montpellier, France

M Chan-Yeung
Department of Medicine, Respiratory Division
Vancouver General Hospital
University of British Columbia
Vancouver, BC
Canada

Kian Chung MD FRCP
Professor of Respiratory Medicine
National Heart and Lung Institute
Imperial College School of Medicine
London, UK

Cochrane Gordon BSC MBBS FRCP
Consultant Physician
Department of Allergy and Respiratory Medicine
Guy's Hospital
London, UK

Donald Cockcroft BSC MD FRCP(C)
Professor and Head of Division of Respiratory
Medicine
Royal University Hospital
Saskatoon, Sasktchewan
Canada

Annalisa Cogo MD
Assistant Professor
Department of Clinical and Experimental
Medicine
Section of Respiratory Disease
University of Ferrara
Ferrara, Italy

Lorenzo Corbetta MD
Consultant Physician
Department of Pulmonary Diseases
University of Modena and Reggio Emilia
Modena, Italy

Jonathon Corne MA PHD MRCP
Consultant Physician
Department of Respiratory Medicine
University Hospital
Queen's Medical Centre
Nottingham, UK

Julian Crane MBBS FRACP
Professorial Research Fellow
Department of Medicine
Wellington School of Medicine
Wellington, New Zealand

G Crompton MBCHB FRCPE FCCP
Consultant Physician (retired)
Respiratory Unit
Western General Hospital
University of Edinburgh
Edinburgh, UK

Barbro Dahlén
Department of Internal Medicine
Asthma and Allergy Research
Division of Pulmonary Medicine
Karolinksa Institute
Stockholm, Sweden

Sven-Erik Dahlén MD PHD
Institute of Environmental Medicine
Division of Experimental Asthma and Allergy
Research
Karolinksa Institute
Stockholm, Sweden

Jeffrey Drazen MD
Parker B Francis Professor of Medicine
Pulmonary Division
Harvard Medical School
Brigham & Women's Hospital
Boston, MA
USA

Wendyl D'Souza MBCHB
HRC Research Fellow
Department of Medicine
Wellington School of Medicine
Wellington, New Zealand

Stephen Durham MA MD MRCP
Professor of Allergy and Respiratory Medicine
Upper Respiratory Medicine
Royal Brompton Hospital/NHLI
London, UK

David Evans MD MRCP
Consultant Physician
Department of Respiratory Medicine
St Mary's Hospital
Portsmouth, UK

Leonardo Fabbri MD
Professor
Department of Pulmonary Diseases
University of Modena and Reggio Emilia
Modena, Italy

Jeff Garrett MBCHB FRACP
Clinical Director Respiratory Medicine
Green Lane Hospital
Respiratory Services
Auckland, New Zealand

Duncan Geddes MD FRCP
Consultant Physician
Department of Respiratory Medicine
Royal Brompton Hospital
London, UK

Peter Gibson MBBS(HONS) FRACP
Staff Specialist
Department of Respiratory and Sleep Medicine
John Hunter Hospital
Newcastle, NSW
Australia

Andrew Greening BSC MBCHB FRCPE
Consultant Physician and Reader in Respiratory
Medicine
Western General Hospital
Lothian University Hospitals NHS Trust
Edinburgh, Scotland
and University of Edinburgh

Frederick Hargreave MBCHB MD FRCP FRCPC
Professor of Medicine
McMaster University
Firestone Regional Chest and Allergy Unit
St Joseph's Hospital
Hamilton, ON
Canada

Brian Harrison MA MB BCHIR FRCP(Lond) FRCP(Edin)
FCCP
Consultant Physician
Department of Respiratory Medicine
Norfolk & Norwich Hospital
Norwich, UK

Bernadette Hickey MBBS FRACP
Senior Specialist
Intensive Care Unit
St Vincent's Hospital
Fitzroy, Victoria
Australia

Stephen Holgate MD DSC FRCP
MCR Clinical Professor of
Immunopharmacology
Department of University Medicine
Southampton General Hospital
Southampton, UK

Peter Howarth BSC(HONS) DM FRCP
Reader in Medicine and Hon Consultant
Physician
Department of Medical Specialities
Southampton General Hospital
Southampton, UK

Philip Ind
Senior Lecturer/Honorary Consultant Physician
Acting Head, Department of Respiratory
Medicine
Department of Respiratory Medicine
Hammersmith Hospital
London, UK

Elliot Israel MD
Associate Professor of Medicine
Harvard Medical School
Director of Clinical Research
Pulmonary Division
Brigham & Women's Hospital
Boston, MA
USA

Dany Jaffuel MD PHD
Hopital Arnaud de Villeneuve
Clinique des Maladies Respiratoires
Centre Hospitalier Universitaire
Montepellier, France

Elizabeth Juniper MCSP MSC
Department of Clinical Epidemiology &
Biostatistics
McMaster University Medical Centre
Hamilton, Ontario
Canada

Victoria Keena BA
Information Manager
Royal Prince Alfred Hospital
Institute of Respiratory Medicine
Camperdown, New South Wales
Australia

Huib Kerstjens MD PHD
Lung Physician
Department of Pulmonology
University Hospital Groningen
Groningen, Netherlands

Kieran Killian MD FRCP(C)
Professor of Medicine
McMaster University Medical Center
Ambrose Cardio-Respiratory Dept
Hamilton, Ontario
Canada

John Kolbe MBBS FRACP
Associate Professor of Medicine, Respiratory
Physician
Respiratory Services
Green Lane Hospital
Auckland, New Zealand

Stephen Lane MB PHD FRCP FRCPI
Consultant Respiratory Physician
Adelaide & Meath Hospital
Dublin, Ireland

Tak Lee MD SCD FRCPATH FRCP
Professor of Respiratory Medicine and
Allergy
Guy's, King's College and St Thomas' School
of Medicine
Guy's Hospital
London, UK

Mark Levy MBCHB FRCGP
General Practitioner
Kenton Bridge Medical Centre
Kenton, Middlesex
UK

Rachel Limbrey MBBS MRCP
Clinical Research Fellow
Department of Medical Specialities
Southampton General Hospital
Southampton, UK

Jan Lötvall MD PHD
Associate Professor
Lung Pharmacology Group
Department of Respiratory Medicine and
Allergology
Göteborg University
Gothenburg, Sweden

Jean-Luc Malo MD
Professor of Medicine
Chest Department
Sacre-Coeur Hospital
Montreal, Quebec
Canada

Richard Martin MD
Professor of Medicine
University of Colorado
Head: Pulmonary Division and Vice Chair
Department of Medicine
National Jewish Medical and Research Center
Denver, CO
USA

Francois Michel
Hopital Arnaud de Villeneuve
Services des Maladies Respiratoires
Centre Hospitalier Universitaire
Montepellier, France

Robert Naclerio MD
Professor and Chief of Surgery
Otolarynglogy/Head and Neck
University of Chicago
Chicago, IL
USA

Michael Newhouse MD MSC FRCP FACP
Visiting Professor of Medicine
Stanford Medical School
Palo Alto, CA
USA

Paul O'Byrne MB FRCPI FRCP(C)
Head of Respiratory Division
McMaster University
Firestone Regional Chest and Allergy Unit
St Joseph's Hospital
Hamilton, Ontario
Canada

Krishnan Parameswaran MBBS MD MNAMS MRCP FCCP
Research Fellow
McMaster University
Firestone regional Chest and Allergy Unit
St Joseph's Hospital
Hamilton, Ontario
Canada

Martyn Partridge MD FRCP
Chest Clinic
Whipps Cross Hospital
London, UK

James Paton MD MRCP
Senior Lecturer in Paediatric Respiratory Disease
Department of Child Health
Royal Hospital for Sick Children
Glasgow, Scotland
UK

Romain Pauwels MD PHD
Professor of Medicine
Department of Respiratory Diseases
University Hospital Ghent
Ghent, Belgium

Jennifer Peat PHD
Senior Lecturer
Department of Paediatrics and Child Health
University of Sydney
Sydney, Australia

Søren Pedersen MD
Professor of Respiratory Pediatric Medicine
University of Southern Denmark
Kolding Hospital
Kolding, Denmark

Thomas Platts-Mills MD PHD FRCP
Department of Internal Medicine
University of Virginia Health System
Division of Asthma & Allergic Diseases Center
Charlottesville, VA
USA

Dirkje Postma MD PHD
Professor of Pulmonary Diseases
Department of Pulmonology Diseases
University Hospital Groningen
Groningen, Netherlands

Patrick Powers MD
Department of Internal Medicine
University of Virginia Health System
Asthma and Allergic Diseases Center
Charlottesville, VA
USA

Scott Ramsey MD PHD
Assistant Professor
Departments of Medicine and Health
Services
University of Washington
Seattle, WA
USA

Richard Ruffin BSC(HONS) MBSS(HONS) MD FRACP
Professor of Medicine
Department of Medicine
University of Adelaide, TQEH Campus
Woodville, SA
Australia

Nicholas Saltos MBBS FRACP FCCP FRCPI FRCP
Senior Staff Specialist
Department of Respiratory and Sleep Medicine
John Hunter Hospital
Newcastle, New South Wales
Australia

Malcolm Sears MB CHB FRACP FRCPC
Professor of Medicine
McMaster University
Director
Firestone Regional Chest and Allergy Unit
St Joseph's Hospital
Hamilton, Ontario
Canada

Anne Marie Southcott MBBS(HONS) FRACP
Physician, Respiratory Medicine
Acting Director, Respiratory Medicine
The Queen Elizabeth Hospital
Woodville
Australia

Sean Sullivan MS PHD
Associate Professor of Pharmacy
Director
Program in Pharmaceutical Outcomes Research
and Policy
School of Pharmacy
University of Washington
Seattle, WA
USA

Nick ten Hacken MD PHD
Lung Physician
Department of Pulmonology
University Hospital Groningen
Groningen, Netherlands

Neil Thomson MD FRCP
Professor of Respiratory Medicine
Department of Respiratory Medicine
Western Infirmary
Glasgow, UK

Amjad Tuffaha MD
Allergy and Clinical Immunology Fellow
University of Wisconsin Medical School
Section of Allergy and Clinical Immunology
Madison, WI
USA

Samantha Walker
Research Fellow
Upper Respiratory Medicine
Royal Brompton Hospital/NHLI
London, UK

Haydn Walters MA DM FRCP FRACP FCCP
Professor of Medicine, Director of Respiratory
Medicine
The Alfred Hospital and Monash University
Medical School
Melbourne, Vic
Australia

Kevin Weiss MD
Associate Professor and Director
Director, Center for Health Services Research
Rush Primary Care Institute
Rush University
Chicago, IL
USA

Ann Woolcock AO MD FAA FRACP
Director, Institute of Respiratory Medicine
Royal Prince Alfred Hospital
Camperdown, New South Wales
Australia

Jennifer Wyman MD
Department of Internal Medicine
University of Virginia Health Sciences Center
Division of Asthma & Allergic Diseases
Charlottesville, VA
USA

Deborah Yates MBBCHIR MA MSC MD AFOM MRCP
FRACP
Senior Lecturer in Medicine
Department of Respiratory Medicine
Royal North Shore Hospital
St Leonards, Australia

Olle Zetterström
Department of Internal Medicine
Karolinska Hospital
Asthma & Allergy Research at the Division of
Pulmonary Medicine
Stockholm, Sweden

Barry Zimmerman MD FRCPC
Gage Occupational & Environmental Health
Unit
St Michael's Hospital
University of Toronto
Toronto, ON
Canada

Preface

Asthma is the commonest chronic disease of children and adults and there is compelling evidence that the prevalence is rising in many western countries. The morbidity and mortality from asthma is considerable. The first edition of this book appeared in 1995 to provide comprehensive, yet practical and easily accessed advice on the key isues of asthma management. Because of advancing knowledge and increasing interest in asthma we believe it is necessary to produce a second edition after only five years. This new edition has involved updating all the chapters and the addition of several new chapters. It is intended that the manual will aid all those involved with the care of asthmatic patients to apply the published national and international guidelines on the diagnosis and treatment of asthma. We hope that the manual will be used to answer day-to-day clinical problems in asthma management and that in this way it will allow an individualised approach to treatment. We have selected internationally recognised experts on asthma as contributors and have asked them to write for a readership of physicians and other health care professionals who are involved in the day-to-day management of patients with asthma. We are grateful for the enthusiastic way they have helped us to undertake this project. We hope that the book will be of value to general internalists, general practitioners and specialists in respiratory medicine, pulmonology, allergy and paediatrics. Finally we wish to thank Maria Khan and Tim Kimber of W. B. Saunders for all their help and encouragement.

Paul O'Byrne
Neil Thomson
2000

Part 1

Epidemiology and Pathogenesis of Asthma

Chapter 1

Definition, Classification, Epidemiology and Risk Factors

Ann Woolcock, Victoria Keena and Jennifer Peat

INTRODUCTION

It is important that results of research studies can be used to facilitate better methods for preventing and managing asthma in both clinical and population settings. To this end, information of the relative importance of risk factors and their impact on prevalence is essential for designing interventions for preventing the development of disease at an early stage and for reducing severity in those subjects in whom airway inflammation is already established.

In the last 20 years, there have been landmark advances from pharmacological and clinical studies in understanding the mechanisms and treatment of asthma. In addition, epidemiological studies conducted in recent years have revealed a great deal of information about the nature, the likely causes and the natural history of asthma. Epidemiological studies provide knowledge of prevalence and morbidity which is important for resource allocation and for population surveillance. However, they are the only tools that can be used to measure the risk factors associated with the development of asthma. Until this knowledge is available, preventive strategies will not be developed.

In order to make the information from research relevant to these goals, it is important to be able to define asthma accurately, to classify the burden of illness according to severity, and to have precise information about both prevalence and risk factors. This chapter discusses:

- the relative merits of different methods of classifying asthma;
- the impact of asthma in communities;
- knowledge of risk factors that may lead to effective preventive strategies for the control of asthma.

DEFINITIONS OF ASTHMA AND ALLERGY

Because many different mechanisms and causal pathways are involved in the development of asthma, an exact definition that encompasses all conditions is not realistic. However, several working definitions have been devised that describe the broad spectrum of asthma phenotypes. It is important that each of these definitions is used in situations in which it is appropriate to the specific purposes of the study. In research studies designed to investigate risk factors, the effects of interventions or the natural history of asthma, inaccuracies or errors in classifications will lead to measurement errors in assessing causation or prognosis.

Clinical Definition

Asthma is an inflammatory disease of the airways that is associated with abnormal response mechanisms of the airway smooth muscles that lead to episodes of airway narrowing. For this reason, asthma is often described as a disease of the airways that makes the airways prone to narrow excessively in response to a variety of provoking stimuli.[1]

Pathological Definition

Asthma is a disease of the airways characterized by chronic inflammation with infiltration of lymphocytes, eosinophils, and mast cells together with epithelial desquamation, thickening, and disorganisation of the tissues of the airway wall.

American Thoracic Society Definition

Asthma is a clinical syndrome characterized by increased responsiveness of the tracheo-bronchial tree to a variety of stimuli. The major symptoms of asthma are paroxysms of dyspnoea, wheezing and cough, which may vary from almost undetectable to mild to severe and unremitting (status asthmaticus). The primary physiological manifestation of this hyperresponsiveness is variable airways obstruction. This can take the form of spontaneous fluctuations in the severity of obstruction following bronchodilators or corticosteroids, or increased obstruction caused by drugs or other stimuli.[2]

Acute Attacks and Exacerbations

Asthma episodes are referred to as "acute attacks" if they are short-lived and easily reversed with reliever medications. However, if the acute symptom episode lasts longer than one day, the attack is referred to as an "asthma exacerbation".

Allergy

Allergy is a condition associated with increased levels of circulating IgE to common environmental allergens. The terms "allergy", "atopy", "atopic status", "atopic sensitization" and "atopic sensitivity" are often used interchangeably. In epidemiological studies and in clinical situations, the presence of allergy is usually measured by skin-prick tests because this is less expensive and less invasive than measurements of serum IgE level.

Airway Hyperresponsiveness

Airway hyperresponsiveness (AHR) is defined as an abnormal response of the airways to a provoking stimulus. As such, AHR is usually defined as a 20% fall in the forced expiratory volume in 1s (FEV_1) in response to a provoking agent such as inhaled methacholine or histamine (direct stimuli) or physical stimuli such as exercise (indirect stimulus). The presence of AHR is considered to be a marker of airway wall abnormality including thickening, inflammation and/or altered contractility of the smooth muscle. The degree of AHR may vary from a severe condition, in which a 20% fall is triggered by very low doses of a provoking agent, to mild, in which a much higher dose of provoking agent is required to bring about a 20% fall in FEV_1.[3,4] Mild AHR is much less likely to be associated with the presence of symptoms than moderate or severe AHR.[5]

CLASSIFICATION OF ASTHMA AND ALLERGY

Classification by Severity

In the clinic, the severity of asthma is usually assessed by a combination of measurements including the severity and frequency of symptoms, variability of peak flow measurements, and lung function tests.[6,7] These measurements provide an invaluable objective assessment of disease severity, as shown in Table 1.1.

There are many problems in classifying asthma according to severity because the signs and symptoms do not remain constant. Asthmatic symptoms can occur transiently or can vary in severity from day to day. In addition, asthma can go into periods of apparent remission or sudden relapse.[8] The defining characteristics of asthma can occur in combination or in isolation from one another[9] and potential predictive factors such as atopy and AHR are not always associated with severity. The following categories of severity are often used to describe asthma.

Table 1.1: Asthma severity during a non-acute episode

Asthma severity	Symptoms	Bronchodilator use	Peak expiratory flow rate	
			Lowest a.m. % Personal best	% Predicted
Episodic	None	Less than once per month	More than 80%	More than or equal to 100%
Mild persistent	Less than once weekly or on exercise only	Less than once per week	70–80%	90–100%
Moderate persistent	More than once weekly, occasional night waking	Most days	60–70%	70–100%
Severe persistent	Waking most nights	More than four times a day	40–60%	60–100%

Persistent Asthma

Persistent asthma is a chronic abnormality of the airways characterized by either decreased lung function or the presence of AHR between attacks. Persistent, severe asthma causes ongoing frequent symptoms that limit life-style. In patients with this illness, the severity of the symptom episodes can be lessened with the use of inhaled corticosteroids. The histological features of mild, persistent asthma have been described.[10,11] There is some evidence that persistent asthma can go into remission at adolescence and that it can return in later life.[12]

Current Asthma

The term "current asthma" is often used as an epidemiological definition to describe subjects who have AHR on presentation and who have had symptoms of wheeze during the previous year.[5,13,14] Longitudinal population studies show that children with "current asthma" have a more severe illness in terms of atopy, medication requirements, activity limitation and disturbed sleep than children with either AHR or wheeze in the absence of each other.[15] Subjects with current asthma may have mild AHR that sometimes reduces into the normal range, when they then become classified as having episodic or intermittent asthma.

Episodic or Intermittent Asthma

Episodic asthma, which is sometimes called intermittent asthma, is characterized by intermittent respiratory symptoms of sufficient severity to require medication. However, subjects with episodic asthma do not have AHR in symptom-free periods[16] and may not be atopic.[17] Episodic asthma is the most common form of asthma in children[18] and in adults with recent onset of occupational asthma.[19] A characteristic of this type of asthma is that episodes of wheezing can be induced by occasional environmental insults such as viral infections or exposure to high pollen loads.[20]

Obstructed Asthma

Obstructed asthma is characterized by asthmatic symptoms, some reversibility of FEV_1, but airflow limitation that persists after maximal treatment with bronchodilators and oral corticosteroids. Usually AHR cannot be measured because of poor lung function. The pathological changes that lead to the irreversible airflow limitation are not known.

Asthma in Remission

In some subjects asthma goes into remission, often for long periods of time. There is a previous history of symptoms and of AHR, and mild AHR may persist even though the subject has had no symptoms or requirement for treatment in the previous year.

Potential Asthma

A subject with normal lung function who has AHR but who has not experienced symptoms of wheeze has potential asthma. The level of AHR may be severe or moderate. Subjects with asymptomatic AHR and atopy are more likely to develop symptoms at some time in the future than non-atopic subjects.[21] Although the presence of atopy and exposure to inhaled allergens may explain the presence of AHR in these subjects, the mechanisms that protect against the development of symptoms are not known.

Trivial Asthma

Trivial asthma is a term coined by the authors to describe subjects who have episodes of wheeze that are intermittent and are not of sufficient severity to warrant preventive treatment. This abnormality, which is more common in infants and in young children, only progresses to a more severe form of asthma in a minority of the subjects.

Cough-Variant Asthma

The term cough-variant asthma was first described in clinical studies, but is a misnomer for most children who have a persistent cough. Population studies show that children who cough persistently at night but who do not have any symptoms of wheeze do not have an illness that has features in common with asthma.[22,23] The aetiology of the persistent cough is not known, but it is more likely to result from irritation of the upper airways than from an inflammatory condition associated with sensitization to common allergens in the lower airways.

EPIDEMIOLOGICAL DEFINITIONS OF ASTHMA, AIRWAY HYPERRESPONSIVENESS AND ALLERGY

Although measurements of lung function and AHR can be collected in population studies, these measurements are time-consuming and expensive to conduct, especially if the sample size is large. Thus, in population studies, questionnaire responses relating to symptom frequency and effects of symptoms on lifestyle are more frequently used to collect information of asthma severity.[24] The questions that delineate symptoms of asthma that are associated with atopy or AHR from those of cough or breathlessness (unassociated with an atopic condition) have been well defined and validated.[25]

Symptom History

Most measurements of asthma in population studies are made using questionnaires, largely because they are cost-effective and simple to administer. In recent years, standardized, worldwide studies conducted by the International Study of Asthma and Allergies in Childhood (ISAAC) and the European Community Respiratory Health Survey (ECHRS) have relied on questionnaire reports to measure the prevalence and severity of asthma in populations.[26,27]

Despite the many advantages with their use, questionnaire responses are subject to recall bias and may therefore lack precision. In addition, questionnaire responses can be influenced by cultural, sociological and psychological factors, and bias in replies may occur because questions of wheeze history are subject to different interpretations of the term, or because parents may be unaware of symptoms in their child. However, questionnaires are important for research because they are the only method of collecting retrospective information of symptoms and current information of exposure to many risk factors. For this reason, it is important that questionnaires are carefully developed, tested and validated prior to their use in research studies.[28]

Objective Measurements

Objective measurements, such as measurements of lung function, peak flow variability and AHR, are preferred to document the nature and severity of asthma because they eliminate the recall and information bias that is inherent in symptom reporting. These types of measurements, which are important indicators of the severity of asthma, can be readily obtained in epidemiological studies. A variety of airway challenge tests have been developed for epidemiological use, including the use of pharmacological agents such as histamine or methacholine, exercise or hyperventilation with cold air.[4,29–31] Although these measurements are subject to less bias and are therefore more reliable than questionnaires, they only provide a "snap-shot" of disease severity at a single point in time and do not give

any information of past illness or of recent fluctuations in severity.

Current Asthma

In population studies, it is not possible to classify asthma solely by AHR status because approximately one-quarter of subjects with AHR do not report any respiratory symptoms, and about half of the subjects who experience some symptoms of wheeze do not have AHR.[5,32] The epidemiological definition of "current asthma" as the presence of both recent symptoms and AHR has proved to be more useful because this identifies the group in the population with the most severe, ongoing abnormality compared to the use of either definition alone.[33] This definition also has better validity against other markers of symptom severity than a doctor diagnosis of asthma or the presence of recent respiratory symptoms.[34] This definition has also proved useful for measuring the risk factors that are associated with a clinically important level of morbidity,[35] and for describing prognosis.[15]

Allergic Status

In epidemiological studies that are designed to measure risk factors for asthma, atopy is usually measured using skin prick tests to a battery of common, inhaled allergens.[36] The allergens associated with asthma vary because local allergen exposure levels vary substantially between and within regions.[37] For this reason, the content of testing panels usually includes some allergens that are found globally and others that are added to accommodate local conditions.

In some regions, measurements of total serum IgE may not be a good guide to allergy that is associated with asthma because total levels are affected by other allergic reactions, including those to parasites that are irrelevant to asthma. However, in other regions, measurements of specific IgE levels have good agreement with skin-prick tests.[38]

When comparing populations, it is important that the allergens used in skin-prick test panels are standardized between studies, have comparable dilutions and that the size of the skin wheal that defines atopy is decided. The mean skin wheal diameter that has the best validity against asthmatic symptoms varies with age. The most commonly used cut-off points that have optimal validity against symptoms are 2 mm as a positive test for infants, 3 mm for children and 4 mm for adults.

PREVALENCE OF ASTHMA

A significant increase in the prevalence of asthma was documented throughout the 1980s and early 1990s, especially in children in affluent countries.[39–41] The concept of a real increase in the prevalence of asthma has been validated by increases in admission rates to hospital[42,43] and in studies that have used objective markers such as airway responsiveness.[44,45] Although the rate of increase does not seem to have been as high in recent years, there has been no indication of a trend for the prevalence of childhood asthma to decrease in any country.

In Australia, the significant increase in prevalence of asthma in the 1980s[46] now seems to have levelled off in the 1990s.[47] However, apart from some evidence that domestic house-dust mite numbers increased during this period,[48] no other information was collected that could be used to identify why the prevalence increased dramatically in the 1980s. Also, we do not know why some countries have more asthma than other countries, although the beginning of worldwide collaborative studies should facilitate the collection of this information in the next decade. There is biological plausibility for the involvement of a wide variety of factors including diet, allergen load, air pollutant levels, infection rates and housing or life-style changes.

International Prevalence Rates

Recent epidemiological studies that have used standardized and validated methods to carefully document the prevalence and severity of asthma symptoms in many communities and ethnic groups throughout the world[49,50] have been a major advance in the population surveillance of asthma. These studies show that there is almost a 6-fold difference in the prevalence of asthma symptoms in children, from approximately 5% in China to almost 30% in various regions in Oceania. Variations in the prevalence of asthma in adults studied in the ECHRS were less marked because the studies were limited to European and allied countries. However, differences between countries in the prevalence rates measured in adults tended to reflect the regional variations found in children. There is a wide acceptance that these variations are almost certainly a result of different environmental exposures, which strongly suggests that asthma is a preventable illness.

Mortality Rates

Mortality statistics provide an estimate of the amount of severe disease in communities and, to some extent, reflect treatment practices. Mortality statistics for the 5–34 year age group are the most reliable because they lack some of the complications in labelling that may occur for deaths in older or younger age groups.[51] Mortality data are useful for alerting countries to epidemics of deaths, in leading to improvements in management, and for investigating gender and age differences to make inferences about treatment patterns. However, mortality rates should only be interpreted in relation to the prevalence and management of asthma in a particular country and, for this reason, cannot be extrapolated to asthma severity and management in a broader context.

The mortality rates for asthma in the 5–34 year old age group in the USA, Canada, England and Wales, Australia, New Zealand and France are shown in Fig. 1.1. From this figure, two epidemics of deaths are evident. The first occurred in the 1960s in England and Wales, Australia and New Zealand and the second occurred in the 1980s in New Zealand only. This second epidemic led to studies that strongly suggested that the regular, long term use of high doses of fenoterol was associated with an increased risk of death.[52] This finding then led to the suggestion that the epidemic in the 1960s was associated with the regular use of isoprenaline forte.[53] A more recent study in Canada suggested that the use of salbutamol, as well as formoterol, may increase the risk of death.[54] However, the data are ecological and therefore are not able to provide good evidence of causation. On the other hand, repeated studies have shown that inhaled corticosteroids, even when administered in low doses, protect against death.[55] It is interesting that mortality rates for a number of western countries have decreased in the last decade even though prevalence of asthma varies and asthma management methods differ widely.[56]

Risk Factors

It is crucial to have good knowledge of the actions of risk factors for asthma in order that prevention can be achieved. There are three types of prevention possible, primary, secondary and tertiary prevention of asthma are shown in Table 1.2. Primary prevention is the manipulation of risk factors that are responsible for asthma onset in order to prevent the allergic-asthmatic process from beginning. Secondary prevention involves

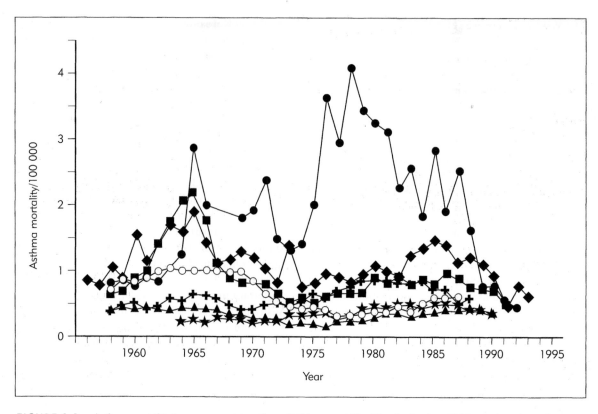

FIGURE 1.1: Asthma mortality in seven countries. (Ages 5–34 years old.) —■—, England and Wales; —◆—, Australia; —●—, New Zealand; —▲—, USA; —✦—, West Germany; —★—, Canada; —○—, Japan.

Table 1.2: Role of risk factors in the development and exacerbation of asthma

Role	Likely process	Application
Primary	Switch on sensitization to inhaled allergens and development of asthmatic processes	Prevent onset using interventions to control environmental risk factors
Secondary	Increase severity of airway inflammation in subjects with elevated serum IgE	Screen for presence of wheeze, allergy (skin-prick test) or eczema to begin early treatment
Tertiary	Trigger acute exacerbations in those who have established illness	Prevent exacerbations and reduce risk of disability in those with symptoms using relevant treatment

the screening of populations for early signs of asthma in order to begin interventions that will prevent the progress to severe disease. Tertiary prevention, involves the manipulation of factors that trigger exacerbations in those who have already developed inflammation of the airways, and has the potential to reduce the risk of disability and improve quality of life. All three types of prevention are essential for reducing the impact of asthma in populations.

To work towards preventing asthma, it is crucial to have precise knowledge of the effects of the risk factors that are potentially open to modification. Although we

Table 1.3: Non-preventable and preventable risk factors

Non-preventable risk factors		Preventable risk factors	
Factor	**Surrogate measurements**	**Factor**	**Surrogate measurements**
Genetic	Family history, gender, ethnicity	Allergen exposure	Sensitization to house-dust mites, moulds, pollens, animals, cockroaches, damp and mould in home
Infections	Vaccination status, maternal infections in pregnancy, exposure to other children	Diet	Omega fatty acids, anti-oxidants, salt, magnesium, selenium
Airway size	Birth weight, head circumference, prematurity, maternal age	Tobacco smoke	Pre- and post-natal maternal smoking, exposure to environmental tobacco smoke
		Breast-feeding	Early introduction of cow's milk
		Outdoor and indoor air pollutants	Industrial air pollutants, gas cooking, diesel exhaust
		Occupational exposures	Western red cedar

do not have any information on the factors responsible for differences in prevalence between countries or for the increased prevalence of asthma in affluent countries in recent years, we have good knowledge of several major risk factors that are associated with the presence of asthma during childhood. Table 1.3 shows examples of the risk factors for asthma categorized into two distinct groups, non-preventable and potentially preventable factors. The non-preventable factors are important for identifying the groups who are most at risk of developing asthma and could be used to identify groups of children in whom early interventions may be most effective. The preventable risk factors, which are environmental in origin, may play a primary role in causing asthma or a secondary or tertiary role in precipitating or triggering asthma symptoms, which suggests that many benefits may derive from prevention of exposures.

Allergen Exposure

The relation between allergic sensitization and the severity of asthma is now well-established. Recent studies of risk factors show that, of all the factors that have been investigated, sensitization to allergens is by far the most important risk factor for asthma in both children and adults.[47,57,58]

House-Dust Mite Allergens In humid regions, house-dust mites provide a potent source of allergens that are associated with asthma severity.[35,59] These allergens are thought to be one of the dominant causes of asthma because they are ubiquitous, occur perennially and release biochemically active enzymes that increase airway permeability and activate inflammatory cells to produce IgE.[60] In regions where house-dust mites are prevalent, most allergic subjects become sensitized to these allergens and up to 50% of children who are sensitized to house-dust mites may develop asthma.[61]

Since a causal relation between exposure to house-dust mite allergens and the severity of asthma in sensitized subjects was first suggested,[62] experimental evidence of a dose–response relationship has been established. Epidemiological studies in Australia have shown that the risk for house-dust mite sensitized children to have current asthma approximately doubles with every doubling of house-dust mite allergen exposure level.[61] A similar relationship has also been demonstrated in a clinical study that was able to control for exposures to pollens and domestic cats.[59] In population terms, these data suggest that the risk of current asthma in sensitized children could be halved, or in clinical terms the severity of asthma could be halved, if levels of house-dust mite allergen exposure could be similarly reduced. Because of this potential for prevention at all levels, many studies to investigate the efficacy and effectiveness of house-dust mite allergen control procedures have been conducted.[63,64]

Reducing House-Dust Mite Allergen Exposures

The effectiveness of various methods in reducing house-dust mite allergen exposure varies considerably. The most expensive methods of removing carpets or altering internal ventilation and heating systems[65] are the most effective, but these methods are clearly unsuitable for large-scale public health interventions. In recent years, less expensive and more practical control methods have been developed and have proved to be effective. These methods include the use of occlusive covers on mattresses and pillows, hot washing of bedding and use of eucalyptus oils or acaracidal laundry additives to kill the mites and remove their allergens.[66] Although these methods have been tested in trials of tertiary prevention, evidence of their effectiveness in primary prevention is only just beginning to emerge.

The primary prevention trials that have been conducted to date have investigated the combined avoidance of inhaled and ingested food allergens. Of these, the most scientifically rigorous study, which was conducted in the UK, found encouraging evidence of a significant reduction in atopy and allergic symptoms in "high risk" infants in each year of study up to age 4 years.[67] A more recent study in Japan showed that the use of occlusive covers could reduce the incidence of house-dust mite sensitization significantly in high-risk babies,[68] but the long-term effectiveness of preventing childhood asthma will not be known for some years.

Moulds and Pollens

The relative importance of different allergens causing allergic disease varies geographically with climate. House-dust mites thrive in humid environments. In Australia for example, allergic sensitization to house-dust mite declines from 34% in children living by the coast to 13% in children living in Broken Hill which is 800 km inland.[69] In contrast, the mould *Alternaria* thrives in hot dry environments so that allergic sensitization to this mould is 23% in the dry, desert environment of Broken Hill compared with 8% in the humid, coastal environment of Sydney.

The role of moulds in asthma is not nearly as well-documented as the role of house-dust mites. *Cladosporium* is commonly reported to be the most abundant mould[70,71] and has been demonstrated to be allergenic, but its role in causing asthma exacerbations has not been well-investigated. However, there is evidence that levels of individual species of moulds in ambient air can reach over 2000 spores m^{-3} and that moulds constitute the largest proportion of respirable allergenic particles in the atmosphere.[72] A study in Minnesota found that exposure to high levels of *Alternaria* were associated with severe asthma exacerbations during summer and autumn.[73] In addition, a study in Tuscon demonstrated that sensitization to *Alternaria* has an important association with asthma in children.[74]

Many studies have found a significant relation between dampness and mould in the home and the presence of asthmatic symptoms and cough in both children and in adults.[75] Home dampness is thought to have health consequences because it has the potential to increase the proliferation of house-dust mites and moulds, both of which are allergenic. A recent study in Munich found that dampness at home was a significant risk factor for persistent AHR and symptoms in children with asthma, and this could not be totally explained by increased exposure to house-dust mites.[76] Similar relationships between mould in the home and respiratory health status have also been demonstrated.[77] The increased risk of children having wheeze or cough if the home is damp or has mould is generally fairly small with an odds ratio that is generally in the range 1.5–3.5.[75] This range is consistent with the measured effect of other environmental exposures such as environmental tobacco smoke and outdoor air pollutants that are considered harmful to respiratory health.

Extensive work has been undertaken, particularly in Europe, in investigating the role of pollens in causing asthma.[78] Pollen-related asthma is highest in spring when pollen levels in the air are highest and in regions where vegetation cover is dense. Pollens from grasses are probably the most important allergens in causing allergic symptoms but exposure to pollens from trees and weeds such as *Betula*, *Olea*, *Ambrosia* and *Parietaria* may also be important. Because of their size, most pollens are thought to be captured in the nose and upper airways where they cause allergic rhinitis. However, intact pollen grains have also been found in the lower respiratory tract.[79] In addition, there is accumulating evidence that extreme weather conditions can cause grains to rupture, thereby releasing allergenic particles which may be easily inhaled.[80,81]

Dietary Risk Factors

There is increasing interest in dietary intakes as risk factors for asthma in both adults and children.[82,83] Epidemiological studies have suggested a relationship between asthma and dietary intakes of salt, magnesium or anti-oxidants[84–86] but the strongest evidence relates to fish intake.[21,82,87] A population based case–control study found that subjects who ate oily fish more than once a week were 30–70% less likely to have asthma.[88]

There is strong biological plausibility for the role of fish oils in the prevention of asthma[89] in that fish oils contain large quantities of omega-3 fatty acids that protect against the airway inflammation which is characteristic of asthma. Nevertheless, trials of fish-oil supplementation in secondary prevention of asthma have not been encouraging in that they have not achieved a significant reduction in symptoms in subjects with established asthma.[90,91] This may be because asthma is an irreversible condition once the mechanisms have become established or because the dose or duration of supplementation may have been insufficient for significant clinical benefits to develop. It seems likely that fish-oil supplementation will need to begin early in life and be sustained over a long period in order to down-regulate the allergic processes that lead to the development of asthma.

Breast-Feeding

There is accumulating evidence from population studies that breast-feeding throughout the first 6 months of life can protect against the development of asthma and allergic symptoms.[92–94] There are several plausible mechanisms for the role of breast-feeding including the presence of long-chain fatty acids that help to prevent against the development of inflammation, and the presence of immunoglobulin A that helps to prevent infection. Interventions to promote prolonged breast-feeding have an important potential to improve many health outcomes including the development of allergic symptoms and asthma in childhood. However, it is not known whether breast-feeding *per se* provides a protective

mechanism or whether the protective effect is conferred by the avoidance of food allergens associated with the early introduction of cow's milk.

Parental Smoking

The role of parental smoking in the aetiology of asthma has been studied more than any other risk factor. A recent series of meta-analyses suggest that there is a causal relationship between parental smoking and the occurrence of respiratory illness in children which cannot be explained by chance, publication bias or other confounding factors.[95–97] These meta-analyses confirm the conclusions of many narrative reviews that there is a small but significant relationship between parental smoking and both respiratory infections and symptoms of airway narrowing in children.

Although the odds ratio for an effect of parental smoking is small compared with other risk factors such as diet and allergen exposure, it is important in population terms because exposure remains high.[98] Recent studies in developed countries such as Australia, the USA and the UK suggest that as many as 25% of women smoke during pregnancy and that between 35–45% of children are exposed to tobacco smoke in their homes. This large proportion of children who are exposed to tobacco smoke on a daily basis from the earliest age are at a significantly increased risk for having impaired respiratory health in later life.

Outdoor Air Pollutants

At high concentrations, sulphur dioxide and, to a lesser extent, nitrogen dioxide and ozone, act as respiratory irritants and may be powerful trigger factors for acute episodes of symptoms.[99,100] Whilst it is tempting to attribute a high prevalence of asthma in some urban regions to the presence of air pollution, there is no evidence that air pollutants in concentrations that are found in industrial cities induce asthma or AHR.

Paradoxically, it seems more likely that particulate air pollutants protect against the development of atopy and asthma. In a study of children living in two regions of Germany, there was a higher prevalence of bronchitis and a lower prevalence of allergic symptoms in the eastern region where levels of sulphur dioxide and total suspended particles were higher than in the western regions.[101] Similar differences have been demonstrated in other regions of Europe.[102] Although causation cannot be attributed, the findings suggest that air pollutants increase the incidence of respiratory infections but that affluent living conditions are a more important risk factor for allergic symptoms and for asthma. In many affluent countries, the prevalence of asthma is equally high in urban and rural regions[69,103] suggesting that factors other than industrial air pollutants are responsible for the high prevalence of asthma in these countries.

It is important to interpret the results of studies that investigate the role of air pollutants in respiratory illness carefully because circumstantial evidence of an association is weak. Air pollutants may act synergistically with allergens by increasing allergic responses, implying that air pollutants have an indirect role in the aetiology of AHR[104,105] and a recent study found that diesel exhaust particles potentiated IgE production in mice.[106] These data, although often quoted, have not been corroborated by large epidemiological studies in which the severity of asthma is well-characterized.

Preventing Asthma

In terms of preventing asthma, the epidemiological evidence shows consistently that asthma is a disease that is associated largely with environmental, and therefore preventable, factors (see Fig. 1.2).[107] Although asthma is perceived as being a disease that is easy to treat and impossible to prevent, better methods of allergen avoidance have become available in the last few years.[64] In public health terms, these preventive methods are likely to provide much greater benefits than treatment with medications.[98] By far the most important and most easily preventable factors are exposures to commonly occurring aeroallergens. It is becoming clear that allergen avoidance from birth, particularly in infants who are most at risk, may have the potential to down-regulate the acquisition of atopic sensitization and to protect airways from developing inflammation.

A good model of effective prevention was demonstrated in epidemics of acute symptoms and consequent hospitalization in Barcelona.[108] These epidemics occurred on days when soya beans were being unloaded from ships into a silo without a filter, which facilitated the release of soya dust into the atmosphere. During the epidemics, those who required hospitalization were

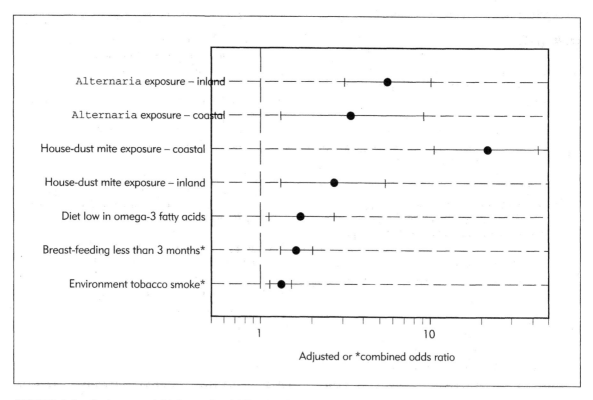

FIGURE 1.2: Environmental risk factors for childhood asthma.

already allergic to soya bean dust which suggests that the allergen was potent enough to cause prior sensitization at relatively low concentrations. In addition, on exposure days, people living many kilometres away from the silo had symptoms. It is of interest that the problem appeared only to affect adults, perhaps because prolonged exposure was needed to build sensitization. Since the silos have been modified so that the dust cannot become airborne, no further epidemics of asthma have occurred.[109]

In practice, the only available options for improving the severity of asthma are long-term treatment with inhaled corticosteroids, and reduction of allergen and other environmental exposures. These methods will be most effective in the groups of children who are most at risk. Recent epidemiological studies suggest that perinatal factors such as low birthweight or pre-term birth,[110,111] a family history of asthma or allergy,[112] exposure to tobacco smoke because of a parent who smokes,[95] or exposure to high levels of indoor allergens in early life[113] confer a high risk for children to develop asthma. Interventions that address these potentially preventable risk factors, especially in high-risk groups, are likely to be effective in both preventing asthma in young children and in reducing the severity of asthma in children and in adults who already have signs of airway inflammation.

KEY POINTS

1. Asthma is best classified into episodic and persistent forms. The former may remit but the latter appears to be an irreversible disease for which there is no cure.

2. Both forms of asthma are increasing in children while death rates in young people (5–34 years) have stabilized or decreased in the last 5 years, indicating improving management.

3. The risk factors for developing asthma are mostly defined making prevention, particularly of persistent disease, the most important approach to management in coming years.

REFERENCES

1. Woolcock AJ. Asthma. In: Murray JF, Nadel J (eds). *Textbook of Respiratory Medicine*. Philadelphia: Saunders, 1994; 1288–330.

2. American Thoracic Society. Standards for the diagnosis and care of patients with chronic obstructive pulmonary disease (COPD) and asthma. *Am Rev Respir Dis* 1987; 136 (Pt 2): 225–43.

3. Cockcroft DW, Killian DN, Mellon JJ, Hargreave FE. Bronchial reactivity to inhaled histamine: a method and clinical survey. *Clin Allergy* 1977; 7: 235–43.

4. Yan K, Salome C, Woolcock AJ. Rapid method for measurement of bronchial responsiveness. *Thorax* 1983; 38: 760–65.

5. Salome CM, Peat JK, Britton WJ, Woolcock AJ. Bronchial hyperresponsiveness in two populations of Australian schoolchildren. I. Relation to respiratory symptoms and diagnosed asthma. *Clin Allergy* 1987; 17: 271–81.

6. ✪ Woolcock A. Assessment of asthma severity. In: Barnes, PJ Grunstein, MM Leff, AR Woolcock, AJ (eds). *Asthma*. Philadelphia: Lippincott-Raven Publishers, 1997; 1499–506.

7. Reddel HK, Salome CM, Peat JK, Woolcock AJ. Which index of peak expiratory flow is most useful in the management of stable asthma? *Am J Resp Crit Care Med* 1995; 151 (5): 1320–25.

8. Strachan DP, Butland BK, Anderson HR. Incidence and prognosis of asthma and wheezing illness from early childhood to age 33 in a national British cohort. *BMJ* 1996; 312: 1195–9.

9. Peat JK. Asthma: a longitudinal perspective. *J Asthma* 1998; 35 (3): 235–41.

10. Laitinen LA, Heino M, Laitinen A, Kava T, Haahtela T. Damage of the airway epithelium and bronchial reactivity in patients with asthma. *Am Rev Respir Dis* 1985; 131: 599–606.

11. Ollerenshaw S, Woolcock AJ. Characteristics of the inflammation in biopsies from large airways of subjects with asthma and subjects with chronic airflow limitation. *Am Rev Respir Dis* 1992; 145: 922–7.

12. Townley RG, Ryo UY, Kolotkin BM, Kang B. Bronchial sensitivity to methacholine in current and former asthmatic and allergic rhinitis patients and control subjects. *J Allergy Clin Immunol* 1975; 56: 429–42.

13. Sears MR, Jones DT, Holdaway MD *et al.* Prevalence of bronchial reactivity to inhaled methacholine in New Zealand children. *Thorax* 1986; 41: 283–9.

14. Backer V, Bach-Mortensen J, Dirksen A. Prevalence and predictors of bronchial hyperresponsiveness in children aged 7–16 years. *Allergy* 1989; 44: 214–19.

15. Peat JK, Toelle B, Salome CM, Woolcock AJ. Predictive nature of bronchial responsiveness and respiratory symptoms in a one year cohort study of Sydney schoolchildren. *Eur Respir J* 1993; 6: 662–9.

16. Stanescu DC, Frans A. Bronchial asthma without increased airway reactivity. *Eur J Respir Dis* 1982; 63: 5–12.

17. Hopp RJ, Townley RG, Biven RE, Bewtra AK, Nair NM. The presence of airway reactivity before the development of asthma. *Am Rev Respir Dis* 1990; 141: 2–8.

18. ❂ Martinez FD, Wright AL, Taussig LM *et al.* Asthma and wheezing in the first six years of life. *N Engl J Med* 1995; 332: 133–8.

19. Chan YM, Lam S. Occupational asthma. *Am Rev Respir Dis* 1986; 133: 686–703.

20. Suphioglu C. Thunderstorm asthma due to grass pollen. *Int Arch Allergy Immunol* 1998; 116 (4): 253–60.

21. Peat JK, Salome CM, Woolcock AJ. Factors associated with bronchial hyperresponsiveness in Australian adults and children. *Eur Respir J* 1992; 5: 921–9.

22. ❂ Faniran AO, Peat JK, Woolcock AJ. Persistent cough: is it asthma? *Arch Dis Child* 1998; 79: 411–14.

23. Wright AL, Holberg CJ, Morgan WJ, Taussig LM, Halonen M, Martinez FD. Recurrent cough in childhood and its relation to asthma. *Am J Respir Crit Care Med* 1996; 153: 1259–65.

24. Burney P, Chinn S. Developing a new questionnaire for measuring the prevalence and distribution of asthma. *Chest* 1987; 91 (6 suppl.): 79S–83S.

25. Bai J, Peat JK, Berry G, Marks GB, Woolcock AJ. Questionnaire items that predict asthma and other respiratory conditions in adults. *Chest* 1998; 114: 1343–8.

26. Worldwide variations in the prevalence of asthma symptoms: the International Study of Asthma and Allergies in Childhood (ISAAC). *Eur Respir J* 1998; 12: 315–35.

27. Burney PGJ, Luczynska S, Jarvis CD. The European community respiratory health survey. *Eur Respir J* 1994; 7: 954–60.

28. Chinn S, Burney PG. On measuring repeatability of data from self-administered questionnaires. *Int J Epidemiol* 1987; 16 (1): 121–7.

29. Britton J, Mortagy A, Tattersfield A. Histamine challenge testing: comparison of three methods. *Thorax* 1986; 41: 128–32.

30. Haby MM, Peat JK, Mellis CM, Anderson SD, Woolcock AJ. An exercise challenge for epidemiological studies of childhood asthma – validity and repeatability. *Eur Respir J* 1995; 8 (5): 729–36.

31. von Mutius E, Fritsch C, Weiland SK, Roll G, Magnussen H. Prevalence of asthma and allergic disorders among children in united Germany: a descriptive comparison. *BMJ* 1992; 305: 1395–9.

32. Burney PG, Chinn S, Britton JR, Tattersfield AE, Papacosta AO. What symptoms predict the bronchial response to histamine? Evaluation in a community survey of the bronchial symptoms questionnaire (1984) of The International Union against Tuberculosis and Lung Disease. *Int J Epidemiol* 1989; 18: 165–73.

33. Toelle BG, Peat JK, Salome CM, Mellis CM, Woolcock AJ. Towards a definition of asthma for epidemiology. *Am Rev Respir Dis* 1992; 146: 633–7.

34. Toelle BG, Peat JK, van den Berg RH, Dermand J, Woolcock AJ. Comparison of three definitions of asthma: a longitudinal perspective. *J Asthma* 1997; 34 (2): 161–7.

35. ❂ Peat JK, Tovey E, Toelle BG *et al.* House dust mite allergens. A major risk factor for childhood asthma in Australia. *Am J Respir Crit Care Med* 1996; 153: 141–6.

36. Sears MR, Herbison GP, Holdaway MD, Hewitt CJ, Flannery EM, Silva PA. The relative risks of sensitivity to grass pollen, house dust mite and cat dander in the development of childhood asthma. *Clin Exp Allergy* 1989; 19: 419–24.

37. Peat JK, Tovey E, Mellis CM, Leeder SR, Woolcock AJ. Importance of house dust mite and Alternaria allergy – an epidemiological study of children living in two climatic areas of Northern NSW. *Clin Exp Allergy* 1993; 23: 812–20.

38. Peat JK, Toelle BG, Dermand J, van den Berg R, Britton WJ, Woolcock AJ. Serum IgE levels, atopy and asthma in young adults: results from a longitudinal cohort study. *Allergy* 1996; 51: 804–810.

39. Burney PG. Asthma mortality in England and Wales: evidence for a further increase, 1974–84. *Lancet* 1986; 2: 323–6.

40. Woolcock AJ, Peat JK, Trevillion LM. Is the increase in asthma prevalence linked to increase in allergen load? *Allergy* 1995; 50: 935–40.

41. Woolcock AJ, Peat JK. Evidence for the increase in asthma worldwide. In: Chadwick D, Cardew G (eds). *The Rising Trends in Asthma*. Ciba Foundation Symposium 206. London: John Wiley, 1997; 206: 122–39; 134–9; 157–9.

42. Vollmer WM, Osborne ML, Buist AS. 20-year trends in the prevalence of asthma and chronic airflow obstruction in an HMO. *Am J Respir Crit Care Med* 1998; 157 (4Pt 1): 1079–84.

43. Kun HY, Oates RK, Mellis CM. Hospital admissions and attendances for asthma – a true increase? *Med J Aust* 1993; 159: 312–13.

44. Peat JK, van den Berg RH, Green WF, Mellis CM, Leeder SR, Woolcock AJ. Changing prevalence of asthma in Australian children. *BMJ* 1994; 308: 1591–6.

45. Burr ML, Butland BK, King S, Vaughan-Williams E. Changes in asthma prevalence: two surveys 15 years apart. *Arch Dis Child* 1989; 64: 1452–6.

46. Robertson CF, Heycock E, Bishop J, Nolan T, Olinsky A, Phelan PD. Prevalence of asthma in Melbourne schoolchildren: changes over 26 years. *BMJ* 1991; 302: 1116–18.

47. ✪ Peat JK, Li J. Reversing the trend: reducing the prevalence of asthma. *J Allergy Clin Immunol* 1999; 103 (1 Pt 1): 1–10.

48. Worldwide variation in prevalence of symptoms of asthma, allergic rhinoconjunctivitis, and atopic eczema: ISAAC. The International Study of Asthma and Allergies in Childhood (ISAAC) Steering Committee. *Lancet* 1998; 351: 1225–32.

49. Asher MI, Pattemore PK, Harrison AC *et al.* International comparison of the prevalence of asthma symptoms and bronchial hyperresponsiveness. *Am Rev Respir Dis* 1988; 138: 524–9.

50. ✪ Burney P, Chinn S, Jarvis D, Luczynska C, Lai E. Variations in the prevalence of respiratory symptoms, self-reported asthma attacks, and use of asthma medication in the European Community Respiratory Health Survey (ECRHS). European Community Respiratory Health Survey. *Eur Respir J* 1996; 9: 687–95.

51. Sears MR, Rea HH, Rothwell RPG *et al.* Asthma mortality: comparison between New Zealand and England. *BMJ* 1986; 293: 1342–5.

52. Crane J, Flatt A, Lackson R *et al.* Prescribed fenoterol and death from asthma in New Zealand, 1981–83: Case-controlled study. *Lancet* 1989; 1: 917–22.

53. Beasley R, Pearce N, Crane J, Windom H, Burgess C. Asthma mortality and inhaled beta agonist therapy. *Aust NZ J Med* 1991; 21: 753–63.

54. Spitzer WO, Suissa S, Ernst P *et al.* The use of β-agonists and the risk of death and near death from asthma. *N Engl J Med* 1992; 326 (8): 501–506.

55. Ernst P, Spitzer WO, Suissa S *et al.* Risk of fatal and near-fatal asthmas in relation to inhaled corticosteroid use. *JAMA* 1992; 268 (24): 3462–4.

56. Beasley R, Pearce N, Crane J. International trends in asthma mortality. *Ciba Found Symp* 1997; 206: 140–50; discussion 150–56, 157–9.

57. ✪ Sears MR, Burrows B, Flannery EM, Herbison GP, Holdaway MD. Atopy in childhood. 1. Gender and allergen related risks for development of hay fever and asthma. *Clin Exp Allergy* 1993; 23: 941–8.

58. Peat JK, Mellis CM, Leeder SR, Woolcock AJ. Differences in airway responsiveness between children and adults living in the same environment: an epidemiological study in two regions of Australia. *Eur Respir J* 1994; 7: 1805–13.

59. Custovic A, Taggart SCO, Francis HC, Chapman MD, Woodcock A. Exposure to house dust mite allergens and the clinical activity of asthma. *J Allergy Clin Immunol* 1996; 98: 64–72.

60. Tovey ER. Allergen exposure and control. *Exp Appl Acarol* 1992; 16: 181–202.

61. Peat JK, Woolcock AJ. Sensitivity to common allergens: relation to respiratory symptoms and bronchial hyperresponsiveness in children from three different climatic areas of Australia. *Clin Exp Allergy* 1991; 21: 573–81.

62. Sporik R, Chapman MD, Platts-Mills TAE. House dust mite exposure as a cause of asthma. *Clin Exp Allergy* 1992; 22: 897–906.

63. Gotzsche PC, Hammarquist C, Burr M. House dust mite control measures in the management of asthma: meta-analysis. *BMJ* 1998; 317 (7166): 1105–1110; discussion 1110.

64. Custovic A, Simpson A, Chapman MD, Woodcock A. Allergen avoidance in the treatment of asthma and atopic disorders. *Thorax* 1998; 53 (1): 63–72.

65. Harving H, Korsgaard J, Dahl R. House-dust mites and associated environmental conditions in Danish homes. *Allergy* 1993; 48 (2): 106–109.

66. Tovey ER, McDonald LG. A simple washing procedure with eucalyptus oil for controlling house dust mites and their allergens in clothing and bedding. *J Allergy Clin Immunol* 1997; 100: 464–6.

67. Hide DW, Matthews S, Tariq S, Arshad SH. Allergen avoidance in infancy and allergy at 4 years of age. *Allergy* 1996; 51: 89–93.

68. Nishioka K, Yasueda H, Saito H. Preventive effect of bedding encasement with microfine fibers on mite sensitization. *J Allergy Clin Immunol* 1998; 101 (1 Pt 1): 28–32.

69. Peat JK, Toelle B, Gray L *et al.* Prevalence and severity of childhood asthma and allergic sensitisation in seven climatic regions of New South Wales. *Med J Aust* 1995; 163: 22–6.

70. Mitakakis T, Ong EK, Stevens A, Guest D, Knox RB. Incidence of *Cladosporium, Alternaria* and total fungal spores in the atmosphere of Melbourne (Australia) over three years. *Aerobiologia* 1997; 13: 83–90.

71. D' Amato G, Spieksma FT. Aerobiologic and clinical aspects of mould allergy in Europe. *Allergy* 1995; 50 (11): 870–77.

72. Bass D, Morgan G. A three year (1993–1995) calendar of pollen and *Alternaria* mould in the atmosphere of south western Sydney. *Grana* 1997; 36: 293–300.

73. O'Hollaren MT, Yunginger JW, Offord KP *et al.* Exposure to an aeroallergen as a possible precipitating factor in respiratory arrest in young patients with asthma. *N Engl J Med* 1991; 324 (6): 359–63.

74. Halonen M, Stern DA, Wright AL, Taussig LM, Martinez FD. *Alternaria* as a major allergen for asthma in children raised in a desert environment. *Am J Respir Crit Care Med* 1997; 155 (4): 1356–61.

75. Peat JK, Dickerson J, Li J. Effects of damp and mould in the home on respiratory health: a review of the literature. *Allergy* 1998; 53 (2): 120–28.

76. Nicolai T, Illi S, von Mutius E. Effect of dampness at home in childhood on bronchial hyperreactivity in adolescence. *Thorax* 1998; 53: 1035–40.

77. Andriessen JW, Brunekreef B, Roemer W. Home dampness and respiratory health status in European children. *Clin Exp Allergy* 1998; 28 (10): 1191–1200.

78. D'Amato G, Spieksma FT, Liccardi G *et al.* Pollen-related allergy in Europe. *Allergy* 1998; 53 (6): 567–78.

79. Michel FB, Marty JP, Quet L, Cour P. Penetration of inhaled pollen into the respiratory tract. *Am Rev Respir Dis* 1977; 115 (4): 609–616.

80. Knox RB. Grass pollen, thunderstorms and asthma. *Clin Exp Allergy* 1993; 23 (5): 354–9.

81. Anto JM, Sunyer J. Thunderstorms: a risk factor for asthma attacks. *Thorax* 1997; 52 (8): 669–70.

82. Vincent D, Weiss ST. Relationship of dietary fish intake to level of pulmonary function (Letter). *Eur Respir J* 1995; 8: 507.

83. Weiss ST. Risk factor diet. In: Barnes PJ, Grunstien MM, Leff AR, Woolcock AJ, (eds.). *Asthma*, vol. 1. Philadelphia: Lippincott-Raven, 1997; 105–119.

84. Britton J, Pavord I, Richards K *et al*. Dietary magnesium, lung function, wheezing, and airway hyperreactivity in a random adult population sample. *Lancet* 1994; 344: 357–62.

85. Britton J, Pavord I, Richards K *et al*. Dietary sodium intake and the risk of airway hyperreactivity in a random adult population. *Thorax* 1994; 49: 875–80.

86. Seaton A, Godden DJ, Brown K. Increase in asthma: a more toxic environment or a more susceptible population? *Thorax* 1994; 49: 171–4.

87. Britton J. Dietary fish oil and airways obstruction. *Thorax* 1995; 50 (suppl. 1): S11–S15.

88. Hodge L, Salome CM, Peat JK, Haby MM, Xuan W, Woolcock AJ. Consumption of oily fish and childhood asthma risk. *Med J Aust* 1996; 164 (3): 137–40.

89. Ritter JM, Taylor JW. Fish oil in asthma. *Thorax* 1988; 43: 81–3.

90. Thien FCK, Mencia-Huerta J-M, Lee TH. Dietary fish oil effects on seasonal hay fever and asthma in pollen-sensitive subjects. *Am Rev Respir Dis* 1993; 147 (5): 1138–43.

91. Hodge L, Salome CM, Hughes JM *et al*. Effect of dietary intake of omega-3 and omega-6 fatty acids on severity of asthma in children. *Eur Respir J* 1998; 11 (2): 361–5.

92. Businco L, Marchetti F, Pellegrini G, Cautani A, Perlini R. Prevention of atopic disease in "at risk new borns" by prolonged breast-feeding. *Ann Allergy* 1983; 51: 296–9.

93. Saarinen VM, Kajosaari M, Backman A, Siimes MA. Prolonged breast-feeding as prophylaxis for atopic disease. *Lancet* 1979; 2: 163–6.

94. Wright AL, Holberg CJ, Martinez FD, Morgan WJ, Taussig LM. Breast feeding and lower respiratory tract illness in the first year of life. Group Health Medical Associates. *BMJ* 1989; 299: 946–9.

95. Cook DG, Strachan DP. Health effects of passive smoking. 3. Parental smoking and prevalence of respiratory symptoms and asthma in school age children. *Thorax* 1997; 52: 1081–94.

96. Cook DG, Strachan DP. Health effects of passive smoking. 7. Parental smoking, bronchial reactivity and peak flow variability in children. *Thorax* 1998; 53 (4): 295–301.

97. Strachan DP, Cook DG. Health effects of passive smoking. 5. Parental smoking and allergic sensitisation in children. *Thorax* 1998; 53 (2): 117–23.

98. Peat JK. Can asthma be prevented? Evidence from epidemiological studies of children in Australia and New Zealand in the last decade. *Clin Exp Allergy* 1998; 28 (3): 261–5.

99. Duhme H, Weiland SK, Keil U. Epidemiological analyses of the relationship between environmental pollution and asthma. *Toxicol Lett* 1998; 102–103: 307–316.

100. Anderson HR, Ponce de Leon A, Bland JM, Bower JS, Emberlin J, Strachan DP. Air pollution, pollens, and daily admissions for asthma in London 1987–92. *Thorax* 1998; 53 (10): 842–8.

101. von Mutius E, Martinez FD, Fritzsch C, Nicolai T, Roell G, Theimann H-H. Prevalence of asthma and atopy in two areas of West and East Germany. *Am J Respir Crit Care Med* 1994; 149: 358–64.

102. Jogi R, Janson C, Bjornsson E, Boman G, Bjorksten B. Atopy and allergic disorders among adults in Tartu, Estonia compared with Uppsala, Sweden. *Clin Exp Allergy* 1998; 28: 1072–80.

103. Fontaine V, Deniaud F, Lefort F, Lecoutour X, Brun J. Epidemiology of childhood asthma in the department of Calvados. [French]. *Rev Pneumol Clin* 1999; 55 (1): 5–11.

104. Ciccone G, Forastiere F, Agabiti N *et al*. Road traffic and adverse respiratory effects in children. SIDRIA Collaborative Group. *Occup Environ Med* 1998; 55 (11): 771–8.

105. Seaton A, MacNee W, Donaldson K, Godden D. Particulate air pollution and acute health effects. *Lancet* 1995; 345 (8943): 176–8.

106. Bayram H, Devalia JL, Sapsford RJ *et al.* The effects of diesel exhaust particles on cell function and release of inflammatory mediators from human bronchial epithelial cells *in vitro. Am J Respir Cell Mol Biol* 1998; 18 (3): 441–8.

107. Peat JK. Prevention of asthma. *Eur Respir J* 1996; 9 (7): 1545–55.

108. Anto JM, Sunyer J. Epidemiologic studies of asthma epidemics in Barcelona. *Chest* 1990; 98 (suppl.): 185S–190S.

109. Anto JM, Sunyer J, Reed CE *et al.* Preventing asthma epidemics due to soybeans by dust-control measures. *N Engl J Med* 1993; 329: 1760–63.

110. Schatz M, Zeiger RS, Hoffman CP, and the Kaiser-Permanente Asthma and Pregnancy Study Group. Intrauterine growth is related to gestational pulmonary function in pregnant asthmatic women. *Chest* 1990; 98: 389–92.

111. Fergusson DM, Crane J, Beasley R, Horwood LJ. Perinatal factors and atopic disease in childhood. *Clin Exp Allergy* 1997; 27 (12): 1394–401.

112. Martinez FD. Maternal risk factors in asthma. *Ciba Found Symp* 1997; 206: 233–9; discussion 239–243.

113. Sporik R, Holgate ST, Platts-Mills TAE, Cogswell JJ. Exposure to house-dust mite allergen (*Der p* 1) and the development of asthma in childhood. A prospective study. *N Engl J Med* 1990; 323: 502–507.

Chapter 2

Natural History

Malcolm Sears

The preceding chapter addresses the definition, classification and epidemiology of asthma, together with risk factors for its development. This chapter describes the natural history of asthma with respect to its evolution over time, both in children and in adults, factors predisposing to remission or persistence of asthma, and risk factors for death from asthma.

ASTHMA IN EARLY CHILDHOOD

There is a relative dearth of information about the natural history of wheezing in infancy and early childhood, as most studies have examined the course of asthma from mid-childhood to adult life. Recently a cohort study in Tucson, Arizona has yielded excellent data regarding development, persistence and remission of asthma in the first 6 years of life.[1] Children born to parents enrolled in a health maintenance organization were studied through questionnaires, while sub-groups of children within this cohort had measurements taken of serum IgE at birth and at age 9 months, and pulmonary function testing in infancy and at age 6 years. The children were reviewed at age 3 and 6 years with respect to symptoms and pulmonary function, with data available for 826 of 1246 children at 6 years. By age six, only 51% had never wheezed, while 20% developed wheezing before age 3 years and remitted by 6 years, 15% first developed wheezing between age 3 and age 6, and 14% developed early wheezing before age 3 with persisting symptoms to age 6. Remission of early childhood wheezing is therefore common, as although 49% of children had reported wheezing by age 6 years, only 29% were still wheezing at 6. Those who remitted were more likely to be exposed to maternal cigarette smoke, had lower lung function on average at age one year and at 6 years, and were less likely to have features of atopy including high IgE levels, positive skin tests, or a family history of asthma. On the other hand, those whose wheezing persisted through early childhood to age 6 more often had a history of maternal asthma, elevated serum IgE at one year and 6 years, and abnormal lung function by age 6 years.

The influence of smaller airways on development of early childhood wheezing was confirmed in a UK study, which found an odds ratio (OR) for wheezing of 2.1 for every unit decline in specific airway conductance.[2] Among those whose mothers smoked during pregnancy, the OR for wheezing was 4.9 (95% CI 1.6–15.0).

In early childhood, factors predicting persistence are both genetic and environmental linked with atopy, whereas early wheezing which subsequently remitted was associated with small airways and cigarette smoke exposure rather than with allergy. Evidence suggests that an immune response to viral infection in early life skewed towards an IgE or an eosinophil-mediated slant is predictive of persisting wheezing to age 6.[3,4]

ASTHMA IN CHILDHOOD

The natural history of childhood asthma after the first 6 years through to adulthood has been examined in several different types of studies, including follow-up from family or consultant practice, university hospital-based practices, and longitudinal population studies, of which there are relatively few. Longitudinal studies which enrol an unselected cohort of subjects among whom the incidence and prevalence of asthma is periodically determined, and the features of asthma re-examined over time, provide the best indication of natural history across the spectrum of asthma. Conversely, those children seen in office or specialty practice are likely to have more severe asthma than children identified with asthma in a population-based study, and therefore different outcomes.

Follow-Up from Office Practices

In Boston, Massachusetts, subjects diagnosed as having asthma in childhood were followed up 20 years later.[5] Of 449 children, four had died of asthma, giving a mortality rate of 0.5 per 1000 children with asthma per annum. Among children whose asthma seemed related to animal exposure, only 17% were symptom free or "cured" as adults, whereas of those with food-related asthma, 44% were cured, as were 57% of those whose asthma was related to pollen allergy. Among children with mixed atopic or unidentified aetiology of asthma, only 25% were fully in remission as adults, 11% were well, provided they avoided known allergens and trigger factors, 30% had mild asthma and also suffered from hay fever, while 30% had persistent asthma. Overall, about half of the group with atopic asthma in childhood had persistent symptoms as adults, and 17% had severe adult asthma.

Blair reviewed UK children initially diagnosed and treated for asthma before age 12 years.[6] Twenty years later, 244 of 267 subjects were available for review, of whom 28% were asymptomatic, 24% had occasional mild symptoms, 27% had gone into remission for at least 3 years but had relapsed, while 21% had had persistent asthma since childhood without remission. Persistence was predicted by the presence of other atopic disease, a family history of asthma, and the severity of asthma in childhood.[7]

Follow-Up from Specialty Practices

Follow-up studies from university clinics have been described from Denmark and the Netherlands. Among 119 children aged 6–14 years seen at a university clinic in the Netherlands between 1966 and 1969, 101 were reviewed after 16 years.[8] At both surveys, investigations included symptom questionnaires, skin allergy testing, spirometry and methacholine challenge testing. As adults, 43% had persisting symptoms, and only 29% showed airway hyperresponsiveness to histamine as adults compared with 82% in childhood. The severity of symptoms and the degree of airway responsiveness was less in adulthood than in childhood. Airway hyperresponsiveness and low lung function in childhood were predictive of persistence of asthma into adulthood. Atopy was not predictive, but 95% of the cohort were

atopic as children and this likely made it difficult to show different outcomes between atopic and non-atopic children.

In another cohort of 406 Dutch children aged 8–12 years seen between 1972 and 1976, 259 were reviewed at age 25 years.[9] Of these, 76% had persistent symptoms as adults (women 85%, men 72%). Over half of the subjects needed regular or intermittent medication as adults. Persistence to adulthood was predicted by several childhood factors including severity of symptoms, airway responsiveness and lung function.

Children seen at a Copenhagen hospital clinic when aged 5–15 years were followed up 10–12 years later.[10] There was improvement in both atopic and non-atopic asthmatics, with decreased severity of symptoms and improved lung function. However, despite this improvement, 86% had had symptoms as adults within the previous 12 months and most required treatment. The severity of lung function abnormality in childhood was again a predictive factor for persistence in both atopic and non-atopic subjects.

In a Swedish study, 92 of 101 children hospitalized with wheezing before age 2 were reviewed at age 10 years.[11] Only 30% had asthma (mild 20%, moderate 8%, severe 2%) while 70% were symptom free. Factors predicting persistent asthma were the severity of the initial airflow obstruction, early onset, other atopic disease, and smoking in the home, but respiratory syncytial virus (RSV) infection was not predictive.

Longitudinal Population Studies

Longitudinal studies of populations drawn randomly from a local community have reported outcomes at intervals varying from 6–28 years. Although the sample sizes, the means of obtaining the original cohort, and the methods of investigations have varied considerably, several findings are common among these studies.

In Scotland, 2511 children were selected as a 1 in 5 sample of primary school children in Aberdeen in 1962.[12] Twenty-five years later, about two-thirds of the 121 with asthma in childhood, and of the 167 with wheezing with infections, together with a sample of control children without wheezing or asthma, were reviewed by questionnaire, lung function and airway responsiveness measurements. Childhood asthma was associated with adult wheezing (OR 14.4) and sputum production (OR 3.3), as well as with a lower FEV_1 and greater airway responsiveness, compared with normals. Childhood wheezing not diagnosed as asthma gave an odds ratio for wheezing as adults of 3.8, and was associated with lesser severities of symptoms with essentially normal lung function and airway responsiveness measurements. Predictors for adult wheezing included childhood symptoms, atopy, and smoking as adults.

An Australian study of the natural history of childhood asthma began in 1969 using a random sample of grade 2 children in Melbourne schools.[13] This cohort included every 7-year-old child with diagnosed asthma or with "wheezy bronchitis" (more than five episodes per year of wheezing associated with infection), every second child with mild wheezy bronchitis (less than five episodes per year associated with infection), and every 20th normal child. These subjects were followed up at ages 10, 14, 21, 28 and 35 years with 86% cohort retention at age 35. The study sample was "enriched" at age 10 with the addition of 67 children with more severe asthma to provide data for outcome of severe asthma. However it is possible to extract data from several publications to look at trends in the original randomly selected population.

At age 35, among the original cohort, 20% had persistent wheezing, and 15% had symptoms occurring less often than once per week in the previous 3 months, so that in total 35% had wheezing symptoms.[14] Among those diagnosed with asthma at age 7, 50% had frequent or persistent symptoms and only 30% were asymptomatic. Among those with "wheezy bronchitis" (wheezing with infections), whether having more or less than five episodes per year, two-thirds were asymptomatic as adults. Hence the likelihood of persistence of childhood wheezing symptoms was strongest in those already labelled as asthmatic at age 7 years. This may well have changed since 1969, as the label of asthma is now used much more readily for childhood wheezing. Present-day wheezing children not diagnosed as asthmatic are more similar to non-wheezing children with respect to lung function, airway hyperresponsiveness, exercise lability and skin test reactivity.[15] Risk factors for persistence of symptoms to age 35 in the Melbourne study included multiple episodes occurring before the age of 2 years, childhood eczema and atopy, and low lung function. The age of onset of symptoms was not an independent risk factor for persistence.

In Tasmania, 8600 children aged 7 years in 1968 were studied by questionnaire and spirometry.[16] At that age, 16% reported asthma. The cohort was followed up some 20 years later. Of those with asthma reported at age 7, 26% had asthma at age 29–32 years. Of those who were asymptomatic at age 7, 10% now had asthma. Current frequent asthma as adults was reported by 5% and 2% respectively of these childhood symptomatic or asymptomatic groups. Adult asthma was associated with a later age of onset, a greater total number of attacks and more frequent attacks. Risk factors for persistence of childhood asthma into adulthood included the personal history of childhood asthma, being female, having eczema, having low lung function as children, and having a family history of asthma.

A longitudinal study was commenced with a cohort of 18 559 UK children all born in one week in March 1958,[17] and reviewed at age 7, 11, 16, 23 and 33 years with respect to respiratory illness. At age 7, 18% reported asthma or wheeze ever, but by age 11 and 16 prevalence had dropped to 12%. The prevalence of asthma or wheezing in the last 12 months at ages 7, 11, 16 and 23 was respectively 8%, 5%, 3% and 4%. The incidence of asthma between age 17 and age 33 was associated with cigarette smoking and with hay fever, and more weakly with female sex and histories of eczema and migraine.[18] Relapse of asthma by age 33 was more common among atopic subjects and current smokers. The prevalence of wheezing attacks in the previous year among the 1880 subjects who had reported asthma or wheezing between birth and age 7 was 50% at age 7 (i.e. half of the early childhood wheezers had already gone into remission), 18% at age 11, 10% at age 16, 10% at age 23, but there was a significant relapse rate with 27% prevalence of symptoms at age 33.

A further longitudinal study of asthma in children was commenced using a cohort of 1037 children born in Dunedin, New Zealand, between April 1972 and March 1973 and still residing in the province of Otago at age 3 years.[19] Respiratory assessments were performed at age 9, 11, 13, 15, 18 and 21 years, together with measurements of spirometry and airway responsiveness to methacholine; tests for allergy included skin testing and IgE measurements. The prevalence of diagnosed asthma at each age was substantially less than the reported prevalence of recurrent wheezing. Atopy (one or more positive skin test weals ≥ 2 mm diameter) was found in 44% of the population at age 13 and 60% at age 21. The prevalence of airway responsiveness (methacholine $PC_{20} \leq 8$ mg ml^{-1} or >10% response to salbutamol in obstructed children) decreased with age from 18% at age 9 to become stable at 8–10% of the population between age 13 and 21. Factors associated with persistence of asthma or recurrent wheezing symptoms from the time of onset to age 21 include house-dust mite and cat sensitivity, airway responsiveness, and current cigarette smoking at age 18 and 21 years.[20]

Strachan, using data from three longitudinal cohort studies, reported a return to normal or near-normal lung function in children who outgrew asthma, while those with persistent symptoms had impaired lung function not fully reversible with bronchodilator.[21]

FACTORS PREDISPOSING TO PERSISTENCE OF CHILDHOOD ASTHMA

Family History

A family history of asthma (particularly if accompanied by a strong family history of atopy) is the dominant risk factor in most studies for development of childhood asthma and personal atopy and for persistence of asthmatic symptoms.[22,23]

Atopy

The great majority of studies, especially those based on a population sample, have shown that personal atopy is a risk factor for persistence of asthma.[14,16,20] Remission occurs less frequently in those with more marked degrees of atopy, especially to indoor allergens such as house-dust mite and cat dander.

Environmental Exposures

Epidemiologically based data supporting the hypothesis that persistent allergen exposure is a risk factor for persistent symptoms, with documentation of levels of exposure correlated with the risk of persistence, are scarce. However, clinical studies of children and young adults attending emergency rooms for management of troublesome asthma have found sensitization to indoor allergens, including house-dust mite and cockroach, is very common, with high exposure levels in their homes.[24]

Smoking

Parental smoking has two apparently conflicting effects. A large part of the excess incidence of wheezing in smoking households is relatively mild and often remits. However, among those with persisting asthma, parental smoking is associated with more severe disease.[25]

Personal smoking is a risk factor for persistence of childhood respiratory symptoms to adulthood. Among Aberdeen children, those who smoked in adolescence and adulthood had more symptoms and lower lung function, but not more airway hyperresponsiveness, than non-smokers.[12] In the UK national cohort, relapse of asthma at age 33 after prolonged remission of childhood wheezing more commonly occurred among current smokers.[18]

Severity of Childhood Asthma

All studies show that the greater the severity of childhood asthma, whether measured by the frequency of episodes in childhood, by lung function abnormality, or by the severity of airway hyperresponsiveness, the more likely it is to persist.

Gender

Childhood asthma is more common among boys than girls, as is the prevalence of atopy, but persistence of childhood asthma into adulthood is more common in girls in virtually all longitudinal studies. The change from male dominance to female dominance at the age of puberty is less evident among studies following clinic populations, because the cohort being followed is biased by including more males with troublesome asthma in childhood. Nevertheless, these studies also show a greater likelihood of persistence among females.

ASTHMA IN ADULTS

Data on the course and prognosis of adult asthma, and the effects of treatment, are few. One major study of adult asthma was undertaken in Tucson, Arizona. Of 1109 adults enrolled in a random population survey, the change in prevalence over an 8-year period was small, from 19.2% to 21.4%, and remission was uncommon.[26] Wheezing in the absence of a cold was related to both smoking and skin test reactivity. Symptoms of wheezing and shortness of breath may be present for some years before asthma is diagnosed, even in younger adults.[27] Hence the natural history of asthma is confounded by the uncertainty over, and delay in making, the diagnosis despite symptoms. In the Tucson cohort, the concurrence of chronic bronchitis with asthma was associated with a steeper decline in lung function measured by FEV_1 than in those in whom asthma was the sole diagnosis. Greater responsiveness to β agonist was also predictive of a steeper decline in FEV_1 in both asthma and bronchitis.[28]

Among younger adults retested 25 years after initial investigations for asthma, 40% were asymptomatic as adults, but 79% still showed airway hyperresponsiveness. Remission of asthma favoured younger subjects, those with less severe disease initially, and those treated relatively early after the onset of asthma.[29] Among older subjects in Tucson, Arizona, aged over 65 years at enrollment, less than 7% went into remission over the next 7 years.[30]

Remission of adult asthma was confirmed to be rare in a Scandinavian study, in that only 3% of those reporting current asthma in 1986 were asymptomatic on review 10 years later.[31] In a Netherlands study, with 24-year follow-up, increased airway responsiveness was not only positively associated with development of chronic respiratory symptoms, but was also negatively associated with remission of symptoms.[32]

In occupational asthma, symptoms, abnormal pulmonary function and airway hyperresponsiveness often persist even when subjects are removed from exposure, though the outcome does depend on the duration of exposure and the nature of the sensitizing agent.[33,34] In a study of 56 subjects with baker's asthma, examined 1–6 months after cessation of exposure, and then 36–48 months later, while there was objective improvement, there was no objective improvement in peak flow rates or FEV_1, and no reduction in airway responsiveness in the majority of subjects.[33]

Irreversible airflow obstruction can occur in asthma, especially in the elderly, without a history of smoking or development of chronic obstructive pulmonary disease through other mechanisms.[35–37] Reed, in a series from the Mayo Clinic in which he reviewed every fourth record of more than 1200 subjects over 65 years treated for asthma, found that the majority had severe asthma which was poorly reversible, despite being non-smokers.[38]

Ulrik has reviewed factors leading to irreversible changes in lung function in asthma. Some are less uncertain, such as the possibility that females have a worse prognosis than males, and the impact of the age of onset and duration of asthma.[39] However, clear correlations have been established between the severity of lung function, the severity of airway responsiveness, response to β agonist, mucus hypersecretion, blood eosinophilia, severity of symptoms, and cigarette smoking, and decrease in reversibility of airflow obstruction.

MORTALITY FROM ASTHMA

The risk of death from asthma in an individual asthmatic is very small. However, over the last three decades, there has been increasing concern about asthma mortality, highlighted by two epidemics which increased mortality rates, particularly among young people, to levels three to five times those seen in the pre-epidemic years. There is now near-consensus that the 1960s epidemic, which occurred in England and Wales, Australia and New Zealand, was linked with use of high-dose isoprenaline as an adrenergic agonist used in the management of asthma, while the second epidemic, which was confined to New Zealand, was linked with the excessive use of a high-dose β-adrenergic agent, fenoterol.[40] These drugs were thought to increase mortality because of cardiac arrhythmias, but clinical trials have demonstrated that frequent use of inhaled short-acting β agonists may increase airway responsiveness to allergen,[41,42] decrease lung function and decrease control of asthma[43,44] leading to greater severity of disease and therefore greater risk of mortality. The rapid decline in not only mortality but also morbidity as measured in hospital admissions, in New Zealand adults after withdrawal of fenoterol is further strong evidence for an increased severity of disease associated with its use, which decreased rapidly after the drug was withdrawn.[45]

There has been a gradual upward trend in mortality worldwide through the 1960s to mid-1980s, but in most countries this has now begun to decline. The recognition that asthma can be fatal, that over-reliance on β agonists may be a direct or indirect risk factor for mortality, and is a marker of uncontrolled asthma which requires urgent attention, have all contributed to reducing the mortality rate from asthma.

Risk factors for mortality other than excessive β agonist use were studied in Copenhagen.[46] Risk factors include age (age over 40, OR 2.5 compared with age under 40), cigarette smoking (OR 2.6 for <20 pack year, 5.9 for >20 pack years), eosinophilia (OR 7.4), moderate rather than severe reduction in lung function (OR 4.9 for FEV_1 40–69% predicted, OR 3.3 for FEV_1 < 40%, relative to FEV_1 >70%), and reversibility (OR 7.0 for reversibility >50% relative to reversibility 15–24%). The latter three risk factors identify the more labile and more atopic individual.

CONCLUSIONS

Childhood asthma is common, but is often mild and frequently remits. Early transient childhood wheezing or "asthma" under the age of 6 years is associated with smaller airways and irritant exposure, including environmental tobacco smoke, together with effects of respiratory infections. Early onset persistent and later onset childhood asthma is influenced by family history and personal atopy, together with allergen exposure. Risk factors for persistence of asthma include the severity of childhood asthma (as indicated by the frequency of symptoms, abnormalities of lung function, and degree of airway hyperresponsiveness), atopy (whether measured by serum IgE or specific skin testing), and gender. Overall about one-third of childhood asthmatics have persistent troublesome asthma in adulthood. Death is rare, but not unknown, and usually reflects severe disease and poor management. Adult asthma may commence at any age, may be related to occupational exposures but often is idiopathic, and is generally persistent throughout adulthood. Remission is more likely in younger adults with less severe disease and less marked airway responsiveness, but overall is infrequent.

KEY POINTS

1 Transient wheezing in infancy may be related to small airways and tobacco smoke exposure.

2 Persistent wheezing in infancy is related to a maternal history of asthma, and development of personal atopy.

3 Two-thirds of children with asthma experience remission, especially those with mild disease, but some will relapse as adults.

4 Persistence of childhood asthma into adulthood is predicted by atopy to indoor allergens, severity of childhood disease, increased airway responsiveness and impaired lung function.

5 Remission of asthma in adults is uncommon.

6 Younger adults with less severe disease may go into remission.

7 Adult asthma may become chronic and irreversible even in the absence of smoking.

8 Mortality from asthma is uncommon. Risk factors include age, smoking, labile asthma, excessive β agonist use, and inadequate long-term care.

REFERENCES

1. ✪ Martinez FD, Wright AL, Taussig LM, Holberg CJ, Halonen M, Morgan WJ. Asthma and wheezing in the first six years of life. *New Engl J Med* 1995; 332: 133–8.

2. ✪ Dezateux C, Stocks J, Dundas I, Fletcher ME. Impaired airway function and wheezing in infancy. The influence of maternal smoking and a genetic predisposition to asthma. *Am J Respir Crit Care Med* 1998; 159: 403–410.

3. Martinez FD. Role of respiratory infection in onset of asthma and chronic obstructive pulmonary disease. *Clin Exp Allergy* 1999; 29: 53–8.

4. Martinez FD, Helms PJ. Types of asthma and wheezing. *Eur Respir J* 1998; 12 (suppl. 27): 3s–8s.

5. Rackemann FM, Edwards MC. Asthma in children: a follow-up study of 688 patients after an interval of twenty years. *N Engl J Med* 1952; 246: 815–23.

6. Blair H. Natural history of childhood asthma. *Arch Dis Child* 1977; 52: 613–19.

7. Blair H. Symposium: the wheezy child. Natural history of wheezing in childhood. *J R Soc Med* 1979; 72: 42–8.

8. Gerritsen J, Koeter GH, Postma DS, Schouten JP, Knol K. Prognosis of asthma from childhood to adulthood. *Am Rev Respir Dis* 1989; 140: 1325–30.

9. Roorda RJ, Gerritsen J, Van Aalderen WMC *et al.* Risk factors for the persistence of respiratory symptoms in childhood asthma. *Am Rev Respir Dis* 1993; 148: 1490–95.

10. Ulrik CS, Backer V, Dirksen A, Pedersen M, Koch C. Extrinsic and intrinsic asthma from childhood to adult age: a 10-year follow-up. *Respir Med* 1995; 89: 547–54.

11. Wennergren G, Amark M, Amark K, Oskarsdottir S, Sten G, Redfors S. Wheezing bronchitis reinvestigated at the age of 10 years. *Acta Paediat* 1997; 86: 351–5.

12. Godden DJ, Ross S, Abdalla M *et al*. Outcome of wheeze in childhood. Symptoms and pulmonary function 25 years later. *Am J Respir Crit Care Med* 1994; 149: 106–112.

13. Williams H, McNicol KN. Prevalence, natural history and relationship of wheezy bronchitis and asthma in children. An epidemiological study. *BMJ* 1969; 4: 321–5.

14. Oswald H, Phelan PD, Lanigan A, Hibbert M, Bowes G, Olinsky A. Outcome of childhood asthma in mid-adult life. *BMJ* 1994; 309: 95–6.

15. Nystad W, Stensrud T, Rijcken B, Hagen J, Magnus P, Carlsen K-H. Wheezing in school children is not always asthma. *Pediat Allergy Immunol* 1999; 10: 58–65.

16. Jenkins MA, Hopper JL, Bowes G, Carlin JB, Flander LB, Giles GG. Factors in childhood as predictors of asthma in adult life. *BMJ* 1994; 309: 90–93.

17. Anderson HR, Pottier AC, Strachan DP. Asthma from birth to age 23: incidence and relation to prior and concurrent atopic disease. *Thorax* 1992; 47: 537–42.

18. Strachan DP, Butland BK, Anderson HR. Incidence and prognosis of asthma and wheezing illness from early childhood to age 33 in a national British cohort. *BMJ* 1996; 312: 1195–9.

19. ✪ Sears MR, Herbison GP, Holdaway MD, Hewitt CJ, Flannery EM, Silva PA. The relative risks of sensitivity to grass pollen, house dust mite and cat dander in the development of childhood asthma. *Clin Exp Allergy* 1989; 19: 419–24.

20. Sears MR, Wiecek E, Willan A *et al*. Persistence, remission, and relapse of childhood asthma: a longitudinal study from age 9 to age 21. *Eur Respir J* 1998; 12: 401s.

21. Strachan D, Gerritsen J. Long-term outcome of early childhood wheezing: population data. *Eur Respir J* 1996; 9: 42s–47s.

22. Gerritsen J, Koeter GH, de Monchy JGR, Knol K. Allergy in subjects with asthma from childhood to adulthood. *J Allergy Clin Immunol* 1990; 85: 116–25.

23. Roorda RJ, Gerritsen J, Van Aalderen WMC, Knol K. Skin reactivity and eosinophil count in relation to the outcome of childhood asthma. *Eur Respir J* 1993; 6: 509–16.

24. Platts-Mills TAE, Carter MC. Asthma and indoor exposure to allergens. *N Engl J Med* 1997; 336: 1382–4.

25. Strachan DP, Cook DG. Parental smoking and childhood asthma: longitudinal and case-control studies. *Thorax* 1998; 53: 204–212

26. Barbee RA, Halonen M, Kaltenborn WT, Burrows B. A longitudinal study of respiratory symptoms in a community population sample. Correlations with smoking, allergen skin-test reactivity, and serum IgE. *Chest* 1991; 99: 20–26.

27. Dodge R, Cline MG, Lebowitz MD, Burrows B. Findings before the diagnosis of asthma in young adults. *J Allergy Clin Immunol* 1994; 94: 831–5.

28. Postma DS, Lebowitz MD. Persistence and new onset of asthma and chronic bronchitis evaluated longitudinally in a community population sample of adults. *Arch Intern Med* 1995; 155: 1393–9.

29. ✪ Panhuysen CIM, Vonk JM, Koeter GH *et al*. Adult patients may outgrow their asthma. A 25-year follow-up study. *Am J Respir Crit Care Med* 1997; 155: 1267–72.

30. Burrows B, Barbee RA, Cline MG, Knudson RJ, Lebowitz MD. Characteristics of asthma among elderly adults in a sample of the general population. *Chest* 1991; 100: 935–42.

31. Rönmark E, Jönsson E, Lundbäck B. Remission of asthma in the middle aged and elderly: report from the Obstructive Lung Disease in Northern Sweden study. *Thorax* 1999; 54: 611–13.

32. ✪ Xu X, Rijcken B, Schouten JP, Weiss ST. Airways responsiveness and development and remission of chronic respiratory symptoms in adults. *Lancet* 1997; 350: 1431–4.

33. Górski P, Kolacinska, Wittczak T. Analysis of the clinical state of patients with occupational asthma following

cessation of exposure to allergens. *Occupat Med* 1999; 49: 285–9.

34. Venables KM, Chan-Yeung M. Occupational asthma. *Lancet* 1997; 349: 1465–9.

35. Brown PJ, Greville HW, Finucane KE. Asthma and irreversible airflow obstruction. *Thorax* 1984; 39: 131–6.

36. Fabbri LM, Caramori G, Beghe B, Papi A, Ciaccia A. Physiologic consequences of long-term inflammation. *Am J Respir Crit Care Med* 1998; 157: S195–S198.

37. Dow L. Asthma versus chronic obstructive pulmonary disease–exploring why "reversibility versus irreversibility" is no longer an appropriate approach. *Clin Exp Allergy* 1999; 29: 739–43.

38. Reed CE. The natural history of asthma in adults: The problem of irreversibility. *J Allergy Clin Immunol* 1999; 103: 539–47.

39. Ulrik CS. Outcome of asthma: longitudinal changes in lung function. *Eur Respir J* 1999; 13: 904–918.

40. Sears MR, Taylor DR. The β_2-agonist controversy.

Observations, explanations and relationship to asthma epidemiology. *Drug Safety* 1994; 11: 259–83.

41. Cockcroft DW, McPaarland CP, Britto SA, Swystun VA, Rutherford BC. Regular inhaled salbutamol and airway responsiveness to allergen. *Lancet* 1993; 342: 833–7.

42. Cockcroft DW, O'Byrne PM, Swystun VA, Bhagat R. Regular use of inhaled albuterol and the allergen-induced late asthmatic response. *J Allergy Clin Immunol* 1995; 96: 44–9.

43. ✪ Sears MR, Taylor DR, Print CG *et al.* Regular inhaled beta-agonist treatment in bronchial asthma. *Lancet* 1990; 336: 1391–6.

44. Taylor DR, Sears MR, Herbison GP *et al.* Regular inhaled β agonist in asthma: effect on exacerbations and lung function. *Thorax* 1993; 48: 134–8.

45. Sears MR. Epidemiological trends in asthma. *Can Respir J* 1996; 3: 261–8.

46. Ulrik CS, Frederiksen J. Mortality and markers of risk of asthma death among 1075 outpatients with asthma. *Chest* 1995; 108: 10–15.

Chapter 3

Pathogenesis

Paul O'Byrne

INTRODUCTION

Asthma was, in the past, identified as the presence of characteristic symptoms and by variable airway narrowing and airway hyperresponsiveness to a variety of inhaled bronchoconstrictor stimuli (Fig. 3.1). Variable airway narrowing is the "sine qua non" of asthma, and while airway hyperresponsiveness is present in virtually all asthmatics with current symptoms[1] it is not specific for asthma, as it can be present in patients with other airway diseases.[2,3] In the past 20 years, there has been a recognition of the central role that airway inflammation plays in the development of the physiological abnormalities of asthma and in the development of symptoms.[4] Interestingly, the importance of airway inflammation in causing (at least severe) asthma has been known for more than 100 years. In the medical textbook, *The Principals and Practice of Medicine*, William Osler described that "bronchial asthma … in many cases is a special form of inflammation of the smaller bronchioles".[5] However, for the next 80 years this was considered to be relevant in only severe, fatal asthma. From the late 1940s the ability to measure lung function easily and reliably and the identification of the presence of airway hyperresponsiveness[6] in almost all asthmatics, as important physiological hallmarks of asthma, were the major focus of research efforts. However, since the early 1980s the pivotal role of acute and/or persisting airway inflammation, and the consequences to the airways of these changes, in causing the physiological abnormalities and asthma symptoms has been identified. Much research effort is now underway to identify the stimuli causing the inflammation; the immunological mechanisms leading to the inflammation; the structural consequences to the airways of persisting inflammation; the relationships between the inflammation and abnormal airway function; the mechanisms causing resolution of the inflammation; and the effects of treatment on the inflammation.

DEFINING AIRWAY INFLAMMATION

Dorlands Medical Dictionary defines inflammation as the "condition into which tissues enter as a reaction to injury". A common manifestation of inflammation is the presence, at some time in the process, of activated inflammatory cells at the affected tissue site. The type of inflammatory cell varies with the type of inflammation. The most important inflammatory cell at sites of acute inflammation is the neutrophil. However, in other more chronic inflammatory conditions, eosinophils, lymphocytes, or mast cells appear to be more prominent. For the purposes of this chapter, airway inflammation will be defined as the presence of activated inflammatory cells in the airways. While this definition is restrictive and excludes other important components of inflammatory events, such as oedema and vasodilation, quantifying numbers and occasionally state of activation of inflammatory cells has been the most commonly used index of airway inflammation in studies of asthma to date. It must also be recognized, however, that the structural consequences of persisting airway inflammation in asthma may be as, or more important than, the presence of the activated inflammatory cells.

AIRWAY HYPERRESPONSIVENESS IN ASTHMA

Measuring airway responsiveness to inhaled bronchoconstrictor stimuli, such as methacholine or histamine, is an important tool in the diagnosis of asthma and in research. This is measured by patients inhaling

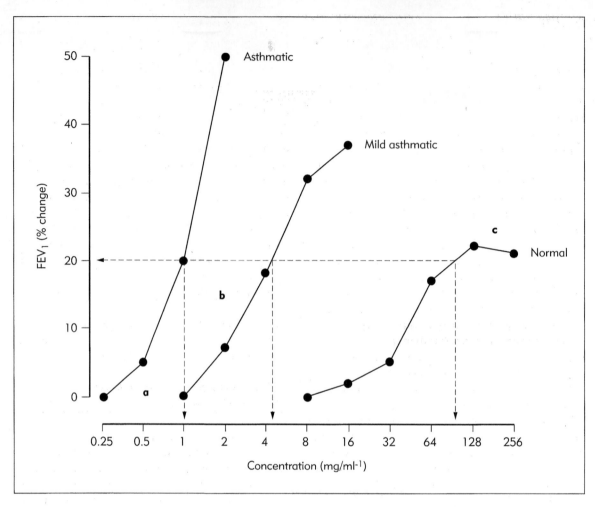

FIGURE 3.1: Dose-response curves to inhaled constrictor agonists in a normal subject, and asthmatic subjects with mildly and severely increased airway hyperresponsiveness. The responses are measured as the fall in FEV_1 from baseline values, and in these examples, the responses are expressed as the provocative concentrations of the agonist causing a 20% fall in FEV_1. The dose-response curves demonstrate the threshold response (a), which is lower in asthmatics, the slope (b), which is steeper in asthmatics, and both the mild asthmatic and normal subjects demonstrate a plateau response (c), which is lost in the more severe asthmatic subject.

increasing doses or concentrations of the bronchoconstrictor stimulus until a given level of bronchoconstriction is achieved, typically a 20% fall in forced expired volume in 1 second (FEV_1). A partial dose-response curve is thereby constructed, and airway responsiveness is then expressed as the provocative dose or concentration of the stimulus required to achieve this degree of bronchoconstriction (PD_{20} and PC_{20} respectively) (Fig. 3.1). The PC_{20} measurement is most often used to express the results, as the PD_{20} value assumes a knowledge of the dose delivered to the lungs, which is, in fact, not known.

Asthmatic patients develop greater degrees of bronchoconstriction to lower inhaled concentrations of the inhaled agonist. Several terms are used, often interchangeably, to describe this phenomenon. These are *hyperresponsiveness*, *hyperreactivity* or *hypersensitivity*. The terms hyperreactivity and hypersensitivity have very specific pharmacological meanings. Hypersensitivity reflects a lower threshold response to an agonist, while hyperreactivity reflects a steeper dose-response curve, once the response has been initiated. This is illustrated in Fig. 3.1, where partial dose response curves to an inhaled bronchoconstrictor agonist from a normal subject, a mild asthmatic and a more severe asthmatic are shown. It can be seen that a decrease in PC_{20} may be due to a steeper dose-response curve, or to a shift in the curve to the left, or both. Also, asthmatics have a greater maximal response to the agonist. For these reasons, the term *airway (or bronchial) hyperresponsiveness* is preferred when discussing PC_{20} measurements, as this is a non-specific term that encompasses the underlying mechanisms that may be responsible for differences in these measurements either between individuals, or within an individual over time.

Airway hyperresponsiveness is present in almost all patients with current symptomatic asthma.[1] Airway hyperresponsiveness is not, however, specific for asthma, being described in patients with allergic rhinitis,[2] cystic fibrosis,[7] and chronic obstructive pulmonary disease.[3] In general, patients with more severe asthma, requiring more medication for treatment, have more severe airway hyperresponsiveness than patients with mild disease.[8] The difference in airway responsiveness between normal individuals and asthmatic patients is substantial, being 4–8 doubling concentrations of inhaled methacholine less than in those normal subjects in whom it can be measured. In fact, no identifiable airway responsiveness can be measured in many healthy individuals, as FEV_1 does not fall by 20%. Within an asthmatic patient, airway responsiveness is generally quite stable when the disease is stable, but can increase during exacerbations of asthma induced by inhaled allergens,[9] or other stimuli.[10]

GENETICS

It has been recognized for many years that familial clustering exists for asthma and, more recently, for airway hyperresponsiveness.[11,12] This could reflect a genetic predisposition for the development of asthma, a shared environmental risk(s), or most likely a combination of both. Efforts have also been made to examine the genetic basis of airway hyperresponsiveness. Studies of monozygotic and dizygotic twins have suggested that there is some genetic basis for the development of airway hyperresponsiveness, but that environmental factors are more important.[13] Also, measurements of airway hyperresponsiveness in young infants (mean age

4.5 weeks) have indicated that airway hyperresponsiveness can be present very early in life, and that a family history of asthma and parental smoking were risk factors for its development.[14] More recently, reports of genetic linkage of airway hyperresponsiveness have been published. One study has identified genetic linkage between histamine airway hyperresponsiveness and several genetic markers on chromosome 5q, near a locus that regulates serum IgE levels.[15] Another study has identified linkage between a highly polymorphic marker of the B subunit of the high affinity IgE receptor on chromosome 11q and methacholine airway hyperresponsiveness, even in patients with nonatopic asthma.[16] Thus, a genetic basis for airway hyperresponsiveness seems very likely; however, the genetic linkage studies need to be confirmed by other investigators in different patient populations. One specific gene polymorphism (Glu 27) of the nine identified of the β_2-adrenoceptor has also been associated with increased methacholine airway hyperresponsiveness,[17] while another polymorphism (Gly 16) was associated with the presence of nocturnal asthma.[18]

TRANSIENT ASTHMA AND AIRWAY INFLAMMATION

The observation that allergen inhalation can cause symptoms of asthma which can last several days was originally made more than 100 years ago by Blackley,[19] who was investigating his own allergy to grass pollen. In the early 1950s, Herxheimer,[20] identified two distinct components to the response to inhaled allergen, which he called the early and late responses. The early asthmatic response is identified as brochoconstriction developing within 10–15 minutes of the inhalation, which reaches a maximum within 30 minutes and generally resolves within 1 to 3 hours. In some subjects, the bronchoconstriction persists and either does not return to baseline values or recurs after 3 to 4 hours and reaches a maximum over 6 to 12 hours. This is the late asthmatic response. The late asthmatic response need not necessarily be preceded by a clinically evident early response. Altounyan[21] described another important consequence of the inhalation of allergen, in that exposure to grass pollen during the grass pollen season could increase airway responsiveness to inhaled histamine in sensitized subjects. Subsequently, Cockcroft and co-workers[22] demonstrated that the increase in histamine and methacholine responsiveness that occurs after inhaled allergen, occurs in association with the allergen-induced late asthmatic response. The magnitudes of the changes in airway responsiveness after inhaled allergen in the research laboratory or during natural pollen exposure are, however, smaller (being 1–2 doubling doses) than the differences described between normals and asthmatics.

The identification of stimuli, such as inhaled allergens, which can cause transient asthma has proven to be important in studies of airway inflammation in asthma. This is because the evidence that the presence of inflammatory cells is causally related to the development of airway hyperresponsiveness and transient asthma in human subjects initially depended on studies which have examined numbers of cells and cellular differentials in bronchoalveolar lavage (BAL) fluid before and after inhalation of ozone,[10] the occupational sensitizing agent toluene diisocyanate (TDI),[23] and allergen,[24] all of which are known to cause airway hyperresponsiveness and transient asthma, or exacerbate persisting asthma. These studies have all demonstrated an acute inflammatory response in the airways associated with the development of variable airflow obstruction, airway hyperresponsiveness, and asthma. In addition, the studies have suggested that the stimulus which initiates the airway hyperresponsiveness determines the type of cellular response. For example, a substantial increase in neutrophils and a smaller increase in eosinophils was described in BAL in subjects with airway hyperresponsiveness following TDI.[23] In contrast, airway challenge with plicatic acid responsible for western red cedar asthma, a different form of occupational asthma, caused increases in eosinophil numbers, but not neutrophils, in BAL.[25] After allergen challenge, some studies describe increases in eosinophils,[24] or eosinophils and neutrophils,[26] or eosinophils, lymphocytes and basophils.[27] However, measurements in these studies have been carried out at different time points, and with different challenge techniques which might explain the varied results.

More recently, a less invasive method than bronchoscopy has been developed, using sputum induced by the inhalation of hypertonic saline, to quantify and characterize inflammatory cells in asthmatic airways. This method has allowed a much more careful examination of the relationship between the development of allergen-induced airway hyperresponsiveness and the influx and efflux of eosinophils and basophils across the inflamed airways.[28,29] These studies have demonstrated

that increases in airway eosinophils occur before 7 hours after allergen inhalation, and are involved in the pathogenesis of the allergen-induced late response. The basophils influx has resolved by 3 days, while the airway eosinophils remain elevated for up to 7 days, the time course of which is correlated to the allergen-induced changes in methacholine airway hyperresponsiveness (Fig. 3.2). Very similar information has been obtained when repeated low doses of inhaled allergens are used as the stimulus, inhaled daily over 5 days.[30] Once again the allergen-induced changes in airway hyperresponsiveness are closely temporally related to the influx and efflux of airway eosinophils. These airway eosinophils are in an activated state in the airways, as indicated by increases in EG2+ cells (EG2 is a monoclonal antibody which recognizes cleaved eosinophilic cationic protein (ECP) in eosinophils), as well as increased amounts of ECP in sputum supernatant. Studies using this method have also demonstrated that eosinophils increase markedly in sputum samples of some asthmatics undergoing an exacerbation of their asthma,[31] while increases in airway neutrophils occur in other asthmatics during an exacerbation.[32]

AIRWAY INFLAMMATION IN PERSISTING ASTHMA

There have been a number of studies which have provided information on cell populations in BAL fluid in mild stable asthmatics with persistent airway hyperresponsiveness and asthma.[33–35] Common findings in all of these studies, as well as in examinations of bronchial mucosal biopsies are the presence of increased numbers of inflammatory cells such as eosinophils, lymphocytes and mast cells compared with normal control subjects with normal airway responsiveness. The eosinophils have shown signs of activation, as indicated by increased levels of granular proteins, major basic protein (MBP)[34] and ECP.[35] In the bronchial mucosa the eosinophils have shown morphological features of activation, as indicated by heterogeneity of the granular structure[36] or as eosinophil granules lying free in the mucosal interstitium.[37] Also, a significant increase in numbers of activated T-lymphocytes has been described.[38] Mast cells in the airway mucosa have exhibited various stages of degranulation[39] suggesting that mediator release is an ongoing process in the airways of stable asthmatics with persistent airway hyperresponsiveness.

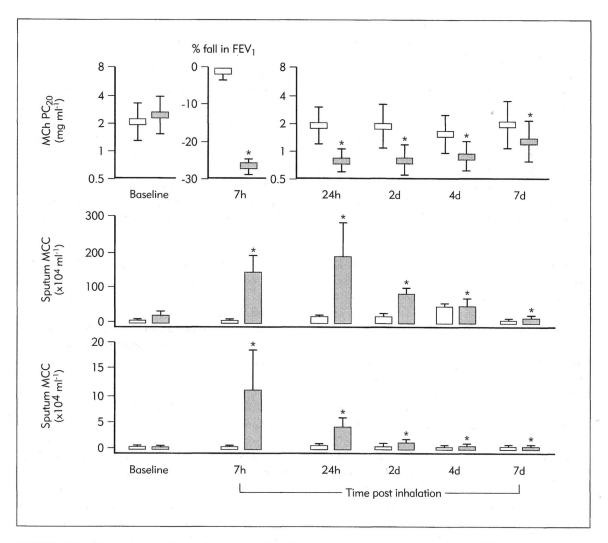

FIGURE 3.2: Time course of changes in methacholine PC_{20} and maximum percentage late fall in FEV_1 (top panel), sputum eosinophils (middle panel) and metachromatic cells (bottom panel) in response to diluent (open bars) and allergen (stippled bars) inhalation challenge (*$P < 0.05$). (From Gauvreau GM, Watson RM, O'Byrne PM. Kinetics of allergen-induced airway eosinophilic cytokine production and airway inflammation. *Am J Respir Crit Care Med* 1999; 160: 640–7, with permission.)

Some studies have correlated numbers of inflammatory cells in BAL fluid with the severity of methacholine airway hyperresponsiveness or clinical severity in stable asthmatics. Kirby et al.[33] demonstrated close correlations between degree of airway hyperresponsiveness in subjects with mild asthma and number of mast cells and eosinophils in lavage fluid. Kelly and co-workers[40] showed correlations between numbers of neutrophils and airway hyperresponsiveness. Others, however, have not been able to find correlations between numbers of airway inflammatory cells and airway hyperresponsiveness.[41] Bousquet et al.[42] have demonstrated that the numbers of eosinophils and levels of ECP in BAL correlated with the severity of asthma as measured by an asthma severity score, and with pulmonary function.

These studies can be summarized as demonstrating the presence of activated inflammatory cells, eosinophils, neutrophils, lymphocytes and mast cells in the airways of asthmatics even at a time when they are considered stable and asymptomatic. The numbers of cells increase following a stimulus which causes airway hyperresponsiveness, as well as in natural exacerbations of asthma. The presence of activated eosinophils appears to be the best correlate with the presence of pulmonary function abnormalities, airway hyperresponsiveness and asthma severity. However, the precise mechanism that eosinophils, and the other cells demonstrated to be increased in asthma, are playing in the pathogenesis is still under very active investigation.

MECHANISMS OF PERSISTING AIRWAY INFLAMMATION

The mechanisms by which the effector cells in asthma, eosinophils, mast cells, basophils, lymphocytes and neutrophils, are recruited into the airways, persist and are activated in the airways, involve important roles for cytokines and chemokines. There are now more than 30 different protein mediators that are classed as cytokines or chemokines. Some of these have been implicated in the pathogenesis of asthma, mainly because of their ability to promote inflammatory cell growth and differentiation, or inflammatory cell migration and activation, or cause changes in the structural cells of the airways. The study of the cytokines in asthma is not yet as developed as for other mediators, such as the leukotrienes, mainly because of the lack of specific antagonists which can be studied in humans. However, the cytokines interleukin (IL)3, IL5, and granulocyte macrophage-colony stimulating factor (GM-CSF) may be important because of their ability to promote eosinophil and mast cell differentiation, recruitment and activation into the airways, and prolong the survival of these cells once in the airways. All of these cytokines, as well as IL4, which is necessary for IgE production, are produced by one type of helper T-cell, the TH_2 cell, which is present in asthmatic airways.[43] In addition, other airway cells may be responsible for the production of these cytokines.[44,45] Increased amounts of GM-CSF, but not IL3, are present in airway biopsies from mild asthmatics,[46] and the levels increase after allergen challenge.[47] Also, IL-5 levels are increased in asthmatics and following allergen inhalation.[30,48] In addition, upregulation of the IL-5 receptor is necessary for increased eosinophil production in the bone marrow following allergen inhalation.[49] The chemokines (small molecular weight, <10 Kd, proteins

which can chemoattract inflammatory cells), eotaxin and RANTES are potent chemoattractants for eosinophils and there are increases in the airways following allergen inhalation,[29] while IL-8 is a potent chemoattractant for neutrophils.[50] It would appear very likely that these, as well as other cytokines, are responsible for the presence of persisting activated eosinophils and mast cells in asthmatic airways; however, further studies with drugs which block the action of specific cytokines will be needed to establish precisely their role in asthma. Finally, IL-10 is an important anti-inflammatory cytokine,[51] whose production may be reduced in asthmatic airways, thereby allowing airway inflammation to persist.

OTHER INFLAMMATORY MEDIATORS IN ASTHMA

Histamine and Acetylcholine

Histamine and acetylcholine have biological effects which are relevant to asthma; both are released in response to appropriate stimuli, acetylcholine from airway nerves and histamine from airway mast cells and basophils; both are potent bronchoconstrictors and histamine has other effects, such as vasodilation and increases vascular permeability. In addition, H_1-receptor antagonists have been demonstrated to partially inhibit some asthmatic responses, such as exercise-induced bronchoconstriction,[52] and allergen-induced early and late responses.[53] However, even very potent and long-acting antihistamines are not effective bronchodilators, nor do they have a useful role in the management of asthma. Atropine and other anticholinergics, such as ipratropium bromide, are bronchodilators and have been used for many years to treat bronchoconstriction, and more recently to treat (together with inhaled β_2 agonists) acute severe asthma.[54] This suggests that acetylcholine is released from airway nerves in asthmatics and causes bronchoconstriction. However, anticholinergics do not modify any other important component of asthma, which indicates that acetylcholine release is not involved in the underlying pathogenesis of asthma.

Prostaglandins and Thromboxane

Prostaglandins (PG) and thromboxane (Tx) in the form of PGD_2 and TxA_2 are potent constrictors of airway smooth muscle, and cause bronchoconstrcition in asthmatics.[55,56] Studies examining the effects of a thromboxane synthetase inhibitor on airway responses after allergen challenge demonstrated slight, but significant, inhibition of the allergen-induced early asthmatic responses by 20–25%, but no inhibition of allergen-induced late asthmatic responses nor allergen-induced histamine airway hyperresponsiveness 24 hours post-allergen.[57] This suggested that thromboxane may be released following allergen challenge, and be partly responsible for the early asthmatic response, but is not important in causing other allergen-induced responses. Anti-thromboxanes are used for asthma treatment in Japan, however, there are no well controlled, double-blind comparisons demonstrating marked clinical efficacy in the management of asthma, and they are not widely available elsewhere.

Inhibitory prostaglandins, particularly PGE_2, play a role in maintaining airway function by causing refractoriness to bronchoconstriction following repeated bouts of exercise.[58] Also, pretreatment with PGE_2 can attenuate allergen-induced airway responses and airway inflammation.[59] This raises the possibility that PGE_2, released in asthmatic airways in association with a worsening airway inflammation, may limit the extent of the inflammation or assist in its resolution.

Cysteinyl Leukotrienes

Cysteinyl leukotrienes $(LT)C_4$ and D_4 are the most potent bronchoconstrictors yet studied in human subjects, being up to 10 000 times more potent than methacholine in some normal subjects,[60] and with a longer duration of action than inhaled histamine.[61] Also, increases in urinary levels of LTE_4, the metabolite of LTC_4 and LTD_4 have been demonstrated following allergen-induced early responses,[62] in patients presenting to hospital with acute severe asthma,[63] and following exercise-induced bronchoconstriction.[64] Studies with potent and specific leukotriene antagonists have supported an important role for the leukotrienes in clinical models of asthma, such as exercise-,[65] allergen-[66,67] (Fig. 3.3) and aspirin-induced asthma.[68] Also, leukotriene release is, in part, responsible for spontaneous bronchoconstriction[69] and possibly for some of the cellular inflammation in asthma.[70] Lastly, the studies of the leukotriene antagonists and synthesis inhibitors have demonstrated clinical efficacy in asthma.[71–73] These results taken together indicate that the cysteinyl leukotrienes are important in the pathogenesis of asthma.

AIRWAY STRUCTURAL CHANGES IN ASTHMA

A number of structural changes have been described in asthmatic airways, which appear to be characteristic of the disease, even in patients with mild persisting asthma, and which may be responsible for the presence of persisting airway hyperresponsiveness in asthma. These changes include patchy desquamated epithelium;[74] goblet cell hyperplasia; increased numbers of mucous glands;[75] thickening of the reticular collagen layer below the basement membrane;[76] new vessel formation;[77] and an increase in airway smooth muscle volume.[75] Both airway epithelial damage and airway smooth muscle hypertrophy have been implicated in the pathogenesis of airway hyperresponsiveness in asthma.

Airway Epithelial Damage

Airway epithelial damage and desquamation is present in airways of patients with asthma.[74] There is also a marked number of goblet cells in the damaged epithelium, which may represent a rapid turnover of the ciliated epithelial cells. One hypothesis to explain epithelial damage and desquamation in asthmatic airways is that basic proteins such as MBP, ECP and EPX released from activated eosinophils damage the epithelium. Levels of MBP have been shown to be increased in BAL from asthmatic patients.[34] Using immunofluorescence, MBP has also been identified in tissue sections from airways of patients dying from severe asthma.[78] Even in sections where identifiable eosinophils could not be seen, evidence showed MBP to be present in epithelium and submucosa giving signs of tissue damage.

Several hypotheses have been proposed to explain how epithelial damage may result in airway hyperresponsiveness in asthma. These have included increased permeability of the airway epithelium; loss of inhibitory mediators generated by the airway epithelium; and loss of neutral endopeptidase. Several studies have compared the permeability of the respiratory epithelium in normal subjects, asthmatics and asymptomatic smokers. These studies demonstrated that the clearance of inhaled radiolabelled aerosols from the lung into the blood was much faster in the asymptomatic smokers with normal airway responsiveness than in either the normal subjects with normal airway responsiveness, or the asthmatic subjects with airway hyperresponsiveness.[79] These results make it very unlikely that increases in airway epithelial permeability is the cause of airway hyperresponsiveness in asthma.

33

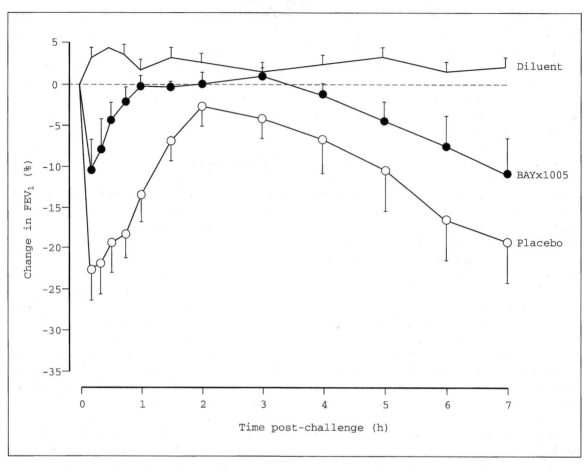

FIGURE 3.3: Mean (± SEM) percent change in FEV_1 from baseline during the early and late asthmatic response to allergen inhalation after treatment with the anti-leukotriene BAY×1005 (closed circles) or placebo (open circles) and after inhaled diluent. (*P < 0.05; **P < 0.001). (From Hamilton AL, Watson RM, Wylie G, O'Byrne PM. A 5-lipoxygenase activating protein antagonist Bay x 1005, attenuates both early and late phase allergen-induced bronchocostriction in asthmatic subjects. *Thorax* 1997; SZ: 348–54, with permission.)

The epithelium has been reported to release a factor which reduces the airway smooth muscle contractile responses to agonists such as histamine and acetylcholine.[80] This mediator has been called epithelium-derived relaxing factor (EpDRF). The hypothesis that loss of an inhibitory EpDRF may be responsible for airway hyperresponsiveness in asthma has not been possible to test in human subjects. Airway epithelial cells are known to release PGE_2,[81] which has potent inhibitory effects in the airways, such as presynaptic modulation and inhibition of acetylcholine release from muscarinic nerves.[82] In addition, PGE is able to reduce contractile responses to inhaled histamine, acetylcholine and methacholine,[83] and reduce bronchoconstrictor res-

ponses to exercise[58] and allergen-induced airway inflammation[59] in asthmatics. The airway epithelium also contains enzymes, neutral endopeptidases, capable of metabolizing tachykinins, such as substance P,[84] which are bronchoconstrictor and pro-inflammatory mediators. Loss of these inhibitory mediators may have important results in asthmatic airways; however, this hypothesis has not yet been tested in asthmatic subjects.

Increases in Extra Cellular Matrix Proteins Below the Basement Membrane

An increase in the "basement membrane" below the airway epithelium has been known for many years to be a characteristic feature of patients with persisting asthma[75] and the extent of the thickness has been correlated to the severity of airway hyperresponsiveness.[85] Changes to the extent found in asthma are not found in other airway diseases, such as chronic obstructive pulmonary disease (COPD). The abnormality is, in fact, increased deposition of extracellular matrix proteins, such as collagen types III and V,[76] reticulin and tenacin.[86] An increase in the number of airway myofibroblasts below the basement membrane has been described in asthmatics, and these cells have the capacity to produce these extracellular matrix proteins.[87] Also, a large increase in airway myofibroblasts has been described in airway biopsies 24 hours after allergen inhalation from asthmatic subjects.[88] These cells may also be progenitor cells for airway myocytes, which may help to explain the increase in volume of the airway smooth muscle in asthma.

Airway Smooth Muscle

Airway hyperresponsiveness in asthma is non-specific. This means that asthmatic airways are more responsive to all bronchoconstrictor mediators acting on airway smooth muscle receptors. One explanation for the lack of specificity is that the underlying abnormality in asthmatic airways resides in the airway smooth muscle. This may be through the increase in airway smooth muscle volume in asthmatics causing airway hyperresponsiveness by a thickening of asthmatic airways. James *et al.*[89] have, by using modelling studies, demonstrated that a small increase in the thickness of the airway wall, which it is not possible to demonstrate by changes in spirometric indices, could result in airway hyperresponsiveness in asthma. The responses of airway smooth muscle from human subjects with airway hyperresponsiveness *in vivo* have been studied by a number of different investigators.[90,91] No consistent increase in smooth muscle responsiveness *in vitro* has been associated with airways hyperresponsiveness *in vivo*. Very few studies have examined smooth muscle *in vitro* from subjects with airway hyperresponsiveness *and* asthma. A small number of studies of airway smooth muscle from asthmatic subjects suggest that the smooth muscle is hyperresponsive to agonists *in vitro*, when compared with airways from non-asthmatic subjects.[92,93] Thus, an inherent defect may exist in asthmatic airway smooth muscle, which would account for airway hyperresponsiveness.

CONCLUSIONS

Airway inflammation appears to be central to the pathogenesis of all of the clinical manifestations of asthma. Many studies have now demonstrated the presence of activated eosinophils and of mast cells in the airway lumen and airway wall of patients with asthma, even those with mild disease. The presence and survival of these inflammatory cells may be promoted by the presence of increased levels of proinflammatory cytokines, such as GM-CSF and IL-5, in asthmatic airways. These cells have the capacity to release potent bronchoconstrictor mediators such as the cysteinyl leukotrienes, which are responsible, in part at least, for airway narrowing in asthma and for allergen-, exercise- and aspirin-induced asthma. Other cells, such as a subset of T-lymphocytes (TH$_2$), may also be important in maintaining the inflammatory cascade. Airway structural changes caused by the persisting inflammation, such as airway epithelial damage, or altered smooth muscle function or volume, are likely important in the pathogenesis of stable long standing airway hyperresponsiveness. Mediators released from the inflammatory cells may be responsible for these changes. Despite the great increase in knowledge about the importance of airway inflammation in the pathogenesis of asthma, the precise sequence of events which leads to the presence of persisting airway inflammatory cells, airway structural changes and airway hyperresponsiveness in asthma remains to be clarified.

KEY POINTS

1. Asthma is a chronic inflammatory disease of the airways.

2. The cellular inflammatory infiltrate most often consists of increased numbers of eosinophils, mast cells and T-lymphocytes (TH_2-subtype).

3. The eosinophilic airway inflammation is likely caused by increased levels of airway cytokines (GM-CSF, IL-3 and IL-5) and chemokines (RANTES and eotaxin).

4. Asthmatic airways demonstrate structural changes, which consist of damaged epithelium, increased numbers of goblet cells and mucous glands, deposition of extra cellular matrix below the basement membrane, increased vascularity, and increased volume of airway smooth muscle.

5. Airway hyperresponsiveness is a characteristic physiological abnormality in asthma.

6. Airway hyperresponsiveness can be further increased by inhalation of environmental allergens, viral respiratory infections, occupational sensitizers, or atmospheric pollutants.

7. Both the underlying airway structural abnormalities and the cellular inflammation contribute to the pathogenesis of airway hyperresponsiveness.

8. Cysteinyl leukotrienes are an important cause of bronchoconstriction in asthmatics.

REFERENCES

1. Cockcroft DW, Killian DN, Mellon JJ, Hargreave FE. Bronchial reactivity to inhaled histamine: a method and clinical survey. *Clin Allergy* 1977; 7: 235–43.

2. Ramsdale EH, Morris MM, Roberts RS, Hargreave FE. Asymptomatic bronchial hyperresponsiveness in rhinitis. *J Allergy Clin Immunol* 1985; 75: 573–7.

3. Ramsdale EH, Morris MM, Roberts RS, Hargreave FE. Bronchial responsiveness to methacholine in chronic bronchitis: relationship to airflow obstruction and cold air responsiveness. *Thorax* 1984; 39: 912–8.

4. Adelroth E, O'Byrne PM. Inflammatory mechanisms in airway hyperresponsiveness. In: Holgate ST, Busse WW (eds). *Asthma and Rhinitis*. Boston, Mass: Blackwell Scientific Publications, 1994: 11067–74.

5. Osler W. *The Principals and Practice of Medicine*. New York, NY: Appleton and Co, 1892: 497.

6. Tiffeneau R, Beauvallet B. Epreuve de bronchoconstriction et de broncholilation par aerosols. *Bull Acad Med* 1945; 129: 165–8.

7. van Haren EH, Lammers JW, Festen J, Heijerman HG, Groot CA, van Herwaarden L. The effects of the inhaled corticosteroid budesonide on lung function and bronchial hyperresponsiveness in adult patients with cystic fibrosis. *Respir Med* 1995; 89: 209–14.

8. Juniper EF, Frith PA, Hargreave FE. Airway responsiveness to histamine and methacholine: relationship to minimum treatment to control symptoms of asthma. *Thorax* 1981; 36: 575–9.

9. Cockcroft DW, Ruffin RE, Dolovich J, Hargreave FE. Allergen-induced increase in non-allergic bronchial reactivity. *Clin Allergy* 1977; 7: 503–13.

10. Stelzer J, Bigby BG, Stulbarg M *et al*. Ozone changes in bronchial reactivity to methacholine and airway inflammation in humans. *J Appl Physiol* 1986; 60: 1321–6.

11. Longo G, Strinati R, Poli F, Fumi F. Genetic factors in nonspecific bronchial hyperreactivity. *Am J Dis Child* 1987; 141: 331–4.

12. Hopp RJ, Bewtra A, Biven R, Nair NM, Townley RG. Bronchial reactivity pattern in nonasthmatic parents of asthmatics. *Ann Allergy* 1988; 61: 184–6.

13. Nieminen MM, Kaprio J, Koskenvuo M. A population based study of bronchial asthma in adult twin pairs. *Chest* 1991; 100: 70–5.

14. Young S, Le Souef PN, Geelhoed GC, Stick SM, Turner KL, Landau LI. The influence of a family history of asthma and parental smoking on airway responsiveness in early infancy. *N Engl J Med* 1991; 324: 1168–73.

15. ✪ Postma DS, Bleeker ER, Amelung PJ, Holroyd KJ, Xu J, Panhyusen CIM *et al.* Genetic susceptibility to asthma-bronchial hyperresponsiveness coinherited with a major gene for atopy. *N Engl J Med* 1995; 333: 894–900.

16. van Herwerden L, Harrap SB, Wong ZY, Abramson MJ, Kutin JJ, Forbes AB *et al.* Linkage of high-affinity IgE receptor gene with bronchial hyperreactivity, even in the absence of atopy. *Lancet* 1995; 346: 1262–5.

17. Hall IP, Wheatley A, Wilding P, Liggett SB. Association of Glu 27 beta 2-adrenoceptor polymorphism with lower airway reactivity in asthmatic subjects. *Lancet* 1995; 345: 1213–4.

18. Turki J, Pak J, Green SA, Martin RJ, Liggett SB. Genetic polymorphism of the beta-2 adrenergic receptor in nocturnal and nonnocturnal asthma. Evidence that Gly 16 correlates with the nocturnal phenotype. *J Clin Invest* 1995; 95: 1635–41.

19. Blackley CH. On the quantity of pollen found floating in the atmosphere during the prevalance of hay fever and its relationship to the intensity of the symptoms. In: *Experimental Researches on the Causes and Nature of Catarrus Aestivus*. London: Baillière, Tindall, Cox, 1873.

20. Herxheimer H. The late bronchial reaction in induced asthma. *Arch Allergy* 1952; 3: 323–8.

21. Altounyan REC. Changes in histamine and atropine responsiveness as a guide to the diagnosis and evaluation of therapy in obstructive airways disease. In: Pepys J, Frankland AW (eds). *Disodium Cromoglycate in Allergic Airways Diseas*. London: Butterworths, 1970: 47–53.

22. Cockcroft DW, Murdock KY. Changes in bronchial responsiveness to histamine at intervals after allergen challenge. *Thorax* 1987; 42: 302–8.

23. Fabbri LM, Boschetto P, Zocca E, Milani G, Pivirotto F, Plebani M *et al.* Bronchoalveolar neutrophilia during late asthmatic reactions induced by toluene diisocyanate. *Am Rev Respir Dis* 1987; 136: 36–42.

24. de Monchy JG, Kauffman HF, Venge P, Koeter GH, Jansen HM, Sluiter HJ *et al.* Bronchoalveolar eosionphilia during allergen-induced late asthmatic reactions. *Am Rev Respir Dis* 1985; 131: 373–6.

25. Lam S, Chan-Yeung M, Le Riche JC, Kijek K, Phillips D. Cellular changes in bronchial lavage fluid following late asthmatic reactions in patients with red cedar asthma. *Am Rev Respir Dis* 1987; 131: 42A.

26. Metzger WJ, Richerson HB, Worden K, Monick M, Hunninghake GW. Bronchoalveolar lavage of allergic asthmatic patients following allergen bronchoprovocation. *Chest* 1986; 89: 477–83.

27. Diaz P, Gonzalez MC, Galleguillos FR *et al.* Leukocytes and mediators in bronchoalveolar lavage during allergen-induced late-phase asthmatic reactions. *Am Rev Respir Dis* 1989; 139: 1383–9.

28. Pin I, Freitag AP, O'Byrne PM, Girgis-Gabardo A, Watson RM, Dolovich *et al.* Changes in the cellular profile of induced sputum after allergen-induced asthmatic responses. *Am Rev Respir Dis* 1992; 145: 1265–9.

29. Gauvreau GM, Watson RM, O'Byrne PM. Kinetics of allergen-induced airway eosinophilic cytokine production and airway inflammation. *Am J Respir Crit Care Med* 1999; 160: 640–7.

30. ✪ Sulakvelidze I, Inman MD, Rerecich TJ, O'Byrne PM. Increases in airway eosinophils and interleukin-5 with minimal bronchoconstriction during repeated low dose allergen challenge in atopic asthmatics. *Eur Respir J* 1998; 11: 821–7.

31. Gibson PG, Wong BJO, Hepperle MJE, Kline P, Girgis-Gabardo A, Guyatt GH *et al.* A research method to induce and examine a mild exacerbation of asthma by withdrawal of inhaled corticosteroid. *Clin Exp Allergy* 1992; 22: 525–32.

32. Turner MO, Hussack P, Sears MR, Dolovich J, Hargreave FE. Exacerbations of asthma without sputum eosinophilia. *Thorax* 1995; 50: 1057–61.

33. Kirby JG, Hargreave FE, Gleich GJ, O'Byrne PM. Bronchoalveolar cell profiles of asthmatic and

nonasthmatic subjects. *Am Rev Respir Dis* 1987; 136: 379–83.

34. Wardlaw AJ, Dunnette S, Gleich GJ, Collins JV, Kay AB. Eosinophils and mast cells in bronchoalveolar lavage in subjects with mild asthma. Relationship to bronchial hyperreactivity. *Am Rev Respir Dis* 1988; 137: 62–9.

35. Adelroth E, Rosenhall L, Johansson SA, Linden M, Venge P. Inflammatory cells and eosinophilic activity in asthmatics investigated by bronchoalveolar lavage. The effects of antiasthmatic treatment with budesonide or terbutaline. *Am Rev Respir Dis* 1990; 142: 91–9.

36. Beasley R, Roche WR, Roberts JA, Holgate ST. Cellular events in the bronchi in mild asthma and after bronchial provocation. *Am Rev Respir Dis* 1989; 139: 806–17.

37. Jeffery PK, Wardlaw AJ, Nelson FC, Collins JV, Kay AB. Bronchial biopsies in asthma. An ultrastructural, quantitative study and correlation with hyperreactivity. *Am Rev Respir Dis* 1989; 140: 1745–53.

38. Azzawi M, Bradley B, Jeffery P *et al.* Identification of activated T-lymphocytes and eosinophils in bronchial biopsies in stable atopic asthma. *Am Rev Respir Dis* 1990; 140: 1407–13.

39. Poston RN, Chanez P, Lacoste JY, Litchfield TM, Lee TH, Bousquet J. Immunohistochemical characterization of the cellular infiltration in asthmatic bronchi. *Am Rev Respir Dis* 1992; 145: 918–21.

40. Kelly C, Ward C, Stenton CS, Bird G, Hendrick DJ, Walters EH. Number and activity of inflammatory cells in bronchoalveolar lavage fluid in asthma and their relation to airway responsiveness. *Thorax* 1988; 43: 684–92.

41. Crimi E, Spanevello A, Neri M, Ind PW, Rossi GA, Brusasco V. Dissociation between airway inflammation and airway hyperresponsiveness in allergic asthma. *Am J Respir Crit Care Med* 1998; 157: 4–9.

42. Bousquet J, Chanez P, Lacoste JY, Barneon G, Ghavanian N, Enander I *et al.* Eosinophilic inflammation in asthma. *N Engl J Med* 1990; 323: 1033–9.

43. ✪ Robinson DS, Hamid Q, Ying S *et al.* Predominant TH-2 like bronchoalveolar T-lymphocyte populations in atopic asthma. *N Engl J Med* 1992; 326: 298–304.

44. Nonaka M, Nonaka R, Woolley K *et al.* Distinct immunohistochemical localization of IL-4 in human inflamed airway tissues. IL-4 is localized to eosinophils *in vivo* and is released by peripheral blood eosinophils. *J Immunol* 1995; 155: 3234–44.

45. Broide DH, Paine MM, Firestein GS. Eosinophils express interleukin 5 and granulocyte macrophage-colony-stimulating factor mRNA at sites of allergic inflammation. *J Clin Invest* 1992; 90: 1414–24.

46. Woolley KL, Adelroth E, Woolley MJ, Ellis R, Jordana M, O'Byrne PM. Granulocyte-macrophage colony-stimulating factor, eosinophils and eosinophil cationic protein in subjects with and without mild, stable, atopic asthma. *Eur Respir J* 1994; 7: 1576–84.

47. Woolley KL, Adelroth E, Woolley MJ, Ellis R, Jordana M, O'Byrne PM. Effects of allergen challenge on eosinophils, eosinophil cationic protein, and granulocyte-macrophage colony-stimulating factor in mild asthma. *Am J Respir Crit Care Med* 1995; 151: 1915–24.

48. Hallden G, Hellman C, Gronneberg R, Lundahl J. Increased levels of IL-5 positive peripheral blood eosinophils and lymphocytes in mild asthmatics after allergen inhalation provocation. *Clin Exp Allergy* 1998; 29: 595–603.

49. Sehmi R, Woods L, Watson RM, Foley R, Hamid Q, O'Byrne PM *et al.* Allergen-induced increases in IL-5 a subunit expression on bone marrow derived CD34+ cells from asthmatic subjects: a novel marker of progenitor cell committment towards eosinophil differentiation. *J Clin Invest* 1997; 100: 2466–75.

50. Smith WB, Gamble JR, Clarke-Lewis I, Vadas MA. IL-8 induces neutrophil transendothelial migration. *Immunology* 1991; 72: 65–72.

51. Lalani I, Bhol K, Ahmed AR. Interleukin-10: biology, role in inflammation and autoimmunity. *Ann Allergy Asthma Immunol* 1997; 79: 469–83.

52. Hartley JPR, Nogrady SG. Effect of an inhaled antihistamine on exercise-induced asthma. *Thorax* 1980; 35: 675–9.

53. Roquet A, Dahlen B, Kumlin M, Ihre E, Aanstren G, Binks S *et al.* Combined antagonist of leukotrienes and histamine produces predominant inhibition of allergen-induced early and late phase airway

obstruction in asthmatics. *Am J Respir Crit Care Med* 1997; 155: 1856–63.

54. Rebuck AS, Chapman KR, Abboud R, Pare PD, Kreisman H, Wolkove N et al. Nebulized anticholinergic and sympathomimetic treatment of asthma and chronic obstructive airways disease in the emergency room. *Am J Med* 1987; 82: 59–64.

55. Beasley R, Varley J, Robinson C, Holgate ST. Cholinergic-mediated bronchoconstriction induced by prostaglandin D2, its initial metabolite 9 alpha, 11 beta-PGF2, and PGF2 alpha in asthma. *Am Rev Respir Dis* 1987; 136: 1140–4.

56. Saroea HG, Inman MD, O'Byrne PM. U46619-induced bronchoconstriction in asthmatic subjects is mediated by acetylcholine release. *J Appl Physiol* 1995; 151: 321–4.

57. Manning PJ, Stevens WH, Cockcroft DW, O'Byrne PM. The role of thromboxane in allergen-induced asthmatic responses. *Eur Respir J* 1991; 4: 667–72.

58. Melillo E, Woolley KL, Manning PJ, Watson RM, O'Byrne PM. Effect of inhaled PGE_2 on exercise-induced bronchoconstriction in asthmatic subjects. *Am J Respir Crit Care Med* 1994; 149: 1138–41.

59. Gauvreau GM, Watson RM, O'Byrne PM. Effect of inhaled prostaglandin E2 on inflammatory responses after inhaled allergen. *Am J Respir Crit Care Med* 1999; 159: 31–6.

60. Adelroth E, Morris MM, Hargreave FE, O'Byrne PM. Airway responsiveness to leukotrienes C4 and D4 and to methacholine in patients with asthma and normal controls. *N Engl J Med* 1986; 315: 480–4.

61. Barnes NC, Piper PJ, Costello JF. Comparative effects of inhaled leukotriene C4, leukotriene D4, and histamine in normal human subjects. *Thorax* 1984; 39: 500–4.

62. Manning PJ, Rokach J, Malo JL, Ethier D, Cartier A, Girard Y et al. Urinary leukotriene E4 levels during early and late asthmatic responses. *J Allergy Clin Immunol* 1990; 86: 211–20.

63. Taylor GW, Black P, Turner N, Taylor I, Maltby NH, Fuller RW et al. Urinary leukotriene E4 after antigen challenge and in acute asthma and allergic rhinitis. *Lancet* 1989; i: 585–7.

64. Kikawa Y, Miyanomae T, Inoue Y, Saito M, Nakai A, Shigematsu Y et al. Urinary leukotriene E4 after exercise challenge in children with asthma. *J Allergy Clin Immunol* 1992; 89: 1111–9.

65. ✪ Manning PJ, Watson RM, Margolskee DJ, Williams VC, Schwartz JI, O'Byrne PM. Inhibition of exercise-induced bronchoconstriction by MK-571, a potent leukotriene D4-receptor antagonist. *N Engl J Med* 1990; 323: 1736–9.

66. Taylor G, Walker J. Charles Harrison Blackley, 1820–1900. *Clin Allergy* 1973; 3: 103–8.

67. Hamilton AL, Watson RM, Wylie G, O'Byrne PM. A 5-lipoxygenase activating protein antagonist, Bay x 1005, attenuates both early and late phase allergen-induced bronchoconstriction in asthmatic subjects. *Thorax* 1997; 52: 348–54.

68. Israel E, Fischer AR, Rosenburg MA, Lilly CM, Callery JC, Shapiro J et al. The pivotal role of 5-lipoxygenase products in the reaction of aspirin-sensitive asthmatics to aspirin. *Am Rev Respir Dis* 1993; 148: 1447–51.

69. Gaddy J, Bush RK, Margolskee D, Williams VC, Busse W. The effects of leukotriene D4 (LTD4) antagonist (MK-571) in mild to moderate asthma. *Am Rev Respir Dis* 1992; 146: 358–63.

70. Wenzel SE, Trudeau JB, Kaminsky DA, Cohn J, Martin RJ, Westcott JY. Effect of 5-lipoxygenase inhibition of bronchoconstriction and airway inflammation in nocturnal asthma. *Am J Respir Crit Care Med* 1995; 152: 897–905.

71. ✪ Israel E, Rubin P, Kemp JP, Grossman J, Pierson W, Siegel SC et al. The effect of inhibition of 5-lipoxygenase by zileuton in mild-to-moderate asthma. *Ann Intern Med* 1993; 119: 1059–66.

72. Spector SL, Glass M, Birmingham BK, Bronsky EA, Dunn KD, Fish JE et al. Effects of 6 weeks of therapy with oral doses of ICI 204,219 a leukotriene D4 receptor antagonist, in subjects with bronchial asthma. *Am J Respir Crit Care Med* 1994; 150: 618–23.

73. Noonan M, Chervinsky P, Brandon M et al. Montelukast, a potent leukotriene receptor antagonist, causes dose-related improvements in chronic asthma. Montelukast Asthma Study Group. *Eur Resp J* 1998; 11: 1232–9.

74. Laitinen LA, Heino M, Laitinen A, Kava T, Haahtela T. Damage of the airway epithelium and bronchial reactivity in patients with asthma. *Am Rev Respir Dis* 1985; 131: 599–606.

75. Dunnill MS, Massarell GR, Anderson JA. A comparison of the quantitive anatomy of the bronchi in normal subjects, in status asthmaticus, in chronic bronchitis and in emphysema. *Thorax* 1969; 24: 176–9.

76. Wilson JW, Li X. The measurement of reticular basement membrane and submucosal collagen in the asthmatic airway. *Clin Exp Allergy* 1997; 27: 363–71.

77. Li X, Wilson JW. Increased vascularity of the bronchial mucosa in mild asthma. *Am J Respir Crit Care Med* 1997; 156: 229–33.

78. Gleich GJ, Frigas E, Loegering DA, Wassom DL, Steinmuller D. Cytotoxic properties of the eosinophil major basic protein. *J Immunol* 1979; 123: 2925–7.

79. O'Byrne PM, Dolovich M, Dirks R, Roberts RS, Newhouse MT. Lung epithelial permeability: relation to nonspecific airway responsiveness. *J Appl Physiol Resp Env Exc Physiol* 1984; 57: 77–84.

80. Flavahan NA, Aarhus LL, Rimele TJ, Vanhoutte PM. Respiratory epithelium inhibits bronchial smooth muscle tone. *J Appl Physiol* 1985; 58: 834–8.

81. Leikauf GD, Ueki IF, Nadel JA, Widdicombe JH. Bradykinin stimulates Cl secretion and prostaglandin E2 release by canine tracheal epithelium. *Am J Physiol* 1985; 248: F48–55.

82. Walters EH, O'Byrne PM, Fabbri LM, Graf PD, Holtzman MJ, Nadel JA. Control of neurotransmission by prostaglandins in canine trachealis smooth muscle. *J Appl Physiol Resp Env Exc Physiol* 1984; 57: 129–34.

83. Manning PJ, Lane CG, O'Byrne PM. The effect of oral prostaglandin El on airway responsiveness in asthmatic subjects. *Pulm Pharmacol* 1989; 2: 121–4.

84. Dusser DJ, Jacoby DB, Djokic TD, Rubinstein I, Borson DB, Nadel JA. Virus induces airway hyperresponsiveness to tachykinins: role of neutral endopeptidase. *J Appl Physiol* 1989; 67: 1504–11.

85. ✪ Boulet LP, Laviolette M, Turcotte H, Cartier A, Dugas M, Malo J et al. Bronchial subepithelial fibrosis correlates with airway responsiveness to methacholine. *Chest* 1997; 112: 45–52.

86. Altraja A, Laitinen A, Virtanen I, Kampe M, Simonsson BG, Karlsson SE et al. Expression of laminins in the airways in various types of asthmatic patients: a morphometric study. *Am J Respir Cell Mol Biol* 1996; 15: 482–8.

87. Brewster CE, Howarth PH, Djukanovic R, Wilson J, Holgate ST, Roche et al. Myofibroblasts and subepithelial fibrosis in bronchial asthma. *Am J Respir Cell Mol Biol* 1990; 3: 507–11.

88. Gizycki M, Adelroth EC, Rogers A, O'Byrne PM, Jeffery PK. Myofibroblast involvement in allergen-induced late responses in mild atopic asthma. *Am J Respir Cell Mol Biol* 1997; 17: 1–8.

89. ✪ James AL, Pare PD, Hogg JC. The mechanics of airway narrowing in asthma. *Am Rev Respir Dis* 1989; 139: 242–6.

90. Vincenc KS, Black JL, Yan K, Armour CL, Donnelly PD, Woolcock AJ. Comparison of *in vivo* and *in vitro* responses to histamine in human airways. *Am Rev Respir Dis* 1983; 128: 875–9.

91. Roberts JA, Raeburn D, Rodger IW, Thomson NC. Comparison of *in vivo* airway responsiveness and *in vitro* smooth muscle sensitivity to methacholine in man. *Thorax* 1984; 39: 837–43.

92. Schellenberg RR, Foster A. *In vitro* responses of human asthmatic airway and pulmonary vascular smooth muscle. *Int Arch Allergy Appl Immunol* 1984; 75: 237–41.

93. ✪ Bai TR. Abnormalities in airway smooth muscle in fatal asthma. *Am Rev Respir Dis* 1990; 141: 552–7.

Part 2

Diagnosis and Investigations
of Asthma

Chapter 4

Triggers of Asthma

Neil Thomson

INTRODUCTION

The diagnosis of asthma based on a history of episodic cough, wheezing, chest tightness or dyspnoea is usually not difficult to make but the clinical presentation may be less straightforward (see Chapter 5 and 6). Asthma attacks can be provoked by different trigger factors and each of these stimuli will be considered briefly in this chapter. The assessment and management of asthma induced by the more important of these triggers is reviewed in Chapters 16, 23 and 33–45.

CLASSIFICATION OF TRIGGER FACTORS

Asthma is a chronic inflammatory disorder of the airways (see Chapter 3). The asthmatic airway exhibits variable airflow obstruction and bronchial hyper-responsiveness to different stimuli (Fig. 4.1, Table 4.1). In susceptible individuals allergens and occupational agents can induce airways inflammation and bronchial hyperresponsiveness as well as trigger symptoms of asthma (inducers of asthma) (see Chapter 3). Viral respiratory tract infections can probably also act as inducers of asthma. Allergens and occupational stimuli as well as non-steroidal anti-inflammatory drugs produce bronchoconstriction only in asthmatics "sensitized" to these agents and even high "doses" of these substances will not produce asthma in non-sensitive patients. Other triggers such as exercise or irritants (inciters of

Table 4.1: Triggers of asthma
Infections[a]
Allergens[a]
Occupational agents[a]
Environmental pollutants[b]
Exercise
Cold air
Hyperventilation
Aerosols of distilled water or hypertonic solutions
Drugs
Foods
Psychological factors

[a] These stimuli can induce the asthmatic state as well as precipitating attacks of asthma.
[b] It is uncertain whether this stimulus can induce asthma in humans.

asthma) produce symptoms of asthma because the airways are inflamed and hyperreactive, but these stimuli probably do not induce chronic airway inflammation. Asthma symptoms will occur in most if not all asthmatic patients provided a high enough "dose" of these latter stimuli is administered.

ALLERGENS

Inhaled, ingested or injected allergens can all precipitate asthma although the inhaled route is the commonest and most important[1,2] (Table 4.2) (see Chapter 16). Allergic factors may be involved in up to 75% of patients with asthma, particularly in children.

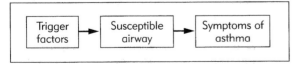

FIGURE 4.1: Trigger factors and asthma.

43

Table 4.2: Inhaled allergens and asthma

Allergen	Comments
Pollens	
Grass	Seasonal asthma (May–July)
Weeds (e.g. ragweed)	Seasonal asthma (Aug.–Oct.); important in North America
Tree	Seasonal asthma (Feb.–May); birch pollen important in Scandinavia
Fungi	
Aspergillus fumigatus	Causes allergic bronchopulmonary aspergillosis
Cladosporium sp., *Alternaria* sp.	Importance in causing asthma unclear; peak spore levels in late summer and early autumn
House-dust mite	
Dermatophagoides spp.	Commonest positive skin-prick test found in asthmatic patients in many countries
Animal danders	
Cats	Symptoms may be related to species, e.g. dogs. Siamese cats and other cats: allergen
Dogs	may persist in household furnishings and cause asthma in sensitive subjects
Birds	
Horses	
Hamsters	
Rabbits	
Mice	
Rats	
Gerbils	
Guinea-pigs	

Asthmatic children with larger numbers of positive immediate skin tests tend to have more severe disease.[3] This relationship does not occur in adults with asthma.[4]

Table 4.3: Assessment of the possible role of allergy in causing attacks of asthma: main points from the history

Are asthma symptoms seasonal or perennial?

Is there an association between allergen exposure and environment, e.g. at home, at work, on holiday, etc.? It should be noted that symptoms may persist for several days after allergen exposure

Are there associated nasal, skin or eye symptoms after exposure to allergen?

Remember that sensitivity to allergens is commoner in children and young adults

The assessment of the possible role of allergy in causing attacks of asthma can often be difficult. The main points to note from the history are summarized in Table 4.3. Sensitivity to a specific allergen can be confirmed by skin-prick testing or *in vitro* determinations of IgE (see Chapter 9).

Specific Allergens Causing Asthma (Table 4.2)

Pollen Allergens Pollens, particularly from grasses, weeds and trees, can cause seasonal symptoms of allergic rhinitis and/or conjunctivitis and asthma[5,6] (Table 4.2). Tree pollens usually cause symptoms in the spring months, grasses in the early and midsummer, and weeds in late summer and autumn. The importance of oil-seed rape in provoking asthma is uncertain.[7]

Fungal Allergens The most important fungus associated with asthma is *Aspergillus fumigatus*. The spores of this organism, which are 2–3 μm in diameter, are almost always found in the atmosphere and counts are highest in late autumn and winter. Allergic bronchopulmonary aspergillosis (ABPA) is characterized by the association of immunological sensitivity to *A. fumigatus*, although other fungi have been implicated, and recurrent pulmonary eosinophilia. The majority of patients have asthma. In the UK and North America approximately 20% of asthmatic patients have positive skin-prick reactions to *A. fumigatus*. The exact percentage of these patients who have ABPA is unknown; estimates range between 2 and 8%. A non-asthmatic form of ABPA has been described in which patients present with non-wheezy dyspnoea often associated with low-grade fever and malaise.[8] The mechanisms by which colonization of the airways with *A. fumigatus* results in disease and the assessment and treatment of ABPA is discussed further in Chapter 35.

The importance of other airborne fungi such as *Cladosporium* sp. and *Alternaria* sp. in causing asthma is uncertain (see Chapter 16).

House-Dust Mites Allergy to the house-dust mites *Dermatophagoides pteronyssinus* or *Dermatophagoides farinae* is an important cause of asthma. *Dermatophagoides pteronyssinus* is the commonest allergen causing IgE-mediated sensitivity in asthma, particularly among asthmatic children. The assessment and treatment of house-dust mite allergy is discussed further in Chapter 16.

Animal and Insect Allergens Household pets can cause asthma due to allergy not only to the animal's dander but also to its saliva, urine or faeces (Table 4.2). Cats are probably the most frequent pet to cause allergic symptoms (see Chapter 16 for more details). The cockroach allergen can cause asthma in sensitive individuals in warm climates and inner city areas in colder climiates[9] (see Chapter 16 for more details).

Types of Asthmatic Response to Inhaled Allergen

Two main types of asthmatic response occur after allergen exposure. The early or immediate asthmatic response peaks at 10–30 minutes after allergen exposure and subsides by 1–2 hours. The late asthmatic response starts 3–4 hours after allergen exposure and usually begins to resolve by 6–12 hours. The possible pathogenic mechanisms involved in allergen-induced asthma are reviewed elsewhere (see Chapter 3).

INFECTIONS

Respiratory tract infections are thought frequently to precipitate attacks of asthma, particularly in children.[10,11] Infections are mainly viral, especially human rhinoviruses but are also caused by respiratory syncytial virus, adenoviruses, parainfluenza and influenza viruses.[12,13] The role of infection in provoking asthma attacks in adults is less certain. Bacterial infections seem rarely to precipitate asthma.[14]

Viral respiratory infections are thought to be involved as "inducers" of asthma although this association is difficult to establish (see Ref. 11). Interestingly a history of a respiratory infection precedes the development of late-onset asthma in adults in up to 50% of cases. The mechanism by which viral infections might exacerbate asthma is unclear but may involve epithelial damage, stimulation of virus-specific IgE antibodies, airway inflammation and/or sensitization of sensory vagal nerve endings.[10,11] Respiratory tract infections can cause transient increases in bronchial reactivity to non-specific stimuli such as histamine, and this effect may last for 6 weeks after the infection.

OCCUPATIONAL AGENTS

Occupational asthma occurs when agents at work cause asthma.[15] It is thought to account for up to 5% of all cases of adult asthma. There are well over 200 reported causes of occupational asthma.[16] Some of the commoner causes are listed in Table 4.4. Atopic subjects are more likely to develop occupational asthma to high molecular weight agents such as animal products, but not to low molecular weight compounds such as isocyanates. Patients diagnosed late and with severe disease are more likely to have persistent asthma symptoms following removal from the offending occupational agent. Thus, early diagnosis and complete removal from the industrial agent is very important. The diagnosis and treatment of occupational asthma is discussed in Chapter 33. Occupational agents can induce airway inflammation and bronchial hyper-responsiveness. This airway response should be differentiated from that caused by "inciters" of asthma that may be encountered at work, e.g. inhaled irritants or exercise.

Table 4.4: Causes of occupational asthma

Agent	Industries
Isocyanates	Plastics, polyurethane foam makers, paints, varnish, adhesives, printing
Grains and flour	Bakers, millers, farmers
Laboratory animals	Laboratory workers exposed to rats, mice, guinea-pigs, rabbits, locusts
Epoxy resins, e.g. phthalic anhydride, triethylene tetramine	Plastics, adhesives and paint workers
Colophony	Electronics
Platinum salts	Platinum metal refiners and in some laboratories
Crustaceans	Processing of crabs, prawns
Woods	Workers using various woods including western red cedar, oak, mahogany, iroka, walnut
Drugs	Manufacturers of pharmaceuticals including cimetidine, psyllium, penicillin, cephalosporins, tetracyclines, sulphathiazole, ispaghula
Ispaghula powder	Manufacture of bulk laxatives
Castor bean dust	Merchant seamen

Other chemicals, e.g.
  Formaldehyde
  Azodicarbonamide
  Ethylenediamine
	
	Plastics; medical staff
	Plastics and rubber
	Photographic processors

Other metals, e.g.
  Cobalt
  Nickel
	
	Hard metal industry
	Metal plating

Reactive dyes, e.g.
  Henna
  Proteolytic enzymes
	
	Hairdressing
	Manufacture of washing powders, also in brewing, baking and leather industries

DRUGS

Many drugs have been reported to lead to exacerbation of asthma[17,18] (Table 4.5). The drugs that most frequently provoke asthma are reviewed below.

Aspirin and Other Non-Steroidal Anti-Inflammatory Drugs

The true incidence of aspirin-induced asthma is unknown. It has been estimated that between 3 and 5% of adult asthmatic patients develop asthma after ingesting aspirin or other non-steroidal anti-inflammatory drugs (NSAIDs), but the incidence is higher when oral aspirin challenges are performed. This condition is rarely seen in children.

Clinical features include acute severe bronchoconstriction that develops within minutes to several hours after ingestion of aspirin or other NSAIDs, such as indomethacin, naproxen, ibuprofen, flurbiprofen or mefenamic acid.[19] The asthmatic symptoms may be

Table 4.5: Drug-induced asthma: some of the drugs reported to cause asthma in susceptible individuals

ACTH

ACE inhibitors

Aminophylline (ethylenediamine)

Aspirin and other non-steroidal anti-inflammatory drugs

β-Adrenoceptor antagonists

Cholinergic drugs, e.g. pilocarpine

Cholinesterase inhibitors, e.g. pyridostigmine

Contrast media

Dextrans

Hydrocortisone

Inhaled agents, e.g.
   Short and long acting β$_2$ agonists
   Corticosteroids
   Hypotonic solutions
   Ipratropium bromide
   Local anaesthetics
   Pentamidine
   Sodium cromoglycate

Pancreozymin

Penicillin

Quinine

Sulphasalazine

associated with rhinorrhoea, flushing and loss of consciousness. Fatal attacks have been recorded. There is often a past history of chronic rhinitis and nasal polyps before asthma develops. These patients often have chronic severe perennial asthma requiring regular oral corticosteroid treatment. A small percentage of these patients also develop urticaria and angio-oedema after aspirin ingestion.

The possible mechanisms involved in aspirin- and other NSAIDs-induced asthma are discussed in Chapter 34.

β-Adrenoceptor Antagonists

Bronchoconstriction is more likely to occur with non-selective than selective β-adrenoceptor antagonists. Nevertheless, severe asthma can occur with selective β-adrenoceptor antagonists such as atenolol or metaprolol and has also been reported with timolol eye drops when used to treat glaucoma.

Fatal attacks of asthma have been reported after the ingestion of β-adrenoceptor antagonists. All β-adrenoceptor antagonists should be avoided in patients with asthma. In the treatment of hypertension or ischaemic heart disease in a patient with asthma, calcium antagonists, nitrates and thiazides can be used safely.

The possible mechanisms involved in β-blocker-induced asthma are unknown. These drugs may block inhibitory presynaptic β receptors on vagal nerves resulting in increased vagal-induced bronchoconstriction.[20]

Angiotensin-Converting Enzyme (ACE) Inhibitors

ACE inhibitors can cause cough. Occasionally cases have been reported of worsening asthma due to these drugs.[21]

Inhaled Drugs

Cough and/or bronchospasm have been reported following the administration of nearly all types of inhaled drugs. Asthmatic patients may develop bronchoconstriction with topical local anaesthetics administered during fibreoptic bronchoscopy[22] or with inhaled pentamidine when used prophylactically for *Pneumocystis carinii* pneumonia.[23] Bronchodilation treatment should be given to prevent these reactions occurring.

FOODS AND DRINKS

Foods and drinks are uncommon causes of asthma in adults and in the majority of children.[24,25] Asthma symptoms are often accompanied by other allergic symptoms, e.g. urticaria, rhinitis. Food allergy may be commoner in asthmatic children of Indian descent. The commonest foods and additives causing asthma include nuts, milk, eggs, tartrazine (yellow colouring agent), cola drinks, metabisulphite (preservative) and possibly monosodium L-glutamate. Alcoholic drinks can cause bronchoconstriction in some patients, and this response is usually due to congeners but can be caused by ethanol itself. The diagnosis and treatment of food allergy is discussed in Chapter 44.

EXERCISE

After sufficient exercise most asthmatic patients develop exercise-induced asthma.[26-28] Exercise-induced asthma is often a problem in children and in adults involved in physical sports and may be the sole symptom in some patients with mild asthma. The maximum degree of bronchoconstriction occurs usually about 5–10 minutes after the cessation of exercise and symptoms subside within 15–30 minutes. There is often a refractory period of around 2 hours after the development of exercise-induced asthma. During this period repeated exercise does not cause bronchospasm. The diagnosis and management of exercise-induced asthma is discussed in Chapter 36.

Exercise-induced asthma is thought to be due to loss of water from the respiratory mucosa possibly also associated with cooling and drying of the airway.[26,28] The ventilation rate appears to be the critical factor causing these effects. The loss of water increases the osmolarity in the lining of the airway and this is thought to result in bronchoconstrictor mediator release from mast cells. Alternatively it has been suggested that bronchoconstriction is due to reactive hyperaemia of the bronchial circulation and associated airway oedema.[29]

HYPERVENTILATION

Voluntary isocapnic hyperventilation and aerosols of distilled or hypertonic solutions may produce bronchoconstriction through similar mechanisms to those of exercise.[28] Crying and laughing can both provoke symptoms of asthma.

ENVIRONMENTAL FACTORS

Indoor irritants

The inhalation of irritants such as cigarette smoke, wood smoke and strong odours and sprays, e.g. perfume, household cleaning agents, fresh paint, can all precipitate attacks of asthma. Environmental tobacco smoke exposure is associated with more acute attacks, worse lung function and increased drug requirements in children with asthma.[30,31]

Air Pollutants

Outdoor pollutants have been implicated as inciters of asthma and as contributing to the rising prevalence of asthma.[32] Ozone, produced by the effect of sunlight on traffic fumes, can cause reductions in lung function and bronchoconstriction in normal and asthmatic individuals taking exercise when atmospheric ozone concentrations are elevated, as can occur during hot summer months.[33] Asthmatic patients are not more likely to be sensitive to the airway effects of ozone than normal individuals. Those asthmatic patients sensitive to ozone, however, are likely to experience more severe respiratory symptoms. Asthmatic patients can experience acute respiratory symptoms including cough, chest tightness and wheeze when exposed to elevated atmospheric concentrations of sulphur dioxide.[34] Elevated concentrations of particulate air pollutants which are emitted mainly from diesel vehicles, have been associated with acute attacks of asthma and with increased morbidity.[35,36] Nitrogen dioxide is thought to have limited direct effects on airway function in asthma.[37] However, recent studies have implicated nitrogen dioxide as contributing towards acute respiratory infection in children.[38]

Atmospheric Temperature

The inhalation of cold air can precipitate symptoms in asthmatic patients. Exercise-induced asthma is more likely to occur when an asthmatic patient is exercising in cold weather. Thunderstorms have been reported to be associated with sudden increases in asthma attacks. Damp housing and mould have been related to increased respiratory symptoms in patients with asthma.[39,40]

NOCTURNAL ASTHMA

Patients with poorly controlled asthma frequently wheeze at night. The cause is not fully established, but appears to involve the effects of increased vagal tone and reduced non-adrenergic non-cholinergic tone acting on a hyperreactive airway. In addition, airway inflammation is increased at night, which may contribute to airway narrowing.[41,42] The assessment and management of nocturnal asthma are discussed in Chapter 37.

PSYCHOLOGICAL FACTORS

Adverse psychological factors may contribute to poor asthma control, but do not cause asthma.[43-45] In susceptible individuals increased anti-asthma treatment usually results in a reduction in the adverse effects of stress, but specific psychological treatments may on occasions also be helpful. An increased mortality from asthma is associated with depression, recent family loss, recent unemployment, schizophrenia and alcohol abuse. Asthma can cause psychological symptoms including panic attacks and low self-esteem. The assessment and management of psychological factors are discussed in Chapter 40.

PREGNANCY AND PRE-MENSES

Approximately one-third of asthmatic patients require more anti-asthma medication during pregnancy and one-third require less therapy.[46] In an individual asthmatic patient the effect of pregnancy on asthma control may differ in successive pregnancies. Asthma control deteriorates in approximately one-third of female asthmatic patients before menses.[47] The management of asthma in pregnancy and pre-menstrual asthma are discussed in Chapter 38.

THYROID DISEASE

The development of hyperthyroidism may result in a worsening of asthma control, with subsequent improvement after treatment of the thyrotoxicosis.[48–50] Conversely the occurrence of hypothyroidism has been reported to be associated with improvement in asthma control.[50] Several possible mechanisms may account for the relationship between asthma and thyroid disease and these include alterations in β-adrenergic function, airway reactivity, arachidonic acid metabolism, hydrocortisone metabolism or respiratory muscle function.

GASTROESOPHAGEAL REFLUX

Gastroesophageal reflux can trigger attacks of asthma although the incidence is unclear. The mechanism is unknown; possibilities include aspiration or an oesophago-bronchial reflex triggered by acid irritation of the oesophageal mucosa. Xanthines relax the lower oesophageal sphincter and may precipitate reflux by this mechanism. The management of gastroesophageal reflux and asthma is discussed in Chapter 41.

KEY POINTS

1 In susceptible individuals, allergens, occupational agents and probably viruses induce airway inflammation and bronchial hyperresponsiveness as well as causing acute symptoms of asthma. These triggers are called inducers of asthma.

2 Other triggers such as exercise or irritants produce symptoms of asthma because the airways are inflamed and hyperresponsive but these stimuli do not induce chronic airway inflammation. These triggers are called inciters of asthma.

REFERENCES

1. ✪ Platts-Mills TAE, Thomas WR, Aalberse RC, Vervloet D, Chapman MD. Dust mite allergens and asthma: report of a second international workshop. *J Allergy Clin Immunol* 1992; 89: 1046–1060.

2. Sporik R, Holgate ST, Platts-Mills TAE, Cogswell JJ. Exposure to house dust mite allergen and the development of asthma in childhood: a prospective study. *N Engl J Med* 1990; 323: 502–7.

3. Zimmerman B, Feanny S, Reisman J *et al.* Allergy in asthma. I. The dose relationships of allergy to severity of childhood asthma. *J Allergy Clin Immunol* 1988; 88: 63–77.

4. Innouye T, Tarlo S, Broder I *et al.* Severity of asthma in skin test-negative and skin test-positive patients. *J Allergy Clin Immunol* 1985; 75: 313–19.

5. Boulet L-P, Cartier A, Thomson NC *et al.* Asthma and increases in non-allergic bronchial responsiveness from seasonal pollen exposure. *J Allergy Clin Immunol* 1983; 71: 399–406.

6. Reid MJ, Moss RB, Hsu Y-P. Seasonal asthma in Northern California: allergy causes and efficacy of immunotherapy. *J Allergy Clin Immunol* 1986; 78: 590–600.

7. McSharry C. New aeroallergens in agricultural and related practice. *Clin Exp Allergy* 1992; 22: 423–6.

8. Berkin KE, Vernon DRH, Kerr JW. Lung collapse caused by allergic bronchopulmonary aspergillosis in non-asthmatic patients. *BMJ* 1982; 285: 552–3.

9. Rosenstreich DL, Eggleston P, Kattan M *et al.* The role of cockroach allergy and exposure to cockroach allergen in causing morbidity among inner-city children with asthma. *N Engl J Med* 1997; 336: 1356–63.

10. ✪ Busse WW, Dick EC, Lemanske RF, Gern JE. Infections. In: Barnes PJ, Rodger IW, Thomson NC (eds). *Asthma: Basic Mechanisms and Clinical Management*, 3rd edn. London: Academic Press, 1998: 547–67.

11. Folkerts G, Busse WW, Nijkamp FP, Sorkness R, Gern JE. Virus-induced airway hyperresponsiveness and asthma. *Am J Respir Crit Care Med* 1998; 157: 1708–1720.

12. Pattemore PK, Johnston SL, Bardin PG. Viruses as precipitants of asthma. I. Epidemiology. *Clin Exp Allergy* 1992; 22: 325–6.

13. Bardin PG, Johnston SL, Pattemore PK. Viruses as precipitants of asthma symptoms. II. Physiology and mechanisms. *Clin Exp Allergy* 1992; 22: 809–22.

14. Berman SZ, Mathison DA, Stevenson DD, Tan EM, Vaughan JH. Trans-tracheal aspiration studies in asthmatic patients in relapse with "infective" asthma and in subjects without respiratory disease. *J Allergy Clin Immunol* 1975; 56: 206–14.

15. Newman-Taylor AJ. Occupational asthma. In: Barnes PJ, Rodger IW, Thomson NC (eds). *Asthma: Basic Mechanisms and Clinical Management*, 3rd edn. London: Academic Press, 1998; 529–45.

16. ✪ Chan-Yeung M, Lam S. Occupational asthma. *Am Rev Respir Dis* 1986; 133: 686–703.

17. Israel-Biet D, Labrune S, Huchon GJ. Drug-induced lung disease: 1990 review. *Eur Respir J* 1991; 4: 465–78.

18. Meeker DP, Widemann HP. Drug-induced bronchospasm. *Clin Chest Med* 1990; 11: 163–75.

19. Szczeklik A, Nizankowska E, Sanak M. New insights into the pathogenesis and management of aspirin-induced asthma. *Clin Asthma Rev* 1998; 2: 79–86.

20. Barnes PJ, Thomson NC. Drug-induced asthma. In: Barnes PJ, Rodger IW, Thomson NC (eds). *Asthma: Basic Mechanisms and Clinical management*, 3rd edn. London: Academic Press, 1998: 597–605.

21. Lunde H, Hedner T, Samuelsson O *et al.* Dyspnoea, asthma and bronchospasm in relation to treatment with angiotensin converting enzyme inhibitors. *BMJ*, 1994; 308: 18–21.

22. McAlpine LG, Thomson NC. Lidocaine-induced bronchoconstriction in asthmatic patients. Relation to histamine airway responsiveness and effect of preservative. *Chest* 1989; 96: 1012–15.

23. Conte JE Jr, Hollander H, Golden JA. Inhaled or reduced dose intravenous pentamidine for *Pneumocystis carinii* pneumonia. *Ann Intern Med* 1987; 107: 495–8.

24. ✪ Metcalfe DD, Sampson HA. Workshop on experimental methodology for clinical studies of adverse reactions to foods and food additives. *J Allergy Clin Immunol* 1990; 86: 421–42.

25. Food Allergy and Intolerance Report of a BSACI Special Interest Group. *Clin Exp Allergy* 1995; 25 (suppl. 1): 1–44.

26. Godfrey S, Bar-Yishay E. Exercise-induced asthma revisited. *Respir Med* 1993; 87: 331–44.

27. ✪ McFadden ER, Gilbert IA. Exercise induced asthma. *N Engl J Med* 1994; 330: 1362–7.

28. Anderson SD. Asthma provoked by exercise, hyperventilation and the inhalation of nonisotonic aerosols. In: Barnes PJ, Rodger IW, Thomson NC (eds). *Asthma: Basic Mechanisms and Clinical Management*, 3rd edn. London Academic Press, 1998: 569–87.

29. McFadden ER. Hypothesis: exercise-induced asthma as a vascular phenomenon. *Lancet* 1990; 335: 880–2.

30. Chilmonczyk BA, Salmun LM, Megathlin KN *et al.* Association between exposure to environmental tobacco smoke and exacerbations of asthma in children. *N Engl J Med* 1993; 328: 1665–9.

31. ✪ Cooke DG, Strachan DP. Summary of effects of parental smoking on the respiratory health of children and implications for research. *Thorax* 1999; 54: 357–66.

32. ✪ Lebowitz MD. Epidemiological studies of the respiratory effects of air pollution. *Eur Respir J* 1996; 9: 1029–1054.

33. Ozone. Advisory Group on Medical Aspects of Air Pollution Exposure. London: HMSO, 1991.

34. Sulphur dioxide, acid aerosols and particulates. Advisory Group on Medical Aspects of Air Pollution Exposure. London: HMSO, 1992.

35. Swartz J, Slater D, Larson TV, Pierson WE, Koenig JQ. Particulate air pollution and hospital emergency room visits for asthma in Seattle. *Am Rev Respir Dis* 1993; 147: 826–31.

36. Roemer W, Hoek G, Brunekreef B. Effect of ambient winter air pollution on respiratory health of children with chronic respiratory symptoms. *Am Rev Respir Dis* 1993; 147: 118–24.

37. Oxides of nitrogen. Advisory Group on Medical Aspects of Pollution Exposure. London: HMSO, 1993.

38. Samet JM, Lambert WE, Skipper BJ *et al.* Nitrogen dioxide and respiratory illness in infants. *Am Rev Respir Dis* 1993; 148: 1258–65.

39. Dales RE, Burnett R, Zevonenburg H. Adverse health effects among adults exposed to home dampness and moulds. *Am Rev Respir Dis* 1991; 143: 505–509.

40. Williamson IJ, Martin CJ, McGill G, Monie RDH, Fennerty AG. Damp housing and asthma: a case-control study. *Thorax* 1997; 52: 229–34.

41. Douglas NJ. Nocturnal asthma. *Thorax* 1993; 48: 100–102.

42. Martin RJ. Nocturnal asthma: circadian rhythms and therapeutic interventions. *Am Rev Respir Dis* 1993; 147: 525–8.

43. ✪ Bosley CM, Corden ZM, Cochrane GM. Psychosocial factors and asthma. *Respir Med* 1996; 90: 453–7.

44. Lask B. Psychological treatments of asthma. *Clin Exp Allergy* 1991; 21: 625–6.

45. Wright RJ, Rodriguez M, Cohen S. Review of psychosocial stress and asthma: an integrated biopsychosocial approach. *Thorax* 1998; 53: 1066–1074.

46. Schatz M, Harden KM, Forsythe A *et al.* The course of asthma during pregnancy, post partum, and with successive pregnancies: a prospective analysis. *J Allergy Clin Immunol* 1988; 81: 509–17.

47. Gibbs CJ, Coutts II, Lock R, Finnegan OC, White RJ. Premenstrual exacerbation of asthma. *Thorax* 1984; 39: 833–6.

48. Ayres J, Clark TJH. Asthma and the thyroid. *Lancet* 1981; ii: 110–11.

49. Lipworth BJ, Dhillon DP, Clark RA, Newton RW. Problems with asthma following treatment of thyrotoxicosis. *Br J Dis Chest* 1988; 82: 310–14.

50. Bush RK, Ehrlick EN, Reed CE. Thyroid disease and asthma. *J Allergy Clin Immunol* 1977; 59: 398–401.

Chapter 5

Diagnosis in Children

Barry Zimmerman

INTRODUCTION

Asthma is defined as a disease of variable airflow obstruction associated with inflammation in the airways and the symptoms of cough, wheeze and dyspnoea.[1] However the diagnosis of asthma in children often relies heavily on history since many children are too young to do the tests that objectively measure airflow obstruction. Several studies have called attention to significant under-diagnosis and under-treatment of childhood asthma.[2-5] Yet there are very few studies documenting airway inflammation in childhood asthma, especially in very young children.[6,7] Children less than 3 years of age who wheeze present a special challenge because of the lack of objective measures of airflow obstruction.

WHEEZING IN CHILDREN LESS THAN 3 YEARS OF AGE

Physicians have felt that young children often "outgrow" intermittent and mild wheezing illnesses and were reluctant to label the child asthmatic resorting to terms such as wheezy bronchitis and asthmatic bronchitis. This reluctance often led to treatment with cough suppressants and antibiotics even when the child had had several episodes of wheezing.[2,3,5] In fact recent studies in infants and toddlers suggest that many, but not all of them, do seem to "outgrow" the wheezing suggesting that the older concept of wheezy bronchitis was not totally misguided. Nevertheless, if "persisting asthma" in childhood commonly begins before age 5,[8-11] and if early management of the inflammation in the airways can result in diminution of the disease and better lung function,[12] then it becomes important to identify the "persisting asthmatics" early and treat them aggressively.

On the other hand, the larger group of infantile wheezers who have a self-limiting condition that is "outgrown", may not need as aggressive therapy. These children may be at more risk from the medication than the disease.

There is now strong evidence that the majority of children who wheeze in the first few years of life will no longer be wheezing by school age.[13-18] It seems likely that there are a group of young infants, more commonly male, who are at risk of wheezing with viral illness based on abnormal lung anatomy[16,17] but who are not atopic. In these infants, eosinophils and perhaps other cellular components of inflammation are not mobilized to the same degree as in "true" asthma. Thus children with asthma symptoms under age 3 seem heterogeneous.[13-23] In one study about 30% of children age three or younger had had wheezing, but almost 60% of them had stopped wheezing by age 6.[17] It is not clear whether such children are at risk for recurrence of the asthma as adults. Stein *et al.*[23] have suggested that very young children with cough and wheeze can be divided into three groups: (1) Infants, usually boys, who have none of the characteristics of asthma such as personal history of atopy or family history of atopy, but who are born with small airways and develop wheezing as a result but "outgrow" this problem as they get older. (2) Young children in the second group present slightly later with symptoms of cough and wheeze during viral illnesses. These children also have no personal or family history of allergy and also tend to outgrow the symptoms. (3) The third group comprises young children with a personal history of atopy and who are more likely to have persisting asthma. These atopic asthmatics seem to present slightly later in infancy[10,17] but unfortunately there is significant overlap in the clinical presentations of the different types of "asthma" in these very young children.

The majority of children with onset of wheeze under age 3 are non-atopic and the episodes are viral-induced.[15,17] By contrast after age 4, wheezing subjects are more likely to be atopic in the majority of instances.[15] These studies are consistent with observations in older children showing that airway hyperresponsiveness as defined by a positive methacholine challenge is related positively to atopy.[24–26] Passive cigarette smoke is also positively related to wheezing in the absence of atopy and this wheezing can persist.[15,17] Maternal smoking has been found to be significantly associated with both transient and persistent wheezing in infants.[17]

VIRAL-INDUCED WHEEZE

The pathophysiology of wheezing in non-atopic viral-induced, episodic asthma is unknown. Bronchial lavage of young children with non-atopic viral-induced wheezing suggests that they have non-eosinophilic inflammation in the airways while atopic asthma is associated with eosinophils in the airways.[7] Other studies using peripheral blood eosinophils and serum eosinophil cationic protein (ECP) as indirect markers for eosinophilic inflammation in childhood asthma suggest that eosinophils and ECP are higher in atopic than non-atopic asthma.[27,28]

A number of studies have documented that following respiratory syncytial virus (RSV)-induced bronchiolitis, a percentage of the children continue to have recurrent wheeze with subsequent respiratory tract infections.[29–35] It has been suggested that RSV infection induces a TH_2 cytokine response that is similar to atopy.[36] Welliver found that wheezing with RSV infection was associated with IgE antibody to the RS virus.[37] Garofalo et al.[38] demonstrated activation of eosinophils during RSV infection. This would suggest that RSV-induced wheezing resembles asthma in the nature of the inflammation in the airways, yet afterwards most of the affected children have only mild symptoms occurring primarily with viral infections for a period of a few years after the original RSV infection.[34] The data suggest that the difference in outcome between post-infectious wheezing and asthma has to do with the presence or absence of atopy[39] and therefore eosinophilic inflammation. An atopic immune system in childhood can lead to greater eosinophilic inflammation resulting in airway reactivity and the possibility of a more persisting chronic asthma.

VIRAL-INDUCED COUGH

Similar considerations apply to the diagnosis of asthma presenting with recurrent or persisting cough in the absence of wheeze. Cough can be the sole manifestation of asthma,[40] an observation that has been confirmed in children.[41–43] Yet persistent cough in childhood is less frequently associated with a positive methacholine or histamine challenge test in children.[44] Similarly cough is associated with less atopy[8] and by inference less eosinophil mobilization and activation.[27] This implies that persistent cough may not always represent asthma[44,45] and might represent a post-infectious phenomenon that has a different outcome from asthma, as suggested by Wright et al.[46] We have studied older children with post-infectious cough using the technique of induced sputum. These children had been coughing for an average of 2 months after a bout of paroxysmal coughing. Such children had mean sputum eosinophils of 0.58% (normal <2.0%) compared with untreated asthmatics (mean sputum eosinophils 22.9%). All of the asthmatic children had a positive methacholine challenge while only 55% of the coughers did.

The distinction between post-infectious cough and asthma-variant cough may prove to be important in the long-term outcome of the illness. Furthermore, if the cough does not clear spontaneously or after institution of treatment with inhaled steroids, then other diagnoses should be considered including: (1) cough due to post-nasal discharge; (2) cough due to acid-reflux and (3) more obscure causes of chronic cough such as tracheo-oesophageal fistula and reflux or aberrant vessel with compression of a bronchus, etc.

ROLE OF ATOPY IN CHILDHOOD ASTHMA

The studies cited to this point all indicate that the outcome of childhood wheezing is very different in non-atopic and atopic individuals. Studies in adults have suggested that activated eosinophils associated with T-lymphocytes producing cytokines of the TH_2 subset are the underlying cause of inflammation in asthmatic airways.[47–50] Permanent airway remodelling and airway hyperresponsiveness may result from this inflammation in the airways. Atopy in childhood seems to be the major source and perhaps the only source of this eosinophilic inflammation which then results in non-specific airway hyperresponsiveness.[51–53] In older children with asthma, the majority, even those who wheeze primarily with respiratory tract infections, are atopic.[15] In contrast infants who wheeze are commonly non-atopic and wheeze only intermittently with viral illnesses.[10,13,17] However, even within infancy, there are a small group of atopic babies who wheeze and are likely to have persisting asthma. It has been shown that infants can demonstrate positive skin tests to airborne allergens[54] and these predicts the development of asthma. Wahn *et al.*[55] have shown that children from high risk families are sensitized to dust mite and cat in infancy and are sensitized by lower quantities of allergens than those children born to non-atopic parents.

DIAGNOSIS OF ASTHMA IN INFANCY

It is generally felt that the youngest wheezy children are the most likely to warrant investigation for diseases other than asthma. Asthma is still by far the commonest cause of these symptoms in infants. Alternative diagnoses are far less common and can usually be excluded by history. A history of failure to thrive, recurrent bacterial infections, significant vomiting or reflux, choking cyanotic episodes or sudden onset of symptoms after possible aspiration with no indication of a viral illness would suggest the need for further investigation. Cystic fibrosis occurs in approximately 1 in 2000 children[56] compared with asthma which occurs in 1 in 10 children.[5] Other diagnoses such as an immune system problem, gastroesophageal reflux and recurrent aspiration, aspiration of a foreign body, tracheobronchiomalacia, bronchial stenosis, and congenital heart disease are also less common than asthma. Physical examination revealing localized chest or cardiovascular abnormalities would also indicate the need for further investigation. Investigation would begin with a simple chest X-ray but could go on to sweat test, immune function tests (primarily quantitative immunoglobulins including IgG subsets), reflux studies and other more specific tests.

Atopy in Infants

Since atopy seems to predict the likelihood of persisting asthma, this history must be carefully sought. Infants usually have not developed many of the symptoms that suggest allergy. A strong family history of atopy or asthma might identify the wheezing toddler more at risk of persisting asthma. A history of an immediate reaction to a food such as egg, and/or the presence of significant atopic dermatitis will suggest the presence of an atopic immune system and identify chil-

dren at risk for persisting asthma. Studies on the formation of IgE antibody in infancy suggest that when children are allergic in the first few years of life, they react to a food protein, commonly milk, egg or peanut.[57–59] This may be associated with a clinical reaction even at the first introduction of the food.[60] Once the child has been identified as allergic, by a reaction to a food for example, it should be assumed that they are becoming sensitized to airborne allergens and dust mite control procedures should be initiated.[61,62] If there is a pet in the home, parents must be actively encouraged to eliminate the animal from the home and undertake procedures to reduce the dander levels.

DIAGNOSIS OF ASTHMA IN PRE-SCHOOL CHILDREN

In an epidemiologic study in the Toronto area we found that 10% of children aged 0 to 5 years had had wheezing in the year prior to the study and a further 8–10% had had significant cough.[5] Other investigators have reported similar prevalences and an increase over the last 10 years.[63] These children have lower respiratory tract symptoms for a week or more with each viral infection. Children of this age can have 6–8 viral respiratory tract infections per year.[64] They are too young to do spirometry correctly and diagnosis relies heavily on the history.

Clinical History

Pre-school children often have cough with or without wheeze during acute viral illness, but then may fail to clear the symptoms completely. They are left with residual coughing especially in the morning when they arise or with exercise or other forms of exertion. These symptoms are especially prominent when the child resides in a household with a smoker or smokers.[65–69] As discussed previously, many of these young children prove to be non-atopic and will outgrow the problem if there is freedom from passive cigarette smoke.[17] As the children get older they tend to develop fewer viral respiratory tract infections and improve. However those children who are atopic now increasingly have an inflammation contributed by this immune response to environmental allergens.

Atopy in Pre-School Children

At around age three, allergic children move from food sensitivity to airborne allergen sensitivity[57,58,59] and it is this sensitivity, especially to the indoor allergens such as dust mite, animal dander, cockroach and mould, that seems to be more important in the development of asthma.[62] These children may have a history of infantile atopic dermatitis or an immediate reaction to a common food such as milk, egg, peanut or nuts, some of which (i.e. to milk and egg) will have been outgrown. They may give a history suggestive of allergic rhinitis with chronic rhinorrhoea, nasal stuffiness, sneezing in the morning and rubbing at the nose. Sneezing and rubbing of the nose are the hallmarks of allergic rhinitis since nasal obstruction and mouth-breathing can also occur with adenoidal hypertrophy. Very young children, even in infancy, are capable of being sensitized to their pet animal. Unfortunately symptoms around the pet are often not noticed by parents, but it should be suspected in any asthmatic child who has other symptoms of allergy despite an apparent absence of symptoms around the pet animal.

Differential Diagnoses

Children who have recurrent lower respiratory tract symptoms with each viral illness are common in the pre-school age and because of the frequency of viral illnesses, they can be almost continuously ill through the winter months. Asthma is by far the commonest cause of these symptoms. Alternative diagnoses are far less common and can usually be excluded by history and a chest X-ray. The symptoms raising red flags are the same as described in infancy, including a history of poor growth, recurrent bacterial infections, significant vomiting or reflux, choking cyanotic episodes, sudden onset of symptoms after possible aspiration. Symptoms of these types along with a poor response to treatment of asthma with adequate doses of steroids would suggest the need for further investigation. Physical examination revealing localized chest or cardiovascular abnormalities would also indicate the need for further investigation. The investigations could include a chest X-ray, tests for cystic fibrosis, immune function tests, primarily quantitative immunoglobulins including IgG subsets, reflux studies and other more specific tests.

Trial of Asthma Therapy

A trial of therapy is often initiated as part of the diagnostic evaluation. Inhaled steroids can be administered even to the youngest children. Failure to respond to a good dose of inhaled steroid within 3 to 4 weeks would suggest the need to re-evaluate the diagnosis. Failure could result from three general possibilities: (1) poor parental compliance with administration of medication either for philosophical or technical reasons; (2) a diagnosis other than asthma; or (3) more significant asthma than first appreciated or an intercurrent respiratory tract infection exacerbating the asthma. In any case, it would not be unreasonable to initiate investigation beginning with a chest X-ray and a review of the history and physical examination seeking alternative diagnoses.

In summary, there are no tests in the pre-school age group that are definitive for the diagnosis of asthma. A chest X-ray should be done in any severe or unusual case to exclude foreign body or congenital anomaly. Allergy testing can help to assess aetiology and prognosis.

DIAGNOSING ASTHMA IN SCHOOL-AGE CHILDREN

At this age the children are able to perform simple spirometry and the diagnosis can be supported with more formal evaluation. All children in this age group should do spirometry or peak flow measurements. Moreover the majority of asthmatic children in this age group, especially those with significant asthma, are atopic[8] and allergy skin tests should be done.

Clinical History

The diagnosis of asthma will be suggested from a characteristic history of recurrent wheeze, shortness of breath and cough, or even recurrent cough by itself. The child often has a history of cough and/or wheeze with each viral illness and a history of similar symptoms on exercise. There may also be symptoms occurring between respiratory tract infections at night or in the morning on arising. Any child with a history of night or morning cough due to asthma would be expected to have symptoms with exercise or in cold air.

Even in this age group a persisting cough may follow an infectious episode particularly if the episode was associated with paroxysmal coughing. This persisting cough is more likely to be asthma if the child has a prior history of symptoms with each viral respiratory tract infection or if the child is allergic. If there is a family history of atopy and/ or asthma there is greater likelihood for expression of asthma with the viral illness. In the presence of these prognostic features, the chance of recurring symptoms increases while in their absence a recurrent asthma becomes less likely.

A positive methacholine or histamine challenge test would increase the possibility that the child has asthma. Similarly the diagnosis would be more likely if variability of FEV_1 or peak flows can be documented, e.g. 20% response to inhaled β_2 agonist. Excessive variability in home peak flow monitoring, either a diurnal variation of 20% or more, or day to day variation of 20% or more, or a 20% response to bronchodilator, would help to confirm the diagnosis of asthma.

Atopic Status

The presence of an atopic immune system in a child with recurrent respiratory symptoms suggests the possibility of asthma. An elevated serum IgE[70] or elevated peripheral eosinophil count (in asthma the elevation is often in the high normal range)[71] might suggest the possibility of atopic asthma. A history suggestive of allergy can be sought. Significant eczema in infancy or an immediate reaction (e.g. hives or swelling) to a food, commonly milk, egg, peanut, nut or fish would suggest the presence of atopy. Symptoms around animals (dog, cat, horse etc) including rhinitis, conjunctivitis, asthma, hives, or symptoms of allergic rhinitis (especially with a seasonal variation) would suggest atopy which in turn heightens the risk of asthma.

Differential Diagnoses

In this age group, asthma is by far the commonest diagnostic possibility for cough and wheeze. Alternative diagnoses might be suggested by physical examination. A chest X-ray, sinus X-ray and possibly a test for cystic fibrosis could be done. At least a third of sinus X-rays will be abnormal in simple uncomplicated asthma and the significance of these abnormalities is a matter of some controversy.[72] The abnormal X-rays are generally not associated with symptoms of sinusitis and may result from the same inflammation occurring in both the upper and lower respiratory tract.[73] Symptomatic sinusitis should be treated and recurring bacterial infections of sinuses and elsewhere would suggest the need for an immunologic work-up, particularly looking for an IgG subset deficiency.[74] IgG subset deficiency is uncommon but can present in very young children beginning with recurrent otitis media, sinusitis and cough. Recurrent or persistent symptomatic sinusitis, nasal discharge and cough might also suggest the need for nasal ciliary studies to rule out dysmotile cilia syndrome. A history of heartburn and reflux would suggest the need for more sophisticated studies of reflux with

a pH probe. A trial of therapy for reflux would be warranted if the diagnosis can be entertained from the history. Occasionally a Mantoux test might be indicated by the history of contact or potential contact with tuberculosis.

Trial of Therapy

Because asthma is by far the commonest diagnosis, a trial of therapy could always be undertaken if a work-up for alternative diagnoses is negative. The therapy should include steroid and home peak flow monitoring along with a symptom diary card. This trial should be undertaken aggressively for a 3–4 week period since most childhood asthma would be expected to show some response to inhaled steroid in that time frame.

KEY POINTS

1 The majority of children who wheeze in the first few years of life will no longer be wheezing by school age.

2 The majority of children with onset of wheeze under age 3 are non-atopic and the episodes are viral induced. By contrast after age 4, wheezing subjects are more likely to be atopic in the majority of instances.

3 The outcome of wheezing in early childhood is very different in non-atopic and atopic individuals. Non-atopic infants and toddlers tend to "outgrow" the wheeze while atopic children tend to have persisting asthma.

4 The youngest wheezy children (infants) are the most likely to warrant investigation for diseases other than asthma. Asthma is still by far the commonest cause of these symptoms in infants. Alternative diagnoses are far less common and can usually be excluded by history.

5 By school-age, children are able to perform simple spirometry and the diagnosis can be supported with more formal evaluation. All children in this age group should do spirometry or peak flow measurements.

CONCLUSION

At any age the diagnosis of asthma includes a wide range of severity from mild intermittent symptoms to continuous severe but atopy clearly plays a significant role in the chronicity. Even in older children there is no one test that will determine the severity of an individual patient's asthma. It is possible that in future tests that reflect airway inflammation, e.g. sputum eosinophil measurements[75] might help to distinguish subtypes of asthma, but at the present they must be managed according to their clinical status.

REFERENCES

1. Sears MR. The definition and diagnosis of asthma. *Allergy* (suppl.) 1993; 48: 12–16.

2. Speight ANP, Lee DA, Hey EN. Underdiagnosis and undertreatment of asthma in childhood. *Br Med J* 1983; 286: 1253–6.

3. Anderson HR, Bailey PA, Cooper JS, Palmer JC. Influence of morbidity, illness label, and social, family and health service factors on drug treatment of childhood asthma. *Lancet* 1981; ii: 1030–32.

4. Clifford RD, Radford M, Howell JB, Holgate ST. Prevalence of respiratory symptoms among 7 and 11 year old school children and association with asthma. *Arch Dis Child* 1989; 64: 1118–25.

5. Kirshner B, Gold M, Zimmerman B. Comparison between the prevalence and treatment of wheezing and coughing in Brampton and Mississauga children. *J Clin Epidemiol* 1990; 43: 765–71.

6. Ferguson AC, Wong FW. Bronchial hyperresponsiveness in asthmatic children. Correlation with macrophages and eosinophils in broncholavage fluid. *Chest* 1989; 96: 988–91.

7. ❂ Stevenson EC, Turner G, Heaney LG, Schock BC, Taylor R, Gallagher T *et al*. Bronchoalveolar lavage findings suggest two different forms of childhood asthma. *Clin Exp Allergy* 1997; 27: 1027–35.

8. Zimmerman B, Feanny S, Reisman J *et al*. Allergy in asthma 1. The dose relationship of allergy to severity of childhood asthma. *J Allergy Clin Immunol* 1988 81: 63–70.

9. Godfrey S. Childhood asthma. In: Clark TJH, Godfrey S (eds). *Asthma*, 2nd edn. London: Chapman and Hall, 1983: 415–56.

10. ❂ Sporik R, Holgate ST, Cogswell JJ. Natural history of asthma in childhood – a birth cohort study. *Arch Dis Child* 1991; 66: 1050–53.

11. Croner S, Kjellman NIM. Natural history of bronchial asthma in childhood. A prospective study from birth up to 12–14 years of age. *Allergy* 1992; 47: 150–57.

12. Pedersen S, Szefler S. Pharmacological interventions. Childhood asthma. *Eur Respir J* (suppl.) 1998; Jul; 27: 40s–45s.

13. Van Asperen PP, Mukhi A. Role of atopy in the natural history of wheeze and bronchial hyper-responsiveness in childhood. *Pediatr Allergy Immunol* 1994; 5: 178–83.

14. Silverman M, Wilson N. Wheezing phenotypes in childhood. *Thorax* 1997; 52: 936–7.

15. Duff AL, Pomeranz ES, Gelber LE *et al*. Risk factors for acute wheezing in infants and children: viruses, passive smoke, and IgE antibodies to inhalant allergens. *Pediatrics* 1993; 92: 535–40.

16. Martinez FD. Definition of pediatric asthma and associated risk factors. *Pediatr Pulmonol* (suppl.) 1997; 15: 9–12.

17. ❂ Martinez FD, Wright AL, Taussig LM, Holberg CJ, Halonen M, Morgan WJ. Asthma and wheezing in the first six years of life. The Group Health Medical Associates. *N Engl J Med* 1995; 332: 133–8.

18. Brooke AM, Lambert PC, Burton PR, Clarke C, Luyt DK, Simpson H. The natural history of respiratory symptoms in preschool children. *Am J Respir Crit Care Med* 1995; 152: 1872–8.

19. Stein RT, Holberg CJ, Morgan WJ *et al*. Peak flow variability, methacholine responsiveness and atopy as markers for detecting different wheezing phenotypes in childhood. *Thorax* 1997; 52: 946–52.

20. Wilson NM. The significance of early wheezing. *Clin Exp Allergy* 1994; 24: 522–9.

21. Hogg C, Bush A. Editorial: Childhood asthma – all that wheezes is not inflammation. *Clin Exp Allergy* 1997; 27: 991–4.

22. Wilson NM, Phagoo SB, Silverman M. Atopy, bronchial responsiveness, and symptoms in wheezy 3 year olds. *Arch Dis Child* 1992; 67: 491–5.

23. Stein RT, Holberg CJ, Morgan WJ *et al.* Peak flow variability, methacholine responsiveness and atopy as markers for detecting different wheezing phenotypes in childhood. *Thorax* 1997; 52: 946–52.

24. Peat JK, Salome CM, Woolcock AJ. Longitudinal changes in atopy during a 4-year period: relation to bronchial hyperresponsiveness and respiratory symptoms in a population sample of Australian schoolchildren. *J Allergy Clin Immunol* 1990; 85: 65–74.

25. Sears MR, Burrows B, Flannery EM, Herbison GP, Hewitt CJ, Holdaway MD. Relation between airway responsiveness and serum IgE in children with asthma and in apparently normal children. *N Engl J Med* 1991; 325: 1067–71.

26. Burrows B, Sears MR, Flannery EM, Herbison GP, Holdaway MD, Silva PA. Relation of the course of bronchial responsiveness from age 9 to age 15 to allergy. *Am J Respir Crit Care Med* 1995; 152: 1302–8.

27. Zimmerman B, Enander I, Zimmerman R, Ahlstedt S. Asthma in children less than 5 years of age: eosinophils and serum levels of the eosinophil proteins ECP and EPX in relation to atopy and symptoms. *Clin Exp Allergy* 1994; 24: 149–55.

28. Takahashi Y, Okamura A, Yasoshima K, Koike A. Serum eosinophil cationic protein in infants during first wheezing episode. *Arerugi* 1996; 45: 1161–5.

29. Young S, Arnott J, Le Souef PN, Landau LI. Flow limitation during tidal expiration in symptom-free infants and the subsequent development of asthma. *J Pediatr* 1994; 124: 681–8.

30. Kattan M, Keens T, Lapierre JG *et al.* Pulmonary function abnormalities in symptom-free children after bronchiolitis. *Pediatrics* 1977; 59: 683–8.

31. Gurwitz D, Mindorff C, Levison H. Increased incidence of bronchial reactivity in children with a history of bronchiolitis. *J Pediatr* 1981; 98: 551–5.

32. Sims DG, Downham MA, Gardner PS, Webb JK, Weightman D. Study of 8 year old children with a history of respiratory syncytial virus bronchiolitis in infancy. *Br Med J* 1978; 1: 11–14.

33. Mok JY, Simpson H. Outcome of acute lower respiratory tract infection in infants: Preliminary report of seven year follow-up study. *Br Med J* 1982; 285: 333–7.

34. Pullan CR, Hey E. Wheezing, asthma and pulmonary dysfunction 10 years after infection with respiratory syncytial virus in infancy. *Br Med J* 1982; 284: 1665–9.

35. Sims D, Gardner PS, Weightman D, Turner MW, Soothill JF. Atopy does not predispose to RSV bronchiolitis or post-bronchiolitic wheezing. *Br Med J* 1981; 282: 2086–8.

36. Martinez FD, Stern DA, Wright AL, Taussig LM, Halonen M. Differential immune responses to acute lower respiratory illness in early life and subsequent development of persistent wheezing and asthma. *J Allergy Clin Immunol* 1998; 102: 915–20.

37. Welliver RC, Wong DT, Sun M *et al.* The development of respiratory syncytial virus-specific IgE and the release of histamine in nasopharyngeal secretions after infection. *N Engl J Med* 1981; 305: 841–6.

38. Garofalo R, Kimpen JL, Welliver RC, Ogra PL. Eosinophil degranulation in the respiratory tract during naturally acquired respiratory syncytial virus infection. *J Pediatr* 1992; 120: 28–32.

39. Zimmerman B, Chambers C, Forsyth S. Allergy in asthma II. The highly atopic infant and chronic asthma. *J Allergy Clin Immunol* 1988; 81: 71–7.

40. McFadden ER. Exertional dyspnea and cough as preludes to acute attacks of bronchial asthma. *N Engl J Med* 1975; 292: 555–9.

41. Cloutier MM, Loughlin GM. Chronic cough in children: a manifestation of airway hyperreactivity. *Paediatrics* 1981; 67: 6–12.

42. Konig P. Hidden asthma in childhood. *Am J Dis Child* 1981; 135: 1053–5.

43. Hannaway PJ, Hopper GD. Cough variant asthma in children. *JAMA* 1982; 247: 206–208.

44. Clifford RD, Howell JB, Radford M, Holgate ST. Association between respiratory symptoms, bronchial response to methacholine, and atopy in two age groups of schoolchildren. *Arch Dis Child* 1989; 64: 1133–9.

45. Clough JB, Williams JD, Holgate ST. Profile of bronchial responsiveness in children with respiratory symptoms. *Arch Dis Child* 1992; 67: 594–9.

46. ❂ Wright AL, Holberg CJ, Morgan WJ, Taussig LM, Halonen M, Martinez FD. Recurrent cough in childhood and its relation to asthma. *Am J Respir Crit Care Med* 1996; 153: 1259–65.

47. Holgate ST. Mediator and cellular mechanisms in asthma. *J Roy Coll Phys Lond* 1990; 24: 304–312.

48. Filley WV, Holley KE, Kephart GM, Gleich GJ. Identification by immunofluorescence of eosinophilic granule major basic protein in lung tissues of patients with bronchial asthma. *Lancet* 1982; 2: 11–16.

49. Venge P, Dahl R, Fredens K, Peterson CG. Epithelial injury by human eosinophils. *Am Rev Respir Dis* 1988; 138: 54–7.

50. Kay AB. Eosinophils as effector cells in immunity and hypersensitivity disorders. *Clin Exp Immunol* 1985; 62: 1–12.

51. Cockcroft DW, Murdock KY, Berscheid BA. Relationship between atopy and bronchial responsiveness to histamine in a random population. *Ann Allergy* 1984; 53: 26–9.

52. Sears MR, Burrows B, Flannery EM, Herbison GP, Hewitt CJ, Holdaway MD. Relation between airway responsiveness and serum IgE in children with asthma and in apparently normal children. *N Engl J Med* 1991; 325: 1067–71.

53. Van Asperen PP, Kemp AS, Mukhi A. Atopy in infancy predicts the severity of bronchial hyperresponsiveness in later childhood. *J Allergy Clin Immunol* 1990; 85: 790–95.

54. Delacourt C, Labbe D, Vassault A, Brunet-Langot D, de Blic J, Scheinmann P. Sensitization to inhalant allergens in wheezing infants is predictive of the development of infantile asthma. *Allergy* 1994; 49: 843–7.

55. Wahn U, Bergmann R, Kulig M, Forster J, Bauer CP. The natural course of sensitisation and atopic disease in infancy and childhood. *Pediatr Allergy Immunol* 1997; 8 (10 suppl): 16–20.

56. Cotton EK. Cystic fibrosis. In: Cherniak RM (ed). *Current Therapy of Respiratory Diseases*. Toronto, BC: Decker, 1989: 184–9.

57. Foucard T. A follow-up study of children with asthmatoid bronchitis. I. skin test reactions and IgE antibodies to common allergens. *Acta Paediat Scand* 1973; 62: 633–44.

58. Zimmerman B, Forsyth S. Diagnosis of allergy in infants: use of mixed allergen RAST disks, Phadiatop and Pediatric mix. *Clin Allergy* 1988; 18: 581–7.

59. Zeiger RS, Heller S, Mellon M, O'Connor R, Hamburger RN. Effectiveness of dietary manipulation in the prevention of food allergy in infants. *J Allergy Clin Immunol* 1986; 78: 224–38.

60. Zimmerman B, Forsyth S, Gold M. Highly atopic children: Formation of IgE antibodies to food protein especially peanut. *J Allergy Clin Immunol* 1989; 83: 764–70.

61. Platt-Mills TA, Tovey ER, Mitchell EB, Moszoro H, Nock P, Wilkins SR. Reduction of bronchial hyperreactivity during prolonged allergen avoidance. *Lancet* 1982; 2: 675–8.

62. ❂ Sears MR, Herbison GP, Holdaway MD, Hewitt CJ, Flannery EM, Silva PA. The relative risks of sensitivity to grass pollen, house dust mite and cat dander in the development of childhood asthma. *Clin Exp Allergy* 1989; 19: 419–24.

63. Warner JO, Gotz M, Landau LI *et al*. Management of asthma: a consensus statement. *Arch Dis Child* 1989; 64: 1065–79.

64. Wright AL, Taussig L, Ray CG, Harrison HR, Holberg CJ. The Tucson children's respiratory study: II. Lower respiratory tract illness in the first year of life. *Am J Epidemiol* 1989; 129: 1232–46.

65. Colley J, Holland W, Corkhill R. Influence of passive smoking and parental phlegm on pneumonia and bronchitis in early childhood. *Lancet* 1974; 2: 1031–34.

66. Fergusson DM, Horwood LJ, Shannon FT. Parental smoking and respiratory illness in infancy. *Arch Dis Child* 1980; 55: 358–61.

67. Bland M, Bewley BR, Pollard V, Banks MH. Effect of children's and parents' smoking on respiratory symptoms. *Arch Dis Child* 1978; 53: 100–105.

68. Murray AB, Morrison BJ. The effect of smoke from the mother on the bronchial responsiveness and severity of symptoms in children with asthma. *J Allergy Clin Immunol* 1986; 76: 575–81.

69. Foratiere F, Agabiti N, Corbo GM *et al.* Passive smoking as a determinant of bronchial responsiveness in children. *Am J Respir Crit Care Med* 1994; 149: 365–70.

70. Sears MR, Burrows B, Flannery EM, Herbison GP, Hewitt CJ, Holdaway MD. Relation between airway responsiveness and serum IgE in children with asthma and in apparently normal children. *N Engl J Med* 1991; 325: 1067–71.

71. Zimmerman B, Lanner A, Enander I, Zimmerman RS, Peterson CGB, Ahlstedt S. Total blood eosinophils, serum eosinophil cationic protein and eosinophil protein X in childhood asthma: relation to disease status and therapy. *Clin Exp Allergy* 1993; 23: 564–70.

72. de Benedictis FM, Bush A. Rhinosinusitis and asthma: epiphenomenon or causal association? *Chest* 1999; 115: 550–6.

73. Dinis PB, Gomes A. Sinusitis and asthma: how do they interrelate in sinus surgery? *Am J Rhinol* 1997; 11: 421–8.

74. DeBaets F, Kint J, Pauwels R, Leroy J. IgG subclass deficiency in children with recurrent bronchitis. *Eur J Pediatr* 1992; 151: 274–8.

75. Hargreave FE. Induced sputum and response to glucocorticoids. *J Allergy Clin Immunol* 1998; 102: S102–5.

Chapter 6

Diagnosis in Adults

Annalisa Cogo, Bianca Beghé, Lorenzo Corbetta and Leonardo Fabbri

INTRODUCTION

In the light of the current knowledge, the latest "Guidelines for Asthma Diagnosis and Management" defines asthma as a chronic inflammatory disorder of the airways.[1] In susceptible individuals this inflammation causes recurrent episodes of wheezing, breathlessness, chest tightness and cough, particularly at night and in the early morning. These symptoms are usually associated with widespread but variable airflow limitation that is at least partly reversible either spontaneously or with treatment. The airway inflammation also causes an associated increase in airway responsiveness to a variety of stimuli.

Airway inflammation is a key factor in asthma and it is likely to account, at least in part, for the pathophysiological characteristic of the disease. Morphological studies of airways from asthmatic patients have shown an infiltration with inflammatory cells, epithelial disruption[2] and thickening of airway wall.[3] This remodelling process, a probable consequence of chronic inflammation, may increase the degree of bronchial obstruction and may even induce a fixed bronchial obstruction. In addition, this chronic inflammation may predispose the airways to hyperreact to exogenous and/or endogenous stimuli and to develop the acute inflammatory reaction that is responsible for the acute airflow limitation associated with asthma attacks.

Unfortunately this definition although excellent for understanding the pathophysiology of asthma, is not very useful in clinical practice. In fact, if one uses the above definition, only a respiratory disease that manifests itself with these symptoms and that is associated with (1) reversible airflow limitation, (2) airway inflam-mation, and (3) airway hyperresponsiveness may be labelled as asthma. Unfortunately airway inflammation can be properly assessed only invasively either with endobronchial biopsies or bronchoalveolar lavage, as the non-invasive measurement of airway inflammation is not yet well standardized. More importantly, while a rather specific airway inflammation is present in most subjects with asthma, it may be absent in some asthmatic subjects, and particularly in mild asthmatics[4] and it may vary in its characteristics over time independently from the activity of asthma.[5,6] The presence of airway hyperresponsiveness, which can be measured with standardized methods,[7] may not accurately reflect the severity of the disease,[8] may be present in asymptomatic subjects and particularly atopics and rhinitics,[9] may be absent out of season reappearing during pollen exposure[10] and thus is not pathognomonic of asthma.[11]

The lack of a "gold standard" for the definition of asthma makes it impossible to assess sensitivity, specificity, and predictive values of features of the medical history, physical examination, and laboratory test. Thus, the clinical diagnosis of asthma still relies on accurate medical history and spirometry. The assessment of reversible airflow limitation represents in fact a simple and objective method to confirm the diagnosis in a subject with symptoms of asthma. While the spontaneous reversibility of airflow limitation may be assessed by monitoring the peak expiratory flow (PEF), the degree of airflow limitation and its reversibility induced by treatment is better assessed by measuring forced expiratory volume in 1 s (FEV_1) before and after a single dose of a bronchodilator, or before and after a short course of full anti-asthma treatment including systemic steroids.

MINIMUM REQUIREMENTS TO ESTABLISH THE DIAGNOSIS OF ASTHMA

The diagnosis of asthma is usually suspected from history, and it is usually confirmed by lung function tests performed to demonstrate reversible airflow limitation.[1]

Medical History

The characteristic symptoms of asthma are recurrent episodes of breathlessness and wheezing, often associated with cough, which reverse partially or completely either spontaneously or after bronchodilators. Other typical symptoms of asthma include non-productive cough, chest tightness and exercise intolerance. Symptoms often first occur at night or early morning, or after non-specific stimuli (Table 6.1).

A typical feature of asthma symptoms is their variability, being more severe on some days or appearing only after exposure to trigger factors. Wheezing even if it is reported as the most characteristic symptom of asthma is non-specific, as it is reported as a principal symptom by 76% of patients suffering from COPD and 28% of cardiac patients.[12]

Cough induced by thermal stimuli, such as exposure to cold, dry air, or by emotional expressions (fear, crying, hard laughing) or by long talking is a sign of bronchial lability and should also be investigated. Some patients, particularly children,[13] complain only of a persistent non-productive cough with no wheezing or dyspnoea (cough-variant asthma). The importance of cough-variant asthma is underlined by the frequency of cough as a complaint, being a very common cause

prompting patients to consult their doctor,[14] and asthma being the cause of cough in a large proportion of these patients. Sputum production is not a frequent symptom reported by asthmatics in stable conditions, but is often reported during exacerbations.

Some patients do not perceive symptoms until their airways are severely narrowed.[15,16] This is especially true in elderly patients whose awareness and attribution of pulmonary symptoms are poor. It is important to keep in mind that asthma in the elderly remains poorly perceived.[17] Thus, breathlessness and wheezing cannot be the only subjective diagnostic criteria since the individual tolerance to a given degree of dyspnoea is variable. Furthermore the severity of symptoms may vary not only from patient to patient but also within the same patient.

Not only the type or severity of symptoms should be carefully investigated but also their onset, duration and frequency. It is in fact important to know the age of the first attack and the pattern of the symptoms, whether they are continuous or episodic, have a seasonal or perennial appearance, or day–night variation (i.e. symptoms at night or early in the morning), whether they worsen outdoors or indoors, at home or in the workplace. Several attempts have been made to find the most valid symptom-based questions to diagnose asthma, particularly for epidemiological studies. Postal questionnaires exist to collect information about the presence and severity of asthma, and these are used for epidemiological studies.[18] Even though these questionnaires have been designed for epidemiological research, the use of some of the questions on current respiratory symptoms can be useful to assess the diagnosis of asthma in an individual. Five simple questions included in the questionnaire developed by the International Union Against Tuberculosis and Lung Diseases (IUATLD) are recommended for assessing the individual patient:

(1) Have you had wheezing or whistling in your chest at any time?
(2) Have you had an attack of shortness of breath that came following strenuous activity at any time?
(3) Have you woken up with an attack of wheezing at any time?
(4) Have you woken up with an attack of cough at any time?
(5) Have you had an attack of shortness of breath that came during the day when you were at rest at any time?

Table 6.1: History and pattern of symptoms in asthma (From Ref. 14.)

Symptoms	Breathlessness, chest tightness, wheezing and cough. May occur singly or in combination.
Pattern	Episodic or variable. Typically worsen nocturnally.
Triggers	Exercise, inhalation of cold air, sulphur dioxide, inhalation to total lung capacity, allergen exposure, viral upper respiratory infection, ingestion of NSAIDs or sulphites.

The sensitivity and specificity of any questionnaire should be tested. Self-reported asthma from a questionnaire has a sensitivity of 36% and a specificity of 94% when using airway hyperresponsiveness as the gold standard of asthma. The sensitivity increases to 68% and the specificity remains 94% when the clinical diagnosis is used as the gold standard of asthma.[19]

The relationship between the answers to a questionnaire and airway hyperresponsiveness has been examined.[20,21] The questions that more strongly predict the presence of airway hyperresponsiveness relate to the appearance of symptoms in response to exercise or dusty environment, and/or development of symptoms at night or early in the morning. This questionnaire has a good sensitivity (65–91%) and specificity (85–96%).[20,21]

A recent analysis examining whether some questions in the IUATLD questionnaire are better for predicting asthma than others reported that the more useful questions are those asking about wheezing in the last 12 months at rest or after exercise, previous asthma attacks and chest tightness.[22] Various scores have been developed to quantify the symptoms. Interestingly if a questionnaire is properly used, it may help to follow single patients and to detect the deterioration of asthma before change in PEF.[23]

In the medical history it is also important to investigate conditions frequently associated with asthma such as nasal, skin or gastric pathologies, as well as precipitating or aggravating factors in order to establish the causes or trigger factors of asthma (see Chapter 4). Among these, correlation with viral respiratory infections, exposure to environmental allergens, occupational sensitizing factors or irritants and consumption of drugs should be investigated. Other important questions concern living conditions in relation to the heating system, the cooking system, the use of air conditioning and the presence of pets.[24–26]

Measures of Airflow Limitation

If the medical history strongly suggests the diagnosis of asthma, efforts should be made to demonstrate the presence of reversible airway limitation. The airflow limitation may be assessed by physical examination, spirometry or peak flow meter.

Physical Examination

Although physical examination remains quite an important diagnostic tool in the diagnosis and assessment of the severity of asthma exacerbations, it is of little help in the diagnosis of intermittent and mild asthma when bronchial obstruction is either absent or very mild.

Expiratory wheezing is the most typical finding of asthma: it is due to the turbulence of airflow in airways which are not uniformly constricted; it is approximately correlated with the severity of bronchial obstruction.[27] However, expiratory wheezing may be absent even when maximal expiratory flows show a reduction of 40–50%.[28] The progression of severity of asthma attacks is characterized by several signs: inability to recline and to speak; use of accessory respiratory muscles; pulsus paradoxus >15 mmHg and reduced intensity of breathing sounds.[29] Tachypnoea, hyperinflation of the chest, prolonged expiration, use of accessory respiratory muscles, hyperresonance of percussion note, wheezing, and inspiratory and/or expiratory rhonchi all reflect airflow limitation.

Spirometry

Lung volumes and expiratory flows can be measured with spirometers.[30,31] Vital capacity (VC) or forced vital capacity (FVC) is the maximum volume of air that can be inhaled or exhaled from the lung. Both VC and FVC may be affected by parenchymal diseases, by chest wall diseases, by neuromuscular diseases, by voluntary effort, and by significant airway diseases. To determine whether an observed reduction in VC is due to restriction or airway obstruction, measurements of flow are obtained. The most common indices of forced expiratory flow are FEV_1, the maximum volume of air expired in the first second from full inspiration; and PEF, the maximum flow rate that can be generated during a forced expiratory manoeuvre.

Spirometry is recommended in the initial assessment of all patients with suspected asthma: a reduction of FEV_1/FVC ratio to <88% predicted is the most sensitive indication of airflow obstruction; the degree of reduction of FEV_1 is used to define the severity of obstruction. Subsequent measurements of PEF are sufficient in the follow-up of most adult patients to assess the severity of symptoms and make therapeutic decisions. Spirometry should be undertaken periodically only in selected patients to confirm the PEF measurements made with a peak flow meter.

While normal expiratory flows do not exclude asthma (asthma often causes only episodic airway narrowing) it should be kept in mind that reduced expiratory flow, even improving significantly after inhaled bronchodilators, is present also in other pulmonary disorders, e.g. chronic obstructive bronchitis, or even in normal subjects following viral upper respiratory infection.[32]

Even though the definition of asthma has improved in recent years it is not yet precise. The diagnosis relies on a triad of clinical history, physical examination, and respiratory function tests (including PEF monitoring and airway hyperresponsiveness). Signs and symptoms are variable and not always present. The lack of a gold standard and the arbitrariness of positivity for tests such as PEF variability and airway responsiveness might lead to the risk of either over-diagnosis or an underestimation of asthma.[33,34]

Peak Expiratory Flow Records and Monitoring

If spirometry does not reveal airflow limitation, home monitoring of PEF for 2–4 weeks may help to diagnose asthma. Peak expiratory flow is the highest flow obtained during a forced expiration starting immediately after a deep inspiration at total lung capacity. It is a simple, reproducible index and can be measured with inexpensive and portable peak flow meters. Daily monitoring of PEF over a period of time is a simple and inexpensive objective lung function test recommended in asthma guidelines to help in establishing the diagnosis of asthma (when spirometry is normal), and to assess the severity of the disease and its response to treatment.

However, PEF measurements have some limitations; PEF is effort dependent, and proper training is required to obtain the best and most reproducible measurements from the individual. Furthermore PEF mainly reflects the calibre of large airways and may therefore underestimate the degree of airflow limitation present in peripheral airways.[35] A single measurement of PEF is therefore not recommended in making the first diagnosis of bronchial obstruction. Predicted values of PEF, related to gender, race, age and height, are available in the literature.[36] These values are useful in assessing individual measurements, but the inter-individual variability is wide and some subjects have PEF values that are very different from the average value of subjects with the same demographic characteristics. Also, some subjects with long-lasting asthma or other chronic obstructive pulmonary diseases may develop irreversible airflow limitation. For these two reasons, in addition to referring to predicted values, it is quite useful to establish the best personal PEF of each patient during a period of

monitoring while the patient is under effective anti-asthma treatment. Thus, one should refer to the personal-best PEF and to the diurnal variability of PEF observed during a period of effective treatment to obtain reference values to use in the assessment of long-term changes. In other words, in clinical practice it is preferable to refer to the patient's personal best and minimum daily variability rather than to a predicted value, particularly for patients with chronically impaired lung function. In assessing the severity of asthma and in reviewing asthma medication a quality control of the measurements and a standardization of conditions for PEF monitoring are very important, especially regarding the timing of the measurement in relationship to the consumption of anti-asthma medication, particularly bronchodilators. Post-bronchodilator PEF, if not indicated, can in fact mask the severity of asthma leading to an inaccuracy in treatment decisions.[36] When the patient is well trained and aware of the importance of accurate records, PEF is very useful in the follow-up, not only to assess the efficacy of asthma therapy but also to discriminate, in presence of a deterioration, between poor asthma control and asthma exacerbations.[37] In fact a high variation of PEF values (>20%) characterizes poorly controlled asthma, whereas during asthma exacerbations a linear fall of PEF values over several days with normal diurnal variability (7.7%) has been observed; the mere observation of variability can therefore lead to misinterpretation of the PEF values during asthma exacerbations.[37]

Sometimes, however, particularly in children, PEF may underestimate the severity of asthma exacerbations and most peak flow meters can be inaccurate.[38] Consequently patients should be informed of these potential biases and advised to perform a spirometry if PEF values do not fit with the clinical severity of asthma.

Peak expiratory flow should be measured at least twice a day, in the morning on waking and again in the evening. Further measurements should be recommended when symptoms develop, or to investigate specific allergen or work-place exposure. Monitoring PEF provides an easy assessment of daily variability of respiratory function and activity of asthma. Diurnal variability is calculated in the following way:

$$\frac{PEF_{max} - PEF_{min}}{PEF_{max} + PEF_{min}/2} \times 100$$

In asthmatic subjects the diurnal variability of PEF is higher than in normal subjects. An arbitrary limit of 20% in diurnal variability is conventionally assumed as normal.[39]

Asthma is a variable condition, and thus even a normal diurnal variation over a short period of time does not exclude asthma. In these cases it might be useful to calculate the diurnal variability from the maximum PEF measured after use of a bronchodilator.

Reversibility of Airflow Limitation Induced by a Single Dose of a Short-Acting Bronchodilator

In subjects with reduced lung function (e.g. FEV_1/FVC less than 88% predicted), the response to a single dose of bronchodilator (e.g. 200 μg salbutamol inhaled from a metered dose inhaler) should be measured. Lung function measurements are usually repeated 15–30 minutes after the inhalation of a β-adrenergic agonist. As measure of reversibility the FEV_1 variation is used: a 12–15% increase in FEV_1 is usually assumed to be evidence of reversible airflow limitation.[1] In some patients, and particularly young patients and athletes with a history of symptoms, a reversibility test is recommended even when baseline lung function is normal, because their normal lung function might be significantly higher than the predicted value. In these cases, a marked improvement in lung function after bronchodilation might reveal airflow limitation even if the observed values of PEF or FEV_1 are within normal limits.

ADDITIONAL CONFIRMATORY TESTS

In subjects with atypical history and symptoms, normal diurnal variability of PEF and/or airflow limitation not reversible by a single dose of bronchodilator, additional confirmatory tests are recommended, including measurement of airway responsiveness to bronchoconstrictor stimuli and the reversibility of airflow limitation after a short course of steroids.

Measurement of Airway Responsiveness (see also Chapter 8)

Airway hyperresponsiveness is an exaggerated response to a large variety of physical, chemical and pharmacological bronchoconstrictor stimuli.[7] Airways narrow too easily and too much to a large variety of stimuli. Virtually all current symptomatic asthmatics show airway hyperresponsiveness. Because, both in asthmatic and non-asthmatic subjects, airflow limitation may by itself be the cause of an exaggerated response to bronchoconstrictor stimuli, the measurement of airway responsiveness for the diagnosis of asthma is usually restricted to subjects with normal lung function.

The degree of airway responsiveness can be measured in the laboratory using various stimuli and methods. Because the airways respond to many stimuli that may cause airflow limitation even in normal subjects, airway hyperresponsiveness is sometimes referred to as non-specific. However, even non-specific stimuli act through very specific mechanisms and some of these stimuli (e.g. exercise, ultrasonically nebulized distilled water) cause airflow limitation only or mainly in asthmatics. The term "non-specific" should therefore be avoided. Airway hyperresponsiveness should be referred to the stimulus used to measure it.

Bronchoconstrictor stimuli may be classified as causing airflow limitation directly by stimulating airway smooth muscles (e.g. methacholine, histamine) or indirectly by releasing pharmacologically active mediators (e.g. exercise, nebulized hypotonic or hypertonic solutions) or stimulating sensory nerves (e.g. metabisulphite, bradykinin and, in part, histamine), or a combination of these mechanisms. Unlike inhalation challenges with indirect stimuli, those with histamine and methacholine have been properly standardized and validated in patients with asthma. Thus they are safe, and should be preferred in the clinical evaluation of patients.[7]

A PC_{20}-FEV_1 methacholine or histamine (the concentration of methacholine and histamine causing a 20% decrease of FEV_1) greater than 16 mg ml^{-1} or a PD_{20}-FEV_1 methacholine or histamine (the concentration of methacholine and histamine causing a 20% decrease of FEV_1) greater than 16 μmol or 1.4 mg are usually considered to be normal.

Airway hyperresponsiveness is present in the great majority of asthmatics, even if it may be absent when the patient is not exposed to the sensitizing agent, e.g. out of the season or away from occupational exposure. Thus a negative inhalation challenge with methacholine or histamine suggests the absence of current asthma. However, in a follow-up study 33 (9%) of 334 subjects with suspected asthma but normal airway responsiveness developed asthma within 10 years. Age, a positive family history of allergy, and FEV_1 values appear to be the best predictors of future development of asthma.[40] On the other hand, up to 10% of normal asymptomatic subjects have an increased response to bronchoconstrictor stimuli and no evidence of asthma. In a 2-year follow-up study, up to 45% of asymptomatic subjects with clear-cut hyperresponsiveness to methacholine (PD_{20} <3.2 μmol) developed asthma within 2 years, suggesting that airway hyperresponsiveness, in addition to being a feature of asthma, might be a risk factor for the development of asthma.[41] The effect of treating asymptomatic airway hyperresponsiveness on the prevention of the subsequent development of asthma remains to be investigated. Interestingly, while an early study showed that monitoring airway responsiveness was useless in the monitoring of asthma,[8] a recent study nicely showed that asthmatic patients treated with the aim of reducing the degree of airway responsiveness instead of just reducing symptoms, had a lower incidence of asthma exacerbations, better improvement of lung function, and a better improvement of the inflammation of the airway mucosa.[42] These results emphasize an interesting role of the measurement of airway responsiveness in the monitoring of the treatment of asthma.

Reversibility of Airflow Limitation Induced by a Course of Steroids

In patients with airflow limitation not relieved by a single dose of a short-acting bronchodilator, the improvement after 2 weeks of treatment with bronchodilators and steroids should be studied, particularly in patients with chronic airflow limitation.[43,44] Corticosteroids may be administered orally (e.g. 40 mg daily prednisone), by aerosol (e.g. 2 mg daily beclomethasone or equivalent) or both. Due to their efficacy and infrequent adverse events, inhaled corticosteroids are increasingly used as first-choice therapy to investigate the reversibility of airflow limitation.[45-47] Some patients with moderate or severe asthma, and up to 20% of patients with chronic obstructive pulmonary diseases, show a significant improvement in airflow limitation that confirms the presence of asthma.[43,44]

Another practical approach to assess the reversibility of airflow limitation not reversed by single administration of inhaled $β_2$ agonists is to measure lung function before and after a 1–3 month course with complete anti-asthma medication, e.g. full doses of inhaled steroids and long acting bronchodilator. Unfortunately no studies have properly examined the sensitivity and specificity of such a simple clinical approach.

Figure 6.1 shows an algorithm for asthma diagnosis.

EVALUATION OF RISK FACTORS

Once the diagnosis of asthma is established, all the potential risk factors should be investigated. The major risk factor for asthma is allergen exposure and the diagnosis of allergy in asthmatic patients is based on the medical history, skin testing and/or *in vitro* determination of specific IgE.

Diagnosis of Allergy (see also Chapter 9)

History The presence of asthma or other allergic disorders in family history should be investigated. History also provides important information about the life-style and the occupation, both influencing exposure to allergens, the time and the factors possibly involved in the onset of asthma, and the exacerbation of asthmatic symptoms in relation to exposure to allergens.

The relationship should be established between exposure to one or more allergens and the occurrence of asthma symptoms and/or ocular and nasal symptoms. The relationship should be assessed with the months of the year (seasonal pollen asthma) and with the presence in the house of pets. A description of the patient's house with special attention to carpets, pillows, and other dust collectors should be obtained.

The identification of one or more allergens is important for the diagnosis and subsequent management of asthma in relation to the first step of treatment, represented, whenever possible, by allergen avoidance.[48]

Allergens are the most important risk factor for asthma. House-dust mite, pollens, animal hair and dander, moulds and, in some countries, cockroaches, are the allergens most frequently involved in asthma. The role of food and food additive allergy remains undetermined, but nevertheless needs to be investigated.

In Vivo and In Vitro Tests for Allergy The choice of the most appropriate test to perform in a patient with suspected allergic asthma depends upon the kind of sensitization and on the nature of the allergen to be tested. Only the combination of history, skin tests and, in a few cases, *in vitro* measurements (allergen-specific IgE antibodies by radioimmunoassay or immunoenzymatic assay) provides the necessary information to establish the importance of a given allergen in the development and maintenance of asthma.

Skin Tests Skin tests with all relevant allergens present in the geographical area of the patient represent the

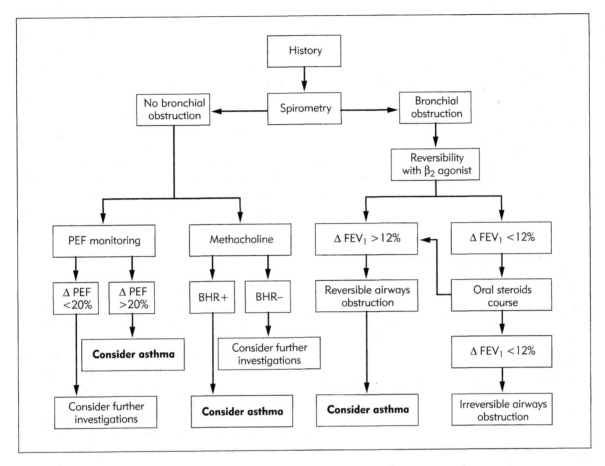

FIGURE 6.1: Algorithm for asthma diagnosis.

first choice test in diagnosis of allergy, because they are simple, easy and rapid to perform, and are highly sensitive and specific. The method most frequently used is represented by the skin test, performed by pricking the skin of the patient through a drop of allergen extract. Skin-prick tests are reproducible and very seldom produce systemic reactions. Although more variable and risky, intradermal tests can be used with low-potency allergen extracts.[49]

In Vitro Tests The *in vitro* measurements of allergen-specific IgE antibodies by immunoassay (RAST) or immunoenzymatic assay (ELISA) are much more expensive than skin-prick tests. They should be used only when skin-prick tests cannot be performed. *In vitro* tests are specific but not as sensitive as the *in vivo* tests. The meas-

urement of total IgE as well as of other immunoglobulins (e.g. IgG_4) provides no additional information.[49-51]

Inhalation Challenges with Allergen, Drugs and Chemical Sensitizers Inhalation challenges with allergens are sometimes required to establish the relevance of single allergens for asthma. Because these tests are risky and demand careful interpretation, they should be performed only in specialized centres. Atopic individuals with airway hyperresponsiveness to methacholine or histamine often also respond to allergens to which they are skin-prick positive, but that may not be relevant for their asthma. The real value of allergen provocation tests in the management of the single patient remains unclear. In general, because these tests are risky and do not provide really useful information on single patients, they should *not* be used in clinical practice.

Inhalation challenges with sensitizing agents such as drugs (e.g. aspirin) or small molecular weight chemical sensitizers (e.g. isocyanates), which cause asthma through a non-IgE-mediated mechanism (and thus cannot be used for skin or *in vitro* tests) may provide the only method that objectively confirms the cause of asthma.

The cost-benefit ratio of performing inhalation tests with allergens or other sensitizing agents should be carefully examined in each single patient, taking into account the high cost and the potential risk involved.[7]

OTHER STUDIES

If the medical history suggests the presence of rhinitis, sinusitis, nasal polyposis (chronic cough, purulent nasal discharge, post-nasal drip)[52,53] a rhinoscopy and a sinus X-ray or sinus CT scan should be undertaken. When a gastroesophageal reflux is suspected (chronic cough, acid reflux, retrosternal burning) the oesophageal pH should be measured and monitored.[54] An appropriate course of anti-reflux therapy may significantly reduce the asthma symptoms,[55] confirming the cause–effect relationship between gastroesophageal reflux and activity of asthma.

Ancillary Tests (see also Chapters 10 and 14)
Cellular and Biochemical Markers of Airway Inflammation
In recent years a growing interest in characterizing the type and intensity of airway inflammation has been observed and many studies have attempted to define the importance of such information for the diagnosis and the assessment of the disease. Even if the best picture of airway inflammation is provided by bronchoscopy and related techniques (bronchial biopsies and bronchoalveolar lavage) this invasive procedure is not yet recommended for the diagnosis of asthma. By contrast, induced sputum may provide a non-invasive method of assessing airway inflammation in asthma.[56]

Induced Sputum
The analysis of cell counts in induced sputum, the characterization of cell activation and the measurement of inflammatory mediators in supernatant (together with the measure in peripheral blood) may provide useful information in the investigation of asthma. The numbers of eosinophils in the sputum are significantly correlated with the degree of airway hyper-

responsiveness, and they decrease after treatment with steroids, reflecting an improvement in asthma.[57,58]

Although these markers may provide quite useful information for the assessment of airway inflammation and the degree of asthma exacerbations, the correlations between sputum, bronchoalveolar lavage and biopsies are not strong enough to be used as interchangeable markers of airway inflammation.[59–61]

Blood and Urinary Level of Inflammatory Mediators
Inflammatory mediators such as eosinophil cationic protein (ECP) and myeloperoxidase (MPO) are increased not only in the bronchoalveolar lavage fluid and sputum of asthmatics but also in the peripheral venous blood, particularly during asthma exacerbations.[60,62–67] Similarly, urinary leukotriene metabolites increase during an asthma attack, and during asthma exacerbations.[68,69] These measures can provide an indirect qualitative index of the presence of airway inflammation but not of the severity of airway inflammation.[70]

Nitric Oxide in Exhaled Air
Nitric oxide (NO), one of the oxides of nitrogen, is formed in the body in a number of cells in contact with the airways. Exhaled NO is considered a biochemical indicator of the function of airways and is increased in asthmatic patients and in the late phase of provoked asthma.[71,72] Recently, significant correlations between exhaled NO, PC_{20} methacholine and sputum eosinophilia have been reported.[73] However, the lack of standardization of methodology reduces the potential use of this marker for monitoring inflammation in asthma.[74] An increased concentration of exhaled NO may help to support the diagnosis of cough-variant asthma in patients with chronic cough.[75]

DIFFERENTIAL DIAGNOSIS

The clinician must be aware of other pathologies inducing symptoms of recurrent cough, dyspnoea and wheezing which could mimic an asthma attack. Differentiation is essential for proper treatment (Table 6.2).

Upper airway obstruction due to laryngeal oedema, vocal cord dysfunction, laryngeal or tracheal stenosis or malacia, primary or secondary neoplasia and foreign bodies should always be considered. In addition to a suggestive history (patients usually complain of paroxysms of cough), patients present with stridor, and physical examination reveals respiratory sounds in the area of the trachea. Laryngoscopy or bronchoscopy may sometimes be useful.[76] Vocal cord dysfunction can sometimes mimic an exercise-induced asthma. When patients complain of atypical exertional symptoms a careful clinical and physiological evaluation must be undertaken.[77,78] When upper airway obstruction is suspected, a complete pulmonary function test, including inspiratory flow volume curves, may be useful.[79]

Chronic obstructive pulmonary diseases should also be considered. Subjects with chronic irreversible airflow limitation may have a transient reversibility of airflow limitation, and may develop acute airflow limitation during exacerbations. A history of smoking, chronic cough and sputum production is suggestive of chronic bronchitis. Imaging of the chest, including chest X-ray and/or high resolution computerized tomography (HRCT) scan of the chest may help to identify specific features of asthma or COPD, particularly in patients with severe symptoms.[80] Physical and radiological signs of irreversible hyperinflation are suggestive of emphysema. The measurement of diffusion capacity of carbon monoxide with the single breath method may help to distinguish between asthma and COPD.[81] Spontaneous and/or induced sputum, and exhaled NO, may also help in the differential diagnosis between asthma and COPD. In fact asthma is associated with sputum eosinophilia and increased concentration of exhaled NO;[60] by contrast COPD is associated with sputum lymphocytosis and neutrophilia,[82,60] and normal or slightly increased concentration of exhaled NO.[83–86] However, most of the cited studies were conducted in groups of patients with well-defined asthma or COPD. In these patients the differential diagnosis between asthma and COPD is quite simple; as there is no problem in distinguishing a young atopic non-smoking individual with recurrent dyspnoea, wheezing or chest tightness and variable and reversible airflow limitation, from a 60-year-old life-long heavy smoker with dyspnoea, chronic cough and sputum, and fixed airflow limitation. The real problem arises when age and risk factors overlap. Unfortunately, no study has been properly conducted so far addressing this population.

When asthma and/or chronic bronchitis, and/or emphysema, occur in the same patient, they should be recognized and treated appropriately.[70,87]

- Congestive heart failure in patients with chronic obstructive pulmonary disease is usually recognizable from signs of left ventricular failure, including basal rales.[88]

- Pulmonary infiltrations with tissue and blood eosinophilia occur in eosinophilic pneumonia, pulmonary parasitic infections, allergic bronchopulmonary aspergillosis and some pulmonary vasculitis syndromes. In these patients, pulmonary eosinophilic infiltrations may be associated with asthma, and therefore they should be properly investigated.[89]

- Pulmonary microembolism or recurrent episodes of pulmonary embolism may mimic asthma attacks because of the sudden development of dyspnoea. The development of dyspnoea is usually unexpected and occurs in patients at risk of pulmonary embolism (venous thrombosis at lower limb, recent surgery). Tests for blood D-dimer levels, a radioisotope lung scan and an angio-CT scan may be necessary to exclude pulmonary embolism in patients at risk.[90]

- Pneumothorax may also cause acute breathlessness, but it is accompanied by acute chest pain, the absence of airflow limitation and, ultimately, a chest X-ray will provide the diagnosis.[91]

- Cardiogenic pulmonary hypertension may both mimic asthma in non-asthmatic cardiopathic subjects and trigger asthma attacks in cardiopathic asthmatic subjects. History, physical and radiological signs of cardiomegaly and/or valvular disease, or additional cardiological examination may be required for the differential diagnosis.[92]

- Bronchial carcinoid tumours may mimic asthma symptoms. Patients with carcinoid tumours may develop the carcinoid syndrome, i.e. flushing of the face and other portions of the body, hyperperistalsis of the gut with diarrhoea, hypotension and tachycardia sometimes associated with wheezing. Facial rash and diarrhoea, in addition to the increase of urinary 5-hydroxyindoleacetic acid, are usually guidelines for a correct diagnosis. A bronchoscopy is necessary for an accurate diagnosis.[93]

MINIMAL REQUIREMENTS TO ESTABLISH THE SEVERITY OF ASTHMA AND ASTHMA EXACERBATIONS

The assessment of severity is based on history, assessment of symptom score, repeated measurement of spirometry and/or PEF and the amount of medication required to keep asthma under control.

Assessment of Severity of Asthma

In clinical practice it is most important to define the severity of asthma, as the physician's decisions on short-term and long-term management depend almost entirely on severity. In addition, a classification of a patient's asthma based on disease severity over the previous years has been shown to relate to pathological indices of airway inflammation.

The descriptions of levels of disease severity based on a combination of symptoms and treatment requirements, as well as objective measurements of lung function, differ little between the guidelines produced in various countries. The most recent classification scheme is presented in Fig. 6.2, and it includes the categories mild intermittent, mild persistent, moderate persistent, and severe persistent. The severity of asthma exacerbations is also based on symptoms, lung function and response to treatment (Fig. 6.2), but must also take into account the time-course and frequency of the exacerbations, which are predictors of outcome.

Table 6.2: Differential diagnosis between asthma and disease causing:

Airflow obstruction
COPD, Upper airway obstruction, vocal cord dysfunction, laryngeal or tracheal stenosis or malacia, primary or secondary neoplasia and foreign bodies

Cough
Rhinitis, sinusitis, bronchitis, airway narrowing, pulmonary fibrosis, gastroesophageal reflux, some drugs

Dyspnoea
COPD, Congestive heart failure, pulmonary microembolism or recurrent episodes of pulmonary embolism, pneumothorax, cardiogenic pulmonary hypertension, carcinoid

Blood and tissue Eosinophilia
Eosinophilic pneumonia, pulmonary parasitic infections, allergic bronchopulmonary aspergillosis and some pulmonary vasculitis syndromes

---

These categories are purely arbitrary; studies to validate them will be important, both as regards their relationship to quality of life and prognosis and, more importantly, as regards the effect of the recommended stepwise approach to treatment. Interestingly, because of the specific features of asthma, which is a syndrome manifesting itself recurrently with asymptomatic periods during which lung volumes might be normal, guidelines have recently been issued that take into account not only symptoms and baseline lung function, but also the degree of airway hyperresponsiveness and the amount of medication required to keep the disease under control.[35,94–96]

Severity of Asthma Exacerbations

Exacerbations of asthma are episodes of worsening shortness of breath, cough, wheezing or chest tightness, or some combination of these symptoms.[87] Exacerbations are usually associated with acute airflow limitation that can be measured with physical examination, spirometry and/or measurements of PEF.

The change of condition is of paramount importance in the evaluation of severity, as absolute values of objective measurements (e.g. blood gases or FEV_1) may be misleading if not compared with the best values of the subject. For instance an FEV_1 of 2 litres or a PaO_2 of 60 mm Hg may be well tolerated by a subject with severe asthma who copes with these values in stable conditions, whereas they may reflect a severe exacerbation for a subject with much higher values, e.g. FEV_1 of 5 litres or a PaO_2 of 80 mm Hg in stable conditions.

Exacerbations usually reflect either a failure in long-term management or exposure to a precipitating stimulus. The severity of asthma exacerbations may range from mild to life-threatening. The deterioration usually progresses over hours or days, but may occasionally occur precipitously over some minutes. Assessment of the patient's pulse, respiratory rate and current symptoms also guides treatment decisions, but objective measurements of lung function are critical.

Previous hospital admission for asthma, especially in an emergency department, must be carefully investigated. Hospital admission in the previous 12 months is reported to be the strongest marker of subsequent risk of asthma death, and the risk increases with the number of previous admissions.[96] Thus, patients with a history of current use of, or recent withdrawal from,

Step 4: Severe persistent

Clinical features before treatment

Continuous symptoms
Frequent exacerbations
Frequent night-time asthma symptoms
Physical activities limited by asthma symptoms
PEF or FEV_1
= †60% predicted;
= variability >30%

Daily medication required to maintain control

Multiple daily controller medications: high doses inhaled corticosteroid, long-acting bronchodilator, and oral corticosteroid long term

Step 3: Moderate persistent

Clinical features before treatment

Symptoms daily
Exacerbations affect activity and sleep
Night-time asthma symptoms > once a week
Daily use of inhaled short-acting β_2-agonist
PEF or FEV_1,
= †60 to <80% predicted;
= variability >30%

Daily medication required to maintain control

Daily controller medications: inhaled corticosteroid and long-acting bronchodilator (especially for night-time symptoms)

Step 2: Mild persistent

Clinical features before treatment

Symptoms ‡ once a week but < once a day
Exacerbations may affect activity and sleep
Night-time asthma symptoms > twice a month
PEF or FEV_1,
= ‡80% predicted;
= variability 20–30%

Daily medication required to maintain control

One daily controller medication: possibly add a long-acting bronchodilator to anti-inflammatory medication (especially for night-time symptoms)

Step 1: Mild intermittent

Clinical features before treatment

Intermittent symptoms < once a week
Brief exacerbations (from a few hours to a few days)
Night-time asthma symptoms < twice a month
Asymptomatic and normal lung function between exacerbations
PEF or FEV_1,
= ‡80% predicted;
= variability <20%

Daily medication required to maintain control

Intermittent reliever medication taken as needed only: inhaled short-acting β_2-agonist. Intensity of treatment depends on severity of exacerbation; oral corticosteroids may be required

FIGURE 6.2: Classification of asthma severity. The presence of one of the features of severity is sufficient to place a patient in that category.

systemic corticosteroids, hospitalization for asthma and/or emergency treatment for asthma in the past year, prior intubation for asthma, psychiatric disease or psychosocial problems and non-compliance with an asthma medication plan are at high risk of asthma-related death. While symptoms may be a sensitive indicator of mild asthma exacerbations, symptoms and physical signs alone cannot be considered accurate indicators of severe airflow limitation. The severity of the exacerbation determines the treatment administered.

Table 6.3 provides a guide to the severity of an exacerbation of asthma at the time the examination is made. Since these are guidelines only, all features in a category need not be present. A more severe grading should be given if the patient has a lack of response to initial treatment, if the attack has progressed quickly or if the patient is at high risk historically as just defined. Indices of severity, particularly PEF (in patients over 5 years old), pulse and respiratory rate should also be monitored during treatment. Any deterioration may require prompt intervention. Initiation of anti-asthma therapy at the earliest possible sign of deteriorating control of asthma is important in the successful management of an exacerbation. Peak expiratory flow monitoring is an integral part of the management. Ideally, all patients should have a written action plan that outlines how to recognize signs of deterioration, how to start treatment and how to ask for medical care.

The assessment of the severity of asthma exacerbations in the hospital requires, in addition to a brief history to document the time-course severity of symptoms, information about the exposure to potential triggering events, a recent change in medication and prior hospitalizations and emergency department visits for asthma. The physical examination will assess severity of exacerbations (Table 6.3), the presence of complications (e.g. pneumonia, atelectasis, pneumothorax or pneumomediastinum). Measurements of PEF and/or FEV_1 should be made at least hourly, with initial measurement made before treatment if possible.

As already mentioned, the knowledge of PEF patient's "personal best" and the way it deteriorated is very important for the management of an exacerbation.

Arterial blood gas measurement provides important information in assessing the severity of asthma exacerbations, particularly when they are severe, e.g. when FEV_1 or PEF are <40% predicted or best personal value, and/or oxygen saturation is decreased, and/or PEF does not increase after the initial treatment. Gas exchange abnormalities, as reflected by arterial hypoxaemia, are common in asthma patients during exacerbation. The degree of ventilation–perfusion mismatching correlates poorly with clinical findings and indices of airflow obstruction and thus alterations of arterial blood gases may be present even when symptoms are mild and/or spirometric indices are normal or borderline.[97] During a mild asthma attack, the usual pattern consists in normal Pao_2, associated with hypocapnia and slight respiratory alkalosis due to compensatory hyperventilation. Normocapnia or hypercapnia associated with normoxaemia or hypoxaemia are poor prognostic evidence of a severe attack. Respiratory failure with hypoxaemia, hypercapnia, respiratory acidosis and the need for intensive care unit (ICU) admission occurs in a minority of patients.

Pulse oximetry provides measurement of oxygen saturation that can monitor a patient's response to acute therapy. The more extensive information obtained from blood gas determinations may be important, particularly if pulse oximetry is normal in the presence of other indications of severe exacerbations. Once initial treatment has been established, clinical examinations may be advisable, e.g. complete blood count, microbiological examinations in patients with purulent sputum, or standard chest X-ray if complicating cardiopulmonary process is suspected.

Acknowledgement

The authors express their gratitude to Dr Elisa Veratelli for her excellent editorial assistance.

Table 6.3: Severity of asthma exacerbations.

	Mild	Moderate	Severe	Respiratory arrest imminent
Breathless	Walking Can lie down	Talking Infant: softer shorter cry; difficulty feeding Prefers sitting	At rest Infant: stops feeding Hunched forward	
Talks in	Sentences	Phrases	Words	
Alertness	May be agitated	Usually agitated	Usually agitated	Drowsy or confused
Respiratory rate	Increased	Increased	Often >30 min^{-1}	
Accessory muscles and suprasternal retractions	Usually not	Usually	Usually	Paradoxical thoraco-abdominal movement
Wheeze	Moderate, often only end expiratory	Loud	Usually loud	Absence of wheeze
Pulse (min^{-1})	<100	100–120	>120	Bradycardia
Pulsus paradoxus	Absent <10 mmHg	May be present 10–25 mmHg	Often present >25 mmHg (adult) 20–40 mmHg (child)	Absence suggests respiratory muscle fatigue
PEF after initial bronchodilator % predicted or % personal best	Over 80%	Approx 60–80%	<60% predicted or personal best (<100 l min^{-1} adults) or response lasts <2 hours	
P_aO_2 (on air)	Normal Test not usually necessary	>60 mmHg	<60 mmHg Possible cyanosis	
and/or P_aCO_2	<45 mmHg	<45 mmHg	>45 mmHg Possible respiratory failure (see text)	
S_aO_2 (on air)	>95%	91–95%	<90%	

Guide to rates of breathing associated with respiratory distress in awake children:

Age	Normal rate
<2 months	<60 min^{-1}
2–12 months	<50 min^{-1}
1–5 years	<40 min^{-1}
6–8 years	<30 min^{-1}

Guide to limits of normal pulse rate in children:

		Normal rate
Infants:	2–12 months	<160 min^{-1}
Pre-school:	1–2 years	<120 min^{-1}
School age:	2–8 years	<110 min^{-1}

Hypercapnia (hypoventilation) develops more readily in young children than in adults and adolescents

KEY POINTS (Fig. 6.1)

1. The gold standard procedure for the clinical diagnosis of asthma consists in (1) an accurate medical history followed by (2) spirometry to confirm the occurrence of airflow obstruction reversible after a single dose of a short-acting bronchodilator. Peak expiratory flow monitoring may be required to asses spontaneous reversibility of airflow limitation, not demonstrable with the bronchodilator test in the laboratory.

2. Hyperresponsiveness to methacholine or histamine or reversibility of airflow limitation after a short course of steroids may be required to demonstrate reversible airflow limitation not revealed by a reversibility test with a single dose of a short acting bronchodilator, nor with peak flow monitoring.

3. Allergy skin tests and/or measurements should be used to diagnose atopy and to identify the allergen(s), if any, involved in the development of asthma, its activity, or causing asthma exacerbations.

4. A differential diagnosis from other conditions mimicking asthma may require other investigations (e.g. chest X-rays, ECG, bronchoscopy).

REFERENCES

1. Guidelines for the Diagnosis and Management of Asthma. US Dept Health and Human Services 1997. 97–4051–A.

2. Busse WW. Inflammation in asthma: the cornerstone of the disease and target of therapy. *J Allergy Clin Immunol* 1998; 102 (4 Pt 2): S17–22.

3. Kuwano K, Bosken CH, Pare PD, Bai TR, Wiggs BR, Hogg JC. Small airways dimensions in asthma and in chronic obstructive pulmonary disease. *Am Rev Respir Dis* 1993; 148 (5): 1220–5.

4. Gizycki MJ, Adelroth E, Rogers AV, O'Byrne PM, Jeffery PK. Myofibroblast involvement in the allergen-induced late response in mild atopic asthma. *Am J Respir Cell Mol Biol* 1997; 16 (6): 664–73.

5. Crimi E, Spanevello A, Neri M, Ind PW, Rossi GA, Brusasco V. Dissociation between airway inflammation and airway hyperresponsiveness in allergic asthma. *Am J Respir Crit Care Med* 1998; 157 (1): 4–9.

6. Brusasco V, Crimi E, Pellegrino R. Airway hyperresponsiveness in asthma: not just a matter of airway inflammation. *Thorax* 1998; 53 (11): 992–8.

7. Sterk PJ, Fabbri LM, Quanjer PH *et al.* Airway responsiveness. Standardized challenge testing with pharmacological, physical and sensitizing stimuli in adults. Report of the Working Party Standardization of Lung Function Tests, European Community for Steel and Coal. Official Statement of the European Respiratory Society. *Eur Respir J* (suppl.) 1993; 16: 53–83.

8. Josephs LK, Gregg I, Mullee MA, Holgate ST. Nonspecific bronchial reactivity and its relationship to the clinical expression of asthma. A longitudinal study. *Am Rev Respir Dis* 1989; 140(2): 350–7.

9. Cockcroft DW, Hargreave FE. Airway hyperresponsiveness. Relevance of random population data to clinical usefulness. *Am Rev Respir Dis* 1990; 142 (3): 497–500.

10. Boulet LP, Cartier A, Thomson NC, Roberts RS, Dolovich J, Hargreave FE. Asthma and increases in nonallergic bronchial responsiveness from seasonal pollen exposure. *J Allergy Clin Immunol* 1983; 71 (4): 399–406.

11. Higgins BG, Britton JR, Chinn S, Lai KK, Burney PG, Tattersfield AE. Factors affecting peak expiratory flow variability and bronchial reactivity in a random population sample. *Thorax* 1993; 48 (9): 899–905.

12. Elliott MW, Adams L, Cockcroft A, MacRae KD, Murphy K, Guz A. The language of breathlessness. Use of verbal descriptors by patients with cardiopulmonary disease. *Am Rev Respir Dis* 1991; 144 (4): 826–32.

13. Doan T, Patterson R, Greenberger PA. Cough variant asthma: usefulness of a diagnostic-therapeutic trial with prednisone. *Ann Allergy* 1992; 69 (6): 505–9.

14. Boushey HA. Clinical diagnosis of asthma. In: Barnes PJ, Leff AR, Woolcock AJ. (eds). *Asthma.* Philadelphia: Lippincott-Raven, 1997; 1391.

15. Bijl-Hofland ID, Cloosterman SG, Folgering HT, Akkermans RP, van Schayck CP. Relation of the perception of airway obstruction to the severity of asthma. *Thorax* 1999; 54 (1): 15–19.

16. Bellia V, Cuttitta G, Cibella F *et al.* Effect of ageing on peak expiratory flow variability and nocturnal exacerbations in bronchial asthma. *Eur Respir J* 1997; 10 (8): 1803–8.

17. Reed CE. The natural history of asthma in adults: the problem of irreversibility. *J Allergy Clin Immunol* 1999; 103 (4): 539–47.

18. Burney PG, Chinn S, Britton JR, Tattersfield AE, Papacosta AO. What symptoms predict the bronchial response to histamine? Evaluation in a community survey of the bronchial symptoms questionnaire (1984) of the International Union Against Tuberculosis and Lung Disease. *Int J Epidemiol* 1989; 18 (1): 165–73.

19. Toren K, Brisman J, Jarvholm B. Asthma and asthma-like symptoms in adults assessed by questionnaires. A literature review. *Chest* 1993; 104 (2): 600–8.

20. Shaw RA, Crane J, Pearce N *et al.* Comparison of a video questionnaire with the IUATLD written questionnaire for measuring asthma prevalence. *Clin Exp Allergy* 1992; 22 (5): 561–8.

21. Venables KM, Farrer N, Sharp L, Graneek BJ, Newman Taylor AJ. Respiratory symptoms questionnaire for asthma epidemiology: validity and reproducibility. *Thorax* 1993; 48 (3): 214–9.

22. Bai J, Peat JK, Berry G, Marks GB, Woolcock AJ. Questionnaire items that predict asthma and other respiratory conditions in adults. *Chest* 1998; 114 (5): 1343–8.

23. Gibson PG, Wong BJ, Hepperle MJ *et al.* A research method to induce and examine a mild exacerbation of asthma by withdrawal of inhaled corticosteroid. *Clin Exp Allergy* 1992; 22 (5): 525–32.

24. Chauhan AJ, Krishna MT, Frew AJ, Holgate ST. Exposure to nitrogen dioxide (NO_2) and respiratory disease risk. *Rev Environ Health* 1998; 13 (1–2): 73–90.

25. Garrett MH, Hooper MA, Hooper BM, Abramson MJ. Respiratory symptoms in children and indoor exposure to nitrogen dioxide and gas stoves. *Am J Respir Crit Care Med* 1998; 158 (3): 891–5.

26. Jarvis D, Chinn S, Luczynska C, Burney P. Association of respiratory symptoms and lung function in young adults with use of domestic gas appliances. *Lancet* 1996; 347 (8999): 426–31.

27. Shim CS, Williams MH Jr. Relationship of wheezing to the severity of obstruction in asthma. *Arch Intern Med* 1983; 143 (5): 890–2.

28. McFadden ER Jr, Kiser R, DeGroot WJ. Acute bronchial asthma. Relations between clinical and physiologic manifestations. *N Engl J Med* 1973; 288 (5): 221–5.

29. Rebuck AS, Read J. Assessment and management of severe asthma. *Am J Med* 1971; 51 (6): 788–98.

30. Lung function testing: selection of reference values and interpretative strategies. American Thoracic Society. *Am Rev Respir Dis* 1991; 144 (5): 1202–18.

31. Guidelines for the evaluation of impairment/disability in patients with asthma. American Thoracic Society. Medical Section of the American Lung Association. *Am Rev Respir Dis* 1993; 147 (4): 1056–61.

32. Busse WW. The role of the common cold in asthma. *J Clin Pharmacol* 1999; 39 (3): 241–5.

33. Britton J. Symptoms and objective measures to define the asthma phenotype. *Clin Exp Allergy* 1998; 1: 2–7.

34. Britton J, Lewis S. Objective measures and the diagnosis of asthma. We need a simple diagnostic test – but don't yet have one [editorial]. *BMJ* 1998; 317 (7153): 227–8.

35. Sawyer G, Miles J, Lewis S, Fitzharris P, Pearce N, Beasley R. Classification of asthma severity: should the international guidelines be changed? *Clin Exp Allergy* 1998; 28 (12): 1565–70.

36. Reddel HK, Ware SI, Salome CM, Marks GB, Jenkins CR, Woolcock AJ. Standardization of ambulatory peak flow monitoring: the importance of recent β_2-agonist inhalation. *Eur Respir J* 1998; 12 (2): 309–14.

37. Reddel H, Ware S, Marks G, Salome C, Jenkins C, Woolcock A. Differences between asthma exacerbations and poor asthma control [published erratum appears in *Lancet* 1999 Feb 27; 353 (9154): 758]. *Lancet* 1999; 353 (9150): 364–9.

38. Miller MR, Pedersen OF, Quanjer PH. The rise and dwell time for peak expiratory flow in patients with and without airflow limitation. *Am J Respir Crit Care Med* 1998; 158 (1): 23–7.

39. Quackenboss JJ, Lebowitz MD, Krzyzanowski M. The normal range of diurnal changes in peak expiratory flow rates. Relationship to symptoms and respiratory disease. *Am Rev Respir Dis* 1991; 143 (2): 323–30.

40. Puolijoki H, Impivaara O, Liippo K, Tala E. Later development of asthma in patients with a negative methacholine inhalation challenge examined for suspected asthma. *Lung* 1992; 170 (4): 235–41.

41. Zhong NS, Chen RC, Yang MO, Wu ZY, Zheng JP, Li YF. Is asymptomatic bronchial hyperresponsiveness an indication of potential asthma? A two-year follow-up of young students with bronchial hyperresponsiveness. *Chest* 1992; 102 (4): 1104–9.

42. Sont JK, Willems LN, Bel EH, van Krieken JH, Vandenbroucke JP, Sterk PJ. Clinical control and histopathologic outcome of asthma when using airway hyperresponsiveness as an additional guide to long-term treatment. The AMPUL Study Group. *Am J Respir Crit Care Med* 1999; 159 (4 Pt 1): 1043–51.

43. Chanez P, Vignola AM, O'Shaugnessy T *et al.* Corticosteroid reversibility in COPD is related to features of asthma. *Am J Respir Crit Care Med* 1997; 155 (5): 1529–34.

44. Callahan CM, Dittus RS, Katz BP. Oral corticosteroid therapy for patients with stable chronic obstructive pulmonary disease. A meta-analysis. *Ann Intern Med* 1991; 114 (3): 216–23.

45. van Grunsven PM, van Schayck CP, Derenne JP *et al.* Long term effects of inhaled corticosteroids in chronic obstructive pulmonary disease: a meta-analysis. *Thorax* 1999; 54 (1): 7–14.

46. Kerstjens HA, Brand PL, Hughes MD *et al.* A comparison of bronchodilator therapy with or without inhaled corticosteroid therapy for obstructive airways disease. Dutch Chronic Non-Specific Lung Disease Study Group. *N Engl J Med* 1992; 327 (20): 1413–9.

47. Pauwels RA, Lofdahl CG, Postma DS *et al.* Effect of inhaled formoterol and budesonide on exacerbations of asthma. Formoterol and Corticosteroids Establishing Therapy (FACET) International Study Group. [Published erratum appears in *N Engl J Med* 1998 Jan 8; 338(2): 139]. *N Engl J Med* 1997; 337 (20): 1405–11.

48. Bessot JC, de Blay F, Pauli G. From allergen sources to reduction of allergen exposure. *Eur Respir J* 1994; 7 (2): 392–7.

49. The use of standardized allergen extracts. American Academy of Allergy, Asthma and Immunology (AAAAI). *J Allergy Clin Immunol* 1997; 99 (5): 583–6.

50. Klink M, Cline MG, Halonen M, Burrows B. Problems in defining normal limits for serum IgE. *J Allergy Clin Immunol* 1990; 85 (2): 440–4.

51. Homburger HA, Mauer K, Sachs MI, O'Connell EJ, Jacob GL, Caron J. Serum IgG_4 concentrations and allergen-specific IgG_4 antibodies compared in adults and children with asthma and nonallergic subjects. *J Allergy Clin Immunol* 1986; 77 (3): 427–34.

52. de Benedictis FM, Bush A. Rhinosinusitis and asthma: epiphenomenon or causal association? *Chest* 1999; 115 (2): 550–6.

53. Osguthorpe JD, Hadley JA. Rhinosinusitis. Current concepts in evaluation and management. *Med Clin North Am* 1999; 83 (1): 27–41, vii–viii.

54. Field SK, Sutherland LR. Does medical antireflux therapy improve asthma in asthmatics with gastroesophageal reflux?: a critical review of the literature. *Chest* 1998; 114 (1): 275–83.

55. Field SK. A critical review of the studies of the effects of simulated or real gastroesophageal reflux on pulmonary function in asthmatic adults. *Chest* 1999; 115 (3): 848–56.

56. Hargreave FE. Induced sputum for the investigation of airway inflammation: Evidence for its clinical application. *Can Respir J* 1999; 6 (2): 169–74.

57. Hargreave FE. Induced sputum and response to glucocorticoids. *J Allergy Clin Immunol* 1998; 102 (5): S102–5.

58. Jatakanon A, Lim S, Chung KF, Barnes PJ. An inhaled steroid improves markers of airway inflammation in patients with mild asthma. *Eur Respir J* 1998; 12 (5): 1084–8.

59. Maestrelli P, Saetta M, Di Stefano A *et al*. Comparison of leukocyte counts in sputum, bronchial biopsies, and bronchoalveolar lavage. *Am J Respir Crit Care Med* 1995; 152 (6 Pt 1): 1926–31.

60. Keatings VM, Evans DJ, O'Connor BJ, Barnes PJ. Cellular profiles in asthmatic airways: a comparison of induced sputum, bronchial washings, and bronchoalveolar lavage fluid. *Thorax* 1997; 52 (4): 372–4.

61. Grootendorst DC, Sont JK, Willems LN *et al*. Comparison of inflammatory cell counts in asthma: induced sputum vs bronchoalveolar lavage and bronchial biopsies. *Clin Exp Allergy* 1997; 27 (7): 769–79.

62. Bousquet J, Chanez P, Lacoste JY *et al*. Eosinophilic inflammation in asthma. *N Engl J Med* 1990; 323 (15): 1033–9.

63. Ulrik CS. Peripheral eosinophil counts as a marker of disease activity in intrinsic and extrinsic asthma. *Clin Exp Allergy* 1995; 25 (9): 820–7.

64. Niimi A, Amitani R, Suzuki K, Tanaka E, Murayama T, Kuze F. Serum eosinophil cationic protein as a marker of eosinophilic inflammation in asthma. *Clin Exp Allergy* 1998; 28 (2): 233–40.

65. Bacci E, Cianchetti S, Ruocco L *et al*. Comparison between eosinophilic markers in induced sputum and blood in asthmatic patients *Clin Exp Allergy* 1998; 28 (10): 1237–43.

66. Grootendorst DC, van den Bos JW, Romeijn JJ *et al*. Induced sputum in adolescents with severe stable asthma. Safety and the relationship of cell counts and eosinophil cationic protein to clinical severity. *Eur Respir J* 1999; 13 (3): 647–53.

67. Grebski E, Wu J, Wuthrich B, Medici TC. Does eosinophil cationic protein in sputum and blood reflect bronchial inflammation and obstruction in allergic asthmatics?. *J Invest Allergol Clin Immunol* 1999; 9 (2): 82–8.

68. Dahlen SE, Kumlin M. Can asthma be studied in the urine? *Clin Exp Allergy* 1998; 28 (2): 129–33.

69. Bellia V, Bonanno A, Cibella F *et al*. Urinary leukotriene E4 in the assessment of nocturnal asthma. *J Allergy Clin Immunol* 1996; 97 (3): 735–41.

70. Jeffery PK. Structural and inflammatory changes in COPD: a comparison with asthma. *Thorax* 1998; 53 (2): 129–36.

71. Kharitonov SA, Yates D, Robbins RA, Logan-Sinclair R, Shinebourne EA, Barnes PJ. Increased nitric oxide in exhaled air of asthmatic patients. *Lancet* 1994; 343 (8890): 133–5.

72. Massaro AF, Gaston B, Kita D, Fanta C, Stamler JS, Drazen JM. Expired nitric oxide levels during treatment of acute asthma. *Am J Respir Crit Care Med* 1995; 152 (2): 800–3.

73. Jatakanon A, Lim S, Kharitonov SA, Chung KF, Barnes PJ. Correlation between exhaled nitric oxide, sputum eosinophils, and methacholine responsiveness in patients with mild asthma. *Thorax* 1998; 53 (2): 91–5.

74. Gustafsson LE. Exhaled nitric oxide as a marker in asthma. *Eur Respir J* (suppl.) 1998; 26: 49S–52S.

75. Chatkin JM, Ansarin K, Silkoff PE, McClean P, Gutierrez C, Zamel N, Chapman KR. Exhaled nitric oxide as a noninvasive assessment of chronic cough. *Am J Respir Crit Care Med* 1999; 159(6): 1810–3.

76. Weiner DJ, Weatherly RA, DiPietro MA, Sanders GM. Tracheal schwannoma presenting as status asthmaticus in a sixteen-year-old boy: airway considerations and removal with the CO_2 laser. *Pediatr Pulmonol* 1998; 25 (6): 393–7.

77. Wolfe JM, Meth BM. Vocal cord dysfunction mimicking a severe asthma attack. *J Emerg Med* 1999; 17 (1): 39–41.

78. Landwehr LP, Wood RP 2nd, Blager FB, Milgrom H. Vocal cord dysfunction mimicking exercise-induced

bronchospasm in adolescents. *Pediatrics* 1996; 98 (5): 971–4.

79. Bucca C, Rolla G, Brussino L, De Rose V, Bugiani M. Are asthma-like symptoms due to bronchial or extrathoracic airway dysfunction? *Lancet* 1995; 346 (8978): 791–5.

80. King GG, Muller NL, Pare PD. Evaluation of airways in obstructive pulmonary disease using high-resolution computed tomography. *Am J Respir Crit Care Med* 1999; 159 (3): 992–1004.

81. Cotton DJ, Soparkar GR, Grahan BL. Diffusing capacity in the clinical assessment of chronic airflow limitation. *Med Clin North Am* 1996; 80 (3): 549–64.

82. Gibson PG. Use of induced sputum to examine airway inflammation in childhood asthma. *J Allergy Clin Immunol* 1998; 102 (5): S100–1.

83. Corradi M, Majori M, Cacciani GC, Consigli GF, de'Munari E, Pesci A. Increased exhaled nitric oxide in patients with stable chronic obstructive pulmonary disease. *Thorax* 1999; 54 (7): 572–5.

84. Maziak W, Loukides S, Culpitt S, Sullivan P, Kharitonov SA, Barnes PJ. Exhaled nitric oxide in chronic obstructive pulmonary disease. *Am J Respir Crit Care Med* 1998; 157 (3 Pt 1): 998–1002.

85. Rutgers SR, van der Mark TW, Coers W *et al.* Markers of nitric oxide metabolism in sputum and exhaled air are not increased in chronic obstructive pulmonary disease. *Thorax* 1999; 54(7): 576–80.

86. Sterk PJ, De Gouw HW, Ricciardolo FL, Rabe KF. Exhaled nitric oxide in COPD: glancing through a smoke screen. *Thorax* 1999; 54 (7): 565–7.

87. Fabbri L, Beghe B, Caramori G, Papi A, Saetta M. Similarities and discrepancies between exacerbations of asthma and chronic obstructive pulmonary disease. *Thorax* 1998; 53 (9): 803–8.

88. Jack CI, Lye M. Asthma in the elderly patient. *Gerontology* 1996; 42 (2): 61–8.

89. Ciaccia A, Ferrari M, Facchini FM, Caramori G, Fabbri L. Pulmonary vasculitis: classification, clinical features, and management. *Clin Rev Allergy Immunol* 1997; 15 (1): 73–95.

90. Marlar RA, Joist JH, Fink LM. Pulmonary embolism. *N Engl J Med* 1998; 339 (21): 1556–7.

91. Delaunois L, el Khawand C. Medical thoracoscopy in the management of pneumothorax. *Monaldi Arch Chest Dis* 1998; 53 (2): 148–50.

92. Ricciardi MJ, Rubenfire M. How to manage secondary pulmonary hypertension. *Postgrad Med* 1999; 105 (2): 183–90; quiz 229.

93. Kulke MH, Mayer RJ. Carcinoid tumors. *N Engl J Med* 1999; 340 (11): 858–68.

94. Rosi E, Ronchi MC, Grazzini M, Duranti R, Scano G. Sputum analysis, bronchial hyperresponsiveness, and airway function in asthma: results of a factor analysis. *J Allergy Clin Immunol* 1999; 103 (2 Pt 1): 232–7.

95. Crane J, Pearce N, Burgess C, Woodman K, Robson B, Beasley R. Markers of risk of asthma death or readmission in the 12 months following a hospital admission for asthma. *Int J Epidemiol* 1992; 21 (4): 737–44.

96. Miller TP, Greenberger PA, Patterson R. The diagnosis of potentially fatal asthma in hospitalized adults. Patient characteristics and increased severity of asthma. *Chest* 1992; 102(2): 515–8.

97. Wagner PD, Hedenstierna G, Rodriguez-Roisin R. Gas exchange, expiratory flow obstruction and the clinical spectrum of asthma. *Eur Respir J* 1996; 9 (6): 1278–82.

Chapter 7

Pulmonary Function Tests

Kieran Killian

INTRODUCTION

Asthma is characterized by a genetic propensity which, combined with external triggering factors, leads to morphological changes in the airways. These changes result in pulmonary impairment which causes distressing symptoms that handicap the patient. The aim of this chapter is to provide an overview of pulmonary function so that some of the interactive effects of this sequence of events can be understood.

STRUCTURE AND FUNCTION

The reliable isolation of asthma from other disorders is recent. The morbid anatomy underlying most of the common diseases date their origin from Morgagni's *The Seats and Causes of Disease Investigated by Anatomy*.[1] Laenneck extended this knowledge of structure using inspection, palpation, percussion and auscultation to recognize the disorders during life.[2] Because of its subtle structural features, bronchial asthma remained an enigma. The recognition by Lavoisier that respiration and combustion were synonymous led to the broader understanding of the function of circulation, respiratory gas exchange, arterial gas concentrations (oxygen and carbon dioxide) and central respiratory control in tissue metabolism.[3] The structural changes found on morbid anatomy, the clinical features found on history and physical examination and their functional consequences could be understood within this system.

ORIGINS OF PULMONARY FUNCTION TESTING

Erasistratus and Herophilus (300 BC) were the first to recognize that contraction of the inspiratory muscles expands the thorax and generates the force required to expand the lungs. In 1844, Hutchinson[4] measured the volume of air that could be displaced between a maximal inspiration and maximal expiration (vital capacity, VC). This measurement was extended to include the pressures generated with maximal voluntary activation of the inspiratory and expiratory muscles against an occluded airway, namely, maximal inspiratory pressure (MIP) and maximal expiratory pressure (MEP). A reduced vital capacity implied a hindrance to breathing (stiff lungs or obstructed airways), a space occupying lesion in the chest (i.e. pleural effusion) and/or reduced muscle contraction and strength. Measurement of VC, MIP and MEP were not adopted by the medical community of his time. Although structure was only as important as its functional consequences, the measurement of function was neglected in favour of structural measurements.

Pulmonary Mechanics

Poiseuille applied the principles underlying fluid mechanics, introduced by the Bernouillis in the eighteenth century, to the circulation yielding his well-known equation:

$$P \, (cmH_2O) = (8 \times l \times V \times \eta) / (981 \times r^2).$$

The application of these principles to ventilation evolved in the following way.

Resistance

Rohrer[5] measured the length (l), the radius (r) of the various generations of human airways and applied Poiseuille's equation to derive resistance. He also added the pressure required to take into account the branching airways and changing cross sectional areas and referred to the additional pressure as extra resistance.

He found that the total resistance in human airways could not be defined as a single number because pressure increased in an accelerating manner relative to flow. The following relationships applied to airflow in the upper and lower airways:

$$P \,(\text{cmH}_2\text{O}) = 0.43 \times V + 0.73 \times V^2 \,(\text{upper})$$

$$P \,(\text{cmH}_2\text{O}) = 0.36 \times V + 0.09 \times V^2 \,(\text{lower}).$$

This polynomial approach to the measurement of resistance continues to be used to the present day.

Elastance

The pressure required to expand isolated mammalian lungs was measured by Carson, Donders, Heynsius and Cloetta.[6] Inspiratory pressure is required to increase lung volume from the resting end expired volume (functional residual capacity, FRC) to total lung capacity (TLC). Expiratory pressure is required to decrease lung volume from FRC to residual volume (RV). Relaxation at any volume above or below FRC against an occluded airway yields the recoil pressure of the lung and chest cage. The elastance of the total respiratory system was measured in this way by Rohrer in 1916.[7] The results are illustrated in Fig. 7.1 as it would appear today in a normal male subject (height 1.80 m and 30 years old). The difference in pressure between the total recoil pressure and the recoil pressure of the lung is the recoil pressure of the thorax. Today we know that 5 cmH$_2$O are required to half inflate the collapsed normal lung; a further 5 cmH$_2$O is required to half inflate it again from 50% to 75% TLC. The relationship is close to

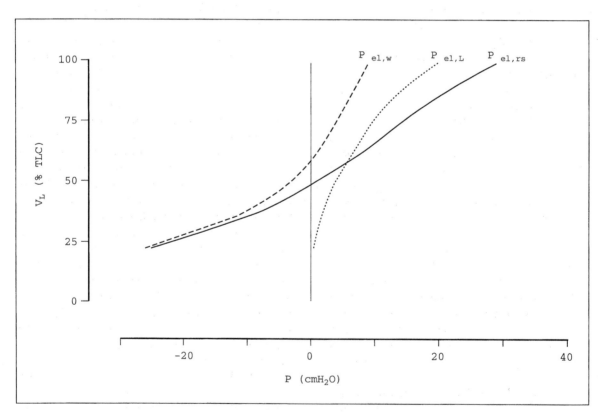

FIGURE 7.1: Lung volume expressed as a percentage of total lung capacity is plotted against pressure in cmH$_2$O. The occlusion pressure measured at the mouth following relaxation of the inspiratory muscles is positive and falls to the right of the zero line; the occlusion pressure following relaxation of the expiratory muscles is negative and falls to the left of the zero line; the solid line represents the elastic characteristics of the respiratory system. The dotted line to the right of the zero line represents the recoil pressure of the lung and is positive at all lung volumes $P_{el, L}$. The dashed line represents the recoil pressure of the chest wall where $P_{el, w} = P_{el, rs} - P_{el, L}$.

exponential with a half inflation pressure of 5 cmH$_2$O and a maximal inflation pressure of 30 cmH$_2$O.

Inertance

Inertance is the relationship between pressure and acceleration (Inertance = Pressure/Acceleration). Pressure is required to accelerate the air from a state of rest to the velocities seen during inspiration and expiration. The acceleration of air molecules is substantial but they have a very small mass and require very little pressure. The lung, chest cage and abdomen have a very large mass but are accelerated minimally and also require very little pressure. Hence, the pressure related to inertance is small and is commonly ignored.

Measurement of the Pressure Required to Drive the Total Respiratory System

Pleural pressure during breathing was first measured in the nineteenth century. The requirement for pleural access and the relative primitive state of measurement techniques precluded precise measurement. Wirz and Von Neergard used the newly invented Fleish pneumotachograph to measure airflow at the mouth and a pleural cannula to measure transpulmonary pressure in human subjects.[8,9] When the respiratory muscles are inactive, as at the end of a normal expiration, the pleural pressure (P_{pl} is equal and opposite to the recoil pressure of the lungs and equal to the recoil pressure of the chest cage: $P_{pl} = P_{alv} - P_{el\,lung} = P_{mus} + P_{el\,thorax}$. The activation of the respiratory muscles either increases or decreases the alveolar pressure. When P_{alv} drops below mouth pressure, inspiratory flow takes place. When P_{alv} exceeds mouth pressure, expiratory flow takes place. There is no airflow when the pressure at the mouth (atmospheric pressure) and the alveolar pressure are equal.

To overcome the need for the measurement of pleural pressure Wirz and Von Neergard transiently occluded the airway during airflow. The pressure at the mouth and alveolar pressure quickly equilibrated yielding the P_{alv}. P_{alv} could then be divided by the flow prior to occlusion yielding airways resistance: Resistance = P_{alv}/Flow. The pressure following airway occlusion continues to decline to a terminal pressure which approximated the elastic pressure. The pressure drop between the early and terminal pressure has since been called viscoelastic. The first mechanical studies performed on asthmatic subjects supported the long suspected idea that asthma was a disorder associated with increased resistance due to airway narrowing.

In 1949, Buytendijk showed that the change in oesophageal pressure is a reasonable estimate of the change in pleural pressure.[10] Advances in electronics and reliable transducers then allowed mechanical principles to be more widely used.

The elastance of the normal respiratory system is 12 cmH$_2$O l^{-1}. Resistance is replaced by an equation describing resistive pressure relative to flow rate. The pressures required to breathe can be measured by adding the static and dynamic pressures:

$$P\,(\text{cmH}_2\text{O}) = \text{Volume (l)} \times 12 + 1.9 \times \text{Flow(l s}^{-1}) + 0.52 \times \text{Flow}^2\,(\text{l s}^{-1}).$$

The pressures generated during breathing can be estimated in normal subjects given the measurements of tidal volumes and flow rates.

RESPIRATORY MUSCLE STRESS

The forces required for a normal inspiration are increased in the presence of cardiac and pulmonary disorders, particularly during exercise. The perception of the increased forces causes exertional dyspnoea (any discomfort experienced and associated with breathing). The intensity of dyspnoea increases with inspiratory pressure and increases, in an accelerating manner, with the stress on the inspiratory muscles. The stress on the inspiratory muscles is defined by the forces generated relative to their capacity. Stress increases with force and increases further as the capacity to generate force declines with the extent and velocity of muscle contraction, intrinsic weakness and muscle fatigue. Patients with profound respiratory muscle weakness are dyspnoeic even in the presence of normal mechanics. The oesophageal pressures from rest to maximal exercise and the capacity to generate pressure are illustrated in Fig. 7.2. The maximal pleural pressure generated is 20 cmH$_2$O while the capacity to generate pressure is 45 cmH$_2$O. The effort required to breathe intensifies with the pleural pressure relative to the maximal dynamic pressure and not the 130 cmH$_2$O that can be developed with airway occlusion at FRC. During exercise, the exertional discomfort related to the stress on the inspiratory muscles becomes intolerable before the maximal capacity to generate pressure is reached.

PULMONARY MECHANICS OF ASTHMA

During an asthmatic attack, resistance increases with bronchoconstriction. The dynamic elastance also

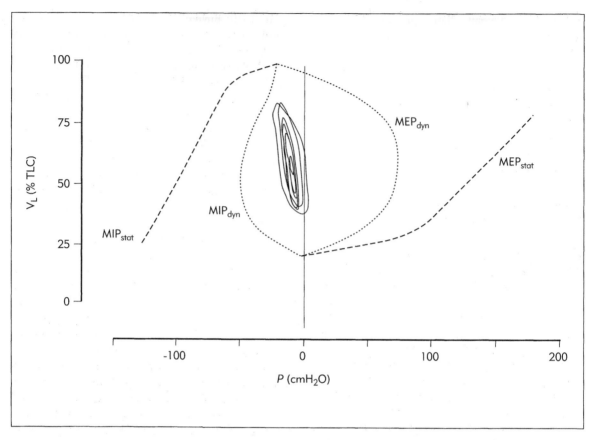

FIGURE 7.2: Lung volume expressed as a percentage of total lung capacity is plotted against pressure in cmH_2O. The pressure–volume loops represent the oesophageal pressure at rest and at increasing levels of work to maximal capacity without a mouthpiece or unidirectional valve. The maximal inspiratory and expiratory oesophageal pressures are shown when the mouth is occluded at all lung volumes (MIP_{stat} and MEP_{stat}) and during a maximal inspiratory and expiatory flow manoeuvre (MIP_{dyn} and MEP_{dyn}). Note that the pressure developed in the pleura at maximal work performance is submaximal.

increases because of the variability in the resistance across lung units ("frequency dependence of compliance"). The asthmatic is handicapped because the force requirements increase, while the capacity to generate inspiratory pressure declines, due to hyperinflation and due to increases in the velocity of inspiratory muscle contraction to compensate for the prolongation of expiration. The contribution due to the increase in force requirements is approximately equal to the decrease in force generating capacity.

DYSPNOEA AND ASTHMA

Normal people can detect very modest increases in resistance (20% of the baseline resistance or $0.6\ cmH_2O\ l^{-1}s^{-1}$).

The "sense of inappropriateness" may be appreciated prior to any detectable reduction in flow rates. Dyspnoea becomes "just noticeable" as resistance and dynamic elastance increase. Dyspnoea intensifies substantially as the magnitude of inspiratory pressure and hyperinflation increases. The intensity of dyspnoea following incrementally increasing bronchoconstriction is illustrated in Fig. 7.3.

PULMONARY FUNCTION TESTING

Mechanical measurement has not been broadly adopted by the medical community. The general principles underlying the commonly used pulmonary function tests date from the 1940s. Cournand and Richards formalized the measurement of cardiorespiratory function aimed at clinical utility.[11-13] They divided function into:

(1) ventilatory function concerned with the mechanical movement of air in and out of the lungs with its characteristic symptom being dyspnoea;
(2) respiratory function concerned with gas exchange with its characteristic sign being hypoxaemia;
(3) cardiocirculatory function with its characteristic sign being congestive failure.

Ventilatory Insufficiency

Maximal breathing capacity (MBC) can be measured by having the patient breathe with maximal respiratory effort for 12–15 seconds (also known as maximal voluntary ventilation). The breathing reserve (BR) was derived by subtracting the ventilation from the maximal voluntary ventilation (MBC). This was then expressed as a percentage of MBC (BR/MBC%). Dyspnoea was unexpected with a BR/MBC% greater than 90%; dyspnoea became more prevalent and intense as the BR/MBC% decreased. These measurements were simple, logical and achieved a broad conceptual appeal. In reality ventilation relative to capacity is essentially similar to force relative to capacity and also represents the stress on the respiratory muscles. Ventilation relative to capacity was easier to understand and continues to be conceptually used as an index of dyspnoea.

The measurement of airflow centred on the MBC. During the measurement, the spirometer trace was noted to drift with a loss in spirometer volume as more air was trapped in the lungs in patients with airflow limitation; the spirometer trace remained unchanged with restrictive disorders. At that time, the measurement of airflow obstruction centred on the reduced MBC, the inspiratory drift during the MBC manoeuvre, high RV/TLC ratio with a high residual nitrogen. The nitrogen washout technique was used to measure lung volume. Nitrogen was rapidly cleared breathing 100% oxygen in normal lungs. Nitrogen fractional concentration greater than 2.5% at the end of 7 minutes was considered as evidence of slow mixing.

Respiratory Insufficiency

Respiratory insufficiency was concerned with the measurement of disturbance in gas exchange. Low V/Q, impaired diffusion, and shunt contributed to the central cyanosis which was the cardinal feature.

Cardiocirculatory Insufficiency

Central venous pressure (CVP) was considered less than $10 \, cmH_2O$ with a normal heart. An increase in CVP with the demonstration of oedema indicated the presence of heart failure. Borderline failure was sought if failure suspected. A decrease in the vital capacity of >8% and a CVP >$10 \, cmH_2O$ following the infusion of 1500 ml of saline (Caughey challenge) was taken as evidence of borderline pulmonary congestion. Calcium gluconate could be injected in the antecubital vein and the time to first taste measured. The circulation time, used as an index of cardiac output, was normally <18 seconds.

TIME BASED SPIROMETRY

In the 1940s Tiffeneau and Beauvallet[14] noted that asthmatics developed bronchoconstriction following the inhalation of acetylcholine and got relief from dyspnoea following the inhalation of epinephrine. Tiffeneau introduced the forced expired volume whereby volume was now assessed relative to the expired time yielding the $FEV_{0.5}$, FEV_1, FEV_2. He also introduced the expression of FEV_1/VC which became known as the Tiffeneau index. The VC, FEV_1 and FEV_1/VC ratio emerged as the standard measurements.

A workable relationship between the FEV_1 and the MBC was intuitively appealing because the FEV_1 is a flow rate and inspiratory flow rates are generally well preserved relative to expiratory flow rates. $FEV_1 \times 35$ was broadly adopted as an approximation of the MBC. Hence, the FEV_1 expressed as a percentage of predicted gave an index of ventilatory capacity relative to normal. The FEV_1 went on to virtually replace the measurement of MBC.

CHRONIC BRONCHITIS, EMPHYSEMA AND ASTHMA

The problem of chronic bronchitis, emphysema and asthma became much more prominent following the successful treatment of pneumococcal pneumonia and tuberculosis. Structural measurement of emphysema using chest radiography proved unreliable. The functional consequences of emphysema and obstructive bronchitis proved easier to measure than its structural features. Functional measurements were broadly appreciated because the contribution of airflow limitation to disability and handicap was quickly recognized.

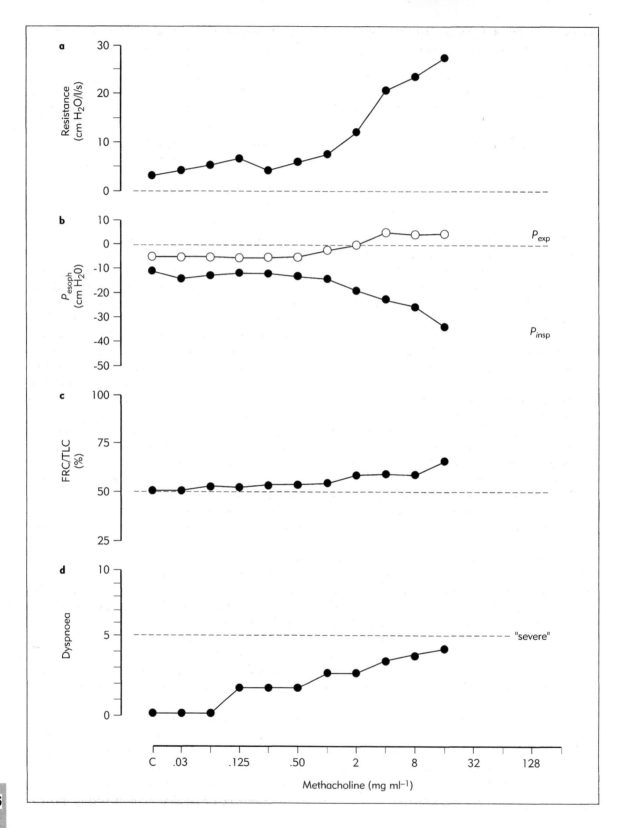

FIGURE 7.3: (a) Measurement of inspiratory resistance, (b) peak oesophageal pressure, (c) functional residual capacity (end-expiratory lung volume), expressed as a percentage of TLC, following incrementally induced bronchoconstriction in an asthmatic subject. The intensity of dyspnoea experienced is shown in (d) where 5 is "severe", 4 is "somewhat severe", 3 is "moderate", 2 is "slight", 1 is "very slight" and 0.5 is "just noticeable".

Chronic obstructive pulmonary disease replaced the terms chronic obstructive bronchitis and emphysema. Confusion between the structure function relationships continues to the present day in the discrimination between asthma, small airways disease and emphysema.

Flow Volume Relationships

Exploration of the mechanisms of airflow limitation in the early 1960s showed that the lung behaved like a Starling resistor with expiratory resistance increasing as expiratory effort increased. The measurement of resistance lost its utility and was replaced by the measurements of flow with increased sensitivity. Measurement of flow relative to volume showed that expiratory flow rates were volume dependent. Maximal expiratory flow rates were achieved with submaximal effort except close to TLC where maximal flow rate was effort dependent. Peak flow rates increase with effort because the equal pressure point is outside the thorax close to TLC. Inspiratory flow rates were effort dependent. The flow volume envelope contained all the information required to estimate the maximal mechanical breathing capacity. The maximal rate at which a given tidal volume could be inspired and expired could be simply calculated by placing the tidal volume within the flow volume envelope. During maximal exercise, the tidal volume normally lies between 50 and 60% of the vital capacity in health and in the presence of pulmonary disease. The maximal rate at which this volume can be expired (T_e) can be approximated by $0.5 \times VC/FEV_1$; the maximal rate at which it can be inspired (T_i) can be approximated by $0.5 \times VC/V_{insp\,max}$. More precise measurements using the range of flow rates seen in the complete flow volume envelope are possible but are laborious and add little to clinical utility. Merely multiplying the $FEV_1 \times 40$ approximates the maximal breathing capacity calculated in this way indicating the rugged reliability of the FEV_1 and its vast clinical acceptance.

In detecting early airflow obstruction, frequency dependence of compliance, maximal mid expiratory flow rates, flow rates at 25, 50% of the vital capacity and airway closure provided sensitive tests. Although useful in detecting airflow limitation early in the course of obstructive diseases, their clinical value is modest.

Peak Flow Rates

Variability in peak flow rates is useful in the detection of variable airflow limitation and the clinical recognition of asthma. Peak flow rates have become very popular in the management of asthma because of the simplicity of the equipment, the ease of measurement and the ability to measure flow rates at home and in the work place. However practical, peak flow rates are not particularly sensitive. As bronchoconstriction increases, peak flow rates are initially maintained while flow rates at lower lung volumes decline. Peak flow rates are dependent on expiratory muscle strength and effort. Hence, they vary within and across subjects. Peak flow rates do not allow an estimate of ventilatory capacity in the same manner as the FEV_1. The measurement of FEV_1 is not as effort dependent as peak flow rates. A submaximal effort is sufficient to generate the FEV_1. Increasing effort causes dynamic compression of airways without increasing flow. Variability in the FEV_1 will only occur with incomplete inspiration or incomplete expiration which is easy to detect because the vital capacity will not be reproduced.

DLCO

Measurement of the uptake of carbon monoxide from the lung, was introduced by the Kroghs to dispel the theory of active transport of oxygen across the alveolar capillary membrane. This measurement has become widely available with improvement in technology. In asthma, the DLCO is generally well preserved but it may be reduced if the inspired gas fails to get to the alveolar capillary membrane. Reductions in diffusion capacity are to be expected in the presence of alveolar destruction due to emphysema or with alveolar disorders such as alveolitis. In the presence of airflow obstruction, reductions in the DLCO are more in keeping with emphysema and alveolar destruction than asthma. No hard and fast rules can be applied because chronic airflow obstruction can also result from airway obstruction in the small airways without advanced alveolar destruction with a relatively well-preserved DLCO. The gas exchange properties of the alveoli seen by the inspired gas can be measured by dividing the DLCO by the alveolar volume measured using an inert gas. This is known as the KCO and a reduced KCO is suggestive of emphysema in the absence of anaemia, high carboxyhaemoglobin levels due to smoking and alveolar disorders.

SUMMARY

If a clinically important question can be answered by a pulmonary function test in an asthmatic patient then it is reasonable to do the test provided that the measurement can be made in a cost effective manner. Asthmatic patients experience symptoms which arise due to impaired pulmonary function. The role of spirometry and peak flow rates in the diagnosis and follow-up of asthmatic patients is well established and requires little further comment. Methacholine and specific allergen challenge tests are acquiring a much broader role. The rating of symptoms during these challenges is particularly useful to calibrate symptom responses in individual patients.

KEY POINTS

1 The ventilatory capacity is proportional to the measured FEV_1.

2 If the FEV_1/VC ratio is > 70%, the mechanism is non-obstructive. If the ratio is <70% the mechanism is obstructive. However, the ratio may increase as airways narrow and actually close. Combined disorders are common.

3 Disability and handicap increase as pulmonary impairment increases.

4 While symptoms are usually sensitive, asthmatics may have severe impairment without symptoms. Repeated and persistent bronchoconstriction leads to adaptation. About 10–15% of asthmatics have poor perception of bronchoconstriction.

5 Asthmatics may become sufficiently inactive to cause muscle weakness and fatigue. A standardized incremental exercise test may be useful in defining the asthmatic patient's capacity to exercise.

6 The absence of airway hyperresponsiveness virtually excludes the presence of asthma. In the presence of normal spirometry a methacholine PC_{20} <8 mg ml^{-1} generally indicates the presence of asthma. However, airway responsiveness may be increased in the presence of any pulmonary impairment. Airway responsiveness in the presence of pulmonary impairment does not necessarily indicate the presence of asthma.

REFERENCES

1. Morgagni JB. *The Seats and Causes of Disease Investigated by Anatomy*. New York: Hafner Publishing, 1769.

2. Laennec R. *A Treatise on the Diseases of the Chest*. (1781–1826). London: Hafner Publishing, 1962; 284–6.

3. Lavoisier AL. Reflexions sur le phlogistique, pour servir de suite a la theorie de la combustion et de la calcination. (Issued with *Hist Acad Roy Sci Paris*, 1777). *Oeuvres de Lavoisier* 1862; 2: 623–55.

4. Hutchinson J. Lecture on vital statistics, embracing an account of a new instrument for detecting the presence of disease in the system. *Lancet* 1844; i: 567–70.

5. Rohrer F. Flow resistance in the human air passages and the effect of irregular branching of the bronchial system on the respiratory process in various regions of the lungs. *Pflüger's Arch Ges Physiol* 1915; 162: 225–99.

6. Wirz K. Changes in the pleural pressure during respiration, and causes of its variability. (Das Verhalten des Druckes in Pleuraraum bei der Atmung und die Ursachen seiner Veranderlichkeit). *Pfluger's Arch Ges Physiol* 1923; 199: 1–56. Reprinted in: West JB (ed). *Translations in Respiratory Physiology*. Stroudsburg, Pennsylvania: Dowden, Hutchinson & Ross, 1975; 174–226.

7. Rohrer F. The correlation of respiratory forces and their dependence upon the state of expansion of the respiratory organs. (Der Zusammenhang der Atemkrafte und ihre Abhangigkeit vom Dehnungszustand der Atmungsorgane). *Pfluger's Arch Ges Physiol* 1916; 165: 419–44. Reprinted in: West JB (ed). *Translations in Respiratory Physiology*. Stroudsburg, Pennsylvania: Dowden, Hutchinson & Ross, 1975; 67–88.

8. Von Neergaard K, Wirz K. Method for measuring lung elasticity in living human subjects, especially in emphysema. (Uber eine Methode zur Messung der Lungenelastizitat am lebenden Menschen, insbesondere beim Emphysem). *Zeitschrift fur klinische Medizin* 1927; 105: 35–50. Reprinted in: West JB (ed). *Translations in Respiratory Physiology*. Stroudsburg, Pennsylvania: Dowden, Hutchinson & Ross, 1975; 227–69.

9. Von Neergaard K, Wirz K. A method for measuring pulmonary elasticity in living man, especially in emphysema. *Z Klin Med* 1927; 105: 43.

10. Buytendijk HJ. Oesophagusdruck en Longelasticiteit. Dissertatie, Univ. Groningen, Netherlands, 1949.

11. Cournand A, Richards DW. Pulmonary insufficiency. I. Discussion of a physiological classification and presentation of clinical tests. *Am Rev Tuberc* 1941; 44: 26–41.

12. Cournand A, Richards DW. Pulmonary insufficiency. II. The effects of various types of collapse therapy upon cardiopulmonary function. *Am Rev Tuberc* 1941; 44: 123–72.

13. Cournand A, Richards DW, Maier HC. Pulmonary insufficiency. III. Cases demonstrating advanced cardiopulmonary insufficiency following artificial pneumothorax and thoracoplasty. *Am Rev Tuberc* 1941; 44: 272–87.

14. Tiffeneau R, Beauvallet M. A synopsis of bronchoconstriction and bronchodilatation test using aerosols: detection, measurement and control in chronic respiratory insufficiency. *Bull Acad Nat Med* 1945; 129: 165–8.

Chapter 8

Provocation Tests

Donald Cockcroft

INTRODUCTION

Bronchoprovocation tests[1–18] have provided great insight into the pathophysiology and pharmacology of asthma.[19–20] Bronchoconstrictor stimuli can be either non-selective (affecting all asthmatics) or selective (affecting only certain asthmatics) (Table 8.1). Selective stimuli can be either sensitizers (allergens and chemical sensitizers) or non-sensitizers [acetylsalicylic acid (ASA), non-steroidal anti-inflammatory drugs (NSAIDs), additives, etc]. Histamine and methacholine (direct-acting, non-selective stimuli) inhalation tests are widely used as a diagnostic aid in asthma. The clinical role of provocation with indirect non-selective stimuli is currently uncertain. Bronchoprovocation with selective stimuli, e.g. chemical sensitizers, ASA, and additives, can occasionally be of value in pinpointing aetiologic agents. Although some controversy still exists, allergen inhalations are primarily a research tool.

NON-SELECTIVE STIMULI

Non-selective stimuli may be either chemical (natural or synthetic) or physical (Table 8.1). An alternate possibly more clinically relevant classification is direct and indirect.[21] Direct stimuli act primarily on specific smooth muscle receptors to cause bronchoconstriction; histamine, cholinergic agonists, and some other naturally-occurring mediators are examples. Indirect stimuli act through intermediate (e.g. neurological reflexes, mediator release etc.) and often incompletely understood pathways to provoke bronchoconstriction; the physical stimuli, AMP, and probably β-adrenergic blockers are examples.[21] Naturally-occurring bronchoconstriction in asthma occurs through "indirect" pathways. Therefore, it is possible that responses to indirect stimuli might be

more specific for asthma and have more clinical relevance.[21] There are some data to support this, particularly in differentiating asthma from chronic airflow limitation.[22,23] This remains an incompletely studied area. Most clinical studies have used the direct stimuli, histamine and methacholine.

Histamine and Methacholine Inhalation Tests

Methods Histamine and methacholine inhalation tests, introduced as early as the 1940s,[24,25] are now widely used for measurement of "non-allergic airway responsiveness" or simply airway responsiveness.[20] Several methods are widely used, including timed tidal breathing from a continuous output nebulizer,[1,2] and counted inspiratory capacity breaths from either a handheld squeeze-bulb nebulizer,[3] or a breath-activated dosimeter.[4] Results are comparable when tests are appropriately standardized. Technical factors requiring regulation are nebulizer type, output, flow rate, particle size etc. Non-technical (subject) factors must also be controlled; these include medications, both non-selective functional antagonists (e.g. bronchodilators) and specific antagonists (e.g. H_1 blockers and anticholinergics), recent respiratory infection, recent allergen exposure and airway calibre. Diluent is inhaled initially, followed by increasing, usually doubling, amounts of the agent, at 1- to 5-minute intervals. Expiratory flow, generally forced expiratory volume in 1 s (FEV_1), is measured initially and from 0.5 to 3 minutes following each inhalation. Tests are continued until the top dose is administered or until the FEV_1 has fallen by $\geq$ 20%. Results are expressed from either the cumulative or non-cumulative log dose–response curve as the provocation concentration or dose required to produce a 20% FEV_1 fall, the PC_{20} (mg ml^{-1}) or PD_{20} (μmol). Other information from the dose–response curve, including the slope,[26] and the plateau,[27] are infrequently

Table 8.1: Stimuli used for provocation tests

Non-selective	Selective
Chemical	*Sensitizers*
Autonomic nervous system	Allergens (inhaled)
Cholinergic agonists	Low molecular weight chemicals
β-Adrenergic antagonists	Foods
α-Adrenergic agonists	
Nicotinic (ganglionic) agonists	*Non-sensitizers*
Amines	ASA/NSAIDs
Histamine	Sulphite/metabisulphite
5 HT, etc.	Other food additives
Lipid metabolites	Foods
$PGF_{2\alpha}$	
Leukotrienes	
PAF	
Peptides	
Bradykinin	
Tachykinins	
AMP, adenosine	
Non-mediator	
SO_2	
KCl, etc.	
Physical	
Exercise/cold air/hyperventilation	
Non-isotonic aerosols	
Hypertonic dry powder (e.g. mannitol)	
"Inert" dusts	

AMP: adenosine monophosphate; ASA: acetylsalicylic acid; 5-HT: 5-hydroxytryptamine; NSAIDs: non-steroidal anti-inflammatory drugs; PAF: platelet activating factor; $PGF_{2\alpha}$: Prostaglandin $F_{2\alpha}$

used clinically, but may be useful in epidemiologic studies; future studies may identify important clinical correlates of these additional features.

Interpretation A number of features noted below are important when interpreting tests of airway responsiveness. Many of these have been recognized recently and are not always appreciated.

UNIMODAL DISTRIBUTION Values of PC_{20} are continuously[28] distributed in a random population probably in a log-normal fashion.[29]

IMPRECISION Histamine and methacholine tests, even with the best of standardization, are not very precise. Tests are repeatable to within ± 1 to 1.6 doubling dilutions.[30,31] This is primarily a measurement imprecision rather than true variability in airway responsiveness.

CUTPOINT Cutpoints used to define airway hyperresponsiveness are arbitrary, and generally selected to have a high sensitivity (i.e. identifying virtually all asthmatics). In a random population, a highly sensitive cutpoint has a fair specificity, but positive predictive value for current asthma symptoms is <50%.[32] Positive tests in subjects denying symptoms occur for several reasons, including failure to encounter natural stimuli potent enough to provoke bronchoconstriction, failure to recognize bronchoconstriction as abnormal, failure to perceive bronchoconstriction, and true false-positive tests.

BORDERLINE AREA Because of the measurement imprecision, and the continuous distribution, there is a "grey zone" of borderline values of PC_{20}; the range is about two doubling concentrations.[33]

VARIABILITY Airway hyperresponsiveness is variable over time and often absent in asthmatics not exposed to a relevant sensitizer.[1,32,34] Therefore, interpretation of these tests *vis-à-vis* a diagnosis of asthma requires the test be done when symptoms/exposures are current i.e. within the past several days.

AIRWAY CALIBRE Subjects with non-asthmatic chronic airflow limitation demonstrate histamine or methacholine airway hyperresponsiveness which is highly correlated to the degree of airflow obstruction.[22,23,35–37] Thus, it is difficult if not impossible to interpret histamine and methacholine tests unless the baseline expiratory flow rates are normal.

SENSITIZERS Subject with normal airway responsiveness can develop bronchoconstriction on exposure to either a chemical sensitizer[38,39] or an allergen[40,41] to which they are highly sensitized, either under natural conditions[38,40] or in the laboratory.[39,41] Therefore, a negative histamine or methacholine inhalation test does not completely exclude naturally-occurring asthma due to high-dose exposure to a sensitizer, especially in highly sensitized individuals.

Clinical Value

DIAGNOSIS Histamine and methacholine inhalation tests are widely recommended as a diagnostic test for asthma. In the absence of variable airflow obstruction, there is no "gold standard" to validate the diagnosis. Therefore, it is impossible to critically assess the diagnostic performance of these tests. Since there is a low positive predictive value for asthma-like symptoms in a random population, the presence of both airway hyperresponsiveness and symptoms cannot prove cause and effect. However, a positive challenge does provide a rationale for a trial of treatment. The high sensitivity and negative predictive value indicate that these tests are particularly useful in ruling out current asthma, keeping in mind the interpretive caveats noted above.

COUGH-VARIANT ASTHMA Asthma presenting with cough alone and normal lung function is common.[42] Some have relied heavily on a positive methacholine challenge to make this diagnosis.[43] Corticosteroid-responsive cough-variant asthma (or the equivalent) can exist, however, without airway hyperresponsiveness.[44] Therefore, a trial of inhaled corticosteroids might be the preferred diagnostic test, regardless of the results of methacholine challenges.[45]

OCCUPATIONAL ASTHMA Measurements of airway responsiveness have several uses in occupational asthma. Firstly, in this condition, it is particularly important to objectively confirm variable airflow obstruction. Secondly, serial measurements of PC_{20} can be used to infer presence to a sensitizer.[46] Thirdly, the tests can be useful in follow-up to assess adequacy of environmental control, and as an objective guide to determining impairment and disability.

ASTHMA SEVERITY In populations, the degree of airway hyperresponsiveness correlates strongly with asthma severity.[1,47,48] However, the scatter in the data precludes relying on this in an individual as an independent measure of severity.

MONITORING TREATMENT Improvement in airway responsiveness can be used to monitor treatment with anti-inflammatory therapies.[49,50] It is not clear that this has any advantages over routine clinical assessment and thus, this is currently a research tool. If it can be shown that treating airway hyperresponsiveness (rather than symptoms) improves outcome, monitoring of airway (hyper-) responsiveness may become a useful clinical tool.

Other Mediators

Inhalation tests with other mediators, serotonin, bradykinin, leukotrienes, prostaglandins, β-blockers, α-agonists, AMP, tachykinins etc, performed with similar methods, are currently research procedures.

Exercise, Cold Air, Hyperventilation

Background Exercise, cold air, hyperventilation and combinations thereof are probably the most potent common natural non-selective bronchoconstrictor stimuli. The precise mechanism(s) whereby large volumes of inspired cool dry air provoke airway narrowing is still a matter of debate.[51,52] These agents are non-selective indirect stimuli for measuring airway responsiveness. Asthmatics with mild airway hyper-responsiveness may develop symptoms only after exercise; the misnomer "exercise-induced asthma" (EIA) should be replaced by "exercise-induced broncho-constriction" (EIB).

Methods

EXERCISE Six to 8 minutes of near maximal exercise, preferably breathing air with <50% relative humidity, are required for induction of bronchoconstriction in subjects with mild airway hyperresponsiveness. Non-standardized techniques such as running up and down the clinic stairs, or a brief run around adjacent fields, have been used by some clinicians as a substitute for standardized exercise challenges (and as a substitute for other measures of airway responsiveness). Standardized exercise challenges[5,6] may be done with either a treadmill or a cycle. The workload is targeted so that subjects achieve approximately 50% of their predicted maximal voluntary ventilation during the last 4 minutes of an 8-minute exercise test. Measurement of FEV_1 is made before, sometimes during (since FEV_1 increases during exercise), and for 15 to 20 minutes after exercise. Results can be expressed as the percentage fall from baseline after exercise, or the maximum variation incorporating the percentage increase during and the percentage reduction following exercise.

COLD AIR Standardized protocols for isocapnic hyperventilation of cold dry air have been developed.[7] Unlike exercise, a dose–response curve can be obtained. A means of producing cold (–10 to 15°C), dry (relative humidity approaching zero) air is necessary; room temperature dry air is sometimes used. End tidal CO_2 must be measured and CO_2 added to the inspired air to prevent hypocapnia. Three-minute periods of doubling ventilation (7.5, 15, 30, 60 l min^{-1}) are used. The FEV_1 is measured before and $\geq$ 5 minutes after each challenge. Results can be expressed similarly to the methacholine challenge with the PD_{20} (or PD_{10}) expressed as ventilation or respiratory heat exchange.

Indications

The use of "natural" stimuli to provoke bronchoconstriction is preferred by some over "chemical" stimuli; however, the implied better safety has not been confirmed. The tests require more expensive equipment and are more tedious for the subject. Because of limitations on the amount of exercise or maximum ventilation that can be achieved, tests with exercise, cold air, and/or hyperventilation are less sensitive than histamine or methacholine inhalation tests; the corollary is that these tests are more specific for asthma. Histamine and methacholine inhalation tests have replaced exercise as the commonest tests to measure airway responsiveness.

Non-Isotonic Aerosols

Background Hypo- and hypertonic aerosols are indirect bronchoconstrictors likely causing bronchoconstriction via the release of mediators from effector cells.

Methods Non-isotonic aerosol inhalation tests[8,9] require high output ($\geq$ 2 ml min^{-1}) ultrasonic nebulizers. A dose response curve is obtained by inhaling distilled water or 4.5% saline for increasing times (0.5, 1, 2, 4, and 8 minutes). An alternate protocol for hypertonic saline inhalation is to use 2-minute inhalations of doubling concentrations of saline up to a top concentration of 14.4% or up to 4.5% followed by doubling inhalation times to 8 minutes. Spirometry is measured before and between 1 and 5 minutes after each inhalation, and the results are expressed similarly to the methacholine challenge with a PD_{15} or PD_{20} expressed in ml.

Indications Non-isotonic aerosol inhalation tests are an alternate way to measure airway responsiveness. Like exercise, cold air and hyperventilation, they are more specific and less sensitive than methacholine challenges. Many subjects develop significant cough which causes both discomfort and a difficulty measuring spirometry. The clinical value of these tests is being actively researched; currently, there are no clear-cut indications to prefer non-isotonic aerosol inhalations over a methacholine challenge.

Hyperosmolar Dry Powder, e.g Mannitol Challenge

A dry powder challenge with mannitol appears to mimic challenge with hyperosmolar aerosols.[17] Capsules of mannitol (5, 10, 20, and 40 mg) are inhaled via dry powder inhaler. With this apparatus, doubling doses of mannitol from 5 to 160 mg are inhaled at 1 to 2 minute intervals followed by measurement of FEV_1. The airway response to mannitol correlates well with airway response to hypertonic saline[17] and to exercise and hyperventilation.[18] The mannitol inhalation test has several advantages; it is cheap, simple to perform, and portable. These practical advantages may make this the ideal provocation test with non-selective indirect-acting stimuli.[18]

SELECTIVE STIMULI

Allergen Inhalation Tests

Background The airway response to allergens (and chemical sensitizers) is much more complex than to the bronchoconstrictors noted above.[53] The early asthmatic response (EAR) is an episode of bronchoconstriction maximal between 20 and 30 minutes after exposure and resolving within 90 to 120 minutes. The late asthmatic response (LAR) is an episode of airway obstruction, involving both bronchoconstriction and airway inflammation, and occurring between 3 and 8 hours after exposure. Approximately half of positive allergen challenges are isolated EARs, half EAR followed by LAR, and a small percentage isolated LARs. Increased airway responsiveness to methacholine can be seen between 3 hours[54] and several days[41] after allergen challenge usually with an LAR.[41] This is likely an indirect indicator of airway inflammation and is generally expressed as the Δ log methacholine PC_{20}.

Methods Carefully standardized allergen inhalation tests[10,53] require measurement of EAR, LAR and Δ log PC_{20}. Subjects must be off all asthma medication and have an $FEV_1 \geq 70\%$ predicted.[51] On a control day, diluent is inhaled by any standardized method three times at 10- to 15-minute intervals, and spirometry is then monitored for 7 hours. This allows the EAR to be differentiated from an irritant response and the LAR to be differentiated from spontaneous fluctuations in FEV_1. On a second day, doubling concentrations of allergen, starting ≥ 4 concentrations below that predicted by skin test endpoint and methacholine PC_{20},[10] are inhaled in similar fashion at 10- to 15-minute intervals, until FEV_1 has fallen $\geq 15\%$. The FEV_1 is then measured every 10 to 15 minutes for the first hour, and hourly for the next 6 hours. Δ log PC_{20} is assessed by comparing methacholine PC_{20} (or PD_{20}) from the day before to the day after allergen challenge, although some have found it more convenient to assess this at 3 hours.[54] The time commitment for a single allergen challenge is almost 20 hours. Unlike the very safe methacholine inhalation tests, allergen inhalation tests pose significant risks to the patient. Tests should be done in hospital with immediate access to bronchodilators and cardiopulmonary resuscitation (CPR)

equipment. Continuous personal attendance of a physician trained in both the challenge procedure and CPR is mandatory throughout the inhalation and the EAR. Precautions must be taken to prevent exposure of laboratory personnel to allergen aerosol.

Indications Clinical indications for allergen inhalation tests are controversial. The most commonly suggested indication is to determine "clinical relevance" of allergens in the polyallergic asthmatic.[55] Other potential indications include a substitute for skin tests when these cannot be performed, and a method to convince patients of a cause and effect relationship.[55] However, the EAR can be predicted from simpler, shorter and safer tests.[10] Because of chronic anti-inflammatory treatment requirements, the LAR is impossible to assess in severe asthmatics, i.e. those in whom the clinical relevance issue is most important. Many investigators thus feel there is no role for allergen inhalation tests in the clinical assessment of asthmatics.[53] Their research use is undisputed; these tests have proved important for investigating the pathophysiology and pharmacology of asthma and are necessary for the conclusive reporting of new allergens. Some investigators, however, maintain that it is important to characterize the complete allergen response in every allergic asthmatic.[56]

Chemical Sensitizers

Background Many low molecular weight chemical sensitizers induce occupational asthma by uncertain, presumably immunological, means. The most common are plicatic acid in Western Red Cedar,[57] and the aromatic diisocyanates.[58] Since the immunologic mechanism has not been identified, specific sensitivity can only be confirmed by provocation tests.

Methods One approach is to do a workplace challenge test in which the subject is sent to work and spirometry and methacholine PC_{20} are monitored.[59] Such a test can implicate the workplace as a cause of bronchoconstriction and/or airway hyperresponsiveness, but frequently cannot pinpoint the specific chemical. Controlled challenges in the laboratory previously used the approach of mimicking work by painting, spraying, sanding, sawing, tipping dusts, etc.[11] However, levels cannot be monitored. Ideally, a well-vented occupational exposure chamber is required where chemical levels (e.g. diisocyanates), or dust levels can be measured continuously.[12] The methods are similar to those

95

outlined for allergens. At least one control day is necessary. Because LARs are common (≥ 90%), the dose must be increased slowly, e.g. doubled or quadrupled at daily intervals. The following sample protocol can be used for TDI. A diluent (e.g. toluene) control day with 7 hours FEV_1 monitoring is followed by a challenge day (TDI 10–15 ppb) commencing with one breath, then doubling exposures from 15 seconds to 4 minutes at 5–10 minute intervals. The cumulative 4-fold increase in exposure times on three TDI exposure days are 8 minutes, 30 minutes, and 2 hours respectively. Assessments are made for EAR, LAR and Δ log methacholine PC_{20} as for allergen. Safety precautions are required as for allergen challenges. A single challenge may require up to 5 days.

Indications These tests should be performed in hospital in specialized centres with an expertise in occupational asthma. Sensitivity to low molecular weight chemical sensitizers can only be confirmed by inhalation tests. However, some investigators will rely on less expensive, less time-consuming indirect diagnostic techniques including a documentation of exposure, objective documentation of variable airflow obstruction, and indirect indicators of occupational asthma such as serial measurements of peak flow rates and methacholine PC_{20} at work and away from work.[46]

ASA/NSAIDs

Background A variable (depending on patient selection) significant proportion (likely about 5%) of adult asthmatics have the aspirin sensitivity–nasal polyp–asthma triad. The mechanism is uncertain; immunologic sensitivity is unlikely.

Methods ASA (or other NSAID) challenges[13] are done by ingesting increasing doses at 3-hour intervals. Sensitivity is often exquisite; the starting dose should be as low as 3 mg. Challenges must be appropriately controlled (as per above challenges) and in some circumstances blinded (either single or double).

Indications The diagnosis of ASA/NSAID sensitivity is often clinically obvious. Prophylactic NSAID avoidance, particularly in asthmatics who are non-atopic and have severe rhinitis or nasal polyps, is often advised. Challenges with NSAID, thus, have relatively infrequent clinical application and are done only in selected centres where there is a special interest.

Sulphite/Metabisulphite

Background Sulphites and metabisulphites (antioxidants added to beer, wine, vegetables, fruits, potatoes, etc.) are the commonest food additives which provoke bronchoconstriction. The mechanism likely involved inhaled SO_2 released in the mouth or stomach. Since SO_2 should provoke symptoms in all asthmatics, the "selective" nature of this stimulus may relate to breathing pattern during chewing, swallowing or eructing in conjunction with the underlying degree of airway responsiveness.

Methods Although ingested capsules of potassium metabisulphite can be used, the most efficient method of controlled dose–response challenge involves drinking a citric fruit beverage in which the chemical is dissolved.[14] Single- or double-blinding may be useful.

Indications Challenges are not routinely done, but may prove useful to clarify what otherwise appears to be single or multiple food sensitivities.

Other Food Additives

Other food or drug additives, such as monosodium glutamate, tartrazine, benzoate, etc. may infrequently provoke asthma. Methods for challenge, done in selected centres, are similar to that for ASA.[15]

Foods

The issue of "food allergy" provokes much controversy. Classic IgE-mediated food sensitivity may be confirmed by skin-prick tests or RAST. Other immunologic or non-immunologic food intolerances require placebo-controlled double-blind food challenges offered in selected centres.[16]

KEY POINTS

1. Provocation with direct-acting non-selective stimuli (histamine/methacholine) are safe, simple and widely used as a diagnostic aid in clinical asthma.

2. Provocation with indirect-acting non-selective stimuli (exercise/hypertonic saline) are more specific but less sensitive than histamine or methacholine (vis-a-vis a diagnosis of asthma).

3. Provocation with allergen remains an important research tool with little or no role in routine clinical assessment of asthma.

REFERENCES

1. Cockcroft DW, Killian DN, Mellon JJA, Hargreave FE. Bronchial reactivity to inhaled histamine: a method and clinical survey. *Clin Allergy* 1977; 7: 235–43.

2. ✪ Juniper EF, Cockcroft DW, Hargreave FE. Histamine and methacholine inhalation tests: tidal breathing method. In: *Laboratory Procedure and Standardisation*, 2nd edn. Lund, Sweden: Astra Draco AB.

3. Yan K, Salome C, Woolcock AJ. Rapid method for measurement of bronchial responsiveness. *Thorax* 1983; 38: 760–65.

4. Fabbri LM, Mapp CE, Hendrick DJ. Standardization of the dosimeter method for measurement of airway responsiveness in man. In: Hargreave FE, Woolcock AJ (eds). *Airway Responsiveness: Measurement and Interpretation*. Astra Pharmaceuticals Canada, 1985: 29–34.

5. Anderton RC, Cuff MT, Frith PA *et al*. Bronchial responsiveness to inhaled histamine and exercise. *J Allergy Clin Immunol* 1979; 63: 315–20.

6. Anderson SD, Schoeffel RE. Standardization of exercise testing in the asthmatic patient: a challenge in itself. In: Hargreave FE, Woolcock AJ (eds). *Airway Responsiveness: Measurement and Interpretation*. Astra Pharmaceuticals Canada, 1985: 51–9.

7. O'Byrne PM, Ryan G, Morris M *et al*. Asthma induced by cold air and its relation to nonspecific bronchial responsiveness to methacholine. *Am Rev Respir Dis* 1982; 125: 281–5.

8. Boulet LP, Legris C, Thibault L, Turcotte H. Comparative bronchial responses to hyperosmolar saline and methacholine in asthma. *Thorax* 1987; 42: 953–8.

9. Smith CM, Anderson SD. Inhalation provocation tests using non-isotonic aerosols. *J Allergy Clin Immunol* 1989; 84: 781–90.

10. Cockcroft DW, Murdock KY, Kirby J, Hargreave FE. Prediction of airway responsiveness to allergen from skin sensitivity to allergen and airway responsiveness to histamine. *Am Rev Respir Dis* 1987; 135: 264–7.

11. Pepys J, Hutchcroft BJ. Bronchial provocation tests in etiologic diagnosis and analysis of asthma. *Am Rev Respir Dis* 1975; 112: 829–59.

12. ✪ Cartier A, Bernstein IL, Sherwood Burge P *et al*. Guidelines for bronchoprovocation on the investigation of occupational asthma: report on the subcommittee on bronchoprovocation for occupational asthma. *J Allergy Clin Immunol* 1989; 84: 823–9.

13. ✪ Stevenson DD. Diagnosis, prevention, and treatment of adverse reactions to aspirin and nonsteroidal anti-inflammatory drugs. *J Allergy Clin Immunol* 1984; 74: 617–22.

14. Bush RK, Taylor SL, Busse W. A critical evaluation of clinical trials in reactions to sulphites. *J Allergy Clin Immunol* 1986; 78: 191–202.

15. ✪ Metcalfe DD, Sampson HA. Workshop on experimental methodology for clinical studies of adverse reactions to foods and food additives. *J Allergy Clin Immunol* 1990; 86: 421–42.

16. Bock SA, Sampson HG, Atkins FM *et al*. Double-blind, placebo-controlled food challenge (DBPCFC) as an office procedure: a manual. *J Allergy Clin Immunol* 1988; 82: 986.

17. ✪ Anderson SD, Brannan J, Spring J *et al*. A new method for bronchial-provocation testing in asthmatic subjects using a dry powder of Mannitol. *Am J Respir Crit Care Med* 1997; 156: 758–65.

18. Brannan JD, Koskela H, Anderson SD, Chew N. Responsiveness to Mannitol in asthmatic subjects with exercise- and hyperventilation-induced asthma. *Am J Resp Crit Care Med* 1997; 158: 1120–26.

19. Cockcroft DW, Murdock KY. Comparative effects of inhaled salbutamol, sodium cromoglycate and beclomethasone dipropionate on allergen-induced early asthmatic responses, late asthmatic responses and increased bronchial responsiveness to histamine. *J Allergy Clin Immunol* 1987; 79: 734–40.

20. Cockcroft DW, Hargreave FE. Airway hyperresponsiveness: definition, measurement, and clinical relevance. In: Kaliner MA, Barnes PJ, Persson CG (eds). *Asthma: Its Pathology and Treatment*. New York: Marcel Dekker, 1991: 51–72.

21. Pauwels R, Joos G, van der Straeten M. Bronchial hyperresponsiveness is not bronchial hyperresponsiveness is not bronchial asthma. *Clin Allergy* 1988; 18: 317–21.

22. Ramsdale EH, Roberts RS, Morris MM, Hargreave FE. Differences in responsiveness to hyperventilation and methacholine in asthma and chronic bronchitis. *Thorax* 1985; 40: 422–6.

23. Du Toit JI, Woolcock AJ, Salome CM, Sundrum R, Black JL. Characteristics of bronchial responsiveness in smokers with chronic airflow limitation. *Am Rev Respir Dis* 1986; 134: 498–501.

24. Dautrebande L, Philippot E. Crise d'asthme experimental par aerosis de carbaminoylcholine cher l'homme. *Press Med*. 1941; 49: 942–6.

25. Curry JJ. The action of histamine on the respiratory tract in normal and asthmatic subjects. *J Clin Invest* 1946; 25: 785–91.

26. Peat JK, Salome CM, Bauman A, Toelle BG, Wachinger SL, Woolcock AJ. Repeatability of histamine bronchial challenge and comparability with methacholine bronchial challenge in a population of Australian schoolchildren. *Am Rev Respir Dis* 1991; 144: 338–43.

27. ○ Woolcock AJ, Salome CM, Yan K. The shape of the dose-response curve to histamine in asthmatic and normal subjects. *Am Rev Respir Dis* 1984; 130: 71–5.

28. Woolcock AJ, Peat JK, Salome CM *et al*. Prevalence of bronchial hyperresponsiveness and asthma in a rural adult population. *Thorax* 1987; 42: 361–8.

29. ○ Cockcroft DW, Berscheid BA, Murdock KY. Unimodal distribution of bronchial responsiveness to inhaled histamine in a random human population. *Chest* 1983; 83: 751–4.

30. Cockcroft DW. Measurement of airway responsiveness to inhaled histamine or methacholine: method of continuous aerosol generation and tidal breathing inhalation. In: Hargreave FE, Woolcock AJ (eds). *Airway Responsiveness: Measurement and Interpretation*. Astra Pharmaceuticals Canada, 1985: 22–8.

31. Dehaut P, Rachiele A, Martin RR, Malo JL. Histamine dose-response curves in asthma: reproducibility and sensitivity of different indices to assess response. *Thorax* 1983; 38: 516–22.

32. Cockcroft DW, Berscheid BA, Murdock KY, Gore BP. Sensitivity and specificity of histamine PC$_{20}$ measurements in a random selection of young college students. *J Allergy Clin Immunol* 1992; 89: 23–30.

33. Woolcock AJ. Expression of results of airway hyperresponsiveness. In: Hargreave FE, Woolcock AJ (eds). *Airway Responsiveness: Measurement and Interpretation*. Astra Pharmaceuticals Canada, 1985: 80–85.

34. Lam S, Wong R, Yeung M. Nonspecific bronchial reactivity in occupational asthma. *J Allergy Clin Immunol* 1979; 63: 28–34.

35. Ramsdale EH, Morris MM, Roberts RS, Hargreave FE. Bronchial responsiveness to methacholine in chronic bronchitis: relationship to airflow obstruction and cold air responsiveness. *Thorax* 1984; 39: 912–18.

36. Verma VK, Cockcroft DW, Dosman JA. Airway hyperresponsiveness to inhaled histamine in chronic obstructive airways disease: chronic bronchitis vs. emphysema. *Chest* 1988; 94: 456–61.

37. Bahous J, Cartier A, Ouimet G, Pineau L, Malo JL. Nonallergic bronchial hyperexcitability in chronic bronchitis. *Am Rev Respir Dis* 1984; 129: 216–20.

38. Hargreave FE, Ramsdale EH, Pugsley SO. Occupational asthma without bronchial hyperresponsiveness. *Am Rev Respir Dis* 1984; 130: 513–15.

39. Cockcroft DW, Mink JT. Isocyanate-induced asthma in an automobile spray painter. *Canadian Med Assoc J* 1979; 121: 602–604.

40. Boulet LP, Cartier A, Thomson NC, Roberts RS, Dolovich J, Hargreave FE. Asthma and increases in nonallergic bronchial responsiveness from seasonal pollen exposure. *J Allergy Clin Immunol* 1983; 71: 399–406.

41. Cockcroft DW, Ruffin RE, Dolovich J, Hargreave FE. Allergen-induced increase in nonallergic bronchial reactivity. *Clin Allergy* 1977; 7: 503–513.

42. McFadden ER Jr. Exertional dyspnea and cough as preludes to acute attacks of bronchial asthma. *N Engl J Med* 1975; 292: 555–9.

43. ○ Irwin RS, Curley FJ, French CL. Chronic cough: the spectrum and frequency of causes, key components of

the diagnostic evaluation, and outcome of specific therapy. *Am Rev Respir Dis* 1990; 141: 640–47.

44. ✪ Gibson PG, Dolovich J, Denburg J, Ramsdale EH, Hargreave FE. Chronic cough: eosinophilic bronchitis without asthma. *Lancet* 1989; 1: 1346–8.

45. Cockcroft DW, Hargreave FE. Airway hyperresponsiveness: relevance of random population data to clinical usefulness. *Am Rev Respir Dis* 1990; 142: 497–500.

46. Cartier A, Pineau L, Malo JL. Monitoring of maximum expiratory peak flow rates and histamine inhalation tests in the investigation of occupational asthma. *Clin Allergy* 1984; 14: 193–6.

47. Juniper EF, Frith PA, Hargreave FE. Airways responsiveness to histamine and methacholine: relationship to minimum treatment to control symptoms of asthma. *Thorax* 1981; 36: 575–9.

48. Murray AB, Ferguson AC, Morrison B. Airway responsiveness to histamine as a test for overall severity of asthma in children. *J Allergy Clin Immunol* 1981; 68: 119–24.

49. Woolcock AJ, Yan K, Salome CM. Effect of therapy on bronchial hyperresponsiveness in the long-term management of asthma. *Clin Allergy* 1988; 18: 165–76.

50. Cockcroft DW. Therapy for airway inflammation in asthma. *J Allergy Clin Immunol* 1991; 87: 914–19.

51. McFadden ER. Hypothesis: exercise-induced asthma as a vascular phenomenon. *Lancet* 1990; 335: 880–83.

52. Anderson SD, Daviskas E. The airway microvasculature and exercise-induced asthma. *Thorax* 1992; 47: 748–52.

53. Cockcroft DW. Bronchial inhalation tests II. *Ann Allergy* 1987; 59: 89–99.

54. Durham SR, Craddock CF, Cookson WO, Benson MK. Increases in airway responsiveness to histamine precede allergen-induced late asthmatic responses. *J Allergy Clin Immunol* 1988; 82: 764–70.

55. Spector SL. Bronchial inhalation challenges with antigen. In: Spector SL (ed). *Provocative Challenge Procedures: Bronchial, Oral, Nasal and Exercise, Vol. I.* Florida: CRS Press, 1983: 97–112.

56. Pelikan Z, Pelikan-Filipek M. The late asthmatic response to allergen challenge – Part I. *Ann Allergy* 1986; 56: 414–20.

57. Chan-Yeung M, Barton GM, MacLean L, Grzybowski S. Occupational asthma and rhinitis due to Western Red Cedar (*Thuja plicata*). *Am Rev Respir Dis* 1973; 108: 1094–1102.

58. Mapp CE, Polato R, Maestrelli P, Hendrick DJ, Fabbri LM. Time course of the increase in airway responsiveness associated with late asthmatic reactions to toluene diisocyanate in sensitized subjects. *J Allergy Clin Immunol* 1985; 75: 568–72.

59. Chan-Yeung M, McMurren T, Catonio-Begley F, Lam S. Clinical aspects of allergic disease: occupational asthma in a technologist exposed to glutaraldehyde. *J Allergy Clin Immunol* 1993; 91: 974–8.

Chapter 9

Investigations of Allergy

Allan Becker

RATIONALE FOR ALLERGY INVESTIGATION

While allergy is usually considered to play an important role in childhood asthma, this has not been generally thought to be true of adults with asthma. However, studies suggest that a "dose-response" relationship exists between allergy and disease severity.[1,2] In a recent multicentre study of patients with moderate to severe asthma a large proportion of adults with asthma were found to be atopic.[3] Therefore, age and severity of disease are important considerations in deciding whether allergy investigations ought to be initiated.

Most national and international guidelines for the treatment of asthma note the importance of control of the environment before introduction of pharmacotherapy. Environmental control measures are without risk to the patient, although when considering the role of animals in asthma pathophysiology, appropriate consideration must be given to emotionally charged personal and family issues. Critical to this issue is the correct diagnosis of the role of allergy for each individual.

GENERAL CONSIDERATIONS

Allergens represent a spectrum of complex antigenic materials. Beginning in 1980, international committees began to agree on international standards for various allergens. Some allergens have proved to be relatively simple with one or two major antigenic proteins, whereas other have proved to be extremely complex with multiple proteins and multiple allergens (for example, various moulds).

A standardized allergen nomenclature has been applied wherein the first three letters of the genus are followed by a space, followed by the first letter of the species name, then a space and an arabic numeral.[4]

For example, Der p 1 refers to *Dermatophagoides pteronyssinus* P_1 Many of these allergens have been sequenced and some cloned materials are available for research purposes.

Better understanding of allergens has allowed us to define their source and their location in our environment. For example, the clinically important allergen in cat (Fel d 1) occurs in hair follicles and is also secreted into saliva and subsequently deposited on cat hair by licking. This material disseminates as an aerosol, tenaciously clinging to surfaces and subsequently widely transferred throughout the environment on clothing.[5] On the other hand, the primary house-dust mite allergens (Der p 1 and Der f 1) are highly concentrated in house-dust mite faeces, are large particles and do not disseminate widely from their source (primarily bedding, mattresses and carpets).

For asthma, it is generally considered that inhalant aeroallergens are relevant whereas food allergens seldom play an important role. However, food allergens may be important for some infants and in a very few older patients (see chapter 44).[6] In general, there are a limited number of groups of important aeroallergens to which patients are exposed. For outdoor aeroallergens, environmental exposure to tree pollens, grass pollens and weed pollens must be considered. Also, mould spores are a concern and specific moulds have a seasonal prevalence in many areas.[7,8] Indoors, perennial aeroallergens also include mould spores as well as house-dust mites, cats and dogs. Cockroach is an increasingly important aeroallergen, particularly in inner city areas. Occupational (or recreational) exposure to other mammals (such as horses, cattle and rodents) and to a number of other allergenic occupational materials will be considered in Chapter 33. Therefore, in general, to assess the role of allergy for any individual patient it is necessary only to consider a limited number of allergens; specifically, mixtures of tree pollens, grass pollens and weed pollens indigenous to the area, plus mixtures of common indoor and outdoor mould spores, in addition to cats, dogs, house-dust mites and possibly cockroach, plus other specific allergens of major local importance. More complete assessment of sensitization to individual pollens or moulds should only be performed if consideration is being given to immunotherapy. There is no rationale to test for aeroallergens to which the patient is not exposed.

PRACTICAL APPROACH TO INVESTIGATION

General Investigation

Some consideration may be given to defining, in general, a patient's "degree of atopy". For this purpose, a complete blood count with differential white blood cell count to determine the number of peripheral blood eosinophils and the concentration of total serum IgE may be considered.

However, these tests tend to be of more value for epidemiological studies than for practical purposes with an individual patient. Assessment of the presence of eosinophils in airway secretions may be helpful.

Specific Allergy Testing

In vivo Testing Skin testing, specifically epicutaneous (prick/puncture) testing, for inhalant aeroallergens remains the gold standard test of choice. This technique has been used since the beginning of the century.

ALLERGEN EXTRACTS Well-standardized extracts, stabilized in 50% glycerol, should be used for epicutaneous tests. If consideration is given to intradermal testing, extracts should contain no more than 2% glycerol.[9] Extracts should be stored at 4°C.

POSITIVE AND NEGATIVE CONTROLS Positive control solutions are used to ensure that a patient exhibits a wheal in response to either histamine (usually histamine hydrochloride 1 mg ml^{-1}) or to a mast cell-activating compound such as codeine (codeine phosphate 30–60 mg ml^{-1}). The rationale for use of the opiate derivatives is to assess the rather more broad response of ensuring the ability of mast cells to become activated; however, this is seldom a specific problem and histamine is most commonly used as the positive control.

The negative control may be the diluent used to preserve the allergen or, more commonly, normal saline is used to assess the impact of the prick/puncture itself. Patients with marked dermatographism will develop wheal and flare reactions from the negative control and this must be carefully defined.

Epicutaneous Testing (Table 9.1)

Interruption of cutaneous integrity will allow for a small amount of fluid applied to the surface to penetrate to the site of cutaneous mast cells. Various techniques have been used, including scratch testing, which is relatively traumatic and highly variable, and prick or puncture tests. The prick/puncture tests are the most commonly used and have the most consistency from test to test in the hands of a well-trained individual.[10] A variety of tools have been proposed to puncture the skin. These include a disposable hypodermic needle (ranging from 18 to 26 gauge) and the standardized Morrow Brown needle.[11] A lancet produced by Pharmacia (the Phazet) was dipped in standardized allergen and allowed to dry. This method was convenient and reproducible[12] albeit somewhat expensive, but is no longer commercially available. Our device of choice is a no. 9 sewing needle, which is inexpensive and can be pre-packaged and sterilized so that it is easily accessible for use. A new needle should be used for each test to avoid any potential "carry-over" of antigen; however, many investigators choose to thoroughly clean a single needle or other puncture device between antigens.

The skin of the forearm or upper back is most convenient for use for testing. We prefer the forearm in

Table 9.1: Important considerations for epicutaneous testing
Antigens   Use good quality, well-defined, standardized antigens wherever possible
Controls   Always use positive and negative controls
Technique   Place tests 2 cm or more apart   Puncture skin cleanly to avoid traumatic testing   Use separate needle for each test   Blot, do not wipe, excess antigen

that it allows the patient the opportunity to observe the testing and the subsequent response. The skin is cleaned with alcohol and dried, and a mark indicating the site for each allergen extract is placed at intervals of no less than 2 cm. A small drop of each allergen extract is placed beside an indicator mark. Positive and negative controls are also applied. The needle is passed through the drop and inserted just into the epidermal surface at approximately a 45° angle. The tip is then lifted upward and withdrawn. After all tests have been performed the allergen extracts may be blotted away with a tissue paper (do not wipe).

Interpretation

The maximal wheal response to histamine is between 5 and 10 minutes and between 10 and 15 minutes for opiates. The maximal wheal response to allergen occurs between 15 and 20 minutes.[13] Practical assessment of the skin test is made in a semi-quantitative fashion by assessing the wheal response.

Wheal Response The wheal may be outlined at the time of its maximal response as may the surrounding flare response. A permanent record of this response may be made using "invisible" tape to transfer the ink outline to paper. The mean wheal diameter may be recorded as a quantitative measure of the response. Commonly, grading of the response is usually semi-quantitative which may relate to the histamine wheal size (+, larger than negative, but less than 50% of histamine wheal; ++, 50%; +++, 100%; and ++++, 200% of the histamine wheal area),[14] or may be referenced to the negative control (+, 1 mm greater; ++, 1–3 min greater; +++, 3–5 mm greater; and ++++, more than 5 mm greater than the negative control). Reactions generally regarded as indicative of clinical allergy are usually 3 mm or more in net mean wheal diameter.[15] This is usually equivalent to the size of the response produced by histamine or an appropriate concentration of opiate.

Intradermal Testing

In general, there is no need to proceed with intradermal testing for the assessment of clinically relevant allergy to inhalant aeroallergens in patients with asthma. Intradermal testing is considered the most sensitive method of skin testing, but is much more capable of producing false-positive reactions because of technique or material used. The additional sensitivity that can be achieved by intradermal testing is indicated for diagnosis of anaphylactic sensitivity to drugs and to stinging insects.

In vitro Testing The prototype *in vitro* assay for antigen-specific IgE was the radioallergo-sorbent test (RAST)[16] initially commercialized by Pharmacia Laboratories. A variety of modified antigen-specific IgE *in vitro* assays are being widely marketed to primary care and specialist physicians for office use. A recent physicians statement by the American Academy of Allergy and Immunology[17] concludes that "In principle, *in vitro* tests for IgE constitute a technically valid method for detection of allergen-specific antibody in serum. When these tests are performed appropriately and interpreted in the light of clinical history and physical examination obtained personally by a physician properly trained in the diagnosis and treatment of allergic and immunologic diseases, *in vitro* tests for IgE can provide a satisfactory alternative to skin testing for confirmation of the diagnosis of most patients with clinical significant aeroallergen disease and IgE-dependent food allergy". *In vitro* tests for IgE are comparable in sensitivity to prick/puncture skin tests. However: "Currently, skin testing is more economical per test than *in vitro* IgE tests, and therefore, properly performed skin testing is the test of choice".[17]

Use of antigen-specific *in vitro* testing should be considered in patients under the following circumstances:

- extensive severe dermatitis,
- marked dermatographism,
- inability to withdraw medications with H_1-receptor antagonism,
- patient preference.

THE ENVIRONMENT

Since the early 1900s, clinicians have had the ability to assess sensitivity of patients to their environment. It is only in the past decade that the ability to measure the potential exposure of patients to aeroallergens in their environment has become available, using immunoassays to quantify concentrations of specific allergens such as Der p 1, Der f 1 and Fel d 1. With this has come improved understanding of the physical, chemical and immunological properties of allergens, particularly of those allergens from domestic animals and the house-dust mites. This, in turn, has allowed appropriate recommendations for environmental control to be provided and has allowed the assessment of the impact of these control measures on the patient's environment.

The seasonality of outdoor aeroallergens has been known for many years. Knowledge of the obvious tree, grass and weed pollen seasons has been helpful; however, exposure to outdoor mould spores has been poorly defined, yet may be critical to patients sensitized to those allergens.[7,8] Measurement of local area outdoor aeroallergens is becoming more common in many areas.

The importance of house-dust mites in allergy and asthma has been the increasing focus of research in recent years.[18,19] We have recently shown a relationship between exposure to house-dust mite allergen, skin test reactivity and asthma.[3] A number of laboratories have begun to offer assays to quantify indoor exposure to such allergens as cat (*Fel d* I), dog (*Can d* I) and house-dust mite (*Der p* I and *Der f* I). For the moment, issues of quality control in such commercial laboratories leave much to be desired.

The importance of aerollergen exposure in both outdoor and indoor environments is just beginning to be understood in terms of primary sensitization issues and secondary triggering of symptoms. In the future it will be increasingly important to define not only an individual patient's sensitivities but also that patient's potential exposure to aeroallergens. Further, it will be critically important to define the impact of attempts at environmental control on the environment and on the individual patient.

KEY POINTS

INVESTIGATIONS OF ALLERGY

Allergy plays an important role in asthma in both children and adults.

- Defining sensitivity to allergens is critical in recommending environmental control measures.
- Epicutaneous testing for inhalant aeroallergen sensitivity remains the gold standard test of choice.
- Assessment of aeroallergen exposure, both outdoors and indoors, will be increasingly important in the future.

REFERENCES

1. ✪ Burrows B, Martinez FD, Halonen M, Barbee RA, Cline MG. Association of asthma with serum IgE levels and skin-test reactivity to allergens. *N Engl J Med* 1989; 320: 271–7.

2. Zimmerman B, Feanny S, Reisman J et al. Allergy in asthma: The dose relationship of allergy to severity of childhood asthma. *J Clin Immunol* 1988; 81: 63–70.

3. ✪ Chan-Yeung M, Manfreda J, Ward H et al. Mite and cat allergen levels in homes and severity of asthma. *Am J Resp Crit Care Med* 1995; 152: 1805–11.

4. Marsh DG, Goodfriend L, King TP, Lowenstein H, Platts-Mills TAE. Allergen nomenclature. *J Allergy Clin Immunol* 1987; 80: 639–45.

5. Quirce S, Dimich-Ward H, Ferguson A, Becker A, Manfreda J, Simons E, Chan-Yeung M. Mite and cat allergens in the homes of asthmatics in two cities in Canada. *Am Rev Respir Dis* 1994; 149: A245.

6. Watson WTA, Simons FER, Roberts JR, Becker AB. Food hypersensitivity and changes in airway function. *J Allergy Clin Immunol* 1992; 89: 184.

7. O'Hollaren MT, Yunginger JW, Offord KP et al. Exposure to an aeroallergen as a possible precipitating factor in respiratory arrest in young patients with asthma. *N Engl J Med* 1991; 324: 359–63.

8. Watson WTA, Al-Malik SM, Lilley MK et al. The association of aeroallergens, precipitation, and environmental pollutants with emergency room visits and hospitalizations for asthma on the Canadian prairies. *J Allergy Clin Immunol* 1993; 91: 304.

9. Lindblad JH, Farr RS. The incidence of positive intradermal reactions and the demonstration of skin sensitizing antibody to extracts of ragweed and dust in humans without history of rhinitis or asthma. *J Allergy* 1961; 32: 392–401.

10. ✪ Demoly P, Bousquet J, Manderscheid J-C, Dreborg S, Dhivert H, Michel F-B. Precision of skin prick and puncture tests with nine methods. *J Allergy Clin Immunol* 1991; 88: 758–62.

11. Brown HM, Su S, Thantrey N. Prick testing for allergens standardized by using a precision needle. *Clin Allergy* 1981; 11: 95–8.

12. Kjellman N-IM, Dreborg S, Fälth-Magnusson K. Allergy screening including a comparison of prick test results with allergen-coated lancets (Phazet®) and liquid extracts. *Allergy* 1988; 43: 277–83.

13. Voorhorst R. Perfection of skin testing technique: a review. *Allergy* 1980; 35: 247–61.

14. Aas K, Belin L. Suggestions for biologic qualitative testing and standardizations of allergen extracts. *Acta Allergol* 1974; 29: 238–40.

15. Dreborg S. Skin tests used in type I allergy testing: Position paper. *Allergy* 1989; suppl. 10: 1–59.

16. Wide L, Bennich H, Johansson SGO. Diagnosis of allergy by an *in vitro* test for allergen antibodies. *Lancet* 1967; ii: 1105–7.

17. ✪ American Academy Executive Committee; The use of *in vitro* tests for IgE antibody in the specific diagnosis of IgE-mediated disorders and in the formulation of allergen immunotherapy. Position statement, American Academy of Allergy and Immunology. *J Allergy Clin Immunol* 1992; 90: 263–7.

18. Sporik R, Chapman MD, Platts-Mills TAE. House dust mite exposure as a cause of asthma. *Clin Exp Allergy* 1992; 22: 897–906.

19. ✪ Platts-Mills TAE, de Weck AL. Dust mite allergens and asthma–a world wide problem. *J Allergy Clin Immunol* 1989; 83: 416–27.

Chapter 10

Examination of Sputum, Nasal Cytology and Exhaled Gases

Peter Gibson, Deborah Yates and Nicholas Saltos

INTRODUCTION

Airway inflammation is a major characteristic of asthma. Investigation of the mechanisms and features of airway inflammation has helped define the pathogenesis of asthma, determine treatment strategies and indicate new directions for therapy. Several non-invasive markers of airway inflammation such as induced sputum and exhaled nitric oxide have been developed for the assessment of asthma. This chapter will review the technique and application of induced sputum and measurement of exhaled gases to assess airway inflammation in asthma (Table 10.1).

INDUCED SPUTUM

Induced sputum analysis was applied to the assessment of asthma in 1992, and has emerged as an important non-invasive marker. Increased mucus production is a principal feature of the inflammatory response in the airway.[1] Since bronchial mucus is often swallowed, sputum expectoration is not a constant feature in asthma. About one in five people with asthma report never having sputum production. Others expectorate during an exacerbation or recovery from an attack.[2] The analysis of spontaneous sputum is therefore limited by unpredictable sampling. This problem can be overcome using induced sputum.

Sputum can be induced from subjects with and without asthma using inhalation of hypertonic saline.[3] This technique can be applied to adults and children (over 7 years), and can be performed on multiple occasions in order to follow disease progression.[4] Airway narrowing due to hypertonic saline can be reduced by pretreatment with a β_2 agonist that does not alter the cellular differential.[5] Since β_2 agonists do not com-

pletely block airways narrowing[6] it is necessary to monitor lung function during sputum induction. An alternative technique is to combine sputum induction and bronchial provocation challenge using hypertonic saline.[7] This combined challenge provides a measure of both airway inflammation and airway responsiveness in a single test.[8,9]

Mechanisms

Inhalation of hypertonic saline causes bronchoconstriction, cough and sputum expectoration. Hypertonic saline causes mast cell degranulation which leads to bronchoconstriction.[10] Cough occurs independently of bronchoconstriction[11] and may be due to stimulation of afferent nerves in the airway. The mechanism of sputum production after hypertonic saline challenge is not established. Mast cell degranulation is unlikely to be the sole mechanism since the pre-treatment with a β_2 agonist does not influence sputum results. The success of the technique may be related to a reduction in the viscosity of tracheobronchial mucus, increased mucociliary clearance, increased mucus production, or an increase in the volume of airway secretions.[12]

Sample Collection and Analysis

Sputum is a variable mixture of tracheobronchial secretions and saliva. Analysis of tracheobronchial secretions can contribute to the investigation of asthma and airway diseases, however saliva is a contaminant that can confound the interpretation of sputum results. The two largest problems to overcome when using sputum for analysis are firstly, how to deal with contaminating saliva, and secondly how to quantify results.[13] Reliable results, which reflect disease severity in asthma, can be obtained when these sources of variability are controlled.[14] Salivary contamination can be minimized by

Table 10.1: Measurement properties of airway sampling techniques

	Sputum	Exhaled NO
Reproducibility		
Within sample time	Good	Good
Over time	Good	Good
Responsiveness		
Does the sample reflect change in response to:		
Allergen exacerbation	Yes	Yes
Asthma exacerbation	Yes	Yes
Corticosteroid therapy	Yes	Yes
Validity		
Relation to objective measures of lung function	Good	Correlates with MCh PC_{20} but not with FEV_1 – not fully evaluated
Adverse events		
Fall in FEV_1	Yes	No
Fall in SaO_2	Yes	No
Subject discomfort	Minor	No
Costs		
Major equipment needs:		
To collect sample	Ultrasonic nebulizer Spirometer	Mouthpieces and Teflon tubing
To process sample	Haemocytometer Cytocentrifuge Microscope	Chemiluminescence analyser

microscopic selection of viscid mucocellular portions of sputum for analysis.[13,14,15]

An alternative method of dealing with salivary contamination is to collect and analyse sputum and saliva together.[16] The salivary results are subtracted from the sputum results to give a "corrected cell count". Both methods have been shown to be useful in assessing airway inflammation, however, the selected sputum method may provide more viable cells, more eosinophils and a higher concentration of eosinophilic cationic protein (ECP).[15,16,17]

Sputum cells need to be dispersed using dithiothreitol prior to cytocentrifugation or flow cytometry. Dispersed cell preparations are useful for cytochemistry and immunocytochemistry. The sputum samples may also be suitable for molecular biological techniques and cell-culture.

Measurement Issues

Reproducibility Sputum total and differential cell counts and fluid-phase markers demonstrate good reproducibility within the same subject on consecutive days,[14,15,18,19] and within a one-week period.[3,14,19]

Effect of Repeated Sputum Induction Studies have noted changes in the composition of sputum in repeated sputum induction within a 24-hour period. There is an increase in neutrophils and a decrease in macrophages, but no significant change in eosinophils or lymphocytes. These changes may limit the utility of repeated inductions within a short time frame.[20,21]

Relationship of Sputum to Bronchoscopy Studies comparing bronchial wash and bronchoalveolar lavage (BAL) to induced sputum show that there is good agreement between the type of cells recovered by sputum and bronchoscopic samples.[22,23,24] Selected sputum is more concentrated than BAL, having a higher density of cell recovery and higher levels of fluid-phase markers.[24]

Relationship to Serum ECP Induced sputum has been found to be a more sensitive and accurate means of detecting airway inflammation than serum ECP.[25,26,27] Measurement of sputum eosinophils can detect the presence of asthmatic inflammation with a better sensitivity (70%) and specificity (90%) than serum ECP which has a sensitivity of 50% and specificity of 50% (Figure 10.1).[26]

Normal Values The normal range for sputum cell counts is now well-established[28] (Table 10.2), and this facilitates clinical use of induced sputum cell counts.

Sputum Eosinophils

Sputum eosinophilia has been associated with asthma since the beginning of this century. Eosinophils arise from a bone marrow derived progenitor cell and circulate via the bloodstream to the airways[29] where they transmigrate across the endothelium to the airway lumen under the influence of cellular adhesion molecules and cytokines (interleukin-5 (IL5), granulocyte/macrophage-colony stimulating factor (GM-CSF)). Sputum eosinophils in asthma are activated, expressing cleaved eosinophil cationic protein[30] and CD11b.[31] The cell adhesion molecules ICAM-1 and HLA-DR are present on sputum (but not blood) eosinophils to allow migration across endothelium and facilitate interaction with other immunocompetent cells such as T-lymphocytes.[32]

The eosinophil has an important role in the pathogenesis of asthma.[33] Eosinophil counts in sputum can reflect disease severity[3] and increase during spontaneous asthma exacerbations,[14,29,34] after allergen inhalation,[4] virus infection[30,35,36] and challenge with occupational sensitizers.[27]

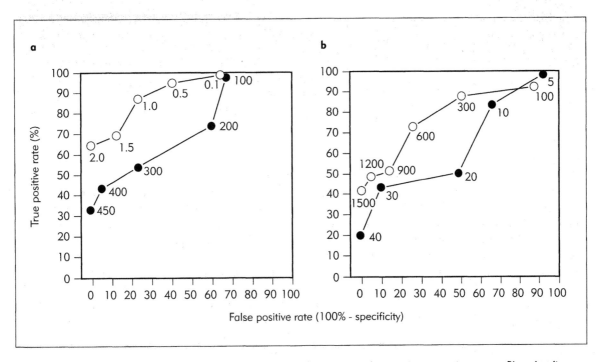

FIGURE 10.1: Operating characteristic of inflammatory markers presented as receiver operating curves. Plots that lie farthest to the "northwest" represent more accurate values. (a) Open circles, sputum eosinophils(%); filled circles, blood eosinophils (%) (b) Open circles, Sputum ECP (µg l⁻¹); filled circles, serum ECP (µg l⁻¹). (From Pizzichini et al. Measuring airway inflammation in asthma: eosinophils and eosinophilic cationic protein in induced sputum compared with peripheral blood. *J Allergy Clin Immunol* 1997; 99: 539–44, with permission.)

Table 10.2: Cell counts in sputum and nasal smears from normal children

	Normal	Atopic normal	Non-atopic normal
Sputum			
TCC × 10^6 cells ml^{-1}			
Mean (95% CI)	5.14 (1.2, 9.08)	1.75 (0.89, 2.6)	8.04 (0.63, 15.5)
Median (IQR)	1.5 (0.8, 3.9)	1.0 (0.55, 2.15)*	1.8 (1.05, 6)*
Eosinophils % sputum	n=70	n=31	n=38
Mean (95% CI)	1.57 (0.62, 2.52)	2.16 (0.83, 3.48)	1.13 (0, 2.54)
Median (IQR)	0.3 (0, 1.05)	0.5 (0, 2.8)	0 (0, 0.6)
Mast cells % sputum	n=70	n=31	n=38
Mean (95% CI)	0.024 (0, 0.05)	0.03 (0, 0.07)	0.02 (0, 0.06)
Median (IQR)	0 (0, 0)	0 (0, 0)	0 (0, 0)
Nasal smear			
Eosinophils % nasal	n=72	n=32	n=39
Mean (95% CI)	1.35 (0.63, 2.07)	2.4 (0.93, 3.89)	0.52 (0.04, 0.99)
Median (IQR)	0 (0, 0.65)	0 (0, 3.68)	0 (0, 0.3)
Mast cell % nasal	n=72	n=32	n=39
Mean (95% CI)	0.033 (0, 0.07)	0.07 (0, 0.15)	0.005 (0, 0.001)
Median (IQR)	0 (0, 0)	0 (0, 0)	0 (0, 0)

TCC: total cell count; IQR: interquartile range; 95%CI: 95% confidence interval; *P<0.05, using Mann–Whitney test.

Clinical Correlates

Several studies have examined sputum analysis in relation to clinical diagnosis in adults and children. Eosinophils[3,9,14,16,28] and the biochemical markers ECP, albumin and fibrinogen[19] are higher in asthmatic sputum than in sputum from normals (Figure 10.2). Similarly, asthmatic sputum has increased eosinophils compared with that of smokers with chronic bronchitis.[14] Children with methacholine airway hyperresponsiveness but no symptoms of current or past asthma do not have increased sputum eosinophils.[37] These studies indicate that eosinophils and their secretory products form the characteristic profile of airway inflammation in asthma (Fig. 10.3).

Sputum eosinophilia may not be a constant feature of asthma but may reflect disease activity (Fig. 10.2). While in controlled asthma, the degree of sputum eosinophilia tends to be no greater than normal,[3] in asthma exacerbations high sputum eosinophil counts were observed.[14] Sputum eosinophilia increases several-fold during exacerbations of asthma[29] and following allergen challenge.[4]

Sputum eosinophils correlate with objective markers of disease severity in asthma. Higher levels of induced sputum eosinophils and ECP are associated with greater airflow obstruction (FEV_1).[3,16,38] The same association holds in severe asthma where sputum eosinophil counts correlated with the degree of airflow obstruction in patients attending the emergency room with status asthmaticus.[39] Following allergen challenge, the increases in sputum eosinophils were correlated with the magnitude of the late response and with the allergen-induced changes in airway responsiveness.[4] These studies indicate a potential role for measuring eosinophils and their degranulation products in monitoring disease severity.

Perhaps one of the most useful and well-established roles for sputum eosinophil examination lies in the prediction of corticosteroid response (Table 10.3). The presence of sputum eosinophils is associated with a good clinical response to corticosteroid while their absence suggests a poor response. This has been demonstrated in subjects with asthma[40] where corti-

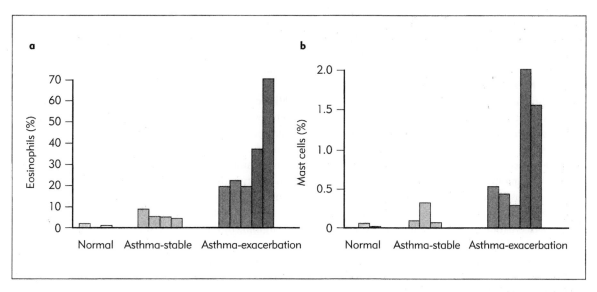

FIGURE 10.2: Sputum eosinophils (a) and mast cells (b) from normal subjects, subjects with stable asthma and subjects with asthma in exacerbation. (Data from Refs 3, 4, 14, 16, 29 for induced sputum and spontaneous sputum samples (last two bars only).)

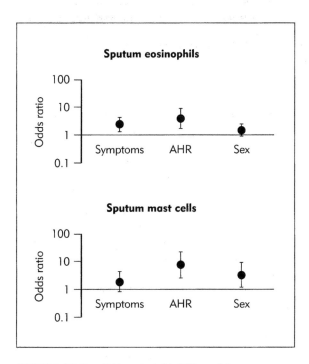

FIGURE 10.3: Odds ratio (with 95% confidence intervals) for the association among sputum eosinophils (top panel), sputum mast cells (bottom panel), and asthma symptoms (P<0.05), airway hyperresponsiveness (AHR) (P<0.05), and sex (P<0.05 for mast cells and male sex).

	Eosinophils and steroid response	No eosinophils and negative response to steroids
Table 10.3: Sputum eosinophilia is associated with a short-term response to corticosteroids in asthma, chronic cough and COPD		
Asthma	Morrow Brown, Ref. 40	No studies
Cough	Gibson, Ref. 42	Pizzichini, in press
COPD	Pizzichini, Ref. 43	Syed, Ref. 44 Pizzichini, Ref. 43 Gibson, Ref. 14

costeroid treatment reduces sputum eosinophils within several days.[30,34,41] The association of eosinophilia and corticosteroid response also holds for subjects with other airway diseases, e.g. chronic cough where there is no airflow obstruction or airway hyperresponsiveness,[42] and chronic obstructive pulmonary disease (COPD).[43] The short term response to corticosteroid is poor when sputum eosinophilia is absent, such as in chronic bronchitis.[14,43,44]

In summary, sputum eosinophilia is a feature of current symptomatic asthma that can be used to predict short-term response to corticosteroid in airway diseases.

Sputum Mast Cells

Both spontaneous and induced sputum samples demonstrate a 10-fold increase in mast cell counts from subjects with asthma when compared with either normals,[3] or smokers with chronic bronchitis.[19] This increase occurs in the formalin-sensitive mast cell population.[14] Formalin-sensitive mast cells are commonly seen at mucosal sites, and stain positive for mast cell tryptase, but not chymase. Mast cell counts are highest during exacerbations of asthma and increase after allergen challenge.[4] Sputum mast cell counts are associated with airway hyperresponsiveness to hypertonic saline.[8]

NASAL CYTOLOGY

Cytologic examination of nasal secretions can be a helpful investigation in subjects with upper respiratory symptoms. Nasal disease frequently coexists with asthma and requires appropriate treatment for symptom control. Nasal secretions may be obtained by nose blowing, nasal scraping with a cotton-tipped swab or plastic scoop, or by nasal lavage with saline. Semi-quantitative cellular differentials from stained smears are often used for clinical assessment, while nasal lavage provides increased precision for research purposes.

Hansel described the use of nasal smears to differentiate allergic from infectious nasal disease.[45] Recent studies describe increased nasal eosinophils in both allergic rhinitis and non-allergic rhinitis, as well as in aspirin sensitivity and nasal polyposis.[45,46] The presence of nasal eosinophilia is associated with a favourable response to topical nasal corticosteroid, while increased neutrophils are seen with infection such as bacterial sinusitis or viral upper respiratory tract infection.[46,47]

Some authors consider untreated upper airway inflammation a trigger for asthma symptoms. In an epidemiological survey of children, high levels of nasal eosinophils were associated with current symptoms of asthma and airway hyperresponsiveness.[8]

EXHALED GASES

Assessment of expired gases in lung disease has considerable appeal because of the direct nature of the reading, the non-invasive nature of the technique, and the rapidity of the test result. It is likely that this area will expand rapidly in the future, but there is much still to be learned about the significance and clinical applicability of such measurements.

Nitric Oxide

The evanescent gas nitric oxide (NO) is formed in the lungs and plays a key role in the regulation of a wide variety of pulmonary functions. Nitric oxide acts as a vasodilator, bronchodilator and non-adrenergic non-cholinergic (NANC) neurotransmitter within the lung and is an important mediator of the inflammatory response.[48] Nitric oxide is formed from the amino acid L-arginine by the action of nitric oxide synthases (NOS). Three main NOS isoforms have now been characterized. The calcium-dependent forms have been isolated from brain and vascular endothelium and comprise neuronal (type 1 or nNOS) and endothelial NOS (type III or eNOS). These are expressed in normal tissue and are responsible for the physiological generation of NO as a signalling molecule. The inducible form (type II or iNOS) is not a normal constituent of healthy cells, and is primarily expressed after exposure to pro-inflammatory cytokines and bacterial endotoxin. The form iNOS has been described in bronchial epithelial and smooth muscle cells, macrophages, fibroblasts, and neutrophils and its induction results in the production of much higher levels of NO than constitutive NOS (cNOS) induction. All three types of NOS have been demonstrated in airway epithelium. *In vitro*, iNOS expression is readily inhibited by corticosteroids, whereas cNOS is unaffected. In mild asthmatic subjects not using inhaled glucocorticosteroids (GCS), bronchial biopsy specimens have shown increased expression of iNOS, whereas cNOS alone is found in normal subjects.[49]

Exhaled NO is increased in asthma and levels are altered by treatment with anti-inflammatory therapy. The increased levels are probably due to induction of iNOS in asthmatic airway inflammation, while levels in normal subjects are likely to reflect basal cNOS expression. This hypothesis is supported by clinical studies which have shown that inhalation of a non-selective NOS inhibitor, L-NMMA, significantly decreases exhaled NO both in normal and asthmatic subjects, while the administration of a selective iNOS inhibitor, aminoguanidine, decreases exhaled NO in asthmatics but not in subjects with normal airways. In keeping with this, administration of oral glucocorticosteroids (GCS), which affect iNOS but not cNOS, will decrease exhaled NO in asthmatic but not in normal subjects.[50] At a cellular level, iNOS can be induced by pro-inflammatory cytokines that are recognized as important in asthma. These include TNFα and IL1-β, which are secreted by activated macrophages and other airway inflammatory cells, and have been shown to upregulate iNOS *in vitro*. The highest NO output appears to be from macrophages and epithelial cells. The large amounts of NO generated by iNOS have been reported to result in suppression of TH_1 cells and reduce levels of IFN-γ, allowing proliferation of TH_2 cells and perpetuation of the inflammatory response.[51] In addition, NO may be autotoxic to the airway epithelium.[52] Exhaled NO level is likely therefore to directly reflect the cytokine-mediated airway inflammation which is characteristic of asthma.

Clinical Studies on Exhaled Nitric Oxide

(Table 10.4)
Studies have shown that exhaled NO is higher in steroid-naïve subjects with asthma compared with normal sub-

jects, both adults and children. Levels are higher in atopic compared with non-atopic normal subjects.[53] Since high concentrations of NO are produced in the nose and paranasal sinuses, the nasal component needs to be excluded from exhaled measurements (see below). Exhaled NO rises during deterioration in asthma control and during acute asthma exacerbation, but returns to baseline levels after initiation of GCS treatment. Exhaled NO is increased by upper respiratory tract infections, and rises if GCS therapy is withdrawn. Studies have shown exhaled NO to decrease in subjects with asthma after use of inhaled or oral GCS.[50,54] Following allergen challenge, exhaled NO does not increase with the early asthmatic response, but rises in parallel with the late asthmatic reaction and the accompanying late inflammatory response.[55] Exhaled nitric oxide correlates with airway hyperresponsiveness in steroid naïve subjects with mild asthma, and with sputum eosinophil counts. After treatment with inhaled budesonide, the resulting improvement in PC_{20} is correlated

Table 10.4: Physiological and pharmacological factors affecting exhaled NO in humans	
Increase exhaled NO	**Decrease exhaled NO**
Pharmacological factors	
Ingested and inhaled L-arginine in normal and asthmatic subjects	Inhaled or i.v. NOS inhibitors (L-NMMA, L-arginine, aminoguanidine etc.)
Isocapnic cold air hyperventilation	Inhaled or oral glucocorticosteroids
Hyperoxia	Isocapnic cold air hyperventilation
	Capsaicin
	Smoking
	Acute alcohol ingestion in asthmatics
Physiological factors	
Menstrual cycle variations	Menstrual cycle variation
Breathholding	Repeated forced expiratory manoeuvre
Physical exercise	
Diseases	
Asthma	Systemic sclerosis with pulmonary hypertension
Allergen challenge (late response)	Cystic fibrosis
Upper respiratory tract infection	COPD
Lower respiratory tract infection	Heart failure
Pollen exposure in sensitized children	
Exposure to occupational aeroallergens	
Hepatopulmonary syndrome	
Active pulmonary TB	
Renal failure	

with the decrease in exhaled NO and with BAL eosinophils.[54,56] The main advantage of exhaled NO is its lack of invasiveness and ease of measurement, and this technique has now been successfully applied to infants, children, the elderly, and in epidemiological studies.[57]

Other Gases

Several gases other than exhaled NO can be assessed. In chronic inflammatory diseases such as asthma, reactive oxygen species (ROS) are produced by airway inflammatory cells. These result in the lipid peroxidation and the production of ethane, pentane and hydrogen peroxide (H_2O_2), all of which can be detected in exhaled air or in breath condensate. Carbon monoxide (CO) is also produced when ROS induce a stress response protein, HO-1, which acts to catalyse the oxidative degradation of heme to bilirubin. Bilirubin is an antioxidant and CO itself has several biological activities. Carbon monoxide is released from heme and can be measured in exhaled air in normal subjects. Two studies to date have demonstrated increased exhaled CO in steroid naive subjects with asthma. Changes in CO concentration were significantly related to the sputum eosinophilia, and corticosteroid use resulted in lower exhaled CO levels. In normals, levels were higher in atopic than in non-atopic subjects. Combined use of exhaled H_2O_2 and NO may be useful in monitoring disease activity in asthma.[58]

Technique of Measurement of Nitric Oxide

Recommendations for both equipment and measurement technique have been published.[57,59] Several sensitive NO analysers are now commercially available and measure exhaled NO by chemiluminescence, which depends on the photochemical reaction between NO and ozone generated by the analyser. These are generally sensitive to NO levels of <1 ppb and the newer analysers have a rapid response time (<7 s). Because plastic absorbs NO, it is important to connect the analyser to a sampling tube made of inert material, usually polytetrafluoroethylene (Teflon).

Nitric oxide can be sampled either directly or into a reservoir. Low positive pressure is required for exhalation (5–20 cm H_2O), achieved by an internal restrictor in the mouthpiece, which is sufficient to close the soft palate and prevent contamination of exhaled air by nasal NO. Subjects should exhale slowly from TLC over 5–30 seconds, and NO is sampled via a side-arm connected to the mouthpiece. Ideally, the oral pressure and exhalation rate should be measured by attaching a sensor to the breathing circuit, and an exhalation flow display will assist subjects to maintain the correct pressure. Carbon dioxide is often also measured simultaneously, and both NO and CO_2 are displayed via a computerised system which also allows choice of the appropriate NO plateau and data storage and analysis. Several technical factors may affect exhaled NO (Table 10.5).

Indirect techniques using reservoirs to collect expired gas are also successful, and several investigators have used impermeable bags, including Tedlar bags, balloons, and Australian wine cask bags. These may be useful for epidemiological field surveys. Preliminary evidence suggests a relatively good correlation between the two techniques.

Table 10.5: Technical factors altering exhaled NO	
Increased NO	**Decreased NO**
Low exhalation rate	High exhalation flow rate
Breathholding	Water vapour
High background concentrations of NO (>20 ppb)	Use of plastic tubing
Contamination by nasal NO	Suboptimal storage from leakage or reservoir
	Poor response time/sensitivity

KEY POINTS

1 Investigation of the mechanisms and features of airway inflammation has helped define the pathogenesis of asthma, determine treatment strategies and indicate new directions for therapy.

2 The presence of sputum eosinophils is associated with a good clinical response to corticosteroid while their absence suggests a poor response.

3 The presence of nasal eosinophilia is associated with a favourable response to topical nasal corticosteroid, while increased neutrophils are seen with infection such as bacterial sinusitis or viral upper respiratory tract infection.

4 The evanescent gas nitric oxide (NO) is formed in the lungs and plays a key role in the regulation of a wide variety of pulmonary functions.

5 High concentrations of NO are produced in the nose and paranasal sinuses, the nasal component needs to be excluded from exhaled measurements.

6 Exhaled NO rises during deterioration in asthma control and during acute asthma exacerbation, but returns to baseline levels after initiation of GCS treatment.

REFERENCES

1. Florey H. Secretion of mucus in the inflammation of mucous membranes. In: Florey H (ed). *General Pathology*, 3rd edn. London: Lloyd Luke Medical Books, 1962; 167–96.

2. Openshaw PJ, Turner-Warwick M. Observations on sputum production in patients with variable airflow obstruction: implications for the diagnosis of asthma and chronic bronchitis. *Respir Med* 1989; 83: 25–31.

3. ✪ Pin I, Gibson PG, Kolendowicz R *et al*. Use of induced sputum cell counts to investigate airway inflammation in asthma. *Thorax* 1992; 47: 25–9.

4. Pin I, Freitag AP, O'Byrne PM *et al*. Changes in the cellular profile of induced sputum after allergen-induced asthmatic responses. *Am Rev Respir Dis* 1992; 145: 1265–9.

5. Pizzichini MM, Kidney JC, Wong BJ *et al*. Effect of salmeterol compared with beclomethasone on allergen-induced asthmatic and inflammatory responses. *Eur Respir J* 1996; 9: 449–55.

6. Wong HH, Fahy JV. Safety of one method of sputum induction in asthmatic subjects. *Am J Respir Crit Care Med* 1997; 156: 299–303.

7. Smith SM, Anderson SD. Inhalation provocation tests using non-isotonic aerosols. *J Allergy Clin Immunol* 1989; 84: 781–90.

8. ✪ Gibson PG, Wlodarczyk JW, Hensley MJ *et al*. Epidemiological association of airway inflammation with asthma sympotoms and airway hyperresponisveness in childhood. *Am J Respir Crit Care Med* 1998; 158: 36–41.

9. Iredale MJ, Wanklyn S, Phillips IP, Krausz T, Ind PW. Non-invasive assessment of bronchial inflammation in asthma: no correlation between eosinophilia of induced sputum and bronchial responsiveness to inhaled hypertonic saline. *Clin Exp Allergy* 1994; 24: 940–5.

10. Finney MJB, Anderson SD, Black JL. Terfenadine modifies airway narrowing induced by the inhalation of nonisotonic aerosols in subjects with asthma. *Am Rev Resp Dis* 1990; 141: 1151–7.

11. Eschenbacher WL, Boushey HA, Sheppard D. Alteration in osmolarity of inhaled aerosols cause bronchoconstriction and cough, but absence of a permanent anion causes cough alone. *Am Rev Respir Dis* 1984; 129: 211–15.

12. Umeno E, McDonald DM, Nadel JA. Hypertonic saline increases vascular permeability in the rat trachea by

producing neurogenic inflammation. *J Clin Invest* 1990; 85: 1905–8.

13. Chodosh S, Zaccheo CV, Segal MS. The cytology and histochemistry of sputum cells. *Am Rev Respir Dis* 1962; 85: 635–48.

14. Gibson PG, Girgis-Gabardo A, Morris MM *et al*. Cellular characteristics of sputum from patients with asthma and chronic bronchitis. *Thorax* 1989; 44: 693–9.

15. Kips JC, Peleman RA, Pauwels RA. Methods of examining induced sputum: do differences matter? *Eur Respir J* 1998; 11: 529–33.

16. Fahy JV, Liu J, Wong H, Boushey HA. Cellular and biochemical analysis of induced sputum from asthmatic and from healthy subjects. *Am Rev Respir Dis* 1993; 147: 1126–31.

17. Spanevello A, Beghe B, Bianchi A *et al*. Comparison of two methods of processing induced sputum: selected versus entire sputum. *Am J Respir Crit Care Med* 1998; 157: 665–8.

18. Belda J, Giner J, Casan P, Sanchis J. Induced sputum in asthma: study of validity and repeatability. *Arch Broncopneumol* 1997; 33: 325–30.

19. ✪ Pizzichini E, Pizzichini MM, Efthinmiadis A *et al*. Indices of airways inflammation in induced sputum: reproducibility and validity of cell and fluid-phase measurements. *Am J Respir Crit Care Med* 1996; 154: 308–17.

20. Nightingale JA, Rogers DF. Effect of repeated sputum induction on cell counts in normal volunteers. *Thorax* 1998; 53: 87–90.

21. Holz O, Richter K, Jorres RA, Speckin P, Mucke M, Magnussen H. Changes in sputum composition between two inductions performed on consecutive days. *Thorax* 1998; 53: 83–6.

22. ✪ Grootendorst DC, Sont JK, Willems LN *et al*. Comparison of inflammatory cell counts in asthma: induced sputum vs bronchoalveolar lavage and bronchial biopsies. *Clin Exp Allergy* 1997; 27: 769–79.

23. Keatings VM, Evans DJ, O'Connor BJ, Barnes PJ. Cellular profiles in asthmatic airways: a comparison of induced sputum, bronchial washings, and bronchoalveolar lavage fluid. *Thorax* 1997; 52: 372–4.

24. Pizzichini E, Pizzichini MM, Kidney JC *et al*. Induced sputum, bronchoalveolar lavage and blood from mild asthmatics: inflammatory cells, lymphocyte subsets and soluble markers compared. *Eur Respir J* 1998; 11: 828–34.

25. Sorva R, Metso T, Turpeinen M, Juntunen-Backman K, Bjorksten F, Haahtela T. Eosinophil cationic protein in induced sputum as a marker of inflammation in asthmatic children. *Pediatr Allergy Immunol* 1997; 8: 45–50.

26. Pizzichini E, Pizzichini MM, Efthimiadis A, Dolovich J, Hargreave FE. Measuring airway inflammation in asthma: eosinophils and eosinophilic cationic protein in induced sputum compared with peripheral blood. *J Allergy Clin Immunol* 1997; 99: 539–44.

27. Di Franco A, Vagaggini B, Bacci E *et al*. Leukocyte counts in hypertonic saline-induced sputum in subjects with occupational asthma. *Respir Med* 1998; 92: 550–57.

28. Cai Y, Carty K, Henry RL, Gibson PG. Persistence of sputum eosinophilia in children with controlled asthma when compared with healthy children. *Eur Respir J* 1998; 11: 848–53.

29. Gibson PG, Wong BJ, Hepperle MJ *et al*. A research method to induce and examine a mild exacerbation of asthma by withdrawal of inhaled corticosteroid. *Clin Exp Allergy* 1992; 22: 525–32.

30. Twaddell SH, Gibson PG, Carty K, Woolley KL, Henry RL. Assessment of airways inflammation in children with acute asthma using induced sputum. *Eur Respir J* 1996; 9: 2140–48.

31. Walker C, Rihs S, Braun RK, Betz S, Bruijnzeal PL. Increased expression of CD11b and functional changes in eosinophils after migration across endothelial monolayers. *J Immunol* 1993; 150: 4061–71.

32. Hansel TT, Braunstein JB, Walker C *et al*. Sputum eosinophils from asthmatics express ICAM-1 and HLA-DR. *Clin Exp Immunol* 1991; 86: 271–7.

33. Frigas E, Gleich GJ. The eosinophil and the pathophysiology of asthma. *J Allergy Clin Immunol* 1986; 77: 527–32.

34. Baigelman W, Chodosh S, Pizzuto D, Cupples LA. Sputum and blood eosinophils during corticosteroid treatment of acute exacerbations of asthma. *Am J Med* 1983; 75: 929–36.

35. Grunberg K, Smits HH, Timmers MC *et al*. Experimental rhinovirus 16 infection. Effects on cell differentials and soluble markers in sputum in asthmatic subjects. *Am J Respir Crit Care Med* 1997; 156: 609–16.

36. Pizzichini MM, Pizzichini E, Efthimiadis A *et al*. Asthma and natural colds. Inflammatory indices in induced sputum: a feasibility study. *Am J Respir Crit Care Med* 1998; 158: 1178–84.

37. Pin I, Radford S, Kolendowicz R *et al*. Airway inflammation in symptomatic and asymptomatic children with methacholine hyperresponsiveness. *Eur Respir J* 1993; 6: 1249–56.

38. Virchow JG Jr, Holscher U, Virchow C Snr. Sputum ECP levels correlate with parameters of airflow obstruction. *Am Rev Respir Dis* 1992; 146: 604–6.

39. Alfaro C, Sharma OP, Navarro L, Glovsky MM. Inverse correlation of expiratory lung flows and sputum eosinophils in status asthmatics. *Ann Allergy* 1989; 63: 251–4.

40. Brown HM. Corticosteroids in asthma. *Lancet* 1958; ii: 1245–7.

41. ✪ Turner MO, Johnston PR, Pizzichini E, Pizzichini MM, Hussack PA, Hargreave FE. Antiinflammatory effects of salmeterol compared with beclomethasone in eosinophilic mild exacerbations of asthma: a randomised, placebo controlled trial. *Can Respir J* 1998; 5: 261–8.

42. ✪ Gibson PG, Dolovich J, Denburg J, Ramsdale EH, Hargreave FE. Chronic cough: eosinophilic bronchitis without asthma. *Lancet* 1989; i: 1346–8.

43. ✪ Pizzichini E, Pizzichini MM, Gibson P *et al*. Sputum eosinophilia predicts benefit from prednisone in smokers with chronic obstructive bronchitis. *Am J Respir Crit Care Med* 1998; 158: 1511–17.

44. Syed A, Hoeppner VH, Cockcroft DW. Predictors of a non-response to corticosteroids in stable chronic airflow limitation. *Clin Invest Med* 1991; 14: 28–34.

45. Hansel FK. Observations on the cytology of the secretions in allergy of the nose and paranasal sinuses. *J Allergy* 1992; 5: 182–9.

46. Lee HS, Majimia Y, Sakakura Y, Shinogi J, Kawaguchi S, Kim BW. Quantitative cytology of nasal secretions under various conditions. *Laryngoscope* 1993; 103: 533–7.

47. Meltzer EO. Evaluating rhinitis: clinical, rhinomanometric and cytologic assessments. *J Allergy Clin Immunol* 1988; 82: 900–8.

48. Barnes PJ, Kharitonov SA. Exhaled nitric oxide: a new lung function test? *Thorax* 1996; 51: 233–7.

49. Hamid Q, Springall DR, Riveros-Moreno V, Polack J. Induction of nitric oxide synthase in asthma. *Lancet* 1993; 342: 1510–3.

50. Yates DH, Kharitonov SA, Robbins RA, Thomas PS, Barnes PJ. Effect of a nitric oxide synthase inhibitor and a glucocorticosteroid on exhaled nitric oxide. *Am J Respir Crit Care Med* 1995; 152: 892–6.

51. Barnes PJ and Liew FY. Nitric oxide and asthmatic inflammation. *Immunol Today* 1995; 16: 128–30.

52. Flak TA, Goldman WE. Autotoxicity of nitric oxide in airway disease. *Am J Respir Crit Care Med* 1996; 154: 5202–6.

53. Kharitonov SA, Chung KF, Evans D, O'Connor BJ, Barnes PJ. The elevated level of exhaled nitric oxide in asthmatic patients is mainly derived from the lower respiratory tract. *Am J Respir Crit Care Med* 1996; 153: 1773–80.

54. ✪ Kharitonov SA, Yates DH, Barnes PJ. Regular inhaled budesonide decreases exhaled nitric oxide concentration in asthma. *Am J Respir Crit Care Med* 1996; 153: 454–7.

55. Kharitonov SA, O'Connor BJ, Evans DJ, Barnes PJ. Allergen-induced late asthmatic reactions are associated with elevation of exhaled nitric oxide. *Am J Respir Crit Care Med* 1995; 151: 1894–9.

56. ✪ Jatakanon A, Lim S, Kharitonov SA, Chung KF, Barnes PJ. Correlation between exhaled nitric oxide, sputum eosinophils, and methacholine responsiveness in patients with mild asthma. *Thorax* 1998; 53: 91–5.

117

57. Kharitonov SA, Alving K, Barnes PJ. Exhaled and nasal nitric oxide measurements: recommendations. *Eur Respir J* 1997; 10: 1683–93.

58. Horvath I, Donnelly LE, Kiss A *et al*. Combined use of exhaled hydrogen peroxide and nitric oxide in monitoring asthma. *Am J Respir Crit Care Med* 1998; 158: 1042–6.

59. American Thoracic Society. Recommendations for standardized procedures for the online and offline measurement of exhaled lower respiratory oxide and nasal nitric oxide in adults and children – 1999. *Am J Respir Crit Care Med* 1999; 160: 2104–2117.

Chapter 11

Bronchoalveolar Lavage and Bronchial Biopsies

Ellinor Ädelroth

INTRODUCTION

When rigid bronchoscopy was first introduced as a means to access the airways it was mainly used for therapeutic reasons, to remove foreign bodies and mucus.[1] In the 1970s, with the development of the flexible, fibreoptic bronchoscope a new era began in the investigation of airway diseases. The fibreoptic bronchoscope was introduced for the investigation of bronchial carcinomas, haemoptysis, for sampling in lung infections, and as an aid in anaesthesiology and so used for years.[2,3] With increased experience in a variety of lung conditions it eventually became evident that fibreoptic bronchoscopy could also be applied in asthmatics with hyperresponsive airways if subjects were carefully selected.

Thus, during the last 20 years numerous research studies involving fibreoptic bronchoscopy with bronchoalveolar lavage (BAL) and/or bronchial biopsies in asthmatics with mild to moderately severe asthma have been performed.[5–20] Results from these studies have greatly increased the knowlegde of asthma pathogenesis and verified that airway inflammation is a characteristic feature of asthma, even early in the course of disease. In addition, the results have contributed to treatment guidelines for asthma which advocate anti-inflammatory therapy as first-line therapy in asthma.[21] The importance of inflammation in asthma has also created a need for ways to reliably evaluate and monitor the airway inflammation and follow effects of treatments.

BRONCHOSCOPY IN ASTHMA

Bronchoscopy in asthmatic patients is *not* a routine investigation in the diagnosis or evaluation of the disease. It is a research procedure and if performed as a part of a research study there are guidelines as to its use which should be adhered to in order to secure the safety of the subject.[22] The guidelines involve suggestions as to the selection of subjects for investigation, pre-procedure investigations (ECG, blood tests, lung function tests, measurement of airway hyperresponsiveness), pre-treatment with a bronchodilator, use of topical anaesthesia, as well as suggestions for monitoring during and after the procedure such as oximetry and spirometry. The bronchoscopy is generally well-tolerated and safe with few complications if the guidelines are followed and the investigation performed by an experienced physician.

BRONCHOALVEOLAR LAVAGE

The bronchoalveolar lavage (BAL) technique was established in the 1970s to sample airway cells and mediators present on the surface of the airway and was used initially to investigate interstitial lung diseases. BAL involves the instillation of saline through the bronchoscope with the tip wedged into a segmental or subsegmental bronchus most often in the right middle lobe or the lingula segment.[4,20] These two locations give the best recovery of the instilled volume when the patient is in the supine position. The saline is instilled in aliquots and each aliquot is gently suctioned back into a vial and analysed for cells and soluble substances. The total volume of the instillate varies between 100–300 ml. Often the first aliquot is analysed separately, as it is considered to sample the proximal airway closest to the tip of the bronchoscope and is sometimes called "bronchial wash", while the subsequent aliquots are pooled and called "bronchoalveolar lavage" or "the larger portion" and they sample the more distal, alveolar part of the airway. The fluid is centrifuged to separate cells from the fluid-phase (supernatant). Total and differential cell counts are made from the cell pellet and various analyses are made on the supernatant. A number of immunochemical techniques can be applied to the cells to, for example, evaluate their state of activation.[11–13,18]

Recommendations for the use of standardized ways for the collection, handling and reporting of BAL data are available to minimize variations of results and facilitate comparisons of results from different studies.[23] An update has recently been published.[24]

BRONCHOALVEOLAR LAVAGE FINDINGS IN ASTHMA

In virtually all BAL studies performed in mild to moderately severe asthmatics increased proportions of eosinophils, mast cells and lymphocytes have been found compared to non-asthmatic control subjects.[6–14] The finding of a predominantly eosinophilic inflammation has been seen in all asthmatics, both in allergic and non-allergic subjects, and also very early in the course of the disease and shortly after the diagnosis of asthma, at a stage when symptoms are occasional and mild.[10–14]

More important than the actual number or proportions of cells is the state of activation of the cells as assessed by a variety of immunochemical methods.[13,17,18] The presence of a number of cytokines has been shown to be important in orchestrating and modulating events in the airways in asthma.[25] Cells from BAL in asthma patients demonstrate a cytokine profile consistent with a TH_2-like phenotype with increased expression of interleukin (IL-)4 involved in local immunoglobulin E regulation and of IL-5 and granulocyte macrophage colony stimulating factor (GM-CSF), which promote eosinophil recruitement and activate and prolong the survival of mature eosinophils, thus contributing to the inflammation seen in asthma.[26,27] Other markers of inflammation such as eosinophilic cationic protein (ECP), major basic protein (MBP), albumin, fibrinogen[6,7,8,10] and mediators such as histamine and sulphidopeptide leukotrienes have all been found in increased concentrations in lavage fluid from asthmatic airways.[28]

The intensity of the eosinophilic inflammation can be related to the severity of asthma,[12] measured as symptom scores,[12] or airway hyperresponsiveness.[29]

The inflammatory picture with BAL eosinophilia and eosinophil activation found in asthmatics under basic non-challenged conditions has been accentuated when BAL has been performed after allergen challenge both endobronchial and by inhalation.[30,31]

Interpretation of BAL Results

The cell findings of a predominantly eosinophil inflammation have been very consistent in all asthma studies in subjects with a mild to moderately severe asthma despite variations in subject characteristics, a number of technical factors pertaining to the BAL procedure and specimen handling.[6–8,10,12,13,18] The interpretation of cell findings has not been difficult. However, interpretation of levels or concentrations of soluble substances measured in BAL fluid has to be made with some caution and results here are not as consistent as those of cell findings.[32–35] The dilution factor for the instilled and recovered BAL fluid is not known. Not all instilled fluid is recovered. There is no satisfactory internal or external marker yet available to accurately assess the BAL dilution factor. Urea has been suggested as internal marker but has been shown to pass very quickly into the newly instilled lavage fluid and is thus unsuitable. The "dwell" time of the instilled fluid should theoretically be standardized, but this is probably not feasible as the most important factor–the lung permeability–likely varies between conditions and also between individuals. Rather, a practical approach should be applied and quantitative results expressed as amounts per ml giving full data on instillate och recovery volumes and thus facilitating interpretation.

BRONCHIAL BIOPSIES IN ASTHMA

The first report on bronchoscopy where bronchial biopsies have been obtained in live asthmatics was published in 1960 by Glynn and Michaels.[36] They described pathological findings in the bronchial mucosa which previously only had been seen in autopsy studies of patients who had died from or with asthma.[37,38] The pathological changes included increased mucus secretion, goblet cell hyperplasia, loss of surface epithelium, a thickened reticular layer of the basement membrane, oedema, an increased smooth muscle mass and an increased cellular infiltrate consisting of eosinophils and lymphocytes.

In the late 1980s, after initial bronchoscopy studies in asthmatics in which BAL had been performed, more widespread study of biopsy material from asthmatics with mild to moderately severe asthma has been undertaken.[5,9,11,12,14–19] These studies have confirmed that a similar pathology as that of autopsy studies is present early in the course of asthma and also in asthmatics without current symptoms of asthma.

With increasing experience of the procedure, studies with multiple biopsies from each event and over time to assess treatment,[10,15,39–41] biopsies from more severe asthmatics[42] and biopsies after allergen challenge[18,30] have been performed. Recently, studies in severe corticosteroid-dependent asthmatics have been undertaken where transbronchial biopsies in addition to endobronchial biopsies have been obtained.[42,43]

Endobronchial mucosal biopsies are obtained from central airways as the carinae of a lobar, segmental or subsegmental bronchus under direct bronchoscopic vision. As the vast majority of studies have used fibreoptic bronchoscopy the biopsies are small, 2–3 mm in diameter, and most often 3–6 biopsies are obtained at the same occasion. Even if multiple mucosal biopsies are obtained during one bronchoscopy the representation of the whole airway surface area can be discussed. There is an intrasubject variability in findings of inflammatory parameters between anatomical sites[44,45]

The handling and fixation of the biopsies should be done immediately according to a predetermined protocol and all vials and solutions for the processing should be prepared in advance. In addition to conventional histological examination, biopsies can be fixed for electron microscopy or *in situ* hybridization or prepared and frozen for immuno-histochemistry.

BIOPSY FINDINGS IN ASTHMA

The results from the bronchial biopsy studies have provided information on airway morphology and confirmed the characteristic pathological picture consisting of a patchy and varied loss of surface epithelium, thickening of the reticular layer of the basement membrane and an increased cellular infiltrate in the mucosa of mainly eosinophils but often mast cells and T-lymphocytes as well.[5,11,14–18,39–43] Activation of eosinophils and T-lymphocytes together with upregulation of several proinflammatory cytokines such as IL-5 and GM-CSF have been found in the bronchial mucosa in parallel to findings in BAL.[11,13,17,18] In the recent studies where transbronchial biopsies have been added to endobronchial biopsies and BAL, a more intense eosinophilia has been noted in the peripheral part of the lung.[43]

The thickening of the reticular layer of basement membrane or the "subepithelial fibrosis" has been shown to be due to an increased deposition of collagens and glucoproteins and, together with the increased muscle mass seen in chronic asthma, is suggested to be a part of the remodelling process, i.e. the structural changes present in longstanding asthma with persistent hyperresponsiveness.[46–48]

Due to the invasive nature of bronchoscopy there have been few studies in which more severe asthmatics have been investigated. In a recent study, severe glucocorticosteroid dependent asthmatics were investigated with BAL, endo- and transbronchial biopsies.[42] The results showed a neutrophilic inflammation and not an eosinophilic predominance. This is seen in BAL, in the endobronchial biopsies from the central airways and in the peripheral airways seen in the transbronchial biopsies. The reasons for this discrepancy are not known. The neutrophilia could be due to the steroid treatment or other unknown reasons and requires further studies.

BRONCHOALVEOLAR LAVAGE VERSUS BRONCHIAL BIOPSIES

The information received from BAL and bronchial biopsies is not identical but rather complementary and dynamic events in the airways can be studied by combining the techniques.[10,11,15,18]

BRONCHOSCOPY IN TREATMENT STUDIES

There are several studies in which the airway inflammation in bronchial biopsies and/or BAL has been evaluated after treatment with anti-inflammatory therapy such as inhaled or oral corticosteroids.[11,14,15,39–42] These studies have shown that the anti-inflammatory treatment can affect certain features of inflammation such as restore the bronchial epithelium, decrease the cellular infiltrate and decrease the number of activated cells, while other features such as the thickening of the reticular layer of the basement membrane have been unaffected. However, in a recent study a decrease in the thickness of the reticular layer of the basement membrane was seen after 6 months of inhaled corticosteroid.[48] In another recent study, one of the glucoproteins shown to be present in the reticular basement membrane – tenascin – and assumed to be involved in the remodelling process in chronic asthma, was shown to be reduced by an inhaled corticosteroid.[49]

Whether treatment indeed can affect all aspects of inflammation even those which to date have been considered not possible to influence, if introduced early in the course of disease, remains to be resolved.

CLINICAL USE OF BRONCHOSCOPY IN ASTHMA?

Bronchoscopy with BAL and/or bronchial biopsy is a research investigation in asthma and not a clinical routine procedure either in the diagnosis or in the evaluation of the disease. A lot of knowledge about asthma pathogenesis has been gained from the many studies which have used this invasive technique to investigate the inflammation in asthma. There is a definite need for means to evaluate and monitor inflammation in asthma, but bronchoscopy is not likely to ever be a routine investigation due to its invasive nature. The examination of induced sputum might be such a method more easily applicable (discussed in Chapters 10 and 14). However, long-term studies will have to show that close monitoring of inflammation by whatever means and change of therapy accordingly, will give a better outcome than thorough clinical assessment with history and lung function.

There are no controlled studies to show the value of BAL and/or bronchial biopsies in the diagnosis and follow-up of asthma. There are exceptional clinical instances where bronchoscopy with BAL or bronchial biopsies might possibly aid the diagnosis and evaluation of asthma. Such exceptions could be the odd patient with difficult to treat asthma where the diagnosis might be challenged, or a patient considered to be "steroid-resistant" where other anti-inflammatory agents (methotrexate or cyclosporin) might be considered. If bronchoscopy is considered the procedure should be performed in accordance with the guidelines of its use in asthma, and at a centre which can provide the proper expertise for both the procedure as such, and for handling and processing the obtained specimens properly.

KEY POINTS

1 Bronchoscopy with bronchoalveolar lavage and/or bronchial biopsies is a research investigation in asthmatics.

2 Results from bronchoscopy studies have greatly increased the knowlegde about airway inflammation in asthma.

3 Cell findings of an eosinophil dominated inflammation in mild to moderately severe asthma have been consistent through many studies.

4 Interpretation of amounts or concentrations of soluble substances in BAL-fluid are difficult and more standardized ways to express results are needed.

5 There is a need for methods to evaluate and monitor inflammation and effects of treatment in an easy and reliable way – bronchoscopy is too invasive to be such a method.

REFERENCES

1. Zöllner F. Gustav Killian, father of bronchoscopy. *Arch Otolaryngol* 1985; 82: 656–9.

2. Ikeda S. Flexible bronchofiberscope. *Ann Otolaryngol* 1970; 79: 916–23.

3. Zavala DC. Diagnostic fiberoptic bronchoscopy. Techniques and results of biopsy in 600 patients. *Chest* 1975; 68 (1): 12–19.

4. Reynolds HY. Bronchoalveolar lavage. *Am Rev Respir Dis* 1987; 135(1): 250–63.

5. Laitinen LA, Heino M, Laitinen A, Kava T, Haahtela T. Damage of the airway epithelium and bronchial reactivity in patients with asthma. *Am Rev Res Dis* 1985; 131: 599–606.

6. DeMonchy JGR, Kauffman HF, Venge P *et al.* Bronchoalveolar lavage eosinophilia during allergen-induced late asthmatic reactions. *Am Rev Respir Dis* 1985; 136: 373–6.

7. Kirby JG, Hargreave FE, Gleich GJ, O'Byrne PM. Bronchoalveolar lavage cell profiles of asthmatic and non-asthmatic subjects. *Am Rev Respir Dis* 1987; 136: 379–83.

8. Wardlaw AJ, Dunnette S, Gleich GJ, Collins JV, Kay AB. Eosinophils and mast cells in bronchoalveolar lavage in subjects with mild asthma. Relationship to bronchial hyperreactivity. *Am Rev Respir Dis* 1988; 137: 62–9.

9. Jeffery PK, Wardlaw AJ, Nelson FC, Collins JV, Kay AB. Bronchial biopsies in asthma. An ultrastructural quantitative study and correlation with hyperreactivity. *Am Rev Respir Dis* 1989; 149: 1745–53.

10. Ädelroth E, Rosenhall L, Johansson SÅ, Linden M, Venge P. Inflammatory cells and eosinophilic activity in asthmatics investigated by bronchoalveolar lavage. The effects of antiasthmatic treatment with budesonide or terbutaline. *Am Rev Respir Dis* 1990; 142: 91–9.

11. ✪ Djukanovic R, Roche WR, Wilson JW *et al*. Mucosal inflammation in asthma. State of the art. *Am Rev Respir Dis* 1990; 142: 434–57.

12. Bousquet J, Chanez P, Lacoste JM *et al*. Eosinophilic inflammation in asthma. *New Engl J Med* 1990; 323: 1016–18.

13. Walker C, Kaegi MK, Braun P, Blaser K. Activated T cells and eosinophilia in bronchoalveolar lavages from subjects with asthma correlated with disease activity. *J Allergy Clin Immunol* 1991; 88: 935–42.

14. Laitinen LA, Laitinen A, Haahtela T. A comparative study of the effects of an inhaled corticosteroid, budesonide, and a β_2-agonist, terbutaline, on airway inflammation in newly diagnosed asthma. A randomized, double-blind, parallel-group controlled trial. *J Allergy Clin Immunol* 1992; 90: 32–42.

15. Jeffery PK, Godfrey RW, Ädelroth E, Nelson F, Rogers A, Johansson SÅ. Effects of treatment on airway thickening of basement membrane reticular collagen in asthma. A quantitative light and electron microscopic study. *Am Rev Respir Dis* 1992; 145: 890–99.

16. Laitinen LA, Laitinen A, Haahtela T. Airway mucosal inflammation even in patients with newly diagnosed asthma. *Am Rev Respir Dis* 1993; 147: 697–704.

17. Bentley AM, Menz G, Storz C *et al*. Identification of T-lymphocytes, macrophages and activated eosinophils in the bronchial mucosa in intrinsic asthma. *Am Rev Respir Dis* 1992; 146: 500–506.

18. Woolley KL, Ädelroth E, Woolley MJ, Ellis R, Jordana M, O'Byrne PM. Granulocyte-macrophage colony-stimulating factor, eosinophils and eosinophilic cationic protein in subjects with and without mild, stable atopic asthma. *Eur Respir J* 1994; 7: 1576–84.

19. Berkman N, Krishnan VL, Gilbey T *et al*. Expression of RANTES mRNA and protein in airways of patients with mild asthma. *Am J Respir Crit Care Med* 1996; 154: 1804–11.

20. ✪ Smith DL, Deshazo RD. Bronchoalveolar lavage in asthma. An update and perspective. *Am Rev Respir Dis* 1993; 148: 523–32.

21. ✪ Global strategy for asthma management and prevention. WHO/NHLB Workshop Report. National Institutes of Health, National Heart, Lung and Blood Institute, 1995. Publication Number 95–3659.

22. ✪ Workshop Summaries and Guidelines. Investigative use of bronchoscopy, lavage, and bronchial biopsies in asthma and other lung diseases. *Clin Exp Allergy* 1991; 21: 533–40.

23. Klech H, Pohl W (eds). Clinical guidelines and indications for bronchoalveolar lavage (BAL): a report of the European Society of Pneumology Task Group on BAL. *Eur Respir J* 1990; 3: 937–74.

24. Haslam PL, Baughman RP (eds). Guidelines for measurement of acellular components and recommendations for standardization of bronchoalveolar lavage. *Eur Respir J* 1999; 14: 245–8.

25. Calhoun WJ, Kelly J. Cytokines in the respiratory tract. In: Chung KF, Barnes PJ (eds). *Pharmacology of the Respiratory Tract*. New York: Marcel Dekker, 1993: 258–88.

26. Walker C, Bode E, Boer L, Hansel TT, Blaser K, Virchow JC Jr. Allergic and nonallergic asthmatics have distinct patterns of T-cell activation and cytokine production in peripheral blood and broncholveolar lavage. *Am Rev Respir Dis* 1992; 146: 109–15.

27. Tang C, Rolland JM, Ward C, Quan B, Walters EH. IL-5 production by bronchoalveolar lavage and peripheral blood mononuclear cells in asthma and atopy. *Eur Respir J* 1997; 10: 624–32.

28. Chung KF. Inflammatory mediators in asthma. In: O'Byrne PM (ed). *Asthma as an Inflammatory Disease*. New York: Marcel Dekker, 1990: 150–83.

29. Bradley BL, Azzawi M, Jacobson M *et al.* Eosinophils, T-lymphocytes, mast cells, neutrophils and macrophages in bronchial biopsy specimens from atopic subjects with asthma: comparison with biopsy specimens from atopic subjects without asthma and normal control subjects and relationship to bronchial hyperresponsiveness. *J Allergy Clin Immunol* 1991; 88: 664–74.

30. Woolley KL, Ädelroth E, Woolley MJ, Ellis R, Jordana M, O'Byrne PM. Effects of allergen challenge on eosinophils, eosinophil cationic protein, and granulocyte-macrophage colony-stimulating factor in mild asthma. *Am J Respir Crit Care Med* 1995; 151: 1915–24.

31. Liu MC, Hubbard WC, Proud D *et al.* Immediate and late inflammatory responses to ragweed antigen challenge of the peripheral airways in allergic asthmatics. Cellular, mediator and permeability changes. *Am Rev Respir Dis* 1991; 144: 51–6.

32. Haslam PL. BAL standardization and measurement of acellular components. *Eur Respir Rev* 1998; 8(64): 1066–71.

33. Kelly CA, Fenwick JD, Corris PA, Fleetwood A, Hendrick DJ, Walters EH. Fluid dynamics during bronchoalveolar lavage. *Am Rev Respir Dis* 1988; 138: 81–4.

34. Ward C, Duddridge M, Fenwich J *et al.* The origin of water and urea sampled at bronchoalveolar lavage in asthmatics and control subjects. *Am Rev Respir Dis* 1992; 146: 444–7.

35. Rennard SI, Aalbers R, Bleeker E *et al.* Bronchoalveolar lavage: performance, sampling procedure, processing and assessment. *Eur Respir J* 1998; 11 (suppl. 26): 13s–15s.

36. Glynn AA, Michaels L. Bronchial biopsy in chronic bronchitis and asthma. *Thorax* 1960; 15: 142–53.

37. Earle BV. Fatal bronchial asthma. *Thorax* 1953; 8: 195–206.

38. Dunnill MS. The pathology of asthma with special reference to changes in the bronchial mucosa. *J Pathol* 1960; 13: 27–33.

39. Booth H, Richmond I, Ward C, Gardiner PV, Harkawat R, Walters EH. Effects of high dose inhaled fluticasone propionate on airway inflammation in asthma. *Am J Respir Crit Care Med* 1995; 152: 45–52.

40. Robinson D, Hamid O, Ying S *et al.* Prednisolone treatment in asthma is associated with modulation of bronchoalveolar lavage cell interleukin-4, interleukin-5 and interferon-γ cytokine gene expression. *Am Rev Respir Dis* 1993; 148: 401–406.

41. Djukanovic R, Homeyard S, Gratziou C *et al.* The effect of treatment with oral corticosteroids on asthma symptoms and airway inflammation. *Am J Respir Crit Care Med* 1997; 155: 826–32.

42. Wenzel SE, Szefler SJ, Leung SY, Sloan SI, Rex MD, Martin RJ. Bronchoscopic evaluation of severe asthma: persistent neutrophilic inflammation associated with high dose glucocorticoids. *Am J Respir Crit Care Med* 1997; 156: 737–43.

43. Kraft M, Djukanovic R, Wilson S, Holgate ST, Martin RJ. Alveolar tissue inflammation in asthma. *Am J Respir Crit Care Med* 1996; 154: 1505–1510.

44. Robinson DS, Faurschou P, Barnes N, Ädelroth E. Biopsies. Bronchoscopic technique and sampling. *Eur Respir J* 1998; 11 (suppl. 26): 16s–19s.

45. Jeffery PK. The value of bronchial biopsies: assessment of inflammation in asthma and COPD. *Eur Respir Rev* 1998; 8 (64): 1079–1085.

46. ✪ Jeffery PK. Pathology of asthma. In: Kay AB (ed). *Allergy and Allergic Disease*, vol 2. Oxford: Blackwell Science, 1997: 1412–28.

47. Brewster CE, Howarth PH, Djukanovic R, Wilson J, Holgate ST, Roche WR. Myofibroblast and subepithelial fibrosis in bronchial asthma. *Am J Respir Cell Mol Biol* 1990; 3: 507–511.

48. Hoshino M, Nakamura Y, Sim J *et al.* Inhaled corticosteroid reduced lamina reticularis of the basement membrane by modulation of insulin-like growth factor (IGF)-I expression in bronchial asthma. *Clin Exp Allergy* 1998; 28: 568–77.

49. Laitinen A, Altraja A, Kämpe M, Linden M, Virtanen I, Laitinen LA. Tenascin is increased in airway basement membrane of asthmatics and decreased by an inhaled steroid. *Am J Respir Crit Care Med* 1997; 156: 951–8.

Part 3

Assessment and Treatment of Asthma

Chapter 12

Assessment of Asthma Control: Symptoms, Drug Use, PEFR

Jonathan Corne, Nicholas Chanarin and Stephen Holgate

The rising mortality from asthma has emphasized the need to monitor closely the state of patients' disease and their response, or lack of response, to treatment. Monitoring of patients has become the hallmark of both patient-directed and physician-directed care. Central to this is observation of the patient's symptoms but a number of studies have highlighted discrepancies between both the patient's and physician's perception of asthma and objective measurements of the state of the disease. Hence symptom monitoring needs to be backed up by more objective measurements of lung function, such as peak expiratory flow rate (PEFR).

SYMPTOMS

Symptoms associated with asthma include wheeze, dyspnoea, cough and nocturnal waking. They all rely on accurate patient reporting and are difficult to quantify, as individual perception of each is highly subjective.

Dyspnoea

This symptom is not a sensitive indicator of asthma severity and its nature remains poorly understood. Airflow obstruction in asthma is greater during expiration than inspiration, yet only 19% of patients perceive their dyspnoea to be expiratory.[1] During an exacerbation a characteristic feature is a sustained increase in inspiratory muscle activity[2] and it may be that it is this that provides the afferent stimulus interpreted centrally as dyspnoea. Therefore the sensation of dyspnoea probably reflects the effort of breathing rather than airflow obstruction itself.

Wheeze

A wheeze is a high-pitched musical sound that may be present in inspiration or expiration and audible with or without a stethoscope. The noise is produced by air moving at a relatively high speed through an airway that is narrowed almost to the point of closure. The walls are thought to flutter so producing a high-pitched musical note.[3] Mathematical models lend support to this theory[3,4] and predict that wheeze is always accompanied by flow limitation but that flow limitation is not always accompanied by wheeze. This is borne out in clinical observation where it is well recognized that episodes of asthma do not always feature wheezing. Baughman and Loudon[5] studied a group of 33 patients in whom wheeze had not been observed and challenged them with histamine or allergen. Two-thirds of these patients showed no wheeze or dyspnoea despite developing marked airflow obstruction.

Patients are not always aware that wheeze is present. Shim and Williams[6] examined 93 patients on 320 occasions. During 165 occasions of patient-reported wheeze, auscultation also demonstrated wheezing on 95% of occasions. During 132 occasions when the patient was not aware of any wheezing, wheeze was heard by auscultation 28% of the time. The presence of wheeze, as determined by auscultation, was significantly associated with lower PEFR, but the range of PEFR was great. The investigators noted that biphasic wheezing was associated with lower PEFR than expiratory wheeze alone. The proportion of the respiratory cycle occupied by wheeze correlates closely with forced expiratory volume in 1 s (FEV_1) ($r=0.893$, $P<0.001$),[5] but unfortunately this index is not accurately assessable by either the patient or clinician. It is the only sign that correlates with airflow obstruction but does not lend itself to subjective assessment.

Cough

Cough is a defence mechanism that protects against aspiration. It is associated with bronchoconstriction and mucous secretion, which enhance its effectiveness. Nerve impulses that originate mainly in the proximal bronchial tree are carried by the vagus nerve.[7,8] The trigeminal, glossopharyngeal and phrenic nerves also carry afferent information. The efferent pathway is mainly autonomic and carried by the recurrent laryngeal, phrenic and spinal nerves. In human subjects with asthma, inhalation challenge produces both bronchoconstriction and cough.[9,10] The two mechanisms appear closely related and can potentiate each other but are not interdependent.[11] For instance, inhaled lignocaine blocks the cough induced by aerosolized water but not the associated bronchoconstriction, while sodium cromoglycate blocks bronchoconstriction but not the cough.[12]

Cough is a very common complaint and not specific to asthma. It has been described as the only symptom in so-called "cough-variant asthma" where it is the sole manifestation of asthma.[13,14] This type of asthma is thought to be characterized by central airways narrowing, the site at which cough receptors are most abundant.[15]

Cough may indicate the presence of asthma but does not correlate with the severity of the underlying disease.

Nocturnal Waking

It is well recognized that circadian rhythms affect pulmonary function in both normal and asthmatic subjects with a decline of pulmonary function being evident in the early hours of the morning. A sign of worsening asthma can be the appearance of symptoms during these hours, typically awakening the patient at night or being present on waking first thing in the morning. A full enquiry into asthma symptoms is not complete until details of night-time and early morning symptoms have been sought. Indeed, the presence of nocturnal asthma correlates strongly with disease activity.

PATIENTS' AND PHYSICIANS' PERCEPTIONS

Several studies have examined the accuracy of patients' perceptions of the severity of their asthma either by artificially changing airway resistance or by comparing patients' estimation of their peak flow with measured values. Rubinfield and Pain[16,17] induced bronchoconstriction through methacholine challenge in 19 asthmatic volunteers. Bronchoprovocation was undertaken to the point when tightness in the chest was just perceived and static lung volumes, spirometric FEV_1 and airway conductance measured and compared with base-

line; 15 of the 19 subjects could detect changes of 25% or less in FEV_1 and four could detect changes of less than 10%. However, four subjects could only detect changes of between 25 and 50% in FEV_1. Changes in small airway resistance (R_{aw}) and lung volumes were perceived in a similar fashion but were proportionally greater than changes in FEV_1 with some subjects experiencing increases of more than 50% in static lung volumes with only a modest development of symptoms. The obvious conclusion was that whereas some asthmatic patients were able to detect changes in R_{aw} greater than 20%, 4 of 19 subjects could not. Presumably this group are at particular risk from the development of unheralded attacks of asthma, making continual and objective measurements of lung function vital.

Other studies have asked asthmatic subjects to assess the severity of their asthma by predicting their PEFR. In a study of 255 patients 60% showed no correlation between visual analogue scores and simultaneous PEFR measurements. In a study of 75 patients Shim and Williams[18] demonstrated a closer correlation between estimated and measured PEFR, with 63% of estimates being within 20% of measured values. However, this study recruited from a hospital- rather than community-based population and the subjects were likely to have had more experience in measuring peak flows and more education about their asthma. Indeed all subjects had had previous experience of using a peak flow meter. An interesting feature of the Shim and Williams study was that 17 patients were examined by physicians whom were then asked to estimate a PEFR. Only 44% of estimates were within 20% of the measured value thus showing the difficulty, outside the acute attack, of predicting PEFR.

In a more recent study Teeter et al.[19] determined the relationship between asthma symptoms and pulmonary function in a cohort of 67 adult patients with chronic asthma. In this study patients graded symptoms of cough, dyspnoea, chest tightness, wheezing, sputum production and nocturnal awakening. There was no significant relationship between total asthma symptom scores and FEV_1 though there was a trend towards significance between FEV_1 and subjective wheeze ($r = 0.237$; $P = 0.089$). Patients tended to overestimate their level of airflow obstruction but also overestimate improvements in PEFR.

A similar result was found in a general practice based study of mild and moderate asthmatic patients.[20] In this study 60% of the participants showed no significant correlation between visual analogue asthma scores and simultaneous PEFR measurements.

PEAK EXPIRATORY FLOW RATE

The nineteenth-century chest physician would conclude his examination by asking the patient to blow out a candle. Donald[21] pointed out that this was a crude means of assessing maximum respiratory velocity and suggested that a "whistle like instrument" be developed to measure this objectively. In 1959 Wright[22] described the Wright peak flow meter (Fig. 12.1), a portable instrument that can be produced commercially and that measures the highest flow rate sustained for at least 10 ms during forced expiration thus providing a measure of large airways resistance. This has subsequently been demonstrated to be easily used and understood by patients.[23]

Several studies have examined the accuracy of peak flow measurements as recorded by the Wright peak flow meter. Meltzer et al.[24] questioned the use of PEFR as a surrogate measurement of FEV_1. They examined 23 stable, treated asthmatic children between 6 and 17 years of age and compared the percentage predicted value of PEFR with the percentage predicted value of FEV_1. Although as a group there was a good correlation between the two (Pearson correlation, coefficient 0.854–0.892) over one-half of patients demonstrated a 10% or greater difference in percentage predicted value between the two measurements and one-third a 20% or greater discrepancy.

A number of investigators have found that certain PEFR meters can give inaccurate measurements of PEFR. For example, the mini-Wright PEFR meter, which is commonly prescribed in the UK, tends to overestimate readings in the mid-range and underestimate readings at the higher range. These errors could in turn lead to errors in the estimate of asthma severity. Indeed Miles et al.[25] studied 127 asthmatic patients for between 15–489 days (median 157.5 days) and showed correction

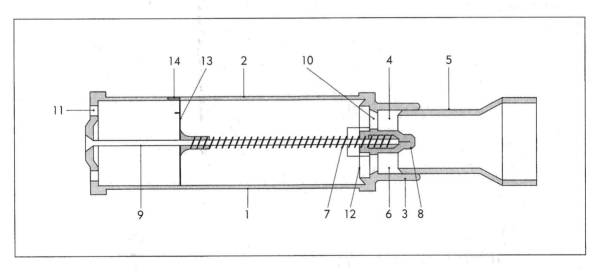

FIGURE 12.1: Diagram of mini-Wright peak-flow meter. The cylindrical body (1) and one end of the instrument are moulded in one piece with a slot (2) down one side. The other end (3) carries a tapered socket (4) which accepts a sterilizable mouthpiece (5) or a disposable cardboard mouthpiece. It has a central hollow boss (6) which houses a tension spring (7). The mouthpiece end is held to the body by a knurled nut (8) screwed on to the threaded end of a central rod (9), the other end of which is secured in the fixed end of the body. Both ends are hexagonal in section to prevent the instrument from rolling and are pierced by a ring of six holes (10, 11) to allow free passage of air. A thin PTFE disc valve (12) is secured to the boss inside the mouthpiece end. The piston (13), which is a light plastic disc with a short sleeve, rides freely on the rod and just clear of the cylinder bore. The scale, which is read vertically, is marked in litres per minute from 60 to 800, but a scale in litres per second to conform with SI units will be available if required. The rider (14) is spring-loaded in the slot with sufficient friction to prevent it overshooting without appreciably affecting movement of the piston. The meter is 5.0 cm in diameter and 15 cm long, and weights 75 g. (Reproduced from Clement Clarke International Ltd, Harlow, Essex, UK).

of PEFR data for the known errors of the meter led to a reduction of the number of days classified as satisfactory asthma control in 72% of participants. The participants in this study all had severe asthma and these results may not be applicable to more mild asthmatic patients.

Further errors in PEFR measurement can be introduced by poor patient technique. Differences in the way the patient blows into the PEFR meter can cause an apparent increase in PEFR measurement.[26] Errors can be reduced by careful observation of patient technique, taking readings with the patient standing, avoiding squeezing the meter and taking the best reading of three.

It is clear from these studies that peak flow meters give a less accurate measure of airway resistance than FEV_1 and should not be used as an alternative. However, they are valuable as a convenient way of monitoring the condition of an asthmatic subject. To do this one needs to look at the changes in PEFR with time.

DIURNAL VARIATION

PEFR has a circadian rhythm both in normal and asthmatic subjects. Hetzel et al.[27] demonstrated PEFR variability in 145 out of 221 normal subjects with a mean amplitude of variation of 8.3% of the mean PEFR. Quackenbass et al.[28] worked out normal limits for variation that were defined in terms of amplitude/mean, this being the amplitude of variation as a percentage of the day's mean PEFR. These limits are shown in Table 12.1. An exaggeration of this diurnal variation is the hallmark of asthma. In the Hertzel study nearly 100% of asthmatic subjects showed diurnal variation

with a mean variation of 50%. In the Quackenbass et al. study there was a very high sensitivity for diagnosed asthma if diurnal variation exceeded the quoted normal limits, with a sensitivity and specificity of 94.5% and 72% respectively for those under 15 years and 70% and 56% for those over 15 years.

Increases in diurnal variation, usually expressed as amplitude of variation as a percentage of mean PEFR, are an important indication of poorly controlled disease. One-third of all patients admitted with asthma show a 50% or greater variation in PEFR. Hertzel et al.[29] studied cases of patients requiring ventilation or dying of their asthma. A feature common to all these patients was the presence of large diurnal swings in PEFR; eight out of the nine patients who sustained a respiratory arrest showed a greater than 50% diurnal variation in PEFR compared with 30% of the total asthma admissions. Interestingly, the standard signs of worsening asthma (heart rate, respiratory rate and absolute PEFR) paralleled the severity of the attack.

Recently the utility of diurnal variation as a measure of asthma severity has been questioned.[30] Most patients are asked to perform PEFR manoeuvres just twice a day yet it has been suggested that recordings need to made at least four times a day if PEFR variation is to be adequately assessed.[31] Furthermore the timing of the recordings is vital and apparent variations in PEFR measurements may be due to small changes in the time the measurement was made rather than reflect genuine changes in asthma control.[31] Also, if monitoring of PEFR is to be of use it requires a level of compliance by the patient which studies have suggested may not be achievable over prolonged periods of time.[32]

Table 12.1: Limits to diurnal changes in PEFR by age group for a reference population. (Adapted from Ref. 28, Official Journal of the American Thoracic Association. ©American Lung Association)

Age group (years)	Diurnal changes (%)	95% percentile	97.5% percentile	Median
6–14	Max./Min.	129.6	140.0	105.0
	Amp./Mean	31.0	37.7	8.2
15–34	Max./Min.	116.7	121.9	102.7
	Amp./Mean	19.0	26.8	5.0
35–65	Max./Min.	118.4	126.0	103.4
	Amp./Mean	19.1	28.8	4.9

DRUG USE

The need for symptom-relieving bronchodilators by patients is a good indicator of the severity of their asthma. Several studies have shown a good correlation between drug use and risk of hospital admission or death; Rea *et al.*[33] showed that the use of three or more categories of drugs was associated with an increased risk of dying of asthma. Nowadays, with asthma management based on the regular use of inhaled steroids, with β_2 agonists reserved for symptomatic relief, the use of the latter, if accurately documented, should provide a reasonable assessment of the patient's clinical state.

PRACTICAL ASSESSMENT

The clinic assessment of the patient must begin with enquiry into symptoms of wheeze, cough, nocturnal awakening and dyspnoea; although not completely reliable, these symptoms will give a good indication of disease severity in many. Nocturnal awakening is a particularly important symptom to elicit.

Regular monitoring of peak flow for a period of at least 3 weeks is an essential part of the diagnosis of asthma and it should be continued if initial results suggest poor control, or suggest low peak flows with little in the way of associated symptoms. Admission to hospital with an asthma attack, recurrent need for oral steroids or persistent symptoms suggest a need for continual peak flow monitoring as an important part of patient assessment. In fact, all patients requiring regular inhaled steroids should undertake monitoring of peak flow since this is the basis of the asthma management plans outlined later. However, many patients find this inconvenient and, if they are asymptomatic, it

is probably reasonable to periodically check 2-week periods of regular peak flows to confirm that their asthma is as well controlled as their symptoms suggest.

Peak flow needs to be checked twice daily if changes in diurnal variation are to be picked up. This is convenient for patients who can keep their peak flow meters by their beds and record readings first thing in the morning and last thing at night, preferably before taking their bronchodilators. The presence of the peak flow meter may also act as useful *aide-mémoire* for the taking of their twice-daily inhaled medication.

ASSESSMENT OF SEVERITY (see Chapter 6)

KEY POINTS

1. Symptoms associated with worsening of asthma are dyspnoea, wheeze, cough and nocturnal wakening, though patients perception of these are not always an accurate reflection of the state of their airways.

2. A small but important group of asthmatic subjects may develop severe airflow limitation without a marked change in symptoms.

3. Changes in peak flow are a convenient way of monitoring the severity of asthma but absolute peak flows are not as reliable as FEV_1.

4. Accurate documentation of medication use may provide useful early warning of an asthma attack.

REFERENCES

1. Morris MJ. Asthma: expiratory dyspnoea? *BMJ* 1981; 283: 838–9.

2. Muller N, Bryan AC, Zamel N. Tonic inspiratory muscle activity as a cause of hyperventilation in asthma. *J Appl Physiol* 1981; 50: 279–82.

3. ✪ Loudon RG, Murphy RLH. Wheezing. In: Weiss EB, Stein M (eds). *Asthma: Mechanisms and Therapeutics*, 3rd edn. Boston: Little, Brown and Co., 1993: 650–4.

4. Grotberg JB, Davis SH. Fluid dynamic flapping of a collapsible channel: sound generation and flow limitation. *J Biomech* 1980; 13: 219–30.

5. Baughman RP, Loudon RG. Lung sound analysis for continuous evaluation of airflow obstruction in asthma. *Chest* 1985; 88: 364–8.

6. Shim CS, Williams HM. Relationship of wheezing to the severity of obstruction in asthma. *Arch Intern Med* 1983; 143: 890–2.

7. Widdicombe JG. Physiology of cough. In: Braga PC, Allegra L (eds). *Cough*. New York: Raven Press, 1989: 3–25.

8. Karlsson JA, Sant-Ambrogio G, Widdicombe J. Afferent neural pathways in cough and reflex bronchoconstriction. *J Appl Physiol* 1988; 65: 1007–23.

9. Chausow AM, Banner AS. Comparison of the tussive effects of histamine and methacholine in humans. *J Appl Physiol* 1983; 55: 541–6.

10. Simonsson BG, Jacobs FM, Nadel JA. Role of autonomic nervous system and the cough reflex in the increased responsiveness of airways in patients with obstructive airways disease. *J Clin Invest* 1967; 46: 1812–8.

11. Editorial. Cough and wheeze in asthma: are they interdependent? *Lancet* 1988; i: 447–8.

12. Sheppard D, Rizk NW, Boushey HA, Bethel RA. Mechanisms of cough and bronchoconstriction induced by distilled water aerosol. *Am Rev Respir Dis* 1983; 127: 691–4.

13. ✪ Corrao WM, Braman SS, Irwin RS. Chronic cough as the sole presenting manifestation of bronchial asthma. *N Engl J Med* 1979; 300: 633–7.

14. Johnson D, Osborn LM. Cough variant asthma: a review of the clinical literature. *J Asthma* 1991; 28: 85–90.

15. McFadden ER. Exertional dyspnoea and cough as preludes to attacks of bronchial asthma. *N Engl J Med* 1975; 292: 555–9.

16. Rubinfield AR. Relationship between bronchial reactivity, airways caliber and severity of asthma. *Am Rev Respir Dis* 1977; 115: 381.

17. ✪ Rubinfield AR, Pain MCF. Perception of asthma. *Lancet* 1976; ii: 822–4.

18. ✪ Shim CS, Williams MH. Evaluation of the severity of asthma: patients versus physicians. *Am J Med* 1980; 68: 11–3.

19. Teeter JG, Bleecker E. Relationship between airway obstruction and respiratory symptoms in adult asthmatics. *Chest* 1998; 113: 272–7.

20. Kendrick AH, Higgs CMB, Whitfield MJ, Laszio C. Accuracy of perception of severity of asthma: patients treated in general practice. *BMJ* 1993; 307: 422–4.

21. Donald KW. *BMJ* 1953; 1: 415.

22. Wright BM, McKerrow CB. Maximum forced expiratory flow rate as a measure of ventilatory capacity. *BMJ* 1959; 1041–7.

23. ✪ Hetzel MR, Williams IP, Shakespeare RM. Can patients keep their own peak flow records reliably? *Lancet* 1979; 1(8116):597–9.

24. Meltzer A, Smolensky MH. D'Alenzo GE, Harrist RB, Scott PH. An assessment of peak expiratory flow as a surrogate measurement of FEV_1 in stable asthmatic children. *Chest* 1989; 96: 329–33.

25. Miles JF, Tunnicliffe W, Cayton RM, Ayres JG, Miller MR. Potential effects of correction of inaccuracies of the mini-Wright peak expiratory flow meter on the use of an asthma self-management plan. *Thorax* 1996; 51: 403–406.

26. Strayhorn V, Leeper K, Tolley E, Self T. Elevation of peak expiratory flow by a "spitting maneuver": Measured with five peak flowmeters. *Chest* 1998; 113: 1134–6.

27. Hetzel MR, Clark TJH. Comparison of normal and asthmatic circadian rhythms in peak expiratory flow rate. *Thorax* 1980; 35: 732–8.

28. Quackenbass JJ, Lebowitz MD, Kryzanowski M. The normal range of diurnal changes in peak expiratory flow rates. *Am Rev Respir Dis* 1991; 143: 323–30.

29. Hetzel MR, Clark TJH, Branthwaite MA. Asthma: analysis of sudden deaths and ventilatory arrests in hospital. *BMJ* 1977; 1: 808–11.

30. Reddel H, Jenkins C, Woolcock A. Diurnal variability-time to change asthma guidelines. *BMJ* 1999; 319: 45–7.

31. Gannon PFG, Newton DT, Pantin CFA, Burge PS. Effect of the number of peak expiratory flow readings per day on the estimation of diurnal variation. *Thorax* 1998; 53: 790–92.

32. Cote J, Cartier A, Malo J-L, Rouleau M, Boulet L-P.

Compliance with peak expiratory flow monitoring in home management of asthma. *Chest* 1998; 113: 968–72.

33. ✪ Rea HR, Scragg R, Jackson R, Beaglehole R, Fenwick J, Sutherland DC. A case-control study of deaths from asthma. *Thorax* 1986; 41: 833–9.

Chapter 13

Assessment of Asthma Control: Quality of Life

Elizabeth Juniper

INTRODUCTION

Many asthma clinicians now recognize the importance of incorporating an assessment of health-related quality of life (HRQL) into their clinical studies and clinical practice. Conventional measures of asthma severity and asthma control, such as spirometry, medication use, symptom severity, airway hyper-responsiveness and sputum analysis, provide valuable information about the status of the airways, but they tell us little about the functional impairments (physical, emotional and social) that are important to asthma patients in their everyday lives. One of the aims of treating patients with asthma should be to ensure that the functional problems that are important to the patients themselves are identified and that improvement of patient well-being is included in the treatment plan.

HEALTH-RELATED QUALITY OF LIFE

The quality of a person's life is usually considered in terms of its richness, completeness and contentedness and there are a number of factors that are important in determining this sense of well-being. These factors include good health, a secure social and occupational environment, financial security, strong spirituality, self-confidence and strong, supportive family relationships. Each factor on its own may be a determinant of a person's quality of life and each factor is also closely interrelated with each of the other factors. For instance, a patient will often be able to cope with asthma better if she has good family support, a strong faith and the financial ability to acquire nourishing food, shelter and treatment.

In recent years, the term "health-related quality of life" (HRQL) has emerged as an important component of health care; HRQL can be considered as that part of a person's overall quality of life that is determined primarily by health status and which can be influenced by clinical interventions. The definition by Schipper and colleagues is both simple and focused:[1] "the functional effects of an illness and its consequent therapy upon a patient, as perceived by the patient". The final phrase is important because it emphasises that these are the impairments that the patients themselves consider important.

THE IMPORTANCE OF HRQL IN ASTHMA

It has been proposed that there are three reasons for treating patients: to prevent mortality; to reduce the probability of future morbidity; and to improve patient well-being.[2] Most conventional clinical measures of asthma control and severity, such as spirometry, medication requirements, symptoms, airway hyper-responsiveness and sputum cells, assess the status of the airways and are primarily used to gauge whether the first two goals are being achieved. In the past, it was frequently assumed that these measures also provided insight into patients' well-being. Certainly, patients with very severe asthma tend to have a worse HRQL than patients with milder disease but there is a growing body of evidence showing that correlations between clinical measures and how patients feel and how they are able to function in daily activities are only weak to moderate[3–6] (Table 13.1). Therefore, to obtain a complete picture of a patient's health status, HRQL must be measured in conjunction with the conventional clinical indices.

Table 13.1: Longitudinal correlations between HRQL and measures of airway function in adults with asthma. (From Juniper EF, Johnston PR, Borkhoff CM et al. Quality of life in asthma clinical trials: comparison of salmeteral and salbutamol. Am J Respir Crit Care Med 1995; 151: 66–70, with permission. Official Journal of the American Thoracic Association. © American Lung Association.)

Change in clinical outcomes	Change in Asthma Quality of Life Questionnaire scores				
	Overall HRQL	Symptoms	Emotions	Activities	Environment
PEF – morning	0.58	0.60	0.56	0.43	0.42
PEF – evening	0.48	0.50	0.43	0.36	0.40
Morning symptoms	0.47	0.49	0.45	0.38	0.28
Disturbance-free nights	0.28	0.30	0.26	0.20	0.17
Daytime symptoms	0.54	0.52	0.54	0.45	0.44
FEV_1	0.38	0.36	0.37	0.33	0.28
Salbutamol use	0.43	0.41	0.46	0.35	0.29

IMPAIRMENTS OF HRQL IN PATIENTS WITH ASTHMA

Adults

Extensive HRQL research has highlighted the functional impairments that are most troublesome to adults with asthma[7–15] (Table 13.2). Certainly, they are bothered by the symptoms themselves, such as shortness of breath, chest tightness, wheeze and cough. Many patients have problems with physical activities such as sports, hurrying, going upstairs and shopping. Allergens may cause difficulties with daily activities such as household chores, outdoor activities and hobbies. Environmental stimuli, such as cigarette smoke, strong smells and troublesome weather conditions, may limit family activities and visiting friends. Asthma patients are bothered by not being able to get a good night's sleep and often feel tired. In addition, they experience

Table 13.2: Functional impairments most important to adults with asthma. (From Juniper EF, Guyatt GH, Epstein RS et al. Evaluation of impairment of health-related quality of life in asthma: development of a questionnaire for use in clinical trials. Thorax 1992; 47: 76–83, with permission)

Symptoms	Emotions	Activities	Environment
Short of breath	Afraid of not having medications available	Exercise/ sports	Cigarettes
Chest tightness	Afraid of getting out of breath	Hurrying	Dust
Wheeze	Concerned about the need to use medications	Social activities	Air pollution
Cough	Frustrated	Pets	Cold air
Tired		Housework	Pollen

fears and concerns about having asthma and become frustrated by not being able to do the things they would like to do. Several studies have now shown that women tend to experience greater impairment of HRQL than men with similar clinical asthma severity.[6,7,9,12,16] Occupational asthma causes its own special problems with HRQL being poorer in these patients than clinically matched patients whose asthma is not of occupational origin.[17]

Children

The burden of illness and functional impairments experienced by children with asthma are similar to those experienced by adults (Table 13.3). In addition, children are troubled because they cannot integrate fully with their peers, they feel isolated and left out and this often causes them to feel frustrated, irritable, sad and angry.[18–25] There is growing evidence that parents of children with asthma often have a poor perception of the problems and emotions that are troubling the child and so it is essential to obtain HRQL information directly from the child.[26–29] Children as young as 6 years have little difficulty understanding HRQL questionnaires and they are able to provide reliable and valid responses.[30,31]

SELECTING AN HRQL INSTRUMENT

We now have a range of instruments for measuring HRQL in both adults and children with asthma. There is no *best* instrument. Each one has been developed for a different purpose and has different measurement properties.

Types of Instrument

Generic Versus Specific Questionnaires There are two types of HRQL questionnaire, generic and specific. Generic health status questionnaires (health profiles) are designed to be applicable to patients in all health states. Among the most commonly used and the best validated in adults are the Sickness Impact Profile (SIP),[32] the Medical Outcomes Survey Short Form 36 (SF-36),[33] the Nottingham Health Profile[34] and the Dartmouth COOP charts.[35] In recent years, shorter versions of these original instruments have become available. For children, there is the Functional Status II (R) Scale [FSII(R)][36] and the Child Health Questionnaire.[37]

A strength of generic instruments is that burden of illness can be compared across different medical conditions.[38,39] However, because these questionnaires are required to be broad in their comprehensiveness to cover all medical conditions, they have very little depth and, as a result, impairments that are important to patients with a specific condition, may not be included. Consequently, in many conditions, including asthma, generic instruments may be unresponsive to small but important changes in HRQL.[4,30] Therefore, the use of generic instruments in clinical trials and clinical practice, where one wants to examine the effect of treatment within individuals or groups of patients, is limited.

This lack of responsiveness of generic instruments has lead to the development of specific instruments. These instruments may be specific for a group of patients (e.g. the elderly), a particular function (e.g. pain, sexual function) or a disease. Disease-specific questionnaires measure the problems and limitations that patients with a specific disease experience in their day-to-day lives. They are developed by asking the patients themselves about the impairments that are most important to them and therefore they focus on the problems for which patients seek help. In asthma, disease-specific instruments are consistently more responsive than generic ones to clinically important changes in HRQL.[4,30]

Utilities These instruments measure the value or utility that either the patient or society places on various health states. They are popular with health economists not only because they provide a single number representing HRQL from 0 = death to 1 = perfect health

Table 13.3: Functional impairments most important to children with asthma. (From Juniper EF, Guyatt GH, Feeny DH et al. Measuring quality of life in children with asthma. Qual Life Res 1996; 5: 35–46, with kind permission fom Kluwer Academic Publishers.)

Symptoms	Activities	Emotions
Short of breath	Sports and games	Feel different and left out
Chest tightness	Activities with friends	Frustrated
Cough	Playing with pets	Angry
Wheeze	School activities	Sad
Tired	Sleeping	Frightened/anxious

but also because the majority of instruments meet the assumptions for utility theory and can be used for estimating Quality Adjusted Life Years (QALYs).[40] For measuring the value that patients themselves place on their own health state, there are the Standard Gamble,[40] the Time Trade Off[40] and the Feeling Thermometer.[40] For measuring the value that society places on various health states, there are the Quality of Well-being Scale,[41] the Multiattribute Health Utilities Index[42] and the EuroQol.[43] For a long time, these instruments were only used in generic form, i.e. to be applicable in all medical conditions and in this form they have the same weakness as the generic health profiles, in that they are unresponsive to important changes.[4,30] Recently, the Standard Gamble and the Feeling Thermometer have been modified for use as disease-specific instruments in children with asthma and appear to have improved measurement properties.[30] Even more recent data have revealed a similar pattern in adults (Juniper *et al.* manuscript in preparation).

INTERPRETING QUALITY OF LIFE DATA

Although much attention has been paid to the methods for developing and validating HRQL questionnaires,[44] little attention has focused on the interpretation of the data they generate. Repeated experience with a wide variety of physiological measures allows clinicians to make meaningful interpretations of results. For instance, the experienced clinician will have little difficulty in interpreting a 0.5 litre increase in FEV_1. In contrast, the meaning of a change in score of 0.5 on a HRQL instrument is less intuitively obvious. Two approaches have been suggested for interpreting HRQL data, these are "anchor-based" and "distribution-based".[45] The former bases interpretation on clinically meaningful changes in other indices, while the latter depends entirely on statistical distribution. The limitation of using the statistical approach is that even if one calculates the effect size, there is no evidence that this magnitude of change is of any importance to the patient.

For our Asthma Quality of Life Questionnaire,[8] the new standardized version of this questionnaire,[46] the Mini Asthma Quality of Life Questionnaire,[47] the Paediatric Asthma Quality of Life Questionnaire[18] and the Paediatric Asthma Caregiver Quality of Life Questionnaire,[48] we have adopted the anchor-based approach and used patient perception of a meaningful change in HRQL as the anchor. We defined a minimal

important difference (MID) as "the smallest difference in score in the domain of interest which patients perceive as beneficial and would mandate, in the absence of troublesome side-effects and excessive cost, a change in the patient's management".[49] A similar anchor-based approach has been used for the St. George's Respiratory Questionnaire.[50]

For many years, statisticians have cautioned against the sole use of mean data and statistical significance for the interpretation of clinical trial data. One reason for this is that patients may be very heterogeneous in their responses to interventions. However, if the MID of the instrument is known, the problem can easily be addressed by presenting the results in terms of the number needed to treat (NNT).[51] The NNT is the number of patients who need to be treated with the new intervention for one patient to have a clinically important improvement over and above that which he/she would have experienced with the control intervention. The NNT is calculated from the proportion of patients who show a clinically important improvement or deterioration (i.e. all those who show a change >MID) on each of the treatments. Presentation of clinical trial results in this manner is more meaningful and easier to interpret than standard deviations and confidence intervals for both clinicians and health policy makers.

For example, in a recent comparison of salmeterol and salbutamol which used the Asthma Quality of Life Questionnaire, the mean difference between the two interventions for the symptom domain was 0.49 ($P < 0.0001$).[3] This value was on the borderline of being clinically important (MID = 0.5). Further analysis revealed an NNT of 4.[51] In other words, four patients need to be treated with salmeterol for one to have a clinically important improvement in asthma-specific quality of life over an above that which he/she would have experienced on salbutamol (i.e. each patient has a 25% chance of having a clinically important improvement). Results in terms of NNT are often quite surprising to those clinicians who expect the majority of patients to respond close to the mean. To put these asthma NNT results into perspective, the use of statins to reduce the risk of stroke is advocated even though the NNT is greater than 200.[52]

HRQL IN RESEARCH

Recognition of the importance of assessing patient well-being, poor correlations between conventional clinical indices and HRQL and the advent of HRQL instruments with strong measurement properties have already ensured that many asthma clinical studies include an assessment of HRQL as one of the primary end-points. Most instruments are short, easily understood and usually in self-administered format making completion very little burden either to the investigator or the patient. We have found that patients enjoy completing HRQL questionnaires because they can relate to the questions and know that the things that are important to them are being taken into consideration. In addition, national pharmaceutical regulatory agencies are beginning to ask for evidence of patient benefit for new product submissions.

HRQL IN CLINICAL PRACTICE

The use of HRQL instruments in clinical practice is growing. Disease-specific quality of life questionnaires provide a standardized and quantified method for taking a simple patient history. They ask the questions that clinicians have been asking for generations:

- does your asthma limit you in your activities?
- Are your symptoms bothering you?
- Is your asthma giving you problems at work?
- Are you concerned about having asthma and the need to take medications?
- Did the new medication help?

The advantages of a questionnaire are that the patient can complete it in the waiting room; a quick scan of the responses will save consultation time; and the interviewer does not have to remember all the important questions. In addition, the questionnaire will often reveal problems not spontaneously identified by the patient (particularly children); the clinician can quickly focus on areas of particular concern; and responses at each clinic visit can be compared to determine whether interventions have been beneficial. Changes over time can be recorded more accurately than by patient recall and long-term data bases can be established.

A limitation to the use of quality of life questionnaires in clinical practice is that they have been developed to measure the problems that are most important to the majority of patients with asthma. Patients are heterogeneous in their experiences and priorities and no questionnaire is going to cover all the problems experienced by all patients. Clinicians should never depend solely on HRQL questionnaires to provide them with a complete and comprehensive picture of the patient's concerns and impairments.

The use of HRQL in clinical practice is in its infancy and we now need good clinical studies to evaluate whether its inclusion benefits patient management and is cost-effective. Until such data are available, the beneficial use of these instrument in clinical practice can only be speculative.

CULTURAL ADAPTATION OF HRQL QUESTIONNAIRES

Adapting quality of life questionnaires to other languages and cultures is considerably more complicated than doing a simple translation.[53] A number of the asthma-specific questionnaires have been translated into a wide range of languages and tested using well established procedures. Information on the availability of the translations can be obtained from the developers.

MODIFICATION OF QUESTIONNAIRES

Health-related quality of life questionnaires are scientific instruments in which the items and response options have been selected using carefully standardized and established psychometric methods.[44] Any modifications may seriously effect the measurement properties and validity of the instrument. Therefore, no changes or adaptations should be made without the permission of the developer.

SOFTWARE

Computerized versions of some questionnaires are now available. These are obviously ideal for clinical trial data collection because they eliminate the problems of "missing data" and transcription errors. They should also prove useful in clinical practice through their ability to provide immediate summary scores and graphical print-outs of longitudinal trends.

CONCLUSION

Asthma-specific quality of life correlates poorly with the conventional clinical measures of asthma control in both adults and children. Since one of the aims of treatment must be to ensure that patients themselves benefit, quality of life must be measured directly. Asthma-specific quality of life questionnaires are now available for both adults and children and can easily be included in both clinical practice and clinical research.

KEY POINTS

1 Health-related quality-of-life assessment captures the aspects of asthma that are most important to the patient.

2 There are only weak to moderate correlations between asthma quality of life and the conventional clinical measures of asthma severity.

3 To ensure that the overall effect of interventions is evaluated, quality-of-life assessments should be included in clinical studies in conjunction with conventional clinical measures.

4 Disease-specific quality-of-life instruments for asthma with strong measurement properties and validity are now available. Most are short and simple and can easily be incorporated into clinical studies.

5 The choice of quality-of-life questionnaire should depend on the study question. Each instrument has different measurement characteristics and these should be matched to the needs of the study.

REFERENCES

1. Schipper H, Clinch J, Powell V. Definitions and conceptual issues. In: Spilker B (ed). *Quality of Life and Pharmacoeconomics in Clinical Trials*. Philadelphia: Lippincott-Raven, 1996: 11–23.

2. ✪ Guyatt GH, Naylor D, Juniper EF, Heyland D, Cook D and the Evidence-Based Medicine Working Group. Users' guides to the medical literature. IX. How to use an article about health-related quality of life. *JAMA* 1997; 277: 1232–7.

3. ✪ Juniper EF, Johnston PR, Borkhoff CM, Guyatt GH, Boulet LP, Haukioja A. Quality of life in asthma clinical trials: comparison of salmeterol and salbutamol. *Am J Respir Crit Care Med* 1995; 151: 66–70.

4. Rutten-van Molken MPMH, Clusters F *et al.* Comparison of performance of four instruments in evaluating the effects of salmeterol on asthma quality of life. *Eur Respir J* 1995; 8: 888–98.

5. Rowe BH, Oxman AD. Peformance of an asthma quality of life questionnaire in an outpatient setting. *Am Rev Respir Dis* 1993; 148: 675–81.

6. Leidy NK, Coughlin C. Psychometric performance of the Asthma Quality of Life Questionnaire in a US sample. *Qual Life Res* 1998; 7: 127–34.

7. ✪ Juniper EF, Guyatt GH, Epstein RS, Ferrie PJ, Jaeschke R, Hiller TK. Evaluation of impairment of health-related quality of life in asthma: development of a questionnaire for use in clinical trials. *Thorax* 1992; 47: 76–83.

8. Juniper EF, Guyatt GH, Ferrie PJ, Griffith LE. Measuring quality of life in asthma. *Am Rev Respir Dis* 1993; 147: 832–8.

9. Marks GB, Dunn SM, Woolcock AJ. A scale for the measurement of quality of life in adults with asthma. *J Clin Epidemiol* 1992; 45: 461–72.

10. Marks GB, Dunn SM, Woolcock AJ. An evaluation of an asthma quality of life questionnaire as a measure of change in adults with asthma. *J Clin Epidemiol* 1993; 46: 1103–11.

11. Hyland ME. The living with asthma questionnaire. *Respir Med* 1991; 85: 13–16.

12. Hyland ME, Finnis S, Irvine SH. A scale for assessing quality of life in adult asthma sufferers. *J Psychomatic Res* 1991; 35: 99–110.

13. ✪ Jones PW, Quirk FH, Baveystock CM, Littlejohns P. A self-complete measure of health status for chronic airflow limitation; the St. George's Respiratory Questionnaire. *Am Rev Respir Dis* 1992; 145: 1321–7.

14. Maille AR, Kaptein AA, Koning CJM, Zwinderman AH. Developing a quality of life questionnaire for patients with respiratory illness. *Monaldi Arch Chest Dis* 1994; 49: 76–8.

15. Creer TL, Wigal JK, Kotses H, McConnaughy K, Winder JA. A life activities questionnaire for adult asthma. *J Asthma* 1992; 29: 393–9.

16. Quirk FH, Baveystock CM, Wilson R, Jones PW. Influence of demographic and disease related factors on the degree of distress associated with symptoms and restrictions on daily living due to asthma in six countries. *Eur Respir J* 1991; 4: 167–71.

17. ✪ Malo JL, Boulet LP, Dewitte JD *et al*. Quality of life of subjects with occupational asthma. *J Allergy Clin Immunol* 1993; 91: 1121–7.

18. ✪ Juniper EF, Guyatt GH, Feeny DH, Ferrie PJ, Griffith LE, Townsend M. Measuring quality of life in children with asthma. *Qual Life Res* 1996; 5: 35–46.

19. Townsend M, Feeny DH, Guyatt GH, Seip AE, Dolovich J. Evaluation of the burden of illness for pediatric asthmatic patients and their parents. *Ann Allergy* 1991; 67: 403–408.

20. Creer TL, Wigal JK, Kotses H, Hatala JC, McConnaughy K, Winder JA. A life activities questionnaire for childhood asthma. *J Asthma* 1993; 30: 467–73.

21. Christie MJ, French D, Sowden A, West A. Development of child-centred disease-specific questionnaires for living with asthma. *Psychosomatic Med* 1993; 55: 541–8.

22. French DJ, Christie MJ, Sowden AJ. The reproducibility of the childhood asthma questionnaires: measures of quality of life for children with asthma aged 4–16 years. *Qual Life Res* 1994; 3: 215–24.

23. Nocon A. Social and emotional impact of childhood asthma. *Arch Dis Child* 1991; 66: 458–60.

24. Usherwood TP, Scrimgeour A, Barber JH. Questionnaire to measure perceived symptoms and disability in asthma. *Arch Dis Child* 1990; 65: 779–81.

25. Osman L, Silverman M. Measuring quality of life for young children with asthma and their families. *Eur Respir J* 1996; 9 (suppl. 21): S35–S41.

26. ✪ Guyatt GH, Juniper EF, Feeny DH, Griffith LE. Children and adult perceptions of childhood asthma. *Pediatrics* 1997; 99: 165–8.

27. Rosenbaum PL, Saigal S. Measuring health-related quality of life in pediatric populations: conceptual issues. In: Spilker B (ed). *Quality of Life and Pharmacoeconomics in Clinical Trials*. Philadelphia: Lippencott-Raven, 1996; 785–91.

28. Wood PR, Hidalgo HA, Prihoda TJ, Kromer ME. Comparison of Hispanic children's and parents' responses to questions about the child's asthma. *Arch Pediatr Adolesc Med* 1994; 148: 43.

29. Theunissen NCM, Vogels TGC, Koopman HM *et al*. The proxy problem: child report versus parent report in health-related quality of life research. *Qual Life Res* 1998; 7: 387–97.

30. Juniper EF, Guyatt GH, Feeny DH, Griffith LE, Ferrie PJ. Minimum skills required by children to complete health-related quality of life instruments: comparison of instruments for measuring asthma-specific quality of life. *Eur Respir J* 1997; 10: 2285–94.

31. Juniper EF, Howland WC, Roberts NB, Thompson AK, King DR. Measuring quality of life in children with rhinoconjunctivitis. *J Allergy Clin Immunol* 1998; 101: 163–70.

32. Bergner M, Bobbitt RA, Carter WB, Gilson BS. The sickness impact profile; development and final revision of a health status measure. *Med Care* 1981; 19: 787–805.

33. Stewart AL, Hays R, Ware JE. The MOS short-form general health survey. Reliability and validity in a patient population. *Med Care* 1988; 26: 724–32.

34. Hunt SM, McKenna SP, McEwen J *et al*. A quantitative approach to perceived health status: a validation study. *J Epidemiol Community Health* 1980; 34: 281–6.

35. Nelson E, Wasson J, Kirk J *et al*. Assessment of function in routine clinical practice: description of the COOP chart method and preliminary findings. *J Chron Dis* 1987; 40 (suppl. 1): S55.

36. Stein RE, Jessop DJ. Functional status II(R): a measure of child health status. *Med Care* 1990; 28: 1041–55.

37. Landgraf JM, Maunsell E, Nixon Speechley K *et al.* Canadian-French, German and UK versions of the Child Health Questionnaire: methodology and preliminary item scaling results. *Qual Life Res* 1998; 7: 433–45.

38. Bousquet J, Bullinger M, Fayol C, Marquis P, Valentin B, Burtin B. Assessment of quality of life in patients with perennial rhinitis with the French version of the SF-36 health status questionnaire. *J Allergy Clin Immunol* 1994; 94: 182–8.

39. Bousquet J, Knani J, Dhivert H *et al.* Quality of life in asthma. 1. Internal consistency and validity of the SF-36 questionnaire. *Am J Respir Crit Care Med* 1994; 149: 371–5.

40. Torrance GW. Measurement of health state utilities for economic appraisal. *J Health Econom* 1986; 5: 1–30.

41. Kaplan RM, Anderson JP, Wu AW, Matthews WC, Kozin F, Orenstein D. The Quality of Well-being Scale: application in AIDS, cystic fibrosis and arthritis. *Med Care* 1989; 27: S27–43.

42. Feeny D, Furlong W, Barr RD, Torrance GW, Rosenbaum P, Weitzman S. A comprehensive multi-attribute system for classifying the health status of survivors of childhood cancer. *J Clin Oncol* 1992; 10: 923–8.

43. The EuroQol Group. A new facility for the measurement of health-related quality of life. *Health Policy* 1990; 16: 199–208.

44. ❍ Juniper EF, Guyatt GH, Jaeschke R. How to develop and validate a new health-related quality of life instrument. In: Spilker B (ed). *Quality of Life and Pharmacoeconomics in Clinical Trials*. Philadelphia: Lippencott-Raven, 1996: 49–56.

45. Lydick E, Epstein RS. Interpretation of quality of life changes. *Qual Life Res* 1993; 2: 221–6.

46. Juniper EF, Buist AS, Cox FM, Ferrie PJ, King DR. Validation of a standardized version of the Asthma Quality of Life Questionnaire. *Chest* 1999; 115: 1265–70.

47. Juniper EF, Guyatt GH, Cox FM, Ferrie PJ, King DR. Development and validation of the Mini Asthma Quality of Life Questionnaire. *Eur Respir J* 1999; 14: 32–8.

48. Juniper EF, Guyatt GH, Feeny DH, Ferrie PJ, Griffith LE, Townsend M. Measuring quality of life in the parents of children with asthma. *Qual Life Res* 1996; 5: 27–34.

49. ❍ Juniper EF, Guyatt GH, Willan A, Griffith LE. Determining a minimal important change in a disease-specific quality of life questionnaire. *J Clin Epidemiol* 1994; 47: 81–7.

50. Jones PW, Lasserson D. Relationship between change in St. George's Respiratory Questionnaire score and patients' perception of treatment efficacy after one year of therapy with nedocromil sodium. *Am J Respir Crit Care Med* 1994; 149: A211.

51. ❍ Guyatt GH, Juniper EF, Walter SD, Griffith LE, Goldstein RS. Interpreting treatment effects in randomised trials. *Br Med J* 1998; 101: 163–70.

52. Crouse JR III, Byington RP, Hoen HM, Furberg CT. Reductase inhibitor monotherapy and stroke prevention. *Arch Intern Med* 1997; 157: 1305–10.

53. Guillemin F, Bombardier C, Beaton D. Cross-cultural adaptation of health-related quality of life measures: literature review and proposed guidelines. *J Clin Epidemiol* 1993; 46: 1417–32.

Chapter 14

Assessment of Asthma Control: Markers of Inflammation

Krishan Parameswaran and Frederick Hargreave

What can be measured can be understood.
What can be understood can be altered.

Pythagoras

INTRODUCTION

Airway inflammation is considered to be the primary cause of asthma, of exacerbations and, through remodelling, of the chronic abnormalities of airway function. Inflammation is the localized protective response caused by tissue injury. In the airways of the lungs it includes cellular infiltration, an increase in vascular flow and permeability, release of various mediators, exudation of serum and mucus secretion. It also causes damage to the epithelium, and deposition of collagen beneath the basement membrane and in the submucosa, as well as hypertrophy and hyperplasia of smooth muscle, which are the components of remodelling. Airway inflammation is therefore responsible for the clinical characteristics of asthma which include symptoms, variable airflow limitation, chronic airflow limitation, and airway hyper-responsiveness. Treating the inflammation is therefore the primary target of treatment.[1]

The control of asthma is currently based on clinical parameters. It is achieved by anti-inflammatory treatment plus the least amount of bronchodilator. It is assumed that the control of clinical features equates with the control of airway inflammation. However, there is evidence that this may not be the case,[2-4] introducing the possibility that the control of asthma should include the reversal of airway inflammation.

In this chapter, we will discuss how airway inflammation can be measured in clinical practice, why direct measurements may be needed to define asthma control, and the evidence that these direct measurements may be needed.

MEASUREMENT OF AIRWAY INFLAMMATION

The presence and severity of airway inflammation can be investigated by indirect or direct methods.[5] The indirect methods include clinical features, blood eosinophils, serum eosinophil cationic protein (ECP) and urinary leukotriene E_4. The direct methods include bronchial washings or bronchoalveolar lavage (BAL), bronchial biopsies, induced or spontaneous sputum, exhaled nitric oxide (NO), carbon monoxide or pentane and exhaled breath condensate of hydrogen peroxide. For the clinical assessment of asthma control, only clinical features, blood eosinophils and serum ECP, induced or spontaneous sputum and exhaled NO need to be considered.

ASTHMA CONTROL BY CLINICAL FEATURES

The definition of the control of asthma is vague. Although optimal control of asthma ideally means the absence of respiratory symptoms, no need for rescue bronchodilator and normal pulmonary function, this may be difficult to achieve in many patients.[1] Therefore, the participants preferred to base treatment needs on what was defined as acceptable control, according to clinical and physiological features (Table 14.1).

The vagueness of the definition immediately suggests that the control of asthma will not correlate closely with the control of airway inflammation. This is supported by a number of observations. For example, the control of asthma by symptoms alone is known to be unsatisfactory with respect to measurements of airway function. While symptoms are usually a sensitive indicator of lack of control or of exacerbations, and precede deterioration in home measurements of peak expiratory flow (PEF)[6] or forced expired volume in 1 s (FEV_1),

Table 14.1: Parameters of asthma control. (From Boulet L-P, Becker A, Bérubé D, Beveridge R, Ernst P. Summary of recommendations from the Canadian Asthma Consensus Report, 1999. CMAJ 1999; 161 (II suppl.): S1–S12, ©Pulsus Group Inc.)

Parameters	Frequency or value
Daytime symptoms	< 4 days per week
Night-time symptoms	< 1 night per week
Physical activity	Normal
Exacerbations	Mild, infrequent
Absenteeism	None
Need for β_2 agonist as required	< 4 doses per week[a]
FEV_1[b] or PEF[c]	≥ 90% personal best
PEF diurnal variation[d] variation	< 15% diurnal

[a] May use one dose per day for prevention of exercise-induced symptoms.
[b] Forced expiratory volume in 1 s.
[c] Peak expiratory flow obtained with a portable peak flow meter.
[d] Diurnal variation is calculated as the highest minus the lowest divided by the highest PEF multiplied by 100.

they can be less sensitive in a minority and they are non-specific. The poor sensitivity and non-specificity was nicely illustrated in family practice by Kendrick and co-workers[7] who found that only 40% could recognize the variability of PEF accurately. Additional measurements of FEV_1 or PEF are therefore required. However, even these measurements are an insensitive indicator of the presence or degree of airway hyperresponsiveness as measured by methacholine inhalation. Thus, the FEV_1 in patients with uncomplicated asthma is usually normal until airway responsiveness to methacholine is moderately increased.[8] Also, when asthma is uncontrolled, treatment results in maximal improvement in FEV_1 before maximal improvement in airway hyperresponsiveness.[9] Furthermore, when asthma deteriorates, airway hyperresponsiveness can worsen before FEV_1. These observations therefore suggest that asthma control based on symptoms and FEV_1 or PEF will not necessarily indicate the best reduction of airway hyper-

responsiveness. Neither do they necessarily indicate the state of control of airway inflammation.

ASTHMA CONTROL BY SPUTUM CELL COUNTS

The introduction of reliable sputum examination, particularly with induced sputum,[10] has provided the only relatively non-invasive method to directly examine airway inflammation. Its relative non-invasive nature means that it can be applied randomly to severe as well as mild disease and repeatedly to monitor and treat airway inflammation in the control of asthma. Sputum induction is safe, providing it is carried out carefully, even in more severe exacerbations of asthma;[11,12] in addition, with trained staff, it is successful more than 90% of the time. The sputum can be processed to examine cell counts and fluid-phase measurements, but only cell counts are of potential use in clinical practice.[13] Two methods have been used, one which selects sputum from the expectorate and the other which processes the whole expectorate.[14] The former method gives better quality cytospins with minimal salivary contamination and the total cell count can be expressed per milligram of sputum which is not influenced by the volume of sputum or salivary contamination. In reporting the counts, the total and differential count are both important as well as the amount of salivary contamination and cell viability. Salivary squamous cell contamination of >20% and cell viability of <50% reduces the reliability of counts.[15] With trained staff, the cell counts are reliable, valid and responsive, the qualities of good measurements.[14] The counts are not acutely influenced by the induction procedure but they can be altered by the duration, later specimens being lower in neutrophils and eosinophils than earlier specimens.[16] Sputum cell counts differ from those in BAL or bronchial biopsies in showing more neutrophils and eosinophils.[17] BAL shows more macrophages and lymphocytes. The predominant cell in biopsies is the lymphocyte. These differences in predominant cell types are due to differences in the compartments of the airway being measured.

The use of sputum cell counts in research has provided evidence that clinical assessment is imprecise with respect to the presence, type and severity of airway inflammation.[13] Sputum cell counts have emphasized the occurrence of three types of inflammation, based on an increase in different cell types. These have different

Table 14.2: Airway inflammation: types and causes		
Eosinophilic	**Neutrophilic**	**Lymphocytic**
Allergens	Smoker's bronchitis	Viral infection
Diisocyanates	Bacterial infection	
Decreased steroid	Pollutants	
"Asthma"	Endotoxin	

causes (Table 14.2), tend to have different clinical presentations and seem to respond differently to corticosteroid treatment. For example, a sputum eosinophilia is usually associated with exacerbations of asthma which respond to treatment with corticosteroid.[11] However, asthma exacerbations can be neutrophilic and non-eosinophilic, and there is increasing evidence that these do not benefit from steroid treatment.[11,18]

Examination of the colour of sputum in patients with asthma shows that purulence indicates a neutrophilia,[19] as previously shown in chronic bronchitis. However, it does not indicate whether there is an eosinophilia or not which can occur in mucoid, mucopurulent or purulent sputum.

Sputum eosinophilia is a sensitive indicator of the control of asthma. It is the first to occur when asthma exacerbates due to reduction of steroid treatment, preceding symptoms, FEV_1, home measurements of PEF, PC_{20} and blood eosinophils.[20,21] When eosinophilic exacerbations of asthma are treated with steroid, symptoms and FEV_1 improve before sputum eosinophils.[11] When asthma is clinically controlled, there can still be sputum eosinophilia[2] which can be reversed by increasing the dose of steroid treatment. The significance of this observation requires investigation.

Sputum cell counts have also illustrated that asthma with considerable variable airflow limitation and airway hyperresponsiveness can occur without sputum eosinophilia and that sputum eosinophilia can occur with normal spirometry and normal or only mild hyperresponsiveness.[22,23] In the former, recurrent symptoms would best be treated with a long-acting bronchodilator or, perhaps, an anti-leukotriene. Symptoms in the latter would need additional steroid treatment with little or no bronchodilator.

These observations indicate that reliable sputum cell counts do have a place in the investigation and treatment of asthma. The extent to which they will be needed or will be useful to monitor anti-inflammatory treatment requires investigation. A problem with their clinical use will be their implementation. We have achieved this in Hamilton, Ontario, by making them available in one centre to which patients can be referred for the measurements. The sputum induction is performed in the pulmonary function laboratory. The fresh specimen is then examined by registered technologists in our research laboratory and the result is available within 2 hours. Quality control checks are implemented once each month. Sputum examination could be performed in the haematology laboratory providing regular quality control checks are made to keep the results reliable.

ASTHMA CONTROL BY OTHER INFLAMMATORY MEASUREMENTS

Blood eosinophils and ECP

Blood eosinophil counts and serum ECP have been advocated as methods of monitoring airway inflammation.[24,25] This is logical since the eosinophils in the airways are derived from the bone marrow via the blood.[26] Blood eosinophils and ECP are raised in uncontrolled asthma and they are reduced after treatment with inhaled or ingested glucocorticoids. However, they are insensitive measurements of eosinophilic airway inflammation, they can be influenced by inflammation elsewhere, e.g. in the nose, and the kinetics of effect of treatment can differ from the airways. For example in one study, the treatment of an exacerbation of asthma with prednisone quickly reduced blood eosinophils and ECP to normal within hours, while sputum eosinophilia was not significantly reduced until the second day of treatment.[11] Therefore, blood eosinophils and serum ECP are not useful measurements for identifying or refining the control of asthma.

Exhaled NO

Exhaled NO is produced by the activation of an inducible form of nitric oxide synthase associated with inflammation. Exhaled NO is easy and quick to measure, it is increased in subjects with asthma compared with healthy subjects and is responsive to treatment with corticosteroids.[27,28] However, exhaled NO is also increased by non-eosinophilic inflammatory responses in bronchiectasis[29] and viral infections[30] and it is reduced to normal by corticosteroids before control

145

of clinical features and sputum eosinophilia.[31] Correlation of exhaled NO with sputum eosinophilia is poor.[32] These observations suggest that the clinical use of exhaled NO is limited and will not be useful in the control of asthma.

CONCLUSIONS

The control of asthma is currently defined and achieved by symptoms and measurements of airway function, particularly FEV_1 and PEF. The methods to achieve control are primarily directed to reverse eosinophilic airway inflammation. While the inflammation is not measured, it is considered that control of clinical features indicates control of airway inflammation. However, the use of induced sputum to measure airway inflammation has indicated that this is not correct and that sputum eosinophilia can still be present when asthma is clinically controlled. This, together with the lack of a close correlation between eosinophilia and the severity of abnormalities of airway function, and the occurrence of non-eosinophilic exacerbations of asthma which seem to be unresponsive to steroid treatment, raises the possibility that reliable sputum cell counts may be needed to optimize anti-inflammatory treatment. This requires further investigation.

KEY POINTS

1 Symptoms and measurement airflow limitation are not sensitive indicators of airway inflammation in asthma.

2 Sputum eosinophilia is a sensitive indicator of the control of asthma.

3 The persistence of sputum eosinophilia when asthma is clinically controlled requires further investigations.

REFERENCES

1. Boulet L-P, Becker A, Bérubé D, Beveridge R, Ernst P. Summary of recommendations from the Canadian Asthma Consensus Report, 1999. *CMAJ* 1999; 161 (II suppl.): S1–S12.

2. Fahy JV, Boushey HA. Effect of low-dose beclomethasone dipropionate on asthma control and airway inflammation. *Eur Respir J* 1998; 11: 1240–7.

3. Cai Y, Carty K, Henry RL, Gibson PG. Persistence of sputum eosinophilia in children with controlled asthma when compared with healthy children. *Eur Respir J* 1998; 11: 848–53.

4. ✪ Parameswaran K, Pizzichini E, Hussack P *et al*. Clinical judgement of airway inflammation versus sputum cell counts in asthma *Eur Respir J* 2000; 15: 486–90.

5. Hargreave FE, Pizzichini E, Pizzichini MMM *et al*. Sputum indices of inflammation in asthma. In: Schleimer R, Busse W, O'Byrne P (eds). *Inhaled Glucocorticoids in Asthma: Mechanisms and Clinical Actions*. New York, NY: Marcel Dekker, 1996: 133–50.

6. Gibson PG, Wong BJO, Hepperle MJE *et al*. A research method to induce and examine a mild exacerbation of asthma by withdrawal of inhaled corticosteroid. *Clin Exp Allergy* 1992; 22: 525–32.

7. ✪ Kendrick AH, Higgs CMB, Whitfield MJ *et al*. Accuracy of perception of severity of asthma: patients treated in general practice. *BMJ* 1993; 307: 422–4.

8. Hargreave FE, Pizzichini MMM, Pizzichini E. Airway hyperresponsiveness as a diagnostic feature of asthma. In: Johansson SGO (ed). *Progress in Allergy and Clinical Immunology*. Toronto, Ontario: Hogrefe and Huber, 1995: 63–7.

9. Juniper EF, Kline PA, Vanzieleghem MA *et al*. Effect of long-term treatment with an inhaled corticosteroid (budesonide) on airway hyperresponsiveness and clinical asthma in nonsteroid-dependent asthmatics. *Am Rev Respir Dis* 1990; 142: 832–6.

10. Pin I, Gibson PG, Kolendowicz R *et al*. Use of induced sputum cell counts to investigate airway inflammation in asthma. *Thorax* 1992; 47: 25–9.

11. ❂ Pizzichini MMM, Pizzichini E, Clelland L *et al.* Sputum in severe exacerbations of asthma: kinetics of inflammatory indices after prednisone treatment. *Am J Respir Crit Care Med* 1997; 155: 1501–8.

12. Vlachos-Mayer H, Leigh R, Sharon RF *et al.* Sputum induction for inflammatory indices: safety and success. *Am J Respir Crit Care Med* 1999; 159 (3): A850.

13. ❂ Hargreave FE. Induced sputum for the investigation of airway inflammation: evidence for its clinical application. *Can Respir J* 1999; 6 (2): 169–74.

14. Kips JC, Peleman RA, Rauwels RA. Methods of examining induced sputum: do differences matter? *Eur Respir J* 1998; 11: 529–33.

15. Ward R, Woltman G, Wardlaw AJ *et al.* Between observer repeatability of sputum differential cell counts: influence of cell viability and squamous cell contamination. *Clin Exp Allergy* 1999; 29: 248–52.

16. Holz O, Richter K, Jorres RA *et al.* Changes in sputum composition between two induction performed on consecutive days. *Thorax* 1998; 53: 83–6.

17. ❂ Maestrelli P, Saetta M, Di Stefano A *et al.* Comparison of leukocyte counts in sputum, bronchial biopsies and bronchoalveolar lavage. *Am J Respir Crit Care Med* 1995; 152: 1926–31.

18. Parameswaran K, Pizzichini MMM, Li D *et al.* Serial sputum cell counts in the management of chronic airflow limitation. *Eur Respir J* 1998; 11: 1405–8.

19. Berlyne GS, Efthimiadis A, Hussack P *et al.* Sputum in asthma: colour versus cell counts. *J Allergy Clin Immunol* 2000; 105: 182–3.

20. Pizzichini MMM, Pizzichini E, Clelland L *et al.* Prednisone dependent asthma: inflammatory indices in induced sputum. *Eur Respir J* 1999; 13: 15–21.

21. Belda J, Kamada D, Lemiére C, Efthimiadis A, Hargreave FE. The kinetics of clinical and inflammatory indices during an exacerbation of asthma induced by inhaled steroid reduction. *Am J Respir Crit Care Med* 1999; 159 (3): A123.

22. Kidney JC, Wong AG, Efthimiadis A *et al.* Elevated B cells in sputum of asthmatics: close correlation with eosinophils. *Am J Respir Crit Care Med* 1996; 153: 540–4.

23. ❂ Gibson PG, Hargreave FE, Girgis-Gabardo A *et al.* Chronic cough with eosinophilic bronchitis and examination for variable airflow obstruction and response to corticosteroid. *Clin Exp Allergy* 1995; 25: 127–32.

24. Horn BR, Robin ED, Theodore J *et al.* Total eosinophil counts in the management of bronchial asthma. *N Engl J Med* 1975; 29: 1152–5.

25. Venge P. Monitoring of asthma inflammation by serum measurements of eosinophil cationic protein: a new clinical approach. *Respir Med* 1995; 89: 1–2.

26. Denburg JA. Bone marrow in atopy and asthma: haemopoietic mechanisms in allergic inflammation. *Immunol Today* 1999; 20: 111–3.

27. ❂ Kharitonov SA, Yates D, Robbins RA *et al.* Increased nitric oxide in exhaled air of asthmatic patients. *Lancet* 1994; 343: 133–5.

28. Kharitonov SA, Yates DH, Chung KF *et al.* Changes in the dose of inhaled steroid affect exhaled nitric oxide levels in asthmatic patients. *Eur Respir J* 1996; 9: 196–201.

29. Kharitonov SA, Wells AU, O'Connor BJ *et al.* Elevated levels of exhaled nitric oxide in bronchiectasis. *Am J Respir Crit Care Med* 1995; 151: 1889–93.

30. Kharitonov SA, Yates D, Barnes PJ. Increased nitric oxide in exhaled air or normal human subjects with upper respiratory tract infections. *Eur Respir J* 1995; 8: 295–7.

31. Jatakanon A, Kharitonov SA, Lim S *et al.* Effect of differing doses of inhaled budesonide on markers of airway inflammation in patients with mild asthma. *Thorax* 1999; 54: 108–114.

32. Berlyne GS, Parameswaran K, Kamada D *et al.* A comparison of exhaled nitric oxide and induced sputum as markers of airway inflammation. *J Allergy Clin Immunol* 2000 (submitted).

Chapter 15

Primary Prevention of Asthma

Allan Becker

FACTORS CRITICAL TO THE DEVELOPMENT OF ASTHMA

Genetic Predisposition

Atopy is the tendency to develop allergic disorders such as asthma, allergic dermatitis, allergic rhinitis and food allergy. Atopic children are at much greater risk for the development of asthma than non-atopic children.[1-5] Given the rapid increase over the last quarter century, it is difficult to ascribe the change in prevalence of asthma to genetic alteration. The gene (or genes) responsible for atopy and/or asthma has (have) not yet been identified. Therefore, the focus has turned to environmental factors.

The Intrauterine Environment

There is increasing evidence that successful pregnancy is a TH_2 phenomenon. In murine studies injection of IL3 or GM-CSF enhances fetal survival and promotes intrauterine growth, whereas injection of IL2, TNF or IFN-γ (TH_1 cytokines) lead to fetal destruction.[6] There is also clinical evidence (summarized in Ref. 6) that "pregnant women undergo immunologic changes consistent of the weakening of cell mediated immunity and strengthening of humoral immunity". This is clinically apparent with improvement during pregnancy in 70% of women who have rheumatoid arthritis (a cell-mediated autoimmune disorder) and worsening of SLE (a humoral driven disorder) in women during pregnancy.[7] Mosmann and colleagues[6] suggest that the placenta acts as an immunoabsorbent which is capable of removing large amounts of anti-fetal antibody without damage, whereas cell-mediated immunity is not well-buffered by the placenta. They suggest that a healthy feto-placental unit primarily supports a humoral immune response and is responsible for driving this TH_2 environment. As a result, at delivery the infant's immune system is preferentially biased toward continuing this intra-uterine established TH_2 immune status. Umbilical cord mononuclear cells stimulated by allergen have a TH_2-like phenotype for cytokine production[8] and the cells responsible for production of these TH_2 cytokines appear to be T-lymphocytes.[8] Further, in atopic children, there appears to be continued TH_2 responses during the first year of life associated with decrease in neonatal IFN-γ (TH_1) production.[9]

Exposure to Allergens

Food Allergens In the first year or two of life, development of allergy is primarily associated with food sensitivity. Breast-feeding has been advocated as a method of preventing allergy and asthma. Studies suggest that atopic dermatitis can be delayed, but not necessarily prevented by breast-feeding infants for the first 4 to 6 months of life.[10] As one component of an allergen avoidance programme, breast-feeding has been shown to decrease "total allergy", eczema, and positive allergy skin tests in children up to 4 years of age. In that study, asthma was decreased at 1 year, but not at 2 years of age in the intervention group compared with the control group.[11] While breast-feeding has not been shown to be effective in preventing the development of asthma, it does decrease the incidence of respiratory infections during infancy.[12]

Of interest, diet may continue to be important in later life. A recent study[13] noted that children who ate fresh, oily fish (greater than 2% fat), had significantly reduced risk of asthma (odds ratio: 0.26; 95% CI 0.09–0.72).

Inhalant Allergens Sensitization to indoor inhalant aeroallergens is more important than sensitization to outdoor aeroallergens in asthma, particularly in Canada where people spend much of their time indoors.

Indoor aeroallergens, including house-dust mites, companion animals and cockroaches appear to be important factors for asthma development. Studies have shown that risk for development of asthma is greater in children whose homes had high dust mite allergen levels during the first year of life.[14] Moreover, the higher the levels of exposure, the earlier children developed symptoms and the more severe were those symptoms.[14–16]

In areas where house-dust mite concentrations are low, asthma and airway hyperresponsiveness tend to better correlate with allergy to cats.[17] Unlike house-dust mite allergens which are present on relatively large particles and settle quickly after being disturbed, cat allergen is present on very small particles which readily become airborne and which are subsequently widely distributed in the community. In low socioeconomic status housing, cockroach allergen plays an important role.[18]

Although there has been some recent debate[19] the preponderance of evidence suggests that in patients with asthma who are sensitized to allergens, environmental control can result in significant improvement of asthma symptoms and lung function.[20–25]

Pollutants/Adjuvants

Environmental tobacco smoke (ETS) is important in development of childhood asthma and in worsening of asthma in children and adults.[26] The earlier, longer and greater the degree of ETS exposure in early childhood, the greater the likelihood of asthma developing in children.[27–30] ETS is by far the single most important pollution exposure factor associated with asthma in infants and children.

Environmental pollutants, other than ETS, may also be a problem.[31] These include noxious gases such as ozone, sulphur dioxide, and nitrous oxides. Exposure to nitrous oxides occurs from a variety of sources, such as incomplete oxidation of natural gas, and is also present in ETS. The classic "visible" pollution which is apparent as overt discolouration of the air is not necessarily associated with increased prevalence of asthma and allergy. Changes which may be far less obvious, particularly in industrialized societies, appear to be rather more important.

Infections

Respiratory viruses may play an important role in the development of asthma.[32,33] The onset of asthma after RSV bronchiolitis in infants has been well-documented,[34,35] however, the role of both viral and bacterial infections is complicated. Certain infections are important in determining the shift from a TH_2 to TH_1 lymphocyte predominance in infancy.[36] Absence of these infections in an industrialized, well-immunized society may not allow for this shift to occur and may influence the increase in allergy and asthma. There are data suggesting that family size and birth order are important factors associated with variation in allergy and asthma prevalence.[37] This may reflect the increased exposure of younger siblings early in life to repeated infections from their older siblings. Immunization and better hygiene in industrialized societies decrease the prevalence of a variety of infectious diseases with resulting decrease in the morbidity and mortality that may have occurred from these diseases.[38]

Bacterial cell wall DNA contains sequences of bases (centred on CpG dinucleotides) which induce TH_1-like responses.[39–41] Mycobacterial infections are particularly capable of inducing this response associated with the presence of an immunostimulatory sequence (ISS) of the oligodeoxynucleotides (ODN) CpG motif in its cell wall.[42] It has been suggested that the primary trigger for a shift to a TH_1-like phenotype is not likely to be from infectious organisms, but rather from "normal" bacterial commensals, particularly those in the gastrointestinal tract (GIT).[43] Holt *et al.* suggest that "microbial products typified by cell wall-derived lipopolysaccharides (LPS) are recognized as "natures TH_1 adjuvant".[43] Avoidance of disease such as measles and tuberculosis and/or modification of the normal gastrointestinal flora perhaps by "better" hygiene and excess use of antibiotics, may allow for perpetuation of a TH_2 phenotype in young children and thus promote development of allergy and asthma. A great deal more information about the positive and negative (in terms of allergy) role of infection is required before any specific recommendations can be made.

APPROACH TO ASTHMA PREVENTION

Primary prevention is the approach to intervening before development of any allergy or allergy-associated disease, including asthma, can occur in any individual.

Asthma Vaccine or Immunization

Several approaches to vaccination/immunization for prevention of allergy and asthma have been suggested.

Holt[44] has suggested a vaccine strategy for asthma and allergies consisting of parenteral vaccination with a cocktail of major inhalant antigens in early childhood. The cocktail would be combined with an adjuvant specifically designed to stimulate the TH_1 response. Hsu and co-workers[45] have studied "allergen gene immunization" in rats. They used intramuscular injection of a plasmid DNA ("naked DNA") encoding a house-dust mite allergen into the leg of rats. This induced a transient IgG response to the gene, but no IgE response which was transferable via $CD8^+$ lymphocytes. These studies are of interest and suggest a number of new potential approaches to control of allergy. In general, these strategies propose an approach to trigger switching of the immune response in infants to a TH_1 phenotype hopefully decreasing the potential for subsequent development of asthma. However, this may not be effective with infants or newborns who are already sensitized to environmental triggers. Similarly, it has been suggested that immunization with BCG may have the potential to shift the immune response balance toward a TH_1 phenotype.[38] However, this may not be true in individuals with a strong, heritable predisposition to atopy.[46]

Dietary intervention

Because of the strong relationship of allergy (albeit more specifically to inhalants) and asthma, attempts to decrease "turn on" of the TH_2 immune process appear logical. Given that allergy to foods is usually the first manifestation of an atopic immune process, consideration should be given to dietary intervention.

Data on the influence of breast-feeding dates to the 1930s with the recognition that breast-fed infants had less atopic dermatitis then bottle-fed infants.[47] Although not all studies of breast-feeding demonstrated a decrease in atopic dermatitis, there appears to be a consensus that breast-feeding for 4 to 6 months will at least delay, if not prevent, atopic dermatitis.[48] Given that allergens such as cow's milk and egg protein are present in breast milk, it was also thought that maternal diet may be important.[49] However, in one study, all breast-fed infants who developed allergy to cow's milk had received supplements of cow's milk formula in the nursery.[49] Thus, "accidental" exposure to cow's milk itself appears to be far more important than the very small amount of cow's milk transmitted through breast milk. Nevertheless, maternal avoidance of highly allergenic foods during breast-feeding has been shown to

delay, but not prevent subsequent development of allergic disease.[10,49] For a variety of sound clinical reasons, breast-feeding for the first 4 to 6 months of life should continue to be encouraged. Delay of exposure of infants to cow's milk and other highly allergenic foods also appears to be helpful.[10,47–49]

Another issue, the use of a maternal exclusion diet during pregnancy, has also been studied. Reduced intake of highly allergenic foods in the last trimester has not been shown to be helpful in the prevention of allergic disease in children at high risk for allergies because of a strong family history.[49–51] Further, an exclusion diet may place mothers at risk for inadequate nutrition intake. One difficulty with studies relating to maternal diet on allergen exposure relates to our lack of understanding as to when the elimination diet should be initiated and to our lack of ability to measure the intrauterine allergen exposure. Both timing and levels of exposure may be critically important in the promotion of allergy and perpetuation of the TH_2 phenotype.

Environment Control: What Can We Do and What Might Be Effective?

Environmental control appears to be important beginning at (or very possibly even before) birth. Data from a limited number of studies suggest that avoidance of allergens, both ingested and inhaled, and avoidance of ETS may at least delay onset of allergy and allergy-associated diseases, including asthma.[10,11]

Allergen Avoidance

INDOOR AEROALLERGENS Given their strong relationship to asthma, avoidance of house-dust mite, companion animals (particularly cat), and cockroach allergens appears to have the greatest potential for benefit.[4,14,17–23,52,53]

Treatment to control house-dust mite is the least controversial and least problematic of this group. House-dust mites thrive in high humidity. Decreasing indoor humidity to less than 50% is associated with lower house-dust mite concentrations. Simply encasing mattresses in a vapour impermeable barrier is effective in decreasing house-dust mite exposure.[54] Laundering bed linens in hot water will also decrease dust mite concentrations.[55] The ability to reduce house-dust mite allergen in carpeting (textile floor coverings) is rather more controversial, but short-term decrease in mite concentrations have been noted with various acaracides and with use of liquid nitrogen to freeze carpeting.[54] Removal of carpeting is the most effective method to decrease the floors house-dust mite concentration.[56]

Removal of the pet from the home is the most effective means to reduce cat or dog allergen.[57] However, this is loaded with psychosocial issues and is not easily dealt with. There are data demonstrating a decrease in airborne cat allergen with the use of high efficiency particular air (HEPA) filters and removal of textile floor covering (which acts as a reservoir for the cat allergen).[23,58] After removal of a cat, it can take more than 6 months for cat allergen levels to return to "baseline".[57] The issue of weekly washing of the cat has not been clearly defined and there is debate as to its value at present. Cat allergen exposure also occurs in public environments such as schools and hospitals associated with upholstered furniture and textile floor coverings. To a widespread degree, cat has become a community-based allergen.

Cockroach infestation is predominantly a socio-economic problem of poor, and often inner city, environments. Decrease in cockroach exposure in those settings will require increased awareness of this community problem at a political level. Changes in housing to impact on this problem will require not only scientific understanding, but also social and political changes.

Out-of-Door Aeroallergens Out-of-door aeroallergens are generally much less of a problem. However, in agricultural, prairie environments, *Alternaria* is a major sensitizer and is often associated with asthma (frequently with severe asthma). This mould spore has marked seasonality with peaks of exposure in the spring, late summer and fall.[59] Air conditioning systems and indoor air filters have the potential to decrease exposure to this allergen.

Pollutants Exposure to ETS in early life must be avoided. Such exposure carries the greatest risk for subsequent development of allergy and asthma.[26,27] The dangers of smoking during pregnancy appear to be well-recognized. However, mothers and other family members must be educated on the importance of avoidance of ETS exposure for infants and toddlers. Societal change should be encouraged through education and increased taxation of cigarettes.

SUMMARY

Given that asthma is a multifactorial disease with complex both genetic and environmental components (Fig. 15.1), it is unlikely that any single intervention currently available will significantly decrease the prevalence of asthma. High-risk populations should be targeted for ongoing research. Pregnancy and the first year of life appears to be a critically important "window" during which time allergy and the potential for asthma develop. In fact, intervention may need to begin even during the pregnancy. Large, well-controlled, multicentre studies should be encouraged in an effort to better understand changing prevalence of asthma in a variety of environmental settings. Primary prevention of allergy and allergy associated diseases including asthma offers the best potential for significant change in the future.

KEY POINTS

1 Genetic predisposition provides a strong heritable drive towards atopy and asthma.

2 The intrauterine environment predisposes all infants to an atopic immune response.

3 Changing conditions in the industrialized world decrease the drive toward balancing the immune response by promoting TH_1 cytokine stimulation.

4 Control of allergen exposure may be important in decreasing the continued TH_2 immune response.

5 Pollutants such as environmental tobacco smoke (indoor) and diesel particulates (outdoor) enhance the atopic response.

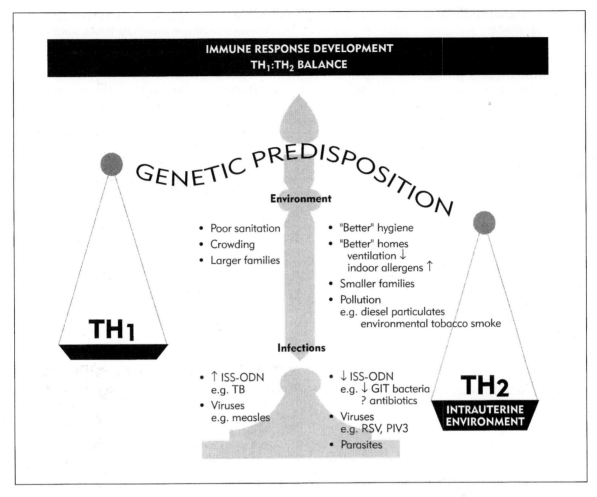

FIGURE 15.1: Genetic predisposition provides a large heritable component to atopy and asthma. With the intrauterine environment predisposing infants to a TH$_2$-like phenotype the impact of the external environment becomes critical. In the industrialized world, infants are protected from a variety of bacterial and viral infections and are exposed to more antibiotics which may decrease the body's "normal" bacterial commensals, particularly in the gastrointestinal tract. This modifies the adjuvant effect of the immunostimulatory sequence of oligodeoxynucleotides (ISS-ODN) from bacteria, which can provide an immune response balance in promoting a TH$_1$-like phenotype.

REFERENCES

1. Horwood IL, Fergusson DM, Hons BA, Shannon FT. Social and familial factors in the development of early childhood asthma. *Pediatrics* 1985; 75: 859–68.

2. Sporik R, Holgate ST, Cogswell JJ. Natural history of asthma in childhood–a birth cohort study. *Arch Dis Child* 1991; 66: 1050–53.

3. Clifford RD, Radford M, Howell JB, Holgate ST.

Associations between respiratory symptoms, bronchial response to methacholine and atopy in two age groups of school children. *Arch Dis Child* 1989; 64: 1153–9.

4. Peat JK, Salome CM, Woolcock AJ. Longitudinal changes in atopy during a 4-year period: Relation to bronchial hyperresponsiveness and respiratory symptoms in a population sample of Australian schoolchildren. *J Allergy Clin Immunol* 1990; 85: 65–74.

5. Martin AJ, Landau LI, Phelan PD. Natural history of

allergy in children followed to adult life. *Med J Aust* 1981; 2: 470–74.

6. ✪ Wegmann TG, Lin H, Guilbert L, Mosmann TR. Bidirectional cytokine interactions in the maternal-fetal relationship: is successful pregnancy a Th2 phenomenon? *Immunol Today* 1993; 14: 353–6.

7. Da Silva JA, Spector TD. The role of pregnancy in the course and aetiology of rheumatoid arthritis. *Clin Rheumatol* 1992; 11: 189–94.

8. Prescott SL, Macaubas C, Holt BJ *et al*. Transplacental priming of the human immune system to environmental allergens: universal skewing of initial T-cell responses towards the Th-2 cytokine profile. *J Immunol* 1998; 160: 4730–37.

9. Prescott SL, Macaubas C, Smallacombe T, Holt BJ, Sly PD, Holt PG. Development of allergen-specific T-cell memory in atopic and normal children. *Lancet* 1999; 353: 196–200.

10. ✪ Zeiger, RS, Heller, S, Sampson, HA. Genetic and environmental factors affecting the development of atopy from birth through age 4 in a prospective randomized controlled study of dietary avoidance. *J Allergy Clin Immunol* 1992; 89: 192.

11. Hide DW, Matthews S, Tariq S, Arshad SH. Allergen avoidance in infancy and allergy at 4 years of age. *Allergy* 1996; 51: 89–93.

12. Woodward A, Douglas RM, Graham NMH, Miles H. Acute respiratory illness in Adelaide children: breast feeding modifies the effect of passive smoking. *J Epid Comm Health* 1990; 44: 224–30.

13. Hodge L, Salome CM, Peat JK, Haby MM, Xuan W, Woolcock AJ. Consumption of oily fish and childhood asthma risk. *Med J Assist* 1996; 164: 137–40.

14. Sporik R, Holgate ST, Platts-Mills TAE, Coswell JJ. Exposure to house-dust mite allergen (*Der p1*) and the development of asthma in childhood. *New Engl J Med* 1992; 323: 502–507.

15. Ehnert B, Lau-Schadendorf S, Weber A, Buettner P, Schou C, Wahn U. Reducing domestic exposure to dust mite allergen reduces bronchial hyperreactivity in sensitive children with asthma. *J Allergy Clin Immunol* 1992; 90: 135–8.

16. Chan-Yeung M, Lam J, Ferguson A *et al*. Relationship between mite allergen levels in the homes, skin test reactivity and asthma. *Am Rev Respir Dis* 1993; 147: A459.

17. Sporik R, Rose G, Muller M *et al*. Allergen sensitization of children with wheeze and bronchial hyperreactivity (BHR) resident at high altitude. *Am Rev Respir Dis* 1993; 147: A458.

18. Rosenstreich DL, Eggleston P, Kattan M *et al*. The role of cockroach allergy and exposure to cockroach allergen in causing morbidity among inner-city children with asthma. *N Engl J Med* 1997; 336: 1356–63.

19. Gotzsche PC, Hammarquist C, Burr M. House dust mite control measures in the management of asthma: meta-analysis. *BMJ* 1998; 317: 1105–10.

20. Murray AB, Ferguson AC. Dust-free bedrooms in the treatment of asthmatic children with house dust or dust mite allergy: a controlled trial. *Pediatrics* 1983; 71: 418–22.

21. Platts-Mills TAE, Mitchell FB, Nock P, Tovey ER, Mosroro H, Wilkins SR. Reduction of bronchial hyper-reactivity during prolonged allergen avoidance. *Lancet* 1982; ii: 675–78.

22. Boner AL, Niero E, Antolini L, Vallotta AE, Gaburro D. Pulmonary function and bronchial hyperreactivity in asthmatic children with house dust mite allergy during prolonged stay in the Italian Alps (Misurina, 1756 m). *Ann Allergy* 1985; 54: 42–5.

23. van der Heide S, Kauffman HF, Dubois AEJ, de Monchy JGR. Allergen reduction measures in houses of allergic asthmatic patients: effects of air-cleaners and allergen-impermeable mattress covers. *Eur Respir J* 1997; 10: 1217–23.

24. Ehnert B, Lau-Schdendorf S, Weber A, Buettner P, Schou C, Wahn U. Reducing domestic exposure to dust mite allergen reduces bronchial hyperreactivity in sensitive children with asthma. *J Allergy Clin Immunol* 1992; 90: 135–8.

25. Custovic A, Simpson A, Chapman MD, Woodcock A. Allergen avoidance in the treatment of asthma and atopic disorders. *Thorax* 1998; 53: 63–72.

26. Weiss ST, Tager IB, Schenker M, Speizer FE. The health effects of involuntary smoking. *Am Rev Respir Dis* 1983; 128: 933–42.

27. Ehrlich RI, Du Toit D, Jordaan E *et al*. Risk factors for childhood asthma and wheezing: importance of maternal and household smoking. *Am J Respir Crit Care Med* 1996; 154: 681–8.

28. Fergusson DM, Horwood LJ. Parental smoking and respiratory illness during early childhood: a six year longitudinal study. *Pediatric Pulmonol* 1985; 1: 99–106.

29. Murray AB, Morrison BJ. The effect of cigarette smoke from the mother on bronchial responsiveness and severity of symptoms in children with asthma. *J Allergy Clin Immunol* 1986; 77: 575–81.

30. Frischer T, Kuehr J, Meinert R *et al*. Maternal smoking in early childhood: a risk factor for bronchial responsiveness to exercise in primary-school children. *J Pediatr* 1992; 121: 17–22.

31. Health Effects of Outdoor Air Pollution. Committee of the Environmental and Occupation Health Assembly of the American Thoracic Society. *Am J Respir Crit Care Med* 1996; 153: 3–50.

32. Weiss ST, Tager IB, Munoz A, Speizer FE. The relationship of respiratory infections in early childhood to the occurrence of increased levels of bronchial responsiveness and atopy. *Am Rev Respir Dis* 1985; 131: 573–8.

33. Busse WW. Respiratory infections: their role in airway responsiveness and the pathogenesis of asthma. *J Allergy Clin Immunol* 1990; 85: 671–83.

34. Johnston SL. Influence of viral and bacterial respiratory infection on exacerbations and symptom severity in childhood asthma. *Pediatr Pulmonol* 1997; 16(suppl.): 88–9.

35. Martinez FD, Wright AL, Taussig LM, Holberg CJ, Halonen M, Morgan WJ. Asthma and wheezing in the first six years of life. The Group Health Medical Associates. *N Engl J Med* 1995; 332: 133–8.

36. ❂ Cookson WOCM, Moffatt MF. Asthma: An epidemic in the absence of infection? *Science* 1997; 275: 41–2.

37. Strachan DP. Hay fever, hygiene, and household size. *BMJ* 1989; 299: 1259–60.

38. Shirakawa T, Enomoto T, Shimazu S, Hopkin J. The inverse association between tuberculin responses and atopic disorder. *Science* 1997; 276: 77–9.

39. Pisetsky DS. The immunologic properties of DNA. *J Immunol* 1996; 156: 421–3.

40. Sato Y, Roman M, Tighe H *et al*. Immunostimulatory DNA sequences necessary for effective intradermal gene immunization. *Science* 1996; 273: 352–4.

41. Kline JN, Waldschmidt TJ, Businga TR *et al*. Cutting edge: modulation of airway inflammation by CpG oligodeoxynucleotides in a murine model of asthma. *Am Assoc Immunol* 1998; 2555–9.

42. Mosmann TR, Sad S. The expanding universe of T-cell subsets: Thl, Th2 and more. *Immunol Today* 1996; 17: 138–46.

43. ❂ Holt PG, Sly PD, Blorksten B. Atopic versus infectious diseases in childhood; a question of balance? *Pediatr Allergy Immunol* 1997; 8: 53–8.

44. Holt PG. A potential vaccine strategy for asthma and allied atopic diseases during early childhood. *Lancet* 1994; 344: 456–8.

45. Hsu CH, Chu KY, Tao MH, *et al*. Immunoprophylaxis of allergen-induced immunoglobulin E synthesis and airway hyperresponsiveness *in vivo* by genetic immunization. *Nat Med* 1996; 2: 540–4.

46. Stannegard IL, Larsson LO, Wennergren G, Strannegard O. Prevalence of allergy in children in relation to prior BCG vaccination and infection with atypical mycobacteria. *Allergy* 1998; 53: 249–54.

47. Grulee, CG, Sanford, HN. The influence of breast and artificial feeding on infantile eczema. *J Pediatr* 1936; 9: 223–5.

48. Kramer, MS. Does breast feeding help protect against atopic disease? Biology, methodology and a golden jubilee of controversy. *J Pediatr* 1988; 112–90.

49. Zeiger RS, Heller S, Mellon MH, *et al*. Effect of combined maternal and infant food-allergen avoidance on development of atopy in early infancy: a randomized study. *J Allergy Clin Immunol* 1989; 84: 72–89.

50. Faith-Magnusson K, Kjellman NIM. Development of atopic disease in babies whose mothers were receiving exclusion diet during pregnancy – a randomized study. *J Allergy Clin Immunol* 1987; 80: 868–75.

51. Faith-Magnusson K, Kjellman NIM. Allergy prevention by maternal elimination diet during late pregnancy – A 5-year follow-up of a randomized study. *J Allergy Clin Immunol* 1992; 89: 709–13.

52. ✪ Arshad SH, Matthews S, Gant C, Hide DW. Effect of allergen avoidance on development of allergic disorders in infancy. *Lancet* 1992; 339: 1439–97.

53. Hide D, Matthews S, Matthews L, *et al*. Effect of allergen avoidance in infancy on allergic manifestations at age of two years. *J Allergy Clin Immunol* 1994; 93: 842–6.

54. Colloff M, Ayres J, Carswell F *et al*. The control of allergens of dust mites and domestic pets. *Clin Exp Allergy* 1992; 22: 1–28.

55. McDonald L, Tovey E. The role of water temperature and laundry procedures in reducing house dust mite populations and allergen content of bedding. *J Allergy Clin Immunol* 1992; 90: 599–608.

56. Becker AB, Chan-Yeung M. Environmental control: an idea whose time has come. *Eur Res J* 1997; 10: 1203–4.

57. Wood R, Chapman M, Adkinson NF, Eggleston P. The effect of cat removal on allergen content in household-dust samples. *J Allergy Clin Immunol* 1989; 83: 730–34.

58. De Blay F, Chapman MD, Platts-Mills TAE. Airborne cat allergen (*Fel d* l): environmental control with cat *in situ*. *Am Rev Respir Dis* 1991; 143: 1334–9.

59. Watson WTA, Al-Malik SM, Lilley MK *et al*. The association of aeroallergens, precipitation, and environmental pollutants with emergency room visits and hospitalizations for asthma on the Canadian prairies. *J Allergy Clin Immunol* 1993; 1991: 304.

Chapter 16

Secondary Allergen Avoidance Measures

Patrick Powers, Jennifer Wyman and Thomas Platts-Mills

INTRODUCTION

Eighty percent of asthmatic children and approximately 50% of asthmatic adults are "atopic".[1] Although many different antigens can give rise to immediate sensitivity, a large percentage of atopic individuals are sensitive to dust mite antigens or other indoor allergens as judged by skin testing.[2–6] While pharmaceutical options for treating asthma have seemingly burgeoned, asthma has become more prevalent, more severe and with an overall increase in mortality. The factors that have contributed to the increase in prevalence or mortality are presently unclear, although an increase in maternal smoking, a gradual tendency to heat and then seal homes (thus increasing humidity), an increase in environmental ozone, a lack of access to timely primary care and even the asthma medications themselves have all been suggested.[2,3,7–10,14] Of these it is changes in temperature (increased) and ventilation rates (decreased) that appear to correlate temporally with increased asthma, and to provide improved conditions for growth of mites and/or fungi.

Studies in the last several years have demonstrated a marked inflammatory component with eosinophils and evidence for T-cell activation in the lungs of chronic asthmatic patients. Inflammatory responses of this kind can be reproduced in the lung following bronchial challenge with relevant allergens, or in skin biopsies following patch testing of atopic dermatitis patients.[15–18] Most asthmatic patients have airway responsiveness to exercise, cold air, or challenge with a wide range of chemicals, e.g. histamine, methacholine, leukotriene D_4 and bradykinin. Bronchoalveolar lavage (BAL) of patients with asthma reveals eosinophilia, sensitized lymphocytes, as well as markers for activation of $CD4^+$ T cells, in addition to interleukin (IL)-4 and IL-5, which

have been linked to the late allergic response.[15,19] A dose–response relationship between allergen exposure and clinical disease in the susceptible atopic patients has been demonstrated and implies a causal relationship to the non-specific inflammation and airway hyper-responsiveness.[20,21] For these reasons, any patient with frequent symptoms requiring regular therapy to control their asthma, including anti-inflammatory medications, should be evaluated for the presence of specific IgE-mediated sensitivity and given advice on allergen avoidance.[20,22–24] In many cases, avoidance of the relevant agent(s) can produce relief in symptoms, decrease in medications, and improved stability of airway and mucosal passages to non-specific stimuli.[25–30]

Indoor aeroallergens have been implicated as an increasingly important source of antigen exposure.[2,20,22,28,31] With the widespread use of wall-to-wall carpets, following the introduction of vacuum cleaners in 1935, general use of central heating, and tighter insulation, houses have changed dramatically over the last 30 years. As a result, household concentrations of airborne allergens have almost certainly increased. Exposure to this environment is repeated and prolonged, with the average person spending 97% of their time indoors with, more significantly, at least one-third of their time at home. Unlike seasonal exposures to pollens and grasses, chronic exposures are often insidious – not necessarily associated with acute conjunctivitis, or rapid onset of nasal symptoms, but more often chronic nasal congestion, and asthma.[31] Some evidence suggests that avoidance measures introduced early in life can help decrease allergen sensitization.[32–34]

Measurement of allergens in house-dust provides information about the reservoir from which allergens become airborne and also an archaeologic record of organic and inorganic matter including accumulations of domestic pet, cockroach or mite allergens. Assays are also very important in assessing the success of avoidance measures. Specific antigens found on dust mite (*Der p* I, *Der f* I), cat (*Fel d* I), and cockroach (*Bla g* II) can be quantified using monoclonal antibody enzyme-linked immunosorbent assay (ELISA).[31,38–40] These assays measure a single protein derived from each source as a marker. This makes standardization of the assays possible and simplifies analysis of the antigens in that maintaining the large pools of human sera containing high levels of specific IgE for radioallergosorbent test (RAST) inhibition is not necessary.

Patient education plays a crucial role in the management of asthma. As we gain an increasingly detailed knowledge of the biology of asthma, it is important that we pass this understanding along to the patient by promoting open communication, emphasizing goals and outcomes, and encouraging family involvement.[41]

DUST MITE

In those areas of the world where the weather is humid for 6 months or more, up to 80% of asthmatic children and young adults have positive skin-prick tests to allergen derived from *Dermatophagoides*. The major dust mites *D. farinae*, *D. pteronyssinus*, *Blomia tropicalis*, and *Euroglyphus maynei* occur with varying distribution worldwide.[42–45] In the USA, *D. farinae*, and *D. pteronyssinus* tend to dominate although *D. farinae* is favoured in climates that have a prolonged dry period and when the relative humidity remains at 60%, i.e. in air conditioned units.[46] *Blomia tropicalis* occurs in tropical and subtropical areas of the world including the USA, Europe, Asia, and South America. Presently its major specific antigens can be assayed with RAST inhibition assay or identified using crossed immunoelectrophoresis. Cross-reactivity with some *D. farinae* and *D. pteronyssinus* antigens has been reported.[47] The mite *Euroglyphus mayneii* has been found predominantly in southern USA and in Europe and has a 30% antigenic homology with *D. pteronyssinus*. Assays using polyclonal antisera for group I dust mite antigens can detect *E. maynei*, but probably underestimate the importance this mite.[48] Two other methods for detecting mite exposure exist: mite counts, which are the gold standard for identifying species, but are time consuming and require a worker trained in the morphologic characteristics of mite species; the other is a kit for revealing guanine in dust which acts as a screen for the presence

of the major nitrogenous waste product of arachnids.[47,49] Although simple and sensitive, guanine detection per se can overestimate mite prevalence due to other sources and the test is not very stable in storage and is not widely available.[30,47,49]

The distribution of dust mite antigens is non-discriminatory, being equally present in urban and suburban houses. However the concentrations found in apartments have been considerably lower presumably reflecting lower humidity. The highest concentrations are found in bedding and mattresses.[25,50] On the basis of multiple studies estimating exposure, it has been proposed that 2 µg of *Der p* 1 per gram of house-dust should be regarded as a threshold for sensitization to the mite, and that 10 µg g^{-1} dust is a level that both increases the risk of asthma and the tendency to develop symptoms earlier in life.[51] Avoidance measures that decrease exposure to < 1.0 µg g^{-1} dust, have been shown to decrease bronchial reactivity in asthmatics.[25,26,51–53]

The source and structure of dust-mite allergens has helped in understanding effective means of avoiding them. *Der p* 1 and *Der f* 1 are enzymes secreted by the gastrointestinal tract of mites. They are found in the mite faecal pellets which are 10–20 µm in diameter.[31] While these particles become airborne with household disturbances such as fans, vacuuming, removing rugs, and changing bedding, they settle rapidly, i.e. in less than 10 minutes.[31,53–55] More prolonged exposure is thought to occur while sleeping or resting on upholstered furniture when the dust source is close to the mouth and inspiration of faecal particles is more likely with quiet respiration.[31,53] Chronic low-dose dust-mite allergen exposure is thought to be the key method of producing bronchial inflammation and may be instrumental in the pathogenesis of chronic allergic asthma.[35] In fact, sensitization to dust mites is felt to be a dominant risk factor for asthma in an adolescent population.[36]

CONTROL OF MITE ALLERGEN

Mite growth requires a humidity greater than 50% and is optimal at a relative humidity of 70–80%, temperatures of 25°C (70–80°F), and requires a supply of organic debris preferably skin scales.[45,56] Therefore mite allergen exposure can be reduced either by relocating to a high altitude and thus low humidity areas, by removing sites where mites can grow, or by creating unfavourable growing conditions.[57] While replacing bedding and mattresses will transiently reduce dust mite to near zero levels, avoidance must be maintained.[58] Mattresses and pillows can be inexpensively enclosed in impermeable plastic covers with the zipper taped shut, or with specially manufactured vapour permeable covers that may be more comfortable and generally last longer.[29,59] These encasements have been shown to prevent leakage of common indoor allergens and are successful at reducing sensitization to dust mite in children with atopic dermatitis.[33,37] Cotton bedding should be washed in hot water (55°C, 130°F) weekly. It has been shown that vacuuming and simply washing bedding and flooring alone is neither effective at decreasing mite counts nor improving pulmonary function.[60] While dry cleaning will kill mites, their antigens are left relatively intact.[61] A number of studies suggest that the addition of benzyl benzoate (to yield an approximate concentration of 0.03%) to a cooler temperature wash is effective at killing mites and washing out the mite allergen.[61,62] Cool water washing alone does not kill mites or remove them from bedding.[60,61] Recent work has shown that benzyl benzoate, when applied to a new mattress, significantly lowered mite and allergen levels as compared with an old mattress, but found no significant difference between the benzyl benzoate and the placebo group.[63] When compared with mattress encasements and placebo, benzyl benzoate was found to cause a small but statistically significant improvement in airway hyperresponsiveness.[70] The question of whether benzyl benzoate adds enough benefit to warrant its use is still under investigation. Benzyl benzoate as a 25% lotion has been safely used for years as a topical treatment for scabies.[65] Its major toxicity being recognized as an irritant effect on eyes or mucosa when used for these indications.[64–66]

Carpets are a major reservoir of mite antigen as well as being an important site of mite growth.[28,29,64,66,67] For patients with moderate to severe asthma, e.g. inadequately controlled or on regular inhaled steroids, removing carpets and installing hardwood or vinyl floors followed by regular damp mopping weekly is essential, especially in the bedroom.[25,26,29] Less satisfactory is covering carpeted flooring with plastic vinyl sheeting and sealing the edges. However, this may be one of few options for the family restricted to a carpeted apartment. It is further recommended that bedroom curtains be washable fabric or venetian-type blinds and that clutter, including clothing, toys, and curios be removed or kept in a closed closet. Upholstered furniture should be replaced with wooden, vinyl, or leather, i.e. dust mite impermeable, washable surfaces.[28,29]

Other important areas where dust mites proliferate are in the family and living rooms. In these rooms, removing carpets and changing furniture is helpful but may not be possible. An attractive proposal has been to treat upholstered furniture and rugs with solutions of aqueous benzyl benzoate, tannic acid, and benzyl derivatives.[64,66–68] While effective at lowering mite counts and allergens in vitro, success has been more varied when these chemicals have been used in homes although they can reduce allergen levels in carpets when applied every 3 months.[64,66,67,69] However the ability of tannic acid to denature allergens is very dependant on the conditions and the benzyl benzoate powder (Acarosan) requires repeated application. In addition, a white powder residue may continue to lift from the carpet after benzyl benzoate treatment.[64] Carpets laid on an unventilated floor, e.g. cement or basement, can be very difficult to dry once exposed to moisture and thus become a source of mite as well as mould and bacterial products. It is particularly important that severely allergic patients do not live or work in such areas. Lifting rugs, mattresses, and upholstered furniture and "beating" them with a rug beater, followed by vigorous vacuuming and airing in strong sunlight, are also effective measures to reduce antigen levels and kill mites.[72]

Reducing relative humidity to below 50% is an effective method for decreasing mite growth. While relative humidity is low during the winter in many areas of the world, during the summer this may require expensive air conditioning.[73,74] In some areas, increasing ventilation rates to one air change per hour for several hours per day is effective and can be accomplished by opening several windows.[74] Air conditioning individual rooms has been shown to decrease mite allergen and is indicated for severely allergic patients[46] (Table 16.1).

COCKROACH

Interest in cockroach allergy has intensified in recent years as more evidence has established that patients living in infested areas have an increased incidence of skin-test positivity and asthma.[75–80] Cockroaches are tropical insects and are found wherever water, warmth, and organic matter are present. Several studies have demonstrated a high prevalence of RAST or skin-test positivity to cockroach among inner-city, especially African–American, asthmatic subjects. In fact, African–American race and low socioeconomic status have been

Table 16.1: Summary of dust mite avoidance measures

1. Enclose mattresses and pillows in a zippered, plastic cover or a special allergen-proof fabric. Tape the zipper, damp wipe the mattress cover every 2 weeks.

2. Wash all bedding, including mattress pad, pillow cases, and blankets in hot water (at least 130° F, 55 C) weekly. Replace quilts with dacron or orlon blankets which are to be washed with the bedding. Alternatively, cover quilt with vapour-permeable, allergen-proof fabric.

3. Remove small objects that accumulate dust, ornaments, books, etc, from the room or place in a closed closet or cabinet. Store clothing in drawers or in a closed cupboard; store unused clothing away from the bedroom.

4. Remove upholstered furniture and replace with leather, plastic, or vinyl furniture.

5. Remove carpets whenever possible, or vacuum weekly using a vacuum cleaner with an effective filter. The patient should avoid being in a room where vacuuming is occurring until at least 20 minutes after it has been completed. If the patient must vacuum, a mask should be worn during this time.
   Remove wall-to-wall carpets on cement slab, and replace with area rugs which are more easily treated, or optimally, install subflooring and hardwood floors.

6. Treat carpets with acaricides, 3% tannic acid, or by airing in strong sunlight after mechanically removing dust.

7. Replace drapes and curtains with washable curtains or venetian blinds. Clean and vacuum approximately every 2 weeks.

8. Control humidity in the house either by increasing ventilation with fresh air when the outside air is dry, using air conditioning (central is best) or using a dehumidifier for very damp areas of the house such as the basement.

9. Replace air filters on air conditioners, or wash with soap and water, approximately every 3 months to remove fungus and airborne debris. Electrostatic filters may also be useful on central air conditioning units for reducing allergens, but will not affect the amount in or produced by reservoirs of dust mites.

shown to be independent significant risk factors for cockroach allergen sensitivity and asthma morbidity and mortality.[81,82] While sensitization is more likely to be seen in patients of deprived socioeconomic status and those living in crowded conditions, it is well worth noting that most of these patients are sensitized to dust mites and other aeroallergens as well.[2,19,22,83–85] As with dust mite and pollen aeroallergens, the prevalence of sensitivity is thought to correlate with exposure.[39,85,86] Some studies show that continued exposure to allergen is an important factor in asthma symptoms.[78,79,85]

Eliciting a history of cockroach exposure in patients can be done with tact. Questions could include: "Do you have a problem with insects in your house?", or "Have you ever seen a cockroach in your house?". Nonetheless, in approximately 20% of houses, with high levels of cockroach allergen the families did not report cockroaches being present and the insects were not seen by the technician visiting the house.[39]

To quantify exposure, sandwich ELISAs to detect *Per a* I or *Bla g* I, produced by American (*Periplaneta americana*) and German (*Blatella germanica*) cockroaches respectively, have been developed. These assays also cross-react with the Asian cockroach (*B. orientalis*) and the brown banded cockroach (*Supella suspellectilium*) which are also common household pests.[87] However, because this cross-reactivity is partial, the assays tend to underestimate exposure to other species.[87] Sensitive monoclonal antibody-based assays specific for *Bla g* I and *Bla g* II, antigens from the German cockroach, have been developed.[39] *Bla g* I and *Bla g* II have been associated with particles of 7–10 μm which can be detected after air disturbance, but like mite faecal particles, are thought to settle rapidly.[55,88] Environmental exposure has been assessed in a number of studies.[39,79,85] In paediatric patients with asthma presenting to an Atlanta emergency department, 9/35 had both cockroach-specific IgE antibodies greater than 50 units and exposure to *Bla g* II in two or more sites, whereas only 1/22 of controls had similar risk factors.[79]

Control of Cockroach Allergen

Studies of American house-dust from Tampa Florida, show levels of *Per a* I ranging from 7 to 200 000 ng *Per a* I equivalents per gram dust with many households having 10–10 000 ng equivalents *Per a* I per gram.[87] *Blatella* allergens are usually found in highest concentration in the kitchen, 50 times the amount elsewhere, with much less in the bedroom, bedding or living rooms of atopic asthmatic subjects. However similar levels are found in the houses of non-atopic control subjects from the same neighbourhood.[39] Avoidance measures, in heavily infested areas, are difficult to maintain, especially in apartment dwellings where cockroaches notoriously evade eradication by moving to surrounding apartments after pesticide application only to re-emerge at a later date. Nonetheless, extermination measures using organophosphates are effective to kill existing cockroaches and to reduce propagation.[89,90] It should be kept in mind that cockroaches often become resistant to any particular extermination method. Cleanliness is most important, by minimizing food or organic debris and careful vacuuming which should be combined with using bait stations or bait paste (hydramethylnon).[89,90] In addition, what are sometimes referred to as "manic mechanical measures" such as careful caulking of all cracks may also be effective both by reducing movement of roaches and by decreasing the spaces for breeding. Preliminary data indicate that these measures reduce cockroach antigens effectively, although the problem tends to reoccur within 3 months if stringent measures are not maintained.[90] (Table 16.2).

CAT

Approximately 3% of the population are allergic to cats.[91] Household cats are present in approximately 28% of American families and are owned by almost one-third of cat-allergic patients (i.e. approximately two million individuals). In emergency room studies, cat-specific IgE antibody has been strongly associated with treatment for asthma.[2,4,22,85] Combining the results for two ER studies, the prevalence of IgE antibody to cat allergen was 30/188 among patients with asthma and 1/202 among controls (odds ratio 38). It has also been demonstrated that airborne cat allergen can precipitate asthma in cat-sensitive patients, when 8–80 ng

Table 16.2: Summary of cockroach avoidance measures

1. Keep kitchen free of food debris and dirty dishes.

2. Caulk all cracks near water sources including bathrooms and kitchen with special attention to areas around taps, pipe fittings at walls, under sinks, around bathtub/shower.

3. Vacuum or carefully sweep kitchen, dining room, and other areas where food is consumed, on a daily basis.

4. Place roach stations in all food areas, concentrating especially on kitchen, and bathroom; replace every 3 months.

5. Spray with organophosphates or other insecticide on a monthly basis. Discard foods and wash dishes after being exposed to the sprays.

of cat allergen *Fel d* 1 is inhaled.[92] An epidemiologic study suggesting that exposure of children to 8 µg *Fel d* 1 per gram house-dust can induce sensitization further supports a causal relation between exposure and the expression of atopy.[73] The fact that many cat-allergic patients know within 15 minutes that they have entered a cat household suggests that significant quantities are airborne. This has been confirmed by studies of airborne *Fel d* 1 in undisturbed cat-containing homes.[20] *Fel d* 1, the major cat allergen, is almost ubiquitous, but levels of >8 µg g^{-1} in reservoir dust or 1–20 ng m^{-3} airborne dust have been found in almost all homes where cats are kept.[73,94] Interestingly, low levels of cat exposure that occurs in many homes without cats may itself cause symptoms in some patients who are sensitive to cats.[93] A recent study examining sensitization to cat allergen as a risk factor of asthma found that airborne *Fel d* 1 was detectable in undisturbed conditions in all homes with cats and in almost a third of homes without cats.[95]

Exposure may be quantified either by measuring *Fel d* 1 in dust or with air sampling devices.[88,91,96] Airborne *Fel d* 1 judged both by falling properties and by particle sizing is carried on particles ranging from 1 to 20 µm.[31] This is quite unlike dust mite antigen which becomes airborne on large particles greater than 8 µm in diameter. In addition, after disturbance of room, airborne particles can reach concentrations of up to 100 ng m^{-3}. Inhaling these levels of allergen it would take only 6 minutes for the sensitized asthmatic to inhale enough antigen to have a significant drop in forced expiratory volume in 1 s (FEV_1).[88,96]

Control of Cat Allergen

The main source of *Fel d* 1 is from the skin in the form of dander, with the saliva being a relatively minor source; the main avoidance measure recommended is complete removal of the cat from the household. However, after removal of the cat, soft furniture, carpeting and even the walls are significant reservoirs of cat allergen.[91] The allergen is easily disturbed by activities such as vacuuming and sweeping and even by small fans.[31,96,97] Consequently, reduction of cat allergen after removal of the cat alone will take up to 12 weeks unless accompanied by vigorous cleaning and removing the major reservoirs.[98]

If the patient or family decides not to remove the cat, allergen levels can be decreased in a number of ways. By washing the cat weekly with 1 litre of water, cat dander and allergen can be reduced under specific circumstances.[91] However this may not be as simple as was originally thought, probably because the cat will reaccumulate allergen both from reservoirs in its environment and from production in the skin.[99] HEPA (high efficiency particulate air) filters can reduce *Fel d* 1 by 90% but only in non-carpeted rooms as the air flow coming out of the filter can cause enough disturbance from a carpet to increase airborne cat allergen.[91] In addition, vacuuming rugs with HEPA-filter vacuum cleaners can reduce 6–20 μm particles of *Fel d* 1 without significantly increasing overall levels of airborne allergen. Recent evidence suggests that high quality bags and/or filters placed before and after the exhaust fan on a vacuum cleaner can greatly reduce the leakage of allergen.[101] There are now several inexpensive brands of vacuum cleaner which trap allergen very well and are useful for reducing cat allergen from this reservoir.[96] Some vacuum cleaners leak allergen far more than others and would not be recommended for controlling exposure.[96,100,101] Lastly, increasing air changes from approximately 0.3 air changes per hour (ACH), a typical flow rate for a modern "tight" house, to 1–2.4 ACH using window or central fan units will help to reduce the particles of <2 μm in diameter, but has little effect on overall airborne cat allergen.[96] The clinical significance of this measure, i.e. changing the distribution of airborne particles, is presently unknown. Patients should be forewarned that reduction of airborne allergen to very low levels, e.g. <2 ng m,[-3] may still be associated with clinical symptoms of sneeze and congestion[102] (Table 16.3).

Due to limitations of space, dog allergen, *Can f* I, will only be discussed in brief. Essentially, as with cats, washing and other measures may be useful to decrease the amount of airborne allergen.[103] The fact that fewer people keep dogs, and that they are often kept outside thus contributing less to indoor aeroallergen load, is thought to be partially responsible for the lack of wide-

Table 16.3: Summary of cat allergen avoidance measures

1. Remove cat from environment, replace upholstered furniture and carpets, steam clean walls.

If cat remains:

2. Keep cat out of bedroom and other rooms where patient spends majority of time.

3. Wash the cat in one litre of water weekly. Kittens treated gently can tolerate this reasonably well, otherwise the veterinarian or pet-grooming service may be preferable to reduce trauma to both owner and cat.

4. Reduce sources of reservoir cat allergen: replace previously exposed upholstered furniture with leather, vinyl, or plastic washable sources. Wash down weekly with water or equivalent.

5. Remove carpets, and replace with washable area rugs or hardwood floors. Clean regularly.

6. Vacuum rugs with HEPA-filter vacuum cleaner to reduce large *Fel d* 1 particles; avoid water reservoir vacuum cleaners as these can disperse *Fel d* 1

7. Increase ventilation rates to 1–2.4 ACH with fans, air-conditioning, or by opening windows, to reduce small *Fel d* 1 particles.

8. Clean air in bedroom or room where patient spends majority of time with use of HEPA-type air cleaner.

9. Electrostatic filters on central air units may have limited value in face of significant exposure from cats and reservoirs, but should otherwise be considered if other measures are instituted.

spread sensitization and clinical symptoms attributed to dogs.[103]

MOULD

Evaluation of sensitization to moulds suggests that between 3 and 10% of the population show sensitivity to moulds.[104] However this is dependent on the extract used for skin testing and there is currently very little evidence about the quality of the majority of mould extracts used. Using aerometric sampling devices, fungus spores are present in very large numbers in the outside air. However, the clinical relevance of these measurements is not clear for several reasons: the measurements show great variability from day to day, many of the spores are difficult to identify visually, while the results of cultures reflect viability rather than allergen content. In addition, house-dust samples reveal a combination of spores and mycelia and it is not clear what these elements contribute to allergen exposure.[105,106,107] It is clear that there is great variability in the optimal growing conditions of different moulds. Changes in growing conditions for a given species can trigger changes in expressed genes and therefore the pattern and distribution of specific allergens. In addition, the paucity of immunoassays for these allergens limits evaluation of exposure.[105,108]

There are four main groups of moulds: Phycomycetes including *Rhizopus* and *Mucor* species; Basidiomycetes including puffballs and gilled mushrooms such as Amanita; Ascomycetes; and the imperfect fungi, so called because they lack a sexual phase of reproduction. The latter includes most of the major fungi traditionally associated with allergy including *Cladosporium, Alternaria, Aspergillus, Helminthosporium* and *Penicillium*. Spores range from 2 to 17 μm in diameter. Fungi have traditionally been identified based on morphological characteristics and growth patterns.[109]

Mould seasons are not defined in the way that pollen seasons are, because most moulds can grow rapidly at any time, when adequate conditions are available. Spore release and distribution depends of wind speed and precipitation.[105] One species may be favoured over another and this may vary both from one site to another or with changes in the weather. Moulds such as *Aspergillus* enjoy warmth; basidiospores are dependent on free water; and *Cladosporium, Alternaria* and *Helminthosporium* are considered "dry spores" and are mobilized with dry windy conditions.[105] The substrate is important. While all moulds are saprophytic if not parasitic, some favour breads (the zygomycete *Rhizopus* and ergot-producing ascomycete *Neurospora*). Damp foundations often harbour *Cladosporium*. Shower areas, air conditioners and humidifier units are important as sources of *Rhizopus, Mucor, Aspergillus,* and *Penicillium*.[105,110] In Hawaii, air conditioned homes are found to have fewer spores of outdoor fungi, but markedly elevated levels of *Aspergillus*.[111] Different *Aspergillus* species are used as a source of enzymes in food production. For example, *Aspergillus oryzae* is used in baking bread; and both *Aspergillus oryzae* and *Saccharomyces cerevesiae* are utilized in sake brewing. *Penicillium* species are used to make some cheeses.[105]

Classically the antigenic determinants of fungi have been detected using crossed-immunoelectrophoresis (CIE). CIE has shown there exists a wide variability of antigen quantity and quality depending on growing and sampling conditions, as well as between the different commercial extracts available for skin testing.[105] While available, CIE is subjective and not presently used to standardize for the specific antigens and would probably not be feasible. Since some of the major spore and mycelial allergens are thought to have important carbohydrate components, characterizing them primarily by protein nitrogen units (PNU) is not accurate. These carbohydrate components also make protein purification difficult. Much of the work to date has focused on the major antigenic determinants of three organisms: *Aspergillus, Trichophyton,* and *Alternaria*.[105,106,112–114] Two of these organisms, *Trichophyton* and *Aspergillus*, are important human pathogens. It is also important to remember that many fungi produce bioactive toxins during normal growth.[105,113]

An association between asthma and positive RAST and/or skin-prick test to several fungi including *Alternaria, Cladosporium,* and *Aspergillus* has been demonstrated.[3,115] Bronchospasm can be induced by controlled inhalation of *Aspergillus* and *Trichophyton* fungal extracts in skin-prick test or RAST-positive asthmatics, but not in skin-prick test negative asthmatic or normal control subjects. Similar studies have documented nasal symptoms using *Alternaria* extracts.[116] In patients with positive bronchoprovocation to *Cladosporium*, symptoms and the use of medications have increased in parallel with increasing spore counts in Denmark, where up to one-third of atopic adults with respiratory allergic diseases are skin-prick test positive to basidiomycete mycelia and/or spore extracts.[117]

Immunoassays using monoclonal antibodies are just becoming available to study the prevalence of specific fungal antigens in the air and dust samples from environment.[113,118] One of the best characterized fungal allergens is *Asp* f I from *Aspergillus fumigatus*. A monoclonal based ELISA has been developed and used to compare levels of *Asp* f I in mycelial extracts, spores and culture media.[113] For example, *Asp* f I, a mycelial antigen, has been found to be absent in most house-dust extracts, but present after culture indicating that spores are present.[119] It is readily detected by aerosampling during outdoor leaf disturbances. This antigen appears to be clinically relevant both in allergic bronchopulmonary aspergillosis (ABPA), and cystic fibrosis (CF). *Asp* f I IgG is found in 98% of cystic fibrosis patients by age 10 implying that *A. fumigatus* mycelia are growing in the bronchi of these patients. *A. fumigatus* has a very wide temperature tolerance and requires high relative humidity (about 80%). The mycelial forms of this organism have been found in pathology specimens and in BAL fluids from these patients.[120]

The genus *Trichophyton* includes a series of fungi that are responsible for chronic or severe cutaneous infections of the groin, feet, or toenails in a large number of patients. What is less clear is how some of these patients become "allergic" to *Trichophyton*. It has been found that *Trichophyton*-sensitive patients, by RAST and skin test, have positive bronchoprovocation tests when challenged with extracts of *Trichophyton*.[116] It is assumed that these patients become sensitized from T-cell mediated reactions to their cutaneous infections as specific IgE and IgG to *Trichophyton* have been measured.[114] Podiatrists have also been known to have *Trichophyton*-induced wheezing, but this was thought to be a result of sensitization from multiple exposures to airborne powders generated during grinding of toenails.[121]

Multiple fungi can occasionally be cultured from patients with allergic sinusitis. These include *Aspergillus*, *Bipolaris*, *Mucor*, *Candida*, and *Rhizopus*.[105,122] While this is an uncommon cause of chronic sinusitis, most of these otherwise immunocompetent patients have a history of steroid or multiple antibiotic use. Increased specific IgG, eosinophilia, and positive skin-prick tests may be seen in these patients. The CT scans from these patients usually reveal sinusitis with or without boney infiltration or radiographic invasion, findings which are confirmed on microscopy of pathology specimens.[24,122]

Control of Mould Exposure

There are three approaches to reducing exposure to mould antigens:(1) avoiding sites where exposure is high i.e. basements, houses with active mould growth and outside sources (e.g. wearing a mask during garden work); (2) reducing humidity in the house to discourage mould growth; (3) cleaning surfaces, with bleach or comparable agents, e.g. shower curtains, refrigerator trays, and sinks. However there are few published controlled trials to support many accepted practices of mould and fungus control.

All allergic patients, and particularly fungus allergic patients, should avoid living or working in basements. Fungal growth is ubiquitous on basement walls and is very difficult to control. Houses with overt mould or in particular active mould in flooring will cause severe problems to most mould allergic patients. In addition, unventilated areas with a high fungus load may be the source of either allergens or toxins especially during the air disturbance of cleaning or renovating.[111,113] Other situations that represent high levels of mould exposure include lawn mowing, moving leaf mould, exposure to compost and rotting wood.[119]

Reducing humidity inside houses is important to control mite or mould growth. Controlling humidity involves reducing sources, and removing the humidity that naturally accumulates in houses.[73] Sources such as clothes dryers or cooking equipment should be vented to the outside.[73,74] In addition, humidifiers and the watering of live plants can contribute to indoor humidity.[110] Reducing humidity can be achieved by opening windows, thus increasing the ventilation to two to three air changes per hour, but this is helpful only when the outside absolute humidity is <6 g kg^{-1}. Alternatively, if the outside humidity is high, then using air conditioning or dehumidifiers is necessary.[74] Portable HEPA filters that reduce airborne particulates of >0.3 μm may also be helpful but have not been tested in relation to clinical symptoms due to moulds.[123]

The primary method of controlling mould growth in the house is to keep surfaces, furniture, etc dry. In addition, no food or other organic matter such as firewood, should be kept in the house. Surprisingly household plants appear to be only a minor source of mould spores. Fungicidal cleaning agents such as bleach in a dilution of 4–6 parts water to 1 part bleach, as well as commercially available fungicides, can be used to clean water soaked areas in the bathroom and kitchen. Nebulizer tubing and humidifiers should be rinsed with a 1:3 parts diluted 5% acetic acid or one-half teaspoonful chlorine bleach in one pint (~0.5 l) of water to discourage fungal growth. Paint additives to inhibit mould growth are also available and can be recommended for areas particularly susceptible to moisture (Table 16.4).

Compliance with avoidance measures has been studied and found to be especially difficult in patients from deprived socioeconomic class. It has been shown that video-taped instructions are useful to improve understanding, but a consistent theme has been that home visits by trained professionals are more effective in ensuring that changes are implemented. Patients often report full compliance when only one or two of several measures have been instituted. Many times there is resistance from the spouse, or the family has not been adequately convinced about the importance of the measures to control the patient's disease.[124]

Table 16.4: Summary of mycelial and spore avoidance measures

1. Fungal allergic patients should avoid sleeping or working for prolonged amounts of time in basements.

2. Wear a mask when disturbing areas where there is high mould growth: when raking leaves, turning mulch, heavy cleaning of basements, etc. Maximize ventilation when working in these areas.

3. Reduce sources of mould in house, keep houseplants free of dead leaves, avoid overwatering, bring in firewood for immediate use only.

4. Reduce general humidity in house as outlined in Table 16.1 and vent kitchen and bathroom as well as any other rooms with water sources, to the outside.

5. Use kitchen fans when cooking.

6. Keep doors closed while showering.

7. Dry clothes outside or vent dryer to outside.

8. Keep areas in kitchen and bathroom clean and dry; use fungicidal cleaners such as bleach diluted 1: 4–6 parts water to eliminate growth on a weekly basis.

9. Clean humidifiers with bleach solution, and rinse out dehumidifiers daily. Reduce other collections of standing water.

10. Allow nebulizer and other moist tubing to completely dry before storing. Rinse with vinegar or bleach solution.

KEY POINTS

1. Association between indoor allergens and asthma has been seen in all parts of the world and appears to be a major cause of the increasing prevalence of asthma.

2. Measurement of exposure to some of the major indoor allergens is now possible and allows for specific monitoring of avoidance measures.

3. Experimental exposure to allergens including mite, cat, or cockroach can induce inflammatory changes in the lung, and it is exactly this form of inflammation that is the hallmark of naturally occurring asthma. Thus allergen avoidance is a logical first line anti-inflammatory treatment for asthma.

4. The detailed way in which avoidance should be incorporated into normal treatment needs more study. However, any patient who requires regular treatment or has had steroid courses should be evaluated for the role of allergens.

5. Avoidance measures are allergen specific and it is not possible to give useful advice without knowing the specific sensitivity of the patient.

6. Avoidance measures require education, encouragement, and repeated reinforcement as with any other form of chronic treatment.

REFERENCES

1. Weiss ST, Sparrow D, O'Connor GT. The interrelationship among allergy, airways responsiveness, and asthma. *J Asthma* 1993; 30: 329–49.

2. Lin RY, LaFrance J, Sauter D. Hypersensitivity to common indoor aeroallergens in asthmatic patients. *Ann Allergy*, 1993; 71: 33–9.

3. O'Hollaren MT, Yunginger J, Offord KP *et al*. Exposure to an aeroallergen as a possible precipitating factor in respiratory arrest in young patients with asthma. *N Engl J Med* 1991; 324: 359–63.

4. Corbo GM, Forastiere F, Dell-Orco V, Pistelli R, Agabiti N, Perucci CA. Effects of environment on atopic status and respiratory disorders in children. *JACI* 1993; 92: 616–23.

5. Canny GJ, Reisman J. Acute asthma: Observations regarding the management of a pediatric emergency room. *Pediatrics* 1989; 83: 507–512.

6. Sly MR, O'Donnell R. Regional distribution of deaths from asthma. *Ann Allergy* 1989; 62: 347–54.

7. Weiss KB, Wagener DK. Changing patterns of asthma mortality: Identifying target populations at high risk. *JAMA* 1990; 264: 1683–7.

8. Jackson R, Sears MR. International trends in asthma mortality 1970–1985. *Chest* 1988; 94: 914–18.

9. NHLBI–Asthma Mortality Institute. Asthma mortality. *JACI* 1991; 88: 447–50.

10. Evans R, Mullally DI, Wilson RW *et al*. National trends in the morbidity and mortality of asthma in the U.S. *Chest* 1987; 91: 65–74S.

11. Boulet L-P, Deschesnes F, Turcotte H, Gignac F. Near-fatal asthma: Clinical and physiologic features, perception of bronchoconstriction, and psychologic profile. *J Allergy Clin Immunol* 1991; 88: 838–46.

12. Chilmoncyzk BA, Salmun LM, Megathin KN, Neveux LM, Palomaki GE. Association between exposure to environmental tobacco smoke and exacerbations of asthma in children. *N Engl J Med* 1993; 326: 1665–9.

13. Gong H Jr. Health effects of air pollution. A review of clinical studies. *Clin Chest Med* 1992; 13: 201–214.

14. Warner JO, Price SA. Aero-allergen avoidance in the prevention and treatment of asthma. *Clin Exp Allergy* 1990; 20: 15–19.

15. Robinson D, Hamid Q, Bentley A, Ying S, Kay AB, Durham SR. Activation of CD4$^+$ T cells, increased TH$_2$-type cytokine mRNA expression, and eosinophil recruitment in bronchoalveolar lavage after allergen inhalation challenge in patients with atopic asthma. *J Allergy Clin Immunol* 1993; 92: 313–24.

16. Platts-Mills TAE, Chapman MD, Mitchell B, Heymann PW, Deuell B. The role of inhalant allergens in atopic dermatitis. In: Ruzicka T, Ring J, Przybilla B (eds). *Handbook of Atopic Eczema*. Berlin: Springer-Verlag, 1991: 192–203.

17. Botey J, Gutierrez V, Pena JM, Eseverri JL, Marin A, Aulesa C. Specific IgE antibodies in nasal secretions: correlation with serum values and clinical tests. *Ann Allergy* 1993; 70: 26–9.

18. Sager N, Feldmann A, Schilling G, Kreitsch P, Neumann C. House dust mite-specific T cells in the skin of subjects with atopic dermatitis: Frequency and lymphokine profile in the allergen patch test. *J Allergy Clin Immunol* 1992; 89: 801–810.

19. Wasserman S, Olivenstein R, Renzi P, Xu L-J, Martin JG. The relationship between late asthmatic responses and antigen-specific immunoglobulin. *J Allergy Clin Immunol* 1992; 90: 661–9.

20. Platts-Mills TAE, Ward GW, Sporik R, Gelber LE, Chapman MD, Heymann PW. Epidemiology of the relationship between exposure to indoor allergens and asthma. *Int Arch Allergy Appl Immunol* 1991; 94: 339–45.

21. Wegner CD, Torcellini CA, Clarke CC, Letts LG, Gundel RH. Effects of single and multiple inhalations of antigen on airway responsiveness in monkeys. *J Allergy Clin Immunol* 1991; 87: 835–41.

22. Pollart SM, Chapman MD, Fiocco GP, Rose G, Platts-Mills TAE. Epidemiology of acute asthma: IgE antibodies to common inhalant allergens as a risk factor for emergency room visits. *J Allergy Clin Immunol* 1989; 83: 875–82.

23. Dodge R, Burrows B, Lebonitz MD. Antecedent features of children in whom asthma develops. *J Allergy Clin Immunol* 1993; 92: 744–9.

24. Newman LF, Platts-Mills TAE, Philips D, Hazen KC, Gross CW. Chronic sinusitis. *J Allergy Clin Immunol* 1994; 271: 363–7.

25. Murray AB, Ferguson AC. Dust-free bedrooms in the treatment of asthmatic children with house dust or house dust mite allergy: a controlled trial. *Pediatrics* 1983; 71: 418–22.

26. ❍ Platts-Mills TAE, Tovey ER, Mitchell EB, Moszoro H, Nock P, Wilkins SR. Reduction of bronchial hyperreactivity during prolonged allergen avoidance. *Lancet* 1982; 2: 675–8.

27. Dorward AJ, Colloff MJ, MacKay NS, McSharry C, Thomson NC. Effect of house dust mite avoidance measures on adult atopic asthma. *Thorax* 1988; 43: 98–105.

28. Korsgaard J. Mite asthma and residency. A case-control study on the impact of exposure to house-dust mites in dwellings. *Amer Rev Respir Dis* 1983; 128: 231–5.

29. Walshaw MJ, Evans CC. Allergen avoidance in house dust mite sensitive adult asthma. *Quart J Med* 1986; 58: 199–215.

30. Sanda T, Yasue T, Oohashi M, Yasue A. Effectiveness of house dust mite allergen avoidance through clean room therapy in patients with atopic dermatitis. *J Allergy Clin Immunol* 1992; 89: 653–7.

31. Platts-Mills TAE, Chapman MD, Pollart S, Luczynska GW, Ward GW Jr. Specific allergens evoking immune reactions in the lung: relationship to asthma. *Eur Respir J* 1991; 4: 68s–77s.

32. ❍ Wahn U, Lau S, Bergmann R, Kulig M, Forster J, Bergmann K, Bauer CP, Guggenmoos-Holzman I. Indoor allergen exposure is a risk factor for sensitization during the first three years of life. *J Allergy Clin Immunol* 1997; 99 (6 Pt 1): 763–9.

33. Nishioka K, Yasueda H, Saito H. Preventive effect of bedding encasement with microfine fibers on mite sensitization. *J Clin Immunol* 1998; 101: 28–32.

34. ❍ Peat JK, Tovey E, Toelle BG *et al*. House dust mite allergens. A major risk factor for childhood asthma in Australia. *Am J Respir Crit Care Med* 1996; 153(1): 141–6.

35. Arshad SH, Hamilton RG, Adkinson NF Jr. Repeated aerosol exposure to small doses of allergen. A model for chronic asthma. *Am J Respir Crit Care Med* 1998; 157(6 Pt 1): 1900–6.

36. ❍ Squillace SP, Sporik RB, Rakes G *et al*. Sensitization to dust mites as a dominant risk factor for asthma among adolescents living in central Virginia. Multiple regression analysis of a population-based study. *Am J Respir Crit Care Med* 1997; 156 (6): 1760–4.

37. Vaughan JW, McLaughlin TE, Perzanowski MS, Platts-Mills TAE. Evaluation of materials used for bedding encasement: Effect of pore size in blocking cat and dust mite allergen. *J Allergy Clin Immunol* 1999; 103 (2): 227–31.

38. Luczynska CM, Li Y, Chapman MD, Platts-Mills TAE. Airborne concentrations and particle size distribution of allergen derived from domestic cats (*Felis domesticus*): Measurements using cascade impactor, liquid impinger and a two site monoclonal antibody assay for *Fel d* I. *Am Rev Respir Dis* 1990; 141: 361–7.

39. Pollart S, Smith TF, Morris EC, Gelber LE, Platts-Mills TAE, Chapman MD. Environmental exposure to cockroach allergens: Analysis with monoclonal antibody-based enzyme immunoassays. *J Allergy Clin Immunol* 1991; 87: 505–510.

40. Chapman MD, Aalberse RC, Brown MJ, Platts-Mills TAE. Monoclonal antibodies to the major feline allergen *Fel d* I. II. Single step affinity purification of *Fel d* I, N-terminal sequence analysis, and development of a sensitive two-site immunoassay to assess *Fel d* I exposure. *J Immunol* 1988; 140: 812–18.

41. National Asthma Education and Prevention Program. *Guidelines for the Diagnosis and Management of Asthma*. NIH Publication No. 97–4051; April 1997.

42. Llerena LP, Fernandez-Caldere ZE, Gracia LRC. Sensitization to *Blomia tropicalis* and *Lepidoglyphus destructor* in *Dermatophagoides* spp-allergic individuals. *J Allergy Clin Immunol* 1991; 88: 943–50.

43. Platts-Mills TAE, Heymann PW, Chapman MD, Hayden ML, Wilkins SR. Cross-reacting and species-specific determinants on a major allergen from *Dermatophagoides pteronyssinus* and *D. farinae*: development of a radioimmunoassay for antigen P1 equivalent in house dust and dust mite extracts. *J Allergy Clin Immunol* 1986; 78: 398–407.

44. Arruda K, Rizzo MC, Chapman MD *et al.* Exposure and sensitization to dust mite allergens among asthmatic children in Sao Paulo, Brazil. *Clin Exp Allergy* 1991; 21: 433–9.

45. Kang C. Allergen exposure of inhaled arthropod material. *Clin Rev Allergy* 1985; 3: 363–75.

46. Linter TJ, Brame KA. The effects of season, climate and air conditioning on the prevalence of dermatophagoides mite allergens in household dust. *J Allergy Clin Immunol* 1993; 91: 862–7.

47. Arlian LG, Vyszenski-Moher DL, Fernandez-Caldas E. Allergenicity of the mite, *Blomia tropicalis*. *J Allergy Clin Immunol* 1993; 91: 1042–50.

48. Arlian LG, Rapp CM, Fernandez-Caldas E. Allergenicity of *Euroglyphus maynei* and its cross reactivity with *Dermatophagoides* species. *J Allergy Clin Immunol* 1993; 91: 1051–8.

49. Chapman MD. Guanine–an adequate index of mite exposure? (Editorial). *Allergy* 1993; 48: 301–2.

50. Rizzo MC, Arruda LK, Chapman MD *et al.* IgG and IgE antibody responses to dust mite allergens among children with asthma in Brazil. *Ann Allergy* 1993; 71: 152–8.

51. ✪ Sporik R, Holgate ST, Platts-Mills TAE, Cogswell J. Exposure to house dust mite allergen (*Der p* I) and the development of asthma in childhood: A prospective study. *N Engl J Med* 1990; 323: 502–507.

52. Price JA, Pollock J, Little SA, Longbottom JL, Warner JO. Measurements of airborne mite allergen in houses of asthmatic children. *Lancet* 1990; 336: 895–7.

53. Tovey ER, Chapman MD, Wells CW, Platts-Mills TAE. The distribution of dust mite allergen in the houses of patients with asthma. *Am Rev Respir Dis* 1981; 124: 630–35.

54. Platts-Mills TAE, Heymann PW, Longbottom JL, Wilkins SR. Airborne allergens associated with asthma: particle sizes carrying dust mite and rat allergens measured with a cascade impactor. *J Allergy Clin Immunol* 1986; 77: 850–57.

55. Swanson MA, Agarwal MK, Reed CE. An immunochemical approach to indoor aeroallergen quantitation with a new volumetric air sampler: studies with mite, roach, cat, mouse and guinea-pig antigens. *J Allergy Clin Immunol* 1987; 76: 724–9.

56. Sporik RB, Chapman MD, Platts-Mills TAE. House dust mite exposure as a cause of asthma (Editorial). *Clin Exp Allergy* 1992; 22: 897–906.

57. Placentini GL, Martinati L, Formari A *et al.* Antigen avoidance in a mountain environment influence on basophil releasability in children with asthma. *J Allergy Clin Immunol* 1993; 92: 644–50.

58. Burr ML, Neale E. Effect of change to mite-free bedding. Thorax 1980; 35: 513–14.

59. Owen S, Morganstern M, Hepworth J, Woodcock A. Control of house dust mite antigen in bedding. *Lancet* 1990; 335: 396–7.

60. Burr ML, Dean BV, Merrett TG, Neale E, St Leger AS, Verrier-Jones ER. Effects of anti-mite measures on children with mite-sensitive asthma: a controlled trial. *Thorax* 1980; 35: 506–512.

61. MacDonald L, Tovey E. The role of water temperature and laundry procedures in reducing house dust mite populations and allergen content of bedding. *J Allergy Clin Immunol* 1992; 90: 599–608.

62. Bischoff ER, Fischer A, Liebenberg B, Kniest FM. Mite control with low temperature washing. I. Elimination of living mites on carpet pieces. *Clin Exp Allergy* 1996; 26 (8): 945–52.

63. Rebmann H, Weber AK, Focke I, Rusche A, Lau S, Ehnert B, Wahn U. Does benzyl benzoate prevent colonization of new mattresses by mites? A prospective study. Allergy: *Eur J Allergy Clin Immunol* 1996; 51(12): 876–82.

64. Hayden ML, Rose G, Diduch KB, Domson P, Chapman MD, Heymann PW, Platts-Mills TAE. Benzyl benzoate moist powder: Investigation of acaricidal activity in cultures and reduction of dust mite allergens in carpets. *J Allergy Clin Immunol* 1992; 89: 536–45.

65. Goodman LS, Gillman A. *The Pharmacologic Basis of Therapeutics*, 6th edn. New York: Macmillan 1980: 985.

66. Greene WF, Nicholas NR, Salome CM, Woolcock AJ. Reduction of house dust mite and mite allergens. *Clin Exp Allergy* 1989; 19: 203–207.

67. Kniest FM, Young E, Van Praag MCG *et al*. Clinical evaluation of a double-blind dust-mite avoidance trial with mite-allergic rhinitis patients. *Clin Exp Allergy* 1990; 21: 39–47.

68. Dietemann A, Bessof JC. A double-blind placebo controlled trial of solidified benzyl benzoate applied in dwellings of asthmatic patient sensitive to mites: clinical efficacy and effect on mite antigens. *J Allergy Clin Immunol* 1993; 91: 738–46.

69. Chang JH, Becker A, Ferguson A *et al*. Effect of application of benzyl benzoate on house dust mite allergen levels. *Ann Allergy Asthma Immunol* 1996; 77: 187–90.

70. ✪ van der Heide S, Kauffman HF, Dubois AE, De Monchy JG. Allergen-avoidance measures in homes of house-dust-mite allergic asthmatic patients: effects of acaricides and mattress encasings. *Allergy*. 1997; 52(9): 921–7.

71. Wolf ST. Suffocating odor and asthma after acarosan powder carpet treatment. *J Allergy Clin Immunol* 1992; 2: 637–8.

72. Tovey ER, Chapman MD, Platts-Mills TAE. Mite faeces are a major source of house dust allergens. *Nature* 1981; 289: 592–3.

73. Korsgaard J. House dust mites and absolute indoor humidity. *Allergy* 1983; 38: 85–92.

74. Korsgaard J. Preventive measures in mite asthma: A controlled trial. *J Allergy Clin Immunol* 38: 93–102.

75. Kang B. Study on cockroach antigen as a probable causative agent in bronchial asthma. *J Allergy Clin Immunol* 1976; 58: 357–65.

76. Bernton HS, McMahon TF, Brown H. Cockroach asthma. *Br J Dis Chest* 1972; 66: 61–6.

77. Kang B, Sulit N. A comparative study of skin hypersensitivity to cockroach and house dust antigens. *Ann Allergy* 1978; 41: 333–6.

78. Kang B, Vellody D, Homburger H, Yunginger JW. Cockroach cause of allergic asthma. Its specificity and immunologic profile. *J Allergy Clin Immunol* 1979; 63: 80–86.

79. Call RS, Smith TF, Morris E, Chapman MD, Platts-Mills TAE. Risk factors for asthma in inner city children. *J Pediatr* 1992; 121: 862–6.

80. ✪ Rosenstreich DL, Eggleston P, Kattan M *et al*. The role of cockroach allergy and exposure to cockroach allergen in causing morbidity among inner-city children with asthma. *N Engl J Med* 1997; 336: 1356–63.

81. Togias A, Horowitz E, Joyner D, Guydon L, Malveaux F. Evaluating the factors that relate to asthma severity in adolescents. *Internat Arch Allergy Immunol* 1997; 113(1–3): 87–95.

82. Sarpong SB, Hamilton RG, Eggleston PA, Adkinson NF Jr. Socioeconomic status and race as risk factors for cockroach allergen exposure and sensitization in children with asthma. *J Allergy Clin Immunol* 1996; 97(6): 1393–401.

83. Fletcher-Bincent SA, Reece ER, Malveaux FJ. Reactivity to cockroach and other allergens in an inner city population with rhinitis and asthma. *J Allergy Clin Immunol* 1994; 93: 174.

84. Neffen HE, Jossen R, Aroaz I *et al*. Socioeconomic status and sensitization to cockroach allergens in asthmatic children in Santa Fe, Argentina. *J Allergy Clin Immunol* 1994; 93: 289.

85. ✪ Gelber LE, Seltzer LH, Bouzoukis JK, Pollart SM, Chapman MD, Platts-Mills TAE. Sensitization and exposure to indoor allergens as risk factors for asthma among patients presenting to hospital. *Am Rev Respir Dis* 1993; 147: 573–8.

86. Lau S, Falkenhorst G, Weber A *et al*. High mite-allergen exposure increases the risk of sensitization in atopic children and young adults. *J Allergy Clin Immunol* 1989; 84: 718–25.

87. Schou C, Fernandez-Caldas E, Lockey RF, Lowenstein H. Environmental assay for cockroach allergen. *J Allergy Clin Immunol* 1991; 87: 828–34.

88. De Blay F, Heymann PW, Chapman MD, Platts-Mills TAE. Airborne dust mite allergens: comparison of group II allergens with group I mite allergen and cat allergen Fel d I. *J Allergy Clin Immunol* 1991; 88: 919–26.

89. Robinson WH, Zungoli PA. Integrated control program for German cockroaches (Dictyoptera: *Blatella*) in multiple-unit dwellings. *J Econ Entomol* 1985; 78: 595–8.

90. Sarpong SB, Wood RA, Eggleston PA. Cockroach allergen (*Bla g* II): Environmental control with extermination and cleaning. *J Allergy Clin Immunol* 1994; 93: 179.

91. De Blay F, Chapman MD, Platts-Mills TAE. Airborne cat allergen (*Fel d* I): Environmental control with the cat *in situ*. *Am Rev Respir Dis* 1991; 143: 1334–9.

92. Ohman JL, Findlay SR, Leitermann SB. Immunotherapy in cat-induced asthma. Double-blind trial with examination of *in vivo* and *in vitro* responses. *J Allergy Clin Immunol* 1984; 74: 230–9.

93. Bollinger ME, Eggleston PA, Flanagan E, Wood RA. Cat antigen in homes with and without cats may induce allergic symptoms. *J Allergy Clin Immunol* 1996; 97 (4): 907–14.

94. Enberg RN, Shamie SM, McCullough J, Ownby DR. Ubiquitous presence of cat allergen in cat-free buildings: probable dispersal from human clothing. *Ann Allergy* 1993; 70: 471–4.

95. ✪ Custovic A, Simpson A, Pahdi H, Green RM, Chapman MD, Woodcock A. Distribution, aerodynamic characteristics, and removal of the major cat allergen *Fel d* I in British homes. *Thorax* 1998; 53: 33–8.

96. Luczynska CM, Li Y, Chapman MD, Platts-Mills TAE. Airborne concentrations and particle size distribution of allergen derived from domestic cats (*Felis domesticus*): Measurements using cascade impactor, liquid impinger and a two site monoclonal antibody assay for *Fel d* I. *Am Rev Respir Dis* 1990; 141: 361–7.

97. Wood RA, Mudd KE, Eggleston PA. The distribution of cat and dust mite allergens on wall surfaces. *J Allergy Clin Immunol* 1992; 89: 126–30.

98. Wood RA, Chapman MD, Adkinson NF Jr, Eggleston PA. The effect of cat removal on allergen content in household-dust samples. *J Allergy Clin Immunol* 1989; 83: 730–34.

99. Klucka CV, Ownby DR, Green J. Cat washings,

100. Woodfolk JA, Luczynska CM, De Blay F, Chapman MD, Platts-Mills TAE. The effect of vacuum cleaners on the concentration and particle size distribution of airborne cat allergen. *J Allergy Clin Immunol* 1993; 91: 829–37.

101. Vaughan JW, Woodfolk JA, Platts-Mills TAE. Assessment of vacuum cleaners and vacuum cleaner bags recommended for allergic subjects. *J Allergy Clin Immunol* 1999; 104: 1079–83.

102. Wood RA, Laheri AN, Eggleston PA. The aerodynamic characteristics of cat allergen. *Clin Exp Allergy* 1993; 23: 733–9.

103. Ingram JM, Sporik R, Rose G, Honsinger R, Chapman MD, Platts-Mills TAE. Quantitative assessment of exposure to dog (*Can f* I) and cat (*Fel d* I) allergens: relationship to sensitization and asthma among children living in Los Alamos, New Mexico. *J Allergy Clin Immunol* 1995; 96: 449–56.

104. Horner WE, Helbling A, Salvaggio JE *et al*. Fungal allergens. *Clin Microbiol Rev* 1995; 8: 161–79.

105. Salvaggio J, Aukrust L. Postgraduate course presentations. Mold-induced asthma. *J Allergy Clin Immunol* 1981; 68: 327–46.

106. Paris S, Fitting C, Latge JP, Herman D, Guinnepain MT, David B. Comparison of conidial and mycelial allergens of *Alternaria alternata*. *Int Arch Allergy Immunol* 1990; 92: 1–8.

107. Fadel R, David B, Paris S, Guesdon JI. *Alternaria* spore and mycelium sensitivity in allergic patients: *in vivo* and *in vitro* studies. *Ann Allergy* 1992; 69: 329–35.

108. Portnoy J, Pacheco F, Barnes C, Upadrashta B, Crenshaw R, Esch R. Selection of representative Alternaria strain groups on the basis of morphology, enzyme profile, and allergen content. *J Allergy Clin Immunol* 1993; 91: 773–82.

109. Al-Doory Y, Ramsey S. *Moulds and Health*. Springfield, IL: CC Thomas, 1987.

110. Solomon WR. Assessing fungus prevalence in domestic interiors. *J Allergy Clin Immunol* 1975; 56: 235.

allerpet or acepromazine do not diminish *Fel d* I shedding. *J Allergy Clin Immunol* 1994; 93: 180.

111. Kodama AM, McGee RI. Airborne microbial contaminants in indoor environments. Naturally ventilated and air-conditioned homes. *Arch Env Health* 1986; 41: 306–311.

112. Paris S, Debeaupuis JP, Prevost MC, Casotto M, Latge JP. The 31 kd major allergen, *Alt a* I, of *Alternaria alternata*. *J Allergy Clin Immunol* 1991; 88: 902–8.

113. Arruda LK, Mann BJ, Chapman MD. Selective expression of a major allergen and cytotoxin, *Asp f* I, in *Aspergillus fumigatus*: Implications for the immunopathogenesis of *Aspergillus* related diseases. *J Immunol* 1992; 149: 3354–9.

114. Deuell BL, Arruda LK, Hayden ML, Chapman MD, Platts-Mills TAE. *Trichophyton tonsurans* allergen I (*Tri t* I): Characterization of a protein that causes immediate but not delayed hypersensitivity. *J Immunol* 1991; 147: 96–101.

115. Malling HF. Diagnosis and immunotherapy of mould allergy. *Allergy* 1986; 41: 342–50.

116. Ward GW Jr, Karlsson G, Rose G, Platts-Mills TAE. *Trichophyton* asthma: sensitisation of bronchi and upper airways to dermatophyte antigen. *Lancet* 1989; 1: 859–62.

117. Lehrer SR, Lopez M, Butcher BT, Olson J, Reed M, Salvaggio JE. Basidiomycete mycelia and spore-allergen extracts: skin test reactivity in adults with symptoms of respiratory allergy. *J Allergy Clin Immunol* 1986; 78: 478–85.

118. Kleine-Tebbe J, Worm M, Jeep S, Matthiesen, Lowenstein H, Kunkel G. Predominance of the major allergen (*Alt a* I) in Alternaria sensitized patients. *Clin Exp Allergy* 1992; 23: 211–18.

119. Sporik RB, Arruda LK, Woodfolk J, Chapman MD, Platts-Mills TAE. Environmental exposure to *Aspergillus fumigatus* (*Asp f* I). *Clin Exp Allergy* 1993; 23: 326–31.

120. El-Dahr J, Fink R, Selden R, Arruda LK, Platts-Mills TAE, Heymann PW. Development of immune responses to *Aspergillus*, including allergen *Asp f* I, at an early age in children with cystic fibrosis. *Am J Respir Crit Care Med* 1994; 150: 1513–8.

121. Goldstein MF, Dvorin DJ, Dunsky EH, Lesser RW, Heuman PJ, Loose JH. Allergic rhizomucor sinusitis. *J Allergy Clin Immunol* 1992; 90: 394–404.

122. Nagda NL, Rector HE, Koontz MD. *Guidelines for monitoring indoor air quality* 1987; Washington: Hemisphere Pub. Co., 1987: 15–24.

123. Denson-Lino JM, Willies-Jacobo LJ, Rosas A, O'Connor RD, Wilson NW. Effect of economic status on the use of house dust mite avoidance measures in asthmatic children. *Ann Allergy* 1993; 71: 130–32.

124. Huss K, Rand CS, Buts AM *et al*. Home environmental risk factors in urban minority asthmatic children. *Ann Allergy* 1994; 72: 173–6.

Chapter 17

Corticosteroids

Peter Barnes

INTRODUCTION

Corticosteroids are the most effective therapy currently available for asthma and improvement with corticosteroids is one of the hallmarks of asthma. Inhaled corticosteroids have revolutionized asthma treatment and have become the mainstay of therapy for patients with chronic disease.[1,2] We now have a much better understanding of the molecular mechanisms whereby corticosteroids suppress inflammation in asthma and this has led to changes in the way corticosteroids are used and may point the way to the development of more specific therapies in the future.[3] This chapter discusses current understanding of the mechanism of action of corticosteroids and how corticosteroids are used in the management of asthma.

MOLECULAR MECHANISMS

Corticosteroids are highly effective anti-inflammatory therapy in asthma and the molecular mechanisms involved in suppression of airway inflammation in asthma are now better understood.[3] Corticosteroids are effective in asthma because they block many of the inflammatory pathways that are abnormally activated in asthma and they have a wide spectrum of anti-inflammatory actions.

Glucocorticoid Receptors

Corticosteroids binding to a single class of glucocorticoid receptors (GR) which are localized to the cytoplasm of target cells. Corticosteroids bind at the C-terminal end of the receptor, whereas the N-terminal end of the receptor is involved in gene transcription. Between these domains is the DNA-binding domain which has two finger-like projections formed by a zinc molecule bound to four cysteine residues that bind to the DNA double helix. The inactive GR is bound to a protein complex that includes two molecules of 90 kDa heat shock protein (hsp90) and various other proteins which act as a "molecular chaperone" preventing the unoccupied GR moving into the nuclear compartment. Once corticosteroids bind to GR, conformational changes in the receptor structure result in dissociation of these molecules, thereby exposing nuclear localization signals on GR which then results in rapid nuclear localization of the activated GR-corticosteroid complex and its binding to DNA (Fig. 17.1). Two GR molecules bind to DNA as a dimer, resulting in changed transcription. Recently a splice variant of GR, termed GR-β, has been identified that does not bind corticosteroids, but binds to DNA and may therefore interfere with the action of corticosteroids.[4]

Effects on Gene Transcription

Corticosteroids produce their effect on responsive cells by activating GR to directly or indirectly regulate the transcription of certain target genes.[5] The number of genes per cell *directly* regulated by corticosteroids is estimated to be between 10 and 100, but many genes are indirectly regulated through an interaction with other transcription factors. Glucocorticoid receptor dimers bind to DNA at consensus sites termed glucocorticoid response elements (GREs) in the 5'-upstream promoter region of steroid-responsive genes. This interaction changes the rate of transcription, resulting in either induction or repression of the gene. Interaction of the activated GR homodimer with GRE usually increases transcription, resulting in increased protein synthesis. GR may increase transcription by interacting with a large coactivator molecule, CREB binding protein, which is bound at the start site of transcription and

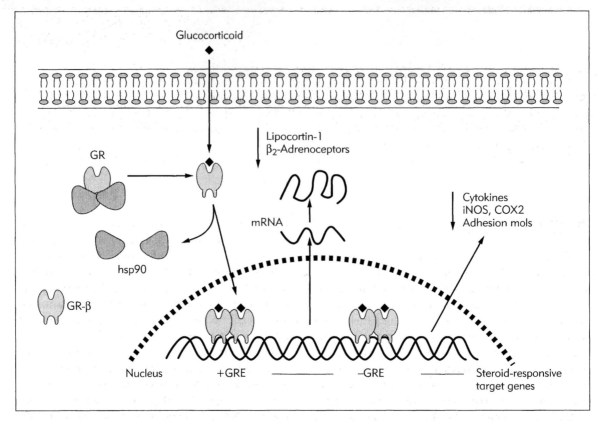

FIGURE 17.1: Classical model of glucocorticoid action. The glucocorticoid enters the cell and binds to a cytoplasmic glucocorticoid receptor (GR) that is complexed with two molecules of a 90 kDa heat shock protein (hsp90). GR translocates to the nucleus where, as a dimer, it binds to a glucocorticoid recognition sequence (GRE) on the 5'-upstream promoter sequence of corticosteroid-responsive genes. GREs may increase transcription and nGREs may decrease transcription, resulting in increased or decreased messenger RNA (mRNA) and protein synthesis. An isoform of GR, GR-β, binds to DNA but is not activated by corticosteroids.

switches on RNA polymerase, resulting in formation of messenger RNA (mRNA) and then synthesis of protein.

However, in controlling inflammation, the major effect of corticosteroids is to inhibit the synthesis of inflammatory proteins, such as cytokines. This was originally believed to be through interaction of GR with a negative GRE, resulting in repression of transcription. However, such negative GREs have rarely been demonstrated. GR may also affect protein synthesis by altering the stability of messenger RNA, through effects on ribonucleases that break down mRNA.

Interaction With Transcription Factors

Activated GRs may bind directly with several other activated transcription factors as a protein–protein inter-

action. This could be an important determinant of corticosteroid responsiveness and is a key mechanism whereby corticosteroids switch off inflammatory genes. Most of the inflammatory genes that are activated in asthma do not appear to have GREs in their promoter regions yet are repressed by corticosteroids. There is increasing evidence that this may be due to a direct interaction between the activated GR and transcription factors that regulate the expression of genes, that code for inflammatory proteins, such as cytokines, inflammatory enzymes, adhesion molecules and inflammatory receptors. These "inflammatory" transcription factors include activator protein-1 (AP-1) and nuclear factor-κB (NF-κB) which may regulate many of the inflammatory genes that are switched on in asthmatic airways.[6,7]

Effects on Chromatin Structure

There is increasing evidence that corticosteroids may have effects on the chromatin structure. DNA in chromosomes is wound around histone molecules in the form of nucleosomes. Several transcription factors interact with large co-activator molecules, such as CBP and the related molecule p300, which bind to the basal transcription factor apparatus. Several transcription factors have now been shown to bind directly to CBP, including AP-1, NF-κB and GR.[8] Since binding sites on this molecule may be limited, this may result in competition between transcription factors for the limited binding sites available, so that there is an indirect rather than a direct protein–protein interaction (Fig. 17.2). At a microscopic level that chromatin may become dense or opaque due to the winding or unwinding of DNA around the histone core. CBP and p300 have histone acetylation activity which is activated by the binding of transcription factors, such as AP-1 and NF-κB. Acetylation of histone residues results in unwinding of DNA coiled around the histone core, thus opening up the chromatin structure, which allows transcription factors to bind more readily, thereby increasing transcription. Repression of genes reverses this process by histone deacetylation.[9] Deacetylation of histone, increases the winding of DNA round histone residues, resulting in dense chromatin structure and reduced access of transcription factors to their binding

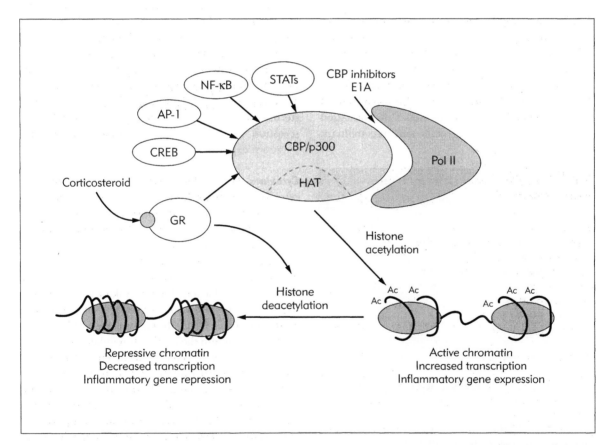

FIGURE 17.2: Effect of corticosteroids on chromatin structure. Transcription factors, such as STATs, AP-1 and NF-κB bind to co-activator molecules, such as CREB binding protein (CBP) or p300, which have intrinsic histone acetyltransferase (HAT) activity, resulting in acetylation (Ac) of histone residues. This leads to unwinding of DNA and this allows increased binding of transcription factors resulting in increased gene transcription. Glucocorticoid receptors (GR) after activation by corticosteroids bind to a glucocorticoid receptor co-activator which is bound to CBP. This results in deacetylation of histone, with increased coiling of DNA around histone, thus preventing transcription factor binding leading to gene repression.

sites, thereby leading to repressed transcription of inflammatory genes. Activated GR may bind to several transcription co-repressor molecules that associate with proteins that have histone deacetylase activity, resulting in deacetylation of histone, increased winding of DNA round histone residues and thus reduced access of transcription factors to their binding sites and therefore repression of inflammatory genes.

Target Genes in Inflammation Control

Corticosteroids may control inflammation by inhibiting many aspects of the inflammatory process through increasing the transcription of anti-inflammatory genes and decreasing the transcription of inflammatory genes (Table 17.1).

Anti-Inflammatory Proteins Corticosteroids may suppress inflammation by increasing the synthesis of anti-inflammatory proteins. For example, corticosteroids increase the synthesis of lipocortin-1, a 37 kDa protein that has an inhibitory effect on phospholipase A_2 (PLA_2), and therefore may inhibit the production of lipid mediators. Corticosteroids induce the formation of lipocortin-1 in several cells and recombinant

lipocortin-1 has acute anti-inflammatory properties. However, lipocortin-1 does not appear to be increased by inhaled corticosteroid treatment in asthma.[10] Corticosteroids increase the expression of other potentially anti-inflammatory proteins, such as interleukin (IL)-1 receptor antagonist (which inhibits the binding of IL-1 to its receptor); secretory leukoprotease inhibitor (which inhibits proteases, such as tryptase); neutral endopeptidase (which degrades bronchoactive peptides such as kinins); CC-10 (an immunomodulatory protein); an inhibitor of NF-κB (IκB-α) and IL-10 (an anti-inflammatory cytokine).

β_2 Adrenoceptors Corticosteroids increase the expression of β_2 adrenoceptors by increasing the rate of transcription and the human β_2-receptor gene has three potential GREs. Corticosteroids double the rate of β_2-receptor gene transcription in human lung *in vitro*, resulting in increased expression of β_2 receptors.[11] This may be relevant in asthma as corticosteroids may prevent down-regulation of β_2 receptors in response to prolonged treatment with β_2 agonists. In rats corticosteroids prevent down-regulation and reduced transcription of β_2 receptors in response to chronic β-agonist exposure.[12]

Cytokines The inhibitory effect of corticosteroids on cytokine synthesis is likely to be of particular importance in the control of inflammation in asthma. Corticosteroids inhibit the transcription of many cytokines and chemokines that are relevant in asthma (Table 17.1). These inhibitory effects are due, at least in part, to an inhibitory effect on the transcription factors that regulate induction of these cytokine genes, including AP-1 and NF-κB. For example, eotaxin which is important in selective attraction of eosinophils from the circulation into the airways is regulated in part by NF-κB and its expression in airway epithelial cells is inhibited by corticosteroids.[13] Many transcription factors are likely to be involved in the regulation of inflammatory genes in asthma in addition to AP-1 and NF-κB. IL-4 and IL-5 expression in T-lymphocytes plays a critical role in allergic inflammation, but NF-κB does not play a role, whereas the transcription factor nuclear factor of activated T-cells (NF-AT) is important.[14] AP-1 is a component of the NF-AT transcription complex, so that corticosteroids inhibit IL-5, at least in part, by inhibiting the AP-1 component of NF-AT.

Table 17.1: Effect of corticosteroids on gene transcription
Increased transcription
Lipocortin-1 (phospholipase A_2 inhibitor)
β_2 Adrenoceptor
Secretory leukocyte inhibitory protein
Clara cell protein (CC10; phospholipase A_2 inhibitor)
IL-1 receptor antagonist
IL-1R2 (decoy receptor)
IκB-α (inhibitor of NF-κB)
Decreased transcription
Cytokines
(IL-1, IL-2, IL-3, IL-4, IL-5, IL-6, IL-11, IL-12, IL-13, TNFα, GM-CSF, SCF)
Chemokines
(IL-8, RANTES, MIP-1α, MCP-1, MCP-3, MCP-4, eotaxin)
Inducible nitric oxide synthase (iNOS)
Inducible cyclooxygenase (COX-2)
Cytoplasmic phospholipase A_2 ($cPLA_2$)
Endothelin-1
NK_1-receptors, NK_2-receptors
Adhesion molecules (ICAM-1, E-selectin)

There may be marked differences in the response of different cells and of different cytokines to the inhibitory action of corticosteroids and this may be dependent on the relative abundance of transcription factors within different cell types. Thus in alveolar macrophages and peripheral blood monocytes GM-CSF secretion is more potently inhibited by corticosteroids than IL-1β or IL-6 secretion.

Inflammatory Enzymes Nitric oxide (NO) synthase may be induced by proinflammatory cytokines, resulting in NO production. NO may amplify asthmatic inflammation and contribute to epithelial shedding and airway hyperresponsiveness through the formation of peroxynitrite. The induction of the inducible form of NOS (iNOS) is inhibited by corticosteroids. In cultured human pulmonary epithelial cells pro-inflammatory cytokines result in increased expression of iNOS and increased NO formation, due to increased transcription of the iNOS gene, and this is inhibited by corticosteroids acting through inhibition of NF-κB. Corticosteroids inhibit the synthesis of several other inflammatory mediators implicated in asthma through an inhibitory effect on the induction of enzymes such as cyclo-oxygenase-2 and cytosolic PLA$_2$

Corticosteroids also inhibit the synthesis of endothelin-1 in lung and airway epithelial cells and this effect may also be via inhibition of transcription factors that regulate its expression.

Inflammatory Receptors Corticosteroids also decrease the transcription of genes coding for certain receptors. Thus the gene for the NK$_1$-receptor, which mediates the inflammatory effects of tachykinins in the airways, has an increased expression in asthma and is inhibited by corticosteroids, probably via an inhibitory effect on AP-1.[15] Corticosteroids also inhibit the transcription of the NK$_2$-receptor which mediates the bronchoconstrictor effects of tachykinins.[16]

Adhesion Molecules Adhesion molecules play a key role in the trafficking of inflammatory cells to sites of inflammation. The expression of many adhesion molecules on endothelial cells is induced by cytokines, and corticosteroids may lead indirectly to a reduced expression via their inhibitory effects on cytokines, such as IL-1β and TNFα. Corticosteroids may also have a direct inhibitory effect on the expression of adhesion molecules, such as ICAM-1 and E-selectin at the level of gene transcription. ICAM-1 and VCAM-1 expression in bronchial epithelial cell lines and monocytes is inhibited by corticosteroids.[17]

Apoptosis Corticosteroids markedly reduce the survival of certain inflammatory cells, such as eosinophils. Eosinophil survival is dependent on the presence of certain cytokines, such as IL-5 and GM-CSF. Exposure to corticosteroids blocks the effects of these cytokines and leads to programmed cell death or apoptosis, although the corticosteroid-sensitive molecular pathways have not yet been defined.[18]

Effects on Cell Function

Corticosteroids may have direct inhibitory actions on several inflammatory cells and structural cells that are implicated in asthma (Fig. 17.3).

Macrophages Corticosteroids inhibit the release of inflammatory mediators and cytokines from alveolar macrophages *in vitro*. Inhaled corticosteroids reduce the secretion of chemokines and pro-inflammatory cytokines from alveolar macrophages from asthmatic patients, whereas the secretion of IL-10 is increased.[19]

Eosinophils Corticosteroids have a direct inhibitory effect on mediator release from eosinophils, although they are only weakly effective in inhibiting secretion of reactive oxygen species and eosinophil basic proteins. More importantly corticosteroids induce apoptosis by inhibiting the prolonged survival due to IL-3, IL-5 and GM-CSF[18] resulting in an increased number of apoptotic eosinophils in induced sputum of asthmatic patients.[20] One of the best described actions of corticosteroids in asthma is a reduction in circulating eosinophils, which may reflect an action on eosinophil production in the bone marrow.

T-Lymphocytes T helper 2 lymphocytes (TH$_2$) play an important orchestrating role in asthma through the release of cytokines such as IL-4 and IL-5 and may be an important target for corticosteroids in asthma therapy.

Mast Cells While corticosteroids do not appear to have a direct inhibitory effect on mediator release from lung mast cells, chronic corticosteroid treatment is associated with a marked reduction in mucosal mast cell number. This may be linked to a reduction in IL-3 and

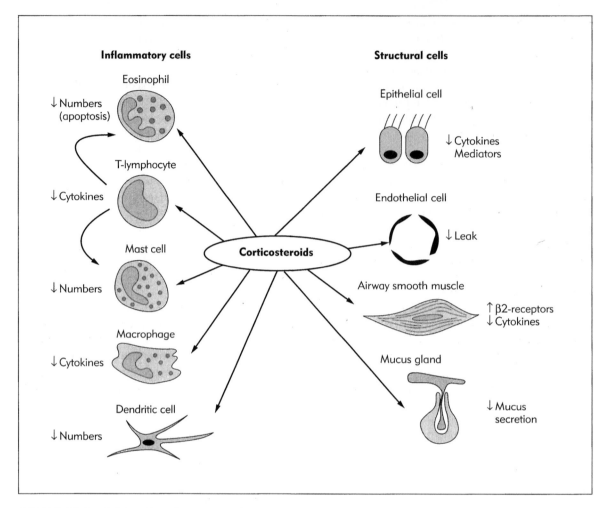

Inflammatory cells

Eosinophil
↓ Numbers (apoptosis)

T-lymphocyte
↓ Cytokines

Mast cell
↓ Numbers

Macrophage
↓ Cytokines

Dendritic cell
↓ Numbers

Corticosteroids

Structural cells

Epithelial cell
↓ Cytokines Mediators

Endothelial cell
↓ Leak

Airway smooth muscle
↑ β2-receptors
↓ Cytokines

Mucus gland
↓ Mucus secretion

FIGURE 17.3: Cellular effect of corticosteroids.

stem cell factor (SCF) production, which are necessary for mast cell expression at mucosal surfaces. Mast cells also secrete various cytokines (TNF-α, IL-4, IL-5, IL-6, IL-8), and this may also be inhibited by corticosteroids.

Dendritic Cells Dendritic cells in the epithelium of the respiratory tract appear to play a critical role in antigen presentation in the lung as they have the capacity to take up allergen, process it into peptides and present it via MHC molecules on the cell surface for presentation to uncommitted T-lymphocytes. In experimental animals the number of dendritic cells is markedly reduced by systemic and inhaled cortico-steroids, thus dampening the immune response in the airways.[21]

Neutrophils Neutrophils, which are not prominent in the biopsies of asthmatic patients, are not sensitive to the effects of corticosteroids. Indeed, systemic corticosteroids increase peripheral neutrophil counts which may reflect an increased survival time due to an inhibitory action of neutrophil apoptosis (in complete contrast to the increased apoptosis seen in eosinophils).[22]

Endothelial Cells Glucocorticoid receptor gene expression in the airways is most prominent in endothelial cells of the bronchial circulation and airway epithelial cells. Corticosteroids do not appear to directly inhibit the expression of adhesion molecules, although they may inhibit cell adhesion indirectly by suppression of cytokines involved in the regulation of adhesion molecule expression. Corticosteroids may have an inhibitory action on airway microvascular leak induced by inflammatory mediators. This appears to be a direct effect on post-capillary venular epithelial cells. The mechanism for this anti-permeability effect has not been fully elucidated, but there is evidence that synthesis of a 100 kDa protein distinct from lipocortin-1 and termed vasocortin may be involved. Although there have been no direct measurements of the effects of corticosteroids on airway microvascular leakage in asthmatic airways, regular treatment with inhaled corticosteroids decreases the elevated plasma proteins found in bronchoalveolar lavage fluid of patients with stable asthma.

Epithelial Cells Epithelial cells may be an important source of many inflammatory mediators in asthmatic airways and may drive and amplify the inflammatory response in the airways through the secretion of proinflammatory cytokines, chemokines and inflammatory peptides. Airway epithelium may be one of the most important targets for inhaled corticosteroids in asthma[23,24] (Fig. 17.4). Inhaled corticosteroids inhibit the increased expression of many inflammatory proteins in airway epithelial cells.[23] An example is iNOS which has an increased expression in airway epithelial and inflammatory cells in asthma and is reduced by inhaled corticosteroids.[25] This is reflected by a reduction in the elevated levels of exhaled NO in asthma after inhaled corticosteroids.[26]

Mucus Secretion Corticosteroids inhibit mucus secretion in airways and this may be a direct action of corticosteroids on submucosal gland cells. Corticosteroids may also inhibit the expression of mucin genes, such as MUC2 and MUC5AC.[27] In addition there are indirect inhibitory effects due to the reduction in inflammatory mediators that stimulate increased mucus secretion.

EFFECTS ON ASTHMATIC INFLAMMATION

Corticosteroids are remarkably effective in controlling the inflammation in asthmatic airways and it is likely that they have multiple cellular effects. Biopsy studies in patients with asthma have now confirmed that

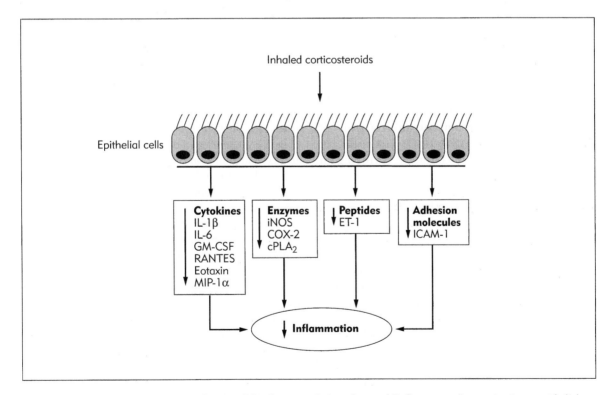

FIGURE 17.4: Inhaled corticosteroids may inhibit the transcription of several "inflammatory" genes in airway epithelial cells and thus reduce inflammation in the airway wall.

inhaled corticosteroids reduce the number and activation of inflammatory cells in the airway mucosa and in bronchoalveolar lavage.[23] These effects may be due to inhibition of cytokine synthesis in inflammatory and structural cells and suppression of adhesion molecules. The disrupted epithelium is restored and the ciliated to goblet cell ratio is normalized after 3 months of therapy with inhaled corticosteroids. There is also some evidence for a reduction in the thickness of the basement membrane, although in asthmatic patients taking inhaled corticosteroids for over 10 years, the characteristic thickening of the basement membrane was still present.

Effects on Airway Hyperresponsiveness

By reducing airway inflammation inhaled corticosteroids consistently reduce airway hyperresponsiveness (AHR) in asthmatic adults and children.[28] Chronic treatment with inhaled corticosteroids reduces responsiveness to histamine, cholinergic agonists, allergen (early and late responses), exercise, fog, cold air, bradykinin, adenosine and irritants (such as sulphur dioxide and metabisulphite). The reduction in AHR takes place over several weeks and may not be maximal until several months of therapy. The magnitude of reduction is variable between patients and is in the order of one to two doubling dilutions for most challenges and often fails to return to the normal range. This may reflect suppression of the inflammation, but persistence of structural changes which cannot be reversed by corticosteroids. Inhaled corticosteroids not only make the airways less sensitive to spasmogens, but they also limit the maximal airway narrowing in response to spasmogens.

CLINICAL EFFICACY OF INHALED CORTICOSTEROIDS

Inhaled corticosteroids are very effective in controlling asthma symptoms in asthmatic patients of all ages and severity[1,29,30] (Table 17.2). Inhaled corticosteroids improve the quality of life of patients with asthma and allow many patients to lead normal lives, improve lung function, reduce the frequency of exacerbations and may prevent irreversible airway changes. They were first introduced to reduce the requirement for oral corticosteroids in patients with severe asthma and many studies have confirmed that the majority of patients can be weaned off oral corticosteroids.[31]

Table 17.2: Effects of inhaled corticosteroids in asthma
Control symptoms
Improve quality of life
Improve lung function
Prevent exacerbations
Reduce mortality (probably)
Prevent irreversible airway changes
Alter natural history of asthma?

Studies in Adults

As experience has been gained with inhaled corticosteroids they have been introduced in patients with milder asthma, with the recognition that inflammation is present even in patients with mild asthma. Inhaled anti-inflammatory drugs have now become first-line therapy in any patient who needs to use a β_2-agonist inhaler more than once a day and this is reflected in national and international guidelines for the management of chronic asthma. In patients with newly diagnosed asthma inhaled corticosteroids (budesonide 600 µg twice daily) reduced symptoms and β_2-agonist inhaler usage and improved peak expiratory flows. These effects persisted over the 2 years of the study, whereas in a parallel group treated with inhaled β_2 agonists alone there was no significant change in symptoms or lung function.[32] In another study patients with mild asthma treated with a low dose of inhaled corticosteroid (budesonide 400 µg daily) showed fewer symptoms and a progressive improvement in lung function over several months and many patients became completely asymptomatic.[33] There was also a significant reduction in the number of exacerbations. Although the effects of inhaled corticosteroids on AHR may take several months to reach a plateau, the reduction in asthma symptoms occurs more rapidly.[34]

High-dose inhaled corticosteroids have now been introduced for the control of more severe asthma. This markedly reduces the need for maintenance oral corticosteroids and has revolutionized the management of more severe and unstable asthma. Inhaled corticosteroids are the treatment of choice in nocturnal asthma, which is a manifestation of inflamed airways, reducing night-time awakening and reducing the diurnal variation in airway function.

High doses of inhaled corticosteroids may also substitute for a course of oral steroids in controlling acute exacerbations of asthma. High-dose fluticasone propionate (2000 µg daily) was as effective as a course of oral prednisolone in controlling acute exacerbations of asthma in general practice.[35]

Inhaled corticosteroids effectively control asthmatic inflammation but must be taken regularly. When inhaled corticosteroids are discontinued there is usually a gradual increase in symptoms and airway responsiveness back to pre-treatment values,[34] although in patients with mild asthma who have been treated with inhaled corticosteroids for a long time, symptoms may not recur.[36]

Studies in Children

Inhaled corticosteroids are equally effective in children. In an extensive study of children aged 7–17 years there was a significant improvement in symptoms, peak flow variability and lung function compared with a regular inhaled β_2 agonist which was maintained over the 22 months of the study,[37] but asthma deteriorated when the inhaled corticosteroids were withdrawn.[38] There was a high proportion of drop-outs (45%) in the group treated with inhaled β_2 agonist alone. Inhaled corticosteroids are more effective than a long-acting β_2 agonist in controlling asthma in children.[39] Inhaled corticosteroids are also effective in younger children. Nebulized budesonide reduces the need for oral corticosteroids and also improved lung function in children under the age of three.[40] Inhaled corticosteroids given via a large volume spacer improve asthma symptoms and reduce the number of exacerbations in pre-school children and in infants.

Dose–Response Studies

Surprisingly, the dose–response curve for the clinical efficacy of inhaled corticosteroids is relatively flat and, while all studies have demonstrated a clinical benefit of inhaled corticosteroids, it has been difficult to demonstrate differences between doses, with most benefit obtained at the lowest doses used.[29,31,41] This is in contrast to the steeper dose–response for systemic effects, implying that while there is little clinical benefit from increasing doses of inhaled corticosteroids the risk of adverse effects is increased. However, the dose–response effect of inhaled corticosteroids may depend on the

parameters measured and, while it is difficult to discern a dose–response when traditional lung function parameters are measured, there may be a dose–response effect in prevention of asthma exacerbations. Thus, in a recent study there was a significantly greater effect of budesonide 800 µg daily compared with 200 µg daily in preventing severe and mild asthma exacerbations.[42] Normally, a four-fold or greater difference in dose has been required to detect a statistically significant (but often small) difference in effect on commonly measured outcomes such as symptoms, PEF, use of rescue β_2 agonist and lung function and even such large differences in dose are not always associated with significant differences in response. These findings suggest that pulmonary function tests or symptoms may have a rather low sensitivity in the assessment of the effects of inhaled corticosteroids. This is obviously important for the interpretation of clinical comparisons between different inhaled corticosteroids or inhalers. It is also important to consider the type of patient included in clinical studies. Patients with relatively mild asthma may have relatively little room for improvement with inhaled corticosteroids, so that maximal improvement is obtained with relatively low doses. Patients with more severe asthma or with unstable asthma may have more room for improvement and may therefore show a greater response to increasing doses, but it is often difficult to include such patients in controlled clinical trials.

More studies are needed to assess whether other outcome measures such as AHR or more direct measurements of inflammation, such as sputum eosinophils or exhaled NO, may be more sensitive than traditional outcome measures such as symptoms or lung function tests.[43–45] A recent study showed that higher doses of inhaled corticosteroids are needed to control AHR than to improve symptoms and lung function, but that this may have a better long-term outcome in terms of reduction in structural changes of the airways.[46]

Prevention of Irreversible Airway Changes

Some patients with asthma develop an element of irreversible airflow obstruction, but the pathophysiological basis of these changes is not yet understood. It is likely that they are the result of chronic airway inflammation and that they may be prevented by treatment with inhaled corticosteroids. There is some evidence that the annual decline in lung function may be slowed by the introduction of inhaled corticosteroids.[47] Increasing evidence also suggests that delay in starting inhaled corticosteroids may result in less overall improvement in lung function in both adults and children.[48-50] These studies suggest that introduction of inhaled corticosteroids at the time of diagnosis is likely to have the greatest impact.[49,50] Several large studies are now underway to assess the benefit of very early introduction of inhaled corticosteroids in children and adults. So far there is no evidence that early use of inhaled corticosteroids is curative and even when inhaled corticosteroids are introduced at the time of diagnosis, symptoms and lung function revert to pre-treatment levels when corticosteroids are withdrawn.[48]

Reduction in Mortality

Inhaled corticosteroids may reduce the mortality from asthma but prospective studies are almost impossible to conduct. In a retrospective review of the risk of mortality and prescribed anti-asthma medication, there was a significant apparent protection provided by regular inhaled BDP therapy (adjusted odds ratio of 0.1), although numbers were small.[51]

Comparison Between Inhaled Corticosteroids

Several inhaled corticosteroids are currently prescribable in asthma, although their availability varies between countries. There have been relatively few studies comparing efficacy of the different inhaled corticosteroids, and it is important to take into account the delivery system and the type of patient under investigation when such comparisons are made. Because of the relatively flat dose–response curve for the clinical parameters normally used in comparing doses of inhaled corticosteroids, it may be difficult to see differences in efficacy of inhaled corticosteroids and most comparisons have concentrated on differences in systemic effects at equally efficacious doses, although it has often proved difficult to establish true clinical efficacy. In the UK beclomethasone dipropionate (BDP), budesonide (BUD) and Fluticasone propionate (FP) are available, whereas in the USA BDP, flunisolide, triamcinolone, FP and BUD are available. There are few studies comparing different doses of inhaled corticosteroids in asthmatic patients. Budesonide has been compared with BDP and in adults and children appears to have comparable anti-asthma effects at equal doses, whereas FP appears to be approximately twice as potent as BDP and BUD. There do appear to be some differences between inhaled corticosteroids in terms of their systemic effects at comparable anti-asthma doses, however.

CLINICAL USE OF INHALED CORTICOSTEROIDS

Inhaled corticosteroids are now recommended as first-line therapy for all patients with persistent symptoms. Inhaled corticosteroids should be started in any patient who needs to use a β_2-agonist inhaler for symptom control more than once daily (or possibly three times weekly). It is conventional to start with a low dose of inhaled corticosteroid and to increase the dose until asthma control is achieved. However, this may take time and a preferable approach is to start with a dose of corticosteroids in the middle of the dose range (400 µg twice daily) to establish control of asthma more rapidly.[52] Once control is achieved (defined as normal or best possible lung function and infrequent need to use an inhaled β_2 agonist) the dose of inhaled corticosteroid should be reduced in a step-wise manner to the lowest dose needed for optimal control. It may take as long as 3 months to reach a plateau in response and any changes in dose should be made at intervals of 3 months or more. This strategy ("start high–go low") is emphasized in the most recent US and UK guidelines.[53,54] When daily doses of ≥ 800 µg daily are needed a large volume spacer device should be used with an MDI and mouth washing with a dry powder inhaler in order to reduce local and systemic side-effects. Inhaled corticosteroids are usually given as a twice daily dose in order to increase compliance. When asthma is more unstable, four times daily dosage is preferable.[55] For patients who require ≤ 400 µg daily, once daily dosing appears to be as effective as twice daily dosing, at least for BUD.[56]

The dose of inhaled corticosteroid should be increased to 2000 µg daily if necessary, but higher doses may result in systemic effects and it may be preferable to add a low dose of oral corticosteroid, since higher doses of inhaled corticosteroids are expensive and have a high incidence of local side-effects. Nebulized budesonide has been advocated in order to give an increased dose of inhaled corticosteroid and to reduce the requirement for oral corticosteroids,[57] but this treatment is expensive and may achieve its effects largely via systemic absorption.

Additional Bronchodilators

Conventional advice was to increase the dose of inhaled corticosteroids if asthma was not controlled, on the assumption that there was residual inflammation of the airways. However it is now apparent that the dose–response effect of inhaled corticosteroids is relatively flat, so that there is little improvement in lung function after doubling the dose of inhaled corticosteroids. An alternative strategy is to add some other call of controller drug. In patients in general practice who were not controlled on BDP 200 µg twice daily, addition of salmeterol 50 µg twice daily was more effective than increasing the dose of inhaled corticosteroid to 500 µg twice daily, in terms of lung function improvement, use of rescue β_2 agonist and symptom control.[58] This surprising result was confirmed in a more severe group of patients who were not controlled on 800–1000 µg BDP daily.[59] Similar results have been found with another long-acting inhaled β_2 agonist, formoterol, which in addition reduced the frequency of mild and severe asthma exacerbations.[42] This has led to the development of fixed combinations of corticosteroids and long-acting β_2 agonists, such as FP and salmeterol (Seretide), which may be more convenient for patients.[60] Recent studies have also shown that addition of low doses of theophylline (giving plasma concentrations of <10 mg l^{-1}) were more effective than doubling the dose of inhaled BUD, either in mild or severe asthma.[61,62] Similar data are now emerging with anti-leukotrienes.[63] The reason why these alternative treatments are more effective than higher doses of inhaled corticosteroids remains to be elucidated, but does suggest that there is a reversible component of asthma that may not be steroid-sensitive inflammation. It is possible that this may be an abnormality in airway smooth muscle itself (as a result of remodelling), oedematous swelling of the airway or production of cysteinyl-leukotrienes that is not sensitive to inhibition by inhaled corticosteroids.[64]

Cost-effectiveness

Although inhaled corticosteroids may be more expensive than short-acting inhaled β_2 agonists, they are the most cost-effective way of controlling asthma, since reducing the frequency of asthma attacks will save on total costs.[65] Inhaled corticosteroids also improve the quality of life of patients with asthma and allow many patients a normal life-style, thus saving costs indirectly.[66]

Corticosteroid-Sparing Therapy (see Chapter 19)

In patients who have serious side-effects with maintenance corticosteroid therapy, there are several treatments which have been shown to reduce the requirement for oral corticosteroids.[67] These treatments are commonly termed corticosteroid-sparing, although this is a misleading description that could be applied to any additional asthma therapy (including bronchodilators). The amount of corticosteroid-sparing with these therapies is not impressive.

Several immunosuppressive agents have been shown to have corticosteroid effects, including methotrexate, oral gold and cyclosporin A. These therapies all have side-effects that may be more troublesome than those of oral corticosteroids, and are therefore only indicated as an additional therapy to reduce the requirement of oral corticosteroids. None of these treatments is very effective, but there are occasional patients who appear to show a good response. Because of side-effects these treatments cannot be considered as a way to reduce the requirement for inhaled corticosteroids. Several other therapies, including azathioprine, dapsone and hydroxychloroquine have not been found to be beneficial. The macrolide antibiotic troleandomycin is also reported to have corticosteroid-sparing effects, but this is only seen with methylprednisolone and is due to reduced metabolism of this corticosteroid, so that there is little therapeutic gain.[68]

PHARMACOKINETICS

The pharmacokinetics of inhaled corticosteroids are important in determining the concentration of drug reaching target cells in the airways and in the fraction of drug reaching the systemic circulation and therefore causing side-effects.[31] Beneficial properties in an inhaled corticosteroid are a high topical potency, a low systemic bioavailability of the swallowed portion of the dose and rapid metabolic clearance of any corticosteroid reaching the systemic circulation. After inhalation a large proportion of the inhaled dose (80–90%) is deposited on the oropharynx and is then swallowed and therefore available for absorption via the liver into the systemic circulation (Fig. 17.5). This fraction is markedly reduced by using a large volume spacer device with a metered dose inhaler (MDI) or by mouth washing and discarding the washing with dry powder inhalers. Between 10 and 20% of inhaled drug enters the respiratory tract, where it is deposited in the airways and this fraction is available for absorption into the systemic circulation. Most of the early studies on the distribution of inhaled corticosteroids were conducted in healthy volunteers, and it is not certain what effect

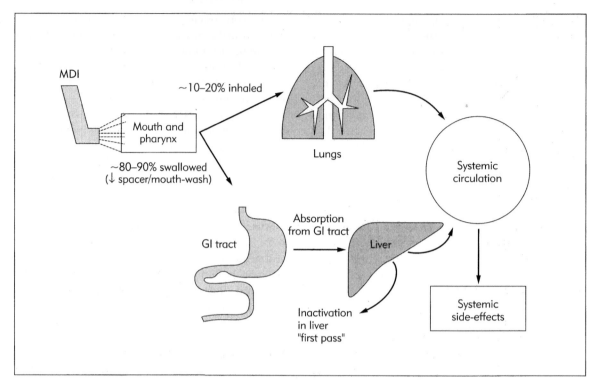

FIGURE 17.5: Pharmacokinetics of inhaled corticosteroids.

inflammatory disease, airway obstruction, age of the patient or concomitant medication may have on the disposition of the inhaled dose. There may be important differences in the metabolism of different inhaled corticosteroids. BDP is metabolized to its more active metabolite beclomethasone monopropionate in many tissues including lung, but there is no information about its absorption or metabolism of this metabolite in humans. Flunisolide and BUD are subject to extensive first-pass metabolism in the liver so that less reaches the systemic circulation. Little is known about the distribution of triamcinolone. FP is almost completely metabolized by first-pass metabolism, which reduces systemic effects.

When inhaled corticosteroids were first introduced it was recommended that they should be given four times daily, but several studies have now demonstrated that twice daily administration gives comparable control, although four times daily administration may preferable in patients with more severe asthma. However, patients may find it difficult to comply with such frequent administration unless they have troublesome symptoms. For patients with mild asthma, who require ≤ 400 µg daily, once daily therapy may be sufficient.

SIDE-EFFECTS OF INHALED CORTICOSTEROIDS

The efficacy of inhaled corticosteroids is now established in short- and long-term studies in adults and children, but there are still concerns about side-effects, particularly in children and when high inhaled doses are needed. Several side-effects have been recognized (Table 17.3).

Local Side-effects
Side-effects due to the local deposition of the inhaled corticosteroid in the oropharynx may occur with inhaled corticosteroids, but the frequency of complaints depends on the dose and frequency of administration and on the delivery system used.

Dysphonia The commonest complaint is of hoarseness of the voice (dysphonia) and may occur in over 50% of

Table 17.3: Side-effects of inhaled corticosteroids
Local side-effects Dysphonia Oropharyngeal candidiasis Cough
Systemic side-effects Adrenal suppression Growth suppression Bruising Osteoporosis Cataracts Glaucoma Metabolic abnormalities (glucose, insulin, triglycerides) Psychiatric disturbances

patients using MDI. Dysphonia is not appreciably reduced by using spacers, but may be less with dry powder devices. Dysphonia may be due to myopathy of laryngeal muscles and is reversible when treatment is withdrawn.[69] For most patients it is not troublesome, but may be disabling in singers and lecturers.

Oropharyngeal Candidiasis Oropharyngeal candidiasis (thrush) may be a problem in some patients, particularly in the elderly, with concomitant oral corticosteroids and more than twice daily administration.[70] Large volume spacer devices protect against this local side-effect by reducing the dose of inhaled corticosteroid that deposits in the oropharynx.

Other Local Complications There is no evidence that inhaled corticosteroids, even in high doses, increase the frequency of infections, including tuberculosis, in the lower respiratory tract. There is no evidence for atrophy of the airway epithelium and even after 10 years of treatment with inhaled corticosteroids there is no evidence for any structural changes in the epithelium. Cough and throat irritation, sometimes accompanied by reflex bronchoconstriction, may occur when inhaled corticosteroids are given via a metered dose inhaler. These symptoms are likely to be due to surfactants in pressurized aerosols as they disappear after switching to a dry powder corticosteroid inhaler device.

Systemic Side-Effects

The efficacy of inhaled corticosteroids in the control of asthma is undisputed, but there are concerns about systemic effects of inhaled corticosteroids, particularly as they are likely to be used over long periods and in children of all ages.[29] The safety of inhaled corticosteroids has been extensively investigated since their introduction 30 years ago.[31] One of the major problems is to decide whether a measurable systemic effect has any significant clinical consequence and this necessitates careful long-term follow-up studies. As biochemical markers of systemic corticosteroid effects become more sensitive, then systemic effects may be seen more often, but this does not mean that these effects are clinically relevant. There are several case reports of adverse systemic effects of inhaled corticosteroids, and these may be idiosyncratic reactions, which may be due to abnormal pharmacokinetic handling of the inhaled corticosteroid. The systemic effect of an inhaled corticosteroid will depend on several factors, including the dose delivered to the patient, the site of delivery (gastrointestinal tract and lung), the delivery system used and individual differences in the patient's response to the corticosteroid.

Effect of Delivery Systems The systemic effect of an inhaled corticosteroid is dependent on the amount of drug absorbed into the systemic circulation. Approximately 90% of the inhaled dose from an MDI deposits in the oropharynx and is swallowed and subsequently absorbed from the gastrointestinal tract. Use of a large volume spacer device markedly reduces the oropharyngeal deposition, and therefore the systemic effects of inhaled corticosteroids, although this is less important when oral bioavailability is minimal, as with FP. For dry powder inhalers similar reductions in systemic effects may be achieved with mouth-washing and discarding the fluid. All patients using a daily dose of ≥ 800 μg of an inhaled corticosteroid should therefore use either a spacer or mouth washing to reduce systemic absorption. Approximately 10% of an MDI enters the lung and this fraction (which presumably exerts the therapeutic effect) may be absorbed into the systemic circulation. As the fraction of inhaled corticosteroid deposited in the oropharynx is reduced, the proportion of the inhaled dose entering the lungs is increased. More efficient delivery to the lungs is therefore accompanied by increased systemic absorption, but this is offset by a reduction in the dose needed for optimal control of airway inflammation. For example, a multiple dry powder delivery system, the Turbuhaler, delivers approximately twice as much corticosteroid to the lungs as other devices, and therefore has increased systemic effects. However this is compensated for by the fact that only half the dose is required.

Hypothalamic–Pituitary–Adrenal Axis Corticosteroids may cause hypothalamic–pituitary–adrenal (HPA) axis suppression by reducing corticotrophin (ACTH) production, which reduces cortisol secretion by the adrenal gland. The degree of HPA suppression is dependent on dose, duration, frequency and timing of corticosteroid administration. There is no evidence that cortisol responses to the stress of an asthma exacerbation or insulin-induced hypoglycaemia are impaired, even with high doses of inhaled corticosteroids. However, measurement of HPA axis function provides evidence for systemic effects of an inhaled corticosteroid. Basal adrenal cortisol secretion may be measured by a morning plasma cortisol, 24-hour urinary cortisol or by plasma cortisol profile over 24 hours. Other tests measure the HPA response following stimulation with tetracosactrin (which measures adrenal reserve) or stimulation with metyrapone and insulin (which measure the response to stress).

There are many studies of HPA axis function in asthmatic patients with inhaled corticosteroids, but the results are inconsistent as they have often been uncontrolled and patients have also been taking courses of oral corticosteroids (which may affect the HPA axis for weeks).[31] BDP, BUD and FP at high doses by conventional MDI (>1600 µg daily) give a dose-related decrease in morning serum cortisol levels and 24-hour urinary cortisol, although values still lie well within the normal range. However, when a large volume spacer is used doses of 2000 µg daily of BDP or BUD have little effect on 24-hour urinary cortisol excretion. Stimulation tests of HPA axis function similarly show no consistent effects of doses of 1500 µg or less of inhaled corticosteroid. At high doses (>1500 µg daily) BUD and FP have less effect than BDP on HPA axis function. In children no suppression of urinary cortisol is seen with doses of BDP of 800 µg or less. In studies where plasma cortisol has been measured at frequent intervals there was a significant reduction in cortisol peaks with doses of inhaled BDP as low as 400 µg daily, although this does not appear to be dose-related in the range 400–1000 µg. The clinical significance of these effects is not certain, however.

Overall, the studies which are not confounded by concomitant treatment with oral corticosteroids have consistently shown that there are no significant suppressive effects on HPA axis function at doses of ≤ 1500 µg in adults and ≤ 400 µg in children.

Effects on Bone Metabolism Corticosteroids lead to a reduction in bone mass by direct effects on bone formation and resorption and indirectly by suppression of the pituitary–gonadal and HPA axes, effects on intestinal calcium absorption, renal tubular calcium reabsorption and secondary hyperparathyroidism.[71] The effects of oral corticosteroids on osteoporosis and increased risk of vertebral and rib fractures are well known, but there are no reports suggesting that long-term treatment with inhaled corticosteroids is associated with an increased risk of fractures. Bone densitometry has been used to assess the effect of inhaled corticosteroids on bone mass. Although there is evidence that bone density is less in patients taking high-dose inhaled corticosteroids, interpretation is confounded by the fact that these patients are also taking intermittent courses of oral corticosteroids.

Changes in bone mass occur very slowly and several biochemical indices have been used to assess the short-term effects of inhaled corticosteroids on bone metabolism. Bone formation has been measured by plasma concentrations of bone-specific alkaline phosphatase, serum osteocalcin or procollagen peptides. Bone resorption may be assessed by urinary hydroxyproline after a 12-hour fast, urinary calcium excretion and pyridinium cross-link excretion. It is important to consider the age, diet, time of day and physical activity of the patient in interpreting any abnormalities. It is also necessary to choose appropriate control groups as asthma itself may have an effect on some of the measurements, such as osteocalcin. Inhaled corticosteroids, even at doses up to 2000 µg daily, have no significant effect on calcium excretion, but acute and reversible dose-related suppression of serum osteocalcin has been reported with BDP and BUD when given by conventional MDI in several studies. Budesonide consistently has less effect than BDP at equivalent doses and only BDP increases urinary hydroxyproline at high doses. With a large volume spacer even doses of 2000 µg daily of either BDP or BUD are without effect on plasma osteocalcin concentrations, however. Urinary pyridinium and deoxypyridinoline cross-links, which are a more accurate and stable measurement of bone and collagen degradation, are not increased with inhaled corticosteroids (BDP >1000 µg daily), even with intermittent courses of oral corticosteroids. It is important to monitor changes in markers of bone formation as well as bone degradation, as the net effect on bone turnover is important.

There has been particular concern about the effect of inhaled corticosteroids on bone metabolism in growing children. A very low dose of oral corticosteroids (prednisolone 2.5 mg) causes significant changes in serum osteocalcin and urinary hydroxyproline excretion, whereas daily BDP and BUD at doses up to 800 μg daily have no effect. It is important to recognize that the changes in biochemical indices of bone metabolism are less than those seen with even low doses of oral corticosteroids. This suggests that even high doses of inhaled corticosteroids, particularly when used with a spacer device, are unlikely to have any long-term effect on bone structure. Careful long-term follow-up studies in patients with asthma are needed.

There is no evidence that inhaled corticosteroids increase the frequency of fractures. Long-term treatment with high-dose inhaled corticosteroids has not been associated with any consistent change in bone density. Indeed, in elderly patients there may be an increase in bone density due to increased mobility.

Effects on Connective Tissue Oral and topical corticosteroids cause thinning of the skin, telangiectasiae and easy bruising, probably as a result of loss of extracellular ground substance within the dermis, due to an inhibitory effect on dermal fibroblasts. There are reports of increased skin bruising and purpura in patients using high doses of inhaled BDP, but the amount of intermittent oral corticosteroids in these patients is not known. Easy bruising in association with inhaled corticosteroids is more frequent in elderly patients[72] and there are no reports of this problem in children. Long-term prospective studies with objective measurements of skin thickness are needed with different inhaled corticosteroids.

Ocular Effects Long-term treatment with oral corticosteroids increase the risk of posterior subcapsular cataracts and there are several case reports describing cataracts in individual patients taking inhaled corticosteroids.[31] In a recent cross-sectional study in patients aged 5–25 years taking either inhaled BDP or BUD no cataracts were found on slit-lamp examination, even in patients taking 2000 μg daily for over 10 years.[73] However, epidemiological studies have identified an increased risk of cataracts in patients taking high dose

inhaled steroids over prolonged periods.[74] A slight increase in the risk of glaucoma in patients taking very high doses of inhaled corticosteroids has also been identified.[75]

Growth There has been particular concern that inhaled corticosteroids may cause stunting of growth and several studies have addressed this issue. Asthma itself (as with other chronic diseases) may have an effect on the growth pattern and has been associated with delayed onset of puberty and decceleration of growth velocity that is more pronounced with more severe disease. However, asthmatic children appear to grow for longer, so that their final height is normal. The effect of asthma on growth makes it difficult to assess the effects of inhaled corticosteroids on growth in cross-sectional studies, particularly as use of oral corticosteroids is a confounding factor. Longitudinal studies have demonstrated that there is no significant effect of inhaled corticosteroids on statural growth in doses of up to 800 μg daily and for up to 5 years of treatment.[31] A meta-analysis of 21 studies, including over 800 children, showed no effect of inhaled BDP on statural height, even with higher doses and long duration of therapy[76] and in a large study of asthmatics treated with inhaled corticosteroids during childhood there was no difference in statural height compared with normal children.[77]

Short-term growth measurements (knemometry) have demonstrated that even a low dose of an oral corticosteroid (prednisolone 2.5 mg) is sufficient to give complete suppression of lower leg growth. However inhaled BUD up to 400 μg is without effect, although some suppression is seen with 800 μg and with 400 μg BDP. The relationship between knemometry measurements and final height are uncertain since low doses of oral corticosteroid that have no effect on final height cause profound suppression.

Metabolic Effects Several metabolic effects have been reported after inhaled corticosteroids, but there is no evidence that these are clinically relevant at therapeutic doses. In adults, fasting glucose and insulin are unchanged after doses of BDP up to 2000 μg daily, and in children with inhaled BUD up to 800 μg daily. In normal individuals high-dose inhaled BDP may slightly increase resistance to insulin. However, in patients with poorly controlled asthma high doses of BDP and BUD paradoxically decrease insulin resistance and improve glucose tolerance, suggesting that the disease itself may lead to abnormalities in carbohydrate metabolism. Neither BDP 2000 µg daily in adults nor BUD 800 µg daily in children have any effect on plasma cholesterol or triglycerides.

Haematological Effects Inhaled corticosteroids may reduce the numbers of circulating eosinophils in asthmatic patients, possibly due to an effect on local cytokine generation in the airways. Inhaled corticosteroids may cause a small increase in circulating neutrophil counts.

Central Nervous System Effects There are various reports of psychiatric disturbance, including emotional lability, euphoria, depression, aggressiveness and insomnia, after inhaled corticosteroids. Only eight such patients have so far been reported, suggesting that this is very infrequent and a causal link with inhaled corticosteroids has usually not been established.

Safety in Pregnancy Based on extensive clinical experience inhaled corticosteroids appear to be safe in pregnancy, although no controlled studies have been performed. There is no evidence for any adverse effects of inhaled corticosteroids on the pregnancy, the delivery or on the foetus.[31,78] It is important to recognize that poorly controlled asthma may increase the incidence of perinatal mortality and retard intra-uterine growth, so that more effective control of asthma with inhaled corticosteroids may reduce these problems.

SYSTEMIC CORTICOSTEROIDS

Oral or intravenous corticosteroids may be indicated in several situations. Prednisolone, rather than prednisone, is the preferred oral corticosteroid as prednisone has to be converted in the liver to the active prednisolone. In pregnant patients prednisone may be preferable as it is not converted to prednisolone in the foetal liver, thus diminishing the exposure of the foetus to corticosteroids. Enteric-coated preparations of prednisolone are used to reduce side-effects (particularly gastric side-effects) and give delayed and reduced peak plasma concentrations, although the bioavailability and therapeutic efficacy of these preparations is similar to uncoated tablets. Prednisolone and prednisone are preferable to dexamethasone, betamethasone or triamcinolone, which have longer plasma half-lives and therefore an increased frequency of adverse effects.

Short courses of oral corticosteroids (30–40 mg prednisolone daily for 1–2 weeks or until the peak flow values return to best attainable) are indicated for exacerbations of asthma, and the dose may be tailed off over 1 week once the exacerbation is resolved. The tail-off period is not strictly necessary, but some patients find it reassuring.

Maintenance oral corticosteroids are only needed in a small proportion of asthmatic patients with the most severe asthma that cannot be controlled with maximal doses of inhaled corticosteroids (2000 µg daily) and additional bronchodilators. The minimal dose of oral corticosteroid needed for control should be used and reductions in the dose should be made slowly in patients who have been on oral corticosteroids for long periods (e.g. by 2.5 mg per month for doses down to 10 mg daily and thereafter by 1 mg per month). Oral corticosteroids are usually given as a single morning dose as this reduces the risk of adverse effects since it coincides with the peak diurnal concentrations. There is some evidence that administration in the afternoon may be optimal for some patients who have severe nocturnal asthma.[79] Alternate day administration may also reduce adverse effects, but control of asthma may not be as good on the day when the oral dose is omitted in some patients.

Intramuscular triamcinolone acetonide (80 mg monthly) has been advocated in patients with severe asthma as an alternative to oral corticosteroids.[80,81] This may be considered in patients in whom compliance is a particular problem, but the major concern is the high frequency of proximal myopathy associated with this fluorinated corticosteroid. Some patients who do not respond well to prednisolone are reported to respond to oral betamethasone, presumably because of pharmacokinetic handling problems with prednisolone.

Acute Severe Asthma

Intravenous hydrocortisone is given in acute severe asthma. The recommended dose is 200 mg i.v..[82] While the value of corticosteroids in acute severe asthma has been questioned, others have found that they speed the resolution of attacks.[83] There is no apparent advantage in giving very high doses of intravenous corticosteroids (such as methylprednisolone 1 g). Indeed, intravenous corticosteroids have occasionally been associated with an acute severe myopathy.[84] In a recent study no difference in recovery from acute severe asthma was seen whether i.v. hydrocortisone in doses of

50, 200 or 500 mg 6-hourly were used[85] and another placebo controlled study showed no beneficial effect of i.v. corticosteroids.[86] Intravenous corticosteroids are indicated in acute asthma if lung function is <30% predicted and where there is no significant improvement with nebulized β_2 agonist. Intravenous therapy is usually given until a satisfactory response is obtained and then oral prednisolone may be substituted. Oral prednisolone (40–60 mg) has a similar effect to intravenous hydrocortisone and is easier to administer.[83,87] Oral prednisolone is the preferred treatment for acute severe asthma, providing there are no contraindications to oral therapy.[53]

CORTICOSTEROID-RESISTANT ASTHMA
(see Chapter 39)

Although glucocorticoids are highly effective in the control of asthma and other chronic inflammatory or immune diseases, a small proportion of patients with asthma fail to respond even to high doses of oral glucocorticoids.[88,89] Resistance to the therapeutic effects of glucocorticoids is also recognized in other inflammatory and immune diseases, including rheumatoid arthritis and inflammatory bowel disease. Corticosteroid-resistant patients, although uncommon, present considerable management problems. Recently, new insights into the mechanisms whereby corticosteroids suppress chronic inflammation has shed new light on the molecular basis of corticosteroid-resistant asthma.

Corticosteroid-resistant asthma is defined as a failure to improve FEV_1 or PEF by >15% after treatment with oral prednisolone 30–40 mg daily for 2 weeks, providing the oral steroid is taken (verified by plasma prednisolone level or a reduction in early morning cortisol level). These patients are not addisonian and they do not suffer from the abnormalities in sex hormones described in the very rare familial glucocorticoid resistance. Plasma cortisol and adrenal suppression in response to exogenous cortisol is normal in these patients, so they suffer from side-effects of corticosteroids.

Complete corticosteroid resistance in asthma is very rare, with a prevalence of <1:1000 asthmatic patients. Much more common is a reduced responsiveness to corticosteroids, so that large inhaled or oral doses are needed to control asthma adequately (corticosteroid-dependent asthma). It is likely that there is a range of responsiveness to corticosteroids and that corticosteroid-resistance is at one extreme of this range.

It is important to establish that the patient has asthma, rather than chronic obstructive pulmonary disease (COPD), "pseudoasthma" (a hysterical conversion syndrome involving vocal cord dysfunction), left ventricular failure or cystic fibrosis which do not respond to corticosteroids. Asthmatic patients are characterized by a variability in PEF and, in particular, a diurnal variability of >15% and episodic symptoms. It is also important to identify provoking factors (allergens, drugs, psychological problems) that may increase the severity of asthma and its resistance to therapy. Biopsy studies have demonstrated the typical eosinophilic inflammation of asthma in these patients.[89]

Mechanisms of Corticosteroid Resistance
There may be several mechanisms for resistance to the effects of glucocorticoids. Certain cytokines (particularly IL-2, IL-4 and IL-13) may induce a reduction in affinity of glucocorticoid receptors in inflammatory cells such as T-lymphocytes, resulting in local resistance to the anti-inflammatory actions of corticosteroids.[89] Another mechanism is an increased activation of the transcription factor AP-1 by inflammatory cytokines, so that AP-1 may consume activated glucocorticoid receptors and thus reduce their availability for suppression of inflammation at inflamed sites[90] (Fig. 17.6). There is an increased expression of c-Fos, one of the components of AP-1.[91] The reasons for this excessive activation of AP-1 by activating enzymes is currently unknown, but may be genetically determined.

FUTURE DIRECTIONS

Inhaled corticosteroids are now used as first-line therapy for the treatment of persistent asthma in adults and children in many countries, as they are the most effective treatments for asthma currently available. The recent trend to start with a relatively high dose of inhaled corticosteroids in order to achieve more rapid control of asthma, before the dose is reduced to the minimum needed to maintain control, may lead to lower overall maintenance doses.[31] While many patients, particularly with more severe asthma, remain undertreated, there is also a danger of over-treatment and many patients with mild asthma who many require very low doses of inhaled corticosteroids are inappropriately treated with high doses. It is essential that inhaled corticosteroids are slowly reduced to the minimal dose required to control asthma. An important clinical

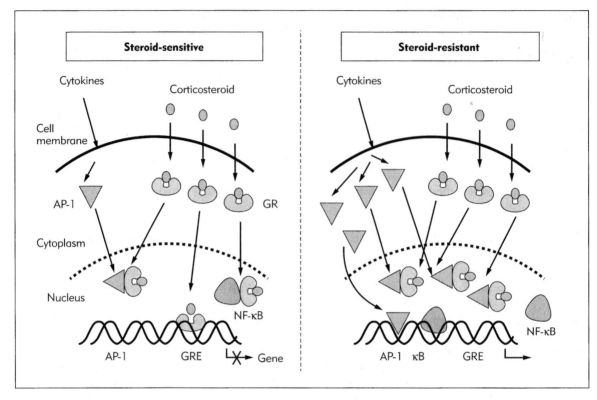

Steroid-sensitive

Steroid-resistant

Cytokines

Corticosteroid

Cell membrane

AP-1

GR

Cytoplasm

Nucleus

NF-κB

AP-1   GRE   Gene

Cytokines

Corticosteroid

NF-κB

AP-1   κB   GRE

FIGURE 17.6: Proposed mechanism of primary corticosteroid-resistance in asthma. Increased activation of activator protein-1 (AP-1) results in the consumption of glucocorticoid receptors (GR), thus preventing the anti-inflammatory action of corticosteroids, either through binding to GREs or through inhibition of NF-κB.

development is the recognition that asthma is better controlled by addition of an alternative class of treatment (long-acting inhaled β₂ agonists, low dose theophylline, anti-leukotrienes) than on increasing the dose of inhaled steroid. However, there may be some patients who are better treated with a higher dose of inhaled corticosteroid and at present it is not possible to identify such patients clinically. Improvement in techniques for the non-invasive monitoring of airway inflammation may be valuable in the future for assessing the requirement for inhaled corticosteroids.[92]

New Corticosteroids

Budesonide and FP have been important advances in inhaled corticosteroid therapy as they have reduced systemic effects because of greater first-pass hepatic metabolism than BDP. There are other inhaled corticosteroids in development, such as mometasone, that show a similar improved profile.[93] However, all cur-

rently available corticosteroids are absorbed from the lungs into the systemic circulation and therefore inevitably have some systemic component. A class of steroids was developed that was metabolized in the lung, but such so called "soft" steroids, such as tipredane and butixocort, did not prove to be clinically effective, probably because they were metabolized too rapidly in the airways. A new soft steroid, ciclesonide, appears to have good efficacy and is now in clinical development.[94] Steroids that are metabolized by enzymes in the circulation may be the safest type of inhaled corticosteroid and novel esterified corticosteroids are now in clinical development. However, it is still not certain whether the anti-inflammatory effects of inhaled corticosteroids in asthma are mediated entirely by local anti-inflammatory effects in the airways, and it is possible that there is a systemic component, for example on bone marrow eosinophil precursors. Furthermore, it is not clear whether inhaled corticosteroids are distributed from their point of deposition in the airways to more peripheral airways via the local circulation. If this is the case then corticosteroids that are degraded by enzymes in the circulation may not reach small airways which are known to be inflamed in asthma.

Understanding the molecular mechanisms of action of corticosteroids has led to the development of a new generation of corticosteroids. As discussed above, a major mechanism of the anti-inflammatory effect of corticosteroids appears to be direct inhibition of transcription factors, such as NF-κB and AP-1 that are activated by pro-inflammatory cytokines (transrepression). By contrast the endocrine and metabolic effects of steroids that are responsible for the systemic side effects of corticosteroids are likely to be mediated via DNA binding (transactivation). This has led to a search for novel corticosteroids that selectively transrepress, thus reducing the potential risk of systemic side-effects. Since corticosteroids bind to the same GR, this seems at first to be an unlikely possibility, but while DNA binding involves a GR homodimer, interaction with transcription factors AP-1 and NF-κB involves only a single GR. A separation of transactivation and transrepression has been demonstrated using reporter gene constructs in transfected cells using selective mutations of the glucocorticoid receptor. Furthermore, some steroids, such as the antagonist RU486, have a greater transrepression than transactivation effect. Indeed, the topical steroids used in asthma therapy today, such as FP and BUD, appear to have more potent transrepression than transactivation effects, which may account for their selection as potent anti-inflammatory agents.[95] Recently, a novel class of steroids has been described in which there is potent transrepression with relatively little transactivation. These "dissociated" steroids, including RU24858 and RU40066 have anti-inflammatory effects *in vivo*.[96] This suggests that the development of steroids with a greater margin of safety is possible and may even lead to the development of oral steroids that do not have significant adverse effects.

New Anti-inflammatory Drugs

There has been a concerted effort to find novel anti-inflammatory drugs that might replace corticosteroids in the future.[30,97] However it has proved very difficult to find classes of drug that are as safe and efficacious as inhaled corticosteroids. More specific anti-inflammatory drugs that selectively inhibit eosinophilic inflammation, such as anti-IL-5 drugs, chemokine receptor (CCR3) inhibitors and adhesion molecule blockers (such as VLA4 inhibitors) are currently in clinical development, but

KEY POINTS

1 Corticosteroids are the most effective treatment for long-term control of asthma.

2 Corticosteroids suppress inflammation in asthmatic airways by repressing multiple inflammatory genes at a transcriptional level and inhibit activation and secretion of multiple inflammatory and structural cells.

3 Airway epithelial cells may be a key cellular target for the effects of inhaled corticosteroids.

4 Inhaled corticosteroids are effective in asthmatic patients of all ages and degrees of severity of asthma.

5 The dose–response effect of inhaled corticosteroids is relatively flat and it is preferable to add another class of drug (long-acting inhaled β₂ agonists, theophylline, anti-leukotrienes) in patients not controlled on moderate doses of inhaled corticosteroids rather than going to high doses.

6 Systemic side-effects of inhaled corticosteroids may occur at high inhaled doses, but are not a problem at doses of ~800 μg daily.

7 Some patients are relatively or completely resistant to the anti-inflammatory actions of corticosteroids and this is explained by a defect in the molecular action of steroid in suppressing inflammatory genes.

whether these more specific drugs will have the efficacy of corticosteroids is not yet known. Drugs that inhibit NF-κB are also in early development, but may prove to be too toxic for use in asthma. More generalized anti-inflammatory drugs, such as phosphodiesterase 4 inhibitors, have proved to be disappointing because of side-effects and immunomodulators, such as cyclosporin A, lack clinical efficacy and have a high degree of toxicity. It is likely that inhaled corticosteroids will remain the mainstay of asthma therapy for many years to come.

REFERENCES

1. ✪ Barnes PJ. Inhaled glucocorticoids for asthma. *New Engl J Med* 1995; 332: 868–75.

2. Barnes PJ. Efficacy of inhaled corticosteroids in asthma. *J Allergy Clin Immunol* 1998; 102: 531–8.

3. ✪ Barnes PJ. Anti-inflammatory actions of glucocorticoids: molecular mechanisms. *Clin Sci* 1998; 94: 557–72.

4. Bamberger CM, Bamberger AM, de Castr M, Chrousos GP. Glucocorticoid receptor b, a potential endogenous inhibitor of glucocorticoid action in humans. *J Clin Invest* 1995; 95: 2435–41.

5. Reichardt HM, Kaestner KH, Tuckermann J *et al*. DNA binding of the glucocorticoid receptor is not essential for survival. *Cell* 1998; 93: 531–41.

6. Barnes PJ, Karin M. Nuclear factor-κB: a pivotal transcription factor in chronic inflammatory diseases. *New Engl J Med* 1997; 336: 1066–71.

7. Barnes PJ, Adcock IM. Transcription factors and asthma. *Eur Respir J* 1998; 12: 221–34.

8. Kamei Y, Xu L, Heinzel T *et al*. A CBP integrator complex mediates transcriptional activation and AP-1 inhibition by nuclear receptors. *Cell* 1996; 85: 403–414.

9. Karin M. New twists in gene regulation by glucocorticoid receptor: is DNA binding dispensable? [comment]. *Cell* 1998; 93: 487–90.

10. Hall SE, Lim S, Witherden IR *et al*. Lung type II cell and macrophage annexin I release: differential effects of two glucocorticoids. *Am J Physiol* 1999; 276: L114–21.

11. Mak JCW, Nishikawa M, Barnes PJ. Glucocorticosteroids increase β_2-adrenergic receptor transcription in human lung. *Am J Physiol* 1995; 12: L41–6.

12. Mak JCW, Nishikawa M, Shirasaki H, Miyayasu K, Barnes PJ. Protective effects of a glucocorticoid on down-regulation of pulmonary β_2-adrenergic receptors *in vivo*. *J Clin Invest* 1995; 96: 99–106.

13. Lilly CM, Nakamura H, Kesselman H *et al*. Expression of eotaxin by human lung epithelial cells: induction by cytokines and inhibition by glucocorticoids. *J Clin Invest* 1997; 99: 1767–73.

14. Rao A, Luo C, Hogan PG. Transcription factors of the NFAT family: regulation and function. *Ann Rev Immunol* 1997; 15: 707–47.

15. Adcock IM, Peters M, Gelder C, Shirasaki H, Brown CR, Barnes PJ. Increased tachykinin receptor gene expression in asthmatic lung and its modulation by steroids. *J Mol Endocrinol* 1993; 11: 1–7.

16. Katsunuma T, Mak JCW, Barnes PJ. Glucocorticoids reduce tachykinin NK_2-receptor expression in bovine tracheal smooth muscle. *Eur J Pharmacol* 1998; 344: 99–107.

17. Atsuta J, Plitt J, Bochner BS, Schleimer RP. Inhibition of VCAM-1 expression in human bronchial epithelial cells by glucocorticoids. *Am J Respir Cell Mol Biol* 1999; 20: 643–50.

18. Walsh GM. Mechanisms of human eosinophil survival and apoptosis. *Clin Exp Allergy* 1997; 27: 482–7.

19. John M, Lim S, Seybold J, Robichaud A, O'Connor B, Barnes PJ, Chung KF. Inhaled corticosteroids increase IL-10 but reduce MIP-1a, GM-CSF and IFN-γ release from alveolar macrophages in asthma. *Am J Respir Crit Care Med* 1998; 157: 256–62.

20. Woolley KL, Gibson PG, Carty K, Wilson AJ, Twaddell SH, Woolley MJ. Eosinophil apoptosis and the resolution of airway inflammation in asthma. *Am J Respir Crit Care Med* 1996; 154: 237–43.

21. Nelson DJ, McWilliam AS, Haining S, Holt PG. Modulation of airway intraepithelial dendritic cells

following exposure to steroids. *Am J Respir Crit Care Med* 1995; 151: 475–81.

22. Cox G. Glucocorticoid treatment inhibits apoptosis in human neutrophils. *J Immunol* 1995; 193: 4719–725.

23. Barnes PJ. Mechanism of action of glucocorticoids in asthma. *Am J Respir Crit Care Med* 1996; 154: S21–7.

24. Schweibert LM, Stellato C, Schleimer RP. The epithelium as a target for glucocorticoid action in the treatment of asthma. *Am J Respir Crit Care Med* 1996; 154: S16–20.

25. Saleh D, Ernst P, Lim S, Barnes PJ, Giaid A. Increased formation of the potent oxidant peroxynitrite in the airways of asthmatic patients is associated with induction of nitric oxide synthase: effect of inhaled glucocorticoid. *FASEB J* 1998; 12: 929–37.

26. Kharitonov SA, Yates DH, Barnes PJ. Regular inhaled budesonide decreases nitric oxide concentration in the exhaled air of asthmatic patients. *Am J Resp Crit Care Med* 1996; 153: 454–7.

27. Kai H, Yoshitake K, Hisatsune A, Kido T, Isohama Y, Takahama K, Miyata T. Dexamethasone suppresses mucus production and MUC-2 and MUC-5AC gene expression by NCI-H292 cells. *Am J Physiol* 1996; 271: L484–8.

28. Barnes PJ. Effect of corticosteroids on airway hyperresponsiveness. *Am Rev Respir Dis* 1990; 141: S70–76.

29. ✪ Kamada AK, Szefler SJ, Martin RJ *et al*. Issues in the use of inhaled steroids. *Am J Respir Crit Care Med* 1996; 153: 1739–48.

30. Barnes PJ. New therapeutic strategies for allergic diseases. *Nature* 1999; 402: B31–8.

31. ✪ Barnes PJ, Pedersen S, Busse WW. Efficacy and safety of inhaled corticosteroids: an update. *Am J Respir Crit Care Med* 1998; 157: S1–53.

32. Haahtela T, Jarvinen M, Kava T *et al*. Comparison of a β_2-agonist terbutaline with an inhaled steroid in newly detected asthma. *New Engl J Med* 1991; 325: 388–92.

33. Juniper EF, Kline PA, Vanzieleghem MA, Ramsdale EH, O'Byrne PM, Hargreave FE. Effect of long-term treatment with an inhaled corticosteroid (budesonide) on airway hyperresponsiveness and clinical asthma in nonsteroid-dependent asthmatics. *Am Rev Respir Dis* 1990; 142: 832–6.

34. Vathenen AS, Knox AJ, Wisniewski A, Tattersfield AE. Time course of change in bronchial reactivity with an inhaled corticosteroid in asthma. *Am Rev Respir Dis* 1991; 143: 1317–21.

35. Levy ML, Stevenson C, Maslen T. Comparison of short courses of oral prednisolone and fluticasone propionate in the treatment of adults with acute exacerbations of asthma in primary care. *Thorax* 1996; 51: 1087–92.

36. Juniper EF, Kline PA, Vanzieleghem MA, Hargreave FE. Reduction of budesonide after a year of increased use: a randomized controlled trial to evaluate whether improvements in airway responsiveness and clinical asthma are maintained. *J Allergy Clin Immunol* 1991; 87: 483–9.

37. van Essen-Zandvliet EE, Hughes MD, Waalkens HJ, Duiverman EJ, Pocock SJ, Kerrebijn KF. Effects of 22 months of treatment with inhaled corticosteroids and/or β_2 agonists on lung function, airway responsiveness and symptoms in children with asthma. *Am Rev Respir Dis* 1992; 146: 547–54.

38. Waalkens HJ, van Essen-Zandvliet EE, Hughes MD, Gerritsen J, Duiverman EJ, Knol K, Kerrebijn KF. Cessation of long-term treatment with inhaled corticosteroids (budesonide) in children with asthma results in deterioration. *Am Rev Respir Dis* 1993; 148: 1252–7.

39. Simons FE. A comparison of beclomethasone, salmeterol, and placebo in children with asthma. Canadian Beclomethasone Dipropionate-Salmeterol Xinafoate Study Group. *N Engl J Med* 1997; 337: 1659–65.

40. Ilangovan P, Pedersen S, Godfrey S, Nikander K, Novisky N, Warner JO. Nebulised budesonide suspension in severe steroid-dependent preschool asthma. *Arch Dis Child* 1993; 68: 356–9.

41. Busse WW, Chervinsky P, Condemi J, Lumry WR, Petty TL, Rennard S, Townley RG. Budesonide delivered by Turbuhaler is effective in a dose-dependent fashion when used in the treatment of adult patients with chronic asthma. *J Allergy Clin Immunol* 1998; 101: 457–63.

42. Pauwels RA, Lofdahl C-G, Postma DS *et al*. Effect of inhaled formoterol and budesonide on exacerbations of asthma. *New Engl J Med* 1997; 337: 1412–18.

43. Lim S, Jatakanon A, John M *et al*. Effect of inhaled budesonide on lung function and airway inflammation. Assessment by various inflammatory markers in mild asthma. *Am J Respir Crit Care Med* 1999; 159: 22–30.

44. Jatakanon A, Lim S, Chung KF, Barnes PJ. An inhaled steroid improves markers of inflammation in asymptomatic steroid-naive asthmatic patients. *Eur Respir J* 1998; 12: 1084–88.

45. Jatakanon A, Kharitonov S, Lim S, Barnes PJ. Effect of differing doses of inhaled budesonide on markers of airway inflammation in patients with mild asthma. *Thorax* 1999; 54: 108–114.

46. Sont JK, Willems LN, Bel EH, van Krieken JH, Vandenbroucke JP, Sterk PJ. Clinical control and histopathologic outcome of asthma when using airway hyperresponsiveness as an additional guide to long-term treatment. The AMPUL Study Group. *Am J Respir Crit Care Med* 1999; 159: 1043–51.

47. Dompeling E, Van Schayck CP, Molema J, Folgering H, van Grusven PM, van Weel C. Inhaled beclomethasone improves the course of asthma and COPD. *Eur Resp J* 1992; 5: 945–52.

48. ☺ Haahtela T, Järvinsen M, Kava T *et al*. Effects of reducing or discontinuing inhaled budesonide in patients with mild asthma. *New Engl J Med* 1994; 331: 700–705.

49. Agertoft L, Pedersen S. Effects of long-term treatment with an inhaled corticosteroid on growth and pulmonary function in asthmatic children. *Resp Med* 1994; 5: 369–72.

50. Selroos O, Pietinalcho A, Lofroos A-B, Riska A. Effect of early and late intervention with inhaled corticosteroids in asthma. *Chest* 1995; 108: 1228–34.

51. Ernst P, Spitzer WD, Suissa S *et al*. Risk of fatal and near fatal asthma in relation to inhaled corticosteroid use. *JAMA* 1992; 268: 3462–4.

52. Barnes PJ. Inhaled glucocorticoids: new developments relevant to updating the Asthma Management Guidelines. *Resp Med* 1996; 90: 379–84.

53. British Thoracic Society. The British Guidelines on Asthma Management. *Thorax* 1997; 52(suppl. 1): S1–21.

54. Expert Panel Report 2. *Guidelines for the Diagnosis and Management of Asthma*. Washington DC: National Institutes of Health, 1997.

55. Malo J, Cartier A, Merland N, Ghezzo H, Burke A, Morris J, Jennings BH. Four-times-a-day dosing frequency is better than twice-a-day regimen in subjects requiring a high-dose inhaled steroid, budesonide, to control moderate to severe asthma. *Am Rev Respir Dis* 1989; 140: 624–8.

56. Jones AH, Langdon CG, Lee PS *et al*. Pulmicort Turbohaler once daily as initial prophylactic therapy for asthma. *Resp Med* 1994; 88: 293–9.

57. Otulana BA, Varma N, Bullock A, Higenbottam T. High dose nebulized steroid in the treatment of chronic steroid-dependent asthma. *Resp Med* 1992; 86: 105–108.

58. Greening AP, Ind PW, Northfield M, Shaw G. Added salmeterol versus higher-dose corticosteroid in asthma patients with symptoms on existing inhaled corticosteroid. *Lancet* 1994; 344: 219–24.

59. Woolcock AJ, Barnes PJ. Asthma: the important questions–Part 3. *Am J Respir Crit Care Med* 1996; 153: S1–31.

60. Chapman KR, Ringdal N, Backer V, Palmqvist M, Saarelainen S, Briggs M. Salmeterol and fluticasone propionate (50/250 mg) administered via combination Diskus inhaler: As effective as when given via separate Diskus inhalers. *Can Respir J* 1999; 6: 45–51.

61. Evans DJ, Taylor DA, Zetterstrom O, Chung KF, O'Connor BJ, Barnes PJ. A comparison of low-dose inhaled budesonide plus theophylline and high-dose inhaled budesonide for moderate asthma. *New Engl J Med* 1997; 337: 1412–18.

62. Ukena D, Harnest U, Sakalauskas R *et al*. Comparison of addition of theophylline to inhaled steroid with doubling of the dose of inhaled steroid in asthma. *Eur Respir J* 1997; 10: 2754–60.

63. Virchow J, Hassall SM, Summerton L, Klim J, Harris A. Reduction of asthma exacerabtions with zafirlukast in patients on inhaled corticosteroids. *Eur Respir J* 1997; 10(suppl. 25): 420S.

64. O'Shaughnessy KM, Wellings R, Gillies B, Fuller RW. Differential effects of fluticasone proprionate on allergen-induced bronchoconstriction and increased urinary leukotriene E_4 excretion. *Am Rev Respir Dis* 1993; 147: 1472–6.

65. Barnes PJ, Jonsson B, Klim J. The costs of asthma. *Eur Respir J* 1996; 9: 636–42.

66. van Schayk CP, Dompeling E, Rutten MP, Folgering H, van den Boom G, van Weel C. The influence of an inhaled steroid on quality of life in patients with asthma or COPD. *Chest* 1995; 107: 1199–1205.

67. Hill SJ, Tattersfield AE. Corticosteroid sparing agents in asthma. *Thorax* 1995; 50: 577–82.

68. Nelson HS, Hamilos DL, Corsello PR, Levesque NV, Buchameier AD, Bucher BL. A double-blind study of troleandamycin and methylprednisolone in asthmatic patients who require daily corticosteroids. *Am Rev Respir Dis* 1993; 147: 398–404.

69. Williamson IJ, Matusiewicz SP, Brown PH, Greening AP, Crompton GK. Frequency of voice problems and cough in patients using pressurised aersosol inhaled steroid preparations. *Eur Resp J* 1995; 8: 590–92.

70. Toogood JA, Jennings B, Greenway RW, Chung L. Candidiasis and dysphonia complicating beclomethasone treatment of asthma. *J Allergy Clin Immunol* 1980; 65: 145–53.

71. Efthimou J, Barnes PJ. Effect of inhaled corticosteroids on bone and growth. *Eur Respir J* 1998; 11: 1167–77.

72. Roy A, Leblanc C, Paquette L *et al.* Skin bruising in asthmatic subjects treated with high doses of inhaled steroids: frequency and association with adrenal function. *Eur Respir J* 1996; 9: 226–31.

73. Simons FER, Persaud MP, Gillespie CA, Cheang M, Shuckett EP. Absence of posterior subcapsular cataracts in young patients treated with inhaled glucocorticoids. *Lancet* 1993; 342: 736–8.

74. Cumming RG, Mitchell P, Leeder SR. Use of inhaled corticosteroids and the risk of cataracts. *New Engl J Med* 1997; 337: 8–14.

75. Garbe E, LeLorier J, Boivin J, Suissa S. Inhaled and nasal glucocorticoids and the risks of ocular hypertension or open-angle glaucoma. *JAMA* 1997; 227: 722–7.

76. Allen DB, Mullen M, Mullen B. A meta-analysis of the effects of oral and inhaled corticosteroids on growth. *J Allergy Clin Immunol* 1994; 93: 967–76.

77. Silverstein MD, Yunginger JW, Reed CE, Petterson T, Zimmerman D, Li JT, O'Fallon WM. Attained adult height after childhood asthma: effect of glucocorticoid therapy. *J Allergy Clin Immunol* 1997; 99: 466–74.

78. Schatz M, Zeiger RS, Harden K, Hoffman CC, Chilingar L, Petitti D. The safety of asthma and allergy medications during pregnancy. *J Allergy Clin Immunol* 1997; 100: 301–306.

79. Beam WR, Ballard RD, Martin RJ. Spectrum of corticosteroid sensitivity in nocturnal asthma. *Am Rev Respir Dis* 1992; 145: 1082–6.

80. McLeod DT, Capewell SJ, Law J, MacLaren W, Seaton A. Intramuscular triamcinolone acetamide in chronic severe asthma. *Thorax* 1985; 40: 840–45.

81. Ogirala RG, Aldrich TK, Prezant DJ, Sinnett MJ, Enden JB, Williams MH. High dose intramuscular triamcinolone in severe life-threatening asthma. *New Engl J Med* 1991; 329: 585–9.

82. British Thoracic Society. Guidelines on the Management of Asthma. *Thorax* 1993; 48S(suppl.): S1–24.

83. Engel T, Heinig JH. Glucocorticoid therapy in acute severe asthma–a critical review. *Eur Respir J* 1991; 4: 881–9.

84. Decramer M, Lacquet LM, Fagard R, Rogiers P. Corticosteroids contribute to muscle weakness in chronic airflow obstruction. *Am J Respir Crit Care Med* 1995; 150: 11–16.

85. Bowler SD, Mitchell CA, Armstrong JG. Corticosteroids in acute severe asthma: effectiveness of low doses. *Thorax* 1992; 47: 584–7.

86. Morell F, Orkiols R, de Gracia J, Curul V, Pujol A. Controlled trial of intravenous corticosteroids in severe acute asthma. *Thorax* 1992; 47: 588–91.

87. Harrison BDN, Stokes TC, Hart GJ, Vaughan DA, Ali NJ, Robinson AA. Need for intravenous hydrocortisone

in addition to oral prednisolone in patients admitted to hospital with severe asthma without ventilatory failure. *Lancet* 1986; i: 181–4.

88. Barnes PJ, Greening AP, Crompton GK. Glucocorticoid resistance in asthma. *Am J Respir Crit Care Med* 1995; 152: 125S–140S.

89. Szefler SJ, Leung DY. Glucocorticoid-resistant asthma: pathogenesis and clinical implications for management. *Eur Respir J* 1997; 10: 1640–47.

90. Adcock IM, Brown CR, Shirasaki H, Barnes PJ. Effects of dexamethasone on cytokine and phorbol ester stimulated c-Fos and c-Jun DNA binding and gene expression in human lung. *Eur Resp J* 1994; 7: 2117–23.

91. Lane SJ, Adcock IM, Richards D, Hawrylowicz C, Barnes PJ, Lee TH. Corticosteroid-resistant bronchial asthma is associated with increased *c-Fos* expression in monocytes and T-lymphocytes. *J Clin Invest* 1998; 102: 2156–64.

92. Barnes PJ, Kharitonov SA. Exhaled nitric oxide: a new lung function test. *Thorax* 1996; 51: 218–20.

93. Prakash A, Benfield P. Topical mometasone. A review of its pharmacological properties and therapeutic use in the treatment of dermatological disorders. *Drugs* 1998; 55: 145–63.

94. Taylor DA, Jensen MW, Kanabar V *et al.* A dose-dependent effect of the novel inhaled corticosteroid ciclesonide on airway responsiveness to adenosine-5'-monophosphate in asthmatic patients. *Am J Respir Crit Care Med* 1999; 160: 237–43.

95. Adcock IM, Barnes PJ. Ligand-induced differentiation of glucocorticoid receptor (GR) trans-repression and transactivation. *Am J Respir Crit Care Med* 1996; 153: A243.

96. Vayssiere BM, Dupont S, Choquart A *et al.* Synthetic glucocorticoids that dissociate transactivation and AP-1 transrepression exhibit anti-inflammatory activity *in vivo*. *Mol Endocrinol* 1997; 11: 1245–55.

97. Barnes PJ. New drugs for asthma. *Clin Exp Allergy* 1996; 26: 738–45.

Chapter 18

Anti-allergic Drugs

André Cartier

Drugs with so-called anti-allergic properties were first developed to control the allergic reaction in asthma, but these same drugs are also used in the management of non-allergic individuals as the inflammatory process seen in the allergic reaction is common to both intrinsic and extrinsic asthma. The aim of this chapter is to describe the old and new anti-allergic agents which are currently used in asthma treatment.

Although corticosteroids have several anti-allergic properties, the term "anti-allergic agents" is reserved here for drugs with anti-inflammatory activity such as cromoglycate and nedocromil or for specific antagonists to mediators of inflammation such as ketotifen.

SODIUM CROMOGLYCATE

First synthesized in 1967, sodium cromoglycate, a derivative of chromone-2- carboxylic acid, was shown to be of benefit value in 1976 by Howell and Altounyan.[1] Since then, several studies have shown its efficacy in the treatment of asthmatic subjects and in the prevention of exercise- and allergen-induced asthma.

Despite its prolonged use in the treatment of child and adult asthma,[2] the mode of action of sodium cromoglycate is not fully understood. Traditionally believed to prevent mast cell degranulation, sodium cromoglycate has a wide variety of other suppressive actions on inflammatory cells; in addition, there is some evidence that it may block neural reflex bronchoconstriction. Sodium cromoglycate is particularly effective in preventing the asthmatic reactions associated with inhaled allergen exposure and the associated increase in airway responsiveness. This is the basis for its important role as a prophylactic anti-inflammatory drug in asthma. However, its effect on airway responsiveness is limited to atopic subjects currently exposed to a rel-

evant allergen, e.g. house-dust mites. Bronchial biopsies of asthmatic subjects treated with sodium cromoglycate have shown reduction of inflammatory cells in the airways.[3] Exerting no bronchodilator activity, sodium cromoglycate is used both on a chronic and on an as-needed basis in the management of asthma in children and adults.

Sodium cromoglycate is a very safe drug being virtually free of systemic side-effects. Occasionally, the potentially irritant nature of the relatively large amount of drug powder or of the aerosol may cause transient bronchoconstriction or cough easily prevented by the prior administration of an inhaled β_2 agonist; it is rarely associated with nausea and headaches.

For the treatment of asthma, sodium cromoglycate is available for inhalation as a powder (20 mg per capsule), as a metered dose inhaler (MDI; 1 or 5 mg per puff, although the latter dosage is not available in all countries) or as a nebulizer solution (10 mg ml^{-1}).

In children, sodium cromoglycate has proven to be effective in controlling mild asthma symptoms, improving spirometry and airway responsiveness.[4-6] It is at least as effective as theophylline in controlling symptoms of asthma, but with fewer side-effects. Studies are lacking to show that it has any corticosparing effects in children with severe asthma or that its combined use with inhaled corticosteroids has any advantage. When given in a child, although symptoms may be controlled within days, its full effect may take several weeks to be achieved during which symptoms may still not be adequately controlled. It is then suggested to combine the use of sodium cromoglycate to inhaled corticosteroids for about 1 month and then try to taper the inhaled corticosteroids; if asthma is not adequately controlled by sodium cromoglycate alone, it should be stopped and replaced by inhaled corticosteroids. The usual

197

dosage is either 20 mg (as a powder) or 2 mg (as an MDI) four times per day, but this should be tapered to the lowest effective dosage once symptoms are under control; some authors recommend higher dosages of the MDI formulation, i.e. 10 mg three times a day. It should be given for at least 4 weeks before it is decided that it is clinically ineffective. While it has been considered the best available first-line prophylactic anti-inflammatory drug in paediatric medicine,[7–9] sodium cromoglycate has been replaced by low-dose inhaled corticosteroids in most guidelines in this setting.

In adults, although studies have shown that sodium cromoglycate does improve control of symptoms in mild to moderate asthmatics,[5,10,11] it is generally replaced by inhaled corticosteroids which are more effective and as safe. Sodium cromoglycate has no place in the treatment of acute asthma either in children or adults.

Used on an as-needed basis, sodium cromoglycate is very effective in preventing the bronchoconstriction induced by exercise or cold air; effective within only a few minutes, it does afford an effective protection for up to 6 hours[12] in the majority of subjects. This protective effect is dose-related.[13] In some subjects, this blocking action is potentiated by inhaled β_2 agonists.[14] Sodium cromoglycate is also particularly effective for preventing the early and late asthmatic reactions following allergen exposure in sensitized individuals; it also prevents the increase in airway responsiveness seen after the late asthmatic reaction.[15] To be effective, it needs to be given before the allergen exposure, e.g. just before exposure, and should be repeated every 2 or 3 hours until end of exposure; if symptoms occur earlier, an inhaled β_2 agonist should be given to relieve symptoms and sodium cromoglycate should be repeated at a more frequent interval.

NEDOCROMIL SODIUM

Nedocromil is a pyrano-quinoline dicarboxylic acid derivative which shares similar pharmacological properties with sodium cromoglycate, although *in vitro* experiments and some clinical studies have shown a broader spectrum of activity. As with sodium cromoglycate, it has no place in the treatment of acute asthma. Nedocromil inhibits mediator release from human lung mast cells, including histamine, prostaglandin D_2 and proinflammatory cytokines such as IL-4, TNF-α. It is also effective in blocking activation of

human blood eosinophils and can modulate reflex bronchoconstriction in the airways. Despite these effects, the regular use of nedocromil does not seem to reduce airway inflammation as assessed by bronchial biospies.[16]

Only available for inhalation as an MDI (2 mg per puff), it has also a very safe profile with virtually no systemic adverse effects; however, many patients feel that it has an unusual or bad taste (up to nearly 30% of patients) that is sometimes associated with nausea. This is, in the experience of the author, a frequent cause of cessation of the drug or of poor compliance. Finally, nedocromil is sometimes associated with throat irritation and/or cough, which may be reduced by the use of a spacer and/or a β_2 agonist prior to its administration, or with headaches.

Few long-term studies have directly compared nedocromil to sodium cromoglycate, although several acute studies have shown that it affords similar or better bronchoprotection against exercise, cold air, irritants such as sodium metabisulphite, or exposure to allergens (preventing the early and late asthmatic reaction as well as the associated increase in airway responsiveness).[17,18] Combined use of nedocromil and a β_2 agonist before exercise may offer additional protection in some subjects. However, in comparison with sodium cromoglycate, there does not appear to exist a dose–response relationship in its bronchoprotection against exercise or cold air, and its duration of action seems to be shorter;[19] 4 mg of nedocromil seems to be equivalent to 8–10 mg of sodium cromoglycate (MDI).

Long-term studies in adults, both atopic and nonatopic, have shown that nedocromil can improve the control of asthma.[17,18,20] Although nedocromil may be given at doses of 4 mg twice daily, the optimal dosage is 4 mg (two puffs) four times per day until maximal improvement has been achieved when it should be tapered slowly in order to keep control of symptoms. Most clinical long-term studies have shown that it improves symptoms in subjects with mild asthma to moderate asthma,[21] but some studies have shown that it offers additional benefit in subjects with severe asthma already taking inhaled corticosteroids (low and high doses).[22–24] Some controversial studies have shown that nedocromil has also some corticosparing effect allowing reduction of oral or inhaled corticosteroids in severe asthmatics.[25–28] However, the drug is not effective in all subjects and should be stopped after 4–6 weeks if no improvement is shown at that time.

In long-term studies in adults, nedocromil was shown to be either superior[29] or similar[30,31] to sodium cromoglycate. In patients with mild to moderate asthma, nedocromil may facilitate reduction in theophylline use or be as effective as theophylline as an add-on treatment.[32] When compared with inhaled corticosteroids given as beclomethasone dipropionate (BDP) 100 μg four times daily, nedocromil 4 mg four times daily allows a similar improvement in symptoms and airway responsiveness, but less improvement in spirometry;[33] this has been confirmed by others. Although nedocromil can be given as a first line anti-inflammatory treatment in asthma, it is the view of most authors and guidelines that inhaled corticosteroids at low doses are the first choice. Indeed, when considering that nedocromil affords a similar protection as low-dose inhaled corticosteroids at doses equivalent to one puff twice daily of the concentrated formulations (e.g. BDP 250 μg per puff or budesonide 200 μg per inhalation), but with a lower rate of success, a lesser improvement in forced expiratory volume in 1 s (FEV_1) and more compliance problems (requiring a four times daily regimen, associated with more local side-effects and no reduction in systemic side-effects), it is easy to choose low-dose inhaled corticosteroids as first-line prophylactic treatment of asthma.

In the last few years, several studies on the use of nedocromil (4 mg four times daily) in children have confirmed its efficacy in improving symptoms and in controlling the need for rescue β_2 agonists in mild to severe asthmatics.[34] Nedocromil also affords effective bronchoprotection against exercise- and fog-induced asthma in children.

KETOTIFEN

Ketotifen is a non-bronchodilating oral anti-asthmatic drug that has some clinical but limited efficacy in the management of asthma.[35] Although *in vitro* studies have shown that it exerts some anti-inflammatory activity, no clinical human studies has confirmed these findings. It is mainly considered as an effective antihistamine. Despite its limited efficacy in the treatment of asthma, ketotifen is widely used around the world.

Ketotifen is a safe drug although frequently associated with drowsiness, particularly in the first 1–2 weeks of treatment, and occasionally with weight gain. Clinical studies with ketotifen were often poorly designed, rendering their interpretation difficult and several studies have shown conflicting results. Most studies have been done in children and have shown only marginal improvement in asthma control.[36] The usual dosage is 1 mg twice daily. One recent placebo-controlled study in adult asthmatics has shown slight improvement in asthma symptom scores, pulmonary function and bronchial responsiveness with reduction in activated eosinophils and T-lymphocytes in the bronchial mucosa with ketotifen 1 mg twice daily.[37]

Two placebo-controlled studies of 1 and 3 years' duration suggested that ketotifen may delay the development of asthma in infants with atopic dermatitis and/or elevated serum IgE and a family history of asthma, who are at high-risk for development of asthma.[38,39] Longer follow-up of these children is needed however, before generalizing the use of ketotifen in this high-risk group.

KEY POINTS

1   The precise mode of action of sodium cromoglycate and nedocromil are still not understood.

2   Sodium cromoglycate and nedocromil are safe drugs and virtually free of systemic side-effects.

3   Sodium cromoglycate and nedocromil can improve asthma control in mild to moderate asthma. They can be used as alternatives to low-dose inhaled corticosteroids where toxicity or fear of toxicity precludes the use of corticosteroids.

4   Sodium cromoglycate is used particularly in children. It should not be added to an established regimen of inhaled or systemic corticosteroids.

5   Both sodium cromoglycate and nedocromil are effective in the prevention of exercise- and allergen-induced asthma.

6   Ketotifen is not recommended for first-line therapy of asthma.

SUMMARY

Among the anti-allergic drugs now available, sodium cromoglycate and nedocromil are the most useful in the treatment of asthma. While they share similar pharmacological activities, nedocromil has a broader sprectum of efficacy both in adults and children, atopic or not, whereas sodium cromoglycate is particularly useful in children, being considered an alternative to low-dose inhaled corticosteroids as first-line prophy-lactic anti-inflammatory treatment. They are particularly effective in the prevention of exercise- or cold air-induced bronchoconstriction and allergen-induced early and late asthmatic reactions. However, for the chronic treatment of asthma, they are less potent than inhaled corticosteroids both in children and adults. Some studies on ketotifen show that this drug may have a place in the treatment of asthma but further well-controlled and well-designed studies are required to clarify this.

REFERENCES

1. Howell JBL, Altounyan REC. A double-blind trial of disodium cromoglycate in the treatment of allergic bronchial asthma. *Lancet* 1976; ii: 539–42.

2. Thomson NC. Asthma. Anti-inflammatory therapies. *Br Med Bull* 1992; 48: 205–220.

3. Hoshino M, Nakamura Y. The effects of inhaled sodium cromoglycate on cellular infiltration into the bronchial mucosa and the expression of adhesion molecules in asthmatics. *Eur Respir J* 1997; 10: 858–65.

4. Norris AA, Holgate ST. Cromolyn sodium and nedocromil sodium. In: Middleton E Jr. (ed). *Allergy: Principles and Practices*, 5th edn. London: Mosby-Year Book, 1998: 661–7.

5. Holgate ST. Inhaled sodium cromoglycate. *Respir Med* 1996; 90: 387–90.

6. König P, Shaffer J. The effect of drug therapy on long-term outcome of childhood asthma: a possible preview of the international guidelines. *J Allergy Clin Immunol* 1996; 98: 1103–1111.

7. ✪ Guidelines on the Management of Asthma. Statement by the British Thoracic Society, the British Paediatric Association, the Research Unit of the Royal College of Physicians of London, the King's Fund Centre, the National Asthma Campaign, the Royal College of General Practitioners, the General Practitioners in Asthma Group, the British Association of Accident and Emergency Medicine, and the British Paediatric Respiratory Group. *Thorax* 1993; 48: S1–24.

8. ✪ Rachelefsky GS, Warner JO. International consensus on the management of pediatric asthma: a summary statement. *Pediatr Pulmonol* 1993; 15: 125–7.

9. International Consensus Report on Diagnosis and Treatment of Asthma. *Clin Exp Allergy* 1992; 22 (suppl. 1): 1–72.

10. Petty TL, Rollins DR, Christopher K, Good JT, Oakley R. Cromolyn sodium is effective in adult chronic asthmatics. *Am Rev Respir Dis* 1989; 139: 694–701.

11. Eigen H, Reid JJ, Dahl R *et al*. Evaluation of the addition of cromolyn sodium to bronchodilator maintenance therapy in the long-term management of asthma. *J Allergy Clin Immunol* 1987; 80: 612–21.

12. ✪ Bar-Yishay E, Gur I, Levy M, Volozni D, Godfrey S. Duration of action of sodium cromoglycate on exercise induced asthma: comparison of 2 formulations. *Arch Dis Child* 1983; 58: 624–7.

13. Tullett WM, Tan KM, Wall RT, Patel KP. Dose–response effect of sodium cromoglycate pressurised aerosol in exercise induced asthma. *Thorax* 1985; 40: 41–4.

14. Latimer KM, O'Byrne PM, Morris MM, Roberts R, Hargreave FE. Bronchoconstriction stimulated by airway cooling. Better protection with combined inhalation of terbutaline sulphate and cromolyn sodium than with either alone. *Am Rev Respir Dis* 1983; 128: 440–43.

15. ✪ Cockcroft DW, Murdock KY. Comparative effects of inhaled salbutamol, sodium cromoglycate, and beclomethasone dipropionate on allergen-induced early asthmatic responses, late asthmatic responses, and increased bronchial responsiveness to histamine. *J Allergy Clin Immunol* 1987; 79: 734–40.

16. Altraja A, Laitinen A, Meriste S *et al*. Effect of regular nedocromil sodium or albuterol on bronchial inflammation in chronic asthma. *J Allergy Clin Immunol* 1996; 98: S58–S64.

17. Brogden RN, Sorkin EM. Nedocromil sodium. An updated review of its pharmacological properties and therapeutic efficacy in asthma. *Drugs* 1993; 45: 693–715.

18. Parish RC, Miller LJ. Nedocromil sodium. *DICP Ann Pharmacother* 1993; 27: 599–606.

19. König P, Hordvik NL, Kreutz C. The preventive effect and duration of action of nedocromil sodium and cromolyn sodium on exercise-induced asthma (EIA) in adults. *J Allergy Clin Immunol* 1987; 79: 64–8.

20. Holgate ST. The efficacy and therapeutic position of nedocromil sodium. *Respir Med* 1996; 90: 391–4.

21. Edwards AM, Stevens MT. The clinical efficacy of inhaled nedocromil sodium (Tilade) in the treatment of asthma. *Eur Respir J* 1993; 6: 35–41.

22. Clancy L, Keogan S. Treatment of nocturnal asthma with nedocromil sodium. *Thorax* 1994; 49: 1225–7.

23. North American Tilade Study Group. A double-blind multicenter group comparative study of the efficacy and safety of nedocromil sodium in the management of asthma. *Chest* 1990; 97: 1299–1306.

24. Rebuck AS, Kesten S, Boulet LP *et al*. A 3-month evaluation of the efficacy of nedocromil sodium in asthma: a randomized, double-blind, placebo-controlled trial of nedocromil sodium conducted by a Canadian multicenter study group. *J Allergy Clin Immunol* 1990; 85: 612–17.

25. Murciano D, Braunstein G, Montagut A, Pariente R. Epargne de la corticothérapie inhalée par le nédocromil sodique dans l'asthme modéré à sévère. Groupe Français d'Etude Tilade. *Rev Mal Respir* 1994; 11: 485–92.

26. Boulet LP, Cartier A, Cockcroft DW *et al*. Tolerance to reduction of oral steroid dosage in severely asthmatic patients receiving nedocromil sodium. *Respir Med* 1990; 84: 317–23.

27. Bone MF, Kubik MM, Keaney NP *et al*. Nedocromil sodium in adults with asthma dependent on inhaled corticosteroids: a double blind, placebo controlled study. *Thorax* 1989; 44: 654–9.

28. ✪ Wong CS, Cooper S, Britton JR, Tattersfield AE. Steroid sparing effect of nedocromil sodium in asthmatic patients on high doses of inhaled steroids. *Clin Exp Allergy* 1993; 23: 370–76.

29. Lal S, Dorow PD, Venho KK, Chatterjee SS. Nedocromil sodium is more effective than cromolyn sodium for the treatment of chronic reversible obstructive airway disease. *Chest* 1993; 104: 438–47.

30. Schwartz HJ, Blumenthal M, Brady R *et al*. A comparative study of the clinical efficacy of nedocromil sodium and placebo. How does cromolyn sodium compare as an active control treatment? *Chest* 1996; 109: 945–52.

31. Boldy DA, Ayres JG. Nedocromil sodium and sodium cromoglycate in patients aged over 50 years with asthma. *Respir Med* 1993; 87: 517–23.

32. Crimi E, Orefice U, De Benedetto F, Grassi V, Brusasco V. Nedocromil sodium versus theophylline in the treatment of reversible obstructive airway disease. *Ann Allergy Asthma Immunol* 1995; 74: 501–508.

33. Bel EH, Timmers MC, Hermans J, Dijkman JH, Sterk PJ. The long-term effects of nedocromil sodium and beclomethasone dipropionate on bronchial responsiveness to methacholine in nonatopic asthmatic subjects. *Am Rev Respir Dis* 1990; 141: 21–8.

34. Armenio L, Baldini G, Bardare M *et al*. Double blind, placebo controlled study of nedocromil sodium in asthma. *Arch Dis Child* 1993; 68: 193–7.

35. Grant SM, Goa KL, Fitton A, Sorkin EM. Ketotifen. A review of its pharmacodynamic and pharmacokinetic properties, and therapeutic use in asthma and allergic disorders. *Drugs* 1990; 40: 412–48.

36. Mylona-Karayanni C, Hadziargurou D, Liapi-Adamidou G, Anagnostakis I, Sinaniotis C, Saxoni-Papageorgiou F. Effect of ketotifen on childhood asthma: a double-blind study. *J Asthma* 1990; 27: 87–93.

37. Hoshino M, Nakamura Y, Shin Z, Fukushima Y. Effects of ketotifen on symptoms and on bronchial mucosa in patients with atopic asthma. *Allergy* 1997; 52: 814–20.

38. Iikura Y, Naspitz CK, Mikawa H. Prevention of asthma by ketotifen in infants with atopic dermatitis. *Ann Allergy* 1992; 68: 233–6.

39. Bustos GJ, Bustos D, Romero O. Prevention of asthma with ketotifen in preasthmatic children: a three-year follow-up study. *Clin Exp Allergy* 1995; 25: 568–73.

Chapter 19

Immunosuppressive Agents

David Evans and Duncan Geddes

INTRODUCTION

The realization that asthma is a disorder characterized by airway inflammation has led to the development of treatment protocols that focus on the use of anti-inflammatory drugs. Specifically inhaled steroids have become central to therapy and there is evidence that supports their use as highly effective agents both in terms of improvements of lung function and symptom control. For disease exacerbations the use of systemic corticosteroids is established and this treatment strategy is also of proven benefit. There are however a small group of asthmatic patients, in the order of 1–2% of sufferers, who despite appropriate inhaled therapy remain dependent on systemic corticosteroids. These individuals consume a disproportionate amount of available resource and are at risk of the longer term side-effects of steroid treatment. This group of individuals has been the subject of considerable research in an effort to find alternative treatments that can be safely used as anti-inflammatory agents either to improve asthma control or to allow systemic steroids to be reduced to a minimum dose. To date the evidence is better for steroid-sparing agents than for asthma control, but both are controversial.

Before considering immunosuppression it is important to re-evaluate a number of issues. The diagnosis needs to be carefully confirmed. Co-existing diagnoses, such as airway tumours or bronchiectasis, should be excluded and appropriately treated. If asthma remains the single diagnosis, the question of appropriate inhaled therapy should be looked at critically and the regimen, including doses and mode of drug delivery to the airway should be optimized. Patient compliance should be confirmed in any individual who remains symptomatic. If despite this approach a patient remains

poorly controlled then it is appropriate to consider systemic corticosteroids and it is this group of individuals who may benefit from a trial of second-line agents.

The combination of second-line agents with systemic steroids in asthma raises interesting problems in the design and method of the trials. It is important to use appropriate outcome measures as an agent may be either efficacious or steroid-sparing but not necessarily both. Under any circumstances all patients with established steroid-dependent asthma should remain on maximal inhaled therapy and be treated with systemic steroids at the lowest possible dose. Therefore the need for steroid dose tapering during the run-in to a trial is essential.

This review will profile the various immunosuppressive agents used as well as outline the results from the key studies reported to date.

METHOTREXATE

Mechanism of Action

Methotrexate has been used for the treatment of malignant diseases for approximately 50 years and more recently for inflammatory diseases of the joints and skin.[1,2] Its mechanism of action in malignant disease is probably via the inhibition of the enzyme dihydrofolate reductase inhibiting nucleic acid synthesis in dividing cells. In inflammatory disease lower doses are thought to work via actions on immune cells. These effects include inhibition of granulocyte chemotaxis as well as blocking histamine release from basophils and inhibiting the actions of IL-1. Indirect evidence suggests this mode of action is unrelated to inhibition of dihydrofolate reductase as the co-administration of folinic acid does not influence its effects in inflammatory diseases. Furthermore at the doses used in the treatment of asthma leucopaenia is rarely observed.[3–5]

203

Clinical Trials

The original observations implying possible benefits of methotrexate were made by Mullarkey. A patient receiving the drug for psoriatic arthropathy showed improvements in asthma control and a reduction in her requirements for corticosteroids. Thereafter a further five patients were reported with improved control or evidence of steroid-sparing benefits from methotrexate.[6] Following on from his own initial observation, Mullarkey reported the effects of methotrexate at doses of 15 mg kg[-1] over a 24-week period in a placebo-controlled cross-over study amongst a group of 14 asthmatics with a mean daily steroid dose of 25 mg. There was a reduction of steroid dose of 36.5% in the active limb compared with placebo with no changes in lung function.[7] However this study did not report doses of inhaled steroids or concomitant asthma treatment. Details of the eight patients who failed to complete the study were not given. Despite these shortfalls the paper suggests a steroid-sparing effect for methotrexate. Subsequently a larger study using a parallel group design has been published. Data from 60 patients were presented and the steroid dependency of the group was confirmed during the run-in period. In fact all the patients had been on a minimum of 7.5 mg of steroid for at least a year prior to the trial. The results showed a significantly greater reduction in the dose of steroid in the methotrexate treated patients (50% versus 14%). In addition, markers of asthma control such as exacerbation rates were fewer in the actively treated group. There were no differences between the groups for measures of lung function.[8]

Three further randomized controlled trials have been published showing steroid reductions in methotrexate treated patients. Dyer studied 12 patients with a mean daily dose of prednisolone of 13 mg and showed a 30% greater reduction in steroid dose compared with placebo over 12-week treatment periods.[9] Stewart reported a significant reduction in steroid dose in the methotrexate treated patients with no change in dose seen during the placebo limb. A total of 21 patients, whose mean daily dose of prednisolone was 24 mg, completed the 9-week treatment phases with a 3-week washout.[10] In a cross-over design, Hedman studied 12 patients with a mean dose of steroid of 10 mg over 12 weeks and found a 38% reduction in steroid dose with no changes seen in the placebo limb.[11]

In contrast there are a number of studies that do not support the use of methotrexate in asthma.

Erzurum failed to show benefits in favour of methotrexate (15 mg per week) over placebo in terms of steroid requirements in a parallel designed trial over 12 weeks amongst 19 asthmatics tapered to a mean level of 20 mg of steroid per day.[12] Clearly the duration of treatment may have been inadequate to allow benefits to emerge given the delayed responses demonstrated by Shiner,[8] although the studies by Dyer and Mullarkey did report responses during similarly brief treatment periods.[7,9]

Studies reported by Taylor and Trigg were negative for steroid-sparing benefits of methotrexate.[13,14] In the first of these the mean daily prednisolone dose for the patients was 16 mg (with no steroid tapering) and in the second 17.5 mg. Both studies were cross-over in design and a possible flaw of them both was lack of adequate washout period between treatment, although the study by Trigg only examined the data from the last 8 weeks of the 12-week treatment period. In favour of the study by Taylor was the duration of treatment at 24 weeks. In the trial by Trigg the dose of methotrexate used was 30 mg per week. Two further studies examining very similar groups of asthmatics with mean daily steroid requirements for prednisolone of 30 mg per day showed no benefit for methotrexate. Coffey studied 11 patients[15] and Kanzow using a parallel group design randomized 21 patients.[16] In this latter trial the reduction in steroid dose was 24% in the active treatment limb compared with 5% in the placebo group. These changes did not reach significance and were not sustained during an 8 week follow-up phase.

An efficacy trial reported by Ogirala looked at the use of methotrexate and triamcinolone compared with placebo amongst a small group of severe asthmatics. This study is difficult to interpret due to its size and failure to taper the steroid doses during run in and showed no benefit for added methotrexate in terms of lung function, airway responsiveness or asthma control.[17]

The possibility that methotrexate may offer benefits when used in the longer term for steroid dependent asthmatics is a further issue that the protagonists for this agent have endeavoured to demonstrate. The questions as to whether a short-term benefit is actually sustained and if there are cumulative later effects over prolonged treatment periods have been the hypotheses of four open trials. In fact the evidence from the earlier steroid sparing trials would suggest that these are not likely added advantages.[8,16] In two of these studies,

Mullarkey and Shiner have published positive effects with 15 out of 31 and 13 of 21 patients respectively weaning from steroids altogether.[18,19] Stanziola recorded mean steroid reductions of 87% in a group of 13 patients, nine of whom discontinued treatment completely, during follow-up for between 54 and 72 weeks.[20] In contrast another trial showed no longer term reductions in steroid doses either during methotrexate treatment over 14 months or during a later 7-month follow-up period.[21] Overall the lack of randomized double-blind placebo-controlled trial evidence makes the results of these studies difficult to interpret.

Only one trial has examined the issue of methotrexate treatment in asthmatic children over any length of time.[22] The remaining reports are either case evidence or open trials of short duration and it is not possible to draw conclusions about steroid-sparing effects, efficacy, or safety.[22-24]

A summary of the trials is shown in Table 19.1.

Adverse Effects

Nausea and abdominal discomfort are common and a consensus from the use of methotrexate in rheumatological disease variously cites these side-effects between 28% and 75% of users.[25] Disordered liver function is frequently observed on treatment and 12 of 60 patients in the study by Shiner showed these abnormalities. Three patients were withdrawn from this study due to abnormalities of liver function although there was no long term damage.[8] No asthma trial has reported liver fibrosis during treatment with methotrexate, although this has occurred during the use of the drug to treat psoriasis and rheumatoid arthritis. Liver biopsy is recommended after a cumulative dose of methotrexate of 1.5 g. Co-morbid conditions such as diabetes, obesity, and alcoholism are all relative contra-indications to the use of the drug as these conditions have been shown to increase the likelihood of liver complications.[26] Mild impairment of renal function, macrocytosis and hypogammaglobulinaemia are recognized on treatment. Interestingly there is at least one report of methotrexate actually precipitating asthma.[27]

Of particular significance is the evidence documenting the phenomenon of drug-induced pneumonitis with methotrexate. Usually this is reversible on stopping methotrexate, although there are reports of an insidious and progressive pneumonitis despite recognition and discontinuation of the drug.[29] Careful monitoring of both the chest X-ray and lung function is required when using this agent for whatever underlying condition.

Methotrexate via its immunosuppressive effect is responsible for increases in infections including *Pneumocystis carinii* pneumonia[30-32] and reactivation of latent herpetic infection.[33]

Methotrexate is teratogenic and should be avoided in pregnancy and in individuals not using adequate contraception. Sulphonamides, non-steroidal anti-inflammatory drugs and diuretics should be avoided in patients taking methotrexate.[34]

Conclusion

The various trials do not support the routine use of methotrexate in the treatment of asthma. There is a meta-analysis showing marginal benefit for the drug in parallel group studies but no overall conclusive benefit.[35] The effect of trial design on the results of this systematic review endorses the possibility of carry-over effects in favour of placebo in the cross-over studies and this should be borne in mind when interpreting studies of this sort. In those instances when methotrexate is used careful monitoring of liver and lung function should be done.

CYCLOSPORIN

Mechanism of Action

Cyclosporin (cyclosporine) is a cyclic undecapeptide metabolite extracted from the fungus *Tolypocladium inflatum*. It is used in the prevention of allograft rejection and has been found to be effective in the treatment of a variety of inflammatory disorders such as rheumatoid arthritis,[36] psoriasis,[37] lichen planus,[38] and nephrotic syndrome.[39]

Its mechanism of action occurs via diffusion into immune cells and inhibition of cell signalling and post-translational protein folding. Cyclosporin binds to cytosolic proteins, for example cyclophilin, whose roles include the regulation of activity of enzymes such as protein kinases and phospholipase A_2.[40] The drug also binds transcription factors involved in inflammatory responses inclusive of activator protein-3 (AP_3),[41] and nuclear factor κB (NFκB).[42] Furthermore cyclosporin inhibits IL-1 via receptor antagonism.[43] As a result of these actions cyclosporin has been shown to inhibit mast cell and basophil secretion of leukotrienes, platelet activating factor (PAF) and histamine,[44] lymphocyte synthesis of cytokines,[45] B-cell synthesis of IgE,[46]

Table 19.1: Placebo-controlled trials for methotrexate

Author	Year	Study design	Patients	Treatment duration	Baseline steroid dose per day	Steroid reduction on methotrexate	Efficacy/other outcomes
Mullarkey[7]	1988	Cross-over	14	12 weeks	25 mg	36.5% greater than placebo	–
Shiner*[8]	1990	Parallel	60	24 weeks	Approx 15 mg	MTX 50%, placebo 14%	Less exacerbations on MTX ($P < 0.05$)
Dyer*[9]	1991	Cross-over	10	12 weeks	8–12 mg	30% greater than placebo	–
Erzurum*[12]	1991	Parallel	18	13 weeks	20 mg	40% reduction for both MTX and placebo	Increases in eosinophil counts
Trigg[14]	1993	Cross-over	12	12 weeks	Median 17.5 mg	No difference between MTX and placebo	Small improvements FEV$_1$ favouring MTX ($P < 0.05$)
Taylor[13]	1993	Cross-over	9	24 weeks	16 mg	16% MTX, 30% placebo (NS)	–
Stewart[10]	1994	Cross-over	21	9 weeks	23 mg	14% reduction in MTX, no change placebo	–
Hedman[11]	1996	Cross-over	12	12 weeks	10 mg	38% reduction on MTX ($P < 0.05$)	Significant improvements in symptoms and β agonists
Coffey*[15]	1994	Cross-over	11	12 weeks	30 mg	20% reduction both MTX and placebo	–
Kanzow*[16]	1995	Parallel	21	16 weeks	Approx 30 mg	24% MTX, 5% placebo (NS)	–

MTX: methotrexate; FEV$_1$: forced expiratory volume in 1 s.
* Steroid tapering during run-in. Six uncontrolled trials[18,19,20,21,23,24] are not detailed above.

eosinophil activation,[47] and macrophage respiratory burst responses.[48]

Cyclosporin is well-tolerated via oral administration and is given in doses in the order of 3 and 7.5 mg kg^{-1}.

Drug monitoring of levels is required and therapeutic ranges lie between 80–150 ng ml^{-1} giving optimum immunomodulatory effects and minimal side-effects.

Clinical Trials

The first cyclosporin trial published was designed to look at possible efficacy in asthma. Alexander randomized 30 patients with a mean daily steroid requirement of 8.5 mg to 12 weeks of treatment in a placebo-controlled cross-over study. The mean cyclosporin level for the active treatment periods was 152 ng ml^{-1}. The results showed significant improvements over placebo in terms of PEF and PEF variability but no differences for symptom scores or rescue medication use. Interestingly a run out period for 11 weeks showed sustained improvements in favour of cyclosporin over placebo for mean morning PEF.[49]

Subsequently, Nizankowska investigated the steroid-sparing qualities and efficacy of cyclosporin. Thirty-two steroid-dependent patients (failed steroid tapers over the previous 6 months – mean daily steroid dose 16 mg) were randomized to receive cyclosporin or placebo in a parallel group study. Initially during the efficacy limb there were improvements in symptoms and rescue medication use in the actively treated patients, but no differences for measures of lung function. A subsequent steroid-sparing phase over 22 weeks showed no benefits for the cyclosporin-treated patients. The mean cyclosporin level in this study was 120 ng ml^{-1}.[50]

Lock treated 39 steroid-dependent asthmatics (mean daily steroid dose 12 mg) in a parallel group trial for 36 weeks. Previous attempts to taper steroids had failed. There were significant reductions in steroid dose within the cyclosporin-treated group although no significant difference between cyclosporin and placebo steroid doses at the end of the treatment period. There was however a significant benefit in favour of cyclosporin over placebo for the lowest dose of steroid during the trial period. In addition there were significant improvements in PEF for the actively treated patients although no other changes for any other measure of lung function or marker of asthma control. The mean cyclosporin level was 144 ng ml^{-1}.[51]

Two other open studies have shown reductions in steroid doses over 3 and 9 months respectively.[52,53] Neither were placebo-controlled studies – in the former there were six non-responders and in the latter there were only data from seven individuals. The cyclosporin levels from each were 105 ng/ml^{-1} and 77 ng/ml^{-1}.

A summary of the trials is shown in Table 19.2.

Adverse Effects

Cyclosporin causes increases in blood pressure and impairment of renal function. Blood pressure was sig-nificantly higher in the actively treated patients in the studies reported by Alexander and Lock.[49,51] Further there was evidence of worsening renal function in both these studies and in the latter the GFR remained decreased during the run out phase indicating lasting damage.[51]

Other adverse effects include hypertrichosis, increased susceptibility to infection, elevation of liver enzymes, neuropathy and gastrointestinal disturbances. The development of inhaled cyclosporin remains a possibility and this would be a potentially safer treatment option.

Conclusion

At best cyclosporin should be reserved for a specific sub-group of patients. Its use should be supervised by experienced physicians and careful monitoring is required.

GOLD

Mechanism of Action

Gold sodium thiomalate, gold thioglucose and aura-nofin are the formulations of gold that are available for use. The latter is a synthetic compound that is lipid soluble and can therefore be administered by mouth unlike the other two parenteral agents. Due to pharmacokinetic differences significantly lower cumulative doses of auranofin are necessary to obtain the same clinical effect compared with parenteral gold therapy. This is clearly an advantage given the cumulative toxicity data that is established for gold therapy.[54]

The mechanism of action for gold salts is not well-understood, and interestingly auranofin probably works in a different way to the parenteral compounds.[55] The putative mechanisms of action for gold are shown on Table 19.3.

Gold is prescribed at a dose of 25–50 mg a week and given by mouth or intramuscular injection.

Clinical Trials

Elemental gold has been used in the treatment of disease for hundreds of years although its use as an anti-inflammatory agent was not appreciated until 1929.[56] The use of gold in the treatment of arthritic conditions is proven following from a number of clinical trials. Interest in its use in the treatment of asthma goes back 50 years,[57–59] and subsequently much of the research interest has arisen from countries such as

Table 19.2: Placebo-controlled trials for cyclosporin A

Author	Year	Study design	Patients	Cyclosporin level (ng ml^{-1})	Treatment duration	Baseline steroid dose per day	Steroid reduction on CsA	Efficacy/other outcomes
Alexander[49]	1992	Cross-over	30	152	12 weeks	8.5 mg	Not documented	Significant improvements for PEFR, FEV$_1$ and exacerbations
Nizankowska*[50]	1995	Parallel	32	120	34 weeks (2 phases; 12 weeks efficacy, 22 weeks steroid reduction)	16 mg	Similar reductions in placebo and CsA groups	No benefit for lung function during efficacy phase, significant improvements in β agonist use and symptoms in favour of CsA
Lock*[51]	1996	Parallel	39	144	36 weeks	12 mg	25% greater reduction in median steroid dose on CsA compared with placebo	Mean PEFR a.m. and p.m. improved with CsA (P < 0.05). No increases in FEV$_1$ or symptom scores compared with placebo

CsA: Cyclosporin A; FEV$_1$: forced expiratory volume in 1s; PEFR: Peak expiratory flow rate. *Steroid tapering. Uncontrolled trials[52,53] are not detailed.

Japan.[60–62] All these trials were uncontrolled and examined the use of parenteral gold. Despite this, these data showed that reductions in steroid dose and improvements in lung function were possible.

As there are probably important differences in the mechanism of action for the various gold preparations notwithstanding differences in route of administration, it is difficult to comment on either steroid-sparing qualities or efficacy from the pooled trial data. Nevertheless for the purpose of this review all the studies for gold will be considered together.

The first study was a parallel group design in 64 steroid-dependent asthmatics with a daily requirement for steroids of 5 mg. No tapering of steroid dose was done during the run-in period. The data were derived from a physician's evaluation of progress and a patient questionnaire. In this way the authors reported a significant improvement in asthma control on parenteral gold.[63]

Another open pilot studied the effects of auranofin over 24 weeks in 24 asthmatics maintained on 15 mg prednisolone daily. There were significant reductions in *ex vivo* IgE-mediated immune responses, but no improvements in asthma control.[64]

Subsequently a number of randomized placebo-controlled trials have been published[64–68] – the first used parenteral gold,[67] and the remainder focusing on auranofin. All used tapering of steroids during run-in.

Table 19.3: Mechanisms of action of gold

Mechanism	Parenteral gold	Auranofin
Inhibition of lymphocyte responses to mitogen	✓	✓
Inhibition of prostaglandin synthesis	✓	
Inhibition of lysozymes	✓	✓
Inhibition of mast cell/basophil mediator release		✓
Inhibition of chemotaxis		✓
Inhibition of antibody synthesis		✓
Inhibition of IL-1 and IL-2 release		✓
Inhibition of allergen-induced contraction of guinea pig trachea		✓

Parenteral gold: gold sodium thiomalate, gold thioglucose.

Whilst these trials demonstrated a steroid-sparing effect of gold (with the exception of the study by Honma which instead achieved its goal of showing a bronchoprotective effect of gold against laboratory airway challenge), they are a diverse group of trials in as much as the severity of the various study groups is too wide to draw a unifying conclusion. In one study only half the patients were receiving inhaled steroids (the other half completely steroid naive),[65] in another the patients were dependent on 7–9 mg of steroid,[66] and in the others the groups were maintained on 25 mg of steroid daily.[67,68]

One open trial showed no benefit of gold over 7–17 months in aspirin-sensitive asthmatic patients.[69] A summary of the trials is shown in Table 19.4.

Adverse Effects
Impairment in renal function is a problem with gold therapy, particularly following longer term treatment. In the studies reported, two patients developed nephrotic syndrome in one trial,[65] and another three patients had lesser degrees of proteinuria that was unsustained following discontinuation of treatment.[61] Bernstein identified gold as the cause of intestinal perforation in two patients and haemorrhage in two others.[64] More usually gold is responsible for milder non-specific gastrointestinal upset. Dermatological problems are documented with gold and eczema, either *de novo* or worsening of pre-existing disease, is the usual manifestation. One patient was withdrawn from a study for this reason.[64] Blood dyscrasias, abnormalities of liver enzymes and pulmonary infiltrates are described during gold treatment.

Conclusion
The data do support a steroid-sparing effect for gold, although the study groups are varied. Gold should be used only for severe asthmatic patients dependent on oral steroids in keeping with published guidelines. The experience with rheumatological disease is that treatment has to be stopped after a period due to side-effects which limits the use of this agent. As some of these side-effects are potentially serious, the likelihood of gold becoming an established treatment for asthma is low.

IMMUNOGLOBULIN

Mechanism of Action
Intravenous immunoglobulin (IVIG) probably has a variety of immunomodulatory roles. Clearly it may be of indirect benefit in the treatment of asthma in those individuals with pre-existing immunoglobulin deficiency by preventing infection. In immunocompetent patients possible effects are more complex. Although interference with the Fc gamma receptor-mediated clearance of IgG-coated particles may be relevant in immune-mediated thrombocytopaenia, this mechanism is unlikely to be important in asthma. Possible alternatives include blockage of IgE-mediated responses and inhibition of B-cell differentiation into antibody secreting cells.[70]

Clinical Trials
The interest in IVIG in the treatment of asthma arose following the realization that asthma was an inflammatory disorder and that IVIG was useful in other inflammatory conditions such as immune thrombocytopaenia and polyneuropathy.

Table 19.4: Clinical trials for gold

Author	Agent	Study design	Patients	Duration	Baseline steroid dose per day	Steroid reduction on gold	Efficacy/other outcomes
Muranaka[63]	Parenteral gold	DBPCT	64	30 weeks	Approx 5 mg	Not documented	Physician's assessment favoured gold ($P < 0.05$)
Bernstein[64]	Auranofin	Open	20	24 weeks	15 mg	34% (NS)	Half doubling dose reduction in PC_{20} (NS) Reduced ex vivo IgE stimulated mediator release ($P < 0.05$)
Honma[65]	Auranofin	DBPCT	25	12 weeks	Inhaled/nil		Reduction PC_{20} auranofin vs placebo
Nierop[66]	Auranofin	DBPCT	28	26 weeks	7–9 mg	33% Auranofin vs 0% placebo	Improved exacerbation rates and FEV_1 ($P <0.05$)
Klaustermeyer[67]	Parenteral gold	DBPCT	8	22 weeks	Approx 23 mg	5/8 patients significantly decreased steroid	
Bernstein[68]	Auranofin	DBPCT	157	8 months	66% 15–20, 35% < 20 mg	60% auranofin vs 32% placebo achieved more than 50% reduction ($P <0.05$)	Mean serum IgE reduced on auranofin ($P < 0.05$), no change lung function cf. placebo
McNeill[69]	Auranofin	Open	9	7–17 months	30–40 mg	Approx 50% reduction	Non-significant improvements in lung function

DBPCT: double-blind placebo-controlled trial; FEV_1: forced expiratory volume in 1 s; PC_{20}: provocative concentration of agonist causing a 20% fall in FEV_1.

Trials of IVIG date back over 30 years and initially targeted episodes of infection often in patients with immunoglobulin deficiency.[71] There are problems in drawing conclusions from the trial data for IVIG because there is a shortage of adult studies and too few of the reported studies have avoided the infection issue. Furthermore the doses of IVIG are too variable to make useful comparisons between results. Finally the design of trials is variable with a lack of data from blinded or placebo-controlled trials.

After initial data showing control of sinopulmonary infection with IVIG, Abernathy evaluated 22 asthmatic children using a double-blind placebo-controlled design. This study found no evidence in favour of IVIG in terms of lung function, symptoms, exacerbations, or indeed infection rates.[72] In contrast an open study by Brown did show improvements in 23 of 29 asthmatics.[73] Both trials used low dose of IVIG–30 mg kg^{-1}. Soon after these studies Fontana published data from a double-blind placebo-controlled study in 41 immunocompetent asthmatics characterized by frequent exacerbations caused by infections. This paper concluded no benefit from the use of IVIG.[74]

Page presented clinical improvements in five asthmatic children with sub-class deficiencies[71] and Smith likewise in a group of 50 asthmatics with chronic infections.[75] Interestingly both these studies showed benefits in asthma control without showing any features suggestive of improvements in terms of infection. As with the other earlier trials neither of these studies examined the issue of steroid-sparing properties.

Mazer has evaluated IVIG in terms of possible steroid-sparing effects in a group of asthmatic children with no evidence of immunodeficiency or active infection. This study was an open trial with only eight subjects. However the trial design was appropriate and employed a 3-month tapering phase during run-in. Despite this the mean daily steroid dose was 32.5 mg. The treatment period was 6 months and the dose of IVIG was 2 g kg^{-1}. The results show a three-fold reduction in maintenance steroid dose and a reduction in the doses of steroids required during exacerbation. Furthermore there were improvements in measures of lung function and reductions in skin prick responses in parallel with significant falls in the levels of IgE. No changes in airway responsiveness were seen.[76] A similar study using five monthly doses of 800 mg kg^{-1} IVIG amongst a group of asthmatics requiring only inhaled steroid at a dose of 720 µg per day was reported by Jakobsson.[77] This study showed significant reductions in steroid requirements compared with placebo, but no changes from control in terms of rescue medication consumption.

Adverse Effects

Apart from frequently reported headaches which are usually mild and self-limiting (although there is one anecdotal report of aseptic meningitis[78]), IVIG is well-tolerated. The other rare adverse event associated with this treatment is allergic reactions and anaphylaxis.

Conclusions

The evidence for a steroid-sparing benefit of IVIG is mixed and there is no convincing data to support a role for efficacy. As IVIG is expensive and requires visits to the clinic for i.v. administration, its use in the treatment of asthma cannot be recommended. Carefully designed controlled trials in adult patients are required to conclusively evaluate this treatment further.

TROLEANDOMYCIN

Mechanism of Action

Troleandomycin (TAO) is a macrolide antibiotic with established benefits in the treatment of infections. A possible role in the treatment of asthma arises from its inhibition of the metabolism of methylprednisolone, hence increasing the effective dose of the steroid. If this is the case then strictly speaking it does not qualify as a second-line agent. Studies in both humans and animals support this mode of action and this effect seems to be specific to methylprednisolone.[79,80] There is some *in vitro* work showing a direct effect on immune mechanisms[81–84] although the consensus is that its effects relate to steroid clearance rather than direct immunomodulatory actions.

Clinical Trials

In 1957 Celmer prepared triacetyloleandomycin, a derivative of oleandomycin.[85] This drug was shown to have superior antibiotic effects compared with its parent drug and was adopted in the treatment of Gram-positive infections. As a result of this work it became clear that asthmatics treated with TAO responded better than expected when compared with those treated with other antibiotics.[86,87] Trials by Itkin[88] and Spector[89] in the 1960s and early 1970s showed benefits in favour of TAO and thereafter a number of other studies have been reported showing steroid-sparing effects of TAO, the results of which are shown in Table 19.5. Initial inspection would suggest an impressive effect for TAO, but the studies are flawed by the absence of placebo limbs and no attempts are made to show a specific anti-inflammatory mechanism. In addition to many of the

Table 19.5: Clinical trials for troleandomycin

Reference	Year	Patients	Design	Duration	Steroid-sparing	Efficacy	Steroid side-effects	TAO side-effects
Itkin[88]	1970	12 Adults	DBPCT	8 weeks	Not examined	↑FEV$_1$ by 22% (placebo↑ 7.4%)	X	✓
Spector[89]	1974	74 Adults	DBPCT	4–8 weeks	67% pts dose ↓ by <50%	↑FEV$_1$ by 0.42 l, (placebo↑ 0.16 l)	✓	✓
Zieger*[90]	1980	16 Adults	Open	4–18 months	MP 29 mg o.d. to 11 mg alt days	↑FEV$_1$ by 39%	✓	✓
Eitches*[91]	1985	11 Children	Open	12–38 months	MP 21.5 mg o.d. to 3.4 mg o.d.	↑FEV$_1$ by 81%	✓	✓
Wald*[92]	1985	15 Adults	Open	12 months	MP 38.9 mg o.d. to 12.6 mg o.d.	↑FEV$_1$ 1.76 to 2.18 l at 3 weeks	X	✓
Ball*[93]	1990	15 Children (3 groups of 5)	DBPCT	2 weeks	50% reduction with MP, pred and placebo	↑FEV$_1$ (% predicted) 73% to 88%; placebo 83% to 91%)	X	✓
Menz[94]	1990	16	Open	4–21 months	Yes, ?degree	11 responders arbitrarily defined	?	✓
Kamada*[95]	1993	18 Children (3 groups of 6)	DBPCT	12 weeks	Reductions, TAO/MP 80%, MP 44%	FEV$_1$ (% predicted) 80% to 75% i.e. worse (NS)	✓	✓
Flotte*[96]	1991	9 Children	Open	4–34 months	MP 15 mg o.d. to 1.4 mg o.d.	X	✓	X
Nelson[97]	1993	75 Adults	DBPCT	2 years	Significant and similar reductions in TAO and placebo	Not examined	✓	X
Siracusa*[98]	1993	14 Adults	Open	14 months	MP dose reduction by 20%	↑FEV$_1$ (% predicted) 60% to 68% (NS)	X	✓

TAO: troleandomycin; DBPCT: double-blind placebo-controlled trial; FEV$_1$: forced expiratory volume in 1 s; MP: methylprednisolone. *Studies with pre-treatment steroid tapering.

other studies discussed already looking at second-line agents in asthma, the trials of TAO are limited by the lack of steroid tapering and the failure to examine for either steroid-sparing effects or measures of efficacy. Furthermore these trials have a number of arbitrary end-points, for example infection and sputum production, and employ short treatment periods often examining too few patients. The studies are a mixture of adult and children asthmatic populations. Only two of the placebo-controlled trials had adequate numbers of patients.[89,97] Unfortunately even these two trials can be criticized as Nelson did not distinguish between efficacy and steroid-sparing properties,[97] and Spector did not randomize treatment sequence.[89]

However, there are two pieces of evidence that might argue in favour of TAO as a steroid-sparing agent. Rosenburg has reported a case study of an asthmatic whose condition improved whilst not taking any systemic glucocorticoid. However the patient remained on inhaled flunisolide and there may be evidence showing inhibitory effects of TAO on this steroid preparation.[99] Secondly there are protagonists of TAO who suggest that the effects on asthma control are in excess of those expected from the relative increase in methylprednisolone levels. This has to be countered by the observation that many patients, despite tapering the dose of steroid, develop Cushingoid side-effects on TAO. Furthermore there appear to be no benefits for those patients who take TAO in parallel with other systemic steroid preparations.

Adverse Effects

Almost without exception patients who take TAO develop steroid-related side-effects when using methylprednisolone. Similar to other macrolide antibiotics, TAO is associated with derangement of liver function and gastrointestinal upset. TAO inhibits the clearance of theophyllines and care should be taken when these drugs are administered together.

Conclusion

The explanation for the improvements seen with TAO are probably secondary to augmented steroid-related effects. Other possible benefits for asthma control may also arise through effects on increased theophylline levels. There are no data to support TAO as having an independent steroid-sparing effect in the treatment of asthma.

ANTI-MALARIALS

Mechanism of action

Chloroquine and hydroxychloroquine have been used in the treatment of asthma. Both these drugs cause inhibition of the enzyme phospholipase A_2. As a consequence of this there is a block in the generation of mediators such as leukotrienes and prostaglandins from membrane phospholipid in inflammatory cells.[100]

Clinical Trials

Following the observed benefits of anti-malarials in the treatment of connective tissue diseases there arose anecdotal evidence from case studies and pilot trials that these drugs may also be of use in the treatment of asthma. These initial data, dating back over 30 years, suggest response rates in the order of 75%.[101,102] Subsequent authors, although reporting results from open-label trials, endorsed the possibility of anti-malarials being effective asthma treatment.[103,104] Tennebaum showed delayed but sustained improvements in asthma control in four subjects treated for 10 weeks, three of whom stopped steroids altogether over the following 6 months.[104]

Thereafter there have three further published studies looking at the effects of anti-malarials in the treatment of asthma. In the first of these Roberts studied nine asthmatics treated for 2 months with hydroxychloroquine 400 mg per day using a double-blinded placebo-controlled cross-over design. The mean steroid requirement of the subjects at baseline was 11.6 mg per day. There were no changes in steroid dose nor improvements in lung function following either treatment limb and the authors concluded that there was no evidence to support the use of hydroxychloroquine in the treatment of asthma.[105]

In contrast, Charous has published two open trials showing improvements in steroid requirements and asthma control. The first of these demonstrated a 15% increase in measures of lung function amongst 11 asthmatics treated over 28 weeks. Seven patients who were steroid-dependent reduced their mean monthly steroid dose from 383 mg to 191 mg. Interestingly the authors also reported a significant reduction in the levels of IgE.[106] The second trial showed sustained improvements in 10 patients for both steroid doses and asthma control over a study period of 22 months.[107]

Adverse Effects

The serious adverse effect of chloroquine relates to its ocular toxicity. The retinopathy caused by chloroquine may be irreversible. Fortunately at the doses of the drug used it is a rare event. However regular formal opthalmological assessments should be made whilst on treatment. The drug should be avoided in epileptic patients, and can cause impairment of liver and renal function. Non-specific gastrointestinal upset is not uncommon and some individuals develop a rash on treatment that is usually well-tolerated and self-limiting. In fact neither Roberts nor Charous reported any untoward effects of the drug in their respective studies.[105–107]

Conclusion

The only data showing benefit of anti-malarials in asthma is derived from open trials. The only blinded placebo-controlled trial, albeit with small numbers of patients, was conclusively negative. At the present there is no evidence to support the use of this class of drug. Further properly controlled studies with adequate numbers of subjects are required. In any event the use of anti-malarials should be accompanied by careful monitoring for adverse effects with specific attention to the possibility of retinopathy.

AZATHIOPRINE

Mechanism of Action

As with the other classes of second-line agents, antimetabolites such as azathioprine have been used in the treatment of various inflammatory disorders for many years. Initially 6-mercaptopurine was used although azathioprine has replaced this drug as a less toxic derivative. Both agents are incorporated into DNA and prevent cell division. The mechanism by which this results in immunosuppression is not understood; however the evidence from the use of these agents in recipients of donor organs does support this conclusion.

Clinical Trials

Interest in the use of these agents evolved from case reports with azathioprine[108] and the previous data with anti-metabolites and alkylating agents in asthma.[109] There are four published trials,[110–113] three of which are placebo-controlled. Unfortunately there are flaws in the design of all of these trials such as lack of washout,[111,112] non-randomization of sequence,[110] and no efforts to taper steroid doses during run-in. Only

one of these trials included subjects all of whom were steroid-dependent.[110] The number of subjects in these trials was small ranging (from four to 13) and the treatment periods were short with the exception of the 12-week open trial reported by Asmundssen.[113] Notwithstanding these observations all of these trials were negative, showing no benefits in favour of the use of azathioprine either in terms of efficacy or steroid-sparing effects. Hodges did identify a sub-group of patients who expectorated large volumes of sputum showing some improvement although no mechanism for this effect has been identified.[112] A summary of the trials is shown in Table 19.6.

Adverse Effects

Azathioprine causes bone marrow suppression and increases susceptibility to infections. Occasional hepatotoxicity occurs. Amongst the trials there were a number of patients who had episodes of gastrointestinal upset and one patient was withdrawn due to this problem.[110]

Conclusion

There is no evidence to recommend the use of azathioprine in the treatment of asthma.

COLCHICINE

Mechanism of Action

Colchicine is central to the treatment of gout. Its mechanism of action is poorly understood and probably multi-factorial and complex. Both *in vitro* and *in vivo* colchicine has been shown to correct the deficiency of concanavalin A-induced supressor cell effect seen in patients with familial Mediterranean fever and primary biliary cirrhosis.[114] As colchicine is an effective treatment for these conditions it has been postulated that this might be the mechanism of its anti-inflammatory effect. The discovery that some patients with asthma also have a deficiency of concanavalin-A suppressor cell function has led investigators to examine the use of colchicine in the treatment of asthma.[115] Interestingly theophylline corrects this deficiency and the effects of colchicine and theophylline are additive with respect to the correction of concanavalin A-induced suppressor cell function. The exact pathway through which colchicine exerts this effect is unknown.

Colchicine inhibits the neutrophil[116] and blocks the release of IL-1 from the lymphocyte.[117] Intracellular

Table 19.6: Clinical trials for azathioprine

Author	Year	Study design	Patients	Duration	Baseline steroid dose per day	Steroid reduction on azathioprine	Efficacy/other outcomes
Kaiser[110]	1966	SBPCT	3	16 weeks	All on steroid, dose not disclosed	No effect	No improvement lung function or symptoms
Arkins[111]	1966	DBPCT	10	3 weeks	Not all receiving steroid, details not disclosed	No effect	No effect on lung function. Non-significant improvement in symptoms in both groups
Hodges[112]	1971	DBPCT	20	7 weeks	Three patients not taking steroid, mean dose of remainder 12 mg	Not evaluated	Two patients with productive cough showed marked improvement. No change lung function
Asmundssen[113]	1971	Open	11	12 weeks	Only six had previously taken steroids. Doses not disclosed	Prednisolone reduced in three patients	Five patients characterized by short duration of asthma improved

SBPCT: single-blind placebo-controlled trial; DBPCT: double-blind placebo-controlled trial.

levels of c-AMP are increased following colchicine treatment.[118] These effects may be a consequence of the binding of the drug to microtubules within the cell.

Clinical Trials

There are four trials looking at the use of colchicine in the treatment of asthma and only one of these looked at possible steroid-sparing qualities. Schwartz reported improvements in symptom scores and use of rescue medication, but did not demonstrate any benefits in terms of lung function. All patients in this study were steroid-naïve.[119] A further trial in 30 children in which all were medicated with theophylline and only nine were on inhaled steroids (none were on oral steroids) showed no improvements in lung function but in parallel with the study by Schwartz did find benefits in symptom scores and β agonist consumption.[120] Newman showed no effects for colchicine in a group of asthmatics taking inhaled steroids over 4 months.[121]

In the fourth trial, Fish has reported the effects of colchicine amongst a group of 71 asthmatics on inhaled steroids. This placebo-controlled study used treatment failure as an end-point following the reduction and discontinuation of the inhaled steroid. The results showed similar failure rates amongst both treatment groups and concluded that colchicine was no better than placebo in the protection against treatment failure in asthma.[122]

Adverse Effects

Colchicine appears to be safe. Diarrhoea is however common. There are sporadic reports of neuropathy and myopathy and these are the only severe adverse effects of this treatment.

Conclusion

There are few trials evaluating colchicine although the data available suggest that it has no added advantage in asthma.

DAPSONE

Mechanism of action

Dapsone (4,4'-diaminodiphenyl sulphone) is established in the treatment of leprosy and rheumatological conditions. The basis for the trial of dapsone in asthma arises from the assumption that the neutrophil may be an important cell type in the generation of asthmatic inflammation. The evidence to support this is limited despite the data from allergen challenge studies in both humans[123,124] and animals.[125] Dapsone inhibits neutrophil respiratory burst[126] and chemotaxis.[127] If the neutrophil were relevant these effects might result in limitation to the tissue injury during the development of airway inflammation.

Clinical trials

Berlow studied 10 patients in an open trial for between 3 and 20 months.[128] The dose of dapsone was 100 mg twice a day. The mean monthly dose of prednisolone was reduced from 428 mg to 82 mg. Five of the patients were able to discontinue steroids altogether. There was no steroid-tapering phase and the group was heterogenous in as much as the ranges of steroid dose varied from 5 mg to 60 mg daily. Furthermore three patients were withdrawn during the study and their data were not included in the analysis.

Adverse effects

Complications of dapsone include haemolytic anaemia (contraindicated in glucose-6-phosphate dehydrogenase deficiency), methaemoglobinaemia, agranulocytosis, gastrointestinal upset, hepatitis, neuropsychiatric reactions, and skin rashes.

Conclusion

The only study published for dapsone shows reductions for steroids; however the evidence in favour for it is outweighed by the potentially toxic adverse effects. Further larger controlled trials are required.

SUMMARY

There is no conclusive evidence in favour of any second-line agent in the routine treatment of asthma. The outcomes of the trials to date give a guide to the appropriate design of further studies with respect to either steroid-sparing effects or markers of efficacy. Meticulous attention to methodology will allow more confident conclusions to be drawn. The onus should be placed on demonstrating evidence in favour of these drugs given their potential side-effects. For the time

KEY POINTS

1 Before considering the use of second-line agents in the treatment of asthma, it is important to confirm the diagnosis and steroid-dependency of asthmatics who remain poorly controlled, establish maximal inhaled therapy and consider issues such as compliance and inhaler technique.

2 Of all the second-line agents, methotrexate has been studied more than any other in the treatment of asthma. There is no conclusive evidence to support its use.

3 The data are limited although there is some evidence for the use of cyclosporin in terms of efficacy. Increases in blood pressure and impairment of renal function are potentially serious side-effects and careful monitoring of drug levels is required.

4 There is some evidence for a steroid-sparing effect for gold. Serious side-effects include impairment of renal function and proteinuria can occur. Use of this agent is limited by the restriction to the duration of its use due to cumulative side-effects.

5 There is no evidence of benefit of immunoglobulin therapy except in the treatment of asthma associated with infection or immunosuppression.

6 The available evidence shows no use for anti-malarials, azathioprine or colchicine in the treatment of asthma.

7 Trial design is crucial to the appropriate evaluation of add-on immunosuppression.

8 The use of immunosuppressive drugs in asthma should be carefully monitored by physicians experienced in their use.

being the use of these agents should be limited to controlled trials and occasional well-monitored therapeutic trials in selected patients. These agents should only be used by experienced specialist physicians.

REFERENCES

1. Gubner R, August S, Ginsberg V. Therapeutic suppression of tissue reactivity. II. Effect of aminopterin in rheumatoid arthritis and psoriasis. *Am J Med Sci* 1951; 221: 176–82.

2. Weinblatt ME, Coblyn JS, Fox DA, Fraser PA. Efficacy of low dose methotrexate in rheumatoid arthritis. *New Engl J Med* 1985; 312: 818–22.

3. O'Callaghan JW, Forrest MJ, Brooks PM. Inhibition of neutrophil chemotaxis in methotrexate treated rheumatoid arthritis patients. *Rheumatol Int* 1988; 8: 41–5.

4. Segal R, Mozes E, Yaron M, Tartakovsky B. The effects of methotrexate on the production and activity of interleukin-1. *Arthritis Rheum* 1989; 32: 370–77.

5. Nolte H, Skov PS. Inhibition of basophil histamine release by methotrexate. *Actions Agents* 1988; 23: 173–6.

6. Mullarkey MF, Webb R, Pardee NE. Methotrexate in the treatment of steroid-dependent asthma. *Ann Allergy* 1986; 65: 347–50.

7. ✪ Mullarkey MF, Blumenstein BA, Andrade WP, Bailey GA, Olason I, Wetzel CE. Methotrexate in the treatment of steroid-dependent asthma. A double blind crossover study. *New Engl J Med* 1988; 318: 603–7.

8. ✪ Shiner RJ, Nunn AJ, Chung KF, Geddes DM. Randomised, double-blind placebo-controlled trial of methotrexate in steroid-dependent asthma. *Lancet* 1990; 336: 137–40.

9. Dyer PD, Vaughan TR, Weber RW. Methotrexate in the treatment of steroid-dependent asthma. *J Allergy Clin Immunol* 1991; 88: 208–12.

10. Stewart GE, Diaz JD, Lockey RF, Seleznick MJ, Trudeau WL, Ledford DK. Comparison of oral pulse methotrexate with placebo in the treatment of severe corticosteroid-dependent asthma. *J Allergy Clin Immunol* 1994; 94: 482–9.

11. Hedman J, Seideman P, Albertioni F, Stenius-Aarniala B. Controlled trial of methotrexate in patients with severe chronic asthma. *Eur J Clin Pharm* 1996; 49: 347–9.

12. Erzurum SC, Leff JA, Cochran JE, Ackerson LM, Szefler SJ, Martin RJ, Cott GR. Lack of benefit of methotrexate in severe, steroid-dependent asthma. *Ann Int Med* 1991; 114: 353–60.

13. Taylor DR, Flannery EM, Herbison GP. Methotrexate in the management of severe steroid-dependent asthma. *NZ Med J* 1993; 106: 409–11.

14. ✪ Trigg CJ, Davies RJ. Comparison of 30 mg methotrexate per week with placebo in chronic steroid-dependent asthma: a 12-week double-blind, crossover study. *Respir Med* 1993; 87: 211–16.

15. Coffey MJ, Sanders G, Eschenbacher WL *et al.* The role of methotrexate in the management of steroid-dependent asthma. *Chest* 1994; 105: 117–21.

16. Kanzow G, Nowak D, Magnussen H. Short term effect of methotrexate in severe steroid-dependent asthma. *Lung* 1995; 173: 223–31.

17. Ogirala RG, Sturm TM, Aldrich TK *et al.* Single high dose intramuscular triamcinolone acetonide versus weekly oral methotrextate in life threatening asthma: a double-blind study. *Am J Respir Crit Care Med* 1995; 152: 1461–6.

18. Mullarkey MF, Lammert JK, Blumenstein BA. Long term methotrexate treatment in corticosteroid-dependent asthma. *Annals Int Med* 1990; 112: 577–81.

19. Shiner RJ, Katz I, Shulimzon T, Silkoff P, Benzaray S. Methotrexate in steroid-dependent asthma: long term results. *Allergy* 1994; 49: 565–8.

20. Stanziola A, Sofia M, Mormile M, Molino A, Carratu L. Long term treatment with methotrexate in patients with corticosteroid-dependent bronchial asthma. *Monaldi Arch Chest Dis* 1995; 50(2): 109–13.

21. Becquart LA, Wallaert B, Lassalle P, Guene-Ribassin C, Tonnel AB. Le methotrexate dans le traitement de l'asthme. *Rev Mal Respir* 1994; 11: 565–71.

22. Stempel DA, Lammert J, Mullarkey MF. Use of methotrexate in the treatment of steroid-dependent adolescent asthmatics. *Ann Allergy* 1991; 67: 346–8.

23. Sole D, Costa-Carvalho BT, Soares FJP, Rullo VV, Naspitz CK. Methotrexate in the treatment of corticodependent asthmatic children. *J Invest Allergol Clin Immunol* 1996; 6(2): 126–30.

24. Guss S, Portnoy J. Methotrexate treatment of severe asthma in children. *Pediatrics* 1992; 89: 635–9.

25. Wilkie WS, Calabrase LH, Segal AM. Incidence of untoward reactions in patients with rheumatoid arthritis treated with methotrexate. *Arthritis Rheum* 1982; 26: S56A.

26. Lewis JH, Schiff E. Methotrexate induced chronic liver injury: guidelines for detection and prevention. *Am J Gastroenterol* 1988; 88: 1337–45.

27. Jones G, Mierins E, Karsha J. Methotrexate induced asthma. *Am Rev Respir Dis* 1991; 143: 179–81.

28. Tsai JJ, Shin JF, Chen CH, Wang SR. Methotrexate pneumonitis in bronchial asthma. *Int Arch Allergy Appl Immunol* 1993; 100: 287–90.

29. Cannon GW, Ward JR, Clegg DO. Acute lung disease associated with low-dose pulse methotrexate therapy in patients with rheumatoid arthritis. *Arthritis Rheum* 1983; 26: 1269–74.

30. Vallerand H, Cossart C, Milsevic D, Lavaud F, Leone J. Fatal pneumocystis pneumonia in an asthmatic patient treated with methotrexate. *Lancet* 1992; 339: 1551–2.

31. Kuitert LM, Harrison AC. *Pneumocystis carinii* pneumonia as a complication of methotrexate treatment in asthma. *Thorax* 1991; 46: 936–7.

32. Wollner A, Mohle-Boetani J, Lambert RE, Perruquet JL, Raffin TA, McGuire JL. *Pneumocystis carinii* pneumonia complicating low dose treatment with methotrexate for rheumatoid arthritis. *Ann Rheum Dis* 1991; 48: 247–9.

33. Reid DJ, Segars LW. Methotrexate for the treatment of chronic corticosteroid-dependent asthma. *Clin Pharm* 1993; 12: 762–7.

34. Bardin PG, Fraenkel DJ, Beasley RW. Methotrexate in asthma; a safety perspective. *Drug Safety* 1993; 9(3): 151–5.

35. Wong E, Lacasse Y, Guyatt GH, Sears MR, Cook DJ. Is methotrexate effective as a steroid sparing agent in steroid-dependent asthmatics? A meta-analysis. *Am J Respir Crit Care Med* 1997; 152: 801A.

36. Tugwell P, Bombardier C, Gent M *et al.* Low-dose cyclosporin versus placebo in patients with rheumatoid arthritis. *Lancet* 1990; 335: 1051–5.

37. Heule F, Meinardi MM, van Joost T, Bos JD. Low-dose cyclosporin is effective in severe psoriasis: a double blind study. *Transplant Proc* 1988; 20(suppl.): 32–41.

38. Eisen D, Ellis EA, Duell CE. Effect of topical cyclosporin rinse on oral lichen planus – a double-blind analysis. *New Engl J Med* 1990; 323: 290–94.

39. Garim EH, Orak JK, Hiott KL, Sutherland SE. Cyclosporin therapy for steroid-resistant nephrotic syndrome: a controlled study. *Am J Dis Child* 1988; 142: 985–8.

40. Takahashi N, Hayano T, Suzuki M. Peptidyl-prolyl *cis-trans* isomerase is the cyclosporin A-binding protein cyclophilin. *Nature* 1989; 337: 473–5.

41. Emmel EA, Verweij CL, Durand BD, Higgins KM, Lacy E, Crabtree GR. Cyclosporin specifically inhibits function of nuclear proteins involved in T cell activation. *Science* 1989; 246: 1617–20.

42. Shimizu H, Mitomo K, Watanabe T, Okamoto S, Yamamoto K. Involvement of a NFκB-like transcription factor in the activation of the interleukin-6 gene by inflammatory lymphokines. *Mol Cell Biol* 1990; 10: 561–8.

43. Bendtzen K, Dinarello CA. Mechanism of action of cyclosporin A. Effect on T cell binding of interleukin-1 and antagonising effect on insulin. *Scand J Immunol* 1984; 20: 43–51.

44. Cirillo R, Triggiani M, Sri L *et al.* Cyclosporin A rapidly inhibits mediator release from human basophils presumably by interacting with cyclophilin. *J Immunol* 1990; 144: 3891–7.

45. Pereira GM, Miller JF, Shevach EM. Mechanism of action of cyclosporin A *in vivo*. *J Immunol* 1990; 144: 2109–16.

46. Renz H, Mazer BD, Gelfand EW. Differential inhibition of T and B cell function in IL-4-dependent IgE by cyclosporin A and methylprednisolone. *J Immunol* 1990; 145: 3641–6.

47. Thomson AW, Milton JI, Aldridge RD. Inhibition of drug-induced eosinophilia by cyclosporin A. *Scand J Immunol* 1986; 24: 163–70.

48. Palay DA, Cluff CW, Wentworth PA, Ziegler HK. Cyclosporin inhibits macrophage-mediated antigen presentation. *J Immunol* 1986; 136: 4348–53.

49. ✪ Alexander AG, Barnes NC, Kay AB. Trial of cyclosporin in cortico-dependent chronic severe asthma. *Lancet* 1992; 339: 324–8.

50. ✪ Nizankowska E, Soja J, Pinis G et al. Treatment of steroid-dependent bronchial asthma with cyclosporin. *Eur Respir J* 1995; 8: 1091–9.

51. Lock SH, Kay AB, Barnes NC. Double-blind placebo-controlled trial of cyclosporin A as a corticosteroid-sparing agent in cortico-dependent asthma. *Am J Respir Crit Care Med* 1996; 153: 509–14.

52. Szczeklik A, Nizankowksa E, Dworski R, Domagala B, Pinis G. Cyclosporin for steroid-dependent asthma. *Allergy* 1991; 46: 312–15.

53. Mungan D, Misirligil Z, Sin B, Kaya A, Demirel Y, Gurbuz L. Cyclosporin in steroid-dependent asthma. *Allergol Immunopathol* 1995; 23(5): 202–6.

54. Blodgett RC. Auranofin; the experience to date. *Am J Med* 1983; 30: 86–9.

55. Bernstein DI, Bernstein IL. Use of gold in the severe asthmatic patient. *Immunol Allergy Clin N Am* 1991; 11: 81–90.

56. Rodnan GP, Benedek TG. The early history of anti-rheumatic drugs. *Arthritis Rheum* 1970; 13: 145–59.

57. Dudan A. Vingt cas d'asthma bronchique traites par la sanocrysine. *Schwiez Med Wochenschr* 1932; 4: 96–100.

58. Montagna CP, Rimoldi AA. Die Goldebehandlung des kindlichem Asthmas. *Deutsch Med Wochenschr* 1936; 50: 2055–8.

59. Von Lebinski. Beitrag zur Goldtherapie. *Ther Ggw* 1936; 77: 564–7.

60. Ishizaki T, Muranaki M, Araki H et al. Clinical study on the effect of aurothioglucose on patients with bronchial asthma. *Diagn Treat* 1965; 53: 750–55.

61. Araki H. Clinical study on the effect of sodium aurothiomalate in bronchial asthma. *Jap J Allergy* 1969; 18: 106–9.

62. Okatani Y. Gold salt therapy on bronchial asthma. *Jap Med J* 1970; 2432: 17–21.

63. Muranaka M, Miyamoto T, Shida T et al. Gold salt in the treatment of bronchial asthma – a double-blind study. *Ann Allergy* 1978; 40: 132–7.

64. Bernstein DI, Bernstein IL, Bodenheimer SS, Pietrusko RG. An open study of auranofin in the treatment of steroid-dependent asthma. *J Allergy Clin Immunol* 1988; 81: 6–16.

65. Honma M, Tamura G, Shirato K, Tkishima T. Effect of an oral gold compound, auranofin, on non-specific bronchial hyperresponsiveness in mild asthma. *Thorax* 1994; 49: 649–51.

66. Nierop G, Gijzel WP, Bel EH, Zwinderman AH, Dijkman JH. Auranofin in the treatment of steroid-dependent asthma. *Thorax* 1992; 47: 349–54.

67. Klaustermeyer WB, Noritake DT, Kwong FK. Chrysotherapy in the treatment of corticosteroid-dependent asthma. *J Allergy Clin Immunol* 1987; 79: 720–25.

68. ✪ Bernstein IL, Bernstein DI, Dubb JW, Faiferman I, Wallin B and Participants of the Auranofin Multi-Center Drug Trial. A placebo-controlled multicenter study of auranofin in the treatment of patients with corticosteroid-dependent asthma. *J Allergy Clin Immunol* 1996; 98: 317–24.

69. McNeill DL. Oral gold therapy in steroid-dependent asthma, nasal polyposis, and aspirin hypersensitivity. *Ann Allergy* 1990; 65: 288–90.

70. Levinson AL, Wheatley LM. Intravenous immunoglobulin: A new therapeutic approach in steroid-dependent asthma? *J Allergy Clin Immunol* 1991; 88: 552–4.

71. Page R, Friday G, Stillwagon P, Skoner D, Calguiri L, Fireman P. Asthma and selective immunoglobulin

deficiency: improvement after immunoglobulin replacement therapy. *J Pediatr* 1988; 112: 127–31.

72. Abernathy RS, Strem EL, Good RA. Chronic asthma in childhood: double-blind controlled study of treatment with gamma-globulin. *Pediatrics* 1958; 21: 908–93.

73. Brown EB, Botstein A. The effect of gamma globulin in asthmatic children. *New York State J Med* 1960; 109: 2539–45.

74. Fontana VJ, Kuttner AG, Wittig HJ, Moreno F. The treatment of infectious asthma in children with gamma globulin. *J Pediatr* 1963; 62: 80–84.

75. Smith TF, Muldoon MF, Bain RP *et al.* Clinical results of a prospective double-blind placebo-controlled trial of intravenous γ-globulin in children with chronic chest symptoms. *Monogr Allergy* 1988; 23: 168–76.

76. Mazer BD, Gelfand EW. An open-label study of high-dose intravenous immunoglobulin in severe childhood asthma. *J Allergy Clin Immunol* 1991; 87: 976–83.

77. Jakobsson T, Croner S, Kjellman N-IM, Petterson A, Vassella C, Bjorksten B. Slight steroid-sparing effect of intravenous immunoglobulin in children and adolescents with moderately severe bronchial asthma. *Allergy* 1994; 49: 413–20.

78. Sekul EA, Cupler EJ, Dalakas MC. Aseptic meningitis associated with high-dose intravenous immunoglobulin therapy: frequency and risk factors. *Ann Intern Med* 1994; 121: 259–62.

79. Selenke WM, Leung GW, Townley RG. Non antibiotic effects of the oleandomycin-erythromycin group with special reference to their steroid-sparing effects. *J Allergy Clin Immunol* 1980; 65: 454–64.

80. Szefler SJ, Rose JQ, Ellis EF, Spector SL, Green AW, Jusko WJ. The effect of troleandomycin on methylprednisolone elimination. *J Allergy Clin Immunol* 1980; 66: 447–51.

81. Greos LS, Szefler SJ, Larsen GL, Irvin CG, Hill MR. Troleandomycin reduces airways inflammation. *Am Rev Respir Dis* 1990; 141: A933.

82. Ong KS, Grieco MH, Rosner W. Enhancement by oleandomycin of the inhibitor effect of methylprednisolone on phytohaemagglutinin-stimulated lymphocytes. *J Allergy Clin Immunol* 1978; 62: 115–18.

83. Mendoza GR, Eitches RW, Orner FB. Direct effects of oleandomycin on histamine release in human basophils. *J Allergy Clin Immunol* 1983; 71: 135A.

84. Goswami SK, Kivity S, Marom Z. Erythromycin inhibits respiratory glyconjugate secretion from human airways *in vitro*. *Am Rev Respir Dis* 1990; 141: 72–8.

85. Celmer WD, Els H, Murai K. Oleandomycin derivatives; preparation and characterization. In: *Antibiotics Annual, 1957–1958*. New York: Interscience Publishers, 1958.

86. Kaplan MA, Goldin M. The use of triacetyloleandomycin in chronic infectious asthma. In: *Antibiotics Annual 1958–1959*. New York: Interscience Publishers, 1959.

87. Fox JL. Infectious asthma treated with triacetyloleandomycin. *Pennsylvania MJ* 1961; 64: 634–8.

88. Itkin IH, Menzel ML. The use of macrolide antibiotic substances in the treatment of asthma. *J Allergy* 1970; 45: 146–62.

89. Spector SL, Katz FH, Farr RS. Troleandomycin: effectiveness in steroid-dependent asthma and bronchitis. *J Allergy Clin Immunol* 1974; 54: 367–79.

90. Zieger RS, Schatz M, Sperling W, Simon RA, Stevenson DD. Efficacy of troleandomycin in outpatients with severe, corticosteroid-dependent asthma. *J Allergy Clin Immunol* 1980; 66: 438–46.

91. Eitches RW, Rachelefsky GS, Katz RM, Mendoza GR, Siegel SC. Methylprednisolone and troleandomycin in treatment of steroid-dependent asthmatic children. *Am J Dis Child* 1985; 139: 264–8.

92. Wald JA, Friedman BF, Farr RS. An improved protocol for the use of troleandomycin (TAO) in the treatment of steroid-requiring asthma. *J Allergy Clin Immunol* 1985; 78: 36–43.

93. Ball BD, Hill MR, Brenner M, Sanks R, Szefler SJ. Effect of low-dose troleandomycin on glucocorticoid

pharmacokinetics and airway hyperresponsiveness in severely asthmatic children. *Ann Allergy* 1990; 65: 37–45.

94. Menz G, Rothe T, Schmitz M, Hauser F, Haack D, Virchow Chr. Erfahrungen mit einer Kombinationtherapie von Methylprednisolon und Troleandomycin (TAO) bei schweren, hochkortoidbedurftigem Asthma bronchiale. *Pneumologie* 1990; 44: 238–40.

95. Kamada AK, Hill MR, Ikle DN, Brenner M, Szefler SJ. Efficacy and safety of low-dose troleandomycin in children with severe steroid-requiring asthma. *J Allergy Clin Immunol* 1993; 91: 873–82.

96. Flotte TR, Loughlin GM. Benefits and complications of troleandomycin (TAO) in young children with steroid-dependent asthma. *Pediatr Pulmonol* 1991; 10: 178–82.

97. ❂ Nelson HS, Hamilos DL, Corsello PR, Levesque NV, Buchmeier AD, Bucher BL. A double-blind study of troleandomycin and methylprednisolone in asthmatics who require daily corticosteroids. *Am Rev Respir Dis* 1993; 147: 398–404.

98. Siracusa A, Brugnami G, Fiordi T, Areni S, Severini C, Marabini A. Troleandomycin in the treatment of difficult asthma. *J Allergy Clin Immunol* 1993; 92: 677–82.

99. Rosenburg SM, Gerhard H, Grunstein MM, Schramm CM. Use of TAO without methylprednisolone in the treatment of severe asthma. *Chest* 1991; 100: 849–50.

100. Kench JG, Seale JP, Temple DM, Tennant C. The effect of non-steroidal inhibitors of phospholipase A_2 on leukotriene and histamine release from human and guinea pig lung. *Prostaglandins* 1985; 30: 199–208.

101. Geshickter CF. A new treatment for bronchial asthma. *Bull Georgetown U Med Ctr* 1953; 7: 39.

102. Engeset A. Therapeutic experiments with anti-malarials in the treatment of bronchial asthma. *Nord Med* 1957; 58: 1904.

103. Goldstein JA. Hydroxychloroquine for asthma. *Am Rev Respir Dis* 1983; 128: 1100–1101.

104. Tennebaum J, Smith R. Anti-malarial therapy for resistant asthma. *Ann Allergy* 1966; 24: 37–40.

105. ❂ Roberts JA, Gunneberg A, Elliott JA, Thompson NC. Hydroxychloroquine in steroid-dependent asthma. *Pulm Pharmacol* 1988; 1: 59–61.

106. Charous BL. Open study of hydroxychloroquine in the treatment of severe symptomatic or corticosteroid-dependent asthma. *Ann Allergy* 1990; 65: 53–8.

107. Charous BL. Effectiveness of long-term treatment of severe asthma with hydroxychloroquine (HCQ). *Ann NY Acad Sci* 1991; 629: 432–3.

108. Cohen EP, Petty TL, Szentivanyi A, Priest RE. Clinical and pathological observations in fatal bronchial asthma. *Ann Int Med* 1965; 62: 103–7.

109. Waldblott GL. Nitrogen mustard in the treatment of bronchial asthma. *Ann Allergy* 1952; 10: 428–9.

110. Kaiser HB, Beall GN. Azathioprine (Imuran) in chronic asthma. *Ann Allergy* 1966; 24: 369–70.

111. Arkins JA, Hirsch SR. Clinical effectiveness of 6-mercaptopurine in bronchial asthma. *J Allergy* 1966; 37: 90–95.

112. Hodges NG, Brewis AL, Howell JBL. An evaluation of azathioprine in severe chronic asthma. *Thorax* 1971; 26: 734–9.

113. Asmundssen T, Kilburn KH, Laszio J, Krock CJ. Immunosuppressive therapy of asthma. *J Allergy* 1971; 47: 136–47.

114. Ilfield D, Theodor E, Delpre G, Kuperman O. *In vitro* correction of a deficiency of Con A-induced suppressor cell function in primary biliary cirrhosis by a pharmacological concentration of colchicine. *Clin Exp Immunol* 1984; 57: 438–42.

115. Hwang KC, Fikrig SM, Friedman HM, Gupta S. Deficient concanavalin A-induced suppressor-cell activity in patients with bronchial asthma, allergic rhinitis, and atopic dermatitis. *Clin Allergy* 1985; 15: 67–72.

116. Spilberg I, Mandell B, Mehta J, Simchowitz L, Rosenburg D. Mechanism of action of colchicine in acute urate crystal-induced arthritis. *J Clin Invest* 1979; 64: 775–80.

117. Kershenobich D, Alcocer J, Quiraga A, Rojkind M. Effect of colchicine on immunoregulatory

T-lymphocytes and monocytes in patients with primary biliary cirrhosis. *Clin Res* 1984; 32: 490A.

118. Rudolph SA, Greengard P, Malawista SE. Effects of colchicine on cyclic AMP levels in human leukocytes. *Proc Natl Acad Sci USA* 1977; 74: 3404–8.

119. Schwartz YA, Kivity S, Ilfield DN *et al.* A clinical and immunological study of colchicine in asthma. *J Allergy Clin Immunol* 1990; 85: 578–82.

120. Adalioglu G, Turktas I, Saraclar Y, Tuncer A. A clinical study of colchicine in childhood asthma. *J Asthma* 1994; 312: 361–6.

121. Newman KB, Mason UG, Buchmeier A, Schmaling KB, Corsello P, Nelson HS. Failure of colchicine to reduce inhaled triamcinolone dose in patients with asthma. *J Allergy Clin Immunol* 1997; 99: 176–8.

122. ✪ Fish JE, Peters SP, Chambers CV *et al.* An evaluation of colchicine as an alternative to inhaled steroids in moderate asthma. *Am J Respir Crit Care Med* 1997; 156: 1165–71.

123. Metzger WJ, Zavala D, Richerson HB. Local allergen challenge and bronchoalveolar lavage of allergic asthmatic lungs. *Am Rev Respir Dis* 1987; 135: 433–40.

124. Carroll M, Durham SR, Walsh G, Kay AB. Activation of neutrophils and monocytes after allergen and histamine-induced bronchoconstriction. *J Allergy Clin Immunol* 1985; 75: 290–96.

125. Murphy K, Wilson M, Irvine C. The requirement of polymorphonuclear leukocytes in the late asthmatic response and heightened airways reactivity in an animal model. *Am Rev Respir Dis* 1986; 134: 62–8.

126. Miyachi Y, Niwa Y. Effects of potassium iodide, colchicine, and dapsone on the generation of polymorphonuclear leukocyte-derived oxygen intermediates. *Br J Dermatol* 1982; 107: 209–14.

127. Harvath L, Yancey K, Katz S. Selective inhibition of human neutrophil chemotaxis to N-formyl-methionyl-leucyl-phenylalanine by sulfones. *J Immunol* 1986; 137: 1305–11.

128. Berlow BA, Liehaber MI, Dyer Z, Spiegal TM. The effect of dapsone on steroid-dependent asthma. *J Allergy Clin Immunol* 1991; 87: 710–15.

Chapter 20

Mediator Antagonists and Other New Agents

Elliot Israel and Jeffrey Drazen

This chapter focuses on the utility of agents whose mechanism of action is to inhibit the synthesis or action of specific chemical mediators in the management of asthma. Over the past several years leukotriene modifiers, agents that antagonize the action or production of leukotrienes, have been shown to be effective in the treatment of asthma. We review their use. In addition, we address the use of agents that inhibit the effects of thromboxane, another derivative of arachidonic acid. Further, we review the utility of antihistamines and platelet activating factor antagonists. Even though inhaled diuretics do not act by inhibiting the synthesis or action of inflammatory mediators, their use in asthma is reviewed in this chapter.

AGENTS AFFECTING METABOLITES OF ARACHIDONIC ACID – LEUKOTRIENE MODIFIERS

Arachidonic acid is cleaved from cell membrane phospholipids as a result of the action of phospholipases. The free arachidonic acid so liberated serves as a substrate for a number of enzyme systems;[1,2] the cyclooxygenase and 5-lipoxygenase systems are those of greatest relevance to the lung. Drugs that inhibit the synthesis or action of the cysteinyl leukotrienes, products of the 5-lipoxygenase enzyme pathway of arachidonic acid metabolism, have been shown to be effective in the treatment of asthma and are reviewed in this section. Additional agents have been discovered or developed whose action is to alter either the metabolism of arachidonic acid or the action of the metabolic products formed from arachidonic acid at specific receptors. Some of these other agents that have been studied in asthma in humans are detailed in Fig. 20.1 and are considered in detail in the next section. The cysteinyl leukotrienes (i.e. leukotrienes that contain the amino acid cysteine) are potent airway smooth muscle constrictors. In addition they attract eosinophils into the airways, promote oedema, and can increase mucus secretion. Of interest to asthma, they can be produced by mast cells and eosinophils. They are synthesized, and can be detected in the airways, to one degree or another, in response to most bronchoprovocative stimuli.[3] Currently, four entities that modify the synthesis or action of these agents are available. One, zileuton (Zyflo™), inhibits cysteinyl leukotriene synthesis by blocking the enzyme 5-lipoxygenase. The family of "lukasts" comprise the other three: montelukast (Singulair™), pranlukast, and zafirlukast (Accolate™). These three antagonize the effects of the cysteinyl leukotrienes at the Cys LT_1 receptor. Studies examining the effects of these agents, known as leukotriene modifiers, are reviewed below.

Studies in Induced Asthma

Exercise/Cold, Dry Air Leukotriene modifiers are effective in reducing responses to most bronchoprovocative stimuli. They reduce the bronchospastic response to exercise and the related stimulus, cold, dry air hyperpnoea, by about 50–60%.[4–9] Exercise-induced responses are inhibited in children as well as adults.[10,11] Depending on the agent used, significant protection may last even 24 hours after dosing[8] and there is no loss of the bronchoprotective effect even after 12 weeks of dosing.[9]

Allergen Allergen-induced responses appear to be more dependent on the elaboration of leukotrienes than exercise-induced airway narrowing. Leukotriene modifiers inhibit the acute response to allergen by 80–90% and significantly inhibit the late response as well.[12–14]

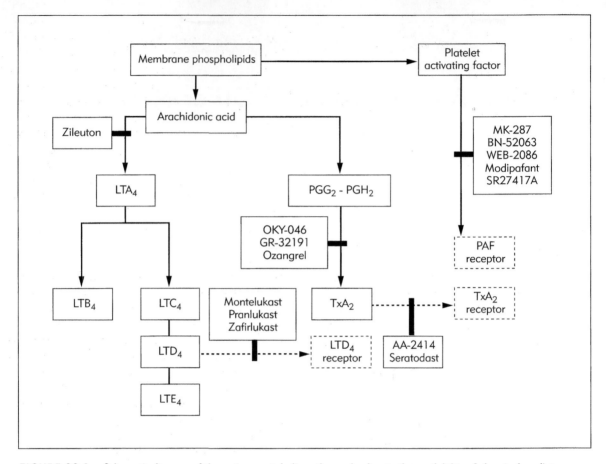

FIGURE 20.1: Schematic diagram of the various metabolic pathways leading to the availability of chemical mediators derived from membrane phospholipid. The agents that have been used in clinical trials are indicated at their site of proposed action. Blockade is indicated by a heavy line. Details about the trials with each agent are given in the appropriate section of the text.

Aspirin/NSAIDs Cysteinyl leukotrienes are critical mediators of aspirin-induced asthmatic responses. Controlled trials have shown that the leukotriene modifiers can significantly inhibit the effects of bronchoprovocative doses of aspirin.[15,16] The extrapulmonary sequelae of aspirin ingestion in sensitive patients are also inhibited by these agents.[15] Chronic treatment can produce improved nasal symptoms and improved pulmonary function even in patients already being treated with corticosteroids.[16] Despite their effectiveness in aspirin-induced asthma, these agents cannot provide absolute protection against aspirin and non-steroidal ingestion.

Other Bronchoprovocations Sulphur dioxide and adenosine-induced airway narrowing have been shown to be blocked by leukotriene modifying drugs as well.[17,18]

Spontaneous Asthma

Global and American guidelines now suggest leukotriene modifiers as alternatives in the chronic treatment of mild, persistent asthmatics.[19,20] These recommendations stem from studies that have shown that, with chronic use, these drugs produced significant improvements in FEV_1, decreased symptoms, decreased β agonist use, decreased night-time awakenings, and diminished the need for oral corticosteroid rescue.[21–27] The mean improvements in FEV_1 that occur range from 8 to 20% above baseline. These effects also occur in patients who are being treated with inhaled corticosteroids.[28,29]

In addition to producing improvements in pulmonary function and symptoms, the leukotriene modifiers also allow a reduction in the use of inhaled corticosteroids. In one study patients had their inhaled corticosteroid dose reduced in half when treated with a leukotriene antagonist – without a significant fall in peak flow.[30] In another study, addition of a leukotriene antagonist allowed further reduction in inhaled corticosteroid dosing.[31]

The leukotriene modifiers have generally been well-tolerated. Zileuton can produce elevations of liver transaminases in 2–3% of patients. Cases of eosinophilic vasculitis (Churg–Strauss syndrome) have been reported in patients treated with these agents. Most of these cases have occurred in patients who were undergoing tapering of oral, or high-dose inhaled, corticosteroids. The incidence of Churg–Strauss is quite rare and appears to be at or near the level of the calculated occurrence of this process in asthma treated with corticosteroids (60 cases per million patient years of treatment).[32]

Summary

Leukotriene modifiers have now become part of the routine armamentarium of agents available for asthma treatment. They are effective in mild asthma and may provide additional relief in patients with more moderate disease. They may be especially useful in treatment of aspirin-sensitive asthma. In addition, they are useful in decreasing responses to environmental stimuli such as exercise. Their availability in an oral form may be a consideration in treatment as well.

OTHER AGENTS MODIFYING THE METABOLISM OF ARACHIDONIC ACID

Thromboxane Synthesis Inhibitors and Receptor Antagonists

Recovery of Thromboxane A_2 Metabolites in Asthma Thromboxane (Tx) A_2 is derived from the PGG_2-PGH_2 complex by the action of thromboxane synthase. Increased amounts of thromboxane metabolites, including TxB_2, 2,3 dinor-TxB_2, and 11-dehydro-TxB_2, have been recovered in the urine from patients during acute severe asthma.[33] However, there is not agreement about whether allergen challenge results in increased urinary recovery of TxA_2 metabolites.[33,34]

Thromboxane Synthesis Inhibitors and Receptor Antagonists in Induced Asthma OKY-046, a thromboxane inhibitor, inhibited exercise-induced asthma in seven out of 11 patients.[35] In contrast GR32191, a structurally distinct thromboxane synthase inhibitor, had no salutary effect on exercise-induced asthma.[36] While ozagrel, another thromboxane synthase inhibitor, had a small but significant effect on allergen-induced early asthmatic responses, neither it or the thromboxane receptor antagonist, seratrodast, had any significant effect on late asthmatic responses or airway hyperresponsiveness; neither agent was nearly as effective as the leukotriene antagonist, pranlukast.[37]

Thromboxane Synthesis Inhibitors and Receptor Antagonists in Spontaneous Asthma GR32191, when given at a dose of 40 mg four times a day failed to exhibit a positive effect on airway physiology, asthma symptoms or asthma medication use in patients with moderate to severe asthma.[38] However, in a small study, the TxA_2 receptor antagonist AA-2414 produced improvements in asthma symptom scores, peak flows, and bronchial responsiveness. These effects were accompanied by decreased numbers of activated eosinophils.[39]

Thromboxane Synthesis Inhibitors and Receptor Antagonists Effects on Airway Hyperresponsiveness Neither OKY-046 nor imidazole salicylate, both thromboxane synthesis inhibitors, were able to significantly decrease airway responsiveness to methacholine.[40,41] However, AA-2414, a TxA_2 receptor antagonist, inhibits the response to aerosol methacholine such that the inhaled concentration required to decrease the FEV_1 by 20% is approximately doubled.[39,42] Seratrodast, another antagonist, decreased airway hyperresponsiveness to methacholine, but did not affect levels of exhaled nitric oxide nor percentage of sputum eosinophils.[43]

Summary These data do not yet indicate a definitive role for thromboxanes in induced or spontaneous asthma. Thromboxanes may, in part, mediate the airway hyperresponsiveness of asthma, but this has yet to be clearly established.

Fish Oils

Fish oils contain eicosapentaenoic acid (EPA) and docosahexaenoic acid (DCHA). EPA can substitute for arachidonic acid as a substrate for the lipoxygenase and cyclooxygenase pathways, diminishes the capacity of neutrophils to respond to chemotactic stimuli and to adhere to endothelial cells, and some of the products derived from the enzymatic processing of EPA and DCHA by lipoxygenase and cyclooxygenase are diminished in biopotency compared with the homologous products derived from arachidonic acid. This spectrum of effects had led to trials in which fish oils, rich in EPA and DCHA, were used in the treatment of asthma and allergic rhinitis.

Treatment with fish oil of patients showing allergen-induced asthmatic responses attenuated the allergen-induced late response, but did not alter their overall asthma severity.[44] The lack of effect of fish oils in chronic stable asthma has been confirmed by another group in a 10-week cross-over study,[45] while Dry and Vincent[46] showed a salutary effect on airflow obstruction in a group of 12 asthmatic subjects treated using a double-blind protocol with fish oil for 1 year.

A placebo-controlled parallel trial in which 25 subjects with pollen sensitivity were treated for 6 months with fish oil failed to show a salutary effect on asthma severity or hayfever symptoms over the 6 months encompassing the pollen season.[47] Taken together these data suggest that fish oil treatment has little to offer in the treatment of asthma or allergic rhinitis.

PLATELET ACTIVATING FACTOR

Platelet activating factor (PAF), 1-*O*-alkyl-2-acetyl-*sn*-glycero-e-phosphocholine, is an inflammatory mediator produced by alveolar macrophages, eosinophils, platelets, mast cells and neutrophils.[48,49] It transduces its effects via specific PAF receptors (Fig. 20.1). A number of agents have been developed with the capacity to inhibit signal transduction by PAF at its receptor. PAF has been implicated in the pathogenesis of asthma because administration of exogenous PAF to humans causes acute bronchoconstriction,[50–52] mucosal oedema,[53] inflammatory cell recruitment,[54] increased mucus production[55] and a possible increase in airway hyperresponsiveness.[50–52] In addition, PAF has been recovered from bronchoalveolar lavage fluid of asthmatics[56] and from the plasma of both asthmatic children[57] and asthmatic adults.[58]

PAF Antagonists in Induced Asthma
Allergen Although daily administration of BN 52063, a potent and selective PAF antagonist, for 3 days, partially attenuated the acute bronchoconstriction induced by the inhalation of allergen,[59] UK-74,505, another PAF antagonist that inhibits PAF-induced broncho-

constriction, failed to inhibit allergen-induced early and late asthmatic responses.[60] BN 52021, a similar compound, produced some inhibition of the early response to allergen but had no effect on methacholine responsiveness,[61] while Y-24180 significantly improved methacholine responsiveness.[62] Another PAF antagonist, WEB-2086, a hetrazepine with proven *in vivo* activity, failed to inhibit the early and late bronchospastic responses to allergen or the hyperresponsiveness to methacholine or histamine that follows antigen exposure.[63,64] MK-287, another antagonist of the *in vivo* effects of PAF, failed to inhibit the response to house-dust mite inhalation.[65] Although a more potent and bioavailable PAF antagonist, SR27417A, modestly attenuated the late asthmatic response, it had no effect on the early asthmatic response, allergen-induced airway responsiveness, or on baseline lung measurement.[66,67]

Exercise and Hyperventilation PAF antagonists have not shown effectiveness in blocking the asthmatic airway response to exercise or the hyperventilation of cold, dry air. BN 52063 failed to inhibit the acute bronchoconstriction following exercise.[68] SCH-37370, a dual PAF and histamine antagonist, did not appear to inhibit the response to cold, dry air isocapnic hyperventilation to any greater degree than would have been expected due to its antihistaminic properties alone.[69]

Clinical Asthma
Modipafant (UK-80,067), a potent and specific antagonist that is the enantiomer of UK-74,505, was used to treat moderate asthma for 4 weeks. It produced no significant improvement in peak flow, FEV_1 symptom scores, or airway responsiveness.[70]

Summary
Although exogenously administered PAF can mimic the physiological events that occur in asthma, the currently available PAF antagonists have not proven effective in preventing induced asthmatic bronchoconstriction or airway hyperresponsiveness. They have failed to decrease asthma symptoms or improve FEV_1. Since several molecular species of PAF exist,[71] several receptors have been identified[72] and PAF may act as an intracellular messenger;[73] it may be necessary to develop antagonists with greater avidity for specific receptor subtypes or greater intracellular activity than those currently available.

HISTAMINE ANTAGONISTS

Histamine has been implicated as a mediator of asthmatic bronchoconstriction since the demonstration that inhaled histamine produced bronchoconstriction in humans. The antihistamines that became available in the 1950s did not permit adequate evaluation of the therapeutic role of histamine antagonism in the treatment of asthma due to their anticholinergic and sedative side-effects. However, the development of H_1-receptor antagonists with markedly reduced side-effects has permitted a re-exploration of the effects of histamine antagonism in asthma. As these new H_1 antagonists frequently possess anti-allergic properties besides their antihistaminic effects, and because various compounds have been shown to inhibit eosinophil migration,[74] histamine release,[75] mast cell degranulation[76,77] and leukotriene release,[78] these agents are increasingly used adjunctively to treat asthma.

Induced Asthma

Allergen Histamine can be detected in biological fluids during allergen-induced early asthmatic responses[79] and antihistamines increase the amount of allergen required to produce an early asthmatic response.[80-83] An inconsistent effect has been noted on the allergen-induced late response. In one study, azelastine was shown to diminish the late response[84] while no such effect was seen in a subsequent examination of the effects of this drug.[85] Cetirizine had been shown to produce a statistically significant reduction in the late response without an effect on the early response.[86] More recent studies have demonstrated that when the antihistamine loratadine was combined with the leukotriene receptor antagonist, zafirlukast, the major part of both the early response (75%) and the late asthmatic response (74%) following exposure to allergen was inhibited. The inhibition produced was greater than that achieved with either agent alone.[87]

Exercise and Hyperventilation Treatment with antihistamines has been shown to attenuate the response to exercise and isocapnic hyperventilation.[88-90] In the case of cetirizine, this effect was only seen when the drug was administered by inhalation rather than by the oral route.[91]

Clinical asthma

Antihistamines have been shown to have effects on resting asthmatic airway tone as evidenced by an improvement to baseline forced expiratory volume in 1 s (FEV_1).[92-94] While studies with chronic use of antihistamines have not demonstrated a significant change in airway responsiveness[95] they have been able to show a reduction in asthma symptom scores, and in the need for β agonists.[95-99] One study has even suggested that they may be effective in reducing the dose of inhaled corticosteroid required to treat asthma.[100] While these results are encouraging, a meta-analysis of placebo-controlled clinical trials utilizing antihistamines for asthma with over 1000 patients failed to demonstrate significant benefits,[101] and a trial with loratadine failed to produce a sustained improvement in pulmonary function in moderate-to-severe asthmatics.[102]

Summary

Histamine appears to play a role in mediating part of the bronchospastic response to allergen, as well as some of the response to exercise and hyperventilation. Antihistamines may be used to attenuate a degree of the response to these asthmogenic stimuli. In mild asthmatics, the third-generation H_1-receptor antagonists improve symptoms as well, but it is not clear that they offer any incremental therapeutic value over currently available treatments. While studies have not demonstrated a significant role for antihistamines in the primary treatment of more chronic and severe asthma, preliminary studies suggest a possible adjunctive role in combination with other mediator antagonists. Their use in patients with asthma and coexisting allergic rhinitis or urticaria is also reasonable.

DIURETICS

Since Bianco and colleagues first reported that inhaled furosemide (frusemide) inhibits the airway narrowing induced by exercise in asthmatic subjects,[103] there have been many studies that have attempted to further define the effect of diuretics in asthma and to investigate their mechanism of action. Aside from the obvious possible effects on the local fluid and electrolyte milieu and resultant alternation of airway liquid, several additional possible mechanisms have been advanced to account for the effects of inhaled diuretics. These include inhibition of mediator release from inflammatory cells,[104,105] stimulation of prostaglandin E_2 production,[106,107] modulation of airway oedema,[108] increased mucociliary clearance,[109] and inhibition of respiratory tract neural responses.[110] While the precise mechanism of the observed effect is unclear, the studies do suggest that the effect is independent of the renal diuretic potency of the drug. In addition, efficacy is dependent on the inhalational route of administration, suggesting that very high local concentrations are required and/or that the target cell is located in the airway epithelium.

Studies in Induced Asthma

The effects of diuretics have been studied extensively in laboratory-induced asthma models in humans. While some of these studies have produced contradictory results, several patterns have emerged. For the most part, diuretics appear to be effective against "indirect" challenges (those that produce their effects via release of bronchoactive mediators) rather than against those that produce direct smooth muscle constriction. Inhaled diuretics have been shown to blunt the early response to inhaled allergen,[111–113] and the reaction to exercise,[103,114–117] hyperventilation,[108,115,118–121] sodium metabisulphite,[122–125] adenosine monophosphate,[123,126,127] hypertonic saline,[128] lysine aspirin[129] and distilled water.[105,130–134] Diuretics have been shown to be generally less effective in preventing the airway response to methacholine, histamine or prostaglandin $F_{2\alpha}$.[107,118,120,122,126]

Summary

Clinical studies of the effects of diuretics in spontaneous asthma are currently underway. A single recent report has suggested that furosemide is effective in the emergency treatment of asthmatic patients with hypercapnia.[135] The studies in induced asthma suggest that the inhaled diuretics may have a prophylactic role in the treatment of asthma similar to that of cromolyn and related compounds. However, in the case of furosemide, such a role may be limited due to the apparent short duration of its effect.[119,127]

KEY POINTS

1. Cysteinyl leukotrienes are important in asthma pathogenesis and anti-leukotrienes are an effective therapy for asthma.

2. Anti-thromboxanes or PAF-antagonists have not shown to be effective asthma treatment.

3. Antihistamines are effective treatment for rhinitis and may have an adjunctive role in combination with other mediator antagonists in treating asthma.

4. Inhaled diuretics attenuate asthmatic responses in induced asthma. Their role in asthma therapy is being investigated.

REFERENCES

1. ○ Samuelsson B, Dahlen SE, Lindgren JA, Rouzer CA, Serhan CN. Leukotrienes and lipoxins: structures, biosynthesis, and biological effects. *Science* 1987; 237: 1171–6.

2. Piper PJ. Formation and actions of leukotrienes. *Physiol Rev* 1984; 64: 744–61.

3. ○ Drazen JM, Israel E, O'Byrne PM. Treatment of asthma with drugs modifying the leukotriene pathway. *N Engl J Med* 1999; 340: 197–206.

4. Israel E, Dermarkarian R, Rosenberg M *et al.* The effects of a 5-lipoxygenase inhibitor on asthma induced by cold, dry air. *N Engl J Med* 1990; 323: 1740–44.

5. Finnerty JP, Wood-Baker R, Thomson H, Holgate ST. Role of leukotrienes in exercise-induced asthma. Inhibitory effect of ICI 204219, a potent leukotriene D4 receptor antagonist. *Am Rev Respir Dis* 1992; 145: 746–9.

6. Makker HK, Lau LC, Thomson HW, Binks SM, Holgate ST. The protective effect of inhaled leukotriene D_4 receptor antagonist ICI 204,219 against exercise-induced asthma. *Am Rev Respir Dis* 1993; 147: 1413–18.

7. Meltzer SS, Hasday JD, Cohn J, Bleecker ER. Inhibition of exercise-induced bronchospasm by zileuton: a 5-lipoxygenase inhibitor. *Am J Respir Crit Care Med* 1996; 153: 931–5.

8. Reiss TF, Hill JB, Harman E *et al.* Increased urinary

excretion of LTE4 after exercise and attenuation of exercise-induced bronchospasm by montelukast, a cysteinyl leukotriene receptor antagonist. *Thorax* 1997; 52: 1030–35.

9. Leff JA, Busse WW, Pearlman D *et al.* Montelukast, a leukotriene-receptor antagonist, for the treatment of mild asthma and exercise-induced bronchoconstriction. *N Engl J Med* 1998; 339: 147–52.

10. Kemp JP, Dockhorn RJ, Shapiro GG *et al.* Montelukast once daily inhibits exercise-induced bronchoconstriction in 6- to 14-year-old children with asthma. *J Pediatr* 1998; 133: 424–8.

11. Pearlman DS, Ostrom NK, Bronsky EA, Bonuccelli CM, Hanby LA. The leukotriene D4-receptor antagonist zafirlukast attenuates exercise-induced bronchoconstriction in children. *J Pediatr* 1999; 134: 273–9.

12. Taylor IK, O'Shaughnessy KM, Fuller RW, Dollery CT. Effect of cysteinyl-leukotriene receptor antagonist ICI 204.219 on allergen-induced bronchoconstriction and airway hyperreactivity in atopic subjects. *Lancet* 1991; 337: 690–94.

13. Findlay SR, Barden JM, Easley CB, Glass M. Effect of the oral leukotriene antagonist, ICI 204,219, on antigen-induced bronchoconstriction in subjects with asthma. *J Allergy Clin Immunol* 1992; 89: 1040–45.

14. Friedman BS, Bel EH, Buntinx A *et al.* Oral leukotriene inhibitor (MK-886) blocks allergen-induced airway responses. *Am Rev Respir Dis* 1993; 147: 839–44.

15. Israel E, Fischer AR, Rosenberg MA *et al.* The pivotal role of 5-lipoxygenase products in the reaction of aspirin-sensitive asthmatics to aspirin. *Am Rev Respir Dis* 1993; 148: 1447–51.

16. Dahlen B, Nizankowska E, Szczeklik A *et al.* Benefits from adding the 5-lipoxygenase inhibitor zileuton to conventional therapy in aspirin-intolerant asthmatics. *Am J Respir Crit Care Med* 1998; 157: 1187–94.

17. Lazarus SC, Wong HH, Watts MJ, Boushey HA, Lavins BJ, Minkwitz MC. The leukotriene receptor antagonist zafirlukast inhibits sulfur dioxide-induced bronchoconstriction in patients with asthma. *Am J Respir Crit Care Med* 1997; 156: 1725–30.

18. van Schoor J, Joos GF, Kips JC, Drajesk JF, Carpentier PJ, Pauwels RA. The effect of ABT-761, a novel 5-lipoxygenase inhibitor, on exercise- and adenosine-induced bronchoconstriction in asthmatic subjects. *Am J Respir Crit Care Med* 1997; 155: 875–80.

19. National Heart Lung and Blood Institute. *NHLBI/WHO Workshop Report: Global strategy for asthma management and prevention.* Global Initiative for Asthma. Bethesda, Maryland. National Heart Lung and Blood Institute (USA). Publication No. 95–3659, 1995.

20. National Heart Lung and Blood Institute. *National Asthma Education and Prevention Program: Guidelines for the diagnosis and management of asthma.* Expert panel report 2. Bethesda, Maryland. NIH publication No. 97–4051, 1997.

21. Spector SL, Smith LJ, Glass M, Accolate Asthma Trialists Group. Effects of 6 weeks of therapy with oral doses of ICI 204, 219, a leukotriene D4 receptor antagonist, in subjects with bronchial asthma. *Am J Respir Crit Care Med* 1994; 150: 618–23.

22. Israel E, Cohn J, Dube L, Drazen J, for the Zileuton Clinical Trial Group. Effect of treatment with zileuton, a 5-lipoxygenase inhibitor, in patients with asthma. *JAMA* 1996; 275: 931–6.

23. Liu MC, Dube LM, Lancaster J, and the Zileuton Study Group. Acute and chronic effects of a 5-lipoxygenase inhibitor in asthma: 6-month randomized multicenter trial. *J Allergy Clin Immunol* 1996; 98: 859–71.

24. Reiss TF, Altman LC, Chervinsky P *et al.* Effects of montelukast (MK-0476), a new potent cysteinyl leukotriene (LTD4) receptor antagonist, in patients with chronic asthma. *J Allergy Clin Immunol* 1996; 98: 528–34.

25. Barnes NC, Pujet J, on behalf of an International Study Group. Pranlukast, a novel leukotriene receptor antagonist: results of the first European, placebo controlled, multicentre clinical study in asthma. *Thorax* 1997; 52: 523–7.

26. Fish JE, Kemp JP, Lockey RF, Glass M *et al.* Zafirlukast for symptomatic mild-to-moderate asthma: A 13-week multicenter study. *Clin Ther* 1997; 19: 675–90.

27. Malmstrom K, Rodriguez-Gomez G, Guerra J A *et al.*

Oral montelukast, inhaled beclomethasone, and placebo for chronic asthma. *Ann Intern Med* 1999; 130: 487–95.

28. Reiss TF, Sorkness CA, Stricker W *et al.* Effects of montelukast (MK-0476), a potent cysteinyl leukotriene receptor antagonist, on bronchodilation in asthmatic subjects treated with and without inhaled corticosteroids. *Thorax* 1997; 52: 45–8.

29. Reiss TF, Chervinsky P, Dockhorn RJ *et al.* Montelukast, a once daily leukotriene receptor antagonist, in the treatment of chronic asthma. *Arch Intern Med* 1998; 158: 1213–20.

30. Tamaoki J, Kondo M, Sakai N *et al.* Leukotriene antagonist prevents exacerbation of asthma during reduction of high-dose inhaled corticosteroid. *Am J Respir Crit Care Med* 1997; 155: 1235–40.

31. Leff JA, Israel E, Noonan MJ *et al.* Montelukast (MK-0476) allows tapering of inhaled corticosteroids (ICS) in asthmatic patients while maintaining clinical stability. *Am J Respir Crit Care Med* 1997; 155(4): A976 Abstract.

32. Wechsler ME, Pauwels R, Drazen JD. Leukotriene modifiers and Churg–Strauss syndrome: Adverse effect or response to corticosteroid withdrawal? *Drug Safety* 1999; 21: 241–51.

33. Taylor IK, Ward PS, O'Shaughnessy KM *et al.* Thromboxane A2 biosynthesis in acute asthma and after antigen challenge. *Am Rev Respir Dis* 1991; 143: 119–25.

34. Sladek K, Dworski R, FitzGerald GA *et al.* Allergen-stimulated release of thromboxane A2 and leukotriene E4 in humans. Effect of indomethacin. *Am Rev Respir Dis* 1990; 141: 1441–1445.

35. Hoshino M, Fukushima Y. Effect of OKY-046 (thromboxane A2 synthetase inhibitor) on exercise-induced asthma. *J Asthma* 1991; 28: 19–29.

36. Finnerty JP, Twentyman OP, Harris A, Palmer JBD, Holgate ST. Effect of GR32191, a potent thromboxane receptor antagonist, on exercise induced bronchoconstriction in asthma. *Thorax* 1991; 46: 190–92.

37. Obase Y, Shimoda T, Matsuo N, Matsuse H, Asai S, Kohno S. Effects of cysteinyl-leukotriene receptor antagonist, thromboxane A2 receptor antagonist, and thromboxane A2 synthetase inhibitor on antigen-induced bronchoconstriction in patients with asthma. *Chest* 1998; 114: 1028–32.

38. Coleman RA. GR32191 and the role of thromboxane A2 in asthma–preclinical and clinical findings. *Agents Actions* (suppl.) 1991; 34: 211–20.

39. Hoshino M, Sim J, Shimizu K, Nakayama H, Koya A. Effect of AA-2414, a thromboxane A2 receptor antagonist, on airway inflammation in subjects with asthma. *J Allergy Clin Immunol* 1999; 103: 1054–61.

40. Peccini F, Dottorini ML, Casucci G, Mezzasoma AM, Sorbini CA, Tantucci C. Ineffectiveness of a four week treatment with the thromboxane synthetase inhibitor, imidazole salycilate, in reducing airway hyperresponsiveness to methacholine in asthmatics. *Monaldi Arch Chest Dis* 1997; 52: 130–37.

41. Kunitoh H, Watanabe K, Nagatomo A, Okamoto H, Nakagawa T. A double-blind, placebo-controlled trial of the thromboxane synthetase blocker OKY-046 on bronchial hypersensitivity in bronchial asthma patients. *J Asthma* 1998; 35: 355–60.

42. Fujimura M, Sakamoto S, Saito M, Miyake Y, Matsuda T. Effect of a thromboxane A2 receptor antagonist (AA-2414) on bronchial hyperresponsiveness to methacholine in subjects with asthma. *J Allergy Clin Immunol* 1991; 87: 23–7.

43. Aizawa H, Inoue H, Nakano H *et al.* Effects of thromboxane A2 antagonist on airway hyperresponsiveness, exhaled nitric oxide, and induced sputum eosinophils in asthmatics. *Prostaglandins Leukot Essent Fatty Acids* 1998; 59: 185–90.

44. ✪ Arm JP, Horton CE, Spur BW, Mencia-Huerta JM, Lee TH. The effects of dietary supplementation with fish oil lipids on the airways response to inhaled allergen in bronchial asthma. *Am Rev Respir Dis* 1989; 139: 1395–400.

45. Stenius-Aarniala B, Aro A, Hakulinen A, Ahola I, Seppala E, Vapaatalo H. Evening primose oil and fish oil are ineffective as supplementary treatment of bronchial asthma. *Ann Allergy* 1989; 62: 534–7.

46. Dry J, Vincent D. Effect of a fish oil diet on asthma: results of a 1-year double-blind study. *Int Arch Allergy Appl Immunol* 1991; 95: 156–7.

47. Thien FCK, Menciahuerta JM, Lee TK. Dietary fish oil effects on seasonal hay fever and asthma in pollen-sensitive subjects. *Am Rev Respir Dis* 1993; 147: 1138–43.

48. Barnes PJ, Chung KF, Page CP. Platelet-activating factor as a mediator of allergic disease. *J Allergy Clin Immunol* 1988; 81: 919–34.

49. ✪ Page CP. The role of platelet-activating factor in asthma. *J Allergy Clin Immunol* 1988; 81: 144–52.

50. Cuss FM, Dixon CMS, Barnes PJ. Effects of inhaled platelet activating factor on pulmonary function and bronchial responsiveness in man. *Lancet* 1986; 2: 189–92.

51. Kaye MG, Smith LJ. Effects of inhaled leukotriene D4 and platelet-activating factor on airway reactivity in normal subjects. *Am Rev Respir Dis* 1990; 141: 993–7.

52. Rubin AH, Smith LJ, Patterson R. The bronchoconstrictor properties of platelet-activating factor in humans. *Am Rev Respir Dis* 1987; 136: 1145–51.

53. Hamasaki Y, Mojarad M, Saga T, Tai HH, Said SI. Platelet-activating factor raises airway and vascular pressures and induces edema in lungs perfused with platelet-free solution. *Am Rev Respir Dis* 1984; 129: 742–6.

54. Archer CB, Page CP, Morley J, MacDonald DM. Accumulation of inflammatory cells in response to intracutaneous platelet activating factor (Paf-acether) in man. *Br J Dermatol* 1985; 112: 285–90.

55. Steiger J, Bray MA, Subramanian N. Platelet activating factor (PAF) is a potent stimulator of porcine tracheal fluid secretion *in vitro*. *Eur J Pharmacol* 1987; 142: 367–372.

56. Stenton SC, Court EN, Kingston WP *et al*. Platelet-activating factor in bronchoalveolar lavage fluid from asthmatic subjects. *Eur Respir J* 1990; 3: 408–413.

57. Hsieh KH, Ng CK. Increased plasma platelet-activating factor in children with acute asthmatic attacks and decreased *in vivo* and *in vitro* production of platelet-activating factor after immunotherapy. *J Allergy Clin Immunol* 1993; 91: 650–57.

58. Kurosawa M, Yamashita T, Kurimoto F. Increased levels of blood platelet-activating factor in bronchial asthmatic patients with active symptoms. *Allergy* 1994; 49: 60–63.

59. Guinot P, Brambilla C, Duchier J, Braquet P, Bonvoisin B, Cournot A. Effect of BN 52063, a specific PAF-acether antagonist, on bronchial provocation test to allergens in asthmatic patients. A preliminary study. *Prostaglandins* 1987; 34: 723–31.

60. Kuitert LM, Hui KP, Uthayarkumar S *et al*. Effect of the platelet-activating factor antagonist UK-74,505 on the early and late response to allergen. *Am Rev Respir Dis* 1993; 147: 82–6.

61. Hsieh KH. Effects of PAF antagonist, BN52021, on the PAF-, methacholine-, and allergen-induced bronchoconstriction in asthmatic children. *Chest* 1991; 99: 877–82.

62. Hozawa S, Haruta Y, Ishioka S, Yamakido M. Effects of a PAF antagonist, Y-24180, on bronchial hyperresponsiveness in patients with asthma. *Am J Respir Crit Care Med* 1995; 152: 1198–1202.

63. Wilkens H, Wilkens JH, Bosse S *et al*. Effects of an inhaled paf-antagonist (web 2086 bs) on allergen-induced early and late asthmatic responses and increased bronchial responsiveness to methacholine. *Am Rev Respir Dis* 1991; 143 (suppl.): A812.

64. Freitag A, Watson RM, Matsos G, Eastwood C, O'Byrne PM. Effect of a platelet activating factor antagonist, WEB 2086, on allergen induced asthmatic responses. *Thorax* 1993; 48: 594–8.

65. Bel EH, De Smet M, Rossing TH, Timmers MC, Dijkman JH, Sterk PJ. The effect of a specific oral paf-antagonist, mk-287, on antigen-induced early and late asthmatic reactions in man. *Am Rev Respir Dis* 1991; 143 (suppl.): A811.

66. Evans DJ, Barnes PJ, Cluzel M, O'Connor BJ. Effects of a potent platelet-activating factor antagonist, SR27417A, on allergen-induced asthmatic responses. *Am J Respir Crit Care Med* 1997; 156: 11–16.

67. Gomez FP, Roca J, Barbera JA, Chung KF, Peinado VI, Rodriguez-Roisin R. Effect of a platelet-activating factor (PAF) antagonist, SR 27417A, on PAF-induced gas exchange abnormalities in mild asthma. *Eur Respir J* 1998; 11: 835–9.

68. Wilkens JH, Wilkens H, Uffmann J, Bovers J, Fabel H,

Frolich JC. Effects of a PAF-antagonist (BN 52063) on bronchoconstriction and platelet activation during exercise induced asthma. *Br J Clin Pharmacol* 1990; 29: 85–91.

69. Dermarkarian RM, Israel E, Rosenberg MA *et al.* The effect of SCH-37370, a dual platelet activating factor (PAF) and histamine antagonist, on the bronchoconstriction induced in asthmatics by cold, dry air isocapnic hyperventilation (ISH). *Am Rev Respir Dis* 1991; 143: A812 (Abstract).

70. Kuitert LM, Angus RM, Barnes NC *et al.* Effect of a novel potent platelet-activating factor antagonist, modipafant, in clinical asthma. *Am J Respir Crit Care Med* 1995; 151: 1331–5.

71. Pinckard RN, Ludwig JC, McManus LM. Platelet activating factors. In: Gallin JI, Goldstein IM, Snyderman R (eds). *Inflammation: Basic Principles and Clinical Correlates* New York: Raven Press, 1988: 139–67.

72. Stewart AG, Dusting GJ. Characterization of receptors for platelet-activating factor on platelets, polymorphonuclear leukocytes and macrophages. *Br J Pharmacol* 1988; 94: 1225–33.

73. Stewart AG, Phillips WA. Intracellular platelet-activating factor regulates eicosanoid generation in guinea-pig resident peritoneal macrophages. *Br J Pharmacol* 1989; 98: 141–8.

74. Fadel R, Herpin-Richard N, Rihoux JP, Henocq E. Inhibitory effect of cetirizine 2HCl on eosinophil migration *in vivo*. *Clin Allergy* 1987; 17: 373–9.

75. Naclerio RM, Kagey-Sobotka A, Lichtenstein LM, Freidhoff L, Proud D. Terfenadine, an H1 antihistamine, inhibits histamine release *in vivo* in the human. *Am Rev Respir Dis* 1990; 142: 167–71.

76. Chand N, Pillar J, Diamantis W, Perhach JL Jr, Sofia RD. Inhibition of calcium ionophore (A23187)-stimulated histamine release from rat peritoneal mast cells by azelastine: implications for its mode of action. *Eur J Pharmacol* 1983; 96: 227–33.

77. Fields DA, Pillar J, Diamantis W, Perhach JL Jr, Sofia RD, Chand N. Inhibition by azelastine of nonallergic histamine release from rat peritoneal mast cells. *J Allergy Clin Immunol* 1984; 73: 400–403.

78. Temple DM, McCluskey M. Loratadine, an antihistamine, blocks antigen- and ionophore-induced leukotriene release from human lung *in vitro*. *Prostaglandins* 1988; 35: 549–54.

79. Busse WW, Swenson CA. The relationship between plasma histamine concentrations and bronchial obstruction to antigen challenge in allergic rhinitis. *J Allergy Clin Immunol* 1989; 84: 658–66.

80. Phillips MJ, Ollier S, Gould C, Davies RJ. Effect of antihistamines and antiallergic drugs on responses to allergen and histamine provocation tests in asthma. *Thorax* 1984; 39: 345–51.

81. Gong H Jr, Tashkin DP, Dauphinee B, Djahed B, Wu TC. Effects of oral cetirizine, a selective H1 antagonist, on allergen- and exercise-induced bronchoconstriction in subjects with asthma. *J Allergy Clin Immunol* 1990; 85: 632–41.

82. Chan TB, Shelton DM, Eiser NM. Effect of an oral H1-receptor antagonist, terfenadine, on antigen-induced asthma. *Br J Dis Chest* 1986; 80: 375–84.

83. Curzen N, Rafferty P, Holgate ST. Effects of a cyclo-oxygenase inhibitor, flurbiprofen, and an H1 histamine receptor antagonist, terfenadine, alone and in combination on allergen induced immediate bronchoconstriction in man. *Thorax* 1987; 42: 946–52.

84. Rafferty P, Ng WH, Phillips G *et al.* The inhibitory actions of azelastine hydrochloride on the early and late bronchoconstrictor responses to inhaled allergen in atopic asthma. *J Allergy Clin Immunol* 1989; 84: 649–57.

85. Twentyman OP, Ollier S, Holgate ST. The effect of H1-receptor blockade on the development of early- and late-phase bronchoconstriction and increased bronchial responsiveness in allergen-induced asthma. *J Allergy Clin Immunol* 1993; 91: 1169–78.

86. Wasserfallen JB, Leuenberger P, Pecoud A. Effect of cetirizine, a new H1 antihistamine, on the early and late allergic reactions in a bronchial provocation test with allergen. *J Allergy Clin Immunol* 1993; 91: 1189–97.

87. Roquet A, Dahlen B, Kumlin M *et al.* Combined antagonism of leukotrienes and histamine produces predominant inhibition of allergen-induced early and late phase airway obstruction in asthmatics. *Am J Respir Crit Care Med* 1997; 155: 1856–63.

88. Hartley JP, Nogrady SG. Effect of an inhaled antihistamine on exercise-induced asthma. *Thorax* 1980; 35: 675–9.

89. Patel KR. Terfenadine in exercise induced asthma. *Br Med J (Clin Res Ed)* 1984; 288: 1496–7.

90. Finnerty JP, Holgate ST. Evidence for the roles of histamine and prostaglandins as mediators in exercise-induced asthma: the inhibitory effect of terfenadine and flurbiprofen alone and in combination. *Eur Respir J* 1990; 3: 540–47.

91. Ghosh SK, De Vos C, McIlroy I, Patel KR. Effect of cetirizine on exercise induced asthma. *Thorax* 1991; 46: 242–4.

92. Kemp JP, Meltzer EO, Orgel HA *et al.* A dose–response study of the bronchodilator action of azelastine in asthma. *J Allergy Clin Immunol* 1987; 79: 893–9.

93. Rafferty P, Holgate ST. Terfenadine (Seldane) is a potent and selective histamine H1 receptor antagonist in asthmatic airways. *Am Rev Respir Dis* 1987; 135: 181–4.

94. Hopp RJ, Townley RG, Agrawal DK, Bewtra AK. Terfenadine effect on the bronchoconstriction, dermal response, and leukopenia induced by platelet-activating factor. *Chest* 1991; 100: 994–8.

95. Rafferty P, Jackson L, Smith R, Holgate ST. Terfenadine, a potent histamine H1-receptor antagonist in the treatment of grass pollen sensitive asthma. *Br J Clin Pharmacol* 1990; 30: 229–35.

96. Taytard A, Beaumont D, Pujet JC, Sapene M, Lewis PJ. Treatment of bronchial asthma with terfenadine; a randomized controlled trial. *Br J Clin Pharmacol* 1987; 24: 743–6.

97. Bruttmann G, Pedrali P, Arendt C, Rihoux JP. Protective effect of cetirizine in patients suffering from pollen asthma. *Ann Allergy* 1990; 64: 224–8.

98. Kemp JP, Bernstein IL, Bierman CW *et al.* Pemirolast, a new oral nonbronchodilator drug for chronic asthma. *Ann Allergy* 1992; 68: 488–91.

99. Chiu CP, Huang JL, Lin TY, Shieh WB, Hsieh KH. Double-blind placebo-controlled study of oxatomide in the treatment of childhood asthma. *Chung Hua Min Kuo Hsiao Erh Ko I Hsueh Hui Tsa Chih* 1997; 38: 14–20.

100. Busse WW, Middleton E, Storms W *et al.* Corticosteroid-sparing effect of azelastine in the management of bronchial asthma. *Am J Respir Crit Care Med* 1996; 153: 122–7.

101. ✪ Van Ganse E, Kaufman L, Derde MP, Yernault JC, Delaunois L, Vincken W. Effects of antihistamines in adult asthma: a meta-analysis of clinical trials. *Eur Respir J* 1997; 10: 2216–24.

102. Ekstrom T, Osterman K, Zetterstrom O. Lack of effect of loratadine on moderate to severe asthma. *Ann Allergy Asthma Immunol* 1995; 75: 287–9.

103. Bianco S, Vaghi A, Robuschi M, Pasargiklian M. Prevention of exercise-induced bronchoconstriction by inhaled frusemide. *Lancet* 1988; 2: 252–5.

104. Anderson SD, He W, Temple DM. Inhibition by furosemide of inflammatory mediators from lung fragments. *N Engl J Med* 1991; 324: 131.

105. Moscato G, Dellabianca A, Falagiani P, Mistrello G, Rossi G, Rampulla C. Inhaled furosemide prevents both the bronchoconstriction and the increase in neutrophil chemotactic activity induced by ultrasonic "fog" of distilled water in asthmatics. *Am Rev Respir Dis* 1991; 143: 561–6.

106. Miyanoshita A, Terada M, Endou H. Furosemide directly stimulates prostaglandin E2 production in the thick ascending limb of Henle's loop. *J Pharmacol Exp Ther* 1989; 251: 1155–9.

107. Polosa R, Rajakulasingam K, Prosperini G, Magri S, Mastruzzo C, Holgate ST. Inhaled loop diuretics and basal airway responsiveness in man: evidence of a role for cyclo-oxygenase products. *Eur Respir J* 1995; 8: 593–9.

108. Daviskas E, Anderson SD, Gonda I, Bailey D, Bautovich G, Seale JP. Mucociliary clearance during and after isocapnic hyperventilation with dry air in the presence of frusemide. *Eur Respir J* 1996; 9: 716–24.

109. Daviskas E, Anderson SD, Brannan JD, Chan HK, Eberl S, Bautovich G. Inhalation of dry-powder mannitol increases mucociliary clearance. *Eur Respir J* 1997; 10: 2449–54.

233

110. Elwood W, Lotvall JO, Barnes PJ, Chung KF. Loop diuretics inhibit cholinergic and noncholinergic nerves in guinea pig airways. *Am Rev Respir Dis* 1991; 143: 1340–44.

111. ✪ Bianco S, Pieroni MG, Refini RM, Rottoli L, Sestini P. Protective effect of inhaled furosemide on allergen-induced early and late asthmatic reactions. *N Engl J Med* 1989; 321: 1069–73.

112. Robuschi M, Pieroni M, Refini M *et al.* Prevention of antigen-induced early obstructive reaction by inhaled furosemide in (atopic) subjects with asthma and (actively sensitised) guinea pigs. *J Allergy Clin Immunol* 1990; 85: 10–16.

113. Verdiani P, Di Carlo S, Baronti A, Bianco S. Effect of inhaled frusemide on the early response to antigen and subsequent change in airway reactivity in atopic patients. *Thorax* 1990; 45: 377–81.

114. Pavord ID, Wisniewski A, Tattersfield AE. Inhaled frusemide and exercise induced asthma: evidence of a role for inhibitory prostanoids. *Thorax* 1992; 47: 797–800.

115. Brannan JD, Koskela H, Anderson SD, Chew N. Responsiveness to mannitol in asthmatic subjects with exercise- and hyperventilation-induced asthma. *Am J Respir Crit Care Med* 1998; 158: 1120–26.

116. Melo RE, Sole D, Naspitz CK. Comparative efficacy of inhaled furosemide and disodium cromoglycate in the treatment of exercise- induced asthma in children. *J Allergy Clin Immunol* 1997; 99: 204–209.

117. Larramendi CH, Chiner E, Calpe JL, Puigcerver MT. Comparative study of inhaled amiloride and inhaled furosemide in exercise-induced asthma. *Allergol Immunopathol (Madr)* 1997; 25: 85–90.

118. Grubbe RE, Hopp R, Dave NK, Brennan B, Bewtra A, Townley R. Effect of inhaled furosemide on the bronchial response to methacholine and cold-air hyperventilation challenges. *J Allergy Clin Immunol* 1990; 85: 881–4.

119. O'Donnell WJ, Rosenberg M, Niven RW, Drazen JM, Israel E. Acetazolamide and furosemide attenuate asthma induced by hyperventilation of cold, dry air. *Am Rev Respir Dis* 1992; 146: 1518–24.

120. Netzel M, Hopp RJ, Buzzas R, Dowling P, Palmeiro E,

Bewtra AK. Effect of inhaled amiloride on the bronchial response to methacholine and cold air hyperventilation challenges. *Chest* 1993; 103: 484–7.

121. Seidenberg J, Dehning J, von der Hardt H. Inhaled frusemide against cold air induced bronchoconstriction in asthmatic children. *Arch Dis Child* 1992; 67: 214–17.

122. Nichol GM, Alton EW, Nix A, Geddes DM, Chung KF, Barnes PJ. Effect of inhaled furosemide on metabisulfite- and methacholine-induced bronchoconstriction and nasal potential difference in asthmatic subjects. *Am Rev Respir Dis* 1990; 142: 576–80.

123. O'Connor BJ, Chung KF, Chen-Worsdell YM, Fuller RW, Barnes PJ. Effect of inhaled furosemide and bumetanide on adenosine 5′-monophosphate- and sodium metabisulfite-induced bronchoconstriction in asthmatic subjects. *Am Rev Respir Dis* 1991; 143: 1329–33.

124. Yeo CT, O'Connor BJ, Chen-Worsdell M, Barnes PJ, Chung KF. Protective effect of loop diuretics, piretanide and frusemide, against sodium metabisulphite-induced bronchoconstriction in asthma. *Eur Respir J* 1992; 5: 1184–8.

125. O'Connor BJ, Yeo CT, Chen-Worsdell YM, Barnes PJ, Chung KF. Effect of acetazolamide and amiloride against sodium metabisulphite- induced bronchoconstriction in mild asthma. *Thorax* 1994; 49: 1096–8.

126. Polosa R, Lau LC, Holgate ST. Inhibition of adenosine 5′-monophosphate- and methacholine-induced bronchoconstriction in asthma by inhaled frusemide. *Eur Respir J* 1990; 3: 665–72.

127. Polosa R, Rajakulasingam K, Prosperini G, Church MK, Holgate ST. Relative potencies and time course of changes in adenosine 5′-monophosphate airway responsiveness with inhaled furosemide and bumetanide in asthma. *J Allergy Clin Immunol* 1993; 92: 288–97.

128. Rodwell LT, Anderson SD, du Toit JI, Seale JP. The effect of inhaled frusemide on airway sensitivity to inhaled 4.5% sodium chloride aerosol in asthmatic subjects. *Thorax* 1993; 48: 208–13.

129. Vargas FS, Croce M, Teixeira LR, Terra-Filho M,

Cukier A, Light RW. Effect of inhaled furosemide on the bronchial response to lysine-aspirin inhalation in asthmatic subjects. *Chest* 1992; 102: 408–11.

130. Bianco S, Robuschi M, Vaghi A, Pieroni MG, Sestini P. Protective effect of inhaled piretanide on the bronchial obstructive response to ultrasonically nebulized H_2O. A dose-response study. *Chest* 1993; 104: 185–8.

131. Robuschi M, Gambaro G, Spagnotto S, Vaghi A, Bianco S. Inhaled frusemide is highly effective in preventing ultrasonically nebulised water bronchoconstriction. *Pulm Pharmacol* 1989; 187–91.

132. Foresi A, Pelucchi A, Mastropasqua B, Cavigioli G, Carlesi RM, Marazzini L. Effect of inhaled furosemide and torasemide on bronchial response to ultrasonically nebulized distilled water in asthmatic subjects. *Am Rev Respir Dis* 1992; 146: 364–9.

133. Siffredi M, Mastropasqua B, Pelucchi A, Chiesa M, Marazzini L, Foresi A. Effect of inhaled furosemide and cromolyn on bronchoconstriction induced by ultrasonically nebulized distilled water in asthmatic subjects. *Ann Allergy Asthma Immunol* 1997; 78: 238–43.

134. Mochizuki H, Shimizu T, Shigeta M, Tokuyama K, Morikawa A, Kuroume T. Effect of inhaled amiloride on water-induced bronchoconstriction in asthmatic children. *Am J Respir Crit Care Med* 1994; 150: 555–7.

135. Tanigaki T, Kondo T, Hayashi Y *et al*. Rapid response to inhaled frusemide in severe acute asthma with hypercapnia. *Respiration* 1997; 64: 108–110.

Chapter 21

Bronchodilators

Jan Lötvall

INTRODUCTION

Asthma is a disease characterized by recurrent bronchoconstriction, and therefore bronchodilators are the most fundamental asthma treatment, which every patient should be prescribed.

β_2 agonist given by aerosol inhalation is a very effective bronchodilator treatment, with limited amount of side-effects. Short-acting drugs, such as salbutamol and terbutaline, are used as rescue medication, whereas long-acting drugs such as salmeterol and formoterol recently have been introduced for regular treatment mainly in combination with inhaled glucocorticoids. Salbutamol and terbutaline can also be given systemically, either by oral, subcutaneous or intravenous route, but this results in more severe systemic side-effects, such as tremor and palpitation.

Other drugs that are used as bronchodilators include inhaled anti-cholinergic drugs (ipratropium bromide) and systemically administered theophylline. Anti-cholinergic drugs have clear limitations, since they only reverse cholinergic bronchoconstriction, and theophylline because of its narrow therapeutic ratio.

In this chapter, the beneficial and adverse effects of all of these treatments will be reviewed, including their mechanisms of action and recommendations for use. In addition, potential future bronchodilator treatments will be mentioned.

SYMPATHICOMIMETICS

Adrenaline and noradrenaline (epinephrine and norepinephrine) are the two endogenous catecholamines with sympathicomimetic activity (Fig. 21.1). Adrenaline is produced in the adrenal medulla, and is a potent stimulant of both α- and β-adrenergic receptors in a non-specific fashion. Thus, adrenaline has multiple effects in many organs. Noradrenaline is produced mainly in post-ganglionic sympathetic neurons, has a slightly different structure, and is more active on β_1 than on β_2 receptors.

There are two major classes of receptor on which catecholamines may act, α and β receptors.[1] In addition, both of these receptor classes have several subtypes. Most important for asthma treatment is the β_2 receptor[2] (Fig. 21.2), which is present in high numbers in the bronchial smooth muscle, bronchial epithelium and in endothelial cells. Furthermore, this receptor is present in relatively high numbers in peripheral blood vascular smooth muscle, and to a lesser extent in the heart. In this chapter, only the effects of activation of the β_2 receptor will be discussed (for detailed discussion of other receptors, see Hardman and Limbird).[3]

Mechanisms of β_2 Receptor Activation

β_2 receptor Signaling The β_2 receptor is a classical seven transmembrane domain receptor, coupled to G-proteins for intracellular signalling (Fig. 21.2). Within the receptor structure, there is a three-dimensional locus for the binding of catecholamines and β_2 agonists (Fig. 21.2).[4–6] When entering the receptor, a pharmacological agonist will form hydrogen bonds to specific amino acids within the receptor protein, which in turn will induce a small confirmational change of the receptor. This conformation change, which occurs principally on the second and third intracellular loops of the receptor protein, allows this part of the receptor to interact with the stimulatory G-protein (Gs: guanine nucleotide-regulatory proteins).[7–9] These events cause the increase of intracellular cAMP (cyclic adenosine monophosphate)[10] with concomitant activation of protein kinase A (PKA), which leads to phosphorylation

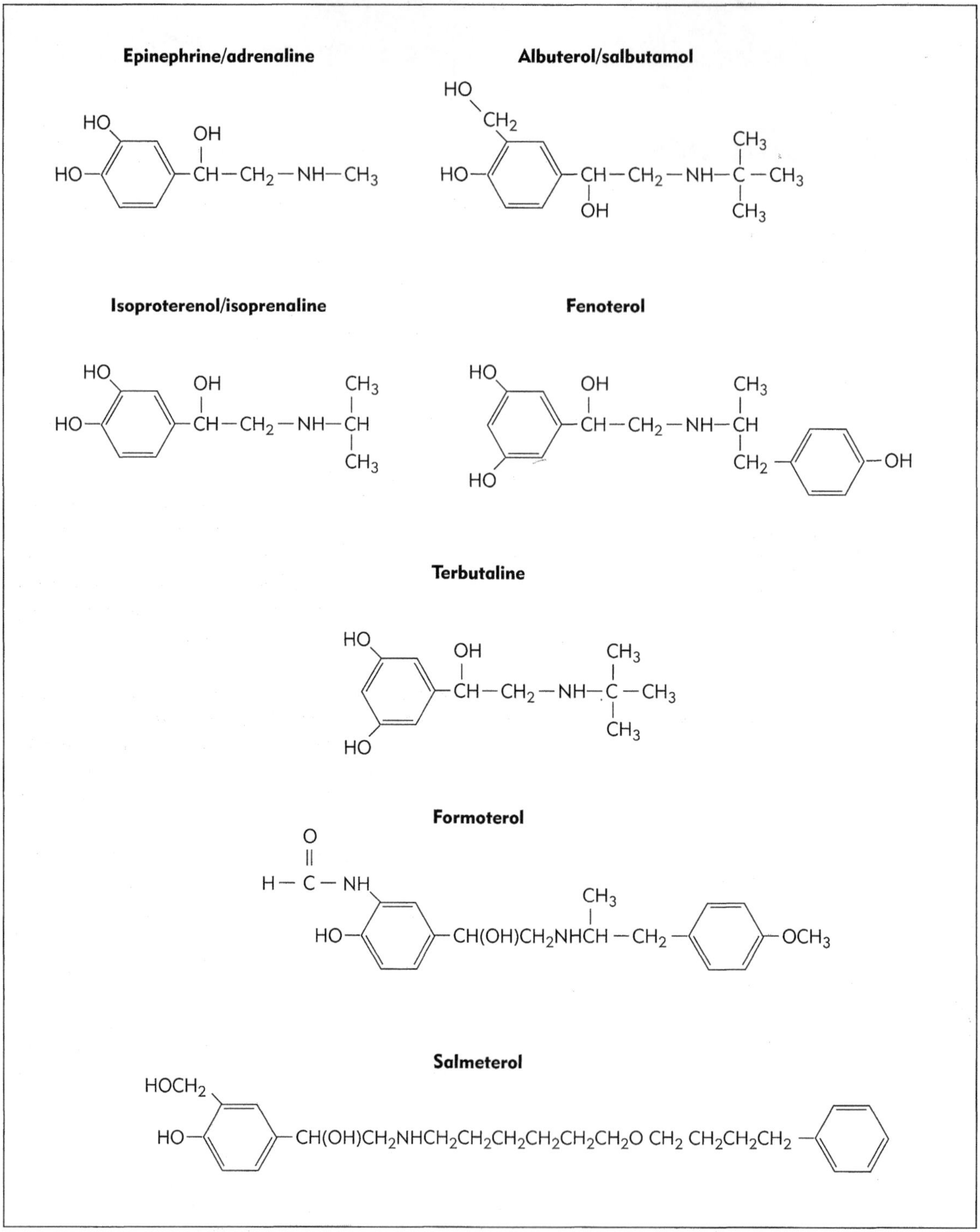

FIGURE 21.1: The chemical structure of adrenaline, isoprenaline, salbutamol, terbutaline, fenoterol, formoterol, and salmeterol. Note that formoterol and salmeterol have a more lipophilic structure than the other drugs, the long aliphatic side-chain of salmeterol makes it the most lipophilic drug.

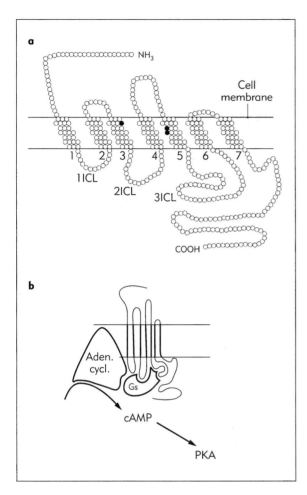

FIGURE 21.2: (a):The structure of the β_2 receptor. This receptor is a seven transmembrane domain receptor (1–7), with three intracellular loops (ICL 1–3). The active site of the receptor is in transmembrane domain 3 and 5, where three amino acids are crucial for agonists mediated receptor activation (b) The β receptor is a G-coupled protein. The G-protein (Gs) binds to ICL 2 and 3, and activates adenyl cyclase (aden. cycl.) to release cyclic AMP (cAMP), which in turn activates protein kinase A (PKA). This cascade of events result in relaxation of bronchial smooth muscle. (see the text.)

of several intracellular proteins, resulting in bronchial smooth muscle relaxation by inhibition of myosin–actin interaction.[11] Thus, cAMP seems to be a major intracellular messenger of β_2 receptors. However, recently it has been proposed that additional pathways may be involved in β_2 receptor function,[11] making the picture more complex. These mechanisms include K^+-channel activation via a sub-unit of the Gs, which has been suggested to induce bronchial smooth muscle relaxation which may be independent of cAMP.[12–16]

It is well-known that the activity of adrenergic receptors will be reduced upon chronic or repeated stimulation in *in vitro* systems.[17,18] This tachyphylaxis of the β_2 receptors (tolerance) is induced by principally three different mechanisms. Firstly, a very rapid phosphorylation and deactivation of the β_2 receptor is induced within seconds of activation, by phosphorylation of the receptor itself via cAMP and cAMP-independent pathways.[19] Secondly, within minutes, the receptor can be sequestrated (internalized), which means that it becomes unavailable for Gs-protein activation.[20] Within hours of activation, the total number of receptors can be down-regulated, either by degradation of receptor protein, instability of mRNA, or by reduced transcription at the gene level.[21,22] In the last 10 years, there has been an intense debate whether chronic treatment with β_2 agonists may be detrimental for asthmatic patients. The clinical implication of this issue is discussed in detail in the sections in this chapter discussing tolerance and risks with β_2 agonists.

Polymorphism of the β_2 Receptor In the last few years, it has been documented that there are several polmorphisms in the human β_2 receptors, and these small differences in receptor amino acid sequence may have implications for β_2 receptor function. In a large study in children with asthma ($n = 269$) it was found that homozygotes for Arg-16 were approximately five times more likely to respond to salbutamol compared with homozygotes for Gly-16.[23] Similarly, in a smaller study in adults ($n = 22$) it was found that the improvement in lung function was more pronounced and more rapid in Arg 16 homozygotes compared with patients with the Gly 16 variant.[24] In this case it was argued that the lower responsiveness was associated with tachyphylaxis (tolerance) in this group of patients. In both studies, the findings in heterozygotes were intermediate. At present, large databases with genotypes of patients with different responsiveness to β_2 agonists are being created, and future data will give us a clearer picture of the exact role of these polymorphisms in the clinical situation.

Biological Effects of β_2 Agonists

Short-acting β_2 agonists such as salbutamol and terbutaline have two isomers, the R- and the S-forms.[25] where the R-form is the active molecule[26] and induces effects in several organs, resulting in a characteristic effect/side-effect profile. Low doses of β_2 agonists given by inhalation evoke effects mainly in the bronchial wall, where the bronchial smooth muscle relaxing properties are the most important. At even higher doses, systemic symptoms will also be induced, including primarily tremor and palpitation. At higher doses, a decrease in serum potassium will be observed, as well as a slight increase in blood glucose.

Side-Effects Most of the side-effects induced by β_2 agonists are mediated by β_2 receptors in respective tissue. Thus, tremor-inducing effects of β_2 agonists are mediated via β_2 receptors on skeletal muscle, and palpitation by β_2 receptors in the heart.[27] In the heart, it has been argued that there may be β_2 receptors in the sympathetic nerves, inducing release of noradrenaline locally when activated, which in turn causes increased heart rate.[28] It cannot be excluded that there also may be some activation by β_1 receptors on cardiac myocytes by β_2 receptor agonists, because of weak activity of these drugs on β_1 receptors.[29] For isoprenaline (isoproterenol), which is still available as a bronchodilator in some countries, the situation is quite different, since this drug activates both β_1 and β_2 receptors in an unspecific way. Thus, the cardiovascular side-effects of this drug are pronounced when given by inhalation in high doses,[30,31] and are much worse than those induced by selective β_2 agonists. In fact, isoprenaline given in high doses has been argued to be associated with the asthma death epidemic that was present in several countries in the late 1960s.[32,33]

Anti-Inflammatory Activity β_2 Agonists are also anti-inflammatory in some respects. Inhaled glucocorticoids are effective in reducing most of the characteristics of inflammation, but most prominently cellular inflammation (the eosinophilia). β_2 agonists have a much narrower anti-inflammatory profile, with effects mainly on the exudation of plasma from the vasculature into the airway wall,[34–36] and inhibition of mediator release from mast cells.[37–40] These effects of β_2 agonists have, in combination with large clinical studies, suggested that combined treatment with inhaled glucocorticoids and inhaled β_2 agonists (long-acting β_2 agonists preferably) has additional therapeutic potential compared with inhaled glucocorticoids alone.[41–44]

Short-acting β_2 Agonists

The most important effect of selective β_2 agonists, as mentioned, is their relaxant effect on bronchial smooth muscle. This leads to dilatation of bronchoconstricted airways,[45–48] as well as functional inhibition of any type of induced bronchoconstriction.[49–51] Worldwide, the most commonly used β_2 agonist is salbutamol (albuterol; Fig. 21.1). In some countries, terbutaline and fenoterol are also used clinically (Fig. 21.1). All these drugs have a rapid onset of action, within minutes after inhalation, but have a relatively short duration of effect, with a peak effect starting to wean off after approximately 2–3 hours,[52,53] and all effects are gone after 5–6 hours. The effect-profile of these drugs is thus optimal for reversal of sudden onset brief bronchoconstriction, and for prophylactic use in situations that the patient knows induces bronchoconstriction (short exercise, exposure to cigarette smoke etc).

Dose Dependency The bronchodilator effect of salbutamol is clearly dose-dependent, but the major part of this dose-dependency is present at quite low doses, lower than those available in the presently used inhalers.[54,55] Thus, patients with relatively stable asthma, with only relatively mild recurrent bronchoconstriction, seldom require doses of salbutamol exceeding 400 μg (terbutaline 500 μg). In acute severe asthma, however, much higher doses of inhaled β_2 agonists may be used.[56–58] For the functional antagonistic effect of inhaled β_2 agonists, it is less clear what the full dose–response curve looks like. It seems that doses of salbutamol between 100–800 μg have a linear dose-dependent protective effect on methacholine responsiveness (PC_{20}), without any clear evidence of the effect reaching a full maximum at the highest doses.[59,60]

Short-Acting β_2 Agonists for Exercise-Induced Asthma Exercise-induced asthma is an example of a clinical sign of bronchial responsiveness that is effectively treated with short-acting β_2 agonists.[61] Thus, a single dose of salbutamol taken just prior to an exercise challenge has been reported to reduce or block the bronchoconstrictor response in 90–100% of patients.[62,63] On a mean basis, the inhibitory effect on the drop in FEV_1 is generally more than 70%.[61] Importantly, the drug should be given just prior to exercise, and not long before, since the duration of protective effect seems to be shorter than the duration of bronchodilation.[62] Lastly, regular treatment with β_2 agonists will slightly reduces the lowest FEV_1 in exercise-induced asthma if no bronchodilator was given as pre-treatment.[64] Still, also after regular treatment, the protective effect of a single dose of salbutamol was substantial.[64] Overall, these data further argue that short-acting β_2 agonists should be used only as needed.

Risks with Regular Use of β_2 Agonists Regular use of β_2 agonists has been associated with worsening of asthma and asthma deaths, especially in New Zealand.[65–67] Thus, a strong association was found between the amount of use of β_2 agonists with the risk of asthma death. Importantly, this association was strongest with the use of fenoterol, which is a more efficacious formulation causing more pronounced side-effects compared with the otherwise used β_2 agonists, such as terbutaline and salbutamol.[68] It has also been argued that the association between the use of β_2 agonists and death in asthma is due to confounding factors, such as higher use of β_2 agonists in patients with severe asthma. Thus, the asthma severity and not the use of drug was the cause of the association with asthma death.[69] Importantly, with inhaled glucocorticoids, the morbidity of asthma is strongly reduced, as well as the risk of asthma deaths.[70–73] The end of the New Zealand asthma death epidemic was also associated with increased use of this type of treatment.[74] This is further supported by the findings that the number of admissions to the hospital due to asthma is strongly reduced when prescription of inhaled glucocorticoids is increased in a population.[75] Thus, it seems to be more important to implement the use of inhaled glucocortcoids in asthma, than to reduce the use of inhaled β_2 agonists.

Tolerance to Short-Acting β_2 Agonists The use of short-acting β_2 agonists as regular treatment has been associated with the induction of tolerance in asthmatic patients. This is not very obvious when evaluating the bronchodilating effects of, for example, salbutamol before and after a period of regular treatment, whereas the side-effects of this treatment show pronounced tolerance (thus fewer side-effects during regular treatment).[31,76–78] However, it seems clearer that regular treatment with salbutamol or terbutaline decrease the protective effect that these drugs have on different provocation models, such as inhaled methacholine, exercise, adenosine or allergen.[64,79–82] Thus, a fixed dose of a short-acting β_2 agonists will to some extent shift the dose–response curve to all of these challenges

after a period of regular β_2 agonist treatment. The tolerance to β_2 agonists is localized to bronchial smooth muscle in the studies of protective effect on methacholine responsiveness, since the dominant mode of action of this bronchoconstrictor is direct bronchial smooth muscle contraction. In the case of adenosine- and allergen-induced bronchoconstriction, part of the inhibitory effect of β_2 agonists may be on the mast cell, and therefore the reduced bronchoprotective effect of such a drug during regular treatment may largely be due to tolerance in mast cells.[81,82] Overall, the tolerance seems to be more pronounced for the mast-cell mediated pathways (adenosine), compared with the direct smooth muscle effect (methacholine).[81] Again, these studies argue against the regular use of short-acting β_2 agonists four times daily in asthma, whereas the effectiveness of these drugs as rescue medication is without question.

β_2 Agonists in Acute Asthma The most important first-line treatment in cases of severe acute asthma in the emergency/casualty ward, as well as for ambulatory patients, is inhaled β_2 agonists such as salbutamol.[58,83–91] The drugs are usually given by nebulizer, although patients with mild symptoms could perhaps also use powder inhalers or pMDI.[92–95] Inhaled β_2 agonists will generally give rapid reversal of bronchoconstriction in most patients with severe asthma exacerbation, and in some studies it has also been shown that repeated inhalations will result in additional improvement of lung function,[96] but more pronounced side-effects.[97] Inhalation with a β_2 agonists should be used as addition to anti-inflammatory therapy, for example i.v. or oral glucocorticoids.[98–103] The role of inhaled anticholinergics in the treatment of acute asthma is discussed below, in a separate section. Inhaled β_2 agonists are often at least as effective, and safer, than i.v. administration of theophylline,[104] which should be used as a second choice.

β_2 Agonist Isomers–Clinical Effects It has been suggested that treatment with the racemate (mixture) of β_2 agonists such as salbutamol may be less safe than treatment with the single R isomer.[26,105–109] Most salbutamol formulations consist of a racemate of the two types of salbutamol (50% R- and 50% S-salbutamol), but recently the single active isomer, R-salbutamol, has been released in some countries for the treatment of asthma.[109] It has been argued that the S-form of salbutamol may be responsible for some of the detrimental effects of salbu-tamol, such as some worsening of bronchial respons-iveness.[107,108] However, recently it has been clarified that the S-salbutamol component does not cause worsening of methacholine responsiveness in asthmatic patients, and that half the total dose of R-salbutamol is as effective as racemic salbutamol.[110] In the same study it was shown that R- and racemic salbutamol were as effective in inducing tolerance to the protective effect of salbutamol on methacholine responsiveness, whereas the S-form was inert in this respect. Lastly, broncho-dilation induced by R- and racemate salbutamol are equipotent, with no signs of any detrimental effects on lung function with the S-form of the molecule.[55] Thus, at this time there seems to be no obvious advantage in using pure R-salbutamol versus the racemic mixture in the treatment of clinical asthma.[109]

Long-acting β_2 Agonists

One of the most important recent improvements in the treatment of asthma has been the introduction of the two inhaled long-acting β_2 agonists, salmeterol and for-moterol.[111–116] Both of these drugs are effective β_2 ago-nists with duration of action for up to at least 12 hours, compared with the 4–5 hour duration of salbutamol. Salmeterol was designed for inhalation, but formoterol was initially an oral bronchodilator invented in Japan, which was, however, shown to be much more long-acting when given by inhalation.[113]

Pharmacology of Formoterol and Salmeterol Salmeterol and formoterol have several similarities in their phar-macological behaviour, but also some substantial differences. Firstly, both drugs are highly lipophilic (Fig. 21.1), but salmeterol is more lipophilic than for-moterol.[117–119] In airway smooth muscle preparations it has been found that salmeterol has a slower onset of action compared with both salbutamol and formoterol, whereas formoterol is almost as rapid in onset as salbu-tamol.[120–122] However, salmeterol and formoterol have very similar duration of action in asthma patients, despite formoterol having a slightly shorter duration of action than salmeterol *in vitro*.[121–124]

The mechanisms of action at the receptor level are somewhat different for formoterol and salmeterol compared with short acting β_2 agonists. Because of its lipophilicity, salmeterol will very rapidly enter into the lipid bilayer of the cell membrane, and probably organize itself along the phospholipids, since it is of similar length as half of the cell membrane thickness (Fig. 21.3). It therefore seems that salmeterol will enter the β_2 receptor from the cell membrane, through the transmembrane domains of the receptor. This is in sharp contrast to other β_2 agonists such as salbutamol, which will enter the receptor from the extracellular space only. Formoterol is not as lipophilic as salme-terol, and will therefore enter the receptor both from the extracellular space, as well as from the cell mem-brane,[118,119,125] which may explain its more rapid onset of action[121,126] (Fig. 21.4). The long durations of action of both formoterol and salmeterol are likely to be explained by both of these drugs are stored in the cell membrane lipid bilayer, in close vicinity to the β_2 recep-tor, allowing them to enter the receptor and reach the active site of the receptor by diffusion laterally, through openings in the transmembrane domains of the recep-tor.[118,125] For salmeterol, an additional mechanism for the long duration of effect has been suggested. In principle, it is argued that the long lipophilic arm of salmeterol (Fig. 21.1) interacts with a specific binding region *within* the β_2 receptor, reducing the possibility of salmeterol leaving the receptor, instead allowing the active portion of the salmeterol molecule to re-engage with the active site of the receptor region (the exosite hypothesis).[125,127–129]

Another potentially important difference between salmeterol and formoterol is that salmeterol is a partial agonist in relation to formoterol. Thus, salmeterol has some intrinsic activity on the β_2 receptor, but does not cause a full smooth muscle dilatation compared with relatively full agonists such as salbutamol or for-moterol.[123] For a pharmacological agent, this would also mean that pre-treatment with the partial agonist could have the capacity to reduce the effect of a full agonist. Such an effect has indeed been shown with salmeterol *in vitro* in relation to several other β_2 agonists.[130–133] In these studies salmeterol acts as an antagonist of other β_2 agonists (blocker of receptor). One study in asthmatic patients suggests that salmeterol may also be clinically a partial agonist in relation to formoterol. In a randomized and blinded study, it was shown that high doses of formoterol result in greater protection against methacholine-induced bronchoconstriction than does salmeterol.[134] Thus, salmeterol showed a maximal bronchoprotective effect of approximately 2.5 doubling doses of methacholine at 250 μg, with no additional effect at 500 μg. By contrast, formoterol showed dose-related protective effects of at least 4.7 doubling doses,

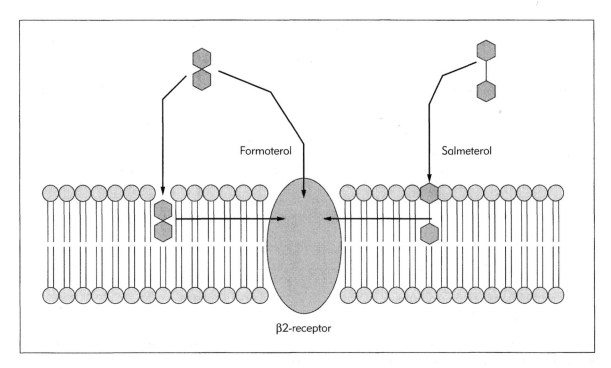

FIGURE 21.3: Salmeterol and formoterol are both long-acting β_2 agonists with slightly different mechanisms of action, and slightly different pharmacological profiles. Formoterol is more rapid in its onset, and salmeterol is slower. The duration of effect in man is similar for both drugs, although the duration of effect seems to be more dose-related for formoterol. The hypothesis for differences in effects are based on the different degree of lipophilicity of the two drugs. Formoterol is less lipophilic than salmeterol, and is proposed to be able to enter the β_2 receptor from the extracellular space. Formoterol will also enter the cell membrane, which will function as a depot of drug. Salmeterol is likely to very rapidly enter the cell membrane, without being able to enter the β_2 receptor from the extracellular space. Both formoterol and salmeterol enter the β_2 receptor also from the cell membrane layer, which explains the long duration of effect of these drugs. (Adapted from Refs 118, 119, 125.)

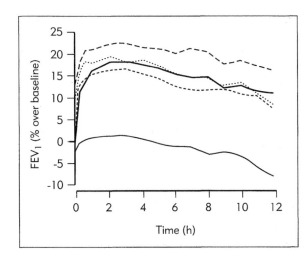

FIGURE 21.4: Onset of action and duration effect of formoterol and salmeterol evaluated in asthmatic patients with reversible airflow obstruction. The study was double-blind and cross-over. Salmeterol had a slower onset of action than formoterol, but the offset of action from maximum effect seem to be similar for salmeterol and all doses of formoterol. Salmeterol 50 µg seems to be equivalent to approximately 9 µg of formoterol. Salmeterol was given by Diskus, and formoterol by Aerolizer. ——salmeterol 50 µg; ----formoterol 6 µg; ········formoterol 12 µg; --- formoterol 24 µg; ——placebo. (From Palmqvist M et al. Inhaled dry-powder formoterol and salmeterol in asthmatic patients: onset of action, duration of effect and potency. *Eur Respir J* 1997; 10: 2484–9, with permission.[121])

with no evidence of a maximum being reached at 120 µg (Fig. 21.5). This higher maximal efficacy of formoterol compared with salmeterol was associated with a higher tremor score on the days with formoterol treatment. It could be concluded from this study that salmeterol is a partial agonist in relation to formoterol in human airways *in vivo*, although the clinical relevance for this remains unclear. Several theoretical consequences of using a partial agonist should be mentioned. Firstly, it is possible that some patients require a full agonist to have any clinical effect. One such case has been described,[135] but it is not clear how common this problem is in a large group of patients. Secondly, a partial agonist could theoretically attenuate the bronchodilating effects of a relatively fuller agonist such as salbutamol.[133] However, no data from asthmatic patients evaluating such a possibility have been published. The implication of a putative finding of salmeterol attenuating salbutamol would be that salmeterol could be detrimental in acute severe asthma, since the effect of nebulized salbutamol could be attenuated. However, this does not seem to be the case, since patients treated with salmeterol do not have reduced effects of salbutamol when experiencing an exacerbation of asthma.[136]

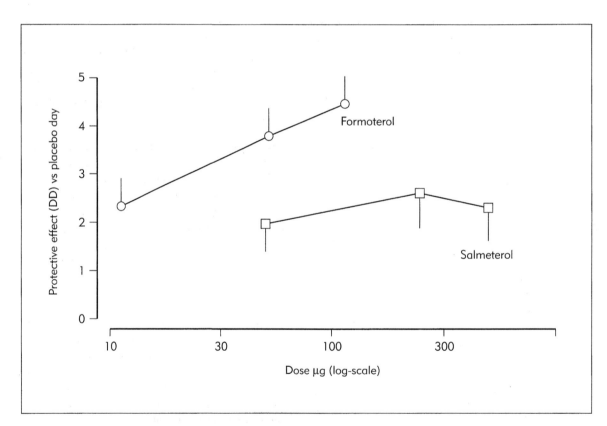

FIGURE 21.5: The degree of protective effect of salmeterol and formoterol on methacholine responsiveness in asthmatic patients. Salmeterol has a maximal protecting effect at 250 µg with no additional effect at 500 µg. Formoterol on the other hand had a continuing dose dependent protective effect all the way up to 120 µg, which was significantly higher than the maximal protective effect of salmeterol. These data show that salmeterol is a partial agonist in relation to formoterol in asthmatic patients *in vivo*, but also that high doses of drugs need to be used to document this difference. (From Palmqvist M, Ibsen T, Mellen A, Lötvall J. Comparison of the relative efficacy of formoterol and salmeterol in asthmatic patients. *Am J Respir Crit Care Med* 1999; 160 (1): 244–9, with permission[134]. Official Journal of the American Thoracic Association. ©American Lung Association.)

Large Multi-Centre Studies Many large multicentre studies have documented the clinical efficacy of both salmeterol and formoterol in asthma patients. Thus, regular treatment with either salmeterol or formoterol produces better control of asthma than salbutamol taken four times daily, using parameters such as lung function, extra bronchodilator use, and asthma symptoms.[137–143] Furthermore, quality of life is improved, as indicated by studies of salmeterol versus placebo.[144]

Long Acting β_2 Agonists as Addition to Inhaled Glucocorticoids A group of asthma patients which is sometimes difficult to treat are those who have symptoms despite adequate treatment with inhaled glucocorticoids. In these patients it seems more effective to add long-acting β_2 agonists rather than increase the dose of inhaled glucocorticoid.[41,42,145] For adding salmeterol, the data are conclusive for improvement in lung function[41,145] (Fig. 21.6), and for adding formoterol it has also been shown that exacerbations of asthma are reduced.[42] Thus, it seems that combining long-acting β_2 agonists with inhaled glucocorticoids gives additional benefit to inhaled glucocorticoids alone. One of these combination treatments is therefore now available with both drugs in one inhaler (salmeterol and fluticasone in the Diskus),[44] although no clear advantage of the combined inhaler versus the concurrent treatment (different inhalers for each drug) have been documented.

It has also been suggested that inhaled long-acting β_2 agonists reduce the required dose of inhaled glucocorticoid.[146] However, tapering inhaled glucocorticoids in patients with concomitant treatment with long-acting β_2 agonists is difficult, since it may be parallel with increased inflammatory processes, despite symptoms being well-controlled.[147] Thus, it cannot be excluded that long-acting β_2 agonists may block the symptoms of worsened asthmatic inflammation,[148] and it is therefore important to maintain an effective dose of inhaled glucocorticoid in patients treated with either inhaled formoterol or salmeterol.

Clinical Comparisons of Salmeterol and Formoterol Few direct comparisons of formoterol and salmeterol have been performed in large patient groups.[149] Overall, smaller clinical studies suggest that 50 μg of salmeterol seems to be equipotent and equally as effective as 12 μg of formoterol;[121,134] this seems to be confirmed in a single dose comparison.[149] However, potency comparisons of formoterol and salmeterol in large patient groups are lacking. The two differences that may be of clinical significance are the more rapid onset of action of formoterol than of salmeterol, and the higher efficacy of formoterol compared with salmeterol (Figure 21.5).[134,150] Because salmeterol is a partial agonist with slow onset of action it is not suitable for rescue medication in asthma,[151] whereas formoterol theoretically could be used in such a way.[152] However, large long-term studies should be performed to document the benefits of using formoterol instead of short-acting β_2 agonists in such a way, from efficacy, safety and pharmacoeconomic perspectives.

Tolerance to Long-Acting β_2 Agonists Regular treatment with the long-acting β_2 agonists salmeterol and formoterol will result in reduced effectiveness of the treatment, as does regular treatment with short-acting β_2 agonists.[79–82,153] The tolerance is not very obvious

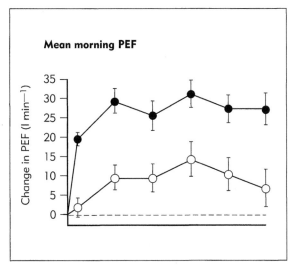

Mean morning PEF

FIGURE 21.6: Change in PEF over a period of treatment with salmeterol in a patient group that had symptoms despite low dose of inhaled glucocorticoid (beclomethasone). The effect of salmeterol was significantly better than doubling the dose of inhaled glucocorticoid. ● Salmeterol/ BDP, ○ Higher-dose BDP. (From Greening AP, Ind PW, Northfield M et al. Added salmeterol versus higher-dose corticosteroid in asthma patients with symptoms an existing inhaled corticosteroid *Lancet* 1994; 344 (8917): 219–24, ©The Lancet Ltd. 1994.[41])

for the bronchodilating effects of short-acting β_2 agonists during regular treatement with salmeterol.[154–157] However, in a large multicentre study evaluating the effect of regular formoterol, baseline lung function was higher after the first doses of drugs, compared with later during regular treatment.[42] Despite this finding on lung function, it is important to note that the formoterol treatment reduced the number of exacerbations of asthma in the same study.[42] There is more evidence that regular long-acting β_2 agonist treatment causes a decrease in the protective effect of these drugs on provoked bronchoconstriction, induced by methacholine,[153] exercise,[158–160] or allergen.[161]

Long-Acting β_2 Agonists versus Anti-Leukotrienes It has recently been shown that an anti-leukotriene is as efficacious as salmeterol in attenuating exercise-induced bronchoconstriction in asthmatic patients. However, the effect of salmeterol is reduced during regular treatment, whereas the protective effect in the group treated with the anti-leukotriene remained stable during regular treatment.[162] Thus, it was proposed that anti-leukotrienes might be more effective than salmeterol in protecting against exercise-induced asthma in the long term. However, it is not clear whether the very high efficacy of a short-acting β_2 agonist on this type of reaction could override the reduced protection seen after regular salmeterol.[61] In addition, large multicentre studies, specifically comparing these treatments, must be performed to give more information on whether long-acting β_2 agonists or anti-leukotrienes are preferred for addition to inhaled glucocorticoids. It is also possible that specific patient groups could be selected for either treatment, but it is not known to date how such selection should be performed. The only reasonable alternative seems to be to test one drug at a time in each patient.

ANTICHOLINERGICS

Mechanisms of Action

Anticholinergics have been used as bronchodilators for several hundred years in Europe. Asthma cigarettes made from *Datura stramonium* (Thornapple) were already marketed in the early 19th century in the UK, although even earlier use of anticholinergic remedies has been documented.[163] Anticholinergic drugs block bronchoconstriction, and perhaps also mucus secretion, induced by endogenous acetylchoine released from parasympathetic nerves in the airways. Acetylcholine induces bronchoconstriction by activating muscarinic M_3 receptors, which are present on airway smooth muscle.[164,165] Two additional types of muscarinic receptors are also present in airways, including M_1 in parasympathetic ganglia in the bronchial wall, and M_2 pre-junctionally on post-ganglionic cholinergic nerves. M_1 receptors are excitatory in ganglia, and M_2 receptors are inhibitory (they reduce acetylcholine release). However, the M_3 receptor is the most important receptor for bronchoconstriction, since blocking it will attenuate all cholinergic responses in the airways.[165,166]

Clinical Effects of Ipratropium Bromide

The most commonly used anticholinergic for asthma treatment is ipratropium bromide, which is used as inhaled aerosol.[167] This drug will cause bronchodilation with a slightly slower onset of action than salbutamol, but the duration of effect is slightly longer.[168] Ipratropium bromide will only reverse one endogenous mediator of airflow obstruction, which is acetylcholine released from nerves, and will not affect bronchoconstriction induced by other mediators, such as leukotrienes. Therefore, it is plausible to hypothesize that functional antagonists of bronchial smooth muscle contractions, such as β_2 agonist, would result in more pronounced bronchodilatation. This is also a finding in several studies,[169–171] as well as in a previously unpublished blinded cross-over study performed by K. Svedmyr and N. Svedmyr in 1984 (data kindly supplied by the investigators; Fig. 21.7). Thus, a full β_2 agonist is more efficacious as a bronchodilator in asthmatic patients. In patients with COPD, it seems that anticholinergics have a better efficacy than in asthmatic patients, probably because the parasympathetic tone contributes to the airway narrowing in these patients.[172,173] However, the maximal effect of a β_2 agonist is still higher in most studies, as is the improvement in bronchial responsiveness.[173–175] For example, inhaled anticholinergics are less effective for exercise-induced asthma compared with β_2 agonists.[176]

The side-effects of inhaled ipratropium bromide are mainly localized to the mouth and airways, with bad taste and dryness as the most commonly reported side-effects. Quite high doses of inhaled ipratropium bromide (up to 1000 µg by nebulization) have been given, without any effects on pupil size, accommodation or intraocular pressure, or on systemic blood pressure.[177–179] Thus, the side-effect profile seems to be better with this type of

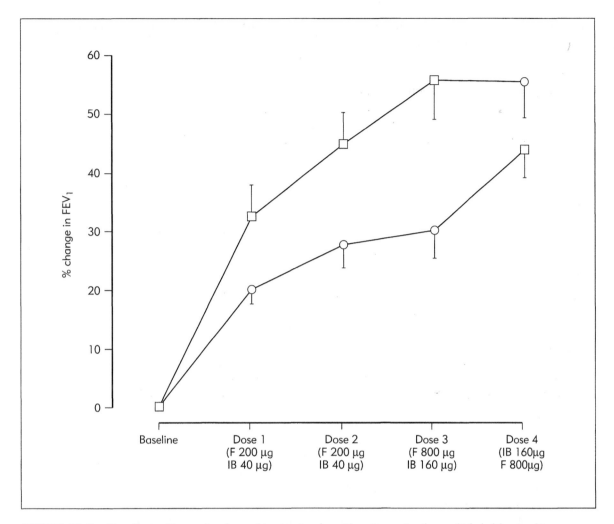

FIGURE 21.7: The effects of increasing doses of ipratropium bromide vs increasing doses of inhaled fenoterol in asthmatic patients with substantial reversible airflow obstruction. With inhaled ipratropium 160 µg, a maximal improvement in lung function is seen, whereas inhaled fenoterol causes significantly better maximal improvement in lung function. Adding fenoterol after the ipratropium bromide dose–response curve improves lung function further, whereas adding ipratropium bromide after the fenoterol dose–response curve does not further improve lung function. Open squares, fenoterol; open circles, pratropium bromide. (Unpublished data from Karin and Nils Svedmyr, presented with their kind permission. The study was performed in 1984.)

drug than with inhaled β_2 agonists, which should be kept in mind when high doses are required.

Oxitropium bromide is another anticholinergic bronchodilator, which was developed in the 1970s, and has, compared with ipratropium bromide, relatively similar pharmacological and clinical properties, although some advantages have been suggested.[180–185]

Tiotropium Bromide

A long-acting inhaled anticholinergic drug, tiotropium bromide,[186–189] has been developed for inhalation use in patients with COPD. It seems that this drug has effect in the airways over 24 hours, and is thus much more long-acting than ipratropium bromide.[187] However, no large-scale clinical studies have been published as full papers to date, and the drug is not registered for clinical use in any country in early 2000.

Anticholinergics in Acute Asthma

The addition of an anticholinergic to high-dose nebulized β[2] agonists in the treatment of acute asthma and exacerbations of COPD does not show any clear additional benefit, at least not on lung function measurements.[190–193] Still, this type of combination treatment is often used in the emergency/casualty ward, because any putative additional effect of the anticholinergic component in an individual patient is without major side-effects.

The combination of salbutamol and ipratropium bromide in one inhaler has recently become available in some countries, and it is argued that a reduced dose of salbutamol will lead to reduced side-effects, with maintained efficacy.[194] However, salbutamol alone is highly effective and well-tolerated in most patients.

XANTHINES

Mechanisms

The most commonly used xanthines are theophylline and aminophylline, which act primarily by increasing the concentration of cAMP intracellularly through reduced degradation of this molecule. This is induced by xanthines inhibiting phosphodiesterases (PD).[195,196] The PD isozymes that are believed to be involved in bronchodilation are type III and IV, whereas the inhibitory effect of theophylline on PDIV has been suggested to exert some anti-inflammatory activity. Theophylline has been suggested to have additional mechanisms of action, including adenosine receptor inhibition.[197,198]

For maintenance treatment, xanthines are preferably given as slow-release tablets. With such treatment, these drugs can be given as a twice daily regimen. However, xanthines have a quite narrow therapeutic ratio. That is, if the dose is increased slightly, or if the concentration of drug in the blood is increased by, for example, interaction with some other drug, severe side-effects may occur. These side-effects include nausea, hypotension, cardiac arrhythmias, and in severe cases seizures.[199–201] Fatal side-effects are not uncommon in places where this treatment is used,[202] and can also occur in children.[203] The narrow therapeutic ratio of xanthines, in combination with the high effectiveness and safety of inhaled β[2] agonist, has limited the use of

this oral bronchodilator treatment to individuals with difficulties in using inhalation, or other uncommon reasons. If this type of drug is selected for an individual patient, careful monitoring of serum concentrations should be implemented.

Toxicology

Intoxication with theophylline should be treated promptly, because of the risk of fatalities. Intravenous access should be established rapidly, and blood taken for electrolyte investigation and measurement of theophylline concentration. Gastric lavage may be performed, and activated charcoal should be given. ECG should be continuously monitored. Charcoal haemoperfusion can also be used in some cases of severe intoxication with life-threatening complications.[200,201]

Importantly, it has been shown that long-acting β[2] agonists such as salmeterol are superior to theophylline in the treatment of chronic asthma, in patients with or without concomitant inhaled glucocorticoid treatment.[204–208]

Anti-inflammatory Activity

In recent years, some experiments in asthma patients have suggested that xanthines, especially theophylline, may have some anti-inflammatory activity in asthmatic patients, as well as in inflammatory cells.[196,209] Thus, it seems that an additional mechanism by which theophylline exerts anti-asthma effects is some mild anti-inflammatory activity.[210] In inflammatory cells, there are several phosphodiesterase enzymes present (PD), which may increase intracellular cAMP if inhibited.[211,212] Novel phosphodiesterase inhibitors have been developed, and it has been suggested that these have more anti-inflammatory activity than theophylline by exerting inhibition of mainly PDIV. However, preliminary clinical studies of such drugs in asthmatic patients have not suggested any improved therapeutic ratio compared with theophylline. Furthermore, the anti-inflammatory effect of inhaled glucocorticoids is obviously greater.

Theophylline in Acute Asthma

Theophylline can be used by i.v. route in patients with acute severe asthma, but should be selected as secondary treatment when nebulized β[2] agonists show insufficient effectiveness. Dosing of i.v. theophylline should always be done with care, but especially so in patients with previous regular oral treatment, since the concentration of drug may be high already at admission. Injections should be given slowly, because of the cardiotoxicity of the drug.

SUMMARY

Overall, for the treatment of asthma, specific β_2 agonists still remain the most effective and most important bronchodilator treatment more than 30 years after their introduction into the marketplace. These drugs are more effective than both inhaled anticholinergics and systemic theophylline in patients with asthma, and much safer than theophylline. The addition of long-acting β_2 agonists to inhaled glucocorticoids in asthma treatment results in long-term improvement in lung function, but has also resulted in improved quality of life and a reduced number of asthma exacerbations.[42,144] Importantly, the risk associated with β_2 agonists seems to be strongly reduced when inhaled glucocorticoid treatment is effective.[42,65]

KEY POINTS

1 β_2 agonists relax bronchial smooth muscle through several intracellular signals, including G-protein associated cAMP production. β_2 agonists may also have some anti-inflammatory effects, including inhibition of plasma exudation, and perhaps also by inhibiting some cellular inflammatory processes. Inhaled glucocorticoids are, however, much more effective in inhibiting airway inflammation than β_2 agonists.

2 The preferred route of treatment with bronchodilators is by inhalation, either by pressurised meter dose (pMDI) inhalers or dry powder inhalers (DPI).

3 The long acting β_2 agonists, salmeterol and formoterol, cause bronchodilation for longer than 12 hours and provide 24 hour coverage when given by regular dosing twice daily. Formoterol has a more rapid onset than salmeterol, and has pharmacologically higher efficacy, and can therefore from a pharmacological standpoint be used as needed.

4 Side effects of β_2 agonists include skeletal muscle tremor and palpitation. Cardiovascular side effects seldom cause risk to the patient, unless the patient has concomitant severe heart disease.

5 β_2 agonists cause tolerance when given as regular treatment. This is seen, for example, by the reduction of side effects such as tremor and palpitation. In the airways, the tolerance is more subtle, but is possible to document by reduced protection on bronchial hyperresponsiveness. Still, clinical efficacy is not reduced during regular treatment, and for example asthma exacerbations are reduced with regular treatment with long acting β_2 agonists.

6 Anticholinergic drugs such as ipratropium bromide block only the endogenous effects of locally released acetylcholine, and will not block bronchoconstriction induced by other mediators. The main effect is localised to M_3 receptors on bronchial smooth muscle. These types of drugs seem to be useful mainly in COPD.

7 Theophylline and other xanthines are considered to act through a non-specific inhibition of phosphodiesterases, but have a narrow therapeutic ratio with high risk of intoxication. Long-acting β_2 agonists are generally preferred as additional treatment to inhaled glucocorticoids.

REFERENCES

1. Ahlquist RP. The adrenergic receptor. *J Pharm Sci* 1966; 55 (4): 359–67.

2. Lands AM, Arnold A, McAuliff JP, Luduena FP, Brown TG Jr. Differentiation of receptor systems activated by sympathomimetic amines. *Nature* 1967; 214 (88): 597–8.

3. Hardman JG, Limbird LE. *Goodman and Gilman's The Pharmacological Basis of Therapeutics*, 9th edn. Maidenhead: McGraw-Hill, 1995.

4. Cascieri MA, Fong TM, Strader CD. Molecular characterization of a common binding site for small molecules within the transmembrane domain of G-protein coupled receptors. *J Pharmacol Toxicol Methods* 1995; 33 (4): 179–85.

5. Strader CD, Sigal IS, Candelore MR, Rands E, Hill WS, Dixon RA. Conserved aspartic acid residues 79 and 113 of the beta-adrenergic receptor have different roles in receptor function. *J Biol Chem* 1988; 263 (21): 10267–71.

6. Tota MR, Strader CD. Characterization of the binding domain of the beta-adrenergic receptor with the fluorescent antagonist carazolol. Evidence for a buried ligand binding site. *J Biol Chem* 1990; 265 (28): 16891–7.

7. O'Dowd BF, Hnatowich M, Regan JW, Leader WM, Caron MG, Lefkowitz RJ. Site-directed mutagenesis of the cytoplasmic domains of the human beta 2-adrenergic receptor. Localization of regions involved in G protein- receptor coupling. *J Biol Chem* 1988; 263 (31): 15985–92.

8. O'Dowd BF, Hnatowich M, Caron MG, Lefkowitz RJ, Bouvier M. Palmitoylation of the human beta 2-adrenergic receptor. Mutation of Cys341 in the carboxyl tail leads to an uncoupled nonpalmitoylated form of the receptor. *J Biol Chem* 1989; 264 (13): 7564–9.

9. Liggett SB, Caron MG, Lefkowitz RJ, Hnatowich M. Coupling of a mutated form of the human beta 2-adrenergic receptor to Gi and Gs. Requirement for multiple cytoplasmic domains in the coupling process. *J Biol Chem* 1991; 266 (8): 4816–21.

10. Mayer SE. Adenyl cyclase as a component of the adrenergic receptor. In: Molecular properties of drug receptors. *Ciba Found Symp* 1970: 43–58.

11. Barnes P. Effects of beta-agonists on airway effector cells. In: Pauwels R, O'Byrne P (eds). *Beta 2-Agonists in Asthma Treatment*. New York: Marcel Dekker, 1997: 35–66.

12. Chung S, Soh H, Uhm D. Beta-adrenergic modulation of maxi-K channels in vascular smooth muscle via Gi through a membrane-delimited pathway. *Pflugers Arch* 1999; 437 (3): 508–10.

13. Nara M, Dhulipala PD, Wang YX, Kotlikoff MI. Reconstitution of beta-adrenergic modulation of large conductance, calcium-activated potassium (maxi-K) channels in *Xenopus* oocytes. Identification of the camp-dependent protein kinase phosphorylation site. *J Biol Chem* 1998; 273 (24): 14920–4.

14. Garcia-Calvo M, Knaus HG, Garcia ML, Kaczorowski GJ, Kempner ES. Functional unit size of the charybdotoxin receptor in smooth muscle. *Proc Natl Acad Sci USA* 1994; 91 (11): 4718–22.

15. Fan SF, Wang S, Kao CY. Enhancement of beta-adrenergic receptor activation of maxi-K+ channels by GM1 ganglioside. *Biochem Biophys Res Commun* 1994; 200 (3): 1341–5.

16. Knaus HG, Garcia-Calvo M, Kaczorowski GJ, Garcia ML. Subunit composition of the high conductance calcium-activated potassium channel from smooth muscle, a representative of the mSlo and slowpoke family of potassium channels. *J Biol Chem* 1994; 269 (6): 3921–4.

17. Fleisch JH, Titus E. The prevention of isoproterenol desensitization and isoproterenol reversal. *J Pharmacol Exp Ther* 1972; 181 (3): 425–33.

18. Marsh JD, Barry WH, Smith TW. Desensitization to the inotropic effect of isoproterenol in cultured ventricular cells. *J Pharmacol Exp Ther* 1982; 223 (1): 60–7.

19. Sibley DR, Benovic JL, Caron MG, Lefkowitz RJ. Regulation of transmembrane signaling by receptor phosphorylation. *Cell* 1987; 48 (6): 913–22.

20. Yu SS, Lefkowitz RJ, Hausdorff WP. Beta-adrenergic receptor sequestration. A potential mechanism of receptor resensitization. *J Biol Chem* 1993; 268 (1): 337–41.

21. Collins S, Caron MG, Lefkowitz RJ. From ligand

binding to gene expression: new insights into the regulation of G-protein-coupled receptors. *Trends Biochem Sci* 1992; 17 (1): 37–9.

22. Nishikawa M, Mak JC, Shirasaki H, Barnes PJ. Differential down-regulation of pulmonary beta 1- and beta 2- adrenoceptor messenger RNA with prolonged *in vivo* infusion of isoprenaline. *Eur J Pharmacol* 1993; 247 (2): 131–8.

23. Martinez FD, Graves PE, Baldini M, Solomon S, Erickson R. Association between genetic polymorphisms of the beta 2-adrenoceptor and response to albuterol in children with and without a history of wheezing. *J Clin Invest* 1997; 100 (12): 3184–8.

24. Tan S, Hall IP, Dewar J, Dow E, Lipworth B. Association between beta 2-adrenoceptor polymorphism and susceptibility to bronchodilator desensitisation in moderately severe stable asthmatics. *Lancet* 1997; 350 (9083): 995–9.

25. Hartley D, Middlemiss D. Absolute configuration of the optical isomers of salbutamol. *J Med Chem* 1971; 14 (9): 995–6.

26. Brittain RT, Farmer JB, Marshall RJ. Some observations on the -adrenoceptor agonist properties of the isomers of salbutamol. *Br J Pharmacol* 1973; 48 (1): 144–7.

27. Löfdahl CG, Svedmyr N. Selectivity of beta-adrenergic stimulating and blocking agents. *Eur J Respir Dis* (suppl.) 1984; 136: 101–13.

28. Newton GE, Azevedo ER, Parker JD. Inotropic and sympathetic responses to the intracoronary infusion of a beta 2-receptor agonist: a human *in vivo* study. *Circulation* 1999; 99 (18): 2402–7.

29. Hool LC, Harvey RD. Role of beta 1- and beta 2-adrenergic receptors in regulation of Cl− and Ca²⁺ channels in guinea pig ventricular myocytes. *Am J Physiol* 1997; 273 (4 Pt 2): H1669–76.

30. Windom HH, Burgess CD, Siebers RW *et al*. The pulmonary and extrapulmonary effects of inhaled beta-agonists in patients with asthma. *Clin Pharmacol Ther* 1990; 48 (3): 296–301.

31. Svedmyr NL, Larsson SA, Thiringer GK. Development of "resistance" in beta-adrenergic

receptors of asthmatic patients. *Chest* 1976; 69 (4): 479–83.

32. Speizer FE, Doll R, Heaf P, Strang LB. Investigation into use of drugs preceding death from asthma. *Br Med J* 1968; 1 (5588): 339–43.

33. Inman WH, Adelstein AM. Rise and fall of asthma mortality in England and Wales in relation to use of pressurised aerosols. *Lancet* 1969; 2 (7615): 279–85.

34. Tokuyama K, Lötvall JO, Löfdahl C-G, Barnes PJ, Chung KF. Inhaled formoterol inhibits histamine-induced airflow obstruction and airway microvascular leakage. *Euro J Pharmacol* 1991; 193: 35–39.

35. Whelan CJ, Johnson M. Inhibition by salmeterol of increased vascular permeability and granulocyte accumulation in guinea-pig lung and skin. *Br J Pharmacol* 1992; 105: 831–8.

36. Proud D, Reynolds CJ, Lichtenstein LM, Kagey-Sobotka A, Togias A. Intranasal salmeterol inhibits allergen-induced vascular permeability but not mast cell activation or cellular infiltration. *Clin Exp Allergy* 1998; 28 (7): 868–75.

37. O'Connor BJ, Fuller RW, Barnes PJ. Nonbronchodilator effects of inhaled beta 2 agonists. Greater protection against adenosine monophosphate- than methacholine-induced bronchoconstriction in asthma. *Am J Respir Crit Care Med* 1994; 150 (2): 381–7.

38. Tomioka K, Yamada T, Ida H. Anti-allergic activities of the beta-adrenoceptor stimulant formoterol (BD 40A). *Arch Int Pharmacodyn Ther* 1981; 250 (2): 279–92.

39. Holgate ST, Benyon RC, Howarth PH *et al*. Relationship between mediator release from human lung mast cells *in vitro* and *in vivo*. *Int Arch Allergy Appl Immunol* 1985; 77 (1–2): 47–56.

40. Cockcroft DW. Inhaled beta 2-agonists and airway responses to allergen. *J Allergy Clin Immunol* 1998; 102 (5): S96–9.

41. Greening AP, Ind PW, Northfield M, Shaw G. Added salmeterol versus higher-dose corticosteroid in asthma patients with symptoms on existing inhaled corticosteroid. Allen and Hanburys Limited UK Study Group. *Lancet* 1994; 344 (8917): 219–24.

42. Pauwels RA, Löfdahl CG, Postma DS *et al*. Effect of inhaled formoterol and budesonide on exacerbations of asthma. Formoterol and Corticosteroids Establishing Therapy (FACET) International Study Group [published erratum appears in *N Engl J Med* 1998 Jan 8; 338(2): 139]. *N Engl J Med* 1997; 337 (20): 1405–11.

43. Eickelberg O, Roth M, Lorx R *et al*. Ligand-independent activation of the glucocorticoid receptor by beta 2-adrenergic receptor agonists in primary human lung fibroblasts and vascular smooth muscle cells. *J Biol Chem* 1999; 274 (2): 1005–10.

44. Chapman KR, Ringdal N, Backer V, Palmqvist M, Saarelainen S, Briggs M. Salmeterol and fluticasone propionate (50/250 microg) administered via combination Diskus inhaler: as effective as when given via separate Diskus inhalers. *Can Respir J* 1999; 6 (1): 45–51.

45. Palmer KN, Diament ML. Effect of salbutamol on spirometry and blood–gas tensions in bronchial asthma. *Br Med J* 1969; 1 (635): 31–2.

46. Bass BH, Disney ME, Morrison-Smith J. Effect of salbutamol on respiratory function in children with asthma. *Lancet* 1969; 2 (7617): 438.

47. Tattersfield AE, McNicol MW. Salbutamol and isoproterenol. A double-blind trial to compare bronchodilator and cardiovascular activity. *N Engl J Med* 1969; 281 (24): 1323–6.

48. Palmer KN, Legge JS, Hamilton WF, Diament ML. Comparison of effect of salbutamol and isoprenaline on spirometry and blood-gas tensions in bronchial asthma. *Br Med J* 1970; 2 (700): 23–4.

49. Casterline CL, Evans R 3rd, Ward GW Jr. The effect of atropine and albuterol aerosols on the human bronchial response to histamine. *J Allergy Clin Immunol* 1976; 58 (5): 607–13.

50. Kraemer R, Duquenne D, Mossay C, Geubelle F. Mode of action of bronchodilating drugs on histamine-induced bronchoconstriction in asthmatic children. *Pediatr Res* 1981; 15 (11): 1433–8.

51. Chung KF, Snashall PD. Methacholine dose-response curves in normal and asthmatic man: effect of starting conductance and pharmacological antagonism. *Clin Sci* 1984; 66 (6): 665–73.

52. Larsson S, Svedmyr N. A comparison of two modes of administering beta 2-adrenoceptor stimulants in asthmatics: tablets and metered aerosol. *Scand J Respir Dis* (suppl.) 1977; 101: 79–83.

53. Svedmyr N, Thiringer G. The effects of salbutamol and isoprenaline on beta-receptors in patients with chronic obstructive lung disease. *Postgrad Med J* 1971; 47 (suppl.): 44–6.

54. Barnes PJ, Pride NB. Dose–response curves to inhaled beta-adrenoceptor agonists in normal and asthmatic subjects. *Br J Clin Pharmacol* 1983; 15 (6): 677–82.

55. Lötvall J, Palmqvist M, Arvidsson P, Mellén A, Ventresca P, Ward J. The therapeutic ratio of racemic-salbutamol is equivalent to R-salbutamol in asthmatic patients. *Eur Respir J* 1999 (abstract); (14) suppl 30: 1575.

56. Beveridge RC, Grunfeld AF, Hodder RV, Verbeek PR. *Guidelines for the emergency management of asthma in adults*. CAEP/CTS Asthma Advisory Committee. Canadian Association of Emergency Physicians and the Canadian Thoracic Society.

57. Bentur L, Canny GJ, Shields MD *et al*. Controlled trial of nebulized albuterol in children younger than 2 years of age with acute asthma. *Pediatrics* 1992; 89 (1): 133–7.

58. Becker AB, Nelson NA, Simons FE. Inhaled salbutamol (albuterol) vs injected epinephrine in the treatment of acute asthma in children. *J Pediatr* 1983; 102 (3): 465–9.

59. Parameswaran KN, Inman MD, Ekholm BP *et al*. Protection against methacholine bronchoconstriction to assess relative potency of inhaled beta 2-agonist. *Am J Respir Crit Care Med* 1999; 160 (1): 354–7.

60. Wong AG, O'Byrne PM, Lindbladh C, Inman MD, Stahl E, Hargreave FE. Dose-response protective effect of salbutamol on methacholine airway responsiveness using pressurized metered dose inhalers and Turbuhalers. *Can Respir J* 1998; 5 (2): 119–23.

61. Anderson SD, Seale JP, Rozea P, Bandler L, Theobald G, Lindsay DA. Inhaled and oral salbutamol in exercise-induced asthma. *Am Rev Respir Dis* 1976; 114 (3): 493–500.

62. Godfrey S, Konig P. Inhibition of exercise-induced asthma by different pharmacological pathways. *Thorax* 1976; 31 (2): 137–43.

63. Anderson S, Seale JP, Ferris L, Schoeffel R, Lindsay DA. An evaluation of pharmacotherapy for exercise-induced asthma. *J Allergy Clin Immunol* 1979; 64 (6 pt 2): 612–24.

64. Inman MD, O'Byrne PM. The effect of regular inhaled albuterol on exercise-induced bronchoconstriction. *Am J Respir Crit Care Med* 1996; 153 (1): 65–9.

65. Crane J, Pearce N, Flatt A *et al.* Prescribed fenoterol and death from asthma in New Zealand, 1981–83: case-control study. *Lancet* 1989; 1 (8644): 917–22.

66. Grainger J, Woodman K, Pearce N *et al.* Prescribed fenoterol and death from asthma in New Zealand, 1981–7: a further case-control study. *Thorax* 1991; 46 (2): 105–11.

67. Sears MR, Taylor DR, Print CG *et al.* Regular inhaled beta-agonist treatment in bronchial asthma. *Lancet* 1990; 336 (8728): 1391–6.

68. Lipworth BJ, Newnham DM, Clark RA, Dhillon DP, Winter JH, McDevitt DG. Comparison of the relative airways and systemic potencies of inhaled fenoterol and salbutamol in asthmatic patients. *Thorax* 1995; 50 (1): 54–61.

69. Rea HH, Garrett JE, Lanes SF, Birmann BM, Kolbe J. The association between asthma drugs and severe life-threatening attacks. *Chest* 1996; 110 (6): 1446–51.

70. Kerstjens HA, Brand PL, Hughes MD *et al.* A comparison of bronchodilator therapy with or without inhaled corticosteroid therapy for obstructive airways disease. Dutch Chronic Non-Specific Lung Disease Study Group. *N Engl J Med* 1992; 327 (20): 1413–9.

71. Ishihara K, Hasegawa T, Okazaki M *et al.* Long-term follow-up of patients with a history of near fatal episodes; can inhaled corticosteroids reduce the risk of death from asthma? *Intern Med* 1995; 34 (2): 77–80.

72. Guite HF, Dundas R, Burney PG. Risk factors for death from asthma, chronic obstructive pulmonary disease, and cardiovascular disease after a hospital admission for asthma. *Thorax* 1999; 54 (4): 301–7.

73. Sears MR. Worldwide trends in asthma mortality. *Bull Int Union Tuberc Lung Dis* 1991; 66 (2–3): 79–83.

74. Pearce N, Beasley R, Crane J, Burgess C, Jackson R. End of the New Zealand asthma mortality epidemic. *Lancet* 1995; 345 (8941): 41–4.

75. Wennergren G, Kristjansson S, Strannegard IL. Decrease in hospitalization for treatment of childhood asthma with increased use of antiinflammatory treatment, despite an increase in prevalence of asthma. *J Allergy Clin Immunol* 1996; 97 (3): 742–8.

76. Nelson HS, Raine D Jr, Doner HC, Posey WC. Subsensitivity to the bronchodilator action of albuterol produced by chronic administration. *Am Rev Respir Dis* 1977; 116 (5): 871–8.

77. Schuster A, Kozlik R, Reinhardt D. Influence of short- and long-term inhalation of salbutamol on lung function and beta 2-adrenoceptors of mononuclear blood cells in asthmatic children. *Eur J Pediatr* 1991; 150 (3): 209–13.

78. Larsson S, Svedmyr N, Thiringer G. Lack of bronchial beta adrenoceptor resistance in asthmatics during long-term treatment with terbutaline. *J Allergy Clin Immunol* 1977; 59 (2): 93–100.

79. Cockcroft DW, Swystun VA, Bhagat R. Interaction of inhaled beta 2 agonist and inhaled corticosteroid on airway responsiveness to allergen and methacholine. *Am J Respir Crit Care Med* 1995; 152 (5 Pt 1): 1485–9.

80. Yates DH, Kharitonov SA, Barnes PJ. An inhaled glucocorticoid does not prevent tolerance to the bronchoprotective effect of a long-acting inhaled beta 2-agonist [published erratum appears in *Am J Respir Crit Care Med* 1997 Apr; 155 (4): 1491]. *Am J Respir Crit Care Med* 1996; 154 (6 Pt 1): 1603–7.

81. O'Connor BJ, Aikman SL, Barnes PJ. Tolerance to the nonbronchodilator effects of inhaled beta 2-agonists in asthma. *N Engl J Med* 1992; 327 (17): 1204–8.

82. Cockcroft DW, McParland CP, Britto SA, Swystun VA, Rutherford BC. Regular inhaled salbutamol and airway responsiveness to allergen. *Lancet* 1993; 342 (8875): 833–7.

83. Cockcroft DW. Management of acute severe asthma. *Ann Allergy Asthma Immunol* 1995; 75 (2): 83–9; quiz 90–3.

84. Emerman CL, Cydulka RK, McFadden ER. Comparison of 2.5 vs 7.5 mg of inhaled albuterol in the treatment of acute asthma. *Chest* 1999; 115 (1): 92–6.

85. Webber BA, Collins JV, Branthwaite MA. Severe acute asthma: a comparison of three methods of inhaling salbutamol. *Br J Dis Chest* 1982; 76 (1): 69–74.

86. Williams S, Seaton A. Intravenous or inhaled salbutamol in severe acute asthma? *Thorax* 1977; 32 (5): 555–8.

87. Turpeinen M, Kuokkanen J, Backman A. Adrenaline and nebulized salbutamol in acute asthma. *Arch Dis Child* 1984; 59 (7): 666–8.

88. Leahy BC, Gomm SA, Allen SC. Comparison of nebulized salbutamol with nebulized ipratropium bromide in acute asthma. *Br J Dis Chest* 1983; 77 (2): 159–63.

89. Robertson CF, Smith F, Beck R, Levison H. Response to frequent low doses of nebulized salbutamol in acute asthma. *J Pediatr* 1985; 106 (4): 672–4.

90. Society BT. Guidelines for the management of asthma: a summary. British Thoracic Society and others [published erratum appears in *BMJ* 1993 Oct 23; 307(6911): 1054]. *BMJ* 1993; 306 (6880): 776–82.

91. Lowhagen O, Ekstrom L, Holmberg S, Wennerblom B, Rosenfeldt M. Experience of an emergency mobile asthma treatment programme. *Resuscitation* 1997; 35 (3): 243–7.

92. Tonnesen F, Laursen LC, Evald T, Stahl E, Ibsen TB. Bronchodilating effect of terbutaline powder in acute severe bronchial obstruction. *Chest* 1994; 105 (3): 697–700.

93. Nana A, Youngchaiyud P, Maranetra N *et al.* Beta 2-agonists administered by a dry powder inhaler can be used in acute asthma. *Respir Med* 1998; 92 (2): 167–72.

94. Robertson CF, Norden MA, Fitzgerald DA *et al.* Treatment of acute asthma: salbutamol via jet nebuliser vs spacer and metered dose inhaler. *J Paediatr Child Health* 1998; 34 (2): 142–6.

95. Morgan MD, Singh BV, Frame MH, Williams SJ. Terbutaline aerosol given through pear spacer in acute severe asthma. *Br Med J (Clin Res Ed)* 1982; 285 (6345): 849–50.

96. Noseda A, Yernault JC. Sympathomimetics in acute severe asthma: inhaled or parenteral, nebulizer or spacer? *Eur Respir J* 1989; 2 (4): 377–82.

97. Bodenhamer J, Bergstrom R, Brown D, Gabow P, Marx JA, Lowenstein SR. Frequently nebulized beta-agonists for asthma: effects on serum electrolytes. *Ann Emerg Med* 1992; 21 (11): 1337–42.

98. Wolfson DH, Nypaver MM, Blaser M, Hogan A, Evans R 3rd, Davis AT. A controlled trial of methylprednisolone in the early emergency department treatment of acute asthma in children. *Pediatr Emerg Care* 1994; 10 (6): 335–8.

99. Hatton MQ, Vathenen AS, Allen MJ, Davies S, Cooke NJ. A comparison of "abruptly stopping" with "tailing off" oral corticosteroids in acute asthma. *Respir Med* 1995; 89 (2): 101–4.

100. Deshpande A, McKenzie SA. Short course of steroids in home treatment of children with acute asthma. *Br Med J (Clin Res Ed)* 1986; 293 (6540): 169–71.

101. Littenberg B, Gluck EH. A controlled trial of methylprednisolone in the emergency treatment of acute asthma. *N Engl J Med* 1986; 314 (3): 150–2.

102. Shapiro GG, Furukawa CT, Pierson WE, Gardinier R, Bierman CW. Double-blind evaluation of methylprednisolone versus placebo for acute asthma episodes. *Pediatrics* 1983; 71 (4): 510–14.

103. Emerman CL, Cydulka RK. A randomized comparison of 100-mg vs 500-mg dose of methylprednisolone in the treatment of acute asthma. *Chest* 1995; 107 (6): 1559–63.

104. Swedish Society of Chest Medicine. High-dose inhaled versus intravenous salbutamol combined with theophylline in severe acute asthma. *Eur Respir J* 1990; 3 (2): 163–70.

105. Cockcroft DW, Swystun VA. Effect of single doses of S-salbutamol, R-salbutamol, racemic salbutamol, and placebo on the airway response to methacholine. *Thorax* 1997; 52 (10): 845–8.

106. Lipworth BJ, Clark DJ, Koch P, Arbeeny C. Pharmacokinetics and extrapulmonary beta 2

adrenoceptor activity of nebulised racemic salbutamol and its R and S isomers in healthy volunteers. *Thorax* 1997; 52 (10): 849–52.

107. Handley DA, McCullough JR, Crowther SD, Morley J. Sympathomimetic enantiomers and asthma. *Chirality* 1998; 10 (3): 262–72.

108. Handley D. The asthma-like pharmacology and toxicology of (S)-isomers of beta agonists. *J Allergy Clin Immunol* 1999; 104 (2 Pt 2): S69–76.

109. Waldeck B. Enantiomers of bronchodilating beta 2-adrenoceptor agonists: is there a cause for concern? *J Allergy Clin Immunol* 1999; 103 (5 Pt 1): 742–8.

110. Cockcroft DW, Davis BE, Swystun VA, Marciniuk DD. Tolerance to the bronchoprotective effect of beta 2-agonists: comparison of the enantiomers of salbutamol with racemic salbutamol and placebo. *J Allergy Clin Immunol* 1999; 103 (6): 1049–53.

111. Ullman A, Svedmyr N. Salmeterol, a new long acting inhaled beta 2 adrenoceptor agonist: comparison with salbutamol in adult asthmatic patients. *Thorax* 1988; 43 (9): 674–8.

112. Arvidsson P, Larsson S, Löfdahl CG, Melander B, Wahlander L, Svedmyr N. Formoterol, a new long-acting bronchodilator for inhalation. *Eur Respir J* 1989; 2 (4): 325–30.

113. Löfdahl CG, Svedmyr N. Formoterol fumarate, a new beta 2-adrenoceptor agonist. Acute studies of selectivity and duration of effect after inhaled and oral administration. *Allergy* 1989; 44 (4): 264–71.

114. Arvidsson P, Larsson S, Löfdahl CG, Melander B, Svedmyr N, Wahlander L. Inhaled formoterol during one year in asthma: a comparison with salbutamol. *Eur Respir J* 1991; 4 (10): 1168–73.

115. Wallin A, Melander B, Rosenhall L, Sandstrom T, Wahlander L. Formoterol, a new long acting beta 2 agonist for inhalation twice daily, compared with salbutamol in the treatment of asthma. *Thorax* 1990; 45 (4): 259–61.

116. Dahl R, Earnshaw JS, Palmer JB. Salmeterol: a four week study of a long-acting beta-adrenoceptor agonist for the treatment of reversible airways disease. *Eur Respir J* 1991; 4 (10): 1178–84.

117. Rabe K, Lindén A. Mechanisms of duration of action of inhaled long-acting beta 2-adrenoceptor agonists. In: Pauwels R, O'Byrne P (eds). *Beta 2-Agonists in Asthma Treatment.* New York: Marcel Dekker, 1997: 131–60.

118. Anderson GP, Linden A, Rabe KF. Why are long-acting beta-adrenoceptor agonists long-acting? *Eur Respir J* 1994; 7 (3): 569–78.

119. Anderson GP. Long acting inhaled beta-adrenoceptor agonists the comparative pharmacology of formoterol and salmeterol. *Agents Actions* (suppl.) 1993; 43: 253–69.

120. Naline E, Zhang Y, Qian Y *et al.* Relaxant effects and durations of action of formoterol and salmeterol on the isolated human bronchus. *Eur Respir J* 1994; 7 (5): 914–20.

121. Palmqvist M, Persson G, Lazer L, Rosenborg J, Larsson P, Lötvall J. Inhaled dry-powder formoterol and salmeterol in asthmatic patients: onset of action, duration of effect and potency. *Eur Respir J* 1997; 10 (11): 2484–9.

122. Anderson P, Lötvall J, Linden A. Relaxation kinetics of formoterol and salmeterol in the guinea pig trachea *in vitro. Lung* 1996; 174 (3): 159–70.

123. Ullman A, Bergendal A, Linden A, Waldeck B, Skoogh BE, Löfdahl CG. Onset of action and duration of effect of formoterol and salmeterol compared to salbutamol in isolated guinea pig trachea with or without epithelium. *Allergy* 1992; 47 (4 Pt 2): 384–7.

124. Linden A, Bergendal A, Ullman A, Skoogh BE, Löfdahl CG. Salmeterol, formoterol, and salbutamol in the isolated guinea pig trachea: differences in maximum relaxant effect and potency but not in functional antagonism. *Thorax* 1993; 48 (5): 547–53.

125. Johnson M, Coleman RA. Mechanisms of action of β_2-adrenoceptor agonists. In: Busse WW, Holgate ST (eds). *Asthma and Rhinitis.* Boston: Blackwell Scientific Publications, 1995: 1278–95.

126. Wegener T, Hedenstrom H, Melander B. Rapid onset of action of inhaled formoterol in asthmatic patients. *Chest* 1992; 102 (2): 535–8.

127. Green SA, Spasoff AP, Coleman RA, Johnson M, Liggett SB. Sustained activation of a G protein-

coupled receptor via "anchored" agonist binding. Molecular localization of the salmeterol exosite within the 2-adrenergic receptor. *J Biol Chem* 1996; 271 (39): 24029–35.

128. Coleman RA, Johnson M, Nials AT, Vardey CJ. Exosites: their current status, and their relevance to the duration of action of long-acting beta 2-adrenoceptor agonists. *Trends Pharmacol Sci* 1996; 17 (9): 324–30.

129. Clark RB, Allal C, Friedman J, Johnson M, Barber R. Stable activation and desensitization of beta 2-adrenergic receptor stimulation of adenylyl cyclase by salmeterol: evidence for quasi-irreversible binding to an exosite. *Mol Pharmacol* 1996; 49 (1): 182–9.

130. Jeppsson AB, Löfdahl CG, Waldeck B, Widmark E. On the predictive value of experiments *in vitro* in the evaluation of the effect duration of bronchodilator drugs for local administration. *Pulmonary Pharmacol* 1989; 2: 81–5.

131. Jeppsson AB, Kallstrom BL, Waldeck B. Studies on the interaction between formoterol and salmeterol in guinea-pig trachea *in vitro*. *Pharmacol Toxicol* 1992; 71 (4): 272–7.

132. Jeppsson AB, Nilsson E, Waldeck B. Formoterol and salmeterol are both long acting compared to terbutaline in the isolated perfused and ventilated guinea-pig lung. *Eur J Pharmacol* 1994; 257 (1–2): 137–43.

133. Kallstrom BL, Sjoberg J, Waldeck B. The interaction between salmeterol and beta 2-adrenoceptor agonists with higher efficacy on guinea-pig trachea and human bronchus *in vitro*. *Br J Pharmacol* 1994; 113 (3): 687–92.

134. Palmqvist M, Ibsen T, Mellen A, Lötvall J. Comparison of the relative efficacy of formoterol and salmeterol in asthmatic patients. *Am J Respir Crit Care Med* 1999; 160 (1): 244–9.

135. Ulrik CS, Kok-Jensen A. Different bronchodilating effect of salmeterol and formoterol in an adult asthmatic. *Eur Respir J* 1994; 7 (5): 1003–5.

136. Korosec M, Novak RD, Myers E, Skowronski M, McFadden ER Jr. Salmeterol does not compromise the bronchodilator response to albuterol during acute episodes of asthma. *Am J Med* 1999; 107 (3): 209–13.

137. Kesten S, Chapman KR, Broder I *et al*. A three-month comparison of twice daily inhaled formoterol versus four times daily inhaled albuterol in the management of stable asthma. *Am Rev Respir Dis* 1991; 144 (3 Pt 1): 622–5.

138. Britton MG, Earnshaw JS, Palmer JB. A twelve month comparison of salmeterol with salbutamol in asthmatic patients. European Study Group [published erratum appears in *Eur Respir J* 1993; 6(1): 150]. *Eur Respir J* 1992; 5 (9): 1062–7.

139. Kesten S, Chapman KR, Broder I *et al*. Sustained improvement in asthma with long-term use of formoterol fumarate. *Ann Allergy* 1992; 69 (5): 415–20.

140. Pearlman DS, Chervinsky P, LaForce C *et al*. A comparison of salmeterol with albuterol in the treatment of mild-to-moderate asthma. *N Engl J Med* 1992; 327 (20): 1420–5.

141. Lundback B, Rawlinson DW, Palmer JB. Twelve month comparison of salmeterol and salbutamol as dry powder formulations in asthmatic patients. European Study Group. *Thorax* 1993; 48 (2): 148–53.

142. Stålenheim G, Wegener T, Grettve L *et al*. Efficacy and tolerance of a 12-week treatment with inhaled formoterol in patients with reversible obstructive lung disease. *Respiration* 1994; 61 (6): 305–9.

143. D'Alonzo GE, Nathan RA, Henochowicz S, Morris RJ, Ratner P, Rennard SI. Salmeterol xinafoate as maintenance therapy compared with albuterol in patients with asthma. *Jama* 1994; 271 (18): 1412–6.

144. Hyland ME. Antiasthma drugs: quality-of-life rating scales and sensitivity to longitudinal change. *Pharmacoeconomics* 1994; 6 (4): 324–9.

145. Woolcock A, Lundback B, Ringdal N, Jacques LA. Comparison of addition of salmeterol to inhaled steroids with doubling of the dose of inhaled steroids. *Am J Respir Crit Care Med* 1996; 153 (5): 1481–8.

146. Wilding P, Clark M, Coon JT *et al*. Effect of long-term treatment with salmeterol on asthma control: a double blind, randomised crossover study. *BMJ* 1997; 314 (7092): 1441–6.

147. McIvor RA, Pizzichini E, Turner MO, Hussack P, Hargreave FE, Sears MR. Potential masking effects of

salmeterol on airway inflammation in asthma. *Am J Respir Crit Care Med* 1998; 158 (3): 924–30.

148. Wong BJ, Dolovich J, Ramsdale EH *et al.* Formoterol compared with beclomethasone and placebo on allergen-induced asthmatic responses. *Am Rev Respir Dis* 1992; 146 (5 Pt 1): 1156–60.

149. Vervloet D, Ekstrom T, Pela R *et al.* A 6-month comparison between formoterol and salmeterol in patients with reversible obstructive airways disease. *Respir Med* 1998; 92 (6): 836–42.

150. Lötvall J, Lunde H, Svedmyr N. Onset of bronchodilation and finger tremor induced by salmeterol and salbutamol in asthmatic patients. *Can Respir J* 1998; 5 (3): 191–4.

151. Lötvall J, Svedmyr N. Salmeterol: an inhaled beta 2-agonist with prolonged duration of action. *Lung* 1993; 171 (5): 249–64.

152. Politiek MJ, Boorsma M, Aalbers R. Comparison of formoterol, salbutamol and salmeterol in methacholine-induced severe bronchoconstriction. *Eur Respir J* 1999; 13 (5): 988–92.

153. Cheung D, Timmers MC, Zwinderman AH, Bel EH, Dijkman JH, Sterk PJ. Long-term effects of a long-acting beta 2-adrenoceptor agonist, salmeterol, on airway hyperresponsiveness in patients with mild asthma. *N Engl J Med* 1992; 327 (17): 1198–203.

154. Ullman A, Hedner J, Svedmyr N. Inhaled salmeterol and salbutamol in asthmatic patients. An evaluation of asthma symptoms and the possible development of tachyphylaxis. *Am Rev Respir Dis* 1990; 142 (3): 571–5.

155. Lötvall J, Lunde H, Ullman A, Tornqvist H, Svedmyr N. Twelve months, treatment with inhaled salmeterol in asthmatic patients. Effects on beta 2-receptor function and inflammatory cells. *Allergy* 1992; 47 (5): 477–83.

156. Grove A, Lipworth BJ. Bronchodilator subsensitivity to salbutamol after twice daily salmeterol in asthmatic patients. *Lancet* 1995; 346 (8969): 201–6.

157. Nelson HS, Berkowitz RB, Tinkelman DA, Emmett AH, Rickard KA, Yancey SW. Lack of subsensitivity to albuterol after treatment with salmeterol in patients with asthma. *Am J Respir Crit Care Med* 1999; 159 (5 Pt 1): 1556–61.

158. Ramage L, Lipworth BJ, Ingram CG, Cree IA, Dhillon DP. Reduced protection against exercise induced bronchoconstriction after chronic dosing with salmeterol. *Respir Med* 1994; 88 (5): 363–8.

159. Nelson JA, Strauss L, Skowronski M, Ciufo R, Novak R, McFadden ER Jr. Effect of long-term salmeterol treatment on exercise-induced asthma. *N Engl J Med* 1998; 339 (3): 141–6.

160. Simons FE, Gerstner TV, Cheang MS. Tolerance to the bronchoprotective effect of salmeterol in adolescents with exercise-induced asthma using concurrent inhaled glucocorticoid treatment. *Pediatrics* 1997; 99 (5): 655–9.

161. Giannini D, Carletti A, Dente FL *et al.* Tolerance to the protective effect of salmeterol on allergen challenge. *Chest* 1996; 110 (6): 1452–7.

162. Villaran C, O'Neill SJ, Helbling A *et al.* Montelukast versus salmeterol in patients with asthma and exercise-induced bronchoconstriction. *J Allergy Clin Immunol* 1999; 104 (3 Pt 1): 547–53.

163. Gandevia B. Historical review of the use of parasympatholytic agents in the treatment of respiratory disorders. *Postgrad Med J* 1975; 51 (suppl. 7): 13–20.

164. Barnes PJ. Muscarinic receptor subtypes: implications for therapy. *Agents Actions* (suppl.) 1993; 43: 243–52.

165. Barnes PJ, Minette P, Maclagan J. Muscarinic receptor subtypes in airways. *Trends Pharmacol Sci* 1988; 9 (11): 412–6.

166. Barnes PJ. Muscarinic receptors in lung. *Postgrad Med J* 1987; 63 (suppl. 1): 13–9.

167. Poppius H, Salorinne Y, Viljanene AA. Inhalation of a new anticholinergic drug, SCH 1000, in asthma and chronic bronchitis: Effect on airway resistance, thoracic gas volume, blood gases and exercise-induced asthma. *Bull Physio Path Resp* 1972; 8: 643–52.

168. Pakes GE, Brogden RN, Heel RC, Speight TM, Avery GS. Ipratropium bromide: a review of its pharmacological properties and therapeutic efficacy in asthma and chronic bronchitis. *Drugs* 1980; 20 (4): 237–66.

169. Petrie GR, Palmer KN. Comparison of aerosol

ipratropium bromide and salbutamol in chronic bronchitis and asthma. *Br Med J* 1975; 1 (5955): 430–2.

170. Ruffin RE, Fitzgerald JD, Rebuck AS. A comparison of the bronchodilator activity of Sch 1000 and salbutamol. *J Allergy Clin Immunol* 1977; 59 (2): 136–41.

171. Ullah MI, Newman GB, Saunders KB. Influence of age on response to ipratropium and salbutamol in asthma. *Thorax* 1981; 36 (7): 523–9.

172. Braun SR, Levy SF. Comparison of ipratropium bromide and albuterol in chronic obstructive pulmonary disease: a three-center study. *Am J Med* 1991; 91 (4A): 28S–32S.

173. Ikeda A, Nishimura K, Koyama H, Izumi T. Comparative dose-response study of three anticholinergic agents and fenoterol using a metered dose inhaler in patients with chronic obstructive pulmonary disease. *Thorax* 1995; 50 (1): 62–6.

174. Britton J, Hanley SP, Garrett HV, Hadfield JW, Tattersfield AE. Dose related effects of salbutamol and ipratropium bromide on airway calibre and reactivity in subjects with asthma. *Thorax* 1988; 43 (4): 300–5.

175. Higgins BG, Powell RM, Cooper S, Tattersfield AE. Effect of salbutamol and ipratropium bromide on airway calibre and bronchial reactivity in asthma and chronic bronchitis. *Eur Respir J* 1991; 4 (4): 415–20.

176. Larsson K. Oxitropium bromide, ipratropium bromide and fenoterol in exercise-induced asthma. *Respiration* 1982; 43 (1): 57–63.

177. Thumm HW. Opthalmic effects of high doses of Sch 1000 MDI in healthy volunteers and patients with glaucoma. *Postgrad Med J* 1975; 51 (suppl. 7): 132–3.

178. Kalra L, Bone MF. Does high dose nebulised atrovent precipitate glaucoma? *Postgrad Med J* 1987; 63 (suppl. 1): A21.

179. Weiser O, Konigshofer R. Dose-response study of Sch 1000 on heart rate, ECG and blood pressure in healthy volunteers. *Postgrad Med J* 1975; 51 (suppl. 7): 125.

180. Peel ET, Anderson G, Cheong B, Broderick N. A comparison of oxitropium bromide and ipratropium bromide in asthma. *Eur J Respir Dis* 1984; 65 (2): 106–8.

181. Taytard A, Auzerie J, Vergeret J, Tozon N, Freour P. Treatment of adult asthma: controlled double-blind clinical trial of oxitropium bromide. *Eur J Clin Pharmacol* 1984; 26 (4): 429–33.

182. Schultze-Werninghaus G. Anticholinergic versus beta 2-adrenergic therapy in allergic airways obstruction: double-blind trials on bronchodilator effect and antiallergic protection of oxitropium bromide and fenoterol. *Respiration* 1981; 41 (4): 239–47.

183. Lulling J, Delwiche JP, Prignot J. Early bronchodilating effect of oxitropium bromide in comparison with ipratropium bromide. *Respiration* 1981; 42 (3): 188–92.

184. Flohr E, Bischoff KO. Oxitropium bromide, a new anticholinergic drug, in a dose-response and placebo comparison in obstructive airway diseases. *Respiration* 1979; 38 (2): 98–104.

185. Minette A, Marcq M. Oxitropium bromide (Ba 253), an advance in the field of anticholinergic bronchodilating treatments. Preliminary results. *Rev Inst Hyg Mines (Hasselt)* 1979; 34 (3): 115–23.

186. Barnes PJ, Belvisi MG, Mak JC, Haddad EB, O'Connor B. Tiotropium bromide (Ba 679 BR), a novel long-acting muscarinic antagonist for the treatment of obstructive airways disease. *Life Sci* 1995; 56 (11–12): 853–9.

187. O'Connor BJ, Towse LJ, Barnes PJ. Prolonged effect of tiotropium bromide on methacholine-induced bronchoconstriction in asthma. *Am J Respir Crit Care Med* 1996; 154 (4 Pt 1): 876–80.

188. Haddad EB, Mak JC, Barnes PJ. Characterization of [3H] Ba 679 BR, a slowly dissociating muscarinic antagonist, in human lung: radioligand binding and autoradiographic mapping. *Mol Pharmacol* 1994; 45 (5): 899–907.

189. Maesen FP, Smeets JJ, Costongs MA, Wald FD, Cornelissen PJ. Ba 679 Br, a new long-acting antimuscarinic bronchodilator: a pilot dose-escalation study in COPD. *Eur Respir J* 1993; 6 (7): 1031–6.

190. McFadden ER Jr, el Sanadi N, Strauss L *et al*. The influence of parasympatholytics on the resc tion of acute attacks of asthma. *Am J Med* 1997; 10 1): 7–13.

191. Zorc JJ, Pusic MV, Ogborn CJ, Lebet R, Duggan AK. Ipratropium bromide added to asthma treatment in the pediatric emergency department. *Pediatrics* 1999; 103 (4 Pt 1): 748–52.

192. Ducharme FM, Davis GM. Randomized controlled trial of ipratropium bromide and frequent low doses of salbutamol in the management of mild and moderate acute pediatric asthma. *J Pediatr* 1998; 133 (4): 479–85.

193. Moayyedi P, Congleton J, Page RL, Pearson SB, Muers MF. Comparison of nebulised salbutamol and ipratropium bromide with salbutamol alone in the treatment of chronic obstructive pulmonary disease. *Thorax* 1995; 50 (8): 834–7.

194. Campbell S. For COPD a combination of ipratropium bromide and albuterol sulfate is more effective than albuterol base. *Arch Intern Med* 1999; 159 (2): 156–60.

195. Rabe KF, Magnussen H, Dent G. Theophylline and selective PDE inhibitors as bronchodilators and smooth muscle relaxants. *Eur Respir J* 1995; 8 (4): 637–42.

196. Dent G, Giembycz MA, Rabe KF, Wolf B, Barnes PJ, Magnussen H. Theophylline suppresses human alveolar macrophage respiratory burst through phosphodiesterase inhibition. *Am J Respir Cell Mol Biol* 1994; 10 (5): 565–72.

197. Persson CG, Erjefalt I, Edholm LE, Karlsson JA, Lamm CJ. Tracheal relaxant and cardiostimulant actions of xanthines can be differentiated from diuretic and CNS-stimulant effects. Role of adenosine antagonism? *Life Sci* 1982; 31 (24): 2673–81.

198. Kroll F, Karlsson JA, Ryrfeldt A, Persson CG. Adenosine-induced bronchoconstriction in the guinea-pig isolated lung: interaction with theophylline and enprofylline. *Pulm Pharmacol* 1988; 1 (2): 85–92.

199. Zwillich CW, Sutton FD, Neff TA, Cohn WM, Matthay RA, Weinberger MM. Theophylline-induced seizures in adults. Correlation with serum concentrations. *Ann Intern Med* 1975; 82 (6): 784–7.

200. Sessler CN. Theophylline toxicity: clinical features of 116 consecutive cases. *Am J Med* 1990; 88 (6): 567–76.

201. Greenberg A, Piraino BH, Kroboth PD, Weiss J. Severe theophylline toxicity. Role of conservative measures, antiarrhythmic agents, and charcoal hemoperfusion. *Am J Med* 1984; 76 (5): 854–60.

202. Shannon M. Life-threatening events after theophylline overdose: a 10-year prospective analysis. *Arch Intern Med* 1999; 159 (9): 989–94.

203. Dunn DW, Parekh HU. Theophylline and status epilepticus in children. *Neuropediatrics* 1991; 22 (1): 24–6.

204. Muir JF, Bertin L, Georges D. Salmeterol versus slow-release theophylline combined with ketotifen in nocturnal asthma: a multicentre trial. French Multicentre Study Group. *Eur Respir J* 1992; 5 (10): 1197–200.

205. Paggiaro PL, Giannini D, Di Franco A, Testi R. Comparison of inhaled salmeterol and individually dose-titrated slow-release theophylline in patients with reversible airway obstruction. European Study Group. *Eur Respir J* 1996; 9 (8): 1689–95.

206. Selby C, Engleman HM, Fitzpatrick MF, Sime PM, Mackay TW, Douglas NJ. Inhaled salmeterol or oral theophylline in nocturnal asthma? *Am J Respir Crit Care Med* 1997; 155 (1): 104–8.

207. Davies B, Brooks G, Devoy M. The efficacy and safety of salmeterol compared to theophylline: meta-analysis of nine controlled studies. *Respir Med* 1998; 92 (2): 256–63.

208. Wiegand L, Mende CN, Zaidel G *et al*. Salmeterol vs theophylline: sleep and efficacy outcomes in patients with nocturnal asthma. *Chest* 1999; 115 (6): 1525–32.

209. Kidney J, Dominguez M, Taylor PM, Rose M, Chung KF, Barnes PJ. Immunomodulation by theophylline in asthma. Demonstration by withdrawal of therapy. *Am J Respir Crit Care Med* 1995; 151 (6): 1907–14.

210. Rabe KF, Dent G. Theophylline and airway inflammation. *Clin Exp Allergy* 1998; 28 (suppl. 3): 35–41.

211. Spina D, Landells LJ, Page CP. The role of theophylline and phosphodiesterase 4 isoenzyme inhibitors as anti-inflammatory drugs. *Clin Exp Allergy* 1998; 28 (suppl. 3): 24–34.

212. Fujii K, Kohrogi H, Iwagoe H *et al*. Novel phosphodiesterase 4 inhibitor T-440 reverses and prevents human bronchial contraction induced by allergen. *J Pharmacol Exp Ther* 1998; 284 (1): 162–9.

Chapter 22

Delivery Systems

G.K. Crompton

Inhaled remedies have been used for many centuries in the treatment of respiratory disorders[1] and bronchodilator aerosols have been used in the treatment of asthma at least since 1935.[2] Various types of inhaler device were used in the early days, many being driven by air generated from the hand-squeezed rubber bulb. The introduction of the pressurized metered dose inhaler (PMDI) in 1956 was a major advance and its popularity with patients and clinicians is reflected by the sales of this device in the decade after its introduction.[3] When corticosteroid therapy became available in the PMDI this allowed topical therapy to replace oral treatment in the majority of adult asthmatic patients – a revolution in the management of asthma in adults. Spacer devices or holding chambers made PMDI therapy available to all but very young children. Dry powder inhalers (DPIs) have provided alternative drug delivery systems and the available choice of PMDI, PMDI plus spacer system or a DPI now makes it possible for the vast majority of patients with reversible airflow limitation to be treated with bronchodilator and anti-inflammatory drugs with inhalation systems they can use efficiently. Nebulizers are less convenient than PMDIs and DPIs, but have an important role in the long-term treatment of some young children, and in the treatment of severe acute asthma.

THE PRESSURIZED METERED DOSE INHALER

The pressurized metered dose inhaler (PMDI) has been used widely in clinical practice since the early 1960s. It consists of a canister and a plastic actuator. When the canister is depressed into the actuator a measured amount of aerosol is released, which is determined by a valve in the actuator into which the canister nozzle is seated. Within the canister is drug either as a suspension or as a solution with fluorocarbon propellants at a pressure of approximately 3 atm (303 kPa). The characteristics of the hydrofluoroalkane propellants (see p. 263) which will replace CFCs will differ. The canister of suspension PMDIs also contains a dispersant or lubricant to ensure accurate functioning of the valve during the multiple actuations of the inhaler. The aerosol released from the PMDI consists of large droplets of propellant within which the drug is enclosed either as a solid crystal or as a liquid.[4] The propellants evaporate rapidly as soon as they leave the canister and this "flashing" breaks up the liquid stream into droplets that continue to evaporate as they move away from the canister at an initial velocity exceeding 30 m s^{-1}.[5] Because of the high velocity of drug particles, the effects of evaporating propellants and the hygroscopicity of the drugs, together with the anatomy of the respiratory tract, the majority of drug impacts in the oropharynx even when a PMDI is used efficiently. Less than 25% of the drug dose reaches the lungs,[6,7] but because all drugs do not possess similar characteristics with regard to hygroscopicity and electrostatic charge the same device will deliver a reproducible amount of the same drug, but it cannot be assumed that a similar proportion of a different drug will reach the intra-pulmonary airways. This is also true of dry powder delivery systems.

The most efficient way of using a PMDI is as follows.[8]

(1) Remove the mouthpiece cap.
(2) Shake the canister thoroughly.
(3) Place the mouthpiece of the actuator between the lips.
(4) Breathe out steadily.
(5) Release the dose while taking a slow, deep breath in.
(6) Hold breath in while counting to 10, or for as long as is comfortable.

These instructions appear to be simple, but many if not the majority of adults cannot use a PMDI efficiently when the only instruction they receive is the manufacturer's package insert.[9-14] Also, more than 10% of patients develop an inefficient inhalation technique simply with continued use of this device,[9,13] the majority of these being those who had difficulty in learning how to use the PMDI initially. The main problem experienced is difficulty in coordinating dose release during inspiration,[13] but a significant proportion of patients cannot continue to inhale through the mouth when the propellants are released into the oropharynx ("cold Freon effect"), and it is rarely possible for these patients to overcome this problem. Children and the elderly have the greatest difficulties using the unmodified PMDI efficiently, and attempts to make this device easier to use have been made; the most successful being the development of holding chambers or "spacers" and modifications of the inhaler to make it breath-actuated.

Spacers or Holding Chambers

The droplet size of aerosols released from pressurized inhalers is dependent on the distance from the actuator orifice, a greater distance allowing more evaporation of propellants. It was found that by attaching tubes to the actuator the total amount of drug lost in the actuator, tube and mouth was reduced.[15] This and subsequent experiments led to the design and development of spacer devices of different sizes. Such devices were found to increase drug availability to the lung and at the same time decrease unwanted drug deposition in the oropharynx,[16,17] although there was considerable initial scepticism about their clinical value.[18] A small-volume extension tube spacer has been shown to improve the efficiency of the PMDI by partially compensating for poor inhalation technique,[19] but large-volume spacers or holding chambers have proved to be of much more clinical value (Table 22.1).[16,20-22] A one-way valve at the mouthpiece of large-volume spacer devices enables them to contain the aerosol before inhalation, and although more particles are lost within the spacer more of the aerosol leaving the device is able to penetrate the lungs. This has been shown to be the case with a 750-ml spacer (Nebuhaler) and a smaller device (Aerochamber),[22] but not all large-volume spacers have been shown to increase pulmonary deposition compared with the PMDI.[7] The efficiency of spacer devices in terms of increasing pulmonary deposition of drug is dependent upon a number of factors

Table 22.1: Some indications for the use of large-volume spacers
1. High-dose steroid therapy to decrease oropharyngeal drug deposition and thereby lessen the risk of candidiasis and systemic activity of drug swallowed. Spacers are not necessary to decrease systemic effects with fluticasone propionate since the swallowed fraction is almost totally inactivated on first pass through the liver
2. Inability to synchronize dose release from a PMDI with inspiration.
3. For the administration of high doses of a β_2 agonist instead of using a nebulizer

including their size, the characteristics of the one-way valve, the drug being used and the electrostatic charge of the plastics used to manufacture the device. The importance of the electrostatic charge has only recently been realized. Static electricity accumulates on many polycarbonate and plastic spacers, attracting drug particles, which become charged when they are produced by the metered dose inhaler. Highly charged spacers deliver less drug than those with an anti-static lining.[23,24] A simple way of reducing the charge on a spacer is to wash it with a detergent[24] and to allow it to drip dry, which has a similar effect on drug delivery as anti-static paint,[23,25] but the charge may re-accumulate. Spacers made of anti-static materials or metals may reduce this problem.[26] Large-volume spacer devices decrease oropharyngeal deposition of drug and their use is recommended for inhaled steroids,[27,28] to decrease systemic effects and oropharyngeal candidiasis.[29-34] Use of spacers for inhaled corticosteroid treatment does not cause much inconvenience since most patients take these drugs twice daily and do not, therefore, have to carry the spacer with them during the day. However, bulky spacers for as-required bronchodilator therapy are much less convenient and are rarely used for such treatment unless the patient is unable to use any of the alternative drug delivery systems. Large-volume spacers are now most often used in young children since many are unable to use the conventional PMDI, the breath-actuated PMDI (p. 263) and the dry powder delivery systems (p. 264). In adults their main use is when PMDI corticosteroid therapy has to be used in high dose.[27] They can be used as an alternative to nebulizers in chronic[35] and severe acute asthma.[36] Spacers do not decrease drug available for deposition in the area of the vocal cords and do not therefore protect against inhaled steroid-related dysphonia.[37]

The Breath-Actuated Metered Dose Inhaler

Attempts have been made to make the conventional PMDI easier to use by making it breath actuated, since the most common problem patients have using this device is co-ordination of dose release with inspiration.[15] Early models were somewhat clumsy and made a loud click when actuated, and were not successful. The first successful breath-actuated PMDI (Autohaler) has design features that have, in the main overcome the problems of its predecessors. The canister is completely enclosed within the body of the actuator; there is a latching level at the top of the inhaler and when this is used to "prime" the device prior to inhalation a blocking system prevents valve actuation. This consists of a vane and a three-compartment triggering mechanism that is housed between the inhaler valve and the inhaler mouthpiece orifice. When "primed" the valve is actuated by an inspiratory flow of about $30 \, l \, min^{-1}$.[38] The Autohaler is easier to use than the conventional PMDI[39,40] and can be triggered by patients with severe airflow obstruction.[41] A breath-actuated PMDI (Easi-Breathe) which is primed simply by opening the mouth piece and is then triggered by an inspiratory flow of less than 30 l per minute is now also in common use and has been found to be very popular in patients already using inhalers and also those who are inhaler-naïve.[42,43] Over 90% of patients have been found to be able to use the breath-actuated PMDIs efficiently, but in the same study one-third of the patients already being treated with the conventional PMDI were unable to use it efficiently.[42] This provides further confirmation of the fact that many adults cannot use the unmodified PMDI.[9–13]

Disadvantages of Metered Dose Inhalers

Problems of coordination of dose release with inspiration can be overcome by the breath-actuated PMDI or a spacer system, and the "cold Freon" effect is not a problem when large-volume spacers are used. However, problems inherent in the basic design of the PMDI have not yet been solved completely. These problems concern the propellants and surfactants/lubricants, which are, of course, essential to allow the device to function. The propellants provide the vehicle in which the drug particles are carried at high velocity from the valve and the surfactant/lubricants are necessary to lubricate the valve and to prevent aggregation of drug particles. The propellants since the introduction of the PMDI some four decades ago have been chlorofluorocarbons (CFCs) and mixtures of two or three of these substances are used to achieve the desired vapour pressure and spray characteristics. There is a numbering system for CFCs that indicates the number of carbon, hydrogen, chlorine and fluorine atoms. The CFCs used in medicinal aerosols are CFC 22, 23 and 114. For many years these were considered to be inert, but in the 1960s their safety was questioned;[44–46] however the majority decision now is that they are safe in the quantities necessary to allow the inhalation of therapeutic doses of drugs.[47–50] Nonetheless, CFCs are now under threat because of their effect on the environment. In the 1980s the ozone "hole" over Antarctica was discovered and in 1987, twenty-seven nations agreed in Montreal to reduce hard CFC consumption by 50% by 1999. Subsequently this was seen to be inadequate and in 1989 representatives of over 80 nations agreed, in principle, to eliminate hard CFCs by the end of the century.[51] In certain Western countries this ban was brought forward to 1995 and in some the ban is now already in force, although exemption for medical aerosols has been allowed on a temporary basis in others. This has stimulated the pharmaceutical industry to find alternative non-CFC propellants for medicinal aerosols, and hydrofluoroalkane (HFA)-134a, which does not contain chlorine, has been produced as an alternative to CFCs. The safety of HFA-134a as a pharmaceutical propellant was established by the pharmaceutical consortium, International Pharmaceutical Aerosol Consortium for Toxicological Testing of HFA 134a (IPACT-1) and HFA-134a has now been globally accepted as a safe alternative for CFCs, in both pharmaceutical and industrial applications.[52–54]

The change-over from CFC propellants to HFA driven devices may cause some confusion to the patient and also to many clinicians. Salbutamol HFA PMDIs will continue to be suspension aerosols and will, therefore, have similar pulmonary deposition profiles and hence similar clinical efficacy dose for dose. The velocity of the aerosol plume and taste of the aerosol may be different, and this is likely to cause some concern in patients who have become used to one brand of PMDI. However, much more concern and confusion is going to be created because at least one beclomethasone dipropionate HFA PMDI is a solution and not a suspension aerosol. This solution PMDI creates smaller respirable particles which allows 55–60% of drug to be deposited in the lungs compared with 4–7% from the CFC PMDI.[55] The amount of drug deposited in the oropharynx is significantly lower with the HFA PMDI[55] and hence spacer systems are unlikely to be necessary if this HFA device is used. The other clinically important disadvantage of many PMDIs is the irritant effects of some of lubricants or surfactants. Cough and decrease in ventilatory function have been shown to be produced by these compounds in up to one-third of patients using PMDIs.[56–58] This is an underestimated clinical problem which has been shown to decrease bronchodilator response[59] and replacement of surfactants should be addressed at the same time as CFC replacement for suspension PMDIs.

DRY POWDER INHALERS

Dry powder inhalation systems depend entirely upon the patient's inspiratory effort and are generally easier to use than PMDIs. The first successful dry powder inhaler (Spinhaler) was introduced in 1969 and it was shown subsequently that the majority of patients unable to use the PMDI were able to cope with the Spinhaler.[9] However, this device was available only for the inhalation of sodium cromoglycate, but in the late 1970s the Rotahaler[60] became available for use with salbutamol and beclomethasone dipropionate. Equipotency of the Rotahaler and the PMDI was demonstrated for salbutamol[50–52] and beclomethasone dipropionate[61–66] and a dry powder inhaler for use with fenoterol (Italseber) was also shown to be at least as effective as the PMDI in asthmatic children.[67] The availability of dry powder inhalers for bronchodilator and steroid therapy made inhaled treatment available to a larger population of patients and was generally welcomed.[68,69] However, the first dry powder inhalers were single-dose devices and had to be re-loaded with a cartridge/capsule containing micronized drug and a lactose or glucose carrier/vehicle each time they were used. However, they are more convenient than large-volume spacers for bronchodilator therapy since they are small and easy to carry.

The second generation of dry powder inhalers contain many doses and are preferred to single dose devices by most patients. The Diskhaler/Rotadisk blister system was designed to be equivalent to the Rotahaler/Rotacaps cartridge system in terms of drug delivery both *in vitro* and in clinical practice.[70] The Diskhaler has been found to be equivalent to the Rotahaler with regard to efficacy and safety for both salbutamol and beclomethasone dipropionate.[70] The numbered blisters, arranged within a circular disc, each contain a unit dose of salbutamol, salmeterol, beclomethasone dipropionate or fluticasone propionate. A needle mechanism in the Diskhaler pierces individual blisters making the powder available for inhalation through the mouthpiece. The device is breath-actuated and claimed to be efficient at low inspiratory flow rates.[70] When required the next dose is made available as lifting the lid rotates the circular blister pack and allows the needle to pierce another blister. The number of doses remaining in the device is visible through a window on its external surface. When all four or eight blisters have been punctured the device has to be opened so that another Rotadisk can be loaded. The aluminium foil blister packs protect the drug and lactose vehicle against adverse effects of moisture. In a Glaxo handling study, 70% of patients preferred the Diskhaler to single-dose dry powder devices and 53% of a large number of patients already using a PMDI expressed a preference for the eight-dose Diskhaler.[70] The 60-dose aluminium blister strip device (Accuhaler/Diskus) and the four-dose Diskhaler are dose-for-dose equipotent and the Accuhaler/Diskus has been well-received by patients.[71]

The Turbuhaler is a 50, 100 or 200-dose dry powder inhaler that has been designed to deliver micronized drug alone, or micronized drug and a minute amount of lactose carrier.[72] It is loaded in the upright position (45° or more from the horizontal) by rotating the turning grip at the bottom of the device. This action fills a cluster of machined conical holes in a rotating dosing disc, scrapers removing surplus drug as the disc revolves beneath them. The numbers and sizes of holes are tailored for dose and different drugs. The Turbuhaler is breath-actuated by the patient breathing in as quickly and as deeply as is comfortable through the mouth-piece after the device is loaded. The inhaler has an in-built resistance to airflow since it has been designed with spiral-shaped channels in the mouthpiece. These create turbulent flow in order to deaggregate drug particles. A dose-indicator window shows when there are 20 or fewer doses remaining in the device, and it is likely that in the future a formal dose counter will be incorporated. A desiccant is stored in the base of the Turbuhaler to ensure that the interior of the device and the drug powder remain dry. When not being used the inhaler must have its watertight cover screwed back in place to protect it against moisture. The spiral channels in the mouthpiece cause inspiratory flow resistance and an inspiratory flow in excess of 30 l min^{-1} is required for the device to function efficiently.[73] The vast majority of adult patients can generate inspiratory flows of 30 l min^{-1} or more[74] during an episode of acute asthma, and the Turbuhaler has been reported to be as effective as the PMDI used with a large volume spacer for the administration of terbutaline in the treatment of patients with acute airways obstruction.[75]

Dry powder inhalers are easier to use than the conventional PMDI since they overcome the PMDI's main problem of synchronizing dose release with inspiration. In general, dry powder inhalers are preferable to the conventional PMDI[76] because of their ease to use and lack of propellants and additives, except for carriers (vehicles) such as lactose. Carrier powders have large particles that are much in excess of the respirable range and are, therefore, deposited in the upper respiratory tract and only rarely cause any adverse effects such as cough.[56,61,64,66] The dry powder devices are less bulky than spacers and are as easy to use as the breath-actuated PMDIs (Autohaler, Easi-Breathe), although some dry powder devices are less convenient because of the need to reload cartridges/capsules or discs frequently. Clinical comparisons of different dry powder inhalers (DPIs) indicate that patients prefer multi-dose devices to single-dose inhalers,[77–79] and a meta-analysis of all available studies showed that 58% of 530 patients preferred a multi-dose DPI to the PMDI.[80] The major drawback of dry powder inhalers is that their efficient use depends upon the patient being able to generate sufficient inspiratory flow to allow drug to reach the bronchi in therapeutic amounts. The various DPIs have different inspiratory resistances and comparisons of intra-pulmonary drug deposition of different devices at inspiratory flow rates between 20 and 140 l per minute reveal major differences,[81] which are likely to be of clinical relevance. Children under the age of 6 years may not be able to generate an inspiratory flow sufficient to use the DPIs such as the Turbuhaler, the younger the child the more likely that this is the case.[61] It is known[73] that the Turbuhaler is less efficient when inspiratory flow is below 30 l min^{-1} compared with 60 l min^{-1}, and the Rotahaler has only about 10% of its maximum bronchodilator effect at inspiratory flow rates of 40 l min^{-1}.[82] Until direct clinical comparisons of all the

dry powder devices have been made and data about optimal inspiratory flow rates for the different devices are available it should be assumed that, unlike the PMDI, the most efficient way of using DPIs is to breathe in from residual volume as quickly and as deeply as possible. There is great need for much more research with dry powder devices,[83] since it cannot be assumed that all have similar characteristics in terms of the proportion of the nominal dose delivered to the target organ, and distribution of drug within the lungs. Compared with the PMDI the Diskhaler is almost 50% less efficient in delivering salbutamol to the lungs and has a pattern of intra-pulmonary deposition similar to that produced by the PMDI without a spacer.[7] According to the manufacturers the Diskhaler was designed to be equivalent to the Rotahaler in terms of drug delivery both *in vitro* and in clinical practice.[70] Distribution of drug and clinical effects of terbutaline sulphate delivered from a Turbuhaler were reported to be similar to those of the PMDI,[84] but more recent studies have found the Turbuhaler to produce a mean lung deposition in the order of twice that of the PMDI with terbutaline[85] and budesonide.[86] Greater efficacy of the Turbuhaler compared with the PMDI is supported by clinical studies of inhaled steroids.[87–89] When dry powder inhalers are used for steroid administration patients should be encouraged to gargle/mouth rinse to decrease systemic effects from drug deposited in the mouth and throat,[90] which can be swallowed and have a varying degree of systemic activity that is dependent on the drug being used.

It is clear that with the proliferation of new delivery systems the clinician has to be aware of major differences in efficacy. It cannot be assumed that all drug delivery systems are the same in terms of the amount of the nominal dose that is delivered to the target organ and deposited in the oropharynx. This is of particular importance with inhaled steroid therapy since a change of inhaler could decrease or increase the amount of drug available to a patient and, therefore, lead to inadequate disease control, or on the other hand the systemic consequences of a dose increase.

NEBULIZERS

Nebulizers are of two types: jet and ultrasonic.

Jet Nebulizers
There are many different makes of jet nebulizer and they have widely differing characteristics with regard to

the generation of drug particles within the respirable range (1–10 μm) that can be inhaled and deposited in the lung.[91,92] The performance of individual nebulizers is influenced by many factors such as the flow rate of the driving gas (air or oxygen), the duration of nebulization, the nature of the solution or suspension being nebulized and the amount of liquid in the chamber of the nebulizer.[93–95] For clinical purposes it is essential to at least be aware of the driving gas flow rate at which a nebulizer functions most efficiently.

Jet nebulizers work by compressed air or oxygen entering a chamber in the nebulizer through a narrow tube. The opening of the gas inlet tube meets that of a liquid inlet tube, and a Venturi effect produces a pressure drop that causes the liquid to flow and break up into droplets of various sizes. Large droplets impact on baffles and a fine aerosol follows the gas stream out of the nebulizer. An increase in gas pressure used to operate the nebulizer will actually decrease particle size.

Ultrasonic Nebulizers

Ultrasonic nebulizers are high-frequency sound waves produced from a piezoelectric crystal. The vibrations are focused on the surface of the liquid in order to create a fountain from which large and small drops are emitted. The particle size of the generated aerosol varies, depending on the frequency of the ultrasonic vibrations. In general, ultrasonic nebulizers are less efficient for drug delivery than jet nebulizers. Indications for the use of nebulizers are listed in Table 22.2.

Table 22.2: Some indications for the use of nebulizers

1. Treatment of severe acute asthma with β_2 agonist and ipratropium bromide in hospital

2. Supervised treatment of severe asthma in the home by general practitioners

3. Treatment of severe acute asthma in ambulances

4. Domiciliary treatment of acute asthma in young children and selected adults with "brittle" asthma

5. Domiciliary treatment of selected patients with chronic obstructive airways disease

6. Administration of antimicrobial drugs in diseases such as cystic fibrosis, bronchiectasis and AIDS

7. Inhalation of hypertonic saline to induce the production of sputum

---

KEY POINTS

1. The pressurized metered dose inhaler has been in clinical use for over 30 years. Only about 50% of adult patients can use it efficiently if the only tuition they have is reading the manufacturer's instruction pamphlet.

2. The main problem patients have using a pressurized metered dose inhaler is coordinating dose-release with inhalation. Some patients cannot continue to breathe in after the dose has been released into the mouth because of the sensation produced by the propellant (cold Freon effect).

3. The most important manoeuvre in the use of a pressurized metered dose inhaler is release of the dose during a slow inspiration.

4. Spacer devices (holding chambers) overcome the problem of coordinating dose-release with inhalation, decrease oropharyngeal deposition and can increase pulmonary deposition of the drug. Spacer devices can be used by the vast majority of patients except for very young children.

5. Plastic spacers develop an electrostatic charge which can reduce considerably the amount of drug available to the patient. Spacers are now being manufactured from materials which do not have a static electrical charge. To decrease the problem with plastic spacers and to increase efficiency, wash with strong detergent solution and allow to drip dry. Never polish or dry a plastic spacer with a cloth.

REFERENCES

1. Miller WF. Aerosol therapy in acute and chronic disease. *Arch Intern Med* 1973; 131: 148–55.

2. Greaser JB, Rowe AH. Inhalation of epinephrine for relief of asthmatic symptoms. *J Allergy* 1935; 6: 415.

3. Inman WHW, Adelstein AM. Rise and fall of asthma mortality in England and Wales in relaion to use of pressurised aerosols. *Lancet* 1969; ii: 279–85.

4. Morén F. Pressurised aerosols for oral inhalation. *Int J Pharm* 1981; 8: 1–10.

5. Newman SP, Clarke SW. Therapeutic aerosols 1 – physical and practical considerations. *Thorax* 1983; 38: 881–6.

6. Newman SP, Morén F, Pavia D, Sheahan NF, Clarke SW. Deposition of pressurised aerosols in the human respiratory tract. *Thorax* 1981; 36: 52–5.

7. Melchor R, Biddiscombe MF, Mak VHF, Short MD, Spiro SG. Lung deposition patterns on directly labelled salbutamol in normal subjects and in patients with reversible airflow obstruction. *Thorax* 1993; 48: 506–11.

8. ✪ Newman SP, Pavia D, Clarke SW. How should a pressurized β-adrenergic bronchodilator be inhaled? *Eur J Respir Dis* 1981; 62: 3–21.

9. Paterson IC, Crompton GK. Use of pressurised aerosols by asthmatic patients. *BMJ* 1976; 1: 76–7.

10. Orehek J, Gayrard P, Grimaud CH, Charpin J. Patient error in use of bronchodilator metered aerosols. *BMJ* 1976; 1: 76.

11. Epstein SW, Manning CPR, Ashley MJ, Corey PN. Survey of the clinical use of pressurised of pressurized aerosol inhalers. *Can Med Assoc J* 1979; 120: 813–6.

12. Gayrard P, Orehek J. Inadequate use of pressurized aerosols by asthmatic patients. *Respiration* 1980; 40: 47–52.

13. ✪ Crompton GK. Problems patients have using pressurized aerosols inhalers. *Eur J Respir Dis* 1982; 63 (suppl. 119): 101–4.

14. de Blaquiere P, Christensen DB, Carter WB, Martin TR. Use and misuse of metered-dose inhalers by patients with chronic lung disease. *Am Rev Respir Dis* 1989; 140: 910–6.

15. Morén F. Drug deposition of pressurized inhalation aerosols 1. Influence of actuator tube design. *Int J Pharm* 1978; 1: 205–12.

16. Lindgren SB, Formgren H, Morén F. Improved aerosol therapy of asthma: effect of actuator tube size on drug availability. *Eur J Respir Dis* 1980; 61: 56–61.

17. Newman SP, Morén F, Pavia D, Little F, Clarke SW. Deposition of pressurized suspension aerosols inhaled through extension devices. *Am Rev Respir Dis* 1981; 124: 317–20.

18. Konig P. Spacer devices used with metered-dose inhalers. Breakthrough or gimmick? *Chest* 1985; 88: 276–84.

19. Bloomfield P, Crompton GK, Winsey NJP. A tube spacer to improve inhalation of drugs from pressurized aerosols. *BMJ* 1979; 2: 1479.

20. Crompton GK. Inhalation devices. *Eur J Respir Dis* 1982; 63: 489–92.

21. Dorrow P, Hidinger KG. Terbutaline aerosol from a metered dose inhaler via a 750 ml spacer. Effect on large and small airways. *Eur J Clin Pharmacol* 1982; 22: 511–4.

22. Newman SP, Millar AB, Lennard-Jones TR, Morén F, Clarke SW. Improvement of pressurised aerosol deposition with Nebuhaler spacer device. *Thorax* 1984; 39: 935–41.

23. Barry PW, O'Callaghan C. The effect of delay, multiple actuations and spacer charge on the *in vitro* delivery of budesonide from the Nebuhaler. *Br J Clin Pharmacol* 1995; 40: 76–8.

24. ✪ Wildhaber JH, Devadason SG, Eber E *et al.* Effect of electrostatic charge, flow, decay and multiple actuations in the *in vitro* delivery of salbutamol from different small volume spacers for infants. *Thorax* 1995; 51: 985–8.

25. Clark DJ, Lipworth BJ. Effect of multiple actuations, delayed inhalation and antistatic treatment on the lung bioavailability of salbutamol via a spacer device. *Thorax* 1996; 51: 981–4.

26. Bisgaard H, Anhøj J, Klug B, Berg EA. A non-electrostatic spacer for aerosol delivery. *Arch Dis Child* 1995; 73: 226–30.

27. The British Guidelines on Asthma Management *Thorax* 1997; 52 (suppl. 1): S1–S21.

28. Sackner MA, Kim CS. Auxiliary MDI aerosol delivery systems. *Chest* 1985; 88 (suppl.): 161s–170s.

29. Prahl P, Jensen T. Decreased adreno-cortical

30. ✪ Brown PH, Blundell G, Greening AP, Crompton GK. Do large volume spacer devices reduce the systemic effects of high dose inhaled corticosteroids? *Thorax* 1990; 45: 736–9.

31. Farrer M, Francis AJ, Pearce SJ. Morning serum cortisol concentrations after 2 mg inhaled beclomethasone dipropionate in normal subjects: effects of a 750 ml spacing device. *Thorax* 1990; 45: 740–2.

32. Brown PH, Matusiewicz SP, Shearng C, Tibi L, Greening AP, Crompton GK. Systemic effects of high dose inhaled steroids: comparison of beclomethasone dipropionate and budesonide in healthy subjects. *Thorax* 1993; 48: 967–73.

33. Toogood JH, Jennings B, Bakerville J, Newhouse M. Assessment of a device for reducing oropharyngeal complications during beclomethasone treatment of asthma. *Am Rev Respir Dis* 1981; 123: 113.

34. Toogood JH, Bakerville J, Jennings B, Lefcoe NM, Johansson SA. Use of spacers to facilitate inhaled corticosteroid treatment of asthma. *Am Rev Respir Dis* 1984; 129: 723–9.

35. O'Reilly JF, Buchanan DR, Sudlow MF. Pressurised aerosol with conical spacer is an effective alternative to nebuliser in chronic stable asthma. *BMJ* 1983; 286: 1548.

36. Morgan MDL, Singh, BV, Frame MH, Williams SJ. Terbutaline aerosol given through pear spacer in acute severe asthma. *BMJ* 1982; 285: 849–50.

37. Toogood JH, Jennings B, Baskerville J, Johansson SA. Clinical use of spacer systems for corticosteroid inhalation therapy: a preliminary analysis. *Eur J Respir Dis* 1982; 63 (suppl. 62): 100–7.

38. Baum EA, Bryant AM. The development and laboratory testing of a novel breath-actuated pressurised inhaler. *J Aerosol Med* 1988; 1: 219–20.

39. Crompton G, Duncan J. Clinical assessment of a new breath-actuated inhaler. *Practitioner* 1989; 233: 268–9.

40. Newman SP, Weisz AWB, Talaee N, Clarke SW. Improvement of drug delivery with a breath actuated

suppression utilising the Nebuhaler for inhalation of steroid aerosols. *Clin Allergy* 1987; 17: 393–8.

pressurised aerosol for patients with poor inhaler technique. *Thorax* 1991; 46: 712–6.

41. Fergusson RJ, Lenny J, McHardy GJR, Crompton GK. The use of a new breath-actuated inhaler by patients with severe airflow obstruction. *Eur Respir J* 1991; 4: 172–4.

42. Lenney J, Innes JA, Crompton GK. Inappropriate inhaler use – assessment of use and patient preference of seven inhalation devices. *Respir Med* 2000; 94: 496–500.

43. Hartung TK, Allbut H, Dewar M, Innes JA, Crompton GK. Hydrofluoroalkane metered dose inhaler – patient acceptability study. 1999 (submitted for publication).

44. Speizer FE, Doll R, Heaf P. Observations on recent increase in mortality from asthma. *BMJ* 1968; 1: 339–43.

45. Speizer FE, Wegman DH, Ramirez A. Palpitation rates associated with fluorocarbon exposure in a hospital setting. *N Engl J Med* 1975; 292: 624–6.

46. Bass M. Sudden sniffing death. *JAMA* 1970; 212: 2075–9.

47. Dollery CT, Williams FM, Draffan GH *et al.* Arterial blood levels of fluorocarbons in asthmatics following the use of pressurized aerosols. *Clin Pharmacol Ther* 1974; 15: 59–66.

48. Thompson PJ, Dhillon P, Cole P. Addiction to aerosol treatment: the asthmatic alternative to glue sniffing. *BMJ* 1983; 287: 1515.

49. Brennan PO. Addiction to aerosol treatment. *BMJ* 1983; 287: 1877.

50. O'Callaghan C, Milner AD. Aerosol treatment abuse. *Arch Dis Child* 1988; 63: 70.

51. Newman SP. Metered dose pressurized aerosols and the ozone layer. *Eur Respir J* 1990; 3: 495–7.

52. Leach CL. Preclinical safety of propellant HFA-134a and Airomir. *Br J Clin Pract* 1995; (suppl.) 79: 10–12.

53. Alexander DJ. Safety of propellants. *J Aerosol Med* 1995; 8: S29–S47.

54. ✪ Leach CL. Safety assessment of the HFA propellant and the new inhaler. *Eur Respir Rev* 1997; 7: 35–6.

55. Leach CL, Davidson PJ, Boudreau RJ. Improved airway targeting with the CFC-free HFA-beclomethasone metered-dose inhaler compared with CFC-beclomethasone. *Eur Respir J* 1998; 12: 1346–53.

56. Yarbrough J, Mansfield L, Ting S. Metered dose inhaler induced bronchospasm in asthmatic patients. *Ann Allergy* 1985; 55: 25–7.

57. Shim CS, Williams MH. Cough and wheezing from beclomethasone dipropionate aerosol are absent after triamcinalone acetonide. *Ann Intern Med* 1987; 106: 700–3.

58. Williamson I, Matusiewicz S, Brown P, Crompton G, Greening AP. Frequency of voice problems and cough in patients using aerosol steroid preparations. *Thorax* 1991; 46: 769P.

59. Selroos O, Löfroos A-B, Pietinalho A, Riska H. Comparison of terbutaline and placebo from a pressurised metered dose inhaler and a dry powder inhaler in a subgroup of patients with asthma. *Thorax* 1994; 49: 1228–30.

60. Hallworth GW. An improved design of powder inhaler. *Br J Clin Pharmacol* 1977; 4: 689–90.

61. Duncan D, Paterson IC, Harris D, Crompton GK. Comparison of the bronchodilator effects of salbutamol inhaled as a dry powder and by conventional pressurised aerosol. *Br J Clin Pharmacol* 1977; 4: 669–71.

62. Hetzel MR, Clark TJH. Comparison of salbutamol Rotahaler with conventional pressurized aerosol. *Clin Allergy* 1977; 7: 563–8.

63. Hartley JP, Nogrady SG, Gibby OM, Seaton A. Bronchodilator effects of dry salbutamol powder administered by Rotahaler. *Br J Clin Pharmacol* 1977; 4: 673–5.

64. Carmichael J, Duncan D, Crompton GK. Beclomethasone dipropionate dry-powder inhalation compared with conventional aerosol in chronic asthma. *BMJ* 1978; 2: 657–8.

65. Morrison Smith J, Gwynn CM. A clinical comparison of aerosol and powder administration of beclomethasone dipropionate in asthma. *Clin Allergy* 1978; 8: 479–81.

66. Edmunds AT, McKenzie S, Tooley M, Godfrey S. A clinical comparison of beclomethasone dipropionate delivered by pressurised aerosol and as a powder from a Rotahaler. *Arch Dis Child* 1979; 54: 233–5.

67. Chambers S, Dunbar J, Taylor B. Inhaled powder compared with aerosol administration of fenoterol in asthmatic children. *Arch Dis Child* 1980; 55: 73–4.

68. Crompton GK. Inhalation devices. *Eur J Respir Dis* 1982; 63: 489–92.

69. Croner S, Hedenskog NI, Odelram H. Salbutamol by powder or spray inhalation in childhood asthma. *Allergy* 1980; 35: 589–92.

70. Meldrum L, Wheeler AWE, Huskisson SC, Palmer JBD. *International Diskhaler Handling Study STC 406.* Greenford: Glaxo Group Research.

71. Gunawardena KA, Pleace KJ, Clay MM, Fuller RW. Salmeterol delivered from a new multi-dose powder inhaler (Diskus/Accuhaler) or Diskhaler inhaler in adult asthmatics. *Am J Resp Crit Care Med* 1994; 149 (4 part 2): A219.

72. Wetterlin K. Turbuhaler: a new powder inhaler for administration of drugs to the airways. *Pharm Res* 1988; 5: 506–8.

73. Pedersen S, Hansen OR, Fugsland G. Influence of inspiratory flow rate upon the effect of a Turbuhaler. *Arch Dis Child* 1990; 65: 308–10.

74. Brown PH, Greening AP, Crompton GK. Peak inspiratory flow rates in acute asthma: are they adequate for efficient use of a Turbuhaler? *Thorax* 1992; 47: 239P.

75. Tonnesen F, Laursen LC, Ibsen T, Evald T, St Åhl E. Terbutaline powder in acute bronchial obstruction. *Lancet* 1991; 337: 1099–1100.

76. Crompton GK. New inhalation devices. *Eur Respir J* 1988; 1: 679–80.

77. Brown PH, Lenney J, Armstrong S, Ning ACWS, Crompton G. Breath-actuated inhalers in chronic asthma: comparison of Diskhaler and Turbohaler for delivery of beta-agonists. *Eur Respir J* 1992; 5: 1143–5.

78. Anani A, Higgins AJ, Crompton GK. Breath-actuated inhalers; comparison of terbutaline Turbuhaler with salbutamol Rotahaler. *Eur Respir J* 1989; 2: 640–2.

79. Stallert RALM. The Bricanyl Turbuhaler, efficacy and acceptability compared to the Ventolin Rotahaler. *Abstract, XIII International Congress of Allergy and Clinical Immunology, Montreux*, October 1988.

80. Sinninghe Damsté HEJ. Turbuhaler – a clinical overview. In: *Turbuhaler – a non-CFC metered dose inhaler*. Report of a symposium held at the 8th Congress of the International Society for Aerosols in Medicine. Davos, Switzerland, April 1991. Amsterdam Excerpta Medica, 1992: 12–3.

81. de Boer AH, Hagerdoorn P, Gjaltema D. Necessary flow rates for maximum fine particle outputs from commercial dry powder inhalers. *Eur Respir J* 1996; 9: (suppl. 23) 206s.

82. Pedersen S. How to use a Rotahaler. *Arch Dis Child* 1986; 61: 11–4.

83. Richards R, Saunders M. Need for a comparative performance standard for dry powder inhalers. *Thorax* 1993; 48: 1186–7.

84. Newman SP, Morén F, Trofast E, Talaee N, Clarke SW. Deposition and clinical efficacy of terbutaline sulphate from Turbuhaler, a new multi-dose powder inhaler. *Eur Respir J* 1989; 2: 247–52.

85. Pauwels R, Derom E. Deposition and pharmacodynamics of terbutaline inhaled via Turbuhaler. *J Aerosol Med* 1991; 4 (suppl. 1): A187.

86. Thorsson L, Edsbäcker S. Lung deposition of budesonide from Turbuhaler is twice that from a pressurised metered dose inhaler (MDI). *Thorax* 1993; 4: 434.

87. Brambilla C, Braunstein G, Lacronique J, Allaert F, Godard P, Duroux P. Comparison between beclomethasone dipropionate by metered dose inhaler and budesonide by Turbuhaler in asthmatic adults. *Am Rev Respir Dis* 1992; 145: A737.

88. Engel T, Heinig JH, Malling H-J, Scharling B, Nikander K, Madsen F. Clinical comparison of inhaled budesonide delivered either via pressurized metered dose inhaler or Turbuhaler. *Allergy* 1989; 44: 220–5.

89. Sinninghe Damsté HEJ, Oostinga P, Heeringa A. Clinical comparison of inhaled budesonide administered via a pressurized metered dose inhaler or via Turbuhaler in patients with bronchial asthma. *Eur Respir J* 1989; 2: (suppl. 8): 861s.

90. Selroos O, Halme M. Effect of a Volumatic spacer and mouth rinsing on systemic absorption of inhaled corticosteroids from a metered dose inhaler and dry powder inhaler. *Thorax* 1991; 46: 891–4.

91. Hardy JG, Newman SP, Knoch M. Lung deposition from four nebulisers. *Respir Med* 1993; 87: 461–5.

92. Thomas SHL, O'Doherty MJ, Graham A *et al.* Pulmonary deposition of nebulised amiloride in cystic fibrosis: comparison of two nebulisers. *Thorax* 1991; 46: 717–21.

93. Clay MM, Pavia D, Newman SP, Clarke SW. Factors influencing the size distribution of aerosols from jet nebulisers. *Thorax* 1983; 38: 755–9.

94. Clay MM, Pavia D, Newman SP, Lennard-Jones T, Clarke SW. Assessment of jet nebulisers for lung aerosol therapy. *Lancet* 1983; ii: 592–4.

95. Newman SP, Pellow PGD, Clarke SW. The flow-pressure characteristics of compressors used for inhalation therapy. *Eur J Respir Dis* 1987; 71: 122–6.

Chapter 23

Immunotherapy

Samantha Walker and Stephen Durham

INTRODUCTION

Allergen immunotherapy involves the weekly subcutaneous injection of increasing concentrations of an allergen extract followed by monthly "maintenance" injections for several years. The aim is to induce a state of immunological and clinical tolerance with a marked reduction (or absence) of clinical symptoms following subsequent natural allergen exposure. The approach is logical and complementary to allergen avoidance strategies. Thus both depend upon an accurate clinical and immunological diagnosis of the cause of symptoms (generally obtained from the clinical history and allergen skin-prick tests) and attempt to alleviate symptoms through either elimination of the cause or modification of the host response to that cause. However, in assessing the potential values of immunotherapy, efficacy must be balanced against side-effects.

Although widely practised in the USA and Europe, the use of immunotherapy in the UK diminished markedly following a report in 1986 by the Committee on Safety of Medicines.[1] The report questioned the safety of this form of therapy in the UK. A position paper of the British Society of Allergy and Clinical Immunology[2] concluded that immunotherapy was indicated in patients with severe seasonal rhinitis unresponsive to pharmacological treatments, but not indicated in patients with asthma because evidence for efficacy was less convincing and the risk of side-effects was greater in asthmatic. Two position statements[3,4] do recommend that specific immunotherapy may be indicated in asthmatics with clearly defined allergies when avoiding allergens is not possible, and when medications fail to control symptoms. A recent meta-analysis of immunotherapy for asthma provided convincing evidence of efficacy. However the risk/benefit ratio is less favorable for asthma[5] than rhinitis. In this review the role of allergen immunotherapy is considered for rhinitis and asthma separately and an attempt made to balance efficacy with side-effects. Possible mechanisms of immunotherapy are considered in the context of future improvements in this form of treatment.

IMMUNOTHERAPY FOR RHINITIS

Seasonal allergic rhinitis in the UK is most commonly due to allergy to grass pollen, although symptoms during the spring may be due to tree pollens whereas late summer and early autumn coincide with symptoms induced by weeds and mould spores.[6] Avoidance of pollen allergens is difficult, although simple advice such as wearing sunglasses and keeping windows shut in cars and buildings may be helpful. Recent advances in treatment include the availability of topical nasal corticosteroids and oral H_1-selective anti-histamines with a low sedative profile. A recent meta-analysis reported superior symptom control by intranasal corticosteroids over H_1 receptor antagonists on nasal blockage, nasal discharge, nasal itch, post-nasal drip and total nasal symptoms.[7] However, as recently highlighted in a GP-based study, many patients (62%) have uncontrolled symptoms despite the availability of these preparations,[8] emphasizing the need for additional treatments such as immunotherapy. Double-blind placebo controlled trials have shown that immunotherapy is effective in patients with seasonal pollinosis due to grass pollen.[9-12] In one study[12] 40 patients with severe symptoms uncontrolled by conventional antiallergic drugs were treated in a double-blind fashion with a biologically standardized alum-precipitated depot grass pollen extract or matched placebo injections. There was a marked reduction in both seasonal

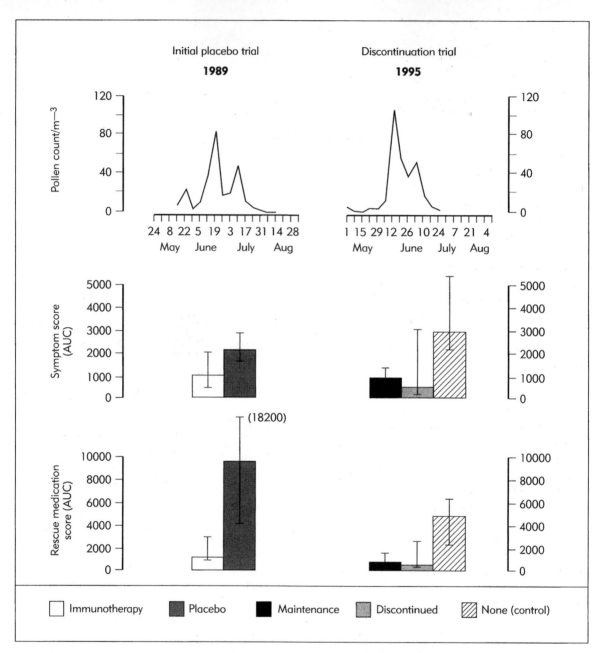

FIGURE 23.1: Symptom scores and rescue medication in 40 adult patients who received immunotherapy or placebo injections for 1 year (1989). After 3–4 years' immunotherapy treatment, the patients were randomized double-blind to receive continued immunotherapy for a further 3 years (maintenance group) or placebo injections (the discontinuation group). Results after the withdrawal phase (1995) are compared with a matched immunotherapy-naïve group. Results are expressed as median area under curve ± interquartile ranges for the peak 11-week pollen season. Grass pollen counts for 1989 and 1995 are expressed as mean weekly counts.

symptoms and the use of rescue medication in the actively-treated group (Fig. 23.1). Systemic side-effects were infrequent (1 in 500 injections) and occurred within 10 minutes of injection. A follow-up study confirmed that clinical efficacy persisted for 3–4 years during continued maintenance injection immunotherapy.[13] Further controlled studies have shown that immunotherapy with birch pollen,[14,15] ragweed[16] and mould allergens[17] may also be effective for rhinitis in carefully selected patients. Perennial rhinitis due to house-dust mite allergy may require long-term use of topical and oral medications. Double-blind placebo-controlled studies using mite immunotherapy have shown efficacy in treating symptoms of perennial allergic rhinitis.[18–20]

Only one study has compared the efficacy of immunotherapy for allergic rhinitis with pharmacotherapy.[21] Treatment with an aqueous topical corticosteroid nasal spray was more effective than treatment with a non-standardized low-potency ragweed extract. Clearly further well-designed comparator studies are needed.

We recently showed that immunotherapy for grass pollen allergy induced prolonged clinical remission.[22] We conducted a randomized double-blind placebo-controlled trial of the discontinuation of immunotherapy in patients in whom 3–4 years' treatment had previously been shown to be effective (Fig. 23.1). A matched group of patients with hayfever who had not received immunotherapy were followed as a control for the natural history of the disease. Seasonal symptoms and use of rescue medication which included short courses of prednisolone remained low for 3 years during the withdrawal phase and there were no significant differences between patients who continued immunotherapy and those who discontinued it (Fig. 23.2). In contrast, symptoms and medication scores were markedly lower for both groups compared to the group who had never received immunotherapy (Fig. 23.1). Other studies of patients with birch,[14] mite,[23] cat[24] or venom[25] allergy who have received 3–5 years' treatment and who were followed up for several years after discontinuation provide further evidence for long-term efficacy. In contrast, in controlled studies of withdrawal of immunotherapy, where the duration of treatment before discontinuation was one year or less, efficacy and objective tests (including the late phase response after allergen inhalation) relapsed within one year.[26–28] One controlled study of withdrawal following 3 years' treat-

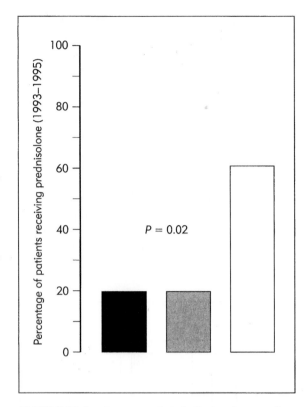

FIGURE 23.2: Long-term clinical efficacy of grass pollen immunotherapy. During the 3-year withdrawal phase (1993–1995), seasonal requirements for short courses of "rescue" predisolone were markedly reduced in both the maintenance and discontinuation groups (3/15 patients in both groups) compared with the immunotherapy-naïve hay-fever group (9/15 patients). (χ^2 test $P = 0.02$.) Key: ■, Maintenance; ▨, discontinued; □, none (control).

ment with a ragweed extract showed recrudescence of nasal responses to allergen at one year, although symptom scores remained low in both active and placebo groups.[29]

IMMUNOTHERAPY FOR ASTHMA

The role of immunotherapy for asthma is controversial. Asthma is frequently multifactorial and only occasionally due to sensitivity to a single inhaled aeroallergen. The exception is grass pollen-induced asthma where several studies have confirmed that injection immunotherapy is effective in reducing asthma symptoms and treatment requirements.[10,28,30,31]

We recently studied 44 adult patients with severe summer hayfever in whom more than half developed peak-seasonal asthma symptoms and increases in bronchial responsiveness to methacholine prior to treatment. Following 2 years' treatment, there was an approximate 50% reduction in hayfever symptoms including chest symptoms (Fig. 23.3) and an 80% reduction in medication scores in the actively treated group. Clinical improvement was accompanied by inhibition of seasonal increases in bronchial methacholine responsiveness. By use of a modified "cluster" regime of grass pollen injections and pre-treatment with antihistamine before injections, the induction period was reduced from 16 to 4 weeks. During this period no immediate systemic reactions were observed.[32]

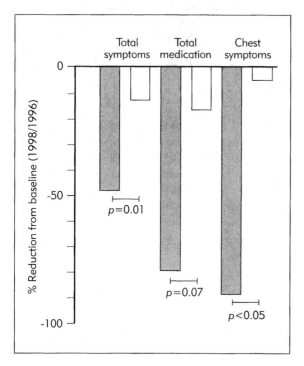

FIGURE 23.3: Reductions in seasonal hayfever symptoms, medication requirements and chest symptoms in 44 adult patients with severe summer hayfever between 1996 and 1998. After the baseline year (1996) patients were stratified for disease severity and randomized double-blind to receive immunotherapy (■) or placebo (□) injections. Results are expressed as the median percentage change of the individual area under curve measurements for the peak 11-week pollen season.

Results following immunotherapy in asthmatic patients with house-dust mite sensitivity have recently been reported in a meta-analysis of optimally designed studies published between 1966 and 1998.[5] Clinical efficacy was measured by asthma symptom scores, asthma medication scores and changes in specific/non-specific bronchial hyperresponsiveness. Of the five mite studies reporting detailed symptom scoring, four showed a significant reduction in asthma symptoms.[18,33-35] The only study not reporting efficacy was not adequately blinded and the authors of the meta-analysis identified methodological problems.[36] Other mite immunotherapy studies with less detailed asthma symptom scoring also favoured immunotherapy. Nine out of 12 blinded studies showed that patients receiving immunotherapy were significantly less likely to report a deterioration in symptoms than those treated with placebo. Asthma medication was also significantly reduced in five out of five studies reporting evaluable results.[34-38] In this analysis, immunotherapy *per se* improved allergen-specific bronchial responsiveness but had no effect on non-specific bronchial hyperresponsiveness or measurement of peak expiratory flow rate/forced expiratory volume in 1 s ($PEFR/FEV_1$). There was significant heterogeneity between mite immunotherapy studies which showed less improvement in symptoms than immunotherapy with pollen and animal dander. Immunotherapy in patients with cat-induced asthma improved asthma symptoms and allergen-specific bronchial responsiveness in one study,[39] but studies have in general focused on the results of bronchial provocation tests[40,41] which may or may not relate to clinical efficacy. A major problem in considering the role of immunotherapy for asthma is that no adequate studies comparing immunotherapy with pharmacotherapy have been performed. Also, it is essential to consider safety aspects (see below) since the risks of immunotherapy with asthma are increased.

IMMUNOTHERAPY IN CHILDREN

Immunotherapy appears to have a greater beneficial effect in children than adults. This is clearly demonstrated in asthmatic children with house-dust mite allergy.[18,42,43] The arbitrary cut-off age below which immunotherapy is not recommended has been set at 5 years. The majority of trials of immunotherapy in children have focused on asthma, as allergic rhinoconjunctivitis tends to be less prominent in this age group. One study has shown that allergen injection immunotherapy in children might reduce the onset of new sensitizations in children.[23] A multicentre study of children with seasonal rhinitis assessed whether or not specific allergen immunotherapy may prevent the onset of allergic asthma in this group. After 3 years' treatment, as well as 2 years after discontinuation of treatment (5 year follow-up) significantly fewer patients developed asthma symptoms in the active group compared with the control group.[44] Although preliminary, this study, which involved standardized allergen extracts, was comparable to a previous 14-year follow-up study in children which suggested that progression from rhinitis to asthma in children may be reduced by specific immunotherapy.[45] Clearly further studies are required; however the available data suggest that in contrast to pharmacological treatment, immunotherapy in children may have a prophylactic effect which persists following discontinuation of treatment. However, there is a tendency for spontaneous improvement of allergic disease in childhood and further more prolonged controlled trials of immunotherapy are required.

SAFETY

Adverse reactions to allergen immunotherapy may occasionally occur. These range from large immediate or delayed local skin responses to immediate systemic reactions, and rarely, life-threatening anaphylaxis. Delayed systemic reactions are less common, in general taking the form of rhinitis, urticaria or lethargy. In patients with asthma delayed bronchospasm may occur. This is important and in all countries immunotherapy guidelines recommend a period of observation following allergen injections. Anaphylaxis (although rare) almost always occurs within minutes, and when recognized early, responds promptly to treatment with adrenaline. In contrast asthmatic patients, particularly those with unstable or poorly controlled asthma are susceptible to the development of delayed bronchospasm which may occur after the patient has left the clinic, in the absence of medical supervision and treatment. This represents the major objection to allergen immunotherapy for asthma. In 1986 the report by the British Committee on Safety of Medicines[1] identified 26 fatalities over the previous 30 years following allergen immunotherapy in the UK. In the 17 patients in whom the indication for injection immunotherapy was known, 16 of these patients received immunotherapy for treatment of asthma (i.e. not rhinitis). Similarly, recent

reports from the USA[46,47] have revealed that between 1987 and 1991, there were 19 deaths associated with immunotherapy of which at least 16 occurred in patients with asthma. Thus patients with asthma are at greater risk of the development of severe systemic reactions.

IMMUNOTHERAPY BY ALTERNATIVE ROUTES

Parenteral allergen injection therapy involves the inconvenience of frequent visits, the discomfort associated with injections and the possibility of adverse reactions. These possibilities have led to renewed interest in using alternative routes of immunotherapy. The best evidence for efficacy comes form the sublingual route, whereby allergen extracts given either daily or several times per week are retained in the mouth for several minutes. One recent study of 2 years' treatment with mite sublingual immunotherapy showed a significant reduction in symptoms in some (but not all) of the winter months[48]; another, using a five-grass pollen mix showed a significant reduction in medication requirements, but no reduction in symptom scores.[49] Several recent well-designed double-blind placebo-controlled trials have also demonstrated clinical efficacy of sublingual–swallow immunotherapy in patients with grass pollen,[50–53] parietaria,[54–56] olive,[57] birch,[58] and mite vaccines[59], although one study in mites showed no difference in symptoms or medication scores between active- and placebo-treated patients. The advantage of this route is the virtual lack of either local or systemic side-effects reported in studies to date. If good efficacy is confirmed, this route provides an attractive alternative, particularly for use in children. The nasal route has also been shown to be effective using pollens[60–62] and mites.[63] Although local side-effects may occur with the nasal route these may be reduced by pre-treatment with nasal cromoglycate. The use of the oral or inhaled route for immunotherapy is not currently recommended.[4]

MECHANISM OF IMMUNOTHERAPY

The mechanisms by which immunotherapy reduces symptoms on re-exposure to allergen are largely unknown. In patients with seasonal pollinosis (hayfever) treated with specific immunotherapy, there is an initial increase in allergen specific IgE concentrations. IgE concentrations subsequently return to baseline although there is a blunting of the usual seasonal increases in IgE during natural pollen exposure.[64] The "blocking antibody theory" is based on the consistent finding of elevated IgG$_4$ concentrations.[65,66] However these changes in serum antibody concentrations do not appear to be related to the clinical response and may possibly represent a "bystander effect" following exposure to high concentrations of allergen during injection immunotherapy. Immunotherapy has also been shown to reduce effector cells including mast cells[66,67] and eosinophils[68,69] in the target organ.[70] For example, ragweed immunotherapy reduced eosinophils in nasal washings following allergen challenge in a dose-dependent manner according to the total dose of allergen given during immunotherapy.[68]

More recent studies have focused on the role of the T-lymphocyte in orchestrating local mast cell migration, tissue eosinophilia and local IgE regulation[70–72] (Fig. 23.4). For example successful grass pollen immunotherapy was associated with a decrease in the late cutaneous response and a decrease in infiltrating CD4$^+$ T-lymphocytes and activated eosinophils in late cutaneous biopsies following intradermal allergen.[73] In situ hybridization studies of both cutaneous[73] and nasal biopsies[71] have suggested that there may be a change in the profile of cytokines produced by infiltrating T-lymphocytes away from that of a "TH$_2$-type" phenotype (with production of IL-4 and IL-5) in favour of a "TH$_1$-type" response with increase in local production of interferon-γ. Other studies based on measurements of peripheral blood T-lymphocytes have suggested that immunotherapy may act by decreasing T-cell proliferation and cytokine production by both TH$_2$ and TH$_1$-type cells.[72,74–76] This may reflect the development of T-lymphocyte tolerance as observed during in vitro studies of immunological tolerance induction.[77] Either or both mechanisms may operate in different individuals and vaccination schedules.[78]

FUTURE DIRECTIONS OF IMMUNOTHERAPY

The above work suggests alternative approaches to immunotherapy. For example immunosuppressive therapy using cyclosporin A has recently been shown to be effective in patients with severe asthma.[79] An alternative strategy may be the use of anti-CD$_4$ monoclonal antibodies, an approach which has been used in rheumatoid disease.[80] Antibodies or antagonists directed against specific cytokines, particularly IL-4[81] and IL-5,[82] may possibly be effective. DNA allergen vaccines have

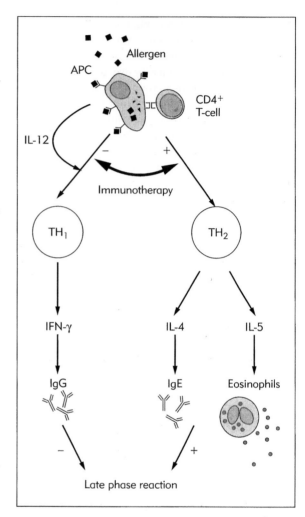

FIGURE 23.4: Hypothesis of mechanism of immunotherapy: shift in favour of a TH$_1$-type response may occur either as a consequence of selective down-regulation (anergy) of the TH$_2$ response or immune deviation under the influence of IL-12. APC: antigen presenting cell; IFN-γ: interferon-γ; IL-4: interleukin 4; IL-5: interleukin 5. (From Durham SR, Till SJ. Immunologic changes associated with allergen immunotherapy. *J Allergy Clin Immunol* 1998; 102: 157–64, with permission.)

been investigated in animal models.[83] An interesting possibility may be the development of peptides which recognize sensitized T-lymphocytes but do not bind IgE.[84] These so-called non-stimulatory peptides may have the potential to modify T-lymphocyte function without provoking IgE-mediated mast cell activation.[85]

The risk of anaphylaxis and other IgE-mediated side-effects might thereby be markedly reduced.

CONCLUSIONS

When considering allergen injection immunotherapy the benefits, side-effects, cost and duration of symptomatic treatment and patient preference must be balanced against those of pharmacotherapy. At present immunotherapy is recommended in the UK in patients with seasonal allergic rhinitis who fail to respond to treatment with topical corticosteroids and antihistamines.[2] In Europe, pollen immunotherapy is considered an adjunct to drug therapy and is introduced earlier.[4] Although immunotherapy for perennial rhinitis due to mite sensitivity is effective, further studies using standardized vaccines should be performed in order to monitor safety and identify safe protocols.

Allergen immunotherapy is a controversial treatment for asthma. It has been shown to be efficacious in pollen asthma and, particularly mite asthma in children. Immunotherapy has not been shown to be effective in patients with perennial allergy and multiple sensitivities. The efficacy of immunotherapy has not been compared with pharmacological treatment. In view of the potential for serious side-effects immunotherapy is not currently indicated within the UK for the treatment of asthma.

Immunotherapy should only be performed with standardized extracts of proven efficacy and in specialist centres with the availability of resuscitated measures.

Important issues for future research include the influence of immunotherapy in modifying disease progression, the evaluation of different immunotherapy protocols, including use of alternative routes of immunotherapy, in terms of efficacy and safety, the optimum duration of immunotherapy and evaluation of factors contributing to adverse reactions. Novel approaches include the use of low molecular weight allergen peptide vaccines which retain the potential to alter T-cell responses whilst avoiding IgE-cross-linking and therefore the possibility of serious IgE-mediated adverse events.

KEY POINTS

1 Allergen immunotherapy is effective in selected patients with IgE-mediated disease and sensitivity to one or a limited number of allergens.

2 Immunotherapy is particularly effective for hayfever and inhibits peak seasonal wheezing and seasonal increases in non-specific bronchial hyperresponsiveness.

3 High-quality, standardized allergen extracts should be used for both diagnosis and treatment.

4 The response to immunotherapy is allergen-specific; mixtures of allergens unrelated to the patient's sensitivity should *not* be used.

5 Treatment should be given for at least 3 years; recent data suggest that an adequate course of treatment (3–4 years) may induce long-term remission for at least 3 years.

6 Immunotherapy in selected patients may be effectively *combined* with allergen avoidance measures and pharmacotherapy.

7 The mechanisms of immunotherapy include changes in allergen-specific antibody levels (increases in IgG, blunting of IgE antibodies), a decrease in the recruitment of effector cells at mucosal sites (mast cells, eosinophils, basophils) and modulation of T-cell responses with alteration of the TH_2/TH_1 balance, either by immune deviation or induction of allergen-specific T-cell unresponsiveness (anergy).

8 Future approaches are likely to include the use of alternative routes of administration and the development of safer vaccines by use of recombinant/modified allergens and allergen peptides.

REFERENCES

1. Committee on Safety of Medicines. Desensitisation vaccines. *BMJ* 1986; 293: 948.

2. BSACI Working Party. Position Paper on Allergen Immunotherapy. *Clin Exp Allergy* 1993; 23: 1–44.

3. WHO/NHLBI Workshop Report. *Global strategy for asthma management and prevention* National Institutes of Health, National Heart, Lung and Blood Institute, 1995; 95–3659.

4. ✪ Bousquet J, Lockey RF, Malling H-J (eds). Allergen immunotherapy: therapeutic vaccines for allergic diseases. *WHO Position Paper* 1998; 53 (44): 1.

5. ✪ Abramson M, Puy R, Weiner J. Immunotherapy in asthma: an updated systematic review. *Allergy* 1999; 54: 1022–41.

6. Varney V. Hayfever in the United Kingdom. *Clin Exp Allergy* 1991; 21:757–62.

7. Weiner JM, Abramson MJ, Puy RM. Intranasal corticosteroids versus oral H_1-receptor antagonists in allergic rhinitis: systemic review of randomised controlled trials. *BMJ* 1998; 317: 1624–9.

8. White P, Smith H, Baker N, Davis W, Frew A. Symptom control in patients with hay fever in UK general practice: how well are we doing and is there a need for allergen immunotherapy? *Clin Exp Allergy* 1998; 28: 266–70.

9. Frankland AW, Augustin R. Prophylaxis of summer hayfever and asthma. A controlled trial comparing crude grass-pollen extracts with the isolated main protein component. *Lancet* 1954; 1055–7.

10. Dolz I, Martinez-Cocera C, Bartolome JM, Cimarra M. A double-blind placebo-controlled study of immunotherapy with grass pollen extract Alutard SQ during a 3-year period with initial rush immunotherapy. *Allergy* 1996; 51: 489–500.

11. Ortolani C, Pastorello E, Moss RB. Grass pollen immunotherapy: A single year double-blind, placebo-controlled study in patients with grass pollen induced asthma and rhinitis. *J Allergy Clin Immunol* 1984; 73: 283–90.

12. ✪ Varney VA, Gaga M, Frew AJ, Aber VR, Kay AB, Durham SR. Usefulness of immunotherapy in patients with severe summer hayfever uncontrolled by antiallergic drugs. *BMJ* 1991; 302: 265–9.

13. Walker SM, Varney VA, Gaga M, Jacobson MR, Durham SR. Grass pollen immunotherapy: A four year follow up study. *Allergy* 1995; 50: 405–413.

14. Jacobsen L, Nuchel Petersen B, Wihl JA, Lowenstein H, Ipsen H. Immunotherapy with partially purified and standardised tree pollen extracts. IV. Results from long-term (6 year) follow-up. *Allergy* 1997; 52: 914–20.

15. Viander M, Koivikko A. The seasonal symptoms of hyposensitised and untreated hayfever patients in relation to birch pollen counts: correlations with nasal sensitivity, prick tests and RAST. *Clin Allergy* 1978; 8: 387–96.

16. Lichtenstein L, Norman P, Winkenwerder L et al. A single year of immunotherapy in ragweed hayfever. *Am J Med* 1971; 44: 514–24.

17. Malling H-J, Dreborg S, Weeke B et al. Diagnosis and immunotherapy of mould allergy. V. Clinical efficacy and side effects of immunotherapy with *Cladosporium herbarum*. *Allergy* 1986; 41:507–19.

18. Pichler CE, Marquardsen A, Sparholt S. Specific immunotherapy with *Dermatophagoides pteronyssinus* and *D. farinae* results in decreased bronchial hyperreactivity. *Allergy* 1997; 52: 274–83.

19. McHugh SM, Lavelle B, Kemeny DM, Patel S, Ewan PW. A placebo-controlled trial of immunotherapy with two extracts of *Dermatophagoides pteronyssinus* in allergic rhinitis, comparing clinical outcome with changes in antigen-specific IgE, IgG and IgG subclasses. *J Allergy Clin Immunol* 1990; 86: 521–31.

20. Ewan PW, Alexander MM, Ind PW, Agrell B, Dreborg S. Effective hyposensitisation in allergic rhinitis using a potent partially purified extract of house dust mite. *Clin Allergy* 1988; 18: 501–508.

21. Juniper EF, Kline PA, Ramsdale EH, Hargreave FE. Comparison of the efficacy and side effects of aqueous steroid nasal spray (budesonide) and allergen-injection immunotherapy (Pollinex-R) in the treatment of seasonal allergic rhinoconjunctivitis. *J Allergy Clin Immunol* 1990; 85: 606–611.

22. ✪ Durham SR, Walker SM, Varga E-M et al. Long-term

clinical efficacy of grass pollen immunotherapy. *N Engl J Med* 1999; 341: 468–75.

23. Des Roches A, Paradis L, Menardo J-L, Bouges S, Daures J-P, Bousquet J. Immunotherapy with a standardised *Dermatophagoides pteronyssinus* extract. VI. Specific immunotherapy prevents the onset of new sensitisations in children. *J Allergy Clin Immunol* 1997; 99: 450–53.

24. Hedlin G, Heilborn H, Lilja G, Norrlind K, Pegelow K-O, Schou C. Long-term follow-up of patients treated with a three year course of cat or dog immunotherapy. *J Allergy Clin Immunol* 1995; 96:879–85.

25. Graft DF, Golden DBK, Reisman RE, Valentine MD, Yunginger JW. The discontinuation of hymenoptera venom immunotherapy. *J Allergy Clin Immunol* 1998; 101: 573–5.

26. Van Bever H, Stevens W. Evolution of the late asthmatic reaction during immunotherapy and after stopping immunotherapy. *J Allergy Clin Immunol* 1990; 86: 141–7.

27. Des Roches A, Paradis L, Knani J *et al.* Immunotherapy with a standardised *Dermatophagoides pteronyssinus* extract. V. Duration of the effects of immunotherapy after its cessation. *Allergy* 1996; 51:430–34.

28. Bousquet J, Hejjaoui A, Michel F-B. Specific immunotherapy in asthma. *J Allergy Clin Immunol* 1990; 86: 292–305.

29. Naclerio RM, Proud D, Moylan BM *et al.* A double-blind study of the discontinuation of ragweed immunotherapy. *J Allergy Clin Immunol* 1997; 100: 293–300.

30. Pastorello EA, Pravettoni V, Incorvaia C *et al.* Clinical and immunological effects of immunotherapy with alum-absorbed grass allergoid in grass-pollen-induced hayfever. *Allergy* 1992; 47: 281–90.

31. Reid MJ, Moss RB. Seasonal asthma in Northern California: allergic causes and efficacy of immunotherapy. *J Allergy Clin Immunol* 1986; 78: 590–600.

32. Walker SM, Pajno G, Torres Lima M, Wilson DW, Durham SR. Grass pollen immunotherapy improves quality of life in seasonal rhinitis and reduces peak

seasonal asthma and bronchial hyperresponsiveness. *J Allergy Clin Immunol* 2000; 105 (1 pt 2) abs 211.

33. Armentia Medina A, Tapias JA, Martin JA, Ventas P, Fernandez A. Immunotherapy with the storage mite *Lepidoglyplus destructor*. *Allergol Immunopathol* 1995; 23: 211–23.

34. Torres Costa JC, Placido JL, Moreira Silva JP, Delgardo L, Vaz M. Effects of immunotherapy on symptoms, PEFR, spirometry, and airway responsiveness in patients with allergic asthma to house-dust mites. *Allergy* 1996; 51: 238–44.

35. Machiels JJ, Somville MA, Lebrun PM, Lebecque SJ, Jacquemin MG, Saint-Remy JM. Allergic bronchial asthma due to *Dermatophagoides pteronsyssinus* hypersensitivity can be efficiently treated by innoculation of allergen-antibody complexes. *J Clin Invest* 1990; 85: 1024–35.

36. Franco C, Barbadori S, Freshwater LL, Kordash TR. A double-blind placebo-controlled study of Alpare mite *D. pteronyssinus* immunotherapy in asthmatic patients. *Allergol Immunopathol* 1995; 23: 58–66.

37. Paranos S, Petrovic S. Early effects of rush immunotherapy with *Dermatophagoides pteronyssinus* in asthmatics. *J Invest Allergol Clin Immunol* 1997; 7: 588–95.

38. Price JF, Warner JO. A controlled trial of hyposensitisation with adsorbed tyrosine *Dermatophagoides pteronyssinus* antigen in childhood asthma: *in vivo* aspects. *Clin Allergy* 1984; 14: 209–219.

39. ✪ Varney VA, Edwards J, Tabbah K, Brewster H, Mavroleon G, Frew AJ. Clinical efficacy of specific immunotherapy to cat dander: a double-blind placebo-controlled trial. *Clin Exp Allergy* 1997; 27: 860–67.

40. Sundin B, Lilja G, Graff-Lonnevig V *et al.* Immunotherapy with partially purified and standardised animal dander extracts I. Clinical results from a double-blind study on patients with animal dander asthma. *J Allergy Clin Immunol* 1986; 77: 478–87.

41. van Metre TE, Marsh DG, Adkinson NF *et al.* Immunotherapy for cat asthma. *J Allergy Clin Immunol* 1988; 82: 1053–8.

42. Warner JO, Price JF. Controlled trial of hyposensitisation to *Dermatophagoides pteronyssinus* in children with asthma. *Lancet* 1978; ii: 912.

43. D'Souza M, Pepys J, Wells I et al. Hyposensitisation with Dermatophagoides pteronyssinus in house dust allergy: a controlled study of clinical immunological effects. Clin Allergy 1973; 3: 177–93.

44. Valovirta E. Capacity of specific immunotherapy in prevention of allergic asthma in children: the Preventive Allergy Treatment Study (PAT). J Invest Allergol Clin Immunol 1999; 7(5): 369–70.

45. Johnstone DE, Dutton DA. The value of hyposensitisation therapy for bronchial asthma in children – a 14 year study. Pediatrics 1968; 42(5): 793–802.

46. Reid MJ, Lockey RF, Turkeltaub PC, Platts-Mills TAE. Fatalities from immunotherapy and skin testing. J Allergy Clin Immunol 1990; 85: 180.

47. Reid MJ, Lockey RF, Turkeltaub PC, Platts-Mills AE. Survey of fatalities from skin testing and immunotherapy 1985–1989. J Allergy Clin Immunol 1993; 92: 6–15.

48. ✪ Passalacqua G, Albano L, Fregonese L et al. Randomised controlled trial of local allergoid immunotherapy on allergic inflammation in mite-induced allergic rhinoconjunctivitis. Lancet 1998; 351: 629–32.

49. Clavel R, Bousquet J, Andre C et al. Clinical efficacy of sublingual swallow immunotherapy: a double-blind placebo-controlled trial of a standardised five-grass-pollen extract in rhinitis. Allergy 1998; 53: 493–8.

50. Feliziania V, Lattuada G, Parmiani S, Dall'Aglio PP. Safety and efficacy of sublingual rush immunotherapy with grass pollen extracts. A double-blind study. Allergol Immunopathol 1995; 23: 224–30.

51. Sabbah A, Hassoun S, Le Sellin J, Andre C, Sicard H. A double-blind placebo-controlled trial by the sublingual route of immunotherapy with a standardised grass pollen extract. Allergy 1994; 49: 309–313.

52. Hordijk GJ, Antvelink JB, Luwema RA et al. Sublingual immunotherapy with a standardised grass pollen extract; a double-blind placebo-controlled study. Allergol Immunopathol 1998; 26: 234–40.

53. Pradalier A, Basset D, Claudel A et al. Sublingual-swallow immunotherapy (SLIT) with a standardised five-grass-pollen extract (drops and sublingual tablets) versus placebo in seasonal rhinitis. Allergy 1999; 54: 819–28.

54. Purello-D'Ambrosio F, Gangemi S, Isola S et al. Sublingual immunotherapy: a double-blind, placebo-controlled trial with Parietaria judaica extract standardised in mass units in patients with rhinoconjunctivitis, asthma or both. Allergy 1999; 54: 968–73.

55. La Rosa M, Ranno C, Andre C, Carat F, Tosca MA, Canonica GW. Double-blind placebo-controlled evaluation of sublingual-swallow immunotherapy with standardised Parietaria judaica extract in children with allergic rhinoconjunctivitis. J Allergy Clin Immunol 1999; 104: 425–32.

56. Troise C, Voltolini S, Canessa A, Pecora S, Negrini AC. Sublingual immunotherapy in Parietaria pollen-induced rhinitis: a double-blind study. J Invest Allergol Clin Immunol 1995; 5: 25–30.

57. Vourdas D, Syrigou E, Potamianou P et al. Double-blind placebo-controlled evaluation of sub-lingual immunotherapy with standardised olive pollen extract in pediatric patients with allergic rhinoconjunctivitis and mild asthma due to olive pollen sensitisation. Allergy 1998; 53: 662–72.

58. Horak F, Stubner P, Berger B, Marks B, Toth J, Jager S. Immunotherapy with sublingual birch pollen extract. A short-term double-blind placebo study. Invest Allergol Clin Immunol 1998; 8(3): 165–71.

59. Tari MG, Mancino M, Monti G et al. Efficacy of sublingual immunotherapy in patients with rhinitis and asthma due to housedust mite. A double-blind study. Allergol Immunopathol 1990; 18: 277–84.

60. Andri L, Senna G, Bettcli C et al. Local nasal immunotherapy with extract in powder form is effective and safe in grass pollen rhinitis. J Allergy Clin Immunol 1996; 97: 34–41.

61. D'Amato G, Lobefalo G, Liccardi G. Cazzola M. A double-blind, placebo-controlled trial of local nasal immunotherapy in allergic rhinitis to Parietaria pollen. Clin Exp Allergy 1995; 25: 141–8.

62. Georgitis JW, Nickelsen JA, Wypych JI, Barde SH, Clayton WF, Reisman RE. Local intranasal immunotherapy with high-dose polymerised ragweed extract. Int Arch Allergy Appl Immunol 1986; 81: 170–73.

63. Andri L, Senna G, Betteli C, Givanni S, Andri G, Falagiani P. Local nasal immunotherapy for *Dermatophagoides*-induced rhinitis: Efficacy of a powder extract. *J Allergy Clin Immunol* 1993; 91: 987–96.

64. Lichtenstein L, Ishikaza K, Norman PS, Sobotka AK, Hill BM. IgE antibody measurements in ragweed hayfever. Relationship to clinical severity and the results of immunotherapy. *J Clin Invest* 1973; 52:(472) 482.

65. Djurup R. The subclass nature and clinical significance of the IgG antibody response in patients undergoing allergen specific immunotherapy. *Allergy* 1985; 40: 469–86.

66. Creticos PS, van Metre TE, Mardingley MR, Rosenberg GL, Adkinson NF. Dose-response of IgE and IgG antibodies during ragweed immunotherapy. *J Allergy Clin Immunol* 1984; 73: 94–104.

67. Otsuka H, Mezawa A, Ohnishi M, Okubo K, Seki H, Okuda M. Changes in nasal metachromatic cells during allergen immunotherapy. *Clin Exp Allergy* 1991; 21: 115–19.

68. Furin MJ, Norman PS, Creticos PS *et al.* Immunotherapy decreases antigen-induced eosinophil migration into the nasal cavity. *J Allergy Clin Immunol* 1991; 88: 27–32.

69. Rak S, Lowhagen O, Venge P *et al.* The effect of immunotherapy on bronchial responsiveness and eosinophil cationic protein in pollen allergic patients. *J Allergy Clin Immunol* 1988; 82: 470–80.

70. Fling JA, Ruff ME, Parker WA *et al.* Suppression of the late cutaneous response by immunotherapy. *J Allergy Clin Immunol* 1989; 83: 101–109.

71. Durham SR, Ying S, Varney VA *et al.* Grass pollen immunotherapy inhibits allergen-induced infiltration of CD4+ T lymphocytes and eosinophils in the nasal mucosa and increases the number of cells expressing messenger RNA for interferon-gamma. *Clin Exp Allergy* 1996; 97: 1356–65.

72. ✪ Durham SR, Till SJ. Immunologic changes associated with allergen immunotherapy. *J Allergy Clin Immunol* 1998; 102: 157–64.

73. Varney VA, Hamid QA, Gaga M *et al.* Influence of grass pollen immunotherapy on cellular infiltration and cytokine mRNA expression during allergen-induced late-phase cutaneous responses. *J Clin Invest* 1993; 92: 644–51.

74. Ebner C, Siemann U, Bohle B, Willheim M, Wiederman U, Schenk S. Immunologic changes during specific immunotherapy of grass pollen allergy: reduced lymphoproliferative responses to allergen and shift from TH$_2$ to TH$_1$ in T cell clones specific to *Phl p* I, a major grass pollen allergen. *Clin Exp Allergy* 1997; 27: 1007–1015.

75. ✪ Akdis CA, Blaser K. IL-10-induced anergy in peripheral T cell and reactivation by microenvironmental cytokines: two key steps in specific immunotherapy. *Faseb J* 1999; 13: 603–609.

76. Secrist H, Chelen CJ, Wen Y, Marshall JD, Umetsu DT. Allergen immunotherapy decreases interleukin 4 production in CD4+ cells from allergic individuals. *J Exp Med* 1993; 178: 2123–30.

77. O'Hehir R, Yssel H, Verma S, de Vries JE, Spits H, Lamb JR. Clonal analysis of differential lymphokine production in peptide and superantigen induced T cell anergy. *Internat Immunol* 1991; 3:(8) 819–26.

78. Lake RA, O'Hehir R, Verhoef A, Lamb JR. CD28 mRNA rapidly decays when activated T cells are functionally anergized with specific peptides. *Internat Immunol* 1993; 5:(5) 461–6.

79. Alexander A, Barnes NC, Kay AB. Trial of cyclosporin in corticosteroid-dependent chronic severe asthma. *Lancet* 1993; 339: 324–8.

80. Herzog C, Walker C, Mullit E. Anti-CD4 antibody treatment of patients with rheumatoid arthritis. I. Effect on clinical course and circulating T cells. *J Autoimmun* 1989; 2: 627–42.

81. Fanslow WC, Clifford KN, Rubin AS, Voice RF, Beckman MP, Widmer MB. Regulation of alloreactivity *in vivo* by IL-4 and the soluble IL-4 receptor. *J Immunol* 1991; 147: 535–40.

82. Chand N, Harrison JE, Rooney S *et al.* Anti-IL5 monoclonal antibody inhibits allergic late phase bronchial eosinophilia in guinea pigs: a therapeutic approach. *Eur J Pharmacol* 1992; 211: 121–3.

83. Tighe H, Corr M, Roman M, Raz E. Gene vaccination: plasmid DNA is more than just a blueprint. *Immunol Today* 1998; 19(2): 89–97.

84. O'Hehir R, Busch R, Rothbard JB, Lamb JR. An *in vitro* model of peptide-mediated immunomodulation of the human T cell response to *Dermatophagoides* spp (house dust mite). *J Allergy Clin Immunol* 1990; 87: 1120–27.

85. Haselden BM, Kay AB, Larche M. IgE-independent MHC-restricted T cell peptide epitope-induced late asthmatic reactions. *J Exp Med* 1999; 189: 1885–94.

Chapter 24

Other Forms of Treatment

Rajesh Bhagat and Donald Cockcroft

INTRODUCTION

This chapter is a brief review of several treatment modalities (pharmacological, surgical and "alternative") (Table 24.1) that currently have limited, uncertain or unproven value in management of asthma. Some of these may improve general well-being (e.g. yoga) while others (e.g. herbal therapy) have been the origin of many of the medicines currently in use for managing asthma (sympathomimetics, anti-cholinergics, cromoglycate, theophylline).

PHARMACOLOGICAL

Calcium Channel Blockers

Calcium is involved in excitation–contraction coupling of muscles and release of mediators/secretions from cells.[1–4] So far, two types of cell membrane calcium channels, the voltage-dependent and receptor operated, have been identified. The voltage-dependent channels, which open in response to a wave of rapid depolarization, are found predominantly in smooth muscle cells of arteries and are blocked by currently

Table 24.1: Other forms of treatment

Treatment	Efficacy
Pharmacological treatments	
Calcium channel blockers	Slight (however "safe" vs β blockers)
Magnesium	Slight
Diuretics	Slight
Heparin	Slight
α-adrenergic antagonists	Limited
Mucolytics	Controversial (may cause bronchospasm)
Immunoglobulins	Uncertain
Alternative treatments	
Acupuncture	Limited
Homeopathy	Probably nil
Yoga	Indirect benefit
Hypnosis	Selected cases
Ionizers	Nil
Spinal manipulation	Nil
Surgery	Not recommended

available calcium blockers.[5-6] There is evidence for presence of voltage-dependent channels in the airway smooth muscle.[7] A very limited success in prevention of exercise-induced bronchospasm,[8-12] and variable results in several trials[8-27] with acute or chronic administration of calcium channel blockers in asthmatic patients, suggest another mechanism or a role for receptor operated channels.[28-30] The recent[4] demonstration of mast cell tryptase potentiated contraction in sensitized bronchi via a calcium-related mechanism is indicative of more complex interaction. The main value of the available data is that calcium channel blockers can be safely used for other indications in asthmatic subjects while, for example, β adrenergic blockers are contraindicated.

Magnesium

During an episode of acute severe asthma, along with other mediators, calcium is involved in mediator release.[1-3] Magnesium, a physiological antagonist to calcium,[31] has been shown to cause a short, rapid, mild, clinically insignificant bronchodilating effect.[32,33] Although there are no data to suggest that patients with asthma have decreased serum magnesium levels, recent studies have suggested that there might be an intracellular deficiency, especially in neutrophils[34] and skeletal muscle cells.[35] The clinical relevance of this finding is still at best ambiguous.[36] Intravenous magnesium sulphate has been used for the management of acute severe asthma[32,33,37,38] and has been shown to shift histamine PC_{20} by almost one doubling dose.[39] However, intravenous magnesium sulphate failed to show benefits in acute severe asthma in two studies.[40,41] More recently, in mild stable asthmatics, short-term increase in oral magnesium intake improved the symptom scores, but failed to improve airflow and airway reactivity.[42]

Diuretics

Inhaled furosemide (frusemide) inhibits bronchoconstriction induced by adenosine monophosphate,[43,44] cold air hyperventilation,[45] and exercise,[46] however, methacholine PC_{20} is unaltered.[45,47] Inhaled furosemide also protects against allergen-induced early and late asthmatic responses.[47] These effects are not seen with oral or intravenous furosemide.[46] The absence of similar responses with bumetanide,[43,44] a stronger Na-K-ATPase inhibitor, suggests an alternative mechanism. Acetazolamide, a carbonic anhydrase inhibitor, has also been shown to reduce cold air hyperventilation-induced

bronchoconstriction.[48] The clinical implications of these effects compared with other asthma medications requires further evaluation.

Heparin

Heparin is known to have anti-inflammatory properties,[49] and was initially tried intravenously for management of asthma in the early 1960s without much success. Recently, studies have shown that inhaled heparin may have a role in preventing asthma. The proposed mechanisms range from direct effect on smooth muscle cells to anti-inflammatory effect on neutrophils and/or mast cells.[50-54] The data are very sketchy and several questions are unanswered, including the clinical significance.

α-Adrenergic Antagonists

There is evidence to support the presence of α-receptors in the airways,[55,56] however, their role in asthma is currently felt to be limited. α-adrenergic antagonists have been shown to partially prevent exercise-induced bronchospasm while studies with histamine- and allergen-induced bronchospasm have shown mixed results.[57-62] The situation is further complicated by a report of reduction of exercise-induced bronchospasm by inhaled α_1-adrenergic agonist, methoxamine,[63] and the bronchodilating effects of α_2 agonists.[64] Thus, the role of α-adrenergic receptors in asthma remains unclear.

Mucolytics

Mucus plugging the tracheobronchial tree in asthmatic subjects is well-recognized; even subjects with mild asthma have some amount of impaired mucociliary clearance.[65] Most studies and reviews on control of mucus secretions have concentrated on pulmonary conditions other than asthma.[66-68] This perhaps is a reflection of the fact that most pharmacological methods for mucus management are already in use for therapy of asthma, i.e. corticosteroids, adrenergic drugs and methylxanthines.[67,69] Recently, rhDNase has been used for cystic fibrosis and there is a study showing benefit in three asthmatic children.[70]

Immunoglobulins

In the past, immunoglobulins have been used for management of asthma, especially in children, but there is no rationale for their use except in hypoimmune states co-existing with asthma. However, a recent open-label study demonstrated that high-dose intravenous immunoglobulins might have a corticosteroid-sparing effect.[71]

ALTERNATIVE MEDICINE

Introduction

"Alternative medicine" encompasses all health and therapeutic practices which owe their origin to region, religion, culture, scriptures, word of mouth, folklore and do not have evidence in the form of scientifically carried out trials, as we understand the term today. The need for this review in the era of evidence-based practice of medicine stems from the fact that over 40% of patients, especially those with allergies, have tried alternative forms of therapy and the out-of-pocket cost to the patients in 1997 was conservatively estimated to be 27 billion dollars.[72] The spectrum of therapies ranges from cupping (application of heated cups on the back),[73] speleotherapy (microenvironment control in the form of cave dwelling),[74] bracelets, Chihuahua sniffing, element-containing syrups,[75] and free medicine dispensed inside a live (expensive) fish[76] to systems like acupuncture, homeopathy, yoga, hypnosis, ionizer therapy and herbal medications.[77,78] Indeed, some of modern asthma therapies are derived from herbal folk remedies, e.g ephedrine from *Ma-huang*, anti-cholinergic alkaloids from *Datura stromanium*, khellin (the basis of cromoglycate) from *Ammi visnaga* and theophylline from tea. A long list of herbs are used for management of asthma by Chinese, East Indians (Ayurveda) and American First Nations Peoples. Potentially, some of these may contain the chemicals for future anti-asthma medications.[78,79] However, these herbs are not all benign and some have been associated with severe toxic effects with occasionally fatal outcomes. A 21st century physician not only needs to safeguard against quacks and unregulated over-the-counter availability of these therapies, but also has to be sensitive enough to know that these health practices may form the regional, religious beliefs of the patient which should not be traumatized. Some of these therapies may provide the "holistic feeling of well-being" – which is still difficult to define and quantify by modern-day medicine.

Acupuncture

Acupuncture is an ancient Chinese art of restoring the "balance of Ying and Yang energies" by stimulating specific nodal points on the body surface at specific depth without local anaesthesia with stainless steel needles that are either rotated or vibrated.[77,78,80,81] It has been shown to relieve chronic osteoarticular pain by release of endogenous endorphin.[82] However, in asthma the results of acupuncture are variable. A meta-analysis of 13 studies found that no study earned more than 72% on the study-quality scale; 8 of the 13 favoured acupuncture.[81] "Din Chuan" is the most widely accepted nodal point;[77,83] it is located approximately 4 cm deep bilaterally on the back 3 cm lateral to midpoint of C7 and T1 spinous processes. Stimulation of Din Chuan may improve expiratory flow rates, but does not affect the airway hyperresponsiveness.[83] The limited efficacy of acupuncture, in reversing acute bronchospasm[83] and exercise-induced bronchospasm,[84,85] is less than that of β agonists. Thus, the current NIH consensus statement[86] suggests that acupuncture may be included as a part of a comprehensive programme.

Homeopathy

The principles of homeopathy include (1) "like cure like" and (2) use of exceedingly weak dilutions of active agents.[77] A substance that causes the symptoms is given in very high dilutions (isopathy). Serial 10- or 100-fold dilutions are repeated along with succussion (intensive shaking) to produce dilutions as weak as $1:100^{12}$ (referred to as C12). Dilutions this weak are unlikely to contain even a single molecule of the original agent.[87] The effect is explained by spatial reorientation of water molecules by succussion with the substance.[88] This has been the source of conflict between the sceptic scientists and proponents of homeopathy.[89,90] The mechanism and clinical relevance of studies with use of dilute oral allergen extracts in hay fever and/or asthma showing mild reproducible statistically significant improvement[87,91] are still uncertain.

Yoga

Yoga is a system of complete health care, consisting of exercises that include asanas (postural exercises), pranayama (breathing exercise), kriyas (neti and vaman dhouti, i.e. nasal and stomach wash) and meditation.[92–94] Several studies on yoga in asthma[93–96] have demonstrated objective improvement in peak flow, symptom score and drug intake in addition to subjective improvement. One study[97] demonstrated a one-dose shift of histamine PC_{20} after practising pranayama for 2 weeks. There is a need for standardization of yogic techniques, and to understand pathophysiological mechanisms.

Hypnosis

Psychological factors, especially emotions and stress, contribute to asthma morbidity and mortality.[98,99] Hypnosis is a technique used for alleviating stress; several trials have demonstrated its benefits in asthmatic subjects.[100–104] However, objective benefits have been small and less than from current modalities which constitute the current standard of care. The situation is further complicated by factors such as: practitioner's experience, patient's susceptibility to hypnosis[105] and, more importantly, the strong placebo effect demonstrated by asthmatics.[106] Hypnosis can help a tense, anxious asthmatic subject and may play a role in changing the neurotic attitude of the subject to the disease.

Ionizer Therapy

Large numbers of negatively or positively charged molecules in the environment inhibit bacterial growth and affect both influenza mortality in rats and their life expectancy.[107] Negative ions deplete serotonin concentration in mice and rabbit trachea.[107,108] Ions are produced artificially by thermionic emission, charge separation, γ-radiation or high voltage discharge[109] and, in nature, by shearing of water as in waterfalls, movements of large masses of air, or by cosmic rays.[107]

Initial data suggested that ionizer use may be of benefit for asthmatic subjects.[110–111] However, two well-controlled studies[109,112] showed no benefit despite a fall in airborne allergen; in fact, one study reported an increase in nocturnal cough. Currently, the evidence is against ionizer use for asthma management, but more objective data are needed before condemning this modality to history.

Spinal Manipulation

Since 1895,[113] spinal manipulation has graduated from a bedside procedure to a school of health for managing not only musculoskeletal disorders but also as therapy for varied disorders such as hypertension, otitis media and asthma. The anecdotal reports of its benefit for asthma lead to two controlled trials[114–115] which did not show any benefit.

SURGERY

Carotid body resection (glomectomy), both unilateral and bilateral, was done in asthmatics during the early 1960s for management of breathlessness. However, the procedures were stopped when unilateral glomectomy was shown to be no better than a sham surgery, while bilateral glomectomy reduced the sensitivity of central nervous system to hypoxaemia and hypercarbia, thus further aggravating the clinical condition although the patient felt less dyspnoeic.[116] Surgery is used only for associated conditions like nasal polyps or chronic sinusitis. Although lungs from donors without asthma have been transplanted in asthmatics without subsequent development of asthma,[117] the role of lung transplant in asthma is more of scientific curiosity.

KEY POINTS

1 Treatments outlined here have limited, uncertain or unproven value.

2 Some treatments may indirectly improve the (or any) condition by improvement in general well-being.

REFERENCES

1. Kirkpatrick CT. Excitation and contraction in bovine tracheal smooth muscle. *J Physiol* 1975; 244: 263–81.

2. Foreman JC, Hallett MB, Mongar JL. The relationship between histamine and $^{45}Ca^{++}$ uptake by mast cells. *J Physiol* 1977; 271: 193–214.

3. Holgate ST, Church MK. Control of mediator release from mast cells. *Clin Allergy* 1982; 12 (suppl.): 5–13.

4. Johnson PR, Ammit AJ, Carlin SM, Armour CL, Caughey GH, Black JL. Mast cell tryptase potentiates histamine-induced contraction in human sensitized bronchus. *Eur Respir J* 1997; 10: 38–43.

5. Triggle DJ, Swamy VC. Pharmacology of agents that affect calcium: agonists and antagonists. *Chest* 1980; 78 (suppl.): 174–9.

6. Braunwald E. Mechanism of action of calcium-channel-blocking agents. *New Engl J Med* 1982; 307: 1618–27.

7. Marthan R, Martin C, Amedee T, Mironneau J. Calcium channel currents in isolated smooth muscle cells from human bronchus. *J Appl Physiol* 1989; 66: 1706–1714.

8. Patel KR. Calcium antagonists in exercise induced asthma. *BMJ* 1981; 282: 932–3.

9. Barnes PJ, Wilson NM, Brown MJ. A calcium antagonist, nifedipine, modifies exercise induced asthma. *Thorax* 1981; 36: 726–30.

10. Cerrina J, Denjean A, Alexandre G, Lockhart A, Duroux P. Inhibition of exercise induced asthma by a calcium antagonist, nifedipine. *Am Rev Respir Dis* 1981; 123: 156–60.

11. Corris PA, Nariman S, Gibson GJ. Nifedipine in the prevention of asthma induced by exercise and histamine. *Am Rev of Respir Dis* 1983; 128: 991–2.

12. McIntyre E, Fitzgibbon B, Otto H, Minson R, Alpers J, Ruffin R. Inhaled verapamil in histamine induced bronchoconstriction. *J Allergy Clin Immunol* 1983; 71: 375–81.

13. Williams DO, Barnes PJ, Vickers HP, Rudolf M. Effect of nifedipine on bronchomotor tone and histamine reactivity in asthma. *BMJ* 1981; 283: 348.

14. Malik S, O'Reilly J, Sudlow MF. Effects of sublingual nifedipine on inhaled histamine and methacholine-induced bronchoconstriction in atopic subjects. *Thorax* 1982; 37: 230.

15. So SY, Lam WK, Yu DYC. Effect of calcium antagonists on allergen induced asthma. *Clin Allergy* 1982; 12: 595–600.

16. Patel KR, Kerr JW. Calcium antagonists in experimental asthma. *Clin Allergy* 1982; 12 (suppl.): 15–20.

17. Miadonna A, Tedeschi A, Leiggieri E, Cootiini M, Restuccia M, Bianchini C. Effect of verapamil on allergen-induced asthma in patients with respiratory allergy. *Ann Allergy* 1983; 51: 201–204.

18. Mathews JI, Richey HM III, Ewald FW Jr, Glending DL. Nifedipine does not alter methacholine induced bronchial reactivity. *Ann Allergy* 1984; 53: 462–7.

19. Popa VT, Somani P, Simon V. The effect of inhaled verapamil on resting bronchial tone and airway contraction induced by histamine and acetylcholine in normal and asthmatic subjects. *Am Rev Respir Dis* 1984; 130: 1006–1013.

20. ✪ Ozenne G, Moore ND, Leprevost A et al. Nifedipine in chronic bronchial asthma: a randomised, double blind, cross over trial against placebo. *Eur J Respir Dis* 1985; 67: 238–43.

21. Moscato G, Danna P, Dorigo N et al. Effect of nifedipine on hyperreactive bronchial responses to methacholine. *Ann Allergy* 1986; 56: 145–9.

22. Schwartzstein RH, Fanta CH. Orally administered nifedipine in chronic stable asthma: comparison with an orally administered sympathomimetic. *Am Rev Respir Dis* 1986; 134: 262–5.

23. Ballester E, Roca J, Rodriguez-Roisin R, Agusti-Vidal A. Effect of nifedipine on arterial hypoxemia occurring after methacholine challenge in asthma. *Thorax* 1986; 41: 468–72.

24. Fish JE, Norman PS. Effect of calcium channel blocker, verapamil, on asthmatic airway responses to muscarinic, histaminergic and allergenic stimuli. *Am Rev Respir Dis* 1986; 133: 730–34.

25. Molho M, Gruzman C, Katz I, Lidgi M, Chaniac A. Nifedipine in asthma: dose related effect on bronchial tone. *Chest* 1987; 91: 667–70.

26. Ferrari M, Oliveri M, Gasperi MD, Lechi A. Differential effects of nifedipine and diltiazem on methacholine-induced bronchospasm in allergic asthma. *Ann Allergy* 1989; 63: 196–200.

27. Kivity S, Brayer M, Topilsky M. Combined effects of nifedipine and diltiazem on methacholine induced bronchoconstriction in asthmatic patients. *Ann Allergy* 1992; 68: 175–9.

28. Murray RK, Kotlikoff MI. Receptor-activated calcium influx in human airway smooth muscle cells. *J Physiol* 1991; 435: 123–44.

29. Murray LE. Effects of a receptor operated channel blocker on intracellular calcium in human airway smooth muscle cells. *Am Rev Respir Dis* 1992; 145: A205.

30. Ritchie DM, Kirschner T, Moore JB et al. Experimental antiasthmatic activity of RWJ 22108: a

bronchoselective calcium entry blocker. *Internat Arch Allergy Immunol* 1993; 100: 274–82.

31. Levine BS, Coburn JW. Magnesium the mimic/antagonist of calcium. *New Engl J Med* 1984; 310: 1253–5.

32. Okayama H, Aikawa T, Okayama M, Sasaki H, Mue S, Takishima T. Bronchodilating effect of intravenous magnesium sulphate in bronchial asthma. *J Am Med Ass* 1987; 257: 1076–78.

33. Rolla G, Bucca C, Caria E *et al*. Acute effect of intravenous magnesium sulfate on airway obstruction of asthmatic patients. *Ann Allergy* 1988; 61: 388–91.

34. Fantidis P, Ruiz Cacho J, Marin M, Jarabo RM, Solera J, Herrero E. Intracellular (polymorphonuclear) magnesium content in patients with bronchial asthma between attacks. *J Roy Soc Med* 1995; 88: 441–5.

35. Gustafson T, Boman K, Rosenhall L, Sandstrom T, Wester PO. Skeletal muscle magnesium and potassium in asthmatics treated with oral beta2-agonists. *Eur Respir J* 1996; 9: 237–40.

36. Durlach J. Commentary on recent clinical advances: magnesium depletion, magnesium deficiency and asthma. *Magnesium Res* 1995; 8: 403–405.

37. Skobeloff EM, Spivey WH, McNamara RM, Greenspon L. Intravenous magnesium sulfate for the treatment of acute asthma in the emergency department. *J Am Med Ass* 1989; 262: 1210–13.

38. ✪ Noppen M, Vanmaele L, Impens N, Schandevyl W. Bronchodilating effect of intravenous magnesium sulfate in acute severe asthma. *Chest* 1990; 97: 373–6.

39. Rolla G, Bucca C, Bugrani M, Arossa W, Spinaci S. Reduction of histamine induced bronchoconstriction by magnesium in asthmatic subjects. *Allergy* 1987; 42: 186–8.

40. ✪ Green SM, Rothrock SG. Intravenous magnesium for acute asthma: failure to decrease emergency treatment duration or need for hospitalization. *Ann Emerg Med* 1992; 21: 260–65.

41. Tiffany BR, Berk WA, Todd IK, White SR. Magnesium bolus or infusion fails to improve expiratory flow in acute asthma exacerbations. *Chest* 1993; 104: 831–4.

42. Hill J, Micklewright A, Lewis S, Britton J. Investigation of the effect of short-term change in dietary magnesium intake in asthma. *Eur Respir J* 1997; 10: 2225–9.

43. O'Connor BJ, Chung KF, Chen-Worsdell YM, Fuller RW, Barnes PJ. Effect of inhaled furosemide and bumetanide on adenosine 5-monophosphate and sodium metabisulphite- induced bronchoconstriction in asthmatic subjects. *Am Rev Respir Dis* 1991; 143: 1329–33.

44. Polosa R, Holgate ST. Inhaled furosemide is more effective than inhaled bumetanide in reducing airway responsiveness to adenosine 5-monophosphate (AMP) in asthma. *Am Rev Respir Dis* 1991; 143 (suppl.): A549.

45. Grubbe RE, Hopp R, Dave NK, Brennan B, Bewtra A, Townley R. Effect of inhaled furosemide on the bronchial response to methacholine and cold air hyperventilation challenges. *J Allergy Clin Immunol* 1990; 85: 881–4.

46. ✪ Bianco S, Vaghi A, Robuschi M, Pasargiklian M. Prevention of exercise induced bronchoconstriction by inhaled furosemide. *Lancet* 1988; ii: 252–5.

47. ✪ Bianco S, Peironi MG, Refini RM, Rottoli L, Sestini P. Protective effect of inhaled furosemide on allergen-induced early and late asthmatic reactions. *New Engl J Med* 1989; 321: 1069–1073.

48. O'Donnell WJ, Rosenberg MA, Niven RW, Drazen JM, Israel E. Inhaled acetazolamide attenuates bronchoconstriction induced by cold-air hyperventilation. *Am Rev Respir Dis* 1991; 143 (suppl.): A211.

49. Martineau P, Vaughn LM. DIAS rounds. Heparin inhalation for asthma. *Ann Pharmacother* 1995; 29: 71–3.

50. Fath MA, Wu X, Hileman RE *et al.* Interaction of secretory leukocyte protease inhibitor with heparin inhibits proteases involved in asthma. *J Biol Chem* 1998; 273: 13563–9.

51. Ceyhan B, Celikel T. Effect of inhaled heparin on methacholine-induced bronchial hyperreactivity. *Chest* 1995; 107: 1009–1012.

52. ✪ Diamant Z, Timmers MC, Veen Hvd, Page CP, Meer FJvd, Sterk PJ. Effect of inhaled heparin on

allergen-induced early and late asthmatic responses in patients with atopic asthma. *Am J Resp Crit Care Med* 1996; 153: 1790–95.

53. ✪ Pavord I, Mudassar T, Bennett J, Wilding P, Knox A. The effect of inhaled heparin on bronchial reactivity to sodium metabisulphite and methacholine in patients with asthma. *Eur Respir J* 1996; 9: 217–19.

54. Polosa R, Magri S, Vancheri C et al. Time course of changes in adenosine 5′-monophosphate airway responsiveness with inhaled heparin in allergic asthma. *J Allergy Clin Immunol* 1997; 99: 338–44.

55. Fleisch JH, Maling HM, Brodie BB. Evidence for existence of alpha adrenergic receptors in mammalian trachea. *Am J Physiol* 1970; 218: 596–9.

56. Barnes PJ, Dollerry CT, Macdermott J. Increased pulmonary α-adrenergic and reduced α-adrenergic receptors in experimental asthma. *Nature* 1980; 285: 569–71.

57. Barnes PJ, Wilson NM, Vickers H. Prazosin, an alpha l-adrenoceptor antagonist partially inhibits exercise induced asthma. *J Allergy Clin Immunol* 1981; 68: 411–15.

58. Walden SM, Bleecker ER, Chahal K, Britt EJ, Mason P, Permutt S. Effect of alpha-adrenergic blockade on exercise-induced asthma and conditioned air. *Am Rev Respir Dis* 1984; 130: 357–62.

59. Barnes PJ, Ind PW, Dollery CT. Inhaled Prazosin in asthma. *Thorax* 1981; 36: 378–81.

60. Jenkins C, Breslin ABX, Marlin GE. The role of alpha and beta-adrenoceptors in airway hyperresponsiveness to histamine. *J Allergy Clin Immunol* 1985; 75: 364–72.

61. Sakai H, Dobashi K, Nakazawa T. Effect of an α₂-adrenoceptor antagonist, Midaglizole, on bronchial responsiveness to histamine in patients with mild asthma. *J Asthma* 1995; 32: 259–64.

62. Sakai H, Dobashi K, Iizuka K, Nakazawa T. Protective effect of an α₂-adrenoceptor antagonist, Midaglizole, against allergen-provoked late asthmatic responses. *J Asthma* 1995; 32: 221–6.

63. Dinh Xuan AT, Chaussain M, Regnard J, Lockhart A. Pretreatment with an inhaled α₁-adrenergic agonist, methoxamine, reduces exercise induced asthma. *Eur Respir J* 1989; 2: 409–414.

64. Din Xuan AT, Lockhart A. Bronchial effects of α₂-adrenoceptor agonist and of other antihypertensive agents in asthma. *Am J Med* 1989; 87 (suppl. 3C): 34s–37s.

65. Bateman JR, Pavia D, Sheahan NF, Agnew JE, Clarke SW. Impaired tracheobronchial clearance in patients with mild stable asthma. *Thorax* 1983; 38: 463–7.

66. Sutton PP, Parker RA, Webber BA et al. Assessment of forced expiratory technique, postural drainage and directed coughing in chest physiotherapy. *Eur J Respir Dis* 1983; 64: 62–8.

67. Clarke SW. Management of mucous hypersecretion. *Eur J Respir Dis* 1987; 71 (suppl. 153): 136–44.

68. Clarke SW. Rationale of airway clearance. *Eur Respir J* 1989; 2 (suppl. 7): 599s–603s.

69. Ziment I. Theophylline and mucociliary clearance. *Chest* 1987; 92 (suppl): 38s–43s.

70. Puterman AS, Weinberg EG. RhDNase in acute asthma. *Pediatric Pulmonol* 1997; 23: 316–17.

71. Mazer BD, Gelfand EW. An open label study of high-dose intravenous immunoglobulin in severe childhood asthma. *J Allergy Clini Immunol* 1991; 87: 976–83.

72. Eisenberg DM, Davis RB, Ettner SL et al. Trends in alternative medicine use in the United States, 1990–97: results of a follow-up national survey. *J Am Med Ass* 1998; 280: 1569–75.

73. Dearlove J, Verguei AP, Birkin N, Latham P. An anachronistic treatment for asthma. *BMJ* 1981; 283: 1684–5.

74. Karakoca Y, Demir AU, Kisacik G, Kalyoncu AF, Findik S. Speleotherapy in asthma and allergic diseases. *Clin Exp Allergy* 1995; 25: 666–7.

75. Kalyoncu AF, Selcuk ZT, Iskendarani A et al. Alternative and complementary medicine. *Thorax* 1992; 47: 762.

76. *India Abroad*, Toronto edn, 1993, 6 August, p. 24.

77. Lane DJ, Lane TV. Alternative and complementary medicine for asthma. *Thorax* 1991; 46: 787–97.

78. Lewith GT, Watkins AD. Unconventional therapies in asthma: an overview. *Allergy* 1996; 51: 761–9.

79. ✪ Ziment I. Unconventional therapy in asthma. *Clin Rev Allergy Immunol* 1996; 14: 289–320.

80. Aldridge D, Pietroni PC. Clinical assessment of acupuncture in asthma therapy: discussion paper. *J R Soc of Med* 1987; 80: 222–4.

81. ✪ Kleijnen J, Reit G, Knipschild P. Acupuncture and asthma: a review of controlled trials. *Thorax* 1991; 46: 798–802.

82. Clement-Jones V, Mcloughlin L, Tomlin S, Besser GM, Rees LH, Wen HL. Increased β-endorphin but not met-enkephalin levels in human cereberospinal fluid after acupuncture for recurrent pain. *Lancet* 1980; ii: 946–8.

83. Yu DYC, Lee SP. Effect of acupuncture on bronchial asthma. *Clin Sci Mol Med* 1976; 51: 503–509.

84. Morton AR, Fazio SM, Miller D. Efficacy of laser-acupuncture in the prevention of exercise-induced asthma. *Ann Allergy* 1993; 70: 295–8.

85. Fung KP, Chow OKW, So SY. Attenuation of exercise-induced asthma by acupuncture. *Lancet* 1986; ii: 1419–21.

86. ✪ NIH Consensus statement *Acupuncture* 1997; 15: 1–22.

87. Kleijnen J, Knipschild P, ter Reit G. Clinical trials of homeopathy. *BMJ* 1991; 302: 316–23.

88. Davenas E, Beauvais F, Amara J *et al.* Human basophil degranulation triggered by very dilute antiserum against IgE. *Nature* 1988; 333: 816–18.

89. Maddox J, Randi J, Stewart WW. "High-dilution" experiments a delusion. *Nature* 1988 334: 287–90. Dr Jacques Benveniste replies *Nature*; 1988; 334: 291.

90. Maddox J. Waves caused by extreme dilution. *Nature* 1988; 335: 760–3. Benveniste on Benveniste affair. *Nature* 1988; 335: 759.

91. Reilly D, Taylor MA, Beattie NGM, Campbell JH, McSharry C, Aitchison TC, Carter R, Stevenson RD. Is evidence for homeopathy reproducible. *Lancet* 1994; 344: 1601–1606.

92. Goyeche JRM, Abo Y, Ikemi Y. Asthma: the yoga perspective. Part II: yoga therapy in treatment of asthma. *J Asthma* 1982; 19: 189–201.

93. Nagendra HR, Nagarathna R. An integrated approach of yoga therapy for bronchial asthma: a 3–54 month prospective study. *J Asthma* 1986; 23: 123–37.

94. Tandon MK. Adjunct treatment with yoga in chronic severe airway obstruction. *Thorax* 1978; 33: 514–17.

95. Nagarathna R, Nagendra HR. Yoga for bronchial asthma: a controlled study. *BMJ* 1985; 291: 1077–9.

96. Jain SC, Rai L, Valecha A, Jha UK, Bhatnagar SOD, Ram K. Effect of yoga training on exercise tolerance in adolescents with childhood asthma. *J Asthma* 1991; 28: 437–42.

97. Singh V, Wisniewski A, Britton J, Tattersfield A. Effect of yoga breathing exercises (pranayama) on airway reactivity in subjects with asthma. *Lancet* 1990; 335: 1381–3.

98. Barnes PJ, Chung FK. Difficult asthma: cause for concern. *BMJ* 1989; 299: 695–8.

99. Strunk RC. Deaths due to asthma: new insights into sudden unexpected deaths, but the focus remains on prevention. *Am Rev Respir Dis* 1993; 148: 550–52.

100. White HC. Hypnosis in bronchial asthma. *J Psychosomat Res* 1961; 5: 272–9.

101. Maher-loughnan GP, MacDonald N, Mason AA, Fry L. Controlled trial of hypnosis in the symptomatic treatment of asthma. *BMJ* 1962; ii: 371–6.

102. Morrison JB. Chronic asthma and improvement with relaxation induced by hypnotherapy. *J Roy Soc Med* 1988; 81: 701–704.

103. A report to the research committee of the British Tuberculosis Association. Hypnosis for asthma–a controlled trial. *BMJ* 1968; 4: 71–6.

104. Ben-Zvi Z, Spohn WA, Young SH, Kattan M. Hypnosis

for exercise-induced asthma. *Am Rev Respir Dis* 1982; 125: 392–5.

105. Ewer TC, Stewart DE. Improvement of bronchial hyperresponsiveness in patients with moderate asthma after treatment with hypnotic technique: a randomized control trial. *BMJ* 1986; 293: 1129–32.

106. Horton DJ, Suda WL, Kinsman RA, Souhrada J, Spector SL. Bronchoconstrictive suggestion in asthma: a role of airways hyperreactivity and emotions. *Am Rev Respir Dis* 1978; 117: 1029–38.

107. Krueger AP, Reed EJ. Biological impact of small air ions. *Science* 1976; 193: 1209–13.

108. Krueger AP, Smith RF. The biological mechanism of air ion action: negative ion effect on the concentration and metabolism of 5HT in the mammalian respiratory tract. *J Gen Physiol* 1960; 44: 269–72.

109. Nogrady SG, Furnass SB. Ionizers in the management of bronchial asthma. *Thorax* 1983; 38: 919–22.

110. Osterballe O, Weeke B, Albrechtsen O. Influence of small atmospheric ions on the airways in patients with bronchial asthma. *Allergy* 1979; 34: 187–94.

111. Ben-Dov I, Amirav I, Shochina M, Amitai I, Bar-Yishay E, Godfrey S. Effect of negative ionisation of inspired air on the response of asthmatic children to exercise and inhaled histamine. *Thorax* 1983; 38: 584–8.

112. Warner JA, Marchant JL, Warner JO. Double blind trial of ionisers in children with asthma sensitive to house-dust mite. *Thorax* 1993; 48: 330–33.

113. Shekelle PG. Editorial: What role for chiropractic in health care. *New Engl J Med* 1998; 339: 1074–75.

114. ✪ Balon J, Aker PD, Crowther ER *et al.* A comparison of active and stimulated chiropractic manipulation as adjunctive treatment for childhood asthma. *New Engl J Med* 1998; 339: 1013–20.

115. Nielsen NH, Bronfort G, Bendix T, Madsen F, Weeke B. Chronic asthma and chiropractic spinal manipulation: a randomized clinical trial. *Clin Exp Allergy* 1995; 25: 80–88.

116. Busey JF, Fenger EPK, Hepper NG *et al.* Current status of the surgical treatment of pulmonary emphysema and asthma: a statement by the committee. *Am Rev Respir Dis* 1968; 97: 486–9.

117. Corris PA, Dark JH. Aetiology of asthma: lessons from lung transplantation. *Lancet* 1993; 341: 1369–71.

Chapter 25

Patient Education

Martyn Partridge

INTRODUCTION

The challenge facing those with an interest in asthma is two-fold. With a rising number suffering from the condition, the prime challenge is to elucidate the reason, and when discovered, implement an effective primary prevention programme. Such a programme may well be possible within the next decade or two. Until then the major challenge is to ensure that all those who have the condition benefit from the excellent treatments which are available. Delivering effective care involves:

- Well-educated health professionals working in an effective well-organized service.
- Adequate funding by State or individual so that optimal treatments and services are available to all.
- Easy-to-take medicines with a good benefit/side-effect profile.
- Effective patient/health professional partnerships in which there is good communication and where a prime goal is the acquisition by patients (and parents) of appropriate self-management skills.

The system by which health care is delivered will vary from country to country, but all involve a mixture of primary care, specialist care, hospital in-patient care and some form of emergency care in emergency rooms and accident and emergency departments. Some patients may only attend one part of a health-care system, for example by avoiding primary care and repetitively seeking assistance in an emergency department.[1] It is therefore important to recognize that "patient education" may need to be offered in an opportunistic manner, and there needs to be good communication between each sector of the health-care system so that care is coordinated and the "at risk" patient identified and targeted.

Within each sector it is also important that each health professional is well trained and offers uniform, evidence-based advice to the patient. International and numerous national guidelines on asthma management[2–4] are now available and offer to all members of the health professional team advice on good management. Production of guidelines alone will not alter health professional behaviour or improve patient outcomes. Production needs to be followed by adequate dissemination of their content by educational activities which are designed to increase health professionals' knowledge and understanding of their recommendations.[5] This in turn needs to be followed by interventions designed to lead to a change in health professional behaviour. Studies of asthma management in primary care have suggested that taking guidelines down to a practice (workplace) level with local education, and the prompting of doctors during consultations about questions to ask of patients and action to be taken, may improve outcomes.[6] The practice of audit of asthma management has also been shown to be associated with alterations in doctor behaviour and improvement in the process of care and outcomes.[7,8] Such dissemination and implementation most often involves local rather than national action. In many areas this task has been taken on by local or district asthma task forces or planning teams.

Suggested members of a local asthma task force are shown in Table 25.1 and the sort of issues that they may tackle are shown in Table 25.2. From such national guidelines may thus be derived departmental or practice protocols and it is at this level that the benefit of guidelines is seen, for example, in improved process of care in emergency departments.[9] Such protocols are essential if a multidisciplinary team approach to the care of those with asthma is adopted and guidelines

295

Table 25.1: Possible members of a local asthma task force set up to adapt national or international guidelines for local use, and to aid their dissemination and implementation

Respiratory physician
Paediatrician
Primary care physician
Practice nurse
Respiratory nurse
Allergist
Pharmacist
Manager
Health planner
Patient support group
Health educationlist

Table 25.2: Possible issues to be considered by a local asthma task force in each district

What is the size of the problem of asthma?
Are mainly children or adults affected?
Who will provide care?
   Primary care–doctor or nurse
   Secondary care
   Other
What arrangements will be made for shared care?
How will we ensure that those attending emergency
   departments because of asthma are followed up in
   either primary care or in specialist care?
Is an "interface" coordinator feasible?
What educational interventions can be offered in the
   Emergency Department?
How can a programme of local workplace (practice-
   based) education be instituted?
Will treatments/inhaler devices/peak flow rates be
   standardized?
Will there be a central educational resource centre?
What public education problems are there in this district
   (e.g. misconceptions about local environmental issues,
   need for training of schoolteachers, cultural minority
   groups etc.)?
How will we audit asthma outcomes in our district?

then provide us with a "common language" with which to communicate with our patients[10] – nothing unsettles the person with asthma more than to appear to be receiving conflicting messages from different members of the health professional team.

Evidence is available which suggests that in addition to under-diagnosis or delayed diagnosis (which may be a particular problem in the elderly[11,12]), many patients still receive too little in the way of treatment and too little regular preventative therapy[13,14] and this may also be a special problem with some cultural minority groups who have been shown to miss out on prompt diagnosis and optimal treatments.[15] Even when the correct diagnosis is made and the correct treatment is given it is suggested that many patients, adults and children, may not take treatment as previously discussed with their health professionals.[16–20] A key factor in determining whether or not a patient complies with therapy relates to the quality of communication between patient, (parent) and health professional.[21] All of the national and international guidelines stress the importance of patient education. What is meant by the term and what does it involve?

COMMUNICATION AND EDUCATION

There are two key parts to the process of education:

(1) The passage of information and the acquisition by the patient (or parent), of certain skills.
(2) A change in behaviour.

It is important to remember that a knowledgeable patient does not automatically use that knowledge to alter their behaviour or their attitude towards illness. A number of barriers to education may exist and these reinforce the cardinal importance of clear communication in patient education. Some potential barriers to education are listed in Table 25.3. In any type of communication there is a sender, a message and a recipient. In an ideal world this is a circular model with the recipient also acting as a sender and the sender, the health professional, also acting as recipient (Fig. 25.1).

The Sender

In the case of patient education the sender may be a person delivering verbal messages, or another transmitter such as the written word, audiovisual material, multi-media, or poster. How the person with asthma may be influenced by multiple outside influences is illustrated in Fig. 25.2. In one study patients expressed a preference to hear information about their condition from a doctor,[22] whilst in a survey of 1631 members of the UK National Asthma Campaign, when asked who they would prefer to see when seeking medical advice,

Table 25.3: Potential barriers to education

Denial and disbelief of the diagnosis
Misconceptions about the nature of the condition
Belief that relieving drugs are best
Distrust of all medications—dislike of dependency
Belief that by altering environment, attacks can be avoided
Feelings of stigmatization
Drugs cause side-effects
"It won't happen to me"
Depression
"Steroid phobia"
Uncertainty and feelings of "not being in control"
Conflicting messages from peers, media, family or health
     professionals

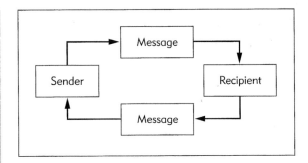

FIGURE 25.1: Clear communication is an essential component of patient education, and involves consideration being paid to the messages and to the recipient so that we match "wants" and "needs".

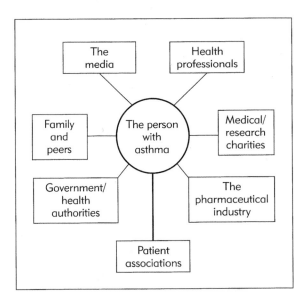

FIGURE 25.2: The person with asthma is subject to numerous influences; sometimes these can be used to reinforce health professional messages (e.g. by the work of patient associations) but sometimes such influences cause confusion and uncertainty (e.g. newspaper scare stories).

5% expressed a preference to see a nurse, 44% a doctor and 48% did not mind which (Personal Communication, National Asthma Campaign, London, 1993). In other situations the sender will be a trained educator or a member of a patient support group.

Patients rarely recall more than 50% of that which they have heard for more than 5 minutes after the end of a consultation and some form of reinforcement of messages is essential. This may be done by the same sender on a subsequent occasion (and by the time the same message has been given more than three times retention approaches 100%), or a verbal message may be reinforced by different routes. Supplementing verbal advice with specific *written* information about a complicated series of proposed treatment changes has been shown to enhance compliance in children[23] and to aid recall of important information about their drug regimen in adults.[24] In one survey of 699 UK health professionals, asthma was the commonest condition for which those in primary care reported that they gave information booklets (asthma 92%, heart disease 84%, diabetes 80%, cancer 34%, epilepsy 17%) but clearly not all with the condition receive such materials.[25] Indeed in the 1993 poll of 1631 members of the UK National Asthma Campaign[25] only 39% had ever received booklets or leaflets and only 4% had ever had the opportunity to see a video on the subject. Two-thirds had had a demonstration of how to use their inhaler devices, but only 27% reported receiving written instructions on how/when to take their medicines. In the UK the Department of Health provides free to health professionals a simple card (Fig. 25.3) developed with the National Asthma Campaign which permits the busy doctor or nurse easily to fill in a patients usual medication regime, and the printed information on the card also provides for the patient some simple information regarding signs that suggest that their asthma is worsening. Giving the written word alone is unlikely to alter patient behaviour[26] and nor

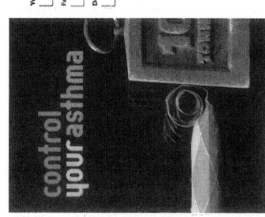

control your asthma

What is asthma?

People with asthma have airways which are almost always inflamed. This makes them more sensitive than normal. Unless this inflammation is minimised with regular anti-inflammatory preventer treatments, triggers such as colds, smoke, pets and dusty environments can act on your airways and cause the symptoms of asthma – coughing, wheezing, breathlessness and a tight chest. Your airways can be inflamed even when you feel well and have no symptoms.

Asthma triggers

An asthma trigger is anything that causes asthma symptoms to appear. Common triggers include viral infections such as flu or colds, house-dust mites, cigarette smoke and animals. Triggers vary from person to person. Most people will have several. It is important that you know what your individual trigger factors are and, where possible, that you try to avoid them.

Your name

Family doctor

Doctor's telephone

Asthma is a common condition. It can be easily controlled with modern treatments. However, in order to look after your asthma properly you need to know a little about your medicines, and you need to know the signs that might suggest your asthma is worsening.

Taking your preventer regularly

- reduces symptoms and the need for reliever medication
- reduces the risk of asthma attacks

and, in the doses usually prescribed, is extremely safe.

If you know that colds often make your asthma worse, it may be sensible to double the dose of your preventer, and continue at that higher dose for a week. Your doctor or nurse will advise you.

Using your reliever

Relievers only rescue you from breathing difficulties as they happen. They do nothing to help reduce the underlying inflammation of the airways.

Preventer inhalers
(usually brown, red or orange)

These are the most important medicines. They help prevent the symptoms of asthma from appearing – coughing, wheezing, tight chest and shortness of breath. Preventers will not work unless they are taken every day, as advised by your doctor or nurse.

Your preventer is

which you should take in a daily dose of

with a (specific device)

Signs that your asthma is worsening include

- needing to use your reliever more often than usual
- waking at night with coughing, wheezing, tight chest or shortness of breath
- finding that your reliever doesn't get rid of your symptoms as effectively, or for as long as usual

If any of these happen, you should seek advice from your doctor or nurse as soon as possible. If you are very breathless and your reliever is not working, you must urgently contact your doctor, who may wish to review your medication.

Reliever inhalers
(usually blue)

These rescue you from asthma symptoms as they happen. You should take your reliever, as advised by your doctor or nurse.

Your reliever is

which you should take with a (specific device)

Other treatments are

Where to go for further information about asthma

The National Asthma Campaign is the independent UK charity working to conquer asthma, in partnership with people with asthma and all who share their concern, through a combination of research, education and support.

National Asthma Campaign Head Office
Providence House
Providence Place
London N1 0NT

NATIONAL ASTHMA CAMPAIGN
conquering asthma

24 hour
information line
0171 971 0444

Registered charity
number 802364

This card has been jointly produced with the **Department of Health**

© Crown Copyright. Produced by Department of Health
H82/003 6683 1P 1M Oct 96 (12)

FIGURE 25.3: An example of a simple pre-printed information card (in this case produced by the UK Department of Health and National Asthma Campaign) on to which a person's individualized medication regimens may easily be added.

will the use of audio tapes.[27] They can only be expected to influence behaviour as part of a wider package. Sometimes materials act only as a source of satisfaction to the patient,[28,29] and sometimes as a means of giving the patient the information they need to enable them to ask more meaningful questions of the health professional. When offering patients leaflets or booklets (and this is preferable to them helping themselves from a rack in the waiting room) it is important to do so in a way which enhances the patient/health professional partnership. This may be done by saying "You may wish to read this booklet about your condition/treatment and make a note of any questions that arise so that we can discuss them again when we next meet".

Preparation of such information materials requires considerable care and a recent review has highlighted how frequently such materials are lacking.[30] A check-list for the production of patient information materials is shown in Table 25.6.

Videotapes represent an alternative to written information, may be particularly appropriate to those with poor literacy skills and are useful for teaching techniques such as use of a metered dose inhaler[31] or peak flow meter. In one study[22] videos were the second most preferred source of information (after the doctor), but preference does not always equate with effectiveness. In another study patients expressed a preference for written information compared with audiotapes, but a simple study of information transfer showed that they actually learnt more from the audiotape.[27] What is important is to have available an array of materials so that the same messages may be given to those with

Table 25.4: Methods of giving information to those with asthma

Verbal (by doctor, nurse or trained educator)

Written (leaflets, booklets, posters)

Audiotapes

Videotapes (for loan, or playing in waiting rooms etc.)

Public lectures

Support group meetings

Newspaper/magazine articles

Drama

Multimedia/Interactive CD ROM

Websites

Table 25.5: Summary of what patients "need" to know about their asthma

The diagnosis and how it was made

How to use an inhaler

The difference between relievers and preventers

Their personal drug regimen

How to use a peak flow meter

Signs and symptoms that suggest worsening asthma and what to do if present

When and where they will be followed up

asthma by several different routes (Table 25.4). All should contain the same core material and some are more suitable for personal use whilst others are effective in giving information to groups.

We should not lose sight of the fact that the individual with asthma does not live in a vacuum (Fig. 25.2). The person with asthma will be under the influence of numerous other factors and his/her illness may also impact upon others around him or her. Eighteen per cent of parents report that their children's asthma has either a great deal, or quite a lot, of influence on their lives, and 20% of cohabitees consider that their own life is influenced to a considerable degree by the asthma of the person with which they live.[32] Furthermore of 397 cohabitees, 12% always made sure that the person with whom they lived was taking their medication, and a further 30% usually, or occasionally, did so. Materials should thus be suitable for sharing, and videos especially can be watched by the whole family together. This may be particularly important in some cultural minority groups where videotapes are popular, and the UK National Asthma Campaign has produced videotapes on asthma in Urdu, Punjabi, Gujerati, Hindi and Bengali. For other audiences, for example schoolchildren, the "sender" may be something innovative such as play-acting or drama, whilst for other recipients, for example physical education teachers, a lecture and demonstration may be more appropriate.

The Message – The "Needs"

Having addressed the "sender" we now need to address the message itself – what might those with asthma "need" to know? Likely needs are listed in Table 25.5 and these are probably non-controversial and require little explanation. As a basic building block for patient

Table 25.6: A checklist for patient information materials. (From Coulter A, Entwhistle V, Gilbert D. Sharing decisions with patients: is the information good enough? BMJ 1999; 318: 318–22, with permission.)

The process

Involve patients throughout the process

Involve a wide range of clinical experts

Be specific about the purpose of the information and the target audience

Consider the information needs of minority groups

Review the clinical research evidence and use systematic reviews wherever possible

Plan how the materials can be used within a wider programme promoting shared decision making

Consider cost and feasibility of distribution and updating when choosing media

Develop a strategy for distribution

Evaluate the materials and their use

Make arrangements for periodic review and updating

Publicize the availability of the information materials

The content

Use patients' questions as the starting point

Ensure that common concerns and misconceptions are addressed

Refer to all relevant treatment or management options

Include honest information about benefits and risks

Include quantitative information where possible

Include checklists and questions to ask the doctor

Include sources of further information

Use non-alarmist, non-patronizing language in active rather than passive voice

Design should be structured and concise with good illustrations

Be explicit about authorship and sponsorship

Include reference to sources and strength of evidence

Include the publication date

education and good compliance, patients and parents do have to have heard and accepted the diagnosis. Some studies do suggest that many are not at ease with the label placed upon them by their doctor. Under such circumstances subsequent educational efforts may be doomed. One qualitative study of those who had a diagnosis of asthma and who had received preventive therapies for asthma for at least a year showed that many made comments which suggested that denial was a prominent feature.[33] Lack of appreciation of this by the health professional may lead to problems as may a failure to appreciate how commonly patients dislike the concept of "regular" medication (of any sort) and the feeling of dependency that it induces.[34] As a prerequisite for good compliance it is important that the patient accepts the diagnosis, understands their treatment, and knows that any risk applies to them and not just to the other person. No person with asthma (or parent of a child with asthma) should be left not knowing what to do in the event of deteriorating asthma and yet the evidence suggests that too few are given explicit instructions about signs that suggest that their asthma is worsening and what to do under those circumstances. Whilst 47% of 1631 National Asthma Campaign members reported having received such advice, in a UK Primary Care Study[35] only 41% of those who had experienced an attack during the previous year had been given a self-management plan. It is not yet possible to define accurately who needs or benefits most from home peak flow monitoring. Many young children lack the physical skills necessary for this and paediatricians remain uncertain as to which older children would benefit most. There is evidence that children may have the same difficulty as adults in perceiving the severity of induced airway narrowing[36] and objective monitoring is therefore likely to be a useful adjunct to advice based upon symptoms. Parents have also been reported to find peak flow monitoring useful in the recognition of severe asthma attacks.[37] In adults studies of induced airway narrowing have shown a poor correlation between subjective and objective parameters of severity[38] and when this was extended to evaluation of perception of day-to-day variation in severity the majority of those with asthma in one community study were shown to be poor discriminators.[39] That this may be important is shown by a Japanese study that showed that perception of airway narrowing may be particularly impaired in those whose asthma deteriorates to the point that they need mechanical ventilation.[40] Table 25.7 outlines some of the current indications for home peak flow monitoring.

The Recipient – The "Wants"

One of the potential barriers to effective patient education is a mismatching of our perception of what the patient "needs" to know, and their list of what they "want" to know. If we believe that a patient needs to

Table 25.7: Possible uses of peak flow monitoring

To aid in the diagnosis of asthma

To delineate possible environmental or occupational triggers

To assess efficacy of treatment

To give warning of impending attacks of asthma

To monitor the stepping down or tailing off of treatment

To gain reassurance as to good control of asthma

know the virtues and mode of action of inhaled steroids and spend valuable time on this subject, when the patient actually *wanted* to know what to avoid so that their asthma would go away, the result is likely to be dissatisfaction, poor compliance and a failure of the patient to alter behaviour in a manner that leads to improved asthma control. It is thus vital that the patient is given adequate opportunity to express their "wants". These are likely to vary considerably in content from patient to patient. They can be elicited by open consultation where it is clear to the patient that the time available is for them, and where they can declare their thoughts and concerns in an open unhurried manner, or they can be elicited by the judicious use of open-ended questions or prompts. Seventy-six percent of a patient's main worries may not be mentioned during a consultation[28] and so it is essential that these are elicited. "How do you feel about having asthma" or "What concerns you most about asthma" may unleash concerns that would not otherwise have been elicited. We know from surveys in general practice that many people with asthma feel different to other people (26% of 210 interviewees); angry (38%); depressed (32%); and unable to enjoy a full life (39%).[41] Others express concern as to the unpredictable nature of the condition, and a feeling of not being in control, and by eliciting specific fears it may be possible to direct management more specifically, for example by giving a self-treatment plan, to enhance a feeling of being in control.

Possible "wants" may also be gleaned by study of issues about which those with asthma call telephone helplines. Questions about side-effects of medicines are part of the reason for the calls in 42% of cases.[42] Knowledge of this means that we can attempt to elicit such unspoken fears during routine consultations. Again open-ended questions are to be preferred. "How do you feel about your treatment?" or "Some people

think steroids are dangerous, what do you think?" may elicit specific concerns which can then be tackled by the provision of both verbal and written information so that the patient may make more informed decisions about whether or not to take a certain treatment.

Reinforcement and Revision

Those with asthma need to be reviewed at regular intervals for the following reasons:

(1) Asthma is usually a long-term condition.
(2) Asthma is a variable condition and advice and management may change.
(3) Much of the information given to the patient will be forgotten, or bad habits and techniques may arise with time.
(4) Giving control to patients does not equal abdication of health professional responsibility. Care should be provided within the context of a partnership. Self-management plans, where issued, should be regarded as plans for *guided* self-management and they require frequent review.
(5) Information needs to be given in a graded, easy-to-assimilate manner, with frequent revision and reinforcement of previously given messages, plus praise to the patient or parent when self-management has been optimal.

It is thus easy to realize that what we are discussing is good communication and the development of a partnership between patient and health professional, where wants and needs are continually matched and where education involves a series of consultations or sessions. The ground that would be covered in such an educational programme is shown in Table 25.8 and it is emphasized that this ground would be covered (and revised) using several adjunctive methods of giving information (verbal, written, videos etc.) with plenty of opportunity for the patient to express their fears and concerns – fears or concerns which need to be addressed as they arise.

Individual or Group Education?

The theme so far has been one of good communication between patient and health professional, and individualized advice. The logic behind such an approach appears to be strong and it is now possible to select a number of published studies to demonstrate support for the approach which has been outlined. It is thus possible to show that intensive education and management

301

Table 25.8: Ground to be covered in an asthma education programme

What is asthma?

What symptoms suggest a diagnosis of asthma?

What signs or symptoms suggest poorly controlled asthma or asthma that is slipping from control

Recognizing triggers:
   Avoidable precipitating factors, and what to do about them
   Non-avoidable factors, such as colds–what to do if they occur

Knowing the different types of medicines:
   Difference between relievers and preventers
   Other treatments for asthma–"long-acting relievers"

Selecting and using an inhaler device (and revision)

Training in the use of a peak flow meter

Using a peak flow meter as part of a guided self-management plan

How to review self-management plans

Specific issues:
   Asthma and pregnancy
   Going on holiday
   Aspirin and other medicines
   Smoking and asthma
   Occupational asthma
   Work and asthma
   Drug interaction
   Why follow-up is necessary
   Where to turn to for help
   CFCs and PMDIs

programmes may reduce admissions for adult asthma in American,[43] Australian,[44] and German[45,46] studies and also in a British study where the educational intervention was by means of computer-assisted personalized booklets being sent to patients.[47] It is also possible to show that such intervention can increase compliance and[48,49] understanding, and improve inhaler technique,[50] children's knowledge and self-management practices of parents.[51] However these studies suggest a certainty which is probably unjustified and there are numerous further areas requiring elucidation and research. In many of the interventions it was difficult to fully separate the effects of more regular supervision and optimized therapy from the educational intervention, and we still have no clear messages as to whether it is preferable to communicate, educate and personalize advice on a one

to one basis or whether there is a benefit for group education as an adjunct to individualized care. One study[52] of group versus individual education versus usual care appears to show a benefit for group education (perhaps by virtue of advanced support, reduction of feelings of stigmatization etc), but recruitment to such groups is not easy and others have highlighted differences in characteristics between those willing and suitable for group education and those who decline to participate.[53] It is also difficult to extrapolate from one health system and culture to another, and programmes based upon 5-day educational courses as an in-patient[45,46] may be neither affordable nor practical in other countries.

What is becoming clear is that the more successful patient education interventions are those involving the patient acquiring skills in self-management – an intervention promoted in some guidelines for a decade or more and promoted before there was actually good evidence of benefit. The subject of self-management is reviewed in Chapter 26 but it is important to note that self-management involves a spectrum of self-care that involves both changes in life-style and changes in medication according to advice received in advance from the health professional. Seminal studies in this area in adults are those from Spain[54] and Finland[55] and the teaching of such skills has now also been shown to reduce the risk of children with asthma being re-admitted to hospital.[56] A recent systematic review of the literature to identify whether education of those with asthma in self-management and regular review by a health practitioner improves health outcomes in adults with asthma has reported positive conclusions. Twenty-two studies comparing self-management education with usual care were identified and showed reduced hospitalization (odds ratio 0.57), days off work or school (odds ratio 0.55) and nocturnal asthma (odds ratio 0.53). The best results were those in which the asthma self-management education allowed patient adjustment of medication based on a written action plan.[57]

The best outcome from patient education is thus likely to result from the development of a partnership between patient (or parent) and health professional, in which communication is of the highest standard and where self-treatment advice is individualized for that patient and written down. The patient will need to be reviewed regularly and messages reinforced, and whilst care may be shared with others in the health professional team, all will give the same message, and verbal advice will be supported by an array of written and audiovisual materials. All patients will be given advice about other sources of information and support associations, and for those who are keen, further education will be offered within a group setting.

PUBLIC EDUCATION AND THE EDUCATION OF OTHERS IN CONTACT WITH THOSE WITH ASTHMA

School Teachers

Children with asthma spend a significant time at school and asthma is the commonest reason for a child to need to take any medication during the school day. Despite this, care for those with asthma at school is often "disorganized"[58] and teachers are often lacking appropriate knowledge to provide for safe care of those in their charge. However 92% of teachers have been shown to want further information[59] and in several countries (e.g. USA, UK and Australia) specific materials or policies have been made available for schools.

Obstetrician and Midwife

Whilst most pregnant ladies with asthma have uneventful pregnancies resulting in the delivery of healthy infants, 42% of patients need increased treatment for their asthma whilst pregnant and there is a higher incidence of pre-eclampsia and neonatal hypoglycaemia.[60] In addition cessation of medication at the onset of pregnancy or fear about its use[42] is common and it is thus important to target antenatal clinics, obstetricians and midwives with appropriate advice and materials[61] so that they may reassure mothers of the safety of asthma therapies.

Employers

Asthma caused by occupational exposure to a variety of sensitizing agents may account for up to 5% of all cases of the disease. Employers need to be aware of this possibility, but health professionals need to be aware that new causes of occupational asthma may present at any time. A numerically larger problem may be that of asthma which is worsened by conditions at work and in one survey of 420 working asthmatics, 9% had to change jobs because of their asthma, 41% felt restricted in the work they could do, 55% had problems with fumes or dust at work, and 74% had problems with the smoking of others in the workplace (personal communication, Workers Poll 1992, National Asthma Campaign, London). Employers thus need to be aware of the importance of, for example, appropriate smoking policies.

Transition to CFC-Free PMDIs

Under the Montreal protocol substances which damage the ozone layer 25 kilometres above the earth's surface are banned. Such substances include the propellants contained within our pressurized metered dose inhalers (PMDIs). Alternatives theoretically include new oral compounds, new hand-held nebulizers, and dry powder devices, but over the last decades manufacturers have been developing new propellants and reformulating the commonly used medicines in redesigned inhalers with the new propellants. PMDIs were designated as essential use of chlorofluorocarbons (CFCs) under the Montreal Protocol to permit the time necessary for this reformulation and redesign. However the new inhalers are now reaching the marketplace and "essentiality" will shortly be removed. Patients therefore need to be forewarned that their new inhalers may have some differences compared with those they replace in that they may weigh different, taste different and impact upon the throat with less force than previously. They also need to be reassured that the previous inhalers were environmentally and not individually damaging.[62]

The Wider Public

Increased awareness of asthma by the general public may be necessary to reduce feelings of stigmatization and to facilitate appropriate domestic and work environments for those with the condition. It is also necessary for the general public and politicians to be educated about the impact of pollution on those with established asthma, but also to be aware of the need for research to highlight which indoor or outdoor factors in the environment are responsible for the increasing prevalence of the condition.

SOURCE OF FURTHER MATERIALS FOR USE WITH THOSE WITH ASTHMA

Australia	National Asthma Campaign, Level 1, Palmerston Crescent, South Melbourne Victoria 3205, Australia.
France	"ASTHME", Programme National de Recherche et d'Education, 10 Rue du Commandant Schloesing, 75116, Paris, France. Tel: 47.55.03.56; fax: 44.05.91.06.

Netherlands	Nederlands Astma fonds, Postbus 5, 3830 AA Leusden, The Netherlands. Tel: 033 94 18 14; fax: 033.95 03 30.
New Zealand	Asthma and Respiratory Foundation of New Zealand, PO Box 1459, 7th Floor, Rossmore House, 123 Molesworth Street, Wellington, New Zealand. Tel: 011 64 4 499 4592; fax: 011 64 4 499 4594.
UK	National Asthma Campaign, Providence House, Providence Place, London, NI 0NT, UK. Tel: 44 20 7226 2260; fax: 44 20 7704 0740. (Materials in English, Welsh, Urdu, Bengali, Gujarati, Punjabi, Hindi.) Telephone Helpline 9 a.m. to 7 p.m. Monday to Friday: 0845 7010203.
USA	AAFA/Asthma and Allergy Foundation of America, 1125 15th Street, NW, Suite 502, Washington, DC 20005, USA. Tel: (202) 466–7643; fax: (202) 466 8940.
	Allergy and Asthma Network, Mothers of Asthmatics, Inc., 2751 Prosperity Avenue, Suite 150, Fairfax, Virginia 22031, USA. Tel: 703–641–9595; fax: 703–573–7794; e-mail: aanma@aol. com.
	National Asthma Education and Prevention Program (NAEPP), PO Box 30105, Bethesda, Maryland 20824–0105, USA. Tel: 301–251–1222; fax: 302–251–1223; e-mail: NHLBIIC@gsys.com.
India	The Asthma Foundation of India, S-82, Anna Nagar, Chennai-600-040, India. Tel: 621–2934.
Belgium	Asthmafonds, Grauwport 9, 9000 Gent, Belgium. Tel. fax: 09/225 65 05.
Denmark	Danish National Association against Lung Disease, 37 Herlufsholmvej, 2720 Vanlose, Denmark. Tel: + 45 38 74 5544; fax: + 45 38 74 0313.
Germany	Deutscher Allergie–Und Asthmabund E.V. (DAAB), Hindenberg Strasse 110,

	D-41061 Moenchengladbach, Germany. Tel: XX 49/2161/814940; fax: XX 49/2161/8149430.
Hungary	Asthmatic and Allergic Children Association of Budapest, H 1192 Budapest XIX, Hungary VT 33. Tel. mobile: 06–30–644–283; fax: 36–1 178–05–44.

KEY POINTS

1 There is more to good asthma management than writing a prescription. Equal or greater attention needs to be paid to the subjects of patient education and self-management.

2 Good communication between patients and health professionals is essential and involves doctors and nurses eliciting from the patient how they feel about their asthma, their fears and concerns, and their goals and expectations from treatment and the consultation.

3 Spoken information should always be reinforced with the written word, including simple instructions regarding the individual's medicine regimen. Other reinforcing methods should also be available including videotapes which may be particularly suitable for demonstrating practical techniques and for those with poor literacy skills.

4 There is now clear evidence that self-management patient education can reduce morbidity and reduce use of health services, and results are best when the education involves the patient receiving a written self-treatment (action) plan.

5 Pregnant asthmatics – reassurance on the safety and efficacy of medication should be offered verbally and by use of printed booklets.

6 CFC transition – As those with asthma are changed from CFC-containing pressurized metered dose inhalers to those containing non-CFC propellants, they should be forewarned that the new inhalers may appear different, the taste may differ and the sensation felt in the throat is likely to be less.

REFERENCES

1. Partridge MR, Latouche D, Trako E, Thurston JGB. A national census of those attending UK accident and emergency departments with asthma. *J Accid Emerg Med* 1997; 14: 16–20.

2. National Heart Lung and Blood Institute. *Global Strategy for Asthma Management and Prevention.* NHLBI/WHO Workshop Report. National Heart, Lung and Blood Institute, 1995. NIH Publication No. 95: 36–59.

3. National Heart Lung and Blood Institute, National Institutes of Health. *International Consensus Report on diagnosis and management of asthma.* 1992; Pub. No. 92–3091.

4. British Thoracic Society, National Asthma Campaign, Royal College of Physicians of London and others. The British Guidelines on Asthma Management. *Thorax* 1997; 52: (suppl. I): 1–20.

5. Grimshaw JM and Russell IT. Achieving health gain through clinical guidelines 11: Ensuring guidelines change medical practice. *Qual Health Care* 1994; 3: 45–52.

6. Feder G, Griffiths C, Highton C, Eldridge S, Spence M, Southgate L. Do clinical guidelines introduced with practice based education improve care of asthmatic and diabetic patients? A randomised controlled trial in general practice in East London. *BMJ* 1995; 311: 1473–8.

7. Neville RG, Hoskins G, Smith B, Clark RA. How general practitioners manage acute asthma attacks. *Thorax* 1997; S2: 153–6.

8. Neville RG, Hoskins G, Smith B, Clark RA. Observations on the structure, process and clinical outcomes of asthma care in general practice. *Br J Gen Pract* 1996; 46: 583–7.

9. Town L, Kwong T, Holst P, Beasley R. Use of a management plan for treating asthma in an emergency department. *Thorax* 1990; 45: 702–706.

10. Lim KL, Harrison BDW. A criteria based audit of inpatient asthma care. *J Roy Coll Phys* 1992; 26: 71–5.

11. Banerjee DC, Lee GS, Malik SR, Daly S. Underdiagnosis of asthma in the elderly. *Br J Dis Chest* 1987; 81: 23–9.

12. Holgate ST, Dow L. Airways disease in the elderly: an easy to miss diagnosis. *J Respir Dis* 1988; 9: 14–22.

13. Gellert AR, Gellert SL, Iliffe SR. Prevalence and management of asthma in a London inner city general practice. *Br J Gen Pract* 1990; 40 (334): 197–201.

14. Blainey AD, Beale A, Lomas D, Partridge MR. The cost of acute asthma–How much is preventable? *Health Trends* 1991; 22: 151–3.

15. Duran-Tularia E, Rona RJ, Chinn S, Burney P. Influencess of ethnic group on asthma treatment in children in 1990–1991–a national cross sectional study. *BMJ* 1996; 313: 148–52.

16. Horn CR, Essex E, Hill P *et al.* Does urinary Salbutamol reflect compliance with inhaled drug regimens by asthmatics? *Resp Med* 1989; 84: 67–70.

17. Spector SL, Kingsman R, Mawhinny H *et al.* Compliance of patients with asthma with an experimental aerolised medication. Implications for controlled clinical trials. *J Allergy Clin Immunol* 1986; 77: 65–70.

18. Cramer JA, Mattson RH, Prevey ML, Scheyer RD, Ovellette GL. How often is medication taken as prescribed? *JAMA* 261: 3273–77.

19. Coutts JA, Gibson NA, Paton JY. Measuring compliance with inhaled medication in asthma. *Arch Dis Child* 1992; 67: 332–3.

20. Rand CS, Wise RA, Nidk S *et al.* Metered dose inhaler adherence in a clinical trial. *Am Rev Resp Dis* 1992; 146: 1559–64.

21. Korsch BM, Negrete VF. Doctor Patient Communication. *Sci Am* 1972; 227: 66–74.

22. Partridge MR. Asthma education: more reading or more viewing? *J R Soc Med* 1986; 79: 326–8.

23. Pedersen S. Ensuring compliance in children. *Eur Resp J* 1992; 5: 143–5.

24. Sandler DA, Heaton C, Garne ST, Mitchell JRA. Giving an information booklet to patients "leaving" hospital. *BMJ* 1989; 298: 870–74.

25. Partridge MR. Asthma: lessons from patient education. *Patient Educ Counsel* 1995; 26: 81–6.

26. Hilton S, Sibbald B, Anderson HR, Freeling P. controlled evaluation of the effects of patient education on asthma morbidity in general practice. *Lancet* 1986; 1: 26–9.

27. Jenkinson D, Davison J, Jones S, Hawtin P. Comparison of effects of a self management booklet and audiocassette for patients with asthma. *BMJ* 1988; 297: 267–70.

28. George CF, Waters WE, Nicholas JA. Prescription information leaflets: a pilot study in general practice. *BMJ* 1983; 287: 1193–6.

29. Gibbs S, Waters WE, George CF. Communicating information to patients about medicines. *J R Soc Med* 1990; 83: 292–7.

30. ✪ Coulter A, Entwhistle V, Gilbert D. Sharing decisions with patients: is the information good enough? *BMJ* 1999; 318: 318–22.

31. Mulloy EMT, Albazzar MK, Warley ARH, Harvey JE. Video education for patients who use inhalers. *Thorax* 1987; 42: 719–20.

32. Applied Research and Communications Ltd. *The Life Quality of Asthmatics*. Uxbridge: Allen and Hanburys, 1990.

33. ✪ Adams S, Pill R, Jones A. Medication, chronic illness and identity: The perspective of people with asthma. *Soc Sci Med* 1997; 45: 189–201.

34. Osman LM. Predicting patients attitudes to medication. *Thorax* 1993; 48: 827–30.

35. Neville RG, Clark RA, Hoskins G, Smith B. First national audit of acute asthma attacks in general practice. *BMJ* 1992; 306: 559–62.

36. Boner AL, DeStefan G, Piacentini GL *et al*. Perception of bronchoconstriction in chronic asthma. *J Asthma* 1992; 19: 323–30.

37. Lloyd BW, Ali MH. How useful do patients find home peak flow monitoring for children with asthma. *BMJ* 1992; 305: 1128–9.

38. Rubinfield AR, Pain MCF. The perception of asthma. *Lancet* 1976; i: 882–4.

39. Kendrick AH, Higgs CMB, Whitfield MJ, Laszlo G.

Accuracy of perception of severity of asthma: patients treated in general practice. *BMJ* 1993; 307: 422–4.

40. Kikuchi Y, Okabe S, Tanura G, Huda W, Homma M, Shirad K, Takashina T. Chemosensitivity and perception of dyspnoea in patients with a history of near fatal asthma. *N Engl J Med* 1994; 330: 1329–34.

41. Sibbald B. Patient self care in acute asthma. *Thorax* 1989; 44: 97–101.

42. Crone S, Partridge M, Mclean F. Launching a national helpline. *Health Visitor* 1993; 66: 94–6.

43. Mayo PH, Richman J, Harris HW. Results of a program to reduce admissions for adult asthma. *Ann Intern Med* 1990; 112: 864–71.

44. Yoon R, McKenzie DK, Nauman A, Miles DA. Controlled trial evaluation of an asthma education programme for adults. *Thorax* 1993; 48: 1110–16.

45. Trautner C, Richter B, Berger M. Cost effectiveness of a structured treatment and teaching programme on asthma. *Eur Resp J* 1993; 6: 1485–91.

46. Worth H. Patient education in asthmatic adults. *Lung* 1990 (Suppl.): 463–8.

47. Osman L, Abdalla MI, Beattie JAG *et al*. Reducing hospital admissions through computer supported education for asthma patients. *BMJ* 1994; 308: 568–71.

48. Bailey WC, Richards JM, Brooks M, Soong S-J, Windsor RA, Manzella BA. A randomized trial to improve self management practices of adults with asthma. *Arch Intern Med* 1990; 150: 1664–8.

49. Windsor RA, Bailey WC, Richards JM, Manzella B, Soong S-J, Brooks M Evaluation of the efficacy and cost effectiveness of health education methods to increase medication adherence amongst adults with asthma. *Am J Pub Health* 1990; 80: 1519–21.

50. Quigley C, Donaghy D, Mulloy E, McNicholas W. Evaluation of patient education in asthma management. *Eur Resp J* (suppl.) 1992; 5: 95.

51. Taggart VS, Zuckerman AE, Sly RM *et al*. You can control asthma: Evaluation of an asthma education program for hospitalized inner city children. *Patient Educ Counsel* 1991; 17: 35–47.

52. Wilson SR, Scamagai P, German DF *et al*. A controlled trial of two forms of self management education for adults with asthma. *Am J Med* 1993; 94: 564–76.

53. Yoon R, McKenzie DK, Miles DA, Barman A. Characteristics of attenders and non attenders at an asthma education programme. *Thorax* 1991; 46: 886–90.

54. Ignacio-Garcia J, Gonzales-Santos P. Asthma self management education program by home monitoring of peak expiratory flow. *Am J Respir Crit Care Med* 1995; 151: 353–9.

55. ✪ Lahdensuo A, Haahtela T, Herrala J *et al*. Randomised comparison of guided self management and traditional treatments of asthma over one year. *BMJ* 1996; 312: 748–52.

56. ✪ Madge P, McColl J, Paton J. Impact of a nurse led home management training programme in children admitted to hospital with acute asthma: a randomised controlled study. *Thorax* 1992; 52: 223–8.

57. ✪ Gibson PG, Coughlan J, Wilson AJ *et al*. Self management education and regular practitioner review for adults with asthma (Cochrane Review). In: *The Cochrane Library*. Issue 1. Oxford: Update Software, 1999.

58. Reynolds MA, Aylward P, Heaf DP. How much do school teachers know about asthma? *Pediatr Rev Commun* 1987; 2: 172–80.

59. Bevis M, Taylor B. What do school teachers know about asthma? *Arch Dis Child* 1990; 65: 622–5.

60. Stenius-Aarniala B, Piirila P, Teramo K. Asthma and pregnancy: a prospective study of 198 pregnancies. *Thorax* 1988; 43: 12–18.

61. National Institutes of Health. Report of the Working Group on Asthma and Pregnancy. *Management of asthma during pregnancy*. Pub US Department of Health, NIH Publication No. 93–3279, 1993.

62. Partridge MR, Woodcock AA, Sheffer AL, Wanner A, Rubinfeld A. Chlorofluorocarbon free inhalers: are we ready for the change? *Eur Respir J* 1998; 11: 1006–1008.

Chapter 26

Self-Management Plans

Wendyl D'Souza, Julian Crane and Richard Beasley

INTRODUCTION

Most asthma attacks are managed by the individual asthmatic in the community without any consultation with the medical profession.[1] This suggests that appropriate self-management by the asthmatic patient could have a major influence on the significant morbidity and mortality associated with this common disease. One way in which this can be achieved is through the use of self-management plans whereby the health professional educates the asthmatic patient to successfully recognize deteriorating asthma and undertake the appropriate therapeutic response(s).

This approach is recommended in national and international guidelines, which state that asthma self-management plans are essential in the long-term treatment of adult asthma.[2–6] Although there are differences in the specific plans recommended, there is a general consensus regarding the basic principles on which this system of self-management should be based. These principles, which are summarized in the Key Points at the end of this chapter, are discussed in detail in many of the other chapters. In many respects, self-management plans simply represent one method whereby the patient and health professional can achieve these principles.

Although asthma education programmes are sometimes considered synonymous with self-management plans,[7] this chapter focuses only on aspects associated with the standardized written self-management guidelines given to adult patients. Although the centrality of asthma education to self-management plans is undisputed and perhaps even impossible to separate, asthma education has been covered in the preceding chapter and will not be specifically discussed.

This chapter attempts to outline the principal components of the self-management plan system of care,

reviews the evidence for its efficacy and discusses its use by subjects with differing asthma severity. Finally, three models will be presented to illustrate how theoretical considerations may be translated into practical examples of self-management plans.

ESSENTIAL COMPONENTS OF SELF-MANAGEMENT PLANS

The basic components of a self-management plan should include the following:

The Recognition of Deteriorating Asthma
(see Table 26.1)
The recognition of unstable asthma requires the educated interpretation of both subjective and objective measures of asthma severity. The need for such an approach is illustrated by the descriptive asthma mortality surveys which have reported the circumstances surrounding asthma deaths.[8–10] The most common and

---

Table 26.1: Simple criteria for the patient to recognize asthma severity

Unstable asthma:
  Nocturnal symptoms
  Pre-bronchodilator PEFR <80–85% of "best"

"Severe" asthma:
  PEFR <60–70% of "best"
  Requirement for frequent use of inhaled β_2 agonist

"Life-threatening" asthma:
  PEFR <40–50% of "best"
  Minimal to no response to frequent high doses of inhaled β_2 agonist

---

important factor associated with a fatal outcome has consistently been an inability of the patient to appreciate the severity of the attack, leading to an inevitable delay in seeking appropriate medical treatment and assistance.

The most likely explanation for these observations is that asthmatic patients base their assessment of the severity of an attack of asthma on their subjective perception of symptoms such as breathlessness, chest tightness and wheeze. However, this practice may be inadequate, as a significant proportion of chronic adult asthmatic patients may have minimal symptoms despite marked airflow obstruction.[11] Poor perception of asthma severity not only occurs in the situation of worsening asthma,[11] but also during recovery from a severe attack[12] and is most marked in patients with greatly increased airway hyperresponsiveness.[13] This suggests that those patients who are at the greatest risk of a severe attack of asthma are those most likely to underestimate the severity of such an attack.

These observations led to the identification of key symptoms to indicate to the patient significant worsening of their asthma. In particular the development of nocturnal asthma was recognized to be a good marker of unstable asthma, and the poor response to the increased use of inhaled β_2 agonist therapy was an important marker of a severe attack requiring medical attention.[14] The use of the latter marker is also supported by the observation that the risk of death increases markedly with the use of more than two β_2 agonist metered dose inhalers (MDIs) per month, which is equivalent to more than 16 puffs per day.[15]

These findings have also led to the introduction and increasing use of peak flow meters to objectively measure the degree of airflow obstruction. While forced expiratory volume in one second (FEV_1) is considered the "gold standard" for the physician, the peak expiratory flow rate (PEFR) is an acceptable alternative for the patient as a portable, simple and practical test of lung function.[16] With education, the PEFR is a highly repeatable measurement[17] with predicted normal values calculated, based on age, sex, and height.[18] Because in many asthmatic patients the PEFR is consistently higher or lower than the mean predicted values, it is recommended that "personal best lung function" is determined, based on a period of preliminary lung function monitoring for 2–4 weeks. In patients with suboptimal lung function, it may be necessary to increase therapy, including a course of oral corticosteroids, to enable the best attainable PEFR to be determined. Although the determination of the "personal best" lung function as the ultimate therapeutic end-point can be time-consuming, it has the advantage of ensuring an objective baseline to gauge any subsequent deterioration in asthma control.

Subsequent asthma exacerbations are then most easily interpreted by patients when expressed as a percentage of this personal best value. The day-to-day variability of PEFR provides an index of asthma stability and/or severity for the physician but has limited use in self-management by the patient because of its complexity, requiring at least two readings and the use of a derived value from a formula.[19,20]

A morning pre-bronchodilator recording is probably the most sensitive method to identify inadequately controlled or deteriorating asthma. As the attack progresses, both pre- and post-bronchodilator recordings will be helpful in determining the response to therapy. In general patients should be encouraged to make recordings more often as their asthma becomes more severe.

Stable Asthma Stable asthma may be defined as a combination of minimal symptoms (ideally none) day and night, no restriction to activities (including work and recreational exercise), infrequent need for inhaled β_2-agonist therapy, optimal pulmonary function (a pre-bronchodilator PEFR >80%), daily variation of PEFR <20% (ideally <10%) and no medication side-effects.[2,5,6]

Unstable Asthma The most reliable markers of unstable asthma are the development of nocturnal symptoms,[21,22] and/or a pre-bronchodilator PEFR <80–85% of best.[5,6] These markers are simple to determine and interpret and should form the basis for the recognition of deteriorating asthma.

Other useful indicators of unstable asthma that are less specific include symptoms of a cold,[23] and an increased need for bronchodilator use. The former recognizes that most exacerbations of asthma are associated with symptoms suggestive of a respiratory tract infection and, conversely, that such symptoms in an asthmatic patient frequently herald the onset of worsening asthma.[24] The latter is more difficult to define, as it depends on the baseline requirements for inhaled bronchodilator therapy. However, both an increased use of inhaled β_2-agonist therapy and an absolute amount of more than 3–4 times daily have been suggested as an indication of deteriorating control.

Severe Asthma Reductions in PEFR to <60–70% predicted or personal best values[25] or requirements for frequent inhaled β_2-agonist therapy[14] are considered to be the key markers of severe asthma. Both have been shown to be associated with sudden death or near-fatal asthma. Once again, the exact amount of inhaled bronchodilator use is difficult to define, however self-administration by the patient more than every 2–4 hours, with the associated feature of reduced magnitude and duration of the bronchodilator effect may be a useful guide.

Life-Threatening Asthma The patient's perception that the attack has deteriorated further, a minimal or no response to bronchodilator medication, or a PEFR less than 40–50% predicted or personal best values should suggest to the patient that their asthma is sufficiently severe to require emergency medical management. Other symptoms or signs, such as an inability to speak in short sentences, cyanosis, or a pulse rate >110–120 beats min[-1] may also indicate a life-threatening attack,[26] however these signs are likely to be too difficult for the patient to measure or interpret in this clinical situation.

The Self-Management of Deteriorating Asthma

Linking the assessment of asthma control with an appropriate therapeutic response represents one of the basic principles of patient self-management (Table 26.2) However, this approach may create problems for the patient, and the scientific validity of some of the treatment guidelines that have been recommended is uncertain. Because of these limitations, what is suggested in this section should be considered as guidelines only; specific treatments should be tailored by the physician to meet the requirements of individual patients.

Stable Asthma The regular use of inhaled anti-inflammatory treatment with inhaled corticosteroids represents the basis of the chronic treatment of adult self-management plans.[2-6] For most patients, this inhaled corticosteroid therapy can be taken according to a twice daily regimen. This has been shown to be as effective as four times daily in stable asthma,[27,28] and has the advantage of improving compliance, especially when linked with a routine twice-daily activity such as teeth-cleaning. Linked with mouth rinsing, this also reduces systemic absorption and the likelihood of developing oral thrush with inhaled corticosteroids. Inhaled sodium cromoglycate and nedocromil sodium represent useful alternatives to inhaled corticosteroids in patients with mild disease.

Inhaled bronchodilator therapy is recommended to be used for relief of symptoms, rather than according to a regularly scheduled regime.[2-6] The use of bronchodilators in this way has stemmed from the concerns that regular inhaled β_2 agonists may make chronic asthma worse.[29] When incorporated in a self-management plan system, it has the advantage of allowing the frequency

Step	Peak flow	Symptoms	Action
		Table 26.2: Adult asthma self-management plan: what to do and when	
1	>80–85% best	Intermittent/few	Continue regular inhaled corticosteroid; inhaled β_2 agonist for relief of symptoms
2	<80–85% best	Waking at night with asthma; symptoms of a "cold"	Increase the dose of inhaled corticosteroid; inhaled β_2 agonist for relief of symptoms
3	<60–70% best	Increasing breathlessness or frequent use of bronchodilator	Start oral corticosteroids and contact a doctor; inhaled β_2 agonist for relief of symptoms
4	<40–50% best	Minimum response to repeated use of bronchodilator	Self-administer high dose inhaled β_2 agonist, call emergency doctor or ambulance urgently

This plan may need to be modified with respect to the amount of detail it provides and the specific drug treatment recommended at each stage. Likewise, the severity of symptoms chosen and the specific peak flow values recommended for each stage may need to be altered in accordance with physician preference and the asthmatic patient's individual needs.

of use and the resulting response to be used as a guide of asthma severity.

Unstable Asthma Although not rigorously tested, the introduction of or increase in the dose of inhaled anti-inflammatory therapy is considered to be one of the therapeutic responses to the recognition of unstable asthma. Thus, in the situation of unstable asthma, the patient is usually instructed to either double the dose of inhaled corticosteroids or start this therapy, if not currently being used. The increased dose is then continued until stable asthma is achieved.

If patients remain unstable, frequently needing to double the dose of their inhaled corticosteroid therapy, then this higher dose becomes the new regular dose. Similarly, if patients have remained stable for a few months, they can be instructed to halve the dose of their inhaled corticosteroid therapy while continuing to use their plan to monitor their response. As patients become more experienced, these dosage adjustments can be done with minimal medical supervision.

This method of varying the dose of inhaled anti-inflammatory therapy over long periods of time is consistent with the recommended guidelines for the long-term management of chronic persistent asthma in adults, in which a step-wise approach to asthma therapy based on the classification of asthma severity is proposed.[2,5] Its incorporation into a self-management plan represents one way in which the recommendations for acute severe and chronic persistent asthma can be brought together within the framework of one system. At this and all other stages, inhaled bronchodilator therapy is recommended for use as required to relieve symptoms, and not according to a regular scheduled regimen.

Severe Asthma Systemic corticosteroids, frequent inhaled bronchodilator use and medical practitioner review are the main components of the management plan for severe asthma. High doses of orally administered corticosteroid (e.g. prednisone 30–40 mg daily), begun early in this way, can prevent a protracted or progressive course, and reduce the requirement for emergency care or hospitalization.[30,31] It is not possible to predict at this stage the likely rate of recovery from the attack and, as a result, how long the patient will need to continue oral corticosteroid therapy.[32] Therefore, the therapeutic response to oral corticosteroids should be used to determine the duration of treatment, with the patient continuing on a high dose until the peak flow

returns to normal values. According to physician and patient preference, the patient would then take either half the dose for the same number of days before stopping, or the dose could be tapered more gradually.

With respect to the frequent use of bronchodilators by patients in the situation of severe asthma, the patient needs to recognize that this is undertaken while medical attention is being sought and should not be considered a substitute for medical assessment and treatment. Should asthma deteriorate further, the patient should be instructed to call the emergency doctor or phone for an ambulance. Other resources such as the availability of oxygen in the patient's home and a nebulizer to administer high doses of a β_2 agonist may be helpful for patients with a previous life-threatening attack.[33] The facility for self-referral and admission to hospital may be organized as part of the self-management programme.[34]

EFFICACY

Despite the consensus on both the necessity and the principles underlying the development of asthma self-management plans, it is only recently that their efficacy has been clearly established. The best assessment of their efficacy can be obtained from the recent systematic review of the literature of the effects of education of the asthmatic in self-management.[35] This review involved 24 randomized controlled trials in which self-management asthma education was studied, of which there were 17 studies which involved the assessment of written action plans. The meta-analysis of these studies identified that self-management involving provision of a written action plan led to a significant reduction in hospitalizations for asthma (odds ratio 0.35) whereas less intensive interventions did not work. Similar findings were observed with respect to emergency hospital visits, in which there was a significant trend for self-management education to reduce the proportion of asthmatics needing such visits, with the additional provision of a written action plan leading to a greater reduction. In those studies in which nocturnal asthma was examined, the greatest reduction was observed in those groups receiving optimal self-management education involving provision of a written plan. In contrast there was no effect on FEV_1 in those studies in which this outcome variable was measured.

In the four studies which compared peak flow with symptom-based management plans, equivalent efficacy was observed in terms of the proportion of subjects requiring hospitalization, emergency room treatment or an unscheduled visit to the doctor. There were no significant differences in efficacy in the five studies in which a comparison was made between those plans in which there was self-adjustment of medication by the patient according to written, predetermined criteria, or on the basis of regular review by a doctor.

Although the efficacy of the asthma self-management plan system of care has been demonstrated, there are a number of issues which have yet to be clarified, as outlined in Table 26.3. While clarification will be obtained for some of these issues when specific studies are undertaken, some features such as which components of the plan lead to its efficacy may prove difficult to unravel, as the different features of the plans are so closely inter-related. The evidence to date suggests that it is likely that the greatest benefit from self-management will be obtained with the close integration of the different features of self-assessment and management.[36–42]

While the implementation of asthma self-management plans has traditionally been considered to be the responsibility of medical practitioners, some of these studies have shown that a nurse practitioner may be a suitable alternative.[37,42]

EXAMPLES OF SELF-MANAGEMENT PLANS

Many different systems of asthma self-management have now been developed reflecting different management and educational practices. It is evident that the needs of all patients cannot be met through the use of one particular version and that different plans will suit different patients. In the following section, three models are briefly presented to provide examples of different self-management plans that have been recommended for use.

The "Credit Card" Asthma Self-Management Plan (see Fig. 26.1)

The "credit card" asthma self-management plan provides guidelines for treatment, based on the assessment of asthma severity, printed on a small plastic card, the size of a standard credit card. In this way, self-management guidelines based on the assessment of peak flows are printed on one side, and those based on the interpretation of symptoms are printed on the reverse side of the card.

For both methods of assessment, there are four general stages in which treatment guidelines are recommended. For each stage of deterioration, clear instructions are written as to what treatment to take and when to seek help. These are tailored to individual patients and their requirements, and are written directly on to the card. Similarly, the patient's individual therapy (inhaled anti-inflammatory drug and bronchodilator) and the name and telephone number of emergency help is also written on to the card.

This card represents the most studied self-management plan available and has been widely promoted by the Health Department and Asthma Foundation of New Zealand; with minor modifications it has also been adopted by the National Asthma Campaign of Australia.

Table 26.3: Issues relating to the structure and implementation of asthma self-management plans that require further clarification

1 Number of stages/levels
 e.g. 2-, 3- vs 4-stage plans

2 Specific peak flow percentages indicating each stage
 e.g. <60% or 70% to start oral steroids

3 Specific symptoms indicating each stage
 e.g. Nocturnal asthma, increasing β_2-agonist use and/or symptoms of a cold for recognizing worsening asthma

4 Role of other medications
 e.g. Long-acting β_2 agonists, leukotriene antagonists, theophylline, sodium cromoglycate/nedocromil

5 The relationship between specific therapeutic responses and outcome
 e.g. Does increasing inhaled steroid dose in worsening asthma prevent further deterioration?

6 Which forms for different patient groups
 e.g. Adults vs children

7 Methods of implementation
 e.g. Doctor vs other health professionals

8 Intensity of implementation
 e.g. How much peak flow and symptoms monitoring is optimal?

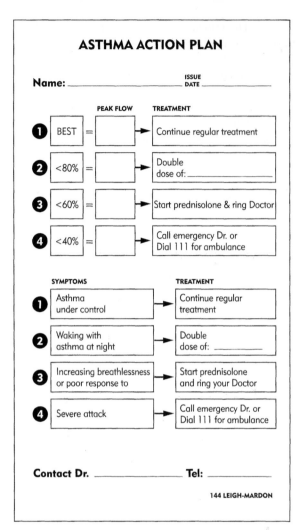

ASTHMA ACTION PLAN

Name: _____ ISSUE DATE _____

PEAK FLOW   TREATMENT

① BEST = [   ] → Continue regular treatment

② <80% = [   ] → Double dose of: _____

③ <60% = [   ] → Start prednisolone & ring Doctor

④ <40% = [   ] → Call emergency Dr. or Dial 111 for ambulance

SYMPTOMS   TREATMENT

① Asthma under control → Continue regular treatment

② Waking with asthma at night → Double dose of: _____

③ Increasing breathlessness or poor response to → Start prednisolone and ring your Doctor

④ Severe attack → Call emergency Dr. or Dial 111 for ambulance

Contact Dr. _____ Tel: _____

144 LEIGH-MARDON

FIGURE 26.1: The Adult "Credit Card" Asthma Self-Management Plan.

National Asthma Campaign: British Plan

(see Fig. 26.2)

This system includes both a detailed and brief (credit card) version of a four-step plan. The detailed version provides considerable information for the patient with respect to guidelines for recognizing deteriorating asthma and the appropriate therapeutic response. No fixed PEFR percentages are recommended to enable doctors to vary the levels at each stage for which treatment guidelines are made according to the requirements of individual patients.

One of the real strengths of this plan is in the method of delivery. This system is part of a comprehensive edu-

cational booklet that is being promoted to both medical and nursing practitioners in general practice. The booklet explains how to undertake PEFR monitoring, the use of medication for chronic and acute asthma and the system of self-management, with the facility for the patient and doctor to work through the booklet and fill in the details of the self-management plan together. The booklet also includes a brief "credit card" version of the plan that can be removed from the main book of instructions and carried by the patient, or kept with a peak flow meter.

International Asthma Management Plan "Zone System" (see Fig. 26.3)

This system probably represents the most complex plan available and as with other systems, uses a step-wise approach in which deteriorating asthma is recognised by reduction in peak flow from best, increasingly severe symptoms, as well as the response to treatment itself. In this way, three "zones" of asthma severity are defined for the patient. The zones have been adapted to a traffic light system to make it simpler for patients to use and remember.[43,44] The recognition of trigger factors is also encouraged through this system. Initiation of oral corticosteroids is more flexible and can be introduced at an earlier level (in the yellow zone). Clinical studies assessing the efficacy of this comprehensive system of self-management are awaited with interest.

RECOMMENDED USE

Whilst there is general acceptance of asthma self-management plans, there is emerging evidence to suggest that certain asthmatics may benefit more than others from this system of care.[45] In particular, it is recognized that the greatest benefit is likely to be obtained in patients with chronic severe asthma, and that compliance is likely to be a major problem in patients with mild asthma. The following serves as a guide to the need for self-management according to asthma severity.

Mild Asthma

In mild asthma, an initial period of assessment with recording of asthma symptoms and peak flow rates is recommended, to educate the patient to recognize changes in asthma severity, to identify those with a poor perception of asthma severity, to determine the best

For your doctor or nurse to complete

Zone 1

Your asthma is under control if:

■ Your peak flow readings are above

_____

and
■ it does not disturb your sleep
and
■ it does not restrict your activities

Action

Continue your normal medicines

3 Your own asthma management plan

This plan helps you to adjust your treatment according to the measurements on your peak flow chart. If you take quick action, you can usually prevent severe attacks.

These instructions are only a guide, so you and your doctor or nurse may need to change them. Although the plan has four 'zones', some doctors prefer to use three and may wish you to ignore Zone 2.

Your doctor will write the ranges of peak flow which relate to each action below.

Your best (target) peak flow is

_____

Zone 2

(Your doctor or nurse may decide not to use this zone)

Your asthma is getting worse if:

■ Your peak flow readings have fallen to between

_____ and _____

■ You are needing to use your

_____

(reliever inhaler) more than usual

■ You are waking at night with asthma symptoms

Action

■ Increase your

_____

(prevent inhaler) to

_____

■ Continue to take your

_____

(reliever inhaler) to relieve your asthma symptoms

FIGURE 26.2: Asthma self-management plan promoted by National Asthma Campaign (UK). Booklet 7: "Self-management and peak flow measurement".

recorded peak flow values, and to monitor the response to the introduction of prophylactic therapy. Following this initial period, it would be possible to develop an asthma self-management plan which simply provides patients with written instructions as to when to seek medical help in the situation of a severe asthma attack. Unless the patient has a poor symptomatic perception of asthma severity, the regular use of a more detailed self-management plan is not recommended at this stage, as it is unlikely to lead to a major improvement in asthma control and is unlikely to be undertaken by the patient (even if recommended).

Patients With Moderate to Severe Asthma

A similar period of assessment is recommended for the same reasons as in mild asthma, and to allow for the development of a more detailed three- or four-stage asthma self-management plan. It is recommended that the amount of detail included will depend on the requirements of the patient and the degree of medical supervision that is deemed to be necessary. Patients should be advised to use the plan preferentially during periods of unstable asthma rather than during periods of good control. Patients who are identified as being poor perceivers of asthma severity on the basis of

For your doctor to complete

Zone 3

Your asthma is severe if:

■ Your peak flow readings have fallen to between

_____ and _____

■ You are getting increasingly breathless

■ You are needing to use your

_____

(reliever inhaler) every

_____

hours or more often

Zone 4

Medical alert/emergency if:

■ Your peak flow readings have fallen to below

_____

■ You continue to get worse

Action

Ring your doctor or nurse

■ Take _____ prednisolone (steroid) tablets (_____ mgs each) and then

_____

_____

_____

■ Discuss with your doctor how to stop taking the tablets

■ Continue to take your

_____

(reliever inhaler) as required

Action

Get help immediately

■ Ring your doctor immediately

(Telephone _____) or call an ambulance

■ Continue to take your

_____

(reliever inhaler) as needed

Do not be afraid of causing a fuss. Your doctor will want to see you urgently.

4 Update your management plan

■ Because your asthma may change as time goes by, your doctor may need to change your plan accordingly. You should visit your doctor or nurse at least twice a year.

■ If you often find yourself in Zones 2 or 3, let your doctor know because your medicines may need to be increased or changed.

■ If you are in Zone 1 all the time it may be possible for your doctor to reduce your medicines.

■ We recommend that a month or so after you start your self-management plan you should review it with your doctor or nurse.

The mini asthma management plan

You might find it helpful to carry this 'credit card' version of your plan with you at all times. It can act as a reminder in case you have unexpected symptoms.

NATIONAL **ASTHMA** CAMPAIGN
getting your health back

Name _____

Best peak flow _____

	Peak flow	Treatment
1		Continue regular treatment
2		Increase dose of
3		Start oral steroids and ring doctor
4		Call emergency medical help

Asthma Helpline 0345 01 02 03, Monday to Friday, 9am to 9pm

FIGURE 26.2   Contd.

symptoms alone are particularly encouraged to use such a self-management plan system of care.

Patients with High-Risk Asthma

For patients with high-risk asthma, for example those with recent hospital admissions, a large diurnal variation of peak flow despite maximal therapy, or known brittle asthma, the regular use of peak-flow monitoring and recording of symptoms in association with an asthma self-management plan is recommended, together with intensive medical and nursing supervision.

CONCLUSION

The need for self-management plans arose as clinicians tried to design better methods by which they could deliver asthma care in an attempt to prevent the significant mortality and morbidity associated with this disease. The basic management principles that resulted have now been universally endorsed with self-management plans now being considered essential in the long-term management of adult asthma.

ASTHMA CONTROL PLAN FOR _____

(name of patient)

Prepared by _____ **M.D.**

This plan will help you control your asthma and do the right thing if you have an asthma episode. Keeping your asthma under control will help you:

- **Be active without having asthma symptoms. This includes being active in exercise or sports.**

- **Sleep through the night without having asthma symptoms.**

- **Prevent asthma episodes (attacks)**

- **Have the best possible peak flow rate.**

- **Avoid side effects from medicines.**

Here are three ways to control your asthma:

■ Follow your medicine plan (see the next page).

- Follow your Green Zone plan every day to keep most asthma symptoms from starting.

- Recognize your symptoms of an asthma attack episode. Act quickly to stop them.

- Follow the Yellow Zone plan to stop asthma symptoms and to keep an asthma episode from getting serious.

- Follow the Red Zone plan to take care of a serious episode. This is an emergency plan!

■ Whenever possible, stay away from things that bring on your asthma symptoms. Follow your asthma trigger control plan to reduce the number of things in your home, workplace, or classroom that bother your asthma.

■ See your doctor regularly. Review this plan with your doctor when you visit him/her. Your doctor will write on the plan what you should do.

Your plan has these medicines:

_____

_____

_____

_____

_____

_____

Important information:

Doctor _____ **Hospital** _____

Telephone _____ Telephone _____

Address _____ Address _____

_____ _____

Ambulance or Emergency Rescue **Friend to call** _____
Squad _____

Telephone _____ Telephone _____

Taxi _____

For more information on Asthma:
National Asthma Education Program
Information Center
P.O. Box 30105
Bethesda, MD 20824-0105
(301) 951-3260

Adapted from National Asthma Education Program "Clinician's Guide: Teaching your Patients About Asthma," National Heart, Lung, and Blood Institute, National Institutes of Health, United States.

FIGURE 26.3: Asthma self-management plan adapted from the National Asthma Education Program "Clinician's Guide: Teaching Your Patients About Asthma", National Heart, Lung and Blood Institute, National Institutes of Health, USA.

ASTHMA CONTROL PLAN FOR _____
(name of patient)

Prepared by _____ **M.D.**

Green Zone: All Clear

This is where you should be every day:

Peak flow between _____
(80-100%
of personal best)*

No symptoms of an asthma episode. You are able to do your usual activities and sleep without having symptoms.

The doctor will check which applies to you.

☐ Take these medicines.

Medicine	How much to take	When to take it
_____	_____	_____
_____	_____	_____
_____	_____	_____
_____	_____	_____

☐ Follow your asthma trigger control plan to avoid things that bring on your asthma.

☐ Take _____ before exercise.
(medicine)

Yellow Zone: Caution

This is not where you should be every day. Take action to get your asthma under control.

Peak flow between _____
(50-80%
of personal best)*

You may be coughing, wheezing, feel short of breath, or feel like your chest is tight. These symptoms may keep you from your usual activities or keep you from sleeping.

☐ _First_, take this medicine:

Medicine	How much to take	When to take it
_____	_____	_____

☐ _Next_, if you feel better in 20 to 60 minutes and your peak flow is over (70% of personal best) then:

☐ Take this medicine

Medicine	How much to take	When to take it
_____	_____	_____
_____	_____	_____

☐ Keep taking your green zone medicine(s).

☐ _But_, if you DO NOT feel better in 20-60 minutes or your peak flow is under _____ **follow the Red Zone Plan.**
(70% of personal best)

Let the doctor know if you keep going into the Yellow Zone. Your Green Zone medicine may need to be changed to keep other episodes from starting.

Red Zone: Medical Alert

This is an emergency! Get help.

Peak flow under _____
(50% of personal best)*

You may be coughing, very short of breath, and/or the skin between your ribs and your neck may be pulled in tight. You may have trouble walking or talking. You may not be wheezing because not enough air can move out of your airways.

* _This is a general guideline only. Some people have asthma that gets worse very fast. They may need to have a yellow zone at 90-100% of personal best._

☐ _First_, take this medicine:

Medicine	How much to take	When to take it
_____	_____	_____
_____	_____	_____

☐ **Next, call the doctor to talk about what you should do next.**

☐ **But, see the doctor RIGHT AWAY or go to the hospital if _any_ of these things are happening:**

– Lips or fingernails are blue

– You are struggling to breathe

– You do not feel any better 20 to 30 minutes after taking the extra medicine and peak flow is still under _____
50% of personal best

– Six hours after you take the extra medicine, you still need an inhaled beta$_2$-agonist medicine every 1 to 3 hours and your peak flow is under _____
70% of personal best

FIGURE 26.3 Contd.

Self-management plans essentially focus on the early recognition of unstable or deteriorating asthma, by monitoring peak expiratory flow recordings (PEFR) or symptoms. Through the use of written guidelines, patients are then able to determine when it is necessary to adjust therapy or obtain medical assistance.

The use of self-management plans by patients with asthma has been shown to lead to improvements in asthma morbidity and requirement for acute medical treatment and hospital admission. However, it is acknowledged that more research is needed to clarify many different issues concerning their structure and implementation.

Many different systems of asthma self-management have now been developed and probably reflect different management and educational practices. It is apparent that the needs of all patients cannot be met through the use of one particular version. Whatever plan is employed written guidelines need to reflect the healthcare system and cultural needs of the respective country, and they must be tailored to meet the specific needs of individual patients.

KEY POINTS

1 Asthma is an inflammatory disease, with the therapeutic implications:
(a) inhaled anti-inflammatory drugs represent the basis of long-term treatment;
(b) systemic corticosteroids are essential in the treatment of severe asthma.

2 Requirement for objective assessment of asthma severity with educated interpretation of:
(a) key symptoms such as nocturnal symptoms and requirement/response to bronchodilator treatment;
(b) peak flow meter recordings.

3 Integration of self-assessment and self-management with written guidelines for both:
(a) long-term treatment of asthma;
(b) treatment of acute severe asthma.

REFERENCES

1. Avery CH, March J, Brook RH. An assessment of the adequacy of self-care by adult asthmatics. *J Comm Health* 1980; 5: 167–81.

2. ❂ British Thoracic Society, Research Unit of Royal College of Physicians, Kings Fund Centre, National Asthma Campaign. Guidelines for management of asthma in adults: I–Chronic persistent asthma. *BMJ* 1990; 301: 651–3.

3. Thoracic Society of Australia and New Zealand. Consensus on asthma: Asthma management plan, 1989. *Med J Aus* 1989; 18: 650–8.

4. Hargreave FE, Dolvich J, Newhouse MT (eds). The assessment and treatment of asthma: A conference report. *J Allergy Clin Immunol* 1990; 85: 1098–1111.

5. Lenfant C. *International Consensus Report on Diagnosis and Management of Asthma*. National Heart, Lung and Blood Institute, National Institute of Health. US Department of Health and Human Services, Bethseda, USA, 1992.

6. ❂ Global Initiative for Asthma. *Global strategy for asthma management and prevention*. NHLBI/WHO Workshop Report. National Institutes of Health, National Heart, Lung and Blood Institute, 1996.

7. Wilson-Pessano SR, Mellins RB. Workshop on asthma self-management: summary of workshop discussion. *J Allergy Clin Immnol* 1987; 80: 487–90.

8. MacDonald JB, Seaston A, Williams DA. Asthma deaths in Cardiff 1963–74: 90 deaths outside hospital. *BMJ* 1976; iii: 1493–5.

9. British Thoracic Association. Death from asthma in two regions of England. *BMJ* 1982; 285: 1251–5.

10. Rea HH, Sears MR, Beaglehole R *et al*. Lessons from the national asthma mortality study: circumstances surrounding death. *NZ Med J* 1987; 100: 10–3.

11. ❂ Rubinfeld AR, Pain MCF. Perception of asthma. *Lancet* 1976; 1: 822–4.

12. McFadden ER, Kiser R, De Groot WJ. Acute bronchial asthma. Relations between clinical and physiological manifestations. *N Engl J Med* 1973; 288: 221–5.

13. Burdon JGW, Juniper EF, Killian KJ, Hargreave FE,

Campbell EJM. The perception of breathlessness in asthma. *Am Rev Respir Dis* 1982; 126: 825–8.

14. Windom HH, Burgess CD, Crane J, Pearce N, Kwong T, Beasley R. The self-administration of inhaled beta agonist drugs during severe asthma. *NZ Med J* 1990; 103: 205–7.

15. Suissa S, Ernst P, Boivin J-F. A cohort analysis of excess mortality in asthma and the use of inhaled β-agonists. *Am J Respir Crit Care Med* 1994; 149: 604–10.

16. Wright BM, Mckerrow CB. Maximum forced expiratory flow rate as a measure of ventilatory capacity: with a description of a new portable instrument for measuring it. *BMJ* 1959; 2: 1041–7.

17. Lal S, Ferguson AD, Campbell EJM. Forced expiratory time: a simple test for airways obstruction. *BMJ* 1964; 1: 814–7.

18. Gregg I, Nunn AJ. Peak expiratory flow in normal subjects. *BMJ* 1973; 3: 282–4.

19. Lebowitz MJ. The use of peak expiratory flow rate measurements in respiratory diseases. *Ped Pneumol* 1991; 11: 166–74.

20. Quackenboss JJ, Lebowitz MD, Krzyzanowski M. The normal range of diurnal changes in peak expiratory flow rates: Relationship to symptoms and respiratory diseases. *Am Rev Respir Dis* 1991; 143: 323–30.

21. Corrao WM, Braman SS, Irwin RS. Chronic cough as the sole presenting manifestation of bronchial asthma. *N Engl J Med* 1979; 300: 633–7.

22. Turner-Warwick M. On observing patterns of airflow obstruction in chronic asthma. *Br J Dis Chest* 1977; 71: 73–86.

23. Partridge MR. Self-care plans for asthmatics. *Practitioner* 1991; 235: 715–21.

24. Pattemore PK, Johnston SL, Bardin PG. Viruses as precipitants of asthma symptoms. I. Epidemiology. *Clin Exp Allergy* 1992; 22: 325–30.

25. Bateman JRM & Clarke SW. Sudden death in asthma. *Thorax* 1979; 34: 40–44.

26. British Thoracic Society (BTS). Guidelines for management of asthma in adults: II–acute severe asthma. *BMJ* 1990; 301: 797–800.

27. Tukiainen H, Vaara J, Terho E, Karttunen P, Silvasti M. Comparison of twice daily and four times daily administration of beclomethasone dipropionate in patients with severe chronic bronchial asthma. *Eur J Clin Pharmacol* 1986; 30: 319–22.

28. Mecoy RJ, Laby B. Beclomethasone dipropionate in twice daily treatment of asthma. *Austral Fam Phys* 1980; 9: 721–8.

29. Sears MR, Taylor DR, Print CG *et al.* Regular inhaled beta agonist treatment in bronchial asthma. *Lancet* 1990; 336: 1391–6.

30. Webb JR. Dose response of patients to oral corticosteroid treatment during exacerbations of asthma. *BMJ* 1986; 292: 1046–7.

31. Fiel SB, Swartz MA, Glanz K, Francis ME. Efficacy of short term corticosteroid therapy in outpatient treatment of acute bronchial asthma. *Am J Med* 1983; 75: 259–62.

32. Smith AP. Patterns of recovery from acute severe asthma. *Br J Dis Chest* 1981; 75: 132–40.

33. Ruffin RE, Latimer K, Schembri DA. Longitudinal study of near fatal asthma. *Chest* 1991; 99: 77–83.

34. Crompton GK, Grant IWB. Edinburgh emergency asthma admission service. *BMJ* 1975; 4: 680–2.

35. ✪ Gibson PG, Coughlan J, Wilson AJ *et al. The effects of self-management education and regular practitioner review in adults with asthma.* The Cochrane Database of Systematic Reviews. The Cochrane Library, Volume 4, 1998.

36. Beasley R, Cushley M, Holgate ST. A self-management plan in the treatment of adult asthma. *Thorax* 1989; 44: 200–4.

37. Charlton I, Charlton G, Broomfield J, Mullee MA. Evaluation of peak flow and symptoms only self-management plans for control of asthma in general practice. *BMJ* 1990; 301: 1355–9.

38. ✪ Lahdensuo A, Haahtela T, Herrala J *et al.* Randomised comparison of guided self-management and traditional treatment of asthma over one year. *BMJ* 1996; 312: 748–52.

39. ✪ Ignacio-Garcia JM, Gonzalez-Santos P. Asthma self-management education program by home monitoring of peak expiratory flow. *Am J Respir Crit Care Med* 1995; 151: 353–9.

40. Mayo PH, Richman J, Harris W. Results of a program to reduce admissions for adult asthma. *Ann Intern Med* 1990; 112: 864–71.

41. D'Souza W, Crane J, Burgess C *et al.* Community-based asthma care: trial of a "credit card" asthma self-management plan. *Eur Respir J* 1994; 7: 1260–5.

42. D'Souza W, Burgess C, Ayson M, Crane J, Pearce N, Beasley R. Trial of a "credit card" asthma self-management plan in a "high risk" group of patients with asthma. *J Allergy Clin Immunol* 1996; 97 (5): 1085–92.

43. Lewis CE, Rachelefsky G, Lewis MA, de la Sota A, Kaplan M. A randomised trial of ACT (asthma care training for kids). *Paediatrics* 1984; 74: 478–6.

44. Mendoza GR, Sander N, Scherrer A. *A User's Guide to Peak Flow Monitoring*. Fairfax, VA: Mothers of Asthmatics, Inc., 1988.

45. ✪ Fishwick D, Beasley R. Use of peak flow-based self-management plans by adult asthmatic patients (editorial). *Eur Respir J* 1996; 9: 861–5.

Chapter 27

Assessment of Compliance

Gordon Cochrane

INTRODUCTION

Non-compliance or poor adherence to medical advice is a significant problem and may account in part for the failure to improve morbidity in the treatment of patients with asthma.[1] The extent of non-compliance with treatment and medical advice in patients with asthma has until recently not been extensively investigated.[2] However, with the recent introduction of oral anti-inflammatory preparations such as the leukotriene antagonists there has been an increase in interest in compliance with therapeutic regimens, particularly in relationship to long-term prophylactic medication in the treatment of asthma. Compliance is defined as "the extent to which the patient's behaviour coincides with medical advice".[3] Full compliance occurs when the patient follows meticulously the medical advice stated. Partial compliance can be when either the patient fails to take the total number of doses of prescribed drug each day, but completes the course with therapy, or has the full number of doses of prescribed medication but fails to complete the prescribed course. The biological effects of partial compliance may therefore differ, particularly in asthma, where more than one preparation is frequently prescribed. Full compliance with bronchodilator "rescue" therapy with partial compliance with corticosteroids "preventer" therapy is likely to lead to a different biological outcome to that where the patient takes most of their "preventer therapy" but fails to take their rescue bronchodilator inhaler.[4] This increased interest in compliance in advice and treatment in asthma has meant that a more critical analysis of the types of non-compliance has been developed, with a better understanding of where educational programmes in asthma should be directed. The role of careful instruction in inhaler technique; the under-standing of the disease process of asthma; and self-management programmes for the patient so that they may be in control of their own disease and treatment regimens, are all now more clearly defined. Factors which may be associated with poor compliance are now becoming better recognized so that physicians can target more at-risk patients, who have severe and potentially life-threatening disease, but for whatever reason find it difficult to follow medical advice. Our greater understanding has also allowed us an insight into the fact that rigid scientific studies, looking at the way patients follow medical advice, may require a new concept of compliance.[5,6] Compliance is to be yielding, complacent and submissive, but in the real world of health care we now require a more concordant approach which incorporates the patient as part of the decision making process in developing an appropriate therapeutic regimen, for the control of the patient's "own" asthma.[7]

TYPES OF NON-COMPLIANCE

There are fundamentally three basic types of non-compliance; identifying the type may well help the physician to identify the most appropriate form of intervention to improve the patient's self-management and control. These are: unwitting non-compliance; erratic compliance; and intentional or so-called "intelligent non-compliance".[8]

Unwitting Non-Compliance
Unwitting non-compliance is where the patient is frequently unaware that they are not complying. The simplest case is the failure of the patient to realize that their inhaler technique is unlikely to deliver any of the dose drug to the lung, such as failure to remove the cap

from the inhaler, to shake the inhaler, or to breath out when actuating a meter dose aerosol. Fortunately, with the introduction of educational programmes, particularly run by health-care professionals, this is less of a problem than it was a few years ago. However, there are other examples of unwitting non-compliance when patients interpret instructions such as "use medication every day" as "use medication every day when wheezing". The reasons for unwitting compliance include misunderstanding the regimen, language barriers and a factor which is frequently overlooked, particularly in the elderly, dementia. Social and cultural differences may have a profound effect on compliance and control of asthma. Studies of doctor–patient communication have often suggested that when leaving their clinician up to 50% of patients do not accurately remember what they are supposed to do, or cannot recount this accurately, and then convert this conversation into a programme of self-management.[9] Unwitting non-compliance can be corrected by improved communication between health-care professional and the patient, and such communication problems are addressed in other chapters.

Erratic Compliance

Patients with erratic compliance know how and when to take their medication, but unfortunately still fail to follow our advice. The response when challenged for the reason for their non-compliance will usually start "I try to take my medicines regularly", and they then continue to discuss that they are too busy, too forgetful or too stressed. Erratic non-compliance has been identified as being more common than previously thought. Greater understanding of poor compliance in asthma therapy certainly led to addressing the problem of complex regimens[10] and improving behavioural strategies such as "cueing", using "simple reminder notes, or programming medication taking into an integral part of the patient's daily activities". An obvious example is to "cue" taking inhaled corticosteroids before cleaning one's teeth morning and night.

Intentional/Intelligent Non-Compliance

Intentional or "intelligent" non-compliance is a pattern of behaviour where the patient deliberately stops or alters the therapy for personal reasons. This type of compliance is the most difficult for the physician or professional health-care worker to understand, but it is associated with complex behaviour responses of the patient to their illness, their surroundings and their

fear of side-effects, perceived ineffectiveness of the therapy, fear of addiction and in certain situations medication cost.[11,12] Intentional non-compliance is the area where the move from compliance to concordance may lead to improved management for individual patients and the acceptance by the physician that compromise may be the best solution for the individual.

METHODS OF ASSESSING PATIENT COMPLIANCE

Assessment of patient compliance can either be by direct or indirect methods (see Table 27.1).

Direct Methods of Assessment

Direct estimation of blood or urine levels to ascertain compliance with therapy are susceptible to error as they only estimate drug consumption in the previous few hours or days and may be anticipated by the patient if used in regular follow-up appointments. As most of the anti-asthma drugs are taken by the inhaled route they are likely to be undetectable in biological fluids. Rescue bronchodilators such as salbutamol have been shown to be both under-used and over-used when measuring urine salbutamol,[13] but this is a complex, expensive estimation and although newer techniques are now available it measures compliance only on the day of estimation. The simplest methods are indirect methods of measuring compliance.

Indirect Methods of Measuring Compliance

The simplest method is patient self-reporting, which is usually considered to be inaccurate and likely to overestimate compliance, with many patients wishing to

Table 27.1: Traditional methods of assessment of compliance

Direct
Blood: single observation
Urine: affected by patient pre-knowledge

Indirect
Patient interview: inaccurate with direct questions
Doctor belief: very inaccurate
Pill counting: rarely applicable in asthma
Aerosol weighing: errors due to "dumping"
Therapeutic outcome: can be affected by variation in asthma severity

please the health-care professional asking the question.[14] However, this is an area where comparative cost of such a simple approach means that in an improved style of questionnaire with open-ended questions, non-interrogative techniques may be important to identify the individual who is likely to be poorly compliant. The newer questionnaires such as that of Horne[15] certainly indicate that those patients who are less compliant with medication and have a poor quality of life can be identified more accurately than previously considered.

Physician impression is cheap but poorly validated, and studies of direct observational techniques using electronic devices show that physician impression of compliance is a poor indicator of non-compliance.[16,17] Canister weighing, although accurate in assessing the number of actuations, tends to be unreliable because patients are aware that they are under scrutiny when asked to retain their inhaler and therefore may "dump" medication before returning the inhaler.[18] Therapeutic response remains the commonest indirect form of assessment of compliance using diary cards and home peak-flow measurement. The development of electronic diary cards which electronically recorded peak-flow measurements and the time the PEFR was actually made showed that such records may suffer falsification. In a study using such electronic diary cards, more than 10% of diary card entries and peak-flow measurements were either mistimed or invented in 17 of the 30 patients.[19] Some patients were in the main compliant and occasionally just forgot, but one-third of patients had invented 25% of the times and measurements. Comparison of written diary cards with the hand-held computer (which did not include peak-flow measurement) again showed that 20% of entries were mistimed and potentially invented.[20] In a more recent study compliance with peak-flow estimation and self-monitoring of home management of asthma showed that short-term compliance was fairly good, but most patients with moderate to severe asthma were not interested in measuring peak-flow twice a day over a long period. Those who had a personal interest in monitoring PEFR regularly did have better asthma control.[21]

OBJECTIVE ASSESSMENT OF COMPLIANCE WITH INHALED THERAPY

The development of electronic recording devices, which record actuation, the time of actuation ("Chronolog")[22] and even whether the drug is inhaled (TIC Turbohaler),[23] has allowed considerably greater insight into the magnitude of non-compliance with inhaled therapy in asthma.

The initial study by Spector[22] using the Chronolog demonstrated the effectiveness of the device, which revealed less than 50% compliance to a four times a day regimen. Mawhinney and co-workers[24] examined compliance in clinical trials of two non-bronchodilator drugs. These workers identified poor compliance even in the clinical trial situation; the level of compliance was adequate in only six out of 34 patients such that drug efficacy could be determined. They also showed that their patients had periods of "multiple simultaneous use" of one or more actuations, i.e. "dumping", so that the canister weight would be nearer the anticipated weight if the patient had been fully compliant. Similar non-compliance was found with ipratropium bromide, a bronchodilator prescribed as two inhalations three times a day.[18] The Chronolog data showed that self-reporting and inhaler canister weighing overestimate adherence and again confirmed that a substantial number of monitored patients deliberately "dump" medication prior to follow-up visits. Braunstein et al.[17] using the Chronolog identified the relative inaccuracies of physician impression, patient admission and canister weighing against electronic MDI use and clearly show the overestimation of physician impression and patient admission.

Bosley and co-workers[23] in conjunction with the research department of Draco, Sweden, developed the Turbohaler inhalation computer (TIC), which recorded the time and date of each inhalation. The inhalations were recorded using a microphone to identify the rotational click and inspiratory flow noise, which had to be sustained for approximately one-third of a second. Thus only "true" inhalations were recorded and "dumping" or multiple simultaneous rotations without inhalation were not recorded, but identified using the number of grip turns on the mechanical counter on the device. This study compared patient compliance with an inhaled corticosteroid (budesonide) and a short-acting inhaled β agonist (terbutaline sulphate) to a Turbohaler inhaler containing a combination of the two drugs.

In this open multicentre parallel group study, over a 100 asthmatic patients were randomly divided into two groups, either receiving the two drugs in separate Turbohalers or combined into one Turbohaler.

325

Table 27.2: Patterns of compliance with asthma therapy

Holiday pattern with "all" or "nothing"

I take everything and a bit more

Surely once not twice a day is enough

Do I really need it?

Back to clinic back on "preventer"

The doctor's wrong, I don't have asthma, and need no treatment

Medication was prescribed as one or two inhalations twice daily over a 12-week period. A number of patients were lost to follow-up, the ultimate form of non-compliance, but those analysed showed the average compliance was between 60 and 70%. Treatment was taken as prescribed on 30–40% of the study days. Only 15% of patients took the drugs prescribed for more than 80% of study days. The combination of inhaled corticosteroid and bronchodilator was not associated with significantly greater compliance. A number of patterns of compliance were identified, some patients taking both drugs only once a day, others having full compliance on and off during the study in a sort of "holiday" pattern, while others tended to be compliant just before and just after clinic visits (see Table 27.2).

FACTORS CONSIDERED NOT TO BE ASSOCIATED WITH POOR COMPLIANCE

Ageing does not increase compliance, but the longer the patient has had asthma there is a tendency to follow advice more precisely. There are no significant gender differences and increased severity of risk of death or "near fatal" attack do not increase compliance. Socioeconomic status alone does not effect compliance, but there is some evidence in the USA that less formally educated and minority groups do have lower compliance with inhaled steroids.[25] Education about the disease process alone without other educational support programmes has little effect on compliance. Combination of short-acting inhaled β agonist with inhaled corticosteroids has not been associated with "electronic" proven increase in compliance[23] but whether the combination of inhaled steroid with long-

acting β agonists will improve compliance is under investigation.

FACTORS AFFECTING COMPLIANCE

Any drug regimen which has greater frequency than twice a day will reduce compliance. There is little difference between once and twice a day drug regimens, and in some cases twice a day is preferable as forgetting a tablet once a day may have a greater therapeutic effect than forgetting a tablet of a twice a day regimen.

Complex drug regimens[17,24] involving multiple drugs with different routes of administration or different inhalers which require alternative inhalation techniques all lead to a reduction in compliance with therapy.

Fear of side-effects alters behaviour whether the fears are genuine or imaginary. Patients and relatives who are well aware of the real side-effects of oral steroids may transfer these fears to inhaled corticosteroids which have far fewer side-effects even when taken over a number of years.[12]

Depression has been identified as a cause of reduced compliance in both a reduction in taking medication as prescribed but also in attendance rates at follow-up clinics.[26]

IMPROVING COMPLIANCE WITH MEDICAL ADVICE

Non-compliance with medical advice, like all human behaviour, results from a complex interaction of many factors.[27] Identifying the presence and type of non-compliance will allow the clinician to develop an appropriate educational and self-management plan for the individual patient. Clinician awareness of the factors, which are associated with poor compliance, should enable the most "at risk" patients to be supported, particularly depressed patients or those with psychosocial problems. However further improvements in compliance and disease management must be associated with patients being actively involved in the process of determining the "therapeutic plan". Recognition that a physician–patient partnership is required rather than the previous authoritarian or paternalistic mode of behaviour is important. This partnership must recognize the patient's own goals, fears, health beliefs and personal circumstances if greater compliance with medical advice is to be obtained, with hopefully a reduction in morbidity and possibly mortality from asthma.

KEY POINTS

1   Non-compliance with medical advice is common and underestimated in clinical trials. It is difficult to assess accurately in asthma, as direct assessment with inhaled therapy is complicated. Improving doctors and health-care communication skills and using non-threatening questionnaires may be a more appropriate way forward than using complicated electronic devices.

2   Causes of non-compliance: these are multifactorial but inappropriate and complex drug regimens are important factors. Depression, shorter duration of illness and lack of family support will all lead to lower levels of compliance with medical advice.

3   Improving compliance: clear written advice with simple drug regimens allied to educational asthma programmes will improve compliance. Consistent advice from health-care professionals and a concordant approach may lead to improved quality of life.

REFERENCES

1. Anon. Are you taking the medicines? *Lancet* 1990; 335: 262–3.

2. Cochrane GM, Horn CR. The management of asthma in the community: Problems of compliance with treatment. *Q J Med* 1991; 81: 797–8.

3. Sackett DL, Snow JC. The magnitude of compliance and non-compliance. In: Hayes RB, Taylor DW, Sackett DI (eds). *Compliance in Health Care*. Baltimore: Johns Hopkins University Press, 1979; 11–22.

4. ✪ Cochrane GM. Compliance and outcomes in patients with asthma. *Drugs* 1996; 52 (suppl. 6): 12–19.

5. Marinker M. The current status of compliance. *Eur Respir J* 1998; (8)56: 235–8.

6. Jarvis ME. Psychological profile of compliance versus non-compliance. *Eur Respir J* 1998; (8)56: 250–54.

7. ✪ Royal Pharmaceutical Society of Great Britain. *From Compliance to Concordance: Towards Shared Goals in Medicine Taking*. London: RPS, 1997.

8. Rand CS, Wise RA. Adherence with asthma therapy in the management of asthma. In: Szaffer SJ, Leung DYM (eds). Severe asthma. Pathogenesis and clinical management. In: *Lung Biology in Health and Disease*, 86th edn. New York: Marcel Decker, 1996; 435–64.

9. ✪ Ley P, Llewellyn S. Improving patients understanding, recall and satisfaction and compliance. In: Broome A, Llewellyn S (eds). *Health Psychology. Process and Applications*, 2nd edn. London: Chapman and Hall, 1995: 75–98.

10. Spector SL, Kinsman RA, Mawhinney M *et al*. Compliance of patients with asthma with an experimental aerosolized medication. Implications for controlled trials. *J Allergy Clin Immunol* 1986; 77: 65–70.

11. Dekker FW, Dieleman FE, Kaptein AA, Mulder JD. Compliance with pulmonary medication in general practice. *Eur Respir J* 1993; 6: 886–90.

12. Bosley CM, Corden ZM, Cochrane GM. Psychosocial factors and asthma. *Respir Med* 1996; 90: 453–7.

13. Horn CR, Essex E, Hill P, Cochrane GM. Does urinary salbutamol reflect compliance with aerosol regimen in patients with asthma? *Respir Med* 1989; 83: 15–18.

14. Morristey EE, Green LW, Levine DM. Concurrent and predictive validity of a self reported measure of medication adherence. *Med Care* 1986; 24: 67–74.

15. ✪ Horne R, Weinman NJ, Hankins M. The beliefs about Medicines questionnaires (BMQ) a new method for assessing cognitive representations of medication. *Psych Health* 1999; 14: 1–24.

16. Mushlin AI, Appel FA. Diagnosing patient non-compliance. *Arch Intern Med* 1977; 137: 318–21.

17. Braunstein GL, Trinquet G, Harper AK and a

Compliance Working Group. Compliance with nedocromil sodium/salbutamol combination. *Eur Respir J* 1996; 9: 393–8.

18. Rand CS, Wise RA, Nides M *et al*. Metered dose inhaler adherence in a clinical trial. *Am Rev Respir Dis* 1992; 146: 1559–64.

19. Chowienczyk PJ, Lawson CP, Morris J, Kermani A, Cochrane GM. Electronic diary card to record physiological measurements. *Lancet* 1992; 339: 251.

20. Hyland ME, Kenyon CAP, Allen R, Howarth P. Diary keeping in asthma: comparison of written and electronic methods. *BMJ* 1993; 306: 487–9.

21. Côté J, Cartier A, Malo JL *et al*. Compliance with peak flow monitoring in home management of asthma. *Chest* 1998; 113: 968–72.

22. Spector SL. Is your asthmatic really complying? *Ann Allergy* 1985; 55: 552–6.

23. ✪ Bosley CM, Parry DT, Cochrane GM. Patient compliance with inhaled medication. Does combining beta agonists with corticosteroids improve compliance? *Eur Respir J* 1994; 7: 504–9.

24. Mawhinney M, Spector SL, Kinsman RA *et al*. Compliance in clinical trials of two non-bronchodilator anti-asthma medications. *Ann Allergy* 1991; 66: 294–9.

25. Williams MV, Baker DW *et al*. Inadequate literacy is a barrier to asthma knowledge and self-care. *Chest* 1998; 114: 1008–1015.

26. Bosley CM, Fosbury JA, Cochrane GM. The psychological problems associated with poor compliance with treatment in asthma. *Am J Crit Care* 1994; 149(4): A248.

27. Mellins RB, Evans D, Zimmerman B, Clarke NM. Patient compliance–are we wasting our time and don't know it? *Am Rev Respir Dis* 1992; 146: 1376–7.

Part 4

Management of Asthma

Chapter 28

General Principles

Andrew Greening

The management of asthma should encompass three component principles: addressing the consequences of the pathophysiology of the disease; recognition of consensus guidelines; and responding to the fact that patients are individuals, not just the group mean of a large clinical trial, and have individual responses and concerns. Interwoven with these principles it is also necessary to differentiate short-term and long-term objectives, and to have appropriate means by which to measure success or failure.

PATHOPHYSIOLOGY OF ASTHMA AND CLINICAL MANAGEMENT

Over the past decade our understanding of the mechanisms underlying asthma has developed considerably. The recognition of the inflammatory processes[1-3] and the resultant airway changes has redirected thoughts on appropriate drug management. Inflammatory exudate and mucosal wall oedema cause greater luminal narrowing than bronchospasm. Thus, in the short- and medium-term corticosteroids can be very effective in resolving airflow obstruction, and the excellent clinical outcomes[4-6] justify the central role that these drugs play in all but occasional asthma. In the long term, however, questions remain to be answered. The concept of "airway remodelling" is relatively new[7-9] and biopsy changes showing deposition of sub-basement membrane collagen may have been overinterpreted as indicative of development of fixed airways obstruction. Nevertheless, there are data to show that some patients do show enhanced decline in lung function over time and develop fixed airways obstruction.[10-12] The evidence is less clear that regular use of inhaled steroids will prevent the development of fixed airways obstruction, although there is an unavoidable logic that sup-

pression of an inflammatory process should help preclude downstream consequences of that process. One could interpret the (limited) data showing benefit of early introduction of inhaled corticosteroids[13,14] as supportive of the idea that these drugs may prevent/limit development of fixed airways obstruction.

Despite the effectiveness of inhaled corticosteroids many patients continue to experience regular symptoms, often generated by bronchospasm superimposed on the airway narrowing caused by the inflammatory processes. Thus, there remains a role for short-acting β_2 agonists. More recently, clinical trials have shown substantial benefit of adding long-acting β_2 agonists to low or moderate doses of inhaled corticosteroids, with such a combination performing better than use of higher doses of inhaled steroids at controlling symptoms, improving lung function and reducing the frequency of asthma exacerbations.[15-19]

Thus, we have seen the asthma management pendulum moving with our understanding of the airway pathophysiology. In the 1960s and 1970s, with the emphasis on bronchospasm, regular short-acting β_2 agonists had the central role. In the 1980s and early 1990s, inflammation was seen as the whole issue and inhaled steroids the whole answer. In the later 1990s we perceived a need for addressing both components. This broader vision, co-incidentally, is aided by the development of newer agents, such as the leukotriene modifiers,[20,21] that affect inflammatory and bronchoconstrictor processes and will, therefore, enhance future therapeutic options. In addition, our evolving understanding of the pathogenetic mechanisms is leading to the development of newer therapies that target specific points in the inflammatory pathways, such as allergen interactions, leukocyte adhesion and eosinophil activation and longevity.

Non-Pharmacological Approaches

Advances in our understanding of the pathogenetic mechanisms of asthma do not necessarily demand a pharmacological response. In addition to well-established evidence that atopy and allergens are of major importance in the initiation and maintenance of asthmatic inflammatory responses,[22,23] we are now beginning to appreciate those environmental factors that favour the development of clinical disease. This creates the potential that we might influence asthma by altering the pre-natal and neonatal environment, for example by altering the smoking behaviour of mothers-to-be or ownership of household pets.[24–27]

On a sensible, day-to-day level allergen avoidance should be of high priority in management plans. However, this is often easier said than done: most patients have multiple allergies; occupational or environmental exposures may be impossible to avoid; removal of domestic allergens such as cats may cause patient distress; the sensitizing agent may be widespread but not obvious, such as additives to foodstuffs.

CONSENSUS GUIDELINES OF ASTHMA MANAGEMENT

Guidelines on the diagnosis and management of asthma first appeared at the end of the 1980s and proliferated rapidly beyond national guidelines, in Australia and the UK, to encompass international consensus statements and latterly "global" views.[28–30] It is important to recognize the reasons for the production of these guidelines when considering their application to patient care. They arose in response to an increasing prevalence of asthma and a slow response by primary care physicians and non-specialists to recognize the importance of anti-inflammatory therapies in the management of the disease. When viewed in this light their introduction can be seen to be successful. In the UK since the introduction of national guidelines in 1990, the asthma death rate has fallen significantly, which appears to be associated with much wider prescribing of inhaled steroids in primary care.

While guidelines are, thus, most helpful in stimulating best practice they do have limitations that are important to recognize. They are more helpful to the generalist than the specialist. They should be evidenced-based, and that can only be as good as the evidence available. They can only provide general guidance and cannot incorporate all variations for individuals. This may be limiting if guidelines are used by health commissioners, such that use of newer or more expensive therapies are prevented. The words used may influence management behaviour. Thus the term "step" in the UK guidelines encourages doctors to start therapy "low" and gradually increase, even if later versions advise "start high and step down". A term such as "level" or "severity" may be more helpful at guiding the "level" of treatment. Finally, the wider based the guidelines (global, international or national) the more all encompassing the guidelines must become to embrace financial and cultural differences.

PATIENTS ARE INDIVIDUALS

The evidence base for management guidelines is a range of well-conducted clinical trials. For historical and scientific reasons the data from such studies are presented as group mean results with the standard error or deviation depicted. This style of presentation inadvertently "conceals" the level or range of responses that individual patients may have to a particular therapy. Thus, such trial data are able to predict the overall likelihood of benefit but not the likelihood of benefit for one individual patient. Physicians with wide experience of clinical practice will immediately recognize the importance of this having observed the range of responses between different individuals. Since, for adults, the benefits of the first 400 μg of inhaled steroid are usually quite substantial, concerns about individual variations in clinical response probably become most pertinent after this level of therapy is achieved. It seems highly likely that future guidelines will acknowledge this and we will find increasing alternatives for therapy added to low doses of inhaled steroid. To support this concept it would be hoped that clinical drug trials in the future display the range of responses encountered.

ASSESSMENT END-POINTS

Clinical trials employ a variety of end-points. Our perception of the benefit of any trial regimen is influenced by the end-points chosen, since the same regimen may have different levels of efficacy for different end-points. In addition the level of benefit from a regimen may be affected by the duration of treatment, for example bronchial hyperresponsiveness or asthma exacerbation rates in response to inhaled steroids. We have to maintain, also, a balance of cynicism when considering the outcomes and end-points chosen, for any particular clinical trial. A substantial number of the important, large-scale trials are pharmaceutical company funded and designed, and the end-points are likely to be selected carefully to show the company's product in the most favourable light.

Trial End-Points

Frequently a balance has to be achieved between externally measured objective end-points, patient recorded "objective" end-points, and patient derived subjective end-points. Thus, trial office FEV_1 recordings will be accurate and objective, but may be only modestly informative since they will be recorded well after the spontaneous improvement from the early morning "dip" in lung function. On the other hand the patient recorded home PEF on waking may capture that "dip", but is affected by patient enthusiasm and memory and is open to fabrication. An electronic recording device with inbuilt peak flow meter can overcome such problems, but expense will limit their use in large trials.

Some end-points may employ various tools that supposedly measure the same thing, yet give somewhat different answers. Quality of life (QoL) assessments[31,32] are "in vogue", and potentially are yielding important information. However, they vary in their ease of administration and in their specificity of information for asthma. For example, a Dutch study[33] compared two asthma-specific and two general QoL measures in 120 mild asthmatics during a 6-week period of drug comparisons, for which lung function and symptoms were also measured. They found that quality of life correlated poorly with lung function on cross-sectional analyses and even worse on longitudinal assessment. All four questionnaires performed differently, with the asthma quality of life questionnaire (AQLQ)[32] perhaps being the best.

Clinical End-Points vs Trial End-Points

Of course, the formal end-points chosen for a clinical trial may be irrelevant or not measurable for the day-to-day clinical management of individual patients in practice. That is not to say that end-points may not be as important in these circumstances; they simply have to meet different needs and facilities. Thus, in contrast to the end-point that is amenable to statistical analysis, for a formal trial, clinical assessment parameters may be set for individual patients. These may include:

• Structured questioning about symptoms (nocturnal

waking; symptoms on waking in the morning; day-time symptoms; rescue bronchodilator use).
• Setting individualized activity/achievement goals.

HEALTH-CARE PROFESSIONALS, PATIENTS AND PERCEPTIONS

As suggested above identifying ideal outcomes and quantifying success in the clinical setting is complex. While health-care professionals' perceptions of a good outcome may in many ways be similar to those of patients, for example "no symptoms", "as little treatment as possible" and "no side-effects from the drugs taken", there are also important differences. While "normal lung function" is a goal for health-care professionals and is cited in guidelines, it is a somewhat nebulous concept for a patient more interested in carrying out their normal daily activities. In addition, most patients harbour expectations that health-care professionals regard as unrealistic – the hope of a cure for their asthma. This may well affect their behaviour towards therapy and adherence to their treatment regimen. When feeling well and symptomatic they will frequently reduce or stop their medication, or if not well and asymptomatic they may embrace alternative medicine.

Perception of Symptoms

Management may have to be modified to take into account different abilities of patients to perceive bronchospasm.[34] Some patients may complain of severe breathlessness when their PEF falls from 500 to 400 l min.$^{-1}$ (This should alert the physician or nurse to alternative explanations than asthma for the symptoms, such as hyperventilation). At the other extreme some patients experience no symptoms at all until their PEF is severely limited. Such people are at risk of death and require additional steps to be taken. This group in particular should use home peak flow monitoring on a daily basis with clear instructions to seek help if their PEF reaches a pre-set level. They should be considered, also, for enrolment into an emergency self-admission service.[35]

In addition, if lung function falls gradually many patients adapt their lifestyle to avoid the associated symptoms. This coping strategy is particularly common among middle-aged and elderly patients who may "expect" to feel breathless through a combination of age, lack of fitness and being overweight. A gradual change in lifestyle, in this manner, can affect symptom perception and alter outcome measures. For example "normal daily activities" can become a highly variable outcome measure and is open to wide misinterpretation.

Perceptions of Treatment

Patients' perceptions of medications may influence their wishes and "compliance" at any level in guidelines of management. Therapies raise a number of patient-centred issues that health-care professionals may often underestimate: the introduction of inhaled cortico-steroids may worry the patient in terms of (frequently misperceived) side-effects; patients may worry that regular use of therapy will lead to gradual loss of efficacy of that treatment (and they would rather "keep it in reserve"); the associated prescription costs for additional drugs/inhalers may induce genuine financial concerns.

Perceptions of Provoking Factors

It is easy to underestimate the impact on quality of life for a patient when the health-care professional pursues "avoidance of provoking factors". The patient may feel that their livelihood is under threat (occupational asthma) or their pleasures are being threatened (domestic pets). On the other side of the coin it is clear that many patients or parents may fail to recognize that the home/work environment is exerting a real influence on the severity of their/their child's asthma. Domestic pets are a good example. The fact that the pets and their allergens are constantly present in the house "conceals" the event of allergen exposure and it is much harder for the patient or parent to appreciate such exposure, in contrast to a similar event in another house or setting. Thus, approximately 20% of our asthma clinic pet owners believe they are allergic to other people's cats or dogs, but not their own!

Perceptions of Life

Psychological factors may affect patients' perceptions of their symptoms and hence, asthma control. This may reflect intrinsic optimism or pessimism ("my glass is half full" vs "my glass is half empty"), but is more likely to reflect the impact of external stresses. These aspects should always be considered, but are most likely to be applicable in patients whose asthma is difficult to control. Questions addressing financial, family, marital and work worries may be revealing and attention at trying to help those issues may improve control of troublesome asthma.

DELIVERY OF ASTHMA CARE

The success of asthma management is frequently dependent upon the mechanisms of delivery of asthma care. Guidelines provide a framework within which the generalist is likely to improve their asthma management. Specialist supervision has much to commend it and can be offered efficiently in the primary care setting by nurse-led asthma clinics. In secondary care clear protocols of management, based on Guidelines, should be readily available (and applied) in the Emergency Admission setting and patient supervision transferred to a respiratory specialist.

The patient focus remains a central key to success. Patients should be empowered to reach decisions about their own care by appropriate information and education, but within the context of ownership of goals and means.

Cost Effectiveness

While asthma management is directed to the individual, physicians have a responsibility to use health-care resources efficiently. This does not necessarily mean that the cheapest drug or inhaler is the correct choice. Good control of the asthma is paramount, since the costs of hospital admissions, emergency room visits, and social security payments will outweigh, considerably, medication costs. The cost-effectiveness of therapy should be considered, but clearly total and not just drug costs must be assessed.

International and Cultural Variations

While GINA has provided a basis for widespread international agreement on asthma management, there remain widespread substantial variations. These may have socioeconomic, cultural or educational reasons. Pricing mechanisms in some countries may favour the use of oral medication or single dose inhalers. In many countries traditional medicines may be favoured as firstline therapy. In some countries, as in Northern Europe, inhaled therapy is much more widely accepted than in others. Education of physicians will influence their practice as will the method of application of healthcare. Both may vary significantly between countries. The future management of asthma worldwide is likely to converge as the evidence base for particular advice increases, and there is greater dialogue between physicians.

KEY POINTS

1 *Asthma Management*
   (a) Should take into account the complex inflammatory pathophysiological mechanisms of the disease.
   (b) Recognize the value of consensus guidelines.
   (c) Should respond to the fact that patients are individuals, not the group mean of a large clinical trial.
   (d) Recognize there are both short-term and long-term objectives.

2 *Environment and Asthma*
   (a) The *in utero* environment is important for the development of childhood asthma (e.g. maternal smoking).
   (b) Allergen exposure in the neonatal period may determine risk of childhood asthma.
   (c) Avoidance of domestic allergens (house-dust mite and domestic pets) can be important for improving asthma control and reducing medication.

3 *Patient Perceptions*
   (a) Patients may perceive falsely that symptoms are due to their asthma (e.g. hyperventilation).
   (b) Older patients may expect to feel breathless through a combination of age, lack of fitness and being overweight, and not equate their symptoms with their asthma.
   (c) External factors, such as financial, family, marital and work worries, may affect adversely patients' perceptions of their asthma symptomatology.

4 *Delivery of Asthma Care*
   (a) Ideally, asthma care should be provided by specialists. In primary care this can be done effectively by nurse-led asthma clinics.
   (b) Protocols of asthma management, based on consensus guidelines, should be available in primary and secondary care.
   (c) Patients should be empowered to reach decisions about their own care by appropriate information and education.
   (d) The cost-effectiveness, not just the cost, of therapy must be considered.

REFERENCES

1. Jeffery PK, Wardlaw AJ, Nelson FC, Collins JV, Kay AB. Bronchial biopsies in asthma. An ultrastructural, quantitative study and correlation with hyperreactivity. *Am Rev Respir Dis* 1989; 140: 1745–53.

2. ✪ Djukanovic R, Roche WR, Wilson JW *et al*. Mucosal inflammation in asthma. *Am Rev Respir Dis* 1990; 142: 434–57.

3. Laitinen LA, Laitinen A, Haahtela T. Airway mucosal inflammation even in patients with newly diagnosed asthma. *Am Rev Respir Dis* 1993; 147: 697–704.

4. Haahtela T, Jarvinen M, Kava T *et al*. Comparison of a beta 2-agonist, terbutaline, with an inhaled corticosteroid, budesonide, in newly detected asthma. *N Engl J Med* 1991; 325: 388–92.

5. Busse WW. What role for inhaled steroids in chronic asthma? *Chest* 1993; 104: 1565–71.

6. ✪ Pedersen S, Hansen OR. Budesonide treatment of moderate and severe asthma in children: a dose-response study. *J Allergy Clin Immunol* 1995; 95: 29–33.

7. Jeffery PK, Godfrey RW, Ädelroth E, Nelson F, Rogers A, Johansson S-A. Effects of treatment on airway inflammation and thickening of basement membrane reticular collagen in asthma: a quantitative light and electron microscopy study. *Am Rev Respir Dis* 1992; 145: 890–99.

8. Bousquet J, Vignola AM, Chanez P, Campbell AM, Bonsignore G, Michel FB. Airways remodelling in asthma: no doubt, no more? *Int Arch Allergy Immunol* 1995; 107: 211–14.

9. Pare PD, Bai TR, Roberts CR. The structural and functional consequences of chronic allergic inflammation of the airways. *Ciba Found Symp* 1997; 206: 71–86.

10. Brown PJ, Greville HW, Finucane KE. Asthma and irreversible airflow obstruction. *Thorax* 1984; 39: 131–36.

11. Peat JK, Woolcock AJ, Cullen K. Rate of decline of lung function in subjects with asthma. *Eur J Respir Dis* 1987; 20: 171–79.

12. Fish JE, Peters SP. Airway remodeling and persistent airway obstruction in asthma. *J Allergy Clin Immunol* 1999; 104: 509–16.

13. ✪ Haahtela T, Jarvinen M, Kava T *et al*. Effects of reducing or discontinuing inhaled budesonide in patients with mild asthma. *N Engl J Med* 1994; 331: 700–705.

14. Selroos O, Pietinalho A, Lofroos AB, Riska H. Effect of early vs late intervention with inhaled corticosteroids in asthma. *Chest* 1995; 108: 1228–34.

15. ✪ Greening AP, Ind PW, Northfield M, Shaw G. Added salmeterol versus higher-dose corticosteroid in asthma patients with symptoms on existing inhaled corticosteroid. *Lancet* 1994; 344: 219–24.

16. Woolcock A, Lundback B, Ringdal N, Jacques LA. Comparison of addition of salmeterol to inhaled steroids with doubling the dose of inhaled steroids. *Am J Respir Crit Care Med* 1996; 153: 1481–8.

17. Wilding P, Clark M, Coon JT *et al*. Effect of long-term treatment with salmeterol on asthma control: a double blind, randomised crossover study. *BMJ* 1997; 314: 1441–6.

18. van Noord JA, Schreurs AJ, Mol SJ, Mulder PG. Addition of salmeterol versus doubling the dose of fluticasone propionate in patients with mild to moderate asthma. *Thorax* 1999; 54: 207–212.

19. ✪ Pauwels RA, Lofdahl CG, Postma DS *et al*. Effect of inhaled formoterol and budesonide on exacerbations of asthma. Formoterol and Corticosteroids Establishing Therapy (FACET) International Study Group. *N Engl J Med* 1997; 337: 1405–1411.

20. Horwitz RJ, McGill KA, Busse WW. The role of leukotriene modifiers in the treatment of asthma. *Am J Respir Crit Care Med* 1998; 157: 1363–71.

21. Wenzel SE. Leukotriene receptor antagonists and related compounds. *Can Respir J* 1999; 6: 189–93.

22. Plaschke P, Janson C, Balder B, Lowhagen O, Jarvholm B. Adult asthmatics sensitized to cats and dogs: symptoms, severity, and bronchial hyperresponsiveness in patients with furred animals at home and patients without these animals. *Allergy* 1999; 54: 843–50.

23. Nelson HS, Szefler SJ, Jacobs J, Huss K, Shapiro G, Sternberg AL. The relationships among environmental allergen sensitization, allergen exposure, pulmonary function, and bronchial hyperresponsiveness in the childhood asthma management program. *J Allergy Clin Immunol* 1999; 104: 775–85.

24. Sears MR, Holdaway MD, Flannery EM, Herbison GP, Silva PA. Parental and neonatal risk factors for atopy, airway hyper-responsiveness, and asthma. *Arch Dis Child* 1996; 75: 392–98.

25. Hu FB, Persky V, Flay BR, Zelli A, Cooksey J, Richardson J. Prevalence of asthma and wheezing in public schoolchildren: association with maternal smoking during pregnancy. *Ann Allergy Asthma Immunol* 1997; 79: 80–84.

26. Burr ML, Merrett TG, Dunstan FD, Maguire MJ. The development of allergy in high-risk children. *Clin Exp Allergy* 1997; 27: 1247–53.

27. Gold DR, Burge HA, Carey V, Milton DK, Platts-Mills T, Weiss ST. Predictors of repeated wheeze in the first year of life: the relative roles of cockroach, birth weight, acute lower respiratory illness, and maternal smoking. *Am J Respir Crit Care Med* 1999; 160: 227–36.

28. British Thoracic Society, Research Unit of Royal College of Physicians, Kings Fund Centre, National Asthma Campaign. Guidelines for management of asthma in adults. I: Chronic persistent asthma. *BMJ* 1990; 301: 651–53.

29. ✪ National Heart Lung and Blood Institute. *Global Strategy for Asthma Management and Prevention*. NHLBI/WHO Workshop Report. National Institutes of Health publication 95-3659. Bethesda, Maryland, US; 1995.

30. Expert Panel Report 2. *Guidelines for the Diagnosis and*

Management of Asthma. National Asthma Education and Prevention Program. National Institutes of Health Publication Number 97-4501, Bethesda, Maryland, US; 1997.

31. Hyland ME, Finnis S, Irvine SH. A scale for assessing quality of life in adult asthma sufferers. *J Psychosom Res* 1991; 35: 99–110.

32. Juniper EF, Guyatt GH, Ferrie PJ, Griffith LE. Measuring quality of life in asthma. *Am Rev Respir Dis* 1993; 147: 832–8.

33. Rutten-van Molken MP, Custers F, van Doorslaer EK

et al. Comparison of performance of four instruments in evaluating the effects of salmeterol on asthma quality of life. *Eur Respir J* 1995; 8: 888–98.

34. Bijl-Hofland ID, Cloosterman SG, Folgering HT, Akkermans RP, van Schayck CP. Relation of perception of airway obstruction to the severity of asthma. *Thorax* 1999; 54: 15–19.

35. Crompton GK, Grant IW, Chapman BJ, Thomson A, McDonald CF. Edinburgh Emergency Asthma Admission Service: report on 15 years' experience. *Eur J Respir Dis* 1987; 70: 266–71.

Chapter 29

Management of Chronic Asthma in Children

James Paton

INTRODUCTION

Asthma is the commonest chronic childhood disease in developed countries. For the children, asthma causes significant sleep disturbance, loss of time from school,[1] interference with activities[2] and hospitalization.[1-4] For their parents, the consequences are significant time off work, restriction of social activities[5] and anxiety, fear and guilt.[3] The economic costs are huge. Although the morbidity is considerable, asthma mortality is rare in children, but the death rate for asthma has fallen very little over a period when other causes of childhood mortality have declined.[3]

The prevalence of childhood asthma appears to have increased,[6,7] although the extent of the increase has been debated.[8,9] The reasons for the increase are not known. Changes in environmental factors or lifestyles are thought the most likely causes.[10,11] There have also been concerns that the severity of asthma has been increasing. In the UK, there is some evidence that the number of severe attacks and chronic disability has fallen[12] and the number of admissions with acute asthma has levelled off[4] and may have started to fall. These encouraging signs may be due to more effective treatment of children with recognized asthma. The willingness of doctors to make the diagnosis is probably one of the most significant factors in improving treatment. Correct diagnosis is likely to lead to appropriate management and treatment.[13] A diagnosis of asthma can relieve parental anxiety rather than cause it.

In the last 20 years, our understanding of asthma has increased greatly. In adults with asthma, the use of fibreoptic bronchoscopy to obtain mucosal lavage and biopsy material to investigate the pathology of asthma during life has led to a picture of asthma as a chronic inflammatory disease of the airways.[14,15] The conse-quences of this inflammatory process are broncho-constriction, oedema, mucus hypersecretion and stimulation of neural reflexes within the airways and in time, fixed airway obstruction – all the features that comprise the clinical syndrome recognized as asthma.[16] Inflammation may also have a key role in the development of bronchial hyperreactivity,[17] which is present in up to 90% of children with frequent wheezing in the previous year, particularly those with atopy.[18,19]

Because of technical difficulties investigating children, and ethical constraints, there is less information on the pathology of asthma in children. The limited pathological studies suggest that airway inflammation is important.[20] In the last 5 years, non-invasive markers of inflammation have been studied in children with asthma.[21-24] Broadly, these studies have confirmed that ongoing eosinophilic airway inflammation is present in children with asthma and atopy. However, there has been increasing recognition that many wheezing episodes in infants and young children are most closely related to viral infection. Eosinophilic inflammation is not evident in bronchoalveolar lavage (BAL) fluid from children with viral associated wheeze.[23] This suggests that there may be different underlying pathophysiological mechanisms depending on the pattern of wheezing (Table 29.1).[25,26] Longitudinal studies have pointed to at least three different wheezing phenotypes in childhood: "transient early wheezing"; "non-atopic wheezing" of the toddler and early school years; and "IgE-associated wheeze/asthma" associated with persistent wheezing at any age.[27]

The concept of asthma as an inflammatory disease has led to a fundamental shift in approach to the treatment of asthma in children. The strategy now used aims to control or prevent the underlying inflammation. Where possible, prevention is achieved by avoidance of factors that induce inflammation ("inducers"),

Table 29.1: Features of the main wheezing disorders of childhood. (From Silverman M. Out of the mouths of babes and sucklings: lessons from early childhood asthma. *Thorax* 1993; 48: 1200–4, with permission)

	Recurrent wheezy LRI in pre-school children	Asthma in school children
Pattern	Episodic	Interval symptoms and episodic
Peak prevalence	6–36 months	5–10 years
Aetiology	Viral infection	Atopic sensitivity (plus viral episodes)
Bronchial responsiveness	Normal	Increased
Prognosis		
Child/young adult	Symptoms largely confined to pre-school era; minor anomalies in early adult life	Persistent
Later life	?Associated with COPD	No relation to COPD

LRI: lower respiratory illness; COPD: chronic obstructive pulmonary disease.

such as known allergens. Currently, avoidance strategies are often ineffective, and control is achieved using anti-inflammatory medication ("preventers"). Broncho-dilators ("relievers") are then used as required for the relief of symptoms.

Despite encouraging signs, there is evidence that asthma in children remains under-diagnosed and inadequately treated.[2,28–30] The principles of diagnosis and treatment have been clearly set out in a number of international guidelines.[31–33] This chapter focuses on the practical aspects of diagnosis and management of asthma in childhood.

INITIAL ASSESSMENT AND DIAGNOSIS OF ASTHMA IN CHILDHOOD (see also Chapter 5)

There is no definitive diagnostic test for asthma at present. The diagnosis in children is essentially clinical. Lung function testing to demonstrate reversible airways obstruction is not usually possible in young children below 4–5 years of age, except in specialist laboratories. The possible role of inflammatory markers in BAL fluid, sputum or exhaled breath, or histological demonstration of inflammation is the subject of active clinical research.

History
A careful, detailed history is the key to diagnosis (Table 29.2). Such a history is likely to be of more value in planning the management than all other investigations.

The cardinal clinical features are wheeze, difficulty breathing, cough and breathlessness. As similar symptoms may occur with viral infections in normal children, a pattern of recurrent episodes or exacerbations is important. Children with three or more episodes of cough, wheeze and/or breathlessness should be considered as having asthma.[34]

Wheeze is frequently described as a whistling noise coming from the chest. However, parents often recognize wheezing in their children by a constellation of features that include wheezing, difficulty breathing and being unwell. Quite often they describe a moist rattly sound ("ruttle" or "crickle") whose relation to asthma is unclear. Occasionally, parents use wheezing as a descriptive term for any respiratory noise, so it is important to ensure they are not describing another respiratory noise such as stridor. Breathlessness may be obvious in older children but can be more difficult to recognize in younger children. A small child may be unable to keep up with their peers, may become tired more easily, may want to be carried or at worst may be reluctant to take part in any activity. In about 5–6% of children with asthma, isolated cough may be the presenting feature.[35] The cough is usually non-productive, but will often be worse at night, and after exercise. Most of these children will have pulmonary function studies consistent with asthma.

When questioned directly, children often report other sensations such as a feeling of tightness in the

Table 29.2: Important areas of inquiry when taking the history in children with asthma. (Adopted from Expert Panel Report, No. 2. *Guidelines for the Diagnosis and Management of Asthma.* NIH Publication No. 97-4051. Bethesda MD: National Institutes of Health, 1997.)

Age at onset

Nature of symptoms
  wheezing–whistling sound when breathing out; difficulty breathing; cough; breathlessness; chest tightness or discomfort; unwell

Triggers
  viral infections; exercise; allergens; changes in weather; laughing or crying; cigarette smoke

Pattern of symptoms
  recurrent or persistent; frequency; nocturnal deterioration; seasonal variation

Severity of symptoms
  previous admissions to hospital or ICU admissions

Exposure to environmental hazards and their effects on disease
  cigarette smoking, active and passive; damp or mouldy housing; house-dust mite; pets

Drug therapy
  past and present therapy including drugs; dose; devices; response and side-effects

Impact of disease on child and family
  sleep disturbance; school performance and attendance; exercise and activity

Family history
  asthma and atopic illnesses in first and second degree relatives

Past illnesses
  bronchiolitis, other significant respiratory infections

Table 29.3: Triggers of asthma in children

Viral infections

Exercise

Exposure to allergens: cats, dogs, house-dust mite, grass

Environmental factors: tobacco smoke, pollution, weather changes

Others: laughing, emotional stress

Another important and diagnostic feature of asthma is the variation with time, both in the short- and long-term. Diurnal variation with symptoms and lung function being worse during the night and first thing in the morning is characteristic.[36,37] Often, there is longer-term variation with acute episodes of respiratory morbidity either superimposed upon perennial symptoms or as the sole manifestation of asthma. Sometimes there are lengthy symptom-free periods between attacks, which may only occur at particular times of year, most commonly in the winter.[26] Many young children only have symptoms with viral respiratory infections and may be completely free of any symptoms between infections.[38] These patterns of disease are important since they may help when deciding the most appropriate treatment. If symptoms are persistent and without variation, alternative diagnoses should be excluded (Table 29.4).

Asthma in children can cause significant morbidity[3] and it is important to inquire specifically about the impact on the child and family. Do symptoms disturb sleep? Are they frequently absent from school?[1] Is academic progress satisfactory? Is asthma interfering with activity or stopping the child doing things they would like to do? Are there frequent emergency visits to the doctor or hospital?

Previous treatments, their effectiveness and side-effects should be reviewed. All too often, a history of recurrent episodes of coughing and wheezing unresponsive to courses of antibiotics is given. What drugs and devices has the child had? Were they effective? If not, are the parents able to offer possible reasons for their failure? What do parents understand about the purpose of the medications and the times when they should be used? Has the child experienced side-effects from the medicines? Have any other steps such as

chest, discomfort or pain. Sometimes the descriptions are quite graphic, for example "like an elephant sitting on my chest".

A diagnosis of asthma is more likely if the cardinal symptoms occur after exposure to certain typical triggers (Table 29.3). Viral infections (particularly with rhinoviruses) and exercise are the most important in children.

Table 29.4: Features that should alert the paediatrician to diagnoses other than asthma

History
Persistent wheeze not responding to appropriate treatment
Wheeze associated with feeding or vomiting
Neonatal onset or wheeze following neonatal lung disease
Acute onset of wheezing/coughing (suggesting foreign body)
Stridor
Productive cough
Steatorrhoea

Examination
Failure to thrive
Finger clubbing
Focal signs

Investigations
Lack of reversibility of airflow obstruction with bronchodilators
Persistent or focal chest X-ray changes

house-dust mite avoidance been taken in an attempt to modify the condition?

Clinical Examination

Abnormalities on clinical examination do not confirm a diagnosis of asthma. As asthma is episodic (and modern treatments now so effective) physical examination is often normal. Clinical features of airway obstruction such as hyperinflation and evidence of chest deformity may indicate chronic, poorly controlled asthma but are not diagnostic. There may be evidence of other atopic diseases, particularly eczema and rhinitis. Drug-related side effects such as tremor due to bronchodilators, or oral candidiasis related to inhaled corticosteroids should always be looked for.

Both asthma, especially when poorly controlled,[39] and its therapy may cause slowing of linear growth.[40] All too often, the inaccuracy of height measuring equipment has confounded the effects of asthma and its treatment on linear growth. It is, therefore, particularly important to measure height accurately using a properly functioning and regularly calibrated device such as a stadiometer. It should always be borne in mind that poor growth might point to another disease such as cystic fibrosis.

Examination is particularly useful when specific features, such as finger clubbing, which point to an alternative diagnosis, are present. Physical abnormalities in asthma should be generalized; recurrent or persistent

focal features may also point to alternative diagnoses. In infants and young children it is especially important to remember that there are other important causes of wheezing and cough and to recognize clinical features that point to alternative diagnoses (Table 29.4). Further investigations (e.g. sweat test, lower oesophageal pH study) may be necessary.

Aids to Diagnosis

When diagnosis is difficult, additional information about the pattern and severity of attacks can be important. There are several useful diagnostic aids.

Diary Cards

Symptom diary cards have been widely used to record the severity and pattern of symptoms over time. In children aged 5 years or over, peak flow can be recorded either alone or in conjunction with symptoms. Unfortunately, diary recording is often inaccurate[41,42] and completion poor. To be valid, diaries should be completed at the time rather than retrospectively. Diaries completed in blocks of uni-coloured ink with unvarying similar neat handwriting should arouse suspicions that the diary has been completed sometime after the recording. Electronic diaries that include a date stamp are becoming available and may be a useful, if expensive, improvement.[43,44]

Lung Function Testing

Simple lung function tests, particularly the peak expiratory flow (PEF), have become an important aspect of asthma management in children old enough to co-operate. Spirometry is increasingly available and can provide a standardized objective measurement of airflow obstruction and its reversibility in children old enough to co-operate. More sophisticated lung function tests in children often provide little additional useful information.

Peak Expiratory Flow Relatively inexpensive portable PEF meters are now widely available and measurement of PEF in children over 5 years is reasonably reproducible.[45] Recent studies have found that many portable PEF meters are non-linear, over-reading by 40–80 l min^{-1} in the mid-range peaking around 300 l min,$^{-1}$ and under-reading by 30–80 l min^{-1} in the high range. This non-linearity is large and of potential clinical relevance in children. It is possible to correct for non-linearity by changing the scale but such linearized PEF meters are not yet widely available.[46] Because of the wide variability between each brand, peak flow meters should be viewed as monitoring devices rather than diagnostic devices.

Many children aged between 3 and 5 years can be persuaded to blow into peak flow meters, although the results are less reproducible.[47] Unfortunately, peak flow meters able to record in the range 20–200 l min^{-1} are not now readily available.

The principle problem with peak expiratory flow is that the measurement is effort-dependent. Poor effort leads to falsely low values. Fortunately, children often enjoy PEF measurement and try very hard to get the best possible value. Occasionally, they even become dispirited if more active asthma leads to levels lower than their best. Older children, particularly boys, can learn to trick the meter by spitting into it and can produce artificially high values.[48] Using a larger mouthpiece placed well into the mouth, and encouraging the child to huff can overcome such cheating.

A single reading is usually of little value unless it is clearly abnormal. Home measurements plotted on a chart can provide evidence of variability and severity of airways obstruction over a period of time (Fig. 29.1). Usually, readings are made twice daily before, and if possible after bronchodilator, with the best of a number of attempts being noted. There are a variety of charts available to allow the values to be recorded for future review. Long-term peak flow measurements should be correlated with other measures of severity such as symptoms.[49]

Predicted values in children are related to height.[50] Ideally, reference values should be specific to each brand of meter, but such brand-specific normative values are generally not available. Where possible the best peak flow, rather than the predicted, should be used as a guide. An exception is those who have persisting airways obstruction. Then the aim should be to improve them to the predicted level. Whether diurnal variability in children with asthma is less than that in adults is not clear.[37,51]

Spirometry Spirometry with flow-volume loops may provide additional information for diagnostic purposes or when assessing the degree of severity of asthma.[52] In

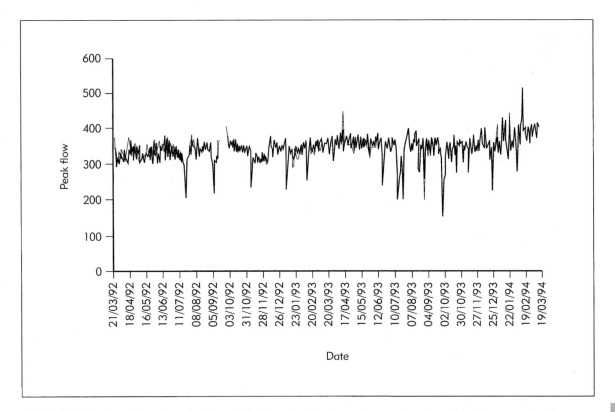

FIGURE 29.1: A peak flow chart showing variation in peak expiratory flow in an asthmatic child. Thick line, a.m.; thin line, p.m.

particular, the maximum expiratory flows from the flow-volume loop are more sensitive to lesser degrees of airway obstruction.[53] However, spirometry test is only practical in children who can perform a forced vital capacity manoeuvre, usually those aged over 5 years. Measurement of functional residual capacity is possible in some pre-school children who may have hyperinflation even when symptoms are controlled.[54]

Reversibility with Bronchodilator In the presence of airway obstruction, an increase in PEF of 15–20% or FEV_1 (usually >12%) after inhalation of a β_2 agonist confirms bronchodilator responsiveness and is typical of asthma. The most appropriate value for reversibility in children is still not clear, and there is no accepted value that can be applied in all cases. Unfortunately, lack of reversibility does not exclude asthma. Both those with near normal lung function and those with fixed airway obstruction may show little improvement.[53]

The measurement of airway resistance by the interrupter technique (Rint) is showing promise as method of demonstrating bronchodilator reversibility in children of 2–5 years of age.[55]

Bronchial Provocation Tests Bronchial hyperresponsiveness is a feature of symptomatic asthma and is usually measured as reduction in FEV_1 of 15 or 20% in response to stimuli such as exercise, histamine/methacholine, cold air, ultrasonically nebulized water or hypertonic saline. It can be present in asymptomatic children and is also found in other conditions such as cystic fibrosis. Community surveys have shown considerable overlap in bronchial responsiveness between children with asthma and symptom-free children[56] making it of limited value in the diagnosis of asthma. It can also occur transiently after upper respiratory infection in normal subjects.[57] Many children experience significant respiratory morbidity in the absence of bronchial hyperresponsiveness.[58,59] Overall, the relation between bronchial reactivity and clinical asthma is not sufficiently close to make it of practical use in diagnosis or management.[60] Occasionally, demonstration of hyperresponsiveness may be of some value in uncommon presentations such as cough-variant asthma; often, a trial of asthma treatment is more useful.

Chest X-ray

There are no characteristic X-ray features of childhood asthma. As with clinical signs, any changes should be generalized. Persistent focal changes should suggest an alternative diagnosis. X-rays of children with more acute symptoms occasionally show areas of atelectasis from mucus plugging of small airways, particularly in the right middle lobe.[61] These infiltrates often clear very rapidly on subsequent chest X-rays but can occasionally be mistaken for recurrent/persistent pneumonia.[62]

A chest X-ray is not always necessary if asthmatic symptoms are mild, the clinical features typical and the disease easily controlled by appropriate therapy. If a chest X-ray is undertaken, it is often best carried out when symptoms are well controlled. Persisting radiological changes then would suggest that an alternative diagnosis should be sought.

Allergy Testing (see also Chapter 9)

Parents are often keen that allergy testing should be carried out, in the hope of identifying the "cause" of their child's asthma. Unfortunately, allergy testing does not diagnose allergic disease. It can only determine the presence of allergen-specific IgE antibodies. The diagnosis rests on a careful clinical and environmental assessment of whether the signs, symptoms and allergy tests are consistent with allergic disease. Determination of sensitivity to perennial indoor allergen is usually not possible from the history alone.[63] The diagnosis may need to be confirmed by exclusion or specific challenge. Allergy tests such as skin-prick tests or radioallergosorbent tests (RASTs) are only part of that diagnostic process.[64] Negative allergy tests exclude clinical allergy with a high degree of reliability but positive results must be correlated with the clinical history.

Skin-prick testing is most commonly used. It is easy to perform, cheap and quick. Usually a limited panel of antigens (house-dust mite, grass pollen, cat or dog dander and moulds, usually *Alternaria*) is all that is required to confirm atopy. Positive and negative controls (saline and histamine) should always be included. Unfortunately, atopy is virtually universal in asthmatic children by school age.[65,66] In the UK, almost all asthmatic children will react to one or more of house-dust mite extract, mixed grass pollen or cat dander. Skin testing has the advantage that positive results are clearly visible to parents and children, a feature that may help encourage compliance with environmental control measures.

RASTs measure the specific quantity of IgE antibodies and are available for a wide range of common antigens. Values correlate well with the size of skin test weals. However, there is no major group of allergens (e.g. pollens, moulds, danders, foods or venoms) in which RAST results are better than those provided by skin tests.[67] They may be useful in the presence of skin disease such as eczema or where there is a risk of anaphylaxis and they are not affected by medications that suppress the immediate skin test such as antihistamines.

Children find both skin-prick testing and blood taking for RAST tests painful and they are not popular.

Direct bronchial challenge with aeroallergen can be undertaken, but because of the possibility of provoking significant asthmatic reactions is limited to clinical research. Indirect challenge where a change in bronchial reactivity is measured after controlled challenge to a natural dose of a suspected allergen may be useful particularly in the investigation of food intolerance.[68]

MANAGEMENT OF CHRONIC ASTHMA IN CHILDHOOD

Once a diagnosis has been reached, an appropriate plan of management can be instituted. In the absence of suitable markers of inflammation, decisions on treatment have to be made on clinical grounds based on the frequency and severity of symptoms. In children over 5 years, lung function tests may provide additional objective information.

The general aims (Table 29.5) of asthma management have been clearly set out in recently published

Table 29.5: Asthma management once a diagnosis has been made – general aims and desirable outcomes. (Based on Refs 31–33)

Aims	Mild/moderate asthma (BTS guidelines steps 1–3)	Severe asthma (BTS guidelines steps 4–5)
	Outcome: Control of asthma	Outcome: Best possible result
Achieve and maintain control of symptoms	Minimally (ideally) no symptoms during the day No nocturnal disturbance Minimal need for relief bronchodilator	Least possible symptoms during the day Minimal nocturnal disturbance Least possible need for relief bronchodilator
Maintain pulmonary function as close to normal as possible	PEF ≥ 80% of predicted or best circadian variation <20%	Best PEF Least possible circadian variation
Maintain normal levels of activity, including no exercise limitation	No limitation on activities or exercise Normal school or nursery attendance	Least possible limitation of activity Least possible time off school or nursery
Maintain normal growth	Normal growth	Least possible growth slowing
Prevent asthma exacerbations	Minimal (infrequent) exacerbations No hospital admissions or emergency room visits	Least possible exacerbations Minimal hospital admissions
Provide optimal pharmacotherapy	Minimal (or no) adverse effects	Least adverse effects
Meet patient's and family's expectations of asthma care		
Prevent asthma mortality		

BTS: British Thoracic Society; PEF: Peak expiratory flow.

Table 29.6: Indications for hospital referral of children with asthma

Referral to a general paediatrician	Referral to respiratory paediatrician
Diagnosis is in doubt	After a life-threatening episode or admission to an intensive care unit
Asthma is unstable	
Asthma interferes with normal life despite treatment	Brittle asthma
Parents or family practitioners want support	Asthma causing severe restriction in normal activity despite treatment
More than 400 μg per day inhaled steroids needed to control asthma	When special investigations are required
	More than 800 μg per day inhaled steroid needed to control asthma

guidelines.[32,33,69] They can be briefly summarized as gaining and maintaining long-term asthma control, and recognizing and managing asthma exacerbations. The key steps are:

- patient education for a partnership in asthma care,
- assessment and monitoring,
- avoidance or control of factors contributing to asthma severity,
- establishing medication plans for chronic management,
- establishing plans for managing exacerbations,
- providing follow-up care.

Most childhood asthma can be managed satisfactorily in the community.[70] More severe cases and cases where problems develop may require specialist referral (Table 29.6).

Education for a Partnership in Asthma Care[32]
(see also Chapters 25 and 27)

Education about managing asthma is an essential and continuing process. It provides the mechanism through which families can learn to carry out the complex behavioural tasks involved in successful asthma management. Recent guidelines highlight the key educational messages (Table 29.7). Parents should not be overwhelmed with information at their first clinic visits and important messages should be be repeated at each contact.

Education begins at diagnosis. Each contact or clinic visit provides an opportunity for further education. Perhaps surprisingly, hospital admissions may be a particularly effective time to deliver education about asthma management.[71] It should involve all members of the health care team. Initially, parents may have a poor understanding of the condition and its treatment

Table 29.7: Key educational messages for patients. (Adapted with permission from Expert Panel Report No. 2. *Guidelines for the diagnosis and Management of Asthma*. NIH Publication No. 97–4051. Bethesda MD: National Institute of Health, 1997)

Check off or document that the following key messages have been covered:

Basic Facts About Asthma

☐ The contrast between asthmatic and normal airways
☐ What happens to the airways in an asthma attack

Roles of Medications

☐ How medications work

    – Long-term control: medications that prevent symptoms, often by reducing inflammation
    – Quick relief: short-acting bronchodilator relaxes muscles around airways

☐ Stress the importance of long-term-control medications and not to expect quick relief from them.

Skills

☐ Inhaler use (patient demonstrate)
☐ Spacer/holding chamber use
☐ Symptom monitoring, peak flow monitoring, and recognizing early signs of deterioration

Environmental Control Measures

☐ Identifying and avoiding environmental precipitants or exposures

When and How To Take Rescue Actions

☐ Responding to changes in asthma severity (daily self-management plan and action plan)

but are usually keen to know more. The aim is to develop a partnership with families to provide them with the confidence, knowledge, skills, and motivation to control their child's asthma. To help promote this partnership the "clinician must be a good listener and a good teacher."[72] As children get older, the emphasis shifts to ensuring that they themselves know about their asthma and take increasing responsibility for their treatment.

Anxieties about asthma are common, yet often poorly dealt with. Partridge reported on a poll of members of the United Kingdom National Asthma Campaign as to their reactions when they or their children were first diagnosed as having asthma. Thirty-eight percent were relieved to have a diagnosis, 32% extremely worried, 23% frightened, 16% bewildered and 10% angry. Only 22% felt that they had had a good discussion with their doctor. Such failures of communication can be costly and may interfere with effective treatment.[73] Fears about the side-effects of inhaled steroids are particularly common and may lead to poor compliance with drug therapy. Appropriate changes in behaviour are only likely when parents and children are given the opportunity to express any fears or concerns and the chance to discuss their expectations of the condition and its treatment.[74] It also important to explore what parents and children want from treatment. Their own goals can then be used as the focus for the development of an individual treatment plan.[32] Sometimes parents' expectations may be inappropriately low and it may be up to the clinician to raise the parents' level of expectations.

There is increasing recognition that, by providing parents and children with asthma management skills enabling them to respond to changes in asthma severity, morbidity[75–77] can be reduced and mortality avoided.[78] The negotiation of an individual tailored "guided self-management plan" is therefore an important educational objective. Once a plan has been developed, it should be written down. National patient support groups often produce excellent action cards for this purpose. Patients need to be encouraged to bring the written plan to reviews so that it can be revised and updated. Over time, plans can be fine-tuned, for example, by noting particular symptoms or peak flow levels that occurred during an exacerbation. Management plans are particularly important for children with more severe asthma or a history of severe exacerbations.

Adherence with treatments is an important issue in any chronic disease and asthma is no exception.[79–81] Clinicians are no better than chance at predicting which patients will adhere.[82,83] Accordingly, strategies to encourage adherence should be built into all patient contacts. Recently, certain clinician behaviours have been shown to be associated with improved health care outcomes and parent satisfaction in children with asthma and their families[84] (Table 29.8). Messages about asthma need to be consistent. Health care teams need to make very sure that there are no conflicting messages in any advice they give about asthma management. Clinics should be organized so that, as far as possible, parents and children do not see a succession of different doctors or nurses. Short clinic waiting times may encourage adherence.[85]

Asthmatic children and their families should be told of any asthma societies, self-help and support groups, or help-lines available. National societies often produce excellent educational material in the form of leaflets, audiotapes and videos which reinforce the physician's message.[86,87] Foreign language material may be particularly useful for ethnic minorities. Schools should be informed and their co-operation enlisted to ensure that the child's attendance and participation in activities is interrupted as little as possible. All educational material must be carefully evaluated to ensure it is appropriate for the educational level of the target audience.

Table 29.8: Behavioural strategies for clinicians to encourage patient adherence. (Adapted from Clark et al. Physician-patient partnership in managing chronic illness. Acad Med 1995; 70: 957–9. ©1995 Academic Medicine.)

Friendly manner:

Show attentiveness (eye contact, attentive listening, etc.)

Give encouragements with non-verbal communication (nodding agreement, smiling, etc.)

Give verbal praise for effective management strategies

Use interactive conversation (e.g. asking open-ended questions)

Reassuring communication:

Elicit patient's underlying concerns about asthma

Allay fears with specific reassuring information

Periodic assessment and monitoring (see also Chapters 12–14)

An important part of the assessment is making a judgement about asthma severity using symptoms, functional status including nocturnal disturbance and loss of time from school, asthma exacerbations, medication requirements and objective measures of lung function (Table 29.9). Detailed examples of useful

Table 29.9: National Heart, Lung and Blood Institute classification of asthma severity. (From Expert Panel Report No 2. *Guidelines for the Diagnosis and Management of Asthma.* NIH Publication No. 97–4051. Bethesda MD: National Institutes of Health, 1997, with permission)

Characteristics	Mild intermittent (Step 1)	Mild persistent (Step 2)	Moderate persistent (Step 3)	Severe persistent (Step 4)
*Clinical features**				
Frequency of symptoms	Intermittent brief symptoms <2 per week. Exacerbations brief – from a few hours to days	Intermittent brief symptoms <1–2 per week	Symptoms > 1–2 times per week. Exacerbation >2 per week – may last days.	Symptoms continuously Frequent exacerbations
Interval symptoms		Asymptomatic between symptoms or exacerbations	Cough and wheeze often present; daily use of β agonists	Cough and wheeze almost always present
Nocturnal asthma	≤ 2 per month	>2 per month	>1 times per week	Frequent
Exercise tolerance		Limitation only on vigorous exercise; exacerbations may affect activity	Diminished exercise tolerance; exacerbations affect activity	Marked limitation of activity
School attendance		Good attendance	Attendance may be affected	Frequent absence from school
Lung function				
PEF	PEF >80% predicted at baseline. PEF variability <20%	PEF >80% predicted at baseline. PEF variability 20–30%	PEF 60–80% PEF variability >30%	PEF <60% PEF variability >30%
Spirometry	Minimal or no airway obstruction. May be little improvement in already normal flows after bronchodilator	Minimal or no airway obstruction. May be little improvement in already normal flows after bronchodilator	Mild airways obstruction present. Reversibility to normal after bronchodilator	Severe airway obstruction. Incomplete reversibility to bronchodilator, i.e. fixed obstruction
Methacholine sensitivity		Methacholine PC_{20} >20 mg ml^{-1}	Methacholine PC_{20} between 2 and 20 mg ml^{-1}	Methacholine PC_{20} <2 mg ml^{-1}

* The National Expert Panel report recommends that the presence of one of the features of severity is sufficient to place a patient in that category. An individual should be assigned to the most severe grade in which any feature occurs. The characteristics may overlap because asthma is highly variable. Furthermore, an individual's classification may change over time. Patients at any level of severity can have mild, moderate, or severe exacerbations. Some patients with intermittent asthma experience severe and life-threatening exacerbations separated by long periods of normal lung function and no symptoms.[32]

questions for all these domains are included in the second US guidelines.[32] For children below 5 years the judgement will, of necessity, be based on clinical information alone. Detailed symptom checking should be limited to a short period of a few weeks before the clinic as recall decreases with time. It may be helpful to provide a diary for parents to record information about symptoms, but in practice many families and children do not use diaries consistently. Where possible, objective measures are desirable because parental or child assessments of symptoms of airways obstruction may be poor.[88] Peak flow measurements, for example, may identify airway narrowing before symptoms develop or wheeze is heard on auscultation.[89]

One of the goals of asthma guidelines has been to promote the use of objective measures of severity in a manner analogous to other chronic diseases such as diabetes.[32] Just as a single blood sugar would be regarded as of little value unless clearly abnormal, so a single peak flow measurement is of little value in isolation. Serial measurements are much more useful with the results noted in a diary card or plotted on one of the available charts. Measured in this way, PEF monitoring can provide objective evidence about the severity of airways obstruction (Fig. 29.1), and can be a useful adjunct in monitoring the response to treatment, detecting exacerbations or facilitating changes in medication. It may also have an educational role in teaching parents about variations in asthma control and their relationship to symptoms.

For most children with mild or moderate asthma, long term PEF recording is an unreasonable expectation. It is usually best confined to those with severe asthma, poor asthma control or previous life-threatening episodes. A practical compromise may be to ask parents to record the PEF for a period of 2–4 weeks before a clinic visit. When compared with supervised measurements at the clinic, diary PEF records may help in developing an individual action plan for exacerbations. The best value needs to be periodically re-evaluated as a child grows.

Parents should bring asthma medications to the clinic so the dosage and their child's device technique can be checked. At each visit, the family's concerns about the child's asthma should be elicited and addressed. Progress on achieving short-term goals should be checked and asthma management plans updated.

Before clinic visits, parents should be encouraged to note down any questions or concerns and to bring their notes to the consultation for discussion. At each visit, the family's concerns about the child's asthma should be addressed. The recent guidelines stress the importance of encouraging open discussion of concerns about and expectations of therapy as well as parent's and child's satisfaction with the asthma care.[32,69]

Avoid or Control Factors Contributing to Asthma Severity (see also Chapter 16)

If specific trigger factors (Table 29.3) have been identified, there may be the potential for controlling or preventing asthma by manipulating the child's environment. The important allergens for children appear to be those that are inhaled. Studies where allergic children have been sent to school at high altitude where house-dust mites, pet allergens, pollens and tobacco smoke were undetectable or absent show that such avoidance can be very effective at reducing evidence of allergy, bronchial reactivity, symptoms of asthma and medication usage.[90] Allergen avoidance is only relevant for those who children who are confirmed to be allergic on testing by skin-prick or RAST test and should be specific for allergens to which the child is sensitive.

There are a number of areas where environmental avoidance approaches have been considered important.

House-Dust Mite While a causal relationship between domestic mites and atopic asthma has not been definitively proved the close association between mite exposure, mite sensitivity and asthma makes it likely that domestic mites are a major contributor to the development and expression of symptoms in atopic asthma.[66,91] The relationship between exposure, sensitization and symptoms has not always been clear due in part to difficulties in measuring mite exposure. It is also not yet known whether long-term average exposure to airborne allergen is more important than intermittent exposure to high dust levels of the type that can occur when beds, carpets or soft furnishings are disturbed.[92]

The two most common mites found in domestic house dust, *Dermatophagoides pteronyssinus* and *D. farinae*, thrive in warm, damp conditions. As the humidity falls, however, they stop reproducing and become immobile, and below 50% relative humidity they are likely to die.[93] Mites are also photophobic; hence, their common habitats in mattresses, bedding, soft furnishings or toys and at the base of carpets.

349

There are many mite allergens, but five or six predominate. Most mite allergens are water-soluble proteins and are found in the faecal pellets of mites. For example, the common Group 1 allergens (*Der p* 1, *Der f* 1) are cysteine proteases associated with mite faecal particles. Mite allergens are predominantly carried on large airborne particles and airborne for brief periods with domestic activity with measurable quantities in the air disappearing within minutes.[94]

Mite sensitivity should be suspected if symptoms coincide with sweeping, vacuuming, dusting or bed-making and improve when outdoors or in dry areas.[63,95] However, patients are often unaware of their sensitivity. Sensitivity can be detected by skin-prick tests or RAST tests. Up to 85% of atopic asthmatics have skin-prick sensitivity to mites in contrast to 5–30% of the non-asthmatic population.[96] Sensitivity to the house-dust mite is the commonest immediate allergic skin-prick reaction in asthmatic children[97] and also the commonest in school children in general.[98]

While avoidance of mites either at high altitude[90,99] or in hospital[100] has been shown to reduce asthmatic symptoms and bronchial reactivity, achieving lower levels of dust mite in the home has proved demanding, time consuming and expensive. Further, it appears that only the most stringent measures produce effective results.[101]

There have been two main approaches to mite avoidance in children with asthma. In the first, attempts have been made to reduce the number of mites in areas most heavily colonized (Table 29.10). Stringent measures such as removing carpets and curtains, increasing the frequency of bed linen laundering, removing soft toys and mite-containing clothing have shown successful results.[101] Newer bed coverings which are impermeable to mite allergen can effectively contain allergen, may prevent mite allergen accumulation and reduce bronchial hyperreactivity in mite-sensitive patients,[102,103] particularly when combined with frequent hot washing of bed linen. However, the coverings are expensive and the duvet, mattress and pillow all have to be covered to achieve a significant reduction in allergen. Synthetic polyester-filled pillows contain more allergens than feather ones.[104]

Simple cleaning and vacuuming alone reduces the mite allergen load but has been shown to be of negligible clinical benefit.[105] Older vacuum cleaners produce an aerosol for mite allergen so a vacuum cleaner with built in high efficiency air filter and double bags should

Table 29.10: Suggested measures to reduce allergic child's exposure to house-dust mites. (From Custovic A, Woodcock A. Environmental manipulation: practical steps in the home to benefit asthma patients. *Asthma J* 1999; 4: 24–7, ©Marcel Dekker inc.).

Essential actions

Encase the mattress, pillow and quilts in an allergen non-permeable cover
Wipe the covers at each change of bedding
Wash the bedding in water of a temperature greater than 130°F or 55°C using a hot cycle weekly

Desirable actions

Reduce indoor humidity to less than 50%
Remove carpets and replace with linoleum or wood
Remove carpets laid on concrete floors
Avoid sleeping or lying on furniture upholstered with fabric; replace with leather
Minimize the number of stuffed toys and hot wash or freeze the toys weekly
Use a vacuum cleaner with an integral high efficiency particulate arrest filter (HEPA) and double bags

be used in sensitive patients.[106] Chemical agents for killing mites are available but the effects are not dramatic or maintained and they are not recommended. Liquid nitrogen on bedding also reduces mite numbers substantially and airway reactivity to histamine when used in the homes of adult asthmatics[107] but is generally not a practical proposition for clinical use. Ionizers, which clean the air electrostatically, can lead to a significant reduction in airborne allergen concentrations, but lead to an increase in night-time cough in asthmatic children[92] and cannot therefore be recommended at present.

The alternative approach is to alter the overall home environment to make it less conducive to mite colonization. This can be achieved by reducing humidity which one Danish study has shown leads to significant improvement in peak expiratory flow.[108] However, increased ventilation usually results in heat loss. The consequent increase in heating bills necessary to maintain the indoor temperature makes this option unaffordable for many.

In practice, the costs and the rigorous nature of the multiple measures necessary to remove house-dust mite mean that, at present, such measures are usually reserved for those with severe asthma and definite sensitivity to house-dust mite.

Pets Pets are the second most common cause of domestic allergen. Over 50% of asthmatic children become sensitive to cat or dog allergen.[109] All warm-blooded pets, including small rodents and birds, produce dander, hair, urine and saliva that can contain allergens. Pet allergens are produced in huge amounts. They are carried on the clothing of pet owners and accumulate and persist in the environment for long periods. In a household with pets, these allergens become widely distributed. A proportion of dog and cat allergen is carried on particles less than 5 μm that easily become airborne and penetrate into the lower respiratory tract.

Exposure to pets can often trigger symptoms. Where there is a clear history of symptoms following exposure and positive allergen tests (skin-prick or RAST), it is best to remove the animal. Unfortunately, animal danders are cleared only slowly from the environment and it can take up to 6 months before beneficial results are seen.[110] Pet owners rarely want to give up their pets. For cats, de Blay *et al.*[111] found that washing the cat regularly reduced the amount *Fel d* 1 allergen present. Twice weekly washings combined with removing carpets, minimizing upholstered furnishings, vacuum cleaning with a high efficiency particulate air filter and air filtration could allow a pet-sensitive patient to live with their pet.

Because of these problems, the introduction of furry or feathered pets into the homes of families with asthma is best discouraged. When a cat or dog is present in a room, airborne allergens are four to five times higher than when the pet is elsewhere in the house. If pets are present, parents should at the very least exclude the pet from their child's bedroom.[106]

Pollens and Moulds Common allergens such as outdoor pollens or moulds are impossible to avoid completely. Indoor levels can be reduced by closing windows and doors, and using air conditioners during peak pollen or mould seasons.[112]

Unfortunately, not all moulds are external. Damp and mouldy housing has been shown to be associated with an increased prevalence and severity of respiratory illnesses in children.[113–115] Whether this is due to the effects of moulds and fungi or to high levels of house-dust mite is not yet clear.[116] However, home dampness

is common and affects 30% or more of the housing stock in some parts of the UK.

Ingested Allergens Foods and dietary additives do not commonly trigger asthmatic symptoms in children. Definite confirmation that an ingested allergen is responsible requires double blind challenge. This may not always be necessary before embarking on avoidance (see section on "Is it due to something in the diet?", p. 377). Drugs such as aspirin and other non-steroidal anti-inflammatory agents, which can cause severe exacerbations in adults, are rarely used in children.

Other Air Pollutants Including Cigarette Smoke Children seem to be very sensitive to respiratory effects from both indoor and outdoor pollutants.[117,118] A number of irritants such as wood smoke or volatile organic substances (e.g. paints and polishes) can cause worsening of asthma. Pollution from road traffic may also be important.[117]

However, by far the most ubiquitous and important pollutant is cigarette smoke. Cook and Strachan recently systematically reviewed the effects of parental smoking on the respiratory health of children[119] (Table 29.11). On present evidence, passive smoking is unlikely to increase the risk of allergic sensitization in children.[120]

Unfortunately, passive smoking is not the sole problem. Active smoking is also common in teenagers with asthma.[121]

All this leaves no doubt that asthmatic children, from the intrauterine period onwards, should not be exposed to cigarette smoke.

General Points about Avoidance Measures Unfortunately, the home is not the only environment where children are exposed to measurable aeroallergens or pollutants. Norwegian studies[122] have shown that children are exposed to measurable levels of domestic allergen at school (house-dust mite, cat, dog). There are also data showing that children who were not exposed to smoking at home had low salivary cotinine concentrations whose level depended on the prevalence of smoking in the community.[123]

The practical difficulties surrounding avoidance strategies mean that for most children they are not, at present, particularly productive approaches to asthma control. Either environmental triggers cannot be identified or they are difficult to avoid completely. Whether allergen avoidance from pregnancy could

351

Table 29.11: Summary of effects of parental smoking on the respiratory health of children (From Cook DG, Strachan DP. Summary of the health effects of parental smoking on the respiratory health of children and implications for research. Thorax 1999; 54: 357–66, with permission)

Outcome	Either parent OR (95% CI)	Mother OR (95% CI)	Father only OR (95% CI)	Both parents OR (95% CI)
Lower respiratory illnesses (LRI) at age 0–2				
All studies	1.57 (1.42 to 1.74)	1.72 (1.55 to 1.91)	1.29 (1.16 to 1.44)	
Community studies of wheeze	1.55 (1.16 to 2.08)	2.08 (1.59 to 2.71)		
Community studies of LRI, bronchitis and/or pneumonia	1.54 (1.31 to 1.80)	1.57 (1.33 to 1.86)		
Hospital admission for LRI, bronchitis, bronchiolitis or pneumonia	1.71 (1.21 to 2.40)	1.53 (1.25 to 1.86)	1.32 (0.87 to 2.00)	
Prevalence rates at age 5–16				
Wheeze	1.24 (1.17 to 1.31)	1.28 (1.19 to 1.38)	1.14 (1.06 to 1.23)	1.47 (1.14 to 1.90)
Cough	1.40 (1.27 to 1.53)	1.40 (1.20 to 1.64)	1.21 (1.09 to 1.34)	1.67 (1.48 to 1.89)
Phlegm	1.35 (1.13 to 1.62)			1.46 (1.04 to 2.05)
Breathlessness	1.31 (1.08 to 1.59)			
Asthma (cross sectional studies)	1.21 (1.10 to 1.34)	1.36 (1.20 to 1.55)	1.07 (0.92 to 1.24)	1.50 (1.29 to 1.73)
Asthma (case–control studies)	1.37 (1.15 to 1.64)			
Bronchial reactivity		1.29[c] (1.10 to 1.50)		
Skin prick positivity		0.87[a] (0.64 to 1.24)		
Incidence of asthma				
Under age 6		1.31[b] (1.22 to 1.41)		
Over age 6		1.13[b] (1.04 to 1.22)		
Middle ear disease				
Acute otitis media	Range 1.0 to 1.6			
Recurrent otitis media	1.48 (1.08 to 2.04)			
Middle ear effusion	1.38[b] (1.23 to 1.55)			
Referral for glue ear	1.21[b] (0.95 to 1.53)			
Sudden infant death		2.13 (1.86 to 2.43)		

[a] Results relate to maternal smoking during pregnancy or exposure to environmental tobacco smoke (ETS) in infancy. Data for ETS exposure during later childhood are too heterogeneous for meta-analysis.

[b] Based on fixed effects estimate.

[c] Relates largely, but not entirely to maternal smoking.

reduce the incidence of asthma is presently under study in several large cohorts. In general, suppressive therapy with preventative anti-inflammatory agents is both less demanding and more effective.

Immunotherapy (see also Chapter 23) The role of immunotherapy in children with asthma as a means of reducing the effects of environmental allergens is controversial. Because of concerns about acute fatal anaphylaxis after allergen injection, immunotherapy is no longer used for asthma in the UK, although it remains widely used in other countries.

The results of clinical trials are variable and conflicting, but a recent meta-analysis of 20 randomized, placebo-controlled studies confirmed the effectiveness of immunotherapy in asthma.[124] It improved asthma symptoms and medication requirements, but had no consistent effect on lung function. It reduced allergen-specific bronchial reactivity to a greater extent than non-specific reactivity. The size of the effect compared with other treatments was not clear.

If immunotherapy is considered it should probably be restricted to selected children with severe asthma triggered by one or a very few specific aeroallergens and poorly responsive to pharmacological and avoidance therapies. A specific extract should be used. It is essential to have an accurate diagnosis based on a convincing history that natural exposure to aeroallergens induces clinically significant symptoms combined with detectable immediate hypersensitivity (skin or RAST testing) to relevant environmental allergen/s. The parents should be fully informed of the nature of the treatment – the need for regular injections, the possibility of reactions to injections, the likelihood of success, the need to continue injections for a protracted period, and the costs. In clinical trials, a high incidence of systemic anaphylactic reactions is usually reported. These are usually mild and not life-threatening but may require adrenaline therapy.[125] However, as more severe reactions can occur, those using immunotherapy should be trained, equipped and ready to manage major systemic anaphylactic reactions. The child should be observed for at least 30 minutes after the treatment. Injections should only be given when the child is asymptomatic since lethal reactions are found more often in asthmatics with severe airway obstruction.[126]

Whatever the present role of immunotherapy, it seems likely that the developments in allergen preparation and a better understanding of the immunology of asthma may lead to a re-evaluation of its role in paediatric asthma in the future.

Establish Medication Plans for Chronic Management

At present, drug treatment is the mainstay of the management of childhood asthma. Establishing a medication plan for an individual child can be broken down into a number of steps:[32]

(1) choosing the drugs to be used;
(2) choosing the route of administration, and for inhaled therapy the appropriate device;
(3) choosing the appropriate drug combinations and doses using a step-wise approach.

Choosing the drugs The understanding of asthma as a chronic inflammatory disorder of the airways has led to a more clearly defined therapeutic strategy, with the emphasis on preventing or controlling the underlying inflammatory process. Usually symptom control is brought about using anti-inflammatory medications ("preventers" or "long-term control medications"). Bronchodilators ("relievers" or "quick relief medications") are then used as required for the relief of symptoms. The drugs commonly prescribed in children are discussed below.

Bronchodilators (see also Chapter 21)
β_2 AGONISTS The selective β_2 agonists are the most potent and widely used bronchodilators available for the treatment of asthma. They have a number of other potentially beneficial actions including enhanced mucociliary clearance, decreased vascular permeability, and modulation of mediator release from mast cells and basophils. The clinical relevance of these actions in childhood asthma is not known at present.

Most of the selective β_2 agonists currently prescribed for children have a relatively short duration of action (4–6 hours). In the various inhaled formulations, they are effective in small doses, rapid in onset, and have a relatively low incidence of adverse effects. They are the preferred treatment for the relief of asthma symptoms, for the prophylaxis of exercise-induced asthma and for the treatment of acute exacerbations.

Side-effects of β_2 agonists are mainly related to stimulation of extra-pulmonary β_2 receptors (Table 29.12). The side-effects are dose-related and are commoner with the larger doses used in oral or intravenous

353

Table 29.12: Side-effects of β₂ agonists. (From Barnes PJ. General pharmacologic principles. In: Murray JF, Nadel JA (eds). *Textbook of Respiratory Medicine.* Philadelphia: WB Saunders, 1994: 1–2739, with permission).

Muscle tremor

Tachycardia

Hypokalaemia

Restlessness, agitation and over-activity

Hypoxaemia due to increased V/Q mismatching

?Worsening of asthma control

therapy. If side-effects such as over-activity or tremor are troublesome, reducing the dosage may be helpful.

There has been vigorous debate as to whether β_2 agonists cause deterioration in asthma control and lead to increased asthma mortality and morbidity ("the β-agonist controversy"). Although available studies have not directly focused on children,[127] they suggested that heavy use of inhaled β_2 agonists, particularly fenoterol, may be associated with an increased risk of death or near-death from asthma.[128,129] There has been some evidence that regular use of β_2 agonists may be associated with decreased control of asthma.[130] More recently, a careful randomized study in patients with mild asthma between 12 and 55 years of age found no deleterious or beneficial effects from the regular use of salbutamol.[131] Nevertheless, present advice for children is that the regular use of short-acting inhaled β_2 agonists is not recommended:[32,132] they should be used on an "as-needed" basis rather than regularly. Increased use (more than 1–2 doses per day) is then a mark of deteriorating asthma control, and points to the need to institute or intensify anti-inflammatory therapy. Tolerance (tachyphylaxis) can occur with chronic β_2 agonist use, but does not appear to be of major clinical importance.[132]

LONG-ACTING INHALED β_2 AGONISTS Long-acting inhaled β_2 agonists (salmeterol, formoterol) with a duration of action of over 12 hours are now available. Salmeterol is not recommended for long-term use alone.[133] However, salmeterol has proved useful in chil-

dren with more severe asthma who are already receiving corticosteroids. In that situation, salmeterol improves lung function, decreases symptoms and use of relief medication.[134,135]

In adults already taking inhaled corticosteroids, adding inhaled long-acting β agonist has produced relatively greater improvement compared with increasing the inhaled corticosteroid.[136,137] However, in children with moderate asthma, taking 200 μg beclomthasone b.d., given either added salmeterol or additional beclomethasone, no improvement occurred over one year in symptom scores, lung function, airway responsiveness or exacerbation rates.[138] The best approach in children with more severe symptomatic asthma needs further study.

Long-acting β_2 agonists are particularly useful for persisting nocturnal symptoms or as prophylaxis against exercise-induced asthma.[139,140] Salmeterol maintains its bronchodilator effects during long-term treatment over at least 4 months. There is no evidence of rebound deterioration in bronchial responsiveness after stopping the drug.[141] The usual long-term dose in children with mild to moderate asthma is 50 μg b.d. It is available as a dry powder in various devices, and as a metered dose inhaler (MDI). Salmeterol is well-tolerated with minimal side-effects.

An oral long-acting β_2 agonist, bambuterol, is available but has not yet been studied in children.

THEOPHYLLINES While theophyllines have been widely used in treatment of both acute and chronic asthma in children for many years, their role has been increasingly questioned.[142,143] Strategies involving the earlier use of inhaled prophylactic treatment (especially inhaled corticosteroids) and the introduction of effective long-acting inhaled bronchodilators, such as salmeterol, have substantially replaced theophylline's traditional role in the treatment of chronic asthma.

Despite extensive studies, the molecular mechanisms responsible for theophylline's therapeutic activity remain poorly defined. Beneficial effects have usually been attributed to bronchodilator action, but more recently there has been interest in possible anti-inflammatory effects.[144] Several groups have shown a significant suppression of the late-phase response to antigen at modest serum levels of theophylline.[145,146] Importantly, these anti-inflammatory effects were achieved at doses that are not associated with unacceptable side-effects and where, in appropriate cases, serum monitoring may not be required.[147] A large clinical study in children with mild/moderate persistent asthma has confirmed that theophylline is effective even when the serum levels are lower than usually recommended.[148]

In children, theophylline now tends to be used later in the therapeutic plan when β_2 agonists and inhaled steroids are proving inadequate. Theophylline is also used in certain well-defined situations such as children with nocturnal asthma,[149] or children who will not take inhaled medications. In corticosteroid-dependent asthma, theophylline, unlike sodium cromoglycate (SCG), can provide clinically useful benefit with a "steroid sparing" effect.[150]

The variable clearance, narrow therapeutic index, high incidence of side-effects, and recognized potential for severe toxic reactions mean that close attention to the details of dosing, and monitoring are important when prescribing theophylline for children. The need to use blood samples for monitoring drug levels when theophylline is used in conventional doses is a significant disadvantage for most children. Recent evidence suggests that theophylline does not usually cause cognitive or behavioural effects in most children although those with pre-existing attention or achievement problems may be more vulnerable.[151,152]

If theophyllines are prescribed for children in conventional doses, slow-release preparations have been found to be convenient, usually requiring only twice daily administration resulting in less fluctuation in serum concentrations. Caffeine-like side-effects such as nausea, nervousness or insomnia occur when initial doses are too high, and can be minimized by starting at a lower dose of around one-half to two-thirds of the expected dose. The dose should be slowly increased at 3-day intervals, only if tolerated, until average doses for age are attained.[153] A peak serum level no higher than the middle of the therapeutic range should be the target (5–15 mg l^{-1}). Parents should be told to stop any dosage that causes adverse side-effects, withholding the drugs until the symptoms have disappeared and then resuming at a lower previously tolerated dose. The final dose should be individualized and should be informed by measurement of peak serum concentration when the dosage has been regular and constant for at least 3 days.

Once the dose is stable, it usually remains stable. Because of the risks of serious toxicity, parents and children should be warned of the early symptoms of intoxication such as nausea and vomiting, and also of factors which might alter the drug level (e.g. prolonged fever or the use of other drugs, particularly erythromycin). If their child has a sustained fever, they should decrease the dose by 50% as a precaution, and they should not administer other medications without obtaining medical device.

ANTICHOLINERGICS Ipratropium bromide is a topically active quaternary ammonium derivative of atropine that acts as a bronchodilator. It is available both as a meter dose aerosol, which can be used with a large volume spacer, and as a nebulizing solution. It achieves its bronchodilating effect by blocking reflex cholinergic bronchoconstriction and has no anti-inflammatory effect. It has a slower onset of action than β_2 agonists, but may have a longer action of up to 8 hours.

Ipratropium has its main role in children with severe acute asthma.[154] In children with chronic asthma, it may be useful as an alternative bronchodilator for those who have significant side-effects to β_2 agonists. It may occasionally be useful as an additional bronchodilator in children with very severe chronic asthma. There is very limited evidence suggesting that it may be particularly useful in treating wheezy babies where β_2 agonists are often not very effective.[155] A recent meta-analysis concluded that the limited evidence did not support the uncritical use of anticholinergics for wheeze in infants and suggested further work was necessary to clarify their role.[156] Side-effects are uncommon because there is virtually no systemic absorption. Paradoxical bronchiconstriction was reported with the nebulized preparation, but was largely explained by the hypotonicity of the nebulizer solution and by the presence of antibacterial additives in the original product.[157]

Anti-Inflammatory Drugs (see also Chapters 17, 18 and 20)

INHALED CORTICOSTEROIDS There is no doubt that inhaled corticosteroids are the most effective treatment for asthma currently available.[158] A number of properly controlled long-term studies in children have shown that regular treatment with inhaled corticosteroids diminishes both day and night-time symptoms, decreases asthma exacerbations and hospital admissions and decreases the need for bronchodilator use.[159–162] Normally, inhaled corticosteroids produce quite marked and rapid clinical improvements and changes in lung function at low doses (around 100 µg) even in children with moderate and severe asthma.[163]

After long-term use, inhaled corticosteroids decrease bronchial reactivity and improve airway calibre in most, although not to normal.[164] Inhaled steroids are effective in children with asthma of all ages. There is an increasing number of controlled trials indicating the effectiveness of inhaled corticosteroids in pre-school children and infants.[165–169] The beneficial effects of inhaled corticosteroids on asthma are greater than for any anti-asthma drug.[133,148,170]

Unfortunately, corticosteroids do not appear to cure asthma. In one series of asthmatic children, 28–36 months of treatment with inhaled corticosteroids and regular bronchodilator improved both symptoms and objective measures of lung function in children.[164] Tapering-off the steroids after that time, while continuing regular bronchodilator use, led to deterioration in asthma control over the next the 4–6 months.[171] This suggests that the underlying inflammatory process is still active even after years on inhaled corticosteroids. Treatment with inhaled corticosteroids is therefore principally aimed at a bringing about symptomatic remission.

Several inhaled steroids are available, although availability varies from country to country. There are differences between steroids in their binding affinity to the glucocorticoid receptor and in their relative potency in skin blanching.[158] Most experience in children has been with inhaled beclomethasone dipropionate (BDP) and budesonide (BUD) but experience with the newer inhaled corticosteroid, fluticasone propionate (FP), is growing rapidly. While a substantial number of comparative studies have been performed, it has proved difficult to come to firm conclusions about the relative efficacy of different inhaled corticosteroids. This is partly due to factors such as the differences in study design, the flat dose–response curve of inhaled corticosteroid and particularly differences between inhaler devices.[158]

The steroid dose required depends on the severity of the disease. In children with mild asthma, substantial improvement in symptoms, lung function and airway responsiveness is seen at doses of inhaled BUD as low as 100 µg daily. There is evidence of a dose-response, with 400 µg per day producing better improvements in FEV_1 than 100 µg per day when given either via an MDI with spacer[163] or as a dry powder.[172] Many children will have no additional benefit with doses above 400 µg per day. However, the plateau on the dose–response curve differs from patient to patient, and according to which response is studied.[173] Pulmonary function tests and symptoms may have rather low sensitivity to the effects of inhaled corticosteroids. In general for all inhaled corticosteroids, the lowest dose has been most effective, producing about 50% of the maximum achievable response.[163] In practice, the vast majority of schoolchildren can achieve optimal control on quite low doses of inhaled corticosteroids of around 100–200 µg per day. Some children with severe asthma responding poorly to conventional doses of inhaled corticosteroids may benefit from doses of 800 µg or above. Because the dose–response curve is quite flat and dose-dependent effects difficult to detect, addition of a drug that acts in a different manner may be a better option than increasing the dose of inhaled corticosteroids when symptoms are not controlled.

Several studies have shown that twice daily use is as effective in controlling stable asthma as four times daily administration for both BDP and BUD, although in severe or poorly controlled asthma four times daily administration may be better.[174] Twice daily administration is likely to be associated with better compliance.[79]

SIDE-EFFECTS Although inhaled steroids for childhood asthma have been used for over 30 years, anxieties about their side-effects continue, especially as they may be used for quite long periods. Inhaled corticosteroids cause systemic effects to the extent that they are absorbed from the gastrointestinal tract and the airways. The amount of steroid absorbed varies with the dose, with the site of deposition and with the metabolism of the particular drug. Most of the newer inhaled corticosteroids have low oral bioavailability.[158] Drugs that are inactivated by first-pass hepatic metabolism are also likely to have fewer systemic effects.

The type of inhaler device used is important because it influences the amount deposited in different sites and therefore changes the amount available for absorption. For example, with metered dose inhalers (MDI) about 80% of the drug is deposited in the oropharynx and can be swallowed and absorbed. The use of a spacer with MDI results in the larger propellant/drug particles becoming smaller and slower moving as the propellant evaporates. The net result is to reduce the amount impacting in the oropharynx, but to maintain or increase the amount reaching the lung. As a consequence the side-effects from systemic absorption can be reduced while the clinical effects, which depend on intrapulmonary deposition, are unaltered. With dry powder inhalers the great majority of the dose is deposited in the oropharynx. The systemic effects can be reduced or abolished by manoeuvres such as mouth washing which remove drug deposited in the oropharnyx.[174] Such manoeuvres will only be relevant for inhaled corticosteroids that are systemically bioavailable after oral dosing. Newer corticosteroids such as fluticasone propionate have negligible bioavailability after oral dosing and their systemic effects arise from absorption across the intrapulmonary airways. Then the characteristics of the inhaler device and the child's inhalation technique are the important factors.[158]

The major concerns about inhaled steroids, particularly in the long term, have centred on their impact on growth. A whole host of factors have made it difficult to measure the impact of inhaled steroids on growth. Asthma, itself, is clearly associated with effects on growth.[40] Children with moderate to severe asthma appear gradually to fall away from their predicted height centile as they approach puberty. The onset of sexual maturation is delayed, and this delay appears to be independent of asthma severity. However, as a result, growth continues for a longer time during the second decade.[175] For the most part, asthmatic children ultimately attain their predicted adult height.[176] The cause of this pattern of growth has been the subject of much speculation but remains unknown. Controlling chronic asthma, even with inhaled corticosteroids, can improve growth.[39] It is quite clear that in treating chronic asthma, substituting oral for inhaled corticosteroids significantly reduces the risk of growth retardation.[177]

Reassuringly, the longitudinal data available suggest that doses up to 800 µg per day of inhaled corticosteroids over 1–5 years does not influence long-term linear growth in asthmatic children when the dose is tailored to the severity of the disease.[158,177] At higher doses, data are more limited. A decrease in height centile was noted in 6 of 50 children receiving 750–1500 µg BDP for an average of 19 months, although four were 10–15 years, an age when the pre-pubertal growth slowing is most marked. In pre-pubertal children, Ninan and Russell found normal growth rates in children taking up to 1600 µg BPD or BUD daily, provided that their symptoms were well-controlled.[39] Longitudinal data on younger children are limited but also reassuring. Two small studies in children age 3–7 years who took inhaled BUD 200 µg per day,[178,179] and doses of 200 µg m^{-2} per day to 1100 µg m^{-2} per day for at least 1 year did not detect any adverse effect on height velocity.[179]

A number of studies using knemometry to measure short-term changes in lower leg growth rate have found reductions in mean growth velocity. In general, however, with inhaled corticosteroid doses below 400 µg per day via spacer or 200 µg per day via dry powder effects have not been seen.[158] As yet, it is not possible to reconcile the short-term knemometry data with data from longitudinal studies, and the long-term implications remain are unclear.[158] Findings from knemometry cannot be used to predict long-term growth.

There have also been concerns about the effects of inhaled corticosteroids on the hypothalamic–pituitary axis. Most studies have not observed significant changes in the (less sensitive) urinary cortisol excretion in children taking up to 400 µg BUD by MDI via spacer or 200 µg per day via Turbohaler.[180] At a doses of BUD 400 µg per day via Turbohaler or 200 µg per day or 400 µg per day of FP via dischaler cortisol excretion was reduced.[180,181] With BDP, some studies[181,182] have found that BDP 300–400 µg per day reduced urinary cortisol excretion but this has not been confirmed in others.[183] There is also evidence of a significant reduction in physiological cortisol secretion measured at frequent intervals in children taking 400–1000 µg BDP during the night or during a 24-hour period.[184] This is a very sensitive test of the hypothalamic–pituitary axis (HPA), however. There are at present no reports of a reduced HPA response to stimulation in children treated with inhaled BUD or BDP up to 400 µg per day, although in some children at doses above 400 µg per day evidence of adrenal suppression was detected.[185] Although there are differences between different inhaled corticosteroids and between different devices at doses below 400 µg per day, treatment with inhaled corticosteroids is normally not associated with significant suppression of the HPA. At higher doses using sensitive tests, changes can be detected. While these changes do not appear to be clinically relevant, the very fact they occur emphasizes the importance of using the minimum dose compatible with good control of asthma.[158] Finally, on a note of caution, these are some recent reports of cases of adrenal suppression occuring with high dose inhaled corticosteroids. A detailed understanding of such cases is not yet available.

Multiple rib or vertebral fractures and generalized osteoporosis are well-recognized effects of long-term oral steroid use, both in children and adults. To date, there is no evidence that inhaled corticosteroids are associated with similar effects. In children, the available data suggest that standard doses of inhaled corticosteroids do not affect markers of bone formation or resorption.[158] There is also, at present, no indication of effects on bone density or increased risk of osteoporosis or fractures in children. However, the bone effects of inhaled corticosteroid in children are still the subject of active investigation. In general, effects on bones have proved very difficult to tease out because of the effects of confounding factors such as the effect of the disease, season, nutrition, heredity, sexual development and exercise.

Central nervous system effects of inhaled corticosteroids have been reported but are in the main rare and confined to case reports. Connett and Lenney reported four young children who developed acute behaviour disturbance, especially hyperactivity and temper tantrums, on BUD via Nebuhaler in doses of 400 µg b.d. or t.d.s.[186] Usually, the reported effects came on rapidly and subsided completely when the dose was reduced or the drug was stopped.

While posterior subcapsular cataracts are a specific and well-recognized complication of long-term oral glucocorticoids, a Canadian study found no evidence that they were associated with the long-term use (median 5 years; range 1–15 years) of inhaled BDP or BUD in moderate to high doses (median 750 µg; range 300–2000 µg) in children and young adults.[187]

Although several metabolic effects have been reported after inhaled steroids, there is little evidence at present that such effects are clinically relevant in children when taking therapeutic doses. In particular, there do not appear to be significant effects on glucose or lipid metabolism. Easy bruising occurs in adults taking inhaled steroids and seems to increase with age and with dose and duration of inhaled steroid, but does not seem to be a problem in children.

In adults, local effects from deposition of inhaled steroid on the upper airway are among the most frequently reported of side-effects, but similar effects tend to be rare in children. In the largest study of children (229 with asthma, 129 taking BDP) clinical candidiasis occurred in only one child. Colonization was found in 40–50% of children taking inhaled steroids compared with 29% of the asthmatic controls. The rate of colonization was not affected by the device used (MDI vs Rotahaler), or by the dose (high vs low). In the same study, sore throat and hoarseness occurred rarely and were not related to the presence of candida or to treatment with inhaled steroid.[188]

The fact that corticosteroid side-effects have been detected with more sensitive tests and at higher doses is perhaps not especially surprising. It is a testimony to the efficacy and safety of inhaled steroids that any effects detected have rarely been of clinical significance.

SYSTEMIC STEROIDS Short courses of oral steroid (prednisolone 1–2 mg kg^{-1} for 5–7 days) are an important component of the treatment of acute exacerbations and may reduce the need for hospital admission.[189–191] While short courses may cause adrenal suppression, rapid recovery in adrenal function occurs.[192] Children receiving more than four courses per year may develop more prolonged adrenal suppression.[193]

Nowadays, oral steroids are rarely used in the chronic treatment of childhood asthma. If they are used, the smallest possible dose compatible with control of symptoms should be used and should be given as a single morning dose. Alternate day use, while preferable, is then often not sufficient to control severe asthma and daily use often necessary. Inhaled steroids should always be continued for their systemic steroid-sparing effect. Apparent (relative) "steroid resistance" is recognized in children with difficult-to-control asthma, and has been shown to be associated with abnormal glucocorticoid pharmacokinetics and glucocorticoid receptor binding.[194]

CROMONES The cromones, sodium cromoglycate and nedocromil, are non-steroidal anti-inflammatory agents with no significant bronchodilator action. Until recently, their precise mode of action was unclear, but they are now thought to block non-specifically the function of a chloride channel involved in cell volume regulation.[195]

Sodium cromoglycate (SCG) has been most widely used for the prophylactic therapy of moderate asthma in children. Given prophylactically, SCG inhibits both early- and late-phase allergen-induced airway narrowing. It also blocks acute airway narrowing due to exercise, fog, cold dry air and methacholine. There is evidence of a dose–response effect, at least for exercise-induced asthma.[139]

The original paediatric study using SCG 20 mg spincaps four times daily showed it was effective in 71% of school age children.[196] When followed up over 3 to 5 years, 65% of 46 children from original study remained well-controlled.[197]

The individual response to SCG is unpredictable. A 4–8 week trial may be necessary to be certain of efficacy. At the start of treatment, SCG is usually given four times a day but, if effective, it may be possible to reduce the dosage to three times a day. Because of its wide safety margin SCG continues to have a role as a first-line prophylactic agent for moderate asthma. However, SCG is not effective for persistently wheezing infants under 1 year of age,[198] except perhaps for those born prematurely.[199] Recently, a randomized controlled trial of SCG 10 mg via Aerochamber three times a day in 1–4 year old children with wheeze found SCG to be no better than placebo,[200] but there were questions as to whether sufficient drug might have reached the intra-pulmonary airways.

Sodium cromoglycate is available as a nebulizer solution (20 mg per vial), a dry powder (20 mg per spincap), and a metered dose aerosol with the most widely used form now the 5 mg MDI. It remains the safest drug developed for the management of asthma. Occasional coughing due to airway irritation can occur after inhaling the dry powder, but may be reduced by pre-treatment with β_2 agonist. Because of this irritant effect, SCG is usually stopped during any acute exacerbations. Transient rashes have also been reported.

Nedocromil sodium has a very similar profile of activity to SCG.[201,202] Nedocromil has been shown to improve daily asthma symptoms and lung function, and to reduce concurrent bronchodilator use, in children with mild to moderately severe disease.[203] Nedocromil is also effective in wheezing in infants born pre-term.[204] It appears to have a fairly rapid onset of action with most of the improvement occurring in the first 4 weeks. The usual dose has been 4 mg two to four times per day. Side-effects of nedocromil are uncommon but headache, sore throat, nausea and a bitter taste have all been reported. A recent report from Finland showed that 70% of children with moderate asthma who needed maintenance therapy could be well-controlled using either SCG or nedocromil.[83]

Either SCG, in a dose of 10 mg, or nedocromil, 4 mg, via MDI provide good protection against exercise challenge in children with an effect that last 2 hours.[205] The degree of protection with SCG has been shown to improve on regular treatment.

LEUKOTRIENE-RECEPTOR MODIFIERS Leukotriene-receptor modifiers (LRMs) are an important new class of orally active non-steroidal anti-asthma therapy. They are a hybrid between preventers (through anatgonism of pro-inflammatory effects of leukotrienes) and relievers (through antagonism of leukotriene-induced bronchoconstriction).[206,207] Currently, two leukotriene-receptor anatagonists are licensed worldwide for treatment of asthma in older children: montelukast (adults and children ≥ 6 years) and zafirlukast (adults and children ≥ 12 years). Licensing differs between the USA and Europe with montelukast approved for use as first-line therapy for persistent asthma in the USA, but only approved as an adjunct treatment to inhaled corticosteroid in Europe. Both drugs are effective over a wide range of asthma severity with a high therapeutic index.

At present, published data on LRMs in children are limited, and confined to relatively short-term studies using montelukast.[208,209] Knorr et al. found a modest improvement in lung function in children with chronic asthma taking montelukast, 5-mg chewable tablet once daily at bedtime for 8 weeks. The response was similar in children taking either as-need β_2 agonist alone or inhaled corticosteroid, was of the same order as reported for other preventive therapies and did not decrease over time. The improvements in asthma control were accompanied by a significant fall in peripheral blood eosinophils suggesting an effect on asthma inflammation.[209]

Leukotriene-receptor antagonists (LRAs) may also be useful for oral prophylaxis against exercise-induced bronchospasm (EIB). Kemp et al.[208] showed that montelukast attenuates EIB in 6–14 year-old children. In adults, the degree of protection from montelukast against EIB did not decrease with time differentiating it from other therapies used for EIB.[210]

The onset of therapeutic action of LRAs is very rapid compared with either inhaled corticosteroids or cromolyn with significant improvements in lung function evident after the first dose of montelukast.[208,209] This and the potential advantage of oral treatment may be important for compliance. To date, side-effects have been no greater than placebo but longer follow-up pharmaco-vigilance data are not yet available. So far, there are no reports of the Churg–Strauss-like syndrome, noted in some adults taking LRAs, occurring in children.

The position of LRAs in asthma management in children is not yet clear. Particular issues are whether they might replace low-dose inhaled corticosteroid as first-line preventative therapy and whether they should be used as an alternative to long-acting bronchodilators

359

as second-line controlling therapy in addition to inhaled corticosteroid.

Furthermore, LRAs are more costly than inhaled corticosteroids. Ultimately patient preference and cost may be more important factors influencing their role in treating mild asthma.

KETOTIFEN Ketotifen is a potent anti-histamine with strong *in vitro* mast-cell stabilizing characteristics. As it is taken orally and lasts for 12 hours, it was hoped that it would be valuable as a long-acting, orally active, anti-asthma compound. A minimum of 8–12 weeks is necessary before any beneficial effects are fully realized. Unfortunately, it has not lived up to its original promise and a long-term placebo-controlled trial in children with mild asthma found that it had no clinical benefit.[211] It has no effect on exercise-induced asthma.[212] It does not have any steroid-sparing effect. Some studies have demonstrated a role in preventing asthma in children at high risk because of a strong family history of atopy or atopic dermatitis.[213]

It has been used in doses of 1 mg twice daily for children over 3 years, and 0.5 mg twice daily for children below 3 years. It appears to be a safe drug, although weight gain and sedation are potential problems.[214]

OTHER AGENTS Other anti-inflammatory agents and immunomodulatory therapies have been used on an experimental basis in severe steroid-dependent asthma in adults.[215] In children with severe asthma taking oral corticosteroids, there are reports of a steroid-sparing effect of both cyclosporin[216] and oral methotrexate.[217] However, there are at present, no proper randomized controlled trials. Because of their potential side-effects, variable effects and the very limited clinical experience in children immunosuppressives should only be used in carefully selected cases by paediatricians with experience of managing very severe asthma. Intravenous infusions of immunoglobulin have also been tried in severe childhood asthma, but a recent randomized placebo-controlled trial in children and adolescents showed no benefit on symptom scores, lung function or bronchial hyperreactivity.[218]

The commonest cause of apparent corticosteroid resistance is lack of compliance with medications. Accordingly, before considering alternative agents for their steroid-sparing effects, efforts should be made to improve asthma control and lower steroid doses by intensive asthma management. A combination of careful diagnostic assessment, frequent evaluation and intensive monitoring can often be surprisingly successful.[219]

COMPLEMENTARY ALTERNATIVE THERAPIES Complementary therapies such as homeopathy, breathing techniques, acupuncture, diets, vitamin supplements and herbal medicines are very widely used. Approximately 55% of children in one study had used alternative therapies for asthma management, most commonly massage, relaxation exercises, diet or vitamins.

At present, there is relatively little scientific evidence about the effectiveness of complementary therapies in childhood asthma. One exception is the addition of chiropractic spinal manipulation where a recent randomized controlled trial found no benefit;[220] another is a special breathing technique (Buteyko breathing technique–BBT) where those practising the technique reduced hyperventilation and use of β_2 agonists.[221]

Choosing the Routes of Administration and Appropriate Inhalation Devices (see also Chapter 22) Since asthma is a disease of airways, treatment via inhalation is generally preferred. The advantages of selective delivery directly to the lungs, rapid onset of action, and particularly reduced dosage and minimal side-effects are important to both doctors and parents. The respiratory tract, however, has a series of physiological defence mechanisms to protect it from particle entry and deposition. While devices suitable for use in childhood are now available, careful training and attention to technique is essential. Unfortunately, because of the range of ages and intelligence no single device at present is appropriate for all ages (Table 29.13).

Failure of inhalation treatment is usually due to inadequate device technique or inappropriate device for that age.[222] Young children, particularly, often co-operate poorly with inhaled therapy. It is then not surprising that choosing the appropriate device and making sure parents and children are properly educated in its use can be as important as the choice of drug.

With development of devices for inhaled therapy, systemic therapy is much less used. Intravenous therapy is now confined to acute asthma. Oral therapy remains an attractive option particularly for some groups such as very young children. There have been no oral prophylactic agents as effective and free from side-effects

Table 29.13: Drug inhalation devices for regular use in children

Age	Appropriate inhaled device
<2.5 years	Spacer device plus facemask
<2.5 years	Nebulizer
2–5 years	Spacer device alone
>4.5–5 years	Dry powder inhaler
>6 years	Breath-actuated device
>10 years	Metered dose inhaler

as those used via inhalers. The introduction of the orally active leukotriene-receptor modifiers is exciting, but their role in asthma management is still to be determined. Oral bronchodilators can occasionally be useful in very young children, but are associated with a slower duration of onset and greater systemic side-effects.

Inhalation Devices There is now a substantial body of evidence about device use in children, identifying the most effective techniques (Table 29.14) and highlighting potential problems. Using these techniques can simply therapy.[223]

At present, four different inhalation systems are in common use in childhood: metered dose inhalers; metered dose inhalers with attached spacers; dry powder inhalers and nebulizers. It is now quite clear

Table 29.14: Techniques of using main inhaled device types in children

Device	Step	Action	Reason
Nebulizer	1	Fill the nebulizer to 4 ml; set flow rate to 6–8 l min^{-1}	Optimal conditions for generating particles of appropriate size
	2	Inhale using tidal breaths	
Dry-powder inhaler	1	Prime the device	
	2	For Rotahaler and Turbohaler hold vertically	Avoids powder falling out
	3	Inhale as quickly as possible	Provide energy to break up the powder into particles of size suitable for inhalation
Metered dose inhaler (MDI)	1	Remove the cap	
	2	Shake the canister	Disperses drug particles uniformaly in the propellant
	3	Hold the canister upright	
	4	Breathe out as far as is comfortable	Conflicting evidence
	5	Place the inhaler between the lips	
	6	Fire the inhaler at the beginning of a slow inspiration	Slow steady inspiration (<30 l min^{-1}) decreases oropharyngeal deposition
	7	Hold the breath for 10 s, or as long as is comfortable	Allows particles to settle on the airways by gravitational sedimentation
	8	If repeating keep upright and shake	Allows the canister to return to thermal equilibrium and the metering chamber to fill
MDI plus large volume spacer	1	Shake the canister and spacer	Disperses drug particles uniformly in the propellant
	2	Actuate the MDI and fill the large volume spacer	
	3	Inhale from the spacer using five tidal breaths	Child breathes in the aerosol Breath holding not necessary

that there are marked differences both within and between each group in factors ranging from design and construction through aerosol generation and output to optimal inhalation technique. It is also clear that one drug delivered by one inhaler may produce quite different results from another drug from the same inhaler. Of particular relevance is the fact that the results from adults may not be predictably transferable to children. In children, drug delivery varies with age and many inhalers cannot be used at all by young children. In choosing a device for a particular child, Pedersen has highlighted a number of issues to consider:[224]

(1) Which is the simplest and easiest for that child to use?
(2) Which inhaler most reproducibly delivers the highest fraction of the delivered dose to the intrapulmonary airways?
(3) Which has the best clinical effect for least systemic effect in day-to-day use? The clinical effect is due to deposition in the airways while systemic effect comes from the amount deposited and systemically absorbed from the intrapulmonary airways and the amount absorbed from the gastrointestinal tract.
(4) Which does the child prefer?

In practice, simple inhalation technique, easy handling and convenient device design may be more important than superior drug delivery to the intrapulmonary airways.

METERED DOSE INHALERS (MDIS) In children under 6 years, more than 50% were noted to have faulty and inefficient MDI technique.[225] (Table 29.15). Particularly significant were co-ordination difficulties, cessation of inhalation when cold particles hit the soft palate ("freon" effect), oral actuation but nasal inspiration and rapid inhalation. Use of a small-volume tube spacer significantly improved problems with co-ordination. Parents co-ordinating the firing of an MDI for their children alone or with a tube spacer did not improve the situation.

With careful tuition children older than 6 years can be taught to use MDIs successfully. However, as a practical rule they are probably best confined to children older than 10 years. If used, the inhalation technique needs to be carefully checked at every clinic visit.

Breath-actuated MDI devices (Autohaler®) can remove the co-ordination difficulties, but do not affect

Table 29.15: Frequency of the most common mistakes observed in 256 children demonstrating the use of an inhaler. (From Pedersen S, Frost L, Arnfred T. Errors in inhalation technique and efficiency in inhaler use in asthmatic children. *Allergy* 1986; 41: 118–24, ©Munksgaard International Publishers Ltd. Copenhagen, Denmark)

	MDI inhaler (n=132)	Tube spacer (n=85)
Forgetting to shake the canister	49%	34%
Forgetting to exhale before firing	45%	51%
Neck flexed during inhalation	12%	14%
Co-ordination problems	55%	17%
Fast inhalation	67%	28%
Breath holding ≤ 7 s	42%	39%
Stopping inspiration when firing aerosol	38%	6%
Inspiration through the nose	24%	32%
Submaximal inspiration	23%	19%
Help from the parents	5%	6%

other problems associated with MDI use, such as rapid inhalation. In a series of over 100 children, Pedersen has shown that even with careful instruction provided by videos and a nurse, only two out of 10 under 5 years old could master the device reliably.[226] Consequently, they should be reserved for children older than 6–7 years.

Until recently, MDIs have used chlorofluorocarbons (CFCs) as propellants. These deplete the ozone layer and have been banned under the Montreal Protocol. At present there is a temporary medical exemption, but CFCs will soon have to be phased out completely from MDIs. Alternative propellants such as hydrofluoroalkanes (HFAs) that do not have ozone-depleting properties have been developed. MDIs using such propellants are appearing. Replacement products will have to demonstrate similar effectiveness and safety to the MDIs they replace. No change in dosage is necessary for salbutamol reformulated with the new propellants, but this will not apply for some inhaled steroids.

SPACERS An MDI with a spacer attached has become an increasingly attractive method of administering inhaled medication to children. The spacer allows the propellant to evaporate leaving smaller, slow-moving respirable particles suitable for inhalation. All spacers reduce the cold "freon effect" and the occurrence of co-ordination problems. The amount of drug deposited in the oropharynx is also reduced, thus decreasing the consequent systemic absorption and increasing lung deposition. This feature makes them particularly suitable when high-dose inhaled corticosteroids are required.

Simple spacers such as a paper cup[227] have been shown to be effective and may be useful in emergencies. However, because of the absence of a valve if the child exhales during the actuation then no drug will be inhaled. Valved spacers (Nebuhaler®, Volumatic®, Aerochamber®, Babyhaler®), which provide a reservoir from which the child can inhale, avoid this problem and are easy for most children to use.

The ideal spacer design volume is not known. Less drug is available for inhalation in smaller spacer devices due to impaction on the walls of the device, but the drug is in a smaller space and hence is more concentrated. At lower tidal volumes, the higher inhaled drug concentration from smaller devices may enhance drug delivery. Smaller devices are also easier to handle while trying to hold a wriggling infant; they are generally less intimidating for the infant and they deliver at least as much if not more drug at these low tidal volumes. Thus a smaller device may be appropriate for infants while a larger device is better for older children.[228] Other aspects of design such as single valve control or separate inlet and outlet valves and minimized dead space also effect dose delivered, especially in very small children.[229] Ideally, spacer devices should be evaluated for each drug prescribed for them in each age group in which they are used.[230]

Static electric charge on plastic spacers has proved an unexpected problem. The charge can lead to marked reduction in the output of respirable particles.[231] Priming a new spacer with up to 15 puffs can reduce this charge and improve output. Washing the inhaler in a detergent and leaving it to dry also reduces the charge and substantially improves output.

Large volume spacers have proved particularly useful for prophylactic medication administration in children between 1 and 4 years of age. For both prophylactic medication and bronchodilator treatment, there is evidence of improvement in symptom scores and lung function, with fewer side-effects.[165,232–234] Small children, and infants, and those with severe airway obstruction, may have difficulties triggering the valves of some spacers[235] because they cannot produce sufficient flow. However, measurements have found the valve of both the Nebuhaler® and Volumatic® opens at flows achievable even by obstructed infants.[236] Tilting the device to allow gravity to keep the valve open may assist. Young children may be unable to seal their lips around the mouthpiece of the device. A spacer with a close-sealing mask (either an attached mask such as Laerdal mask or one built into the device such as an Aerochamber®) allows multiple breaths to be taken with less aerosol escape and can provide effective therapy for children under three.[237]

The usual manufacturer's instructions for a large volume spacer (slow, deep, inhalation followed by a 5–10 second breath hold) are not practical for young children. Gleeson and Price found that five tidal breaths from a Nebuhaler® with no breath-hold resulted in greater bronchodilation than a more conventional inhalation technique.[238] This "five breath technique" is much more practical for young children. Only one actuation per five breaths is recommended[228] because multiple actuations decrease the final dose available for inhalation. Inhalation should also take place as soon after firing as possible since a delay allows the drug to settle on the spacer walls, and again decreases the dose.[231] The reduction in delivery after multiple actuations or any delay before inhalation can be markedly reduced by using either a spacer with an ionic detergent coating or a metal spacer.[239] Plastic spacers should be washed in detergent, rinsed and air dried once a week.[31] They should not be wiped dry as this increases the static charge.

Large volume spacers are bulky and difficult to carry making them unsuitable for self-administration in school-age children. The physical size of some spacers (Nebuhaler®, Volumatic®) can make it difficult for parents to use the device in a struggling toddler. In this situation, smaller spacers such as the Aerochamber® may be easier for a parent to handle.[228]

Small volume ("tube") spacers are also available. They have been shown to lead to greater bronchodilation than an MDI alone. They reduce, but do not abolish, the numbers of inhalation errors that occur with MDIs[240] and they are not now much used.

DRY POWDER INHALERS Dry powder inhalers (DPIs) are now the mainstay of asthma treatment in school children. They are particularly useful in this age group

363

because they are discreet and easy to carry around. Since they are breath-actuated they eliminate the problems of co-ordination seen with MDIs. The newer DPIs such as the Turbohaler and Accuhaler (Diskus) now have multiple doses. The Turbohaler has proved to be a particularly effective device with intra-bronchial deposition twice that of a correctly used MDI.[241]

In DPIs, the drug is provided in a fine powder either alone or in combination with a carrier such as lactose. The turbulent air stream in the device during inhalation causes the powder aggregates to break up into particles small enough to be carried into the lower airways. DPIs, therefore need a certain minimum amount of energy from the inhalation to produce the correct particle size. Up to a certain point, their effectiveness increases with inspiratory flow rate because the increased flow rate will increase the number of particles within the "respirable range". While the flow rate required to generate an optimum effect varies from one device to another, most require the child to develop an inspiratory flow rate of approximately 20–60 l min[-1] (Table 29.16). On average, peak inspiratory flow rate is about a third of peak expiratory flow rate.[242] With an average 4-year-old having a mean peak expiratory flow of 100 l min,[-1] it is obvious that pre-school children particularly if wheezy may have difficulty generating sufficient inspiratory flow to gain full benefit from a dry powder device.[242] An important advantage of the newer "second generation" multi-dose devices such as the Turbohaler® and the Diskhaler® is that they require much lower peak inspiratory flow rates to be effective. Indeed, the Turbohaler® retains about 33% of its effect at flow rates around 13 min l[-1].[243] This

may allow these devices to be used in younger children. Agertoft and Pedersen recently showed that the vast majority of 4 and 5-year-old children could use the Turbohaler correctly after careful instruction.[244] The optimum technique for all DPIs is to inhale as rapidly as possible. Breath-holding, tilting the head back or inhalation from functional residual capacity instead of residual volume does not assist.[242] This technique is simple and easily taught.

With dry powder inhalers the vast majority of the drug is deposited in the oropharynx; only a small proportion enters the lung. Parents and children sometimes need to be reassured that the drug will be effective, even when most of it seems to be deposited in the mouth. With inhaled corticosteroids, mouth washing after use can reduce the systemic effects.[174] One practical suggestion is to take the medication just before tooth brushing and mouth rinsing. Agertoft and Pedersen found a higher intra-bronchial deposition of BUD from a Turbohaler than from a MDI and Nebuhaler and thus in some cases an increase in systemic effect with dry powder inhalers may actually arise because of increased deposition in the airways.[245]

Since young children and older children during exacerbations may not be able to generate sufficient inspiratory flow rates,[243] DPIs are not recommended for children much below 5 years and when first used are likely to be better for the administration of prophylactic medication. If prescribing dry powder bronchodilator in younger children, it may be sensible to anticipate the fact that some may need an alternative device for delivering bronchodilator during acute wheezing.

Table 29.16: Peak inspiratory flow rates necessary to operate inhaled devices in children

Device		Example	Necessary inspiratory flow
Large-volume spacers		Nebuhaler	>30 l min[-1]
		Volumatic	>30 l min[-1]
Dry-powder inhalers	"First generation"	Spinhaler	>80 l min[-1]
		Rotahaler	>60 l min[-1]
	"Second generation"	Diskhaler	>30 l min[-1]
		Turbohaler	>30 l min[-1]
Breath-actuated inhaler		Autohaler	30–55 l min[-1]

Peak inpiratory flow rate is between one-third and one-half peak expiratory flow.[242]

NEBULIZERS[246] Nebulizers allow the delivery of large concentrations of medication and avoid problems with co-ordination. In the acute situation, oxygen can be administered through the nebulizer at the same time. As a result, they are suitable for the very young and the acutely ill. They have been the mainstay of hospital treatment for children with acute asthma. In the home, nebulizers are useful for the delivery of prophylactic medication in young children unable to use other devices because of their age or their intelligence. They are also useful in the severely asthmatic child or in those with frequent severe asthma attacks where they may reduce the need for hospital admission.[247] Unfortunately, compressors suitable for home use are quite bulky, expensive and need a power source. There is no doubt they are overused, particularly with the development of effective alternatives. All too frequently, a request for a home nebulizer arises because of the failure to treat chronic asthma properly.

Two main types are available, jet nebulizers and ultrasonic nebulizers. The most commonly used are jet nebulizers, which work by using the Bernoulli effect to draw drug solution into a gas stream forcing it onto an impaction plate and forming aerosol droplets by impaction and gas turbulence. Drug output varies according to the type of nebulizer, the fill volume, the driving gas pressure and the residual volume remaining after nebulization. Minor changes in the details of administration can have dramatic effects on drug output. For example, a close fitting mask is often used. A gap of only 2 cm between mask and face may result in an 85% reduction in the dose delivered.[248]

The use of a mouthpiece improves lung deposition and reduces deposition on the face, but young children may not use a mouthpiece properly. They may inhale through the nose, block the mouthpiece with the tongue or blow through the mouthpiece, so the best delivery method needs to be individually determined. If a face mask is used for nebulized corticosteroids the eyes and face should be washed after each treatment. Holes in the mask should be covered if the drug used is potentially harmful to the eyes.[249]

The issue of whether the dose of nebulized drug needs to be corrected for size in children has been a matter of concern. Young children with small tidal volumes will inhale pure aerosol from a nebulizer. As they grow, their peak inspiratory flow exceeds the nebulizer output and they entrain air. As a result, older children will inspire the same dose as adults once their inspiratory flow exceeds nebulizer flow and the entire nebulizer output is inhaled. Detailed studies of nebulized cromoglycate[250] and budesonide in young children[251] suggest that children can receive the same dose as adults and scaling of the dose to take account of differing body weights is not necessary.

Before starting nebulizer treatment, parents should be given clear verbal and written instructions in the use of the nebulizer and compressor and their cleaning and maintenance. A maximum duration of treatment should be specified for the prescribed drug/nebulizer/compressor combination. Keeping the nebulization times short may help to improve compliance.[246] Parents should have a clear understanding that they should seek medical help if their child fails to respond to nebulized bronchodilator.[247] The child should be monitored by a specialist clinic.

GENERAL POINTS ABOUT INHALER DEVICE USE It is now quite clear that the device and patient factors influencing intra-pulmonary drug deposition can be complex and vary greatly depending on the child's age, the drug and its formulation, the device used and the inhalation technique. There is often surprisingly little clinical or scientific information about such factors. Uncritical introduction of new devices into clinical practice should be avoided until their effects, and side-effects, have been clearly established in the target population both for the devices and for each drug prescribed for them.

Whatever device is chosen, careful education in its use and repeated checks on technique are important. Technique should be checked every time an asthmatic child is reviewed. If the technique is poor and cannot be improved, then the device should be changed to one that can be used reliably. Regrettably, the education of clinical staff in the use of inhalers is still often neglected. Clinical staff should know which device is likely to be appropriate for a particular child and how to instruct the child in the use of the chosen device. Nowadays, children often know about different inhaled devices because they know of other children using them. Allowing a child to choose the one they like best may help to improve compliance. Failure to observe these simple rules frequently compromises the therapeutic effectiveness of inhalation treatment in children.

Choosing the Appropriate Drug Combinations and Doses using a Stepwise Approach[32] The choice of pharmacological treatment should take account of the severity of the disease and the child's current treatment. Successful drug management aims to reduce or abolish symptoms (Table 29.5) with minimum therapy. Whether it is better to give more aggressive treatment at the outset and then step therapy down when control is achieved or start with moderate therapy and then gradually step-up if control is not achieved is not yet clear. It is argued that more aggressive initial therapy will result in more rapid suppression of airway inflammation and allow for eventual asthma control at lower doses of anti-inflammatory therapy. One retrospective study found that starting therapy with inhaled corticosteroids earlier led to better lung function and less cumulative corticosteroid dose over the long term.[252] An initial "rescue" course of oral corticosteroids can be useful in bringing about rapid control of symptoms, which may be important in gaining the confidence of the family, and encouraging future adherence to treatment. Set against this, many parents are concerned about drug side-effects, particularly from inhaled corticosteroids. The use of higher corticosteroid doses may then influence their compliance adversely. Whichever approach is adopted, therapy should start at a level broadly in keeping with the severity of the asthma. Since asthma is dynamic as well as chronic, treatment should change to accommodate the variations that occur over time.

The current approach to treatment of childhood asthma of differing severity is well-summarized in national and international guidelines.[32,33,69] However, the treatment should then be tailored for each particular child. If control is not achieved with the chosen step within a month or so, it may be appropriate to increase treatment to the next appropriate step. Before any increase, it is essential to check that the child is using the inhaled device properly, and that the present prescription has been understood and correctly taken. It may also be appropriate to reconsider the initial diagnosis. Once satisfactory control has been sustained for a period of weeks or months, consideration can be given to a cautious reduction in therapy ("step down") to the minimum necessary to maintain control. This is usually down gradually every 2–3 months to the lowest dose necessary to maintain asthma control.

MILD INFREQUENT ASTHMA – STEP 1 (Table 29.9) About 60% of children have mild, infrequent symptoms of coughing and wheezing. For such children, the bronchodilator is to be used as required when symptoms are present and this is usually sufficient. Bronchodilator delivery by inhalation is preferable. For children between the ages of 2 and 5 years, an MDI with large volume spacer (and mask, if necessary) is effective. School-age children usually find a dry powder inhaler more convenient. Oral bronchodilators are less effective and have more systemic side-effects, but may be useful for younger children with mild infrequent symptoms. Oral bronchodilators may occasionally be sufficient in slightly older children with mild asthma where the infrequent use of a bronchodilator makes inhalation skills difficult to maintain.

Some children may be symptom-free most of the time, but develop occasional acute exacerbations following viral respiratory infections. The parents often recognize a clear pattern of deterioration which can alert them to the need to start medication (Table 29.17). Bronchodilators alone are often insufficient: a short course of oral steroids started early may help to bring the symptoms under control.[190] Regular use of inhaled corticosteroids in children with viral episodic wheezing does not appear to reduce the frequency or severity of viral induced exacerbations.[253,254] Intermittent inhalation of high-dose corticosteroids from a large volume spacer has also been tried, but the benefits have been modest.[255,256] Parents of children who experience marked exacerbations with viral respiratory infections should, therefore, have a detailed written plan with instructions on when to start a short course of oral corticosteroids. It is often helpful to provide the parents with a store of oral steroids to start in such circumstances.

Treatment with SCG on a seasonal basis may be useful for some children. For pollen-related problems, treatment should be commenced 4–6 weeks before the pollen season and then continued throughout the season. SCG may also be helpful in children with animal-sensitive asthma when taken 15–30 minutes before exposure to the animal(s).

MODERATE ASTHMA – STEPS 2 AND 3 (Table 29.9) About 30% of children suffer more frequent and troublesome symptoms. These children may require daily inhaled prophylactic anti-inflammatory treatments. Prior to starting any prophylactic treatment, it is necessary to explain the plan clearly to the parents so that they appreciate the need for regular treatment.

Table 29.17: Initial prodromal symptoms of asthma and their time-relation to an overt attack of asthma (From Beer S, Laver J, Karpuch J et al. Prodromal features of asthma. *Arch Dis Child* 1987; 62: 345–8, with permission.)

Symptom	No. of patients	Interval (hours) between initial symptom and onset of overt attack	
		Mean (SD)	Range
Rhinorrhoea	39	26.76 (12.0)	6–60
Cough	23	20.73 (0.42)	6–48
Irritability	7	28.28 (4.53)	12–36
Apathy	7	28.28 (4.13)	12–36
Anxiety	3	30	24–36
Sleep disorders	2	18	12–24
Fever (above 38°C)	5	16.2 (4.0)	6–24
Abdominal pain	2	13.5 (6.4)	6–24
Loss of appetite	2	18	12–24
Itching	3	9	6–12
Skin eruption	1	9	6–12
Toothache	1	9	6–12

Published guidelines still suggest starting preventative inhaled treatment in children with SCG which has the advantage of virtually no side-effects. In practice, many paediatricians start with low-dose inhaled corticosteroids. If SCG is used, an initial 4–8 week trial of SCG, administered either via MDI with large volume spacer (10 mg four times per day) or, for older children, via a dry powder inhaler (Spincaps 20 mg four times per day) is appropriate. Parents should be told that 4–6 weeks may be necessary for the treatment to become effective. Some children will respond well to SCG, but it is not possible to predict beforehand which will respond best. Clinically, children with mild symptoms but a particularly prominent cough often seem to benefit most. If SCG is successful, it may be possible to reduce the frequency of administration to three times a day.

If, after 4–8 weeks of SCG, the response to treatment is inadequate, then an inhaled steroid (beclomethasone or budesonide) should be substituted, usually in a dose of 100–200 µg twice daily. At this point, there is generally no benefit in continuing SCG.[257]

With continuing symptoms, or a continuing requirement for a bronchodilator two or three times daily for symptom relief, there are a number of options now available. These include a further increase in steroid dose to 400–800 µg twice a day, the addition of a long-acting bronchodilator such as salmeterol, the use of an oral leukotriene antagonist or low-dose theophylline preparations. While studies in adults suggest that addition of salmeterol to a moderate dose of inhaled corticosteroid results in better symptom control and higher PEF,[136,258] there are less data in children. A large Dutch study found no significant additional benefit of adding either salmeterol or more beclomethasone to a daily dose of 400 µg beclomethasone although growth was significantly slower at the higher dose of BDP.[259] In adults, the addition of low dose theophyllines has been shown to produce similar effects to doubling inhaled corticosteroids in moderate asthma[260,261] although salmeterol may be more effective and associated with fewer side-effects.[262] Similar studies are not yet available in children. Further evidence is also needed about the positioning of leukotriene antagonists in stepwise therapy in children.

SEVERE ASTHMA – STEPS 4 AND 5 (Table 29.9) Fewer than 10% of children with asthma fall into the most severe category.

If a small increase in inhaled steroids and the sequential addition of long-acting bronchodilators, leukotriene antagonists and oral theophylline produces no benefit, higher doses of inhaled corticosteroids (up to 1600–2000 µg per day) may be tried. However, before any step up in treatment, particularly to high-dose inhaled corticosteroids, it is important to check the child's device technique, to ensure, as far as possible, that the child is actually receiving, or taking, the prescribed medicine and to address any factors that may be contributing to poor compliance (Table 29.18). A period of regular peak flow monitoring may be useful. Close attention should be paid to existing or new environmental factors, such as parental smoking, pets, or psychosocial problems that may compromise the effectiveness of treatment. Inhaled short-acting bronchodilators should continue to be used as needed for symptom control, although, by this stage, quite high doses are frequently being used regularly. At this level of treatment, referral to an asthma specialist is strongly advised.

With higher doses of inhaled corticosteroids (above 800 µg per day of BDP or BUD), the use of a spacer device to decrease oropharyngeal deposition and systemic absorption[174,263] may be appropriate; both BDP via a spacer (Volumatic®) and budesonide via spacer (Nebuhaler®) have less systemic activity than the same dose delivered from an MDI or dry powder inhaler (Diskhaler® or Turbohaler), although mouth rinsing after the Turbohaler seems to reduce or abolish this difference. Whatever device is used, it would seem advisable to rinse out the mouth after administration to remove any corticosteroid remaining in the oropharynx. At higher doses of inhaled BDP, using inhaled FP instead is associated with fewer systemic side-effects.

If control remains poor, the administration of inhaled corticosteroids four times per day may help.[264] The use of high-dose nebulized budesonide (up to 2000 µg per day) is also worth considering. If control still remains poor despite maximum doses of inhaled corticosteroids and bronchodilators, oral corticosteroids may be necessary. Often prednisolone 5–10 mg per day will be sufficient and should be used concurrently with high-dose inhaled steroid. Where possible, oral corticosteroids should be administered on alternate days to diminish side-effects, but daily administration is often required for asthma control.

When oral steroids are taken side-effects are likely, and families should be warned to expect them. Early dietary advice may avoid some of the weight gain that should be expected. Careful monitoring of height and weight, blood pressure, urine for glucose and eyes for cataract development, is necessary. A steroid card, containing instructions to increase the steroid dose with intercurrent medical problems, should be issued.

It is a rare child whose asthma genuinely cannot be controlled. Where there is apparent continuing inability to control asthma, the diagnosis should be carefully reviewed. Poor compliance is often at the root of the problem.[265] Relative "steroid resistance" can occur,[194] but is uncommon. Careful education and meticulous attention to all aspects of asthma care by one experienced clinician can often lead to improved control. The clinician should aim to provide consistent support and to keep the therapeutic plan as simple as possible. Periods of inpatient care may help to re-establish control.

STEP DOWN When satisfactory asthma control is achieved, a step down in treatment should be carefully considered. This should be done slowly in 4–6 monthly steps. With older children, a period of peak flow monitoring over the period of the reduction of dose may be helpful.

If control deteriorates, the parents should return to the previous treatment. At any stage, a short course of oral prednisolone may be effective in re-establishing control of asthma. If asthma symptoms do not recur and lung function remains satisfactory no other change in therapy may be indicated.

Table 29.18: Possible reasons for non-compliance. (From Partridge MR. Problems with asthma care delivery. In: Mitchell DM (ed.). *Recent Advances in Respiratory Medicine No. 5.* **London: Churchill Livingstone, 1991: 61–78, with permission)**

Misunderstanding

Lack of confidence in efficacy of the drug

Fear of side-effects/dislike of drugs

Complacency

Rebellion

Difficulties with method of administration

Difficulties with the timing of administration

Developing Plans for Managing Exacerbations and Dealing with Variations in the Disease (see also Chapter 26)

Devising a strategy with parents to cope with asthma exacerbations is an important element in any treatment plan. The parents must be able to recognize deterioration early and change the medicine quickly, without necessarily involving their doctor. The aim is to abort any exacerbation before it becomes severe, and in so to doing avoid hospital admission.

To achieve such an aim, both parents and children must have a clear understanding of the role of the various medicines, and be fully competent in the use of any inhalation device. They should be able to identify early signs of loss of control, such as more frequent nocturnal waking or increased need for relievers. While the necessary education and training are the responsibility of the clinician, they can often be successfully delegated to nurses and physiotherapists. The education and advice should be consistent, repeated and reinforced by written guidelines.

For children under 5 years, plans will be solely symptom-based. Fortunately, exacerbations do not usually happen without warning. In up to 70% of children a sequence of prodromal findings, which is constant in a particular child, is present for approximately 24 hours before the onset of wheezing[266] (Table 29.17). Recognition of such patterns facilitates the early introduction of treatment. In children over 5 years, these early findings can be combined with PEF monitoring.

A number of zone or colour coded ("traffic light") systems have been developed to make management plans easier to use; one example is outlined in Table 29.19. Studies of children show that such approaches are effective in improving asthma control and decreasing morbidity, and enhance the likelihood of a correct response to an exacerbation.[76] In some approaches the essence of the plan is written on a small asthma "credit card" which can be carried around with the patient or parent.[267]

The levels of peak flow at which certain interventions should be initiated have not been validated. For

---

Table 29.19: An example of a colour-coded asthma zone plan. (From Charlton I, Antoniov AG, Atkinson J et al. Asthma at the interface: bridging the gap between general practice and a district general hospital. *Arch Dis Child* 1994; 70: 313–8, with permission)

Green zone
Your peak flow is above 70% of normal or your symptoms score is under 6:
...continue "maintenance therapy" of...

Yellow zone
Your peak flow is less than 70% of normal or your symptoms score is between 6 and 9:
(a) Double your dose of ... until you return to your highest reading
(b) Continue on this dose for the same number of days
(c) Return to the previous dose of "maintenance therapy"

Amber zone
Your peak flow is less than 50% of normal or your symptoms score is less than 9:
(a) Start oral prednisolone immediately ... mg daily and contact GP within 24 hours
(b) Continue on this dose until you return to your highest reading
(c) Reduce oral prednisolone to ... mg daily for the same number of days
(d) Stop prednisolone

Red zone
Your peak flow is less than 30% of normal or your symptoms score is over 12:
(a) Call GP urgently, or if unavailable
(b) Go directly to hospital or if unable
(c) Call ambulance

example, Charlton *et al.* instructed their patients to increase treatment at a PEF of 70% of best, but thought the effect might have been better if 80% of best PEF had been used.[76] There is debate about most effective amount of instruction[76,268] and the optimal intensity of follow-up.[269,270]

As part of the emergency plan, parents should be provided with a course of oral corticosteroids. Oral corticosteroids have been shown to be effective in accelerating the recovery and preventing dangerous deterioration in acute exacerbations.[189, 271] Parents should be instructed to initiate a course if the attack fails to respond to the usual treatment.[78] For those using PEF meters, steroids are usually started at a PEF of 50% [76] to 60% of best. An oral steroid course begun at home by parents at the onset of an exacerbation triggered by a viral URTI has also been shown to be effective.[190,191]

There is little evidence to support starting or altering inhaled corticosteroids during acute exacerbations. Research in adults has demonstrated that doubling twice daily inhaled steroids if asthma deteriorates can be effective.[75,272] In children, Charlton *et al.* found a trend towards improvement in children who doubled their inhaled steroid at 70% of best peak flow compared with those who only used bronchodilators, but the numbers studied were small.[76] However, in two recent randomized trials in children with mild to moderate asthma doubling inhaled corticoteroids at the start of exacerbations was not effective.[273,274] In the second study, the plan was only adequately followed by a quarter of the parents. In children with wheezing triggered only by viral URTIs, high-dose inhaled corticosteroids begun at the onset of symptoms showed only modest effects on symptoms.[255,256,275,276] More research is needed to establish whether treatment in this way is ever beneficial, particularly for those already on prophylactic treatment.

The other essential treatment during an exacerbation is increased repetitive administration of inhaled short acting β_2 agonists. With more severe exacerbations, higher doses of β_2 agonists will usually be needed. In acute asthma in children, large volume spacers have been shown to be as effective as nebulizers.[277–282] Ten to twenty puffs may be needed to produce appropriate bronchodilation. It should be remembered that one nebule of 2.5 mg salbutamol contains the equivalent of 25 puffs from an MDI. In an emergency, a coffee cup can be used as a spacer.[227] If the child improves, treatment can be continued at home. Full recovery from

Table 29.20: Indications for seeking early medical help in an exacerbation
High-risk patient (see Table 29.26)
Severe exacerbation (e.g. PEF less than 50% of predicted or personal best)
Response to bronchodilator lasts less than 3 hours
β_2 agonists every 3–4 hours are needed for more than 24–48 hours
No improvement within 2–6 hours of starting oral corticosteroids
Further deterioration

an exacerbation may be gradual and increased medication may be required for several days.

A plan for managing exacerbations should also set limits so that parents know clearly when treatment is failing and medical advice should be sought (Table 29.20). It is easier to treat a severe exacerbation successfully at an early stage. A brief hospital admission for frequent inhaled bronchodilators and oral steroids is likely to be much less stressful than a period of ventilation in ICU.

Providing Regular Follow-Up Care

Parents and children need regular supervision and support by a physician who is knowledgeable about asthma and its treatment. For a successful therapeutic partnership, families and clinicians must "jointly develop and agree both short- and long-term treatment goals".[32,283] Management plans should be subject to a joint "process of continuing but orderly review" at every clinic visit.[32,284] There is no doubt that parents prefer to see one doctor or nurse and, wherever possible, clinics should be organized to achieve this goal. Good communication skills in the doctor can have a direct influence on both patient satisfaction and outcome.[84]

There are a number of specific tasks to be completed at any review session (Table 29.21). The central task is to assess whether a child's asthma is well-controlled. General questions such as "how have you been?" rarely produce the necessary information. Questions should be directed to specific areas, such as nocturnal disturbance, loss of time from school, problems with exercise,

Table 29.21: A checklist of points to cover at clinic review. (From Guidelines on the management of asthma. *Thorax* 1993; 48: S1–S24.)

Points to review	Possible questions
Asthma – severity and control	How does asthma interfere with your/your child's activities?
Trigger – factors and their avoidance	What makes the asthma worse?
Drugs – effects and side-effects, compliance, fears	What medicines are you taking? Can you explain to me what the drugs do? How often do you take your drugs? Do you ever miss any doses? Can I see your asthma card? Some people think steroids are harmful – what do you think?
Devices – correct technique	Show me how you use your inhaler.
Monitoring – symptom diary cards, peak flow charts	Can I look at your diary card/peak flow charts?
Acute exacerbations – recognition, treatment, when to get help	When would you call your doctor?
Specific anxieties	What do you expect from asthma treatment?

and any exacerbations that have occurred. If a peak flow record is available, it can be a useful basis for discussion, and is particularly helpful when discussing the triggers for, and management of, any exacerbations. Useful insights into parent/child perceptions of the disease can be obtained and an individual child's management plan fine-tuned.

The drug therapy being used should be ascertained and noted, in particular the specific drugs, their doses and the actual devices. All too frequently parents (or other medical carers), for whatever reason, have changed the drugs, the dosages or the devices. It may be appropriate to reinforce the understanding of the purpose of particular drugs. It is also necessary to gauge whether the treatment is being taken appropriately. Non-adherence is difficult to detect by direct questioning. It is usually better to acknowledge that a degree of non-compliance is normal. This helps to avoid implications of criticism and may allow an exploration of why medicines are not been taken.

Inhalation skills should be checked. If they are inadequate and cannot be improved, a change in device may be indicated. The most appropriate device for a child will change with time: e.g. when a child reaches school age, a more easily portable device such as a dry powder inhaler may be better. Children may have

friends with asthma who are using different inhalers, and as a result may have clear ideas about which device they would prefer. Where appropriate, such preferences should be met.

In follow-up, examination usually plays only a limited role. Children with severe asthma taking larger doses of inhaled or oral steroids should be accurately measured, and their height plotted on an appropriate centile chart. Other signs of corticosteroid side-effects should be looked for (Table 29.22). With modern treatments, the chest will usually be clear on auscultation. Both chronic chest deformity and interval wheezing are important signs of more severe asthma and should be noted.[285] Most paediatricians will have encountered an occasional child labelled as asthmatic with respiratory symptoms due to a disorder other than asthma so it is always worth checking for signs, such as finger clubbing, which point to an alternative diagnosis. Anxieties about drug side-effects are common and should be fully aired, since latent anxieties may compromise management. Finally, it is important to update the action to be taken in the event of an acute deterioration.

Most children with asthma can be managed without referral to a specialist but referral may be necessary when asthma is severe, or when the parents need reassurance (Table 29.6).

Table 29.22: Potential side-effects of inhaled corticosteroids to look for when examining children at follow-up. (From Paton JY. The safety of inhaled steroids in childhood asthma. *The Practioner* 1994; 238: 322–6)

Potential problem	Conclusion	Clinical advice
Growth	No evidence from longitudinal studies of impact on long-term growth	Monitor linear growth carefully and regularly at higher inhaled corticosteroid doses
Hypothalamic–pituitary effects	Effects of inhaled steroids can be found but do not appear to be clinically relevant	–
Bones	Below 800 µg of BUD or BDP and 200 µg fluticasone, there does not appear to be an effect on bones	–
Psychiatric effects	Acute behavioural disturbances (hyperactivity or temper tantrums) reported	Ask about any change in behaviour. May need to reduce dose or discontinue
Eyes	No association with subcapsular cataracts on long-term use	–
Metabolic effects	No evidence of clinically relevant effects	–
Connective tissues	Easy bruising does not appear to be a problem in children	Check skin for any signs of unusual bruising
Oral candidiasis	Uncommon in children, but does occur	Check mouth for oral candidiasis. Using large volume spacers and changing dosage to four times daily may help
Sore throat and hoarseness	Rare in children	Ask about (and listen for) any change in voice or occurrence of sore throats. May be less of a problem with dry powder inhalers

In addition to specific points above, it is important to always keep the dose as low as possible (preferably <800 µg of BUD or BDP per day.) BDP: beclomethasone dipropionate; BUD: budesonide.

SPECIAL PROBLEMS AND COMMON QUESTIONS

Asthma in Infants and Young Children

Wheezing in young children is very common. Fifteen per cent of infants in the first year of life, and up to 25% of under-fives, attend their family practitioners with wheezing lower respiratory illnesses. Many more have milder symptoms.[286] Most childhood asthma begins in infancy, with 80% of children who develop asthma having their first episode of wheeze before the age of 3 years.[287] Admissions to hospital are common. Indeed, much of the increase in asthma admissions between 1961 and 1990 has been in children under the age of 4[4,288] (Fig. 29.2).

Despite the frequency of symptoms such as wheezing, difficulty breathing and cough in young children, the diagnosis of asthma in infants and young children remains difficult. In recent years, all wheezing in early childhood has tended to be labelled as "asthma". This

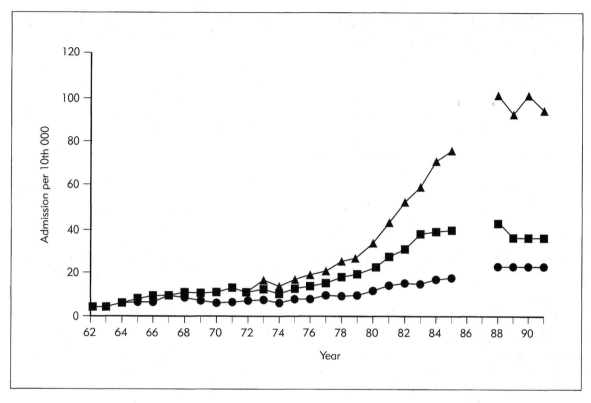

FIGURE 29.2: Age-specific hospital admission rates for asthma in children in England and Wales 1962–91 Key: triangles, 0–4 years; squares, 5–9 years; circles 10–14 years. (From Lung and Asthma Information Agency Factsheet 95/1. Source: OPCS and Welsh Health Common Services Authority).

practice arose because of the failure to demonstrate significant differences between populations of children with "classic" asthma and those with "wheezy bronchitis"[289,290] and in an attempt to act upon the under-diagnosis and under-treatment of asthma.[2] There is increasing evidence challenging this approach[25] (Table 29.1). In particular in infants, there is evidence that lower levels of lung function predispose to wheezing lower respiratory illness.[291] Thus, factors associated with diminished lung function (such as maternal smoking during pregnancy[292,293] and low birth weight[294]) increase the risk of a child's developing wheezing. Wheezing in this situation is very commonly triggered by viral respiratory infections:[295] allergic triggers are relatively unimportant. Nearly 20% of wheezy children will only have one attack[296] and almost all wheezy infants will have outgrown their symptoms between the ages of six and 11 years.[297] Attacks can be frequent, however, with 20% or more of wheezy children having ≥ 5 episodes of wheeze in the preceding year.[3]

The likelihood of a doctor diagnosing asthma increases with an increase in the number of episodes per year, and with the severity of shortness of breath suffered during attacks. Asthma is also more likely to be diagnosed where the episodes are triggered by factors other than colds.[296] Finally, a diagnosis of asthma is to some extent dependent on a child's age, being more likely to be made in older children. Failure to diagnose asthma remains common. Many infants still arrive at paediatric clinics with a history of recurrent "colds", with coughing and wheezing, which have proved unresponsive to antibiotics. Bronchodilators may never have been tried.

Quite apart from the difficulty in diagnosis, management of wheezing is also troublesome (Table 29.23). The response to treatments, particularly bronchodilators, is often variable especially in the first year of life though there is strong evidence that functional β_2 adrenoreceptors are present in the infant airway.[298–301] The unpredictable and often limited effects of β_2 agonists are

Table 29.23: Problems in the management of infants and very young children with wheezing (from Wilson NM,[348] ©Paediatr Respir Med.)

Recurrent wheeze and cough are associated with viral respiratory infections, often without a family history of asthma or atopy

Diagnosis rests almost entirely on symptoms which may be variable, rather than on objective lung function tests

Paucity of suitable designed and tested inhaler devices specific for this age group

Few controlled trials of treatment have been carried out

Treatment response to inhaled therapy differs with age and pattern of disease

Bronchodilator response is variable in the first year of life, but bronchodilators should still be tried

The younger the child the more other disorders may mimic asthma

thought to relate more to airflow limitation due to inflammatory oedema and excess mucus production.[302] In general, anti-asthmatic medications are likely to be more effective than other treatments. Antibiotics, in particular, are not effective.

Inhalation therapy in very young children is difficult and the resulting pulmonary deposition of drugs very poor.[303] Spacer devices with face masks[237] are now most commonly used, but nebulizers may still be necessary in the very young or poorly co-operative child. For children unable to tolerate a facemask, an MDI with a polystyrene coffee cup is effective and may be particularly useful in emergencies.[227]

Treatment of chronic or recurrent symptoms in young children has tended to follow a step treatment plan similar to that adopted for older children. Oral β_2 agonists may suffice for the treatment of very mild and infrequent symptoms. More usually, β_2 agonists via a spacer are used for acute wheezing. There is no clear evidence that ipratropium bromide is effective in children under 1 year.[156]

For recurrent or chronic symptoms, prophylactic medication is appropriate. Recent placebo-controlled studies have suggested that SCG is generally not effective in this age group,[198,200] although it may have a role in symptomatic children born prematurely.[199] Slow-

release theophylline preparations may be tried when inhaled therapy proves impractical; however, compliance is poor and side-effects common.[304] There are no data yet on whether the leukotriene anatgonists will be effective and safe in very young children. When the response to these treatments is inadequate, inhaled steroids, usually via a large volume spacer or occasionally nebulized, are the next step. The most appropriate dose levels are not clearly established, but available data suggest that doses in the range of 200–400 μg per day are effective[167,169,305] and not associated with side-effects.[306] Children as young as one have been shown to benefit.[165] Nebulized BDP proved very disappointing in practice,[307] and is no longer available in the UK; nebulized budesonide has been more successful.[169,308,309] Regular oral steroids may very rarely be indicated. In young children with wheezing associated only with viral URTIs, inhaled corticosteroids, either continuously or at the start of the infection do not appear to be very effective.[253,255,276,310]

Adolescents and Asthma

Asthma is common in teenagers and is often under-diagnosed.[311,312] For children with long-standing symptoms, asthma usually improves during puberty;[313,314] for many, symptoms will disappear completely. However, those with more severe asthma may continue to suffer symptoms throughout adolescence.

For children with asthma, the teenage years may be particularly difficult. The normal features of adolescence such as growth of autonomy, indifference to risk, and peer group identification, may all conspire to make management of asthma particularly difficult. Rebellion against the restrictions of the disease, a denial of symptoms and non-compliance with medication are all common and may have serious consequences if persistent and severe symptoms go unrecognized. Identification with peers frequently leads to a high incidence of teenage smoking. Conflict with authority may result in a perception that the physician is siding with the parents, thus placing the doctor–patient relationship under strain.

The delivery of medical care may also cause problems. Teenagers require services that recognize their autonomy and address their specific needs. Good communication is the key. This may be best achieved by having separate clinics for teenagers where they can be seen alone without their parents. A perceived lack of confidentiality has been highlighted as an important barrier to adolescents' use of health care services.[315]

Physicians need to gain and keep their young patients' trust by being consistent, reasonable and realistic in their therapeutic goals. Simple practical approaches such as exploring health beliefs and goals of the teenager, tailoring treatment, providing individualized written plans and "decriminalizing non-compliance and life-style behaviours such as smoking" may all be useful.[316]

Exercise-Induced Bronchoconstriction (see also Chapter 36)

Exercise-induced bronchoconstriction (EIB) is seen most commonly in children, as their high levels of physical activity causes high levels of ventilation, which in children with heightened airway reactivity triggers acute airway narrowing.[317] Exercise-induced bronchoconstriction is not a separate disorder, but merely one of the commoner stimuli leading to airflow limitation in children.[318,319]

Children with EIB can usually undertake and finish vigorous activity, because the brief, intense bursts of exercise typical of childhood produce fewer problems than sustained exercise. Usually, airway obstruction begins shortly after vigorous exercise stops, peaks in 5–10 minutes at levels between 15 and 50% below baseline and then remits spontaneously and completely within 30–60 minutes. The more strenuous the effort, the greater the ventilation and the more intense the resultant bronchospasm. Running causes more severe airways limitation than jogging, and jogging more than walking (Figure 29.3). Airway obstruction is also greater when the inspired air is dry and cold, and less when the air is warm and moist. Thus exercise on cold, winter days will cause symptoms when similar activity on warm humid, summer days will not. The asthma attacks precipitated by exercise appear no different from those caused by other triggers with symptoms including wheeze, difficulty breathing, chest tightness and cough. However, exercise does not cause prolonged or intense airway obstruction. The problem is not so much the severity of attacks as the limitation of activity that results. This may lead many children to avoid taking part in exercise.

Usually, exercise-induced asthma is easy to recognize. A careful history should elicit the fact that symptoms typically occur not during exercise, but when the workload decreases at the end of exercise. Sometimes cough may be the only presenting feature. Vocal cord dysfunction may rarely masquerade as EIB but then

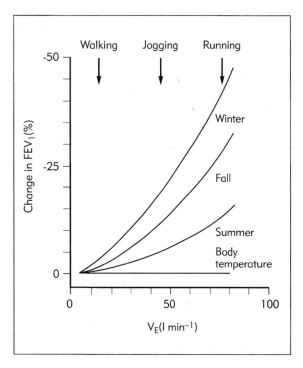

FIGURE 29.3: Effect of the interaction between the intensity of exercise and the thermal environment on the pulmonary mechanical response. (From McFadden ER Jr, Gilbert IA. Exercise-induced asthma. *N Engl J Med* 1994; 330: 1362–7, Copyright 1994 Massachusetts Medical Society. All rights Reserved.)

the development of symptoms is not consistent, breathing difficulties start during exercise, and there is a poor responses to anti-asthma medication.[320] The diagnosis of EIB can be confirmed by a fall in PEF or FEV_1 of ≥ 15% after exercise. In children, treadmill or free running tests are most widely used,[321] but the type of exercise is immaterial as long as the workload is sufficiently high to cause an adequate level of ventilation. In pre-school children, the history may be less obvious. The child may be reluctant to take exercise or want to be carried. Formal exercise testing may not be possible, and a therapeutic trial may be necessary to confirm the diagnosis.

Exercise does not induce increased airway reactivity[322] or long-term deterioration in lung function. Accordingly, continuous therapy is not needed as treatment. However, the sensitivity to exercise and the intensity of symptoms induced by exercise are related to the underlying airway reactivity.[323] Prophylactic therapy may be beneficial by decreasing bronchial hyperreactivity and allowing a greater degree of exercise to occur before airway obstruction develops. Exercise is unique in that it is the only natural trigger that induces tachphylaxis so that with bouts of exercise performed repeatedly within a period of 40 minutes or less, the bronchial narrowing progressively decreases ("refractory period").[324] This is of practical importance for children, especially those taking part in competitive games, because they may be able to limit the inevitable airways obstruction by a short warm up period before planned physical activity.

The primary aim of therapy is prevention using appropriate drug therapy. β_2 agonists, SCG and nedocromil used 10–15 minutes before exercise are all effective. β_2 agonists also work after exercise on symptoms which are slow to resolve whereas SCG and nedocromil only attenuate the response to exercise and must be used before exercise.[317] With adequate treatment, most children can take part in regular activities. Indeed, physical activity is beneficial and has been shown to improve exercise tolerance and cardiorespiratory performance.[325] Asthma, adequately treated, does not preclude high athletic performance.

Children often forget, or, more commonly, do not choose to use inhaled treatment before exercise. Sometimes, they are reluctant to be seen taking medication. In such circumstances, the long acting β_2 agonist, salmeterol, which is effective in preventing exercise-induced asthma for 10–12 hours after a single inhalation, may be useful.[139] Treatment given before leaving home may allow participation in exercise or play without symptoms or limitation. If the child is going to be physically active for more than 30 to 60 minutes then a second dose of salmeterol several hours after they begin exercising may be used. As intensity of exercise increases or the air becomes colder and drier, the effectiveness of all drugs falls. Then, combining a β_2 agonist with SCG or nedocromil may be useful and may allow higher levels of ventilation before symptoms occur. This can be important for children taking part in competitive games who need a greater degree of prevention to allow them to compete successfully. There is no evidence that β_2 agonists are performance enhancing in normal children[326] although there are some data that pre-medication may enhance submaximal running economy in asthmatic children.[327]

While the protection against EIB is maintained with long-term use, the duration of protection decreases.[328] Recent studies in adults have shown that leukotriene antagonists provide substantial protection against EIB for many but not all patients with mild stable asthma. For montelukast, at least, this benefit persists long-term during daily use without measurable tachyphylaxis.[329]

Cough-Variant Asthma (see also Chapter 42)
Recurrent wheeze and/or cough are typical of asthma, and often occur together. For example, parents frequently describe coughing and wheezing after exercise in asthmatic children. Coughing may also lead to wheezing.[330] In the past, cough was under-recognized as a symptom of asthma. In recent years children with recurrent cough as the sole respiratory symptom have increasingly been labelled as having asthma.[331] However, there is evidence from epidemiological studies,[34,332,333] blocking studies[334] and from measurement of the time of occurrence of coughing[335] that they are separate entities. While the mechanisms of cough and wheezing are related, they have distinct pathways and may be triggered independently.[336]

Although cough is a common symptom, it has been difficult to assess objectively. Diary cards have proved unreliable.[41] More objective cough counting systems used in research studies are starting to lead to a better understanding of cough and its treatment.[336]

Cough alone is a poor marker of asthma. Only about 5–6% of children with asthma present with cough as the only symptom,[337] and most will also have evidence of abnormal pulmonary function tests in keeping with asthma. Cough caused by asthma will usually respond quickly to relatively straight forward asthma medications; if it does not, then the diagnosis of asthma should be reconsidered and further investigations undertaken. In children with recurrent cough without other evidence of airway function, neither inhaled salbutamol nor beclomethasone is beneficial.[338] In a few children with cough, a short therapeutic trial of asthma treatment may be indicated. However, it is important to stop such treatment if it is not beneficial and not to increase the dose. There is no objective evidence to support the use of high doses or prolonged courses of inhaled corticosteroids in children with cough alone. In infants, cough as the only symptom warrants comprehensive investigation.

Nocturnal Disturbance and Waking with
Asthma (see also Chapter 37)
Nocturnal disturbance is common in asthmatic children. About three-quarters of asthmatic children are affected, one-third on a regular basis and a small pro-

portion nearly every night. Such disturbance has a substantial impact on well-being and mental functioning.[339] Many children feel sleepy in school the next day, or stay at home because they are too tired.[3] Nocturnal disturbance is also frequently disruptive for parents and siblings. During acute exacerbations, children frequently deteriorate in the early hours of the morning, leading to contact with family practitioners or attendance at emergency departments.

Continuing nocturnal symptoms generally indicate more severe asthma,[340,341] and poor asthmatic control.[342] Nocturnal symptoms are not always reported spontaneously.[341] Since they predict more severe disease, it is, therefore, important to ask specifically about nocturnal symptoms, medication use during the night and the impact of nocturnal disturbance on both child and family. PEF charting may show excessive diurnal variation. However, diary cards may not accurately reflect nocturnal symptoms.[41]

For mild nocturnal symptoms, a nocturnal bronchodilator may be sufficient. However, usually it will be necessary to increase prophylactic treatment, often by means of inhaled corticosteroids.[343] If inhaled steroids do not control the symptoms, then a long-acting bronchodilator should be introduced. Long-acting inhaled β_2 agonists such as salmeterol are probably the best choice, and have been shown to improve the nocturnal symptoms of children with mild-to-moderate asthma.[344] Oral slow-release bronchodilators are an alternative, but may have a high incidence of side-effects[345] and do not improve objective sleep quality in adults; indeed theophyllines may even worsen it.[346] With appropriate treatment it is usually possible to improve a child's nocturnal asthma.

Unfortunately, nocturnal cough – often the most troublesome symptom[347] – can be difficult to settle. Generally, it is not necessary to look for other diagnoses. However, where nocturnal symptoms respond poorly to asthma treatment other possible diagnoses such as pertussis should be considered. Improving nasal symptoms due to allergic rhinitis may also help.

Is It Due to Something in the Diet? (see also Chapter 44)

Ingested substances can occasionally affect airway function (Table 29.24)[348] and may be identified by parents and children as exacerbating asthma.

Typically, two situations arise. In the first, the parents or child spontaneously give a clear history that a par-

Table 29.24: Dietary ingestants causing diet-related asthma. (Adapted from Wilson NM. Diet related asthma in children. Paediatr Respir Med 1993; 1: 14–20.)

Type	Examples
Ingested protein allergens	Eggs, milk, fish, wheat, nuts
Food additives Metabisulphite and sulphur dioxide Artificial colourings and other preservatives Aspirin and acetylsalicylic acid	Tartrazine, sodium benzoate
Physical agents	Cold drinks Fizzy drinks with low pH (e.g. cola)

ticular ingestant has precipitated asthmatic symptoms, often accompanied with other acute allergic features such as urticaria. The child may have other atopic features such as eczema. Ethnic differences occur; for example, Asian children are more sensitive to cola drinks, ice and fried foods.[68] The parents may already have carried out simple food challenges, and may already have instituted dietary avoidance, especially if the substance is not a common dietary constituent. In these situations, further objective confirmation is usually unnecessary, and the parents should continue to avoid the substance.

A second more difficult situation arises where parents worry that food is a factor in their child's symptoms, but cannot identify any particular culprit. In this situation, a link between asthmatic symptoms and oral ingestants is often not confirmed objectively.[349] Immunological markers such as skin tests or RASTs are not particularly useful in diagnosing asthma associated with food allergy. Many asthmatic children are atopic and can have positive responses to foods without any evidence that the food causes asthmatic symptoms. Objective confirmation then depends on a formal food challenge, which should be blind and placebo-controlled. Unfortunately, food challenges give rise to a number of problems. Firstly, variations of lung function over time may confound the effect of the ingestant, making it difficult to demonstrate reactions occurring anything more than a few hours after ingestion. Secondly, asthma prophylaxis may attenuate or abolish a response to an ingestant. More difficult problems arise if repeated doses are required or where the response to the substance is enhanced by an additional stimulus such as exercise. In some cases, a change in bronchial responsiveness has been clearly documented without a change in baseline lung function.[68]

Where a particular dietary substance is clearly identified as causing asthmatic symptoms, eliminating the item from the child's diet may be possible. Accidental ingestion, if it occurs, can be treated symptomatically. As children grow out of food allergies, periodic re-testing may be useful, particularly where the substance is a basic or frequently encountered dietary constituent, such as milk or eggs, the exclusion of which makes the diet unduly complicated.

Where children present with mild asthma but no clear history of ingestant-related symptoms, a search for hidden dietary factors is usually not worthwhile. Even if the symptoms are rather more troublesome, pro-phylactic asthma treatment may prevent or substan-tially alleviate the problem without the necessity of resorting to formal food challenges.

Children with more severe asthma that is difficult to control may be considered for an elimination diet to screen for unrecognized food allergies, but only after all other factors have been excluded. Such diets are often very restrictive and unpalatable, and may be nutrition-ally deficient. A dietitian should always carefully super-vise them. It should be remembered that drugs often have preservatives or colourings that may have to be excluded. If clinical improvement occurs, the diet can be gradually liberalized, preferably one item at a time. If deterioration occurs, the provoking substance can be avoided. If improvement does not occur within a defined period, the diet should be discontinued.

Is It Psychological? (see also Chapter 40)

The clear consensus is that childhood asthma is a phys-ical disease. There are nevertheless related psychosocial factors. Emotions such as anger or excitement can trigger asthmatic symptoms.[350] The asthma itself may have psychological side-effects such as stigma, loss of self-esteem, and strained family relationships. In chil-dren who died from asthma, psychosocial factors, par-ticularly depression, have been more frequent.[351,352] Further, asthma may affect family dynamics: mani-pulative children may use the illness to get their own way;[353] parents may be over-protective or unwilling

to discipline an asthmatic child. Finally, psychological factors such as fear of observing the symptoms or the threat of serious complications may lead to denial of the condition, and may compromise the success of treatment.[354]

Many of these psychosocial factors give rise to poor communication and poor compliance, and are associ-ated with feelings of hopelessness about the illness. Such factors must, therefore, be addressed in order to achieve successful treatment. Clinicians should be exceptionally wary when high-risk psychological features are present in children with severe asthma (Table 29.25).

Occasionally, a functional laryngeal obstruction causes or aggravates asthmatic symptoms[355] resulting in wheezing which is resistant to treatment. The diag-nosis can be difficult, but there may be clinical clues. The child, often an adolescent, may be mostly free of wheeze when asleep at night or during anaesthesia. There may be variable dyspnoea when awake, often increased by stress or anxiety (caused sometimes by the mere approach of the physician). On auscultation, the wheezing may be poorly heard in the lower lung fields, and appear to be localized in the extra-thoracic trachea. Management is likely to involve consultation with a mental health professional.

Effective management of asthma should always recognize the psychosocial adjustment of the child and family, particularly where the child has severe asthma and high-risk psychological features or risk factors for death from asthma (Table 29.26). Such children should have regular follow-up with specific concentration on risk factors. For example, intensive education may help to address poor self-care, and tailoring the medication to the child's routine may aid compliance. Intervention by a child psychiatrist or social worker may be necessary and can result in improvement in asthma control.[352,356] Behavioural approaches (extending to the child's family) can modify the reaction to emotional triggers, deal with manipulative behaviour and improve compliance. Residential schooling may occasionally be helpful for children with severe asthma who fail to respond to out-patient management and psychosocial care.[357]

What About Heating and Housing?

During the last 30 years, substantial changes in indoor environment, including heating and insulation and the more widespread use of fitted carpets, have combined to produce an environment that is ideal for the house-dust mite.

Table 29.25: High-risk psychological variables (From Strunk RC. Identification of the fatality-prone subject with asthma. *J Allergy Clin Immunol* 1989; 83: 477–85, with permission)

Wheezing with stress
    Parents and/or physician consider stress a frequent factor for acute episodes

Problems in self-care
    Parents and/or physician state that there are regular problems
    Child's inability to respond appropriately to asthma symptoms
    Child's inability to attend to routine prophylactic care

Disregard of perceived symptoms
    No action taken to recognized asthma symptoms

Conflict between parent and physician, child and physician or parent–child
    Positive when perceived by either parent or physician
    Ongoing
        Disagreement
        Frustration
        Dissatisfaction with performance of either of identified persons involved

Family dysfunction
    Marital discord
    Lack of parental support to child
    Parental drug or alcohol abuse
    Financial stress
    Inappropriate use of resources

Reaction to separation or loss
    Child frequently has excessive and developmentally inappropriate responses to separation from parent or carer
    A significant loss from which the child has not recovered symptoms, e.g. death of a parent

Emotional disturbance
    Severe enough to require referral for psychiatric treatment

Manipulative use of asthma
    Use of asthma symptoms to:
        Avoid unpleasant tasks
        Place pressure on others to respond to child's wishes

Depression
    Specific psychiatric disturbance (diagnosed from symptoms, affect and functioning)
    Hopelessness/despair (expressed emotional state and direct/indirect references to suicide)

Another significant health hazard that has been recognized in the last 15 years is damp housing. There is now considerable evidence that damp and mouldy housing has a detrimental effect on the respiratory health of children.[114,358,359] There is also evidence that damp and mouldy housing is associated with symptomatic asthma.[115] The effects appear to be related to mould and is not clearly related to other factors such as exposure to house-dust mite antigen.[116,360] Reducing indoor humidity has been shown to lead to significant improvement in peak expiratory flow.[108] However, decreased humidity usually requires increased ventilation, which leads to heat loss and increased fuel bills.

Table 29.26: Factors which point to a high risk for asthma mortality. (From Refs 78, 351, 375–377. with permission)

Previous history of acute life-threatening attacks

Hospitalization within the previous year

Psychosocial problems

Recent reduction or cessation of corticosteroids

Non-compliance with recommended medical therapy (especially in teenagers)

Socioeconomic factors – low income, inner city, poor access to medical care, cultural differences

The best type of heating for an asthmatic child is not known. Recent evidence relating to adults suggests that those with moderate to severe asthma should reduce their exposure to indoor sources of combustion such as gas stoves, fireplaces or wood stoves. Evidence relating to children suggests that symptoms of respiratory tract irritation are commoner in homes heated by wood stoves.[361]

Overall, present evidence suggests that asthmatic children are best housed in dry, warm accommodation with some form of closed heating.

What Happens at School?

Asthma is now so common, affecting 1 in 10 children or more, that an average school class is likely to have two or three children with asthma. An asthmatic child may be absent from school as a result of the disease on average 7–10 days per year.[1] In more severe cases, 30 days absence per year is not uncommon.[362] Help may be needed to allow a child to keep up with schoolwork. There is still evidence of under-diagnosis and under-treatment of asthma in school children.[28,29]

Teachers are responsible for asthmatic children during school hours, and may have to take decisions about physical activities and treatment, both emergency and regular. All too often teachers have a limited understanding of the condition; few receive training and, not surprisingly, many feel inadequate to cope with an asthmatic child.[363] Teachers should be informed of the stimuli which can precipitate attacks; the standard anti-asthma medicines; and the steps to take if a child has an acute attack.

The school environment may present a problem. Guinea pigs, hamsters, birds and rabbits may have to be removed from the classroom if there are asthmatics in the class. Fumes from experiments or glues can also trigger symptoms.

Medications to be taken at school often cause problems. Many children do not like carrying their medication with them, and find it embarrassing to use inhalers at school or in front of their friends.[3] The use of twice-daily prophylactic treatment and long-acting bronchodilators before school may help.[139] Coping with inhaled medication is also a problem for many schools because of anxieties about other children taking the medication inappropriately. Fortunately, the inhaled drugs available today are not toxic in normal children, even in very large doses.

Children with asthma usually know when they need their inhalers and should have easy access to them. Regrettably, but all too often, children are not allowed to keep their own inhalers and, in some cases, parents would even be expected to come to school to administer medications to their children.[364] Ideally, older children (above 7 years) should keep their inhalers with them and be responsible for taking them. A responsible adult should supervise younger children. If there are difficulties, assistance from the school nurse or local community health services should be sought.

Exercise-induced symptoms can interfere with school games and sport. Prolonged outdoor running on a cold, dry winter day is an activity particularly likely to provoke wheezing but even swimming, which is generally well-tolerated, may provoke symptoms.[3] Accordingly, while the use of appropriate warm-up exercises and β_2 agonists before activities may help avoid symptoms, children should carry their medication with them and use it if they become symptomatic.

Minor attacks need not interrupt a child's school day. Rapid use of reliever should help to control the problem and allow the child to continue. If the attack is severe with marked distress or inability to talk, or if the reliever does not work within 5–10 minutes, or if the child is getting exhausted urgent medical advice must be called. Ten to twenty puffs of bronchodilator via a large volume spacer may be given while awaiting medical help.

Can I Take My Child On Holiday?

Parents often worry that asthma exacerbations may occur away from home, and are not sure whether it is safe to go on holiday. Such anxieties restrict their choice of holiday.[3]

Planning ahead is important, particularly where the holiday involves a foreign country. Asthma societies frequently provide useful information pamphlets about going on holiday. Travelling, particularly by air, is not usually a problem, but for long journeys avoiding cigarette smoke can be important.

Unfortunately, there is no guaranteed safe or best place for asthmatics to go on holiday. It is sensible to avoid trigger factors but not always possible to predict all possible hazards in advance. Damp or mouldy accommodation, exposure to unusual aero-allergens such as pollens or animal danders in country areas, house-dust mite in hotel rooms or certain weather conditions can all exacerbate asthma. Air pollution is a problem in some countries. Cigarette smoke can sometimes be difficult to avoid.

A clinic appointment just before a holiday provides an opportunity to review the child's treatment plan. A letter from the physician outlining the diagnosis and treatment may be useful, both for negotiating customs and advising local physicians in the event of an attack. Regular preventive treatment should help to avoid most problems. Stepping-down treatment just before departure should be avoided.

Parents should take sufficient quantities of both routine and emergency medications to cover the period of the holiday. A medical pack for emergencies including a written emergency action plan, adequate "relieving" treatment including a large volume spacer and a full MDI, and a course of steroids, should be carried. Children aged over 5 years should take their peak flow meter. Parents should be given specific instruction on multi-dosing using a spacer for emergencies. In an emergency, a plastic coffee cup and β_2 agonist can provide effective and portable bronchodilation. Where the child is dependent on a nebulizer, it is important to check the electrical voltage in the foreign country and to make sure that the nebulizer will work there. Any necessary electrical adapters should be purchased in advance. Some nebulizers can handle multiple voltages; alternatively, a hand or foot pump nebulizer or battery operated compressor may be used.

Since medical care abroad can be expensive, adequate insurance cover or the appropriate certificate to allow reciprocal health care is essential. If asthma is severe and an exacerbation likely, it is sensible find out in advance how and where to obtain medical atten-

tion. Happily, problems with asthma on holidays are rare.

Will It Get Better?

Parents frequently want to know what will happen in the longer term. There are as yet few population-based and longitudinal cohort studies of the natural course of asthma from childhood to adult life.[343] Most of the published studies start at around 7 years of age[70,313,365,366] or later.[367] Most studies have also been based on moderate or severe asthmatics and, therefore, provide limited information on the full range of the disease.[368]

Despite these limitations, the evidence is reassuring. Over 20–25 years about two-thirds of children with asthma will outgrow their disease and be symptom-free as adults, especially those with mild disease. About a third with more severe disease will have persistent symptoms in adult life. Asthma usually improves during the teenage years, although less so for girls than boys.[313,314] The amount of wheezing in early adolescence seems to be a guide for severity in later life; about 70% of those with few symptoms at age 14 continue to have little or no asthma at age 28 and conversely about 70% of those with frequent symptoms at age 14 are still having recurrent symptoms at age 28.[366] Other risk factors have been identified (Table 29.27) and may provide targets for preventive and/or more aggressive treatment strategies in the future. Interestingly, about

Table 29.27: Risk factors for persistence of childhood asthma	
Sex	Conflicting evidence
Age of onset	Yes; early onset
Severity of asthma	Yes; more severe
Eczema	Yes
Family history of atopy	Yes
Smoking (active/passive)	Yes
Level of lung function	Yes; impaired lung function at age 7 predicts asthmatic symptoms
Treatment	Not known

one in nine children not reported as having asthma at 7 years will have developed asthma by age 30, with female sex, family history of asthma and lower lung function at age 7 being important risk factors.[365]

Other outcomes also seem generally favourable. Although growth may be delayed, particularly during puberty, final height appears to be normal.[175,176,313] The social outcome, too, in terms of education, employment, housing and social class is not greatly affected, at least for mild or moderate asthma.[369,370] One recurrent finding is that smoking is no less common in asthmatics than in the general population, even though asthmatic smokers are more likely to be symptomatic.[367]

Does treatment influence outcome? In particular, can a prolonged remission from asthma be achieved by long-term use of inhaled corticosteroids? Evidence from children is limited. van Essen-Zandvliet et al.[164] showed that 28–36 months of treatment with inhaled corticosteroids and regular bronchodilator improved both symptoms and objective measures of lung function in almost all children. Mean PD_{20} histamine stabilized after 20 months, but usually did not normalize, and even after 36 months on inhaled corticosteroids airway responsiveness remained abnormal in the majority. Cessation of inhaled corticosteroids was followed by a rapid decrease in lung function and a deterioration in lung function,[171] suggesting that the underlying inflammatory process was still present even after years on inhaled corticosteroids, and thus that the asthma had not been "cured". Treatment should, therefore, be aimed principally at symptomatic remission, i.e. normalization in symptoms, without the need for additional bronchodilator.

The long-term relationship between asthma in children and chronic obstructive lung disease remains unclear.[371]

CONCLUSION

In the main, childhood asthma is a simple and rewarding disease to treat. Effective treatments with a low incidence of side-effects are now available. Children can be cared for in the community, and their symptoms and ability to lead a normal life substantially improved by appropriate treatment. Referral to a hospital paediatrician will only be required in certain circumstances. Despite this, under-diagnosis and poor symptom control are still all too common. Comprehensive guidelines summarizing the best in present practice are

KEY POINTS

1 *Diagnosis*
   (a) Diagnosis depends on a detailed history.
   (b) Recurrent episodes of cough, wheeze and difficulty breathing are the key symptoms.
   (c) Viral infections and exercise are the main triggers.
   (d) Physical signs, if present, should be generalized not focal, and are not essential for diagnosis.
   (e) Be careful when diagnosing asthma in children under one year, especially if cough is the only symptom or growth is poor.

2 *Management*
   (a) Effective management requires an informed partnership between parents, children and doctors.
   (b) Avoid trigger factors, particularly passive cigarette smoking, where possible.
   (c) Plan ahead – agree clear written plans for treating chronic asthma and managing exacerbations.
   (d) Devices are critical to the success of inhaled therapy in children – choose carefully and check frequently.
   (e) Attainment of final height may be delayed but is usually normal.

3 *Special problems*
   (a) Treating children under two asthma is often difficult – for everyone.
   (b) Expect poor compliance with medication, at all ages.
   (c) Aim to achieve normal exercise performance.
   (d) Nocturnal disturbances are common and can be difficult to prevent completely.
   (e) Beware of asthmatic children with depression.
   (f) Asthma usually improves around puberty, particularly for boys – it may recur in the twenties.
   (g) Current evidence suggests asthma can be controlled but not cured.

available, but successful treatment requires careful implementation of what is already known. Problem areas remain. A better understanding of wheezing illnesses in infants and young children is still needed, particularly the relationship between asthma and viral respiratory infections. The factors that cause or contribute to asthma must also be better understood if effective preventive measures are to be developed.

REFERENCES

1. Hill RA, Standen PJ, Tattersfield AE. Asthma, wheezing and school absence in primary schools. *Arch Dis Child* 1989; 64: 246–51.

2. Speight ANP, Lee DA, Hey EW. Underdiagnosis and undertreatment of asthma in childhood. *BMJ* 1983; 286: 1253–6.

3. Lenney W, Wells NEJ, O'Neil BA. Burden of paediatric asthma. *Eur Respir Rev* 1994; 4: 49–62.

4. Hyndman SJ, Williams DRR, Merrill SL, Lipscombe JM, Palmer CR. Rates of admission to hospital for asthma. *BMJ* 1994; 308: 1596–600.

5. Nocon A, Booth T. The social impact of asthma. *Fam Pract* 1991; 8: 37–41.

6. Omran M, Russell G. Continuing increase in respiratory symptoms and atopy in Aberdeen schoolchildren. *BMJ* 1996; 312: 34.

7. Venn A, Lewis S, Cooper M, Hill J, Britton J. Increasing prevalence of wheeze and asthma in Nottingham primary schoolchildren 1988–1995. *Eur Respir J* 1998; 11: 1324–8.

8. Phelan PD. Asthma in childhood: epidemiology. *BMJ* 1994; 308: 1584–5.

9. Magnus P, Jaakkola JJ. Secular trend in the occurrence of asthma among children and young adults: critical appraisal of repeated cross sectional surveys. *BMJ* 1997; 314: 1795–9.

10. Cullinan P, Newman Taylor AJ. Asthma in children: environmental factors. *BMJ* 1994; 308: 1585–6.

11. Woolcock AJ, Peat JK. Evidence for the increase in asthma worldwide. *Ciba Found Symp* 1997; 206: 122–34.

12. Anderson HR, Butland BK, Strachan DP. Trends in prevalence and severity of childhood asthma. *BMJ* 1994; 308: 1600–1604.

13. Anderson HR, Bailey PA, Cooper JS, Palmer JC. Influence of morbidity, illness label, and social, family, and health service factors on drug treatment of childhood asthma. *Lancet* 1981; ii: 1030–32.

14. Laitinen LA, Heino M, Laitinen A, Kava T, Haahtela T. Damage of the airway epithelium and bronchial reactivity in patients with asthma. *Am Rev Respir Dis* 1985; 139: 599–606.

15. Djukanovic R, Roche WR, Eilson JW *et al*. State of the art. Mucosal inflammation in asthma. *Am Rev Respir Dis* 1990; 142: 434–57.

16. Barnes PJ. New concepts in asthma and the implications for therapy. In: Mitchell DM (ed). *Recent Advances in Respiratory Medicine No. 5*. London: Churchill Livingstone, 1991: 45–60.

17. Snapper JR. Inflammation and airway function: the asthma syndrome. *Am Rev Respir Dis* 1990; 141: 531–3.

18. Lee DA, Winslow NR, Speight ANP, Hey EW. Prevalence and spectrum of asthma in childhood. *BMJ* 1983; 286: 1256–8.

19. Clough JB, Williams JD, Holgate ST. Effect of atopy on the natural history of symptoms, peak expiratory flow, and bronchial responsiveness in 7- and 8-year-old children with cough and wheeze. A 12-month longitudinal study. *Am Rev Respir Dis* 1991; 143: 755–60.

20. Cutz E, Levison H, Cooper DM. Ultrastructure of airways in children with asthma. *Histopathology* 1978; 2: 407–21.

21. Lanz MJ, Leung DY, McCormick DR, Harbeck R, Szefler SJ, White CW. Comparison of exhaled nitric oxide, serum eosinophilic cationic protein, and soluble interleukin-2 receptor in exacerbations of pediatric asthma. *Pediatr Pulmonol* 1997; 24: 305–11.

22. Cai Y, Carty K, Henry RL, Gibson PG. Persistence of sputum eosinophilia in children with controlled asthma when compared with healthy children. *Eur Respir J* 1998; 11: 848–53.

23. Stevenson EC, Turner G, Heaney LG *et al.* Bronchoalveolar lavage findings suggest two different forms of childhood asthma. *Clin Exp Allergy* 1997; 27: 1027–35.

24. Gibson PG. Use of induced sputum to examine airway inflammation in childhood asthma. *J Allergy Clin Immunol* 1998; 102: S100–S101.

25. ❂ Silverman M. Out of the mouths of babes and sucklings: lessons from early childhood asthma. *Thorax* 1993; 48: 1200–4.

26. Clough JB, Holgate ST. Episodes of respiratory morbidity in children with cough and wheeze. *Am J Respir Crit Care Med* 1994; 150: 48–53.

27. Stein RT, Holberg CJ, Morgan WJ *et al.* Peak flow variability, methacholine responsiveness and atopy as markers for detecting different wheezing phenotypes in childhood. *Thorax* 1997; 52: 946–52.

28. Spee-van der Wekke J, Meulmeester JF, Radder JJ, Verloove-Vanhorick SP. School absence and treatment in school children with respiratory symptoms in the Netherlands: data from the Child Health Monitoring System. *J Epidemiol Community Health* 1998; 52: 359–63.

29. Momas I, Dartiguenave C, Fauroux B *et al.* Prevalence of asthma or respiratory symptoms among children attending primary schools in Paris. *Pediatr Pulmonol* 1998; 26: 106–112.

30. Clifford RD, Radford M, Howell JB, Holgate ST. Prevalence of respiratory symptoms among 7 and 11 year old schoolchildren and association with asthma. *Arch Dis Child* 1989; 64: 1118–125.

31. The British Guidelines on Asthma Management–1995 review and position statement. *Thorax* 1997; 52: Suppl. 1.

32. ❂ Expert Panel Report, No. 2. *Guidelines for the Diagnosis and Management of Asthma*. NIH Publication No. 97–4051. Bethesda, MD: National Institutes of Health, 1997.

33. Warner JO, Naspitz CK, Cropp GJA. Third international pediatric consensus statement on the management of childhood asthma. *Pediatr Pulmonol* 1998; 25: 1–17.

34. Luyt DK, Burton PR, Simpson H. Epidemiological study of wheeze, doctor diagnosed asthma, and cough in preschool children in Leicestershire. *BMJ* 1993; 306: 1386–9.

35. Johnson D, Osborne LM. Cough variant asthma: a review of the clinical literature. *J Asthma* 1991; 28: 85–90.

36. Hetzel MR, Clark TJH. Comparison of normal and asthmatic circadian rhythms in peak expiratory flow rate. *Thorax* 1980; 35: 732–8.

37. Henderson AJW, Carswell F. Circadian rhythm of peak expiratory flow rate in asthmatic children. *Thorax* 1989; 44: 410–14.

38. Wilson NM. Wheezy bronchitis revisited. *Arch Dis Child* 1989; 64: 1194–9.

39. Ninan TK, Russell G. Asthma, inhaled corticosteroid treatment, and growth. *Arch Dis Child* 1992; 67: 703–705.

40. Ferguson AC, Murray AB, Wah-Jun T. Short stature and delayed skeletal maturation in children with allergic disease. *J Allergy Clin Immunol* 1982; 69: 461–6.

41. Archer LNJ, Simpson H. Night coughs and diary card scores in asthma. *Arch Dis Child* 1985; 60: 473–4.

42. Lister J, Budin-Jones S, Palmer J, Cochrane GM. How accurate are asthma diary cards? *Arch Dis Child* 1994; 44: 343.

43. Hyland ME, Kenyon CAP, Allen R, Howarth P. Diary keeping in asthma: comparison of written and electronic methods. *BMJ* 1993; 306: 487–9.

44. Chowienczyk PJ, Lawson CP, Morris J, Kermani A, Cochrane GM. Electronic diary to record physiological measurements. *Lancet* 1992; 339: 251.

45. Nairn JR, Bennett AJ, Andrew JD, MacArthur P. A study of respiratory function in normal school children; the peak flow rate. *Arch Dis Child* 1961; 36: 253–6.

46. Burge PS. Peak flow measurement. *Thorax* 1992; 47: 903.

47. Milner AD, Ingram D. PEFRs in children under 5 years of age. *Arch Dis Child* 1970; 45: 820–23.

48. Connolly CK. Falsely high peak expiratory flow readings due to acceleration in the mouth. *BMJ* 1987; 294: 285.

49. Brand PL, Duiverman EJ, Waalkens HJ, van Essen-Zandvliet EE, Kerrebijn KF. Peak flow variation in childhood asthma: correlation with symptoms, airways obstruction, and hyperresponsiveness during long-term treatment with inhaled corticosteroids. Dutch CNSLD Study Group. *Thorax* 1999; 54: 103–107.

50. Godfrey S, Kamburoff PL, Nairn JR. Spirometry, lung volumes and airway resistance. *Br J Dis Chest* 1970; 64: 15–24.

51. Sly PD, Hibbert ME, Landau LI. Diurnal variation of peak expiratory flow rate in asthmatic children. *Pediatr Pulmonol* 1986; 2: 141–6.

52. Linna OV. Twice-daily peak expiratory flow rate monitoring for the assessment of childhood asthma. *Allergy Proc* 1993; 14: 33–6.

53. Landau LI. The value of lung function in guiding drug therapy in childhood asthma. *Eur Respir Rev* 1994; 4: 10–14.

54. Pool JB, Greenough A, Price JF. Abnormalities of functional residual capacity in symptomatic and asymptomatic young asthmatics. *Acta Paediatr Scand* 1988; 77: 419–23.

55. Bridge PD, Ranganathan S, McKenzie SA. Measurement of airway resistance using the interrupter technique in preschool children in the ambulatory setting. *Eur Respir J* 1999; 13: 792–6.

56. Pattemore PK, Innes Asher M, Harrison AC, Mitchell EA, Rea HH, Stewart AW. The interrelationship among bronchial hyperresponsiveness, the diagnosis of asthma, and asthma symptoms. *Am Rev Respir Dis* 1990; 142: 549–54.

57. Empey DW, Laitinen LA, Jacobs L, Gold WM, Nadel JA. Mechanisms of bronchial hyperreactivity in normal subjects after upper respiratory tract infection. *Am Rev Respir Dis* 1976; 113: 131–9.

58. Clifford RD, Radford M, Howell JB, Holgate ST. Prevalence of respiratory symtpoms among 7 and 11 year old schoolchildren and association with asthma. *Arch Dis Child* 1989; 64: 1118–25.

59. Clough JB, Williams JD, Holgate ST. The profile of bronchial responsiveness in children with respiratory symptoms. *Arch Dis Child* 1992; 67: 574–9.

60. Josephs LK, Gregg I, Mullee MA, Holgate ST. Nonspecific bronchial reactivity and its relationship to the clinical expression of asthma. A longitudinal study. *Am Rev Respir Dis* 1989; 140: 350–57.

61. Altamirano HG, McGready SJ, Mansmann HC. Right middle lobe syndromes in asthmatic children. *Pediatr Asthma Allergy Immunol* 1991; 5: 33–7.

62. Eigen H, Laughlin JJ, Homrighausen J. Recurrent pneumonia in children and its relationship to bronchial hyperreactivity. *Pediatrics* 1982; 70: 698–704.

63. Murray AB, Milner RA. The accuracy of features in the clinical history for predicting atopic sensitization to airborne allergens in children. *J Allergy Clin Immunol* 1995; 96: 588–96.

64. Ownby DR. Allergy testing: *in vivo* versus *in vitro*. *Pediatr Clin North Am* 1988; 35: 995–1009.

65. Burrows B, Mortimer FD, Halonen M, Barbee RA, Cline MG. Association of asthma with serum IgE levels and skin-test reactivity to allergens. *N Engl J Med* 1989; 320: 271–7.

66. Sporik R, Holgate ST, Platts-Mills TAE, Cogswell JJ. Exposure to house-dust mite allergen (Der p 1) and the development of asthma in childhood: A prospective study. *N Engl J Med* 1990; 323: 502–507.

67. Adkinson NF. The radioallergosorbent test in 1981–limitations and refinements. *J Allergy Clin Immunol* 1981; 67: 87–9.

68. Wilson NM, Silverman M. Diagnosis of food sensitivity in childhood asthma. *J R Soc Med* 1985; 78: 11–16.

69. The British guidelines on asthma management. *Thorax* 1997; 52(suppl. 1): S1–S21.

70. Oswald H, Phelan PD, Lannigan A, Hibbert ME, Bowes G, Olinsky A. Outcome of childhood asthma in mid-adult life. *BMJ* 1994; 309: 95–6.

71. Madge P, McColl J and Paton J. Impact of a nurse-led home management training programme in children

admitted with acute asthma: a randomised controlled study. *Thorax* 1997; 52: 223–8.

72. Evans D. To help patients control asthma the clinician must be a good listener and teacher. *Thorax* 1993; 48: 685–7.

73. Korsch BM, Negrete VF. Doctor patient communication. *Sci Am* 1972; 227: 66–72.

74. Roter DL, Hall JA, Kern DE, Barker LR, Cole KA, Roca RP. Improving physicians' interviewing skills and reducing patients' emotional distress. A randomized clinical trial. *Arch Intern Med* 1995; 155: 1877–84.

75. Beasley CRW, Cushley M, Holgate ST. A self management plan in the treatment of adult asthma. *Thorax* 1989; 44: 200–204.

76. Charlton I, Antoniou AG, Atkinson J et al. Asthma at the interface: bridging the gap between general practice and a district general hospital. *Arch Dis Child* 1994; 70: 313–8.

77. Klingelhofer EL, Gershwin ME. Asthma self management programs: Premises, not promises. *J Asthma* 1988; 25: 89–101.

78. Fletcher HJ, Ibrahim SA, Speight ANP. Survey of asthma deaths in the Northern region 1970–1985. *Arch Dis Child* 1990; 65: 163–7.

79. Coutts JA, Gibson NA, Paton JY. Measuring compliance with inhaled medication in asthma. *Arch Dis Child* 1992; 67: 332–3.

80. Gibson NA, Ferguson AE, Aitchison TC, Paton JY. Compliance with inhaled asthma medication in preschool children. *Thorax* 1995; 50: 1274–9.

81. Milgrom H, Bender B, Ackerson L, Bowry P, Smith B, Rand C. Noncompliance and treatment failure in children with asthma. *J Allergy Clin Immunol* 1996; 98: 1051–7.

82. Sackett DL, Haynes RB. *Compliance with Therapeutic Regimens*. Baltimore and London: John Hopkins University Press, 1976.

83. Korhonen K, Korppi M, Remes ST, Reijonen K, Remes K. Lung function in school-aged children with inhaled cromoglycate, nedocromil and corticosteroid therapy. *Eur Respir J* 1999; 13: 82–6.

84. Clark NM, Gong M, Schork MA et al. Impact of education for physicians on patient outcomes. *Pediatrics* 1998; 101: 831–36.

85. Geertsen HR, Gray RM, Ward JR. Patient non-compliance within the context of seeking medical care for arthritis. *J Chronic Dis* 1973; 26: 689–98.

86. Partridge MR. Asthma education: More reading or more viewing? *J R Soc Med* 1994; 79: 326–8.

87. Mulloy EMT, Albazzaz MK, Warley ARH, Harvey JE. Video education for patients who use inhalers. *Thorax* 1987; 42: 719–20.

88. Sly PD, Landau LI, Weymouth R. Home recording of peak expiratory flow rates and perception of asthma. *Am J Dis Child* 1985; 139: 479–82.

89. Shim CS, Williams H. Relationship of wheezing to the severity of airway obstruction in asthma. *Arch Intern Med* 1992; 1983; 890–92.

90. Peroni DG, Boner AL, Vallone G, Antolini I, Warner JO. Effective allergen avoidance at high altitude reduces allergen-induced bronchial hyperresponsiveness. *Am J Respir Crit Care Med* 1994; 149: 1442–6.

91. Korsgaard J. Mite allergy and residence: a case controlled study on the impact of exposure to house-dust mites in dwellings. *Am Rev Respir Dis* 1983; 128: 231–5.

92. Warner JA, Marchant JL, Warner JO. Double blind trial of ionisers in children with asthma sensitive to the house dust mite. *Thorax* 1993; 48: 330–33.

93. Report of international workshop. Dust mite allergens and asthma–a worldwide problem. *J Allergy Clin Immunol* 1989; 83: 416–27.

94. Platts-Mills TAE, Heymann PW, Longbottom JL, Wilkins SR. Airborne allergens associated with asthma: particle sizes carrying dust mite and rat allergens measured with a cascade impactor. *J Allergy Clin Immunol* 1986; 77: 850–57.

95. Murray AB, Ferguson AC, Morrison AJ. Diagnosis of house dust mite allergy in asthmatic children: What constitutes a positive history? *J Allergy Clin Immunol* 1983; 71: 21–8.

96. Feather IH, Warner JA, Holgate ST, Thompson PJ, Stewart GA. Cohabiting with domestic mites. *Thorax* 1993; 48: 5–9.

97. Sarsfield JK, Gowland G, Toy R, Norman ALE. Mite-sensitive asthma of childhood: trial of avoidance measures. *Arch Dis Child* 1974; 49: 716–21.

98. Godfrey RC, Griffiths M. The prevalence of immediate positive skin test to *Dermatophagoides pteronyssinus* and grass pollen in school children. *Clin Allergy* 1976; 6: 79–82.

99. Charpin D, Birnbaum J, Haddi E. Altitude and allergy to house dust mites. *Am Rev Respir Dis* 1991; 143: 983–6.

100. Platts-Mills TAE, Mitchell EB, Nock P, Tovey ER, Moszoro H, Wilkins SR. Reduction of bronchial hyperreactivity during prolonged allergen avoidance. *Lancet* 1982; ii: 675–8.

101. Murray AB, Ferguson AC. Dust free bedrooms in the treatment of children with house dust mite allergy: a controlled trial. *Pediatrics* 1983; 71: 418–22.

102. Owen S, Morganstern M, Hepworth J, Woodcock A. Control of house dust mite antigen in bedding. *Lancet* 1990; 335: 396–7.

103. Ehnert B, Lau-Schadendorf S, Weber A, Buettner P, Wahn E. Reducing domestic exposure to dust mite allergen reduces bronchial hyperreactivity in sensitive children with asthma. *J Allergy Clin Immunol* 1992; 90: 135–8.

104. Kemp TJ, Siebers RW, Fishwick D, O'Grady GB, Fitzharris P, Crane J. House dust mite allergen in pillows. *BMJ* 1996; 313: 916.

105. Carswell F, Robinson DW, Oliver J, Clark J, Robinson P, Wadsworth J. House dust mites in Bristol. *Clin Allergy* 1982; 12: 533–45.

106. Custovic A, Woodcock A. Environmental manipulation: practical steps in the home to benefit asthma patients. *Asthma J* 1999; 4: 24–7.

107. Collof MJ. Use of liquid nitrogen in the control of house dust mite populations. *Clin Allergy* 1986; 16: 411–17.

108. Korsgaard J, Iversen M. Epidermiology of house dust mite allergy. *Allergy* 1991; 46 (suppl. 11): 14–18.

109. Warner JA. Environmental changes and asthma control in paediatrics. *Paediatric Resp Med* 1993; 1: 9–13.

110. Wood RA, Chapman MD, Adkinson NF, Eggleston PA. The effect of cat removal on allergen content in household-dust samples. *J Allergy Clin Immunol* 1989; 83: 730–34.

111. de Blay F, Chapman MD, Platts-Mills TAE. Air-borne cat allergen (*Fel d* 1): Environmental control with the cat *in situ*. *Am Rev Respir Dis* 1991; 143: 1334–9.

112. Solomon LOR, Burge HA, Bloise JR. Exclusion of particulate allergens by window air conditioners. *J Allergy Clin Immunol* 1980; 65: 305–308.

113. Platt SD, Martin CJ, Hunt SM, Lewis CW. Damp housing, mould growth, and symptomatic health state. *BMJ* 1989; 298: 1673–8.

114. Strachan DP. Damp housing, mould allergy and childhood asthma. *Proc R Coll Physicians Edinb* 1991; 21: 140–46.

115. Williamson IJ, Martin CJ, McGill G, Monie RDH, Fennerty AG. Damp housing: a case-control study. *Thorax* 1997; 52: 229–34.

116. Nicolai T, Illi S, von Mutius E. Effect of dampness at home in childhood on bronchial hyperreactivity in adolescence. *Thorax* 1998; 53: 1035–40.

117. Wjst M, Reitmeir P, Dold S *et al*. Road traffic and adverse effects on respiratory health. *BMJ* 1993; 307: 596–600.

118. Samet JM. Learning about air pollution and asthma. *Am J Respir Crit Care Med* 1994; 149: 1398–9.

119. Cook DG, Strachan DP. Summary of the health effects of parental smoking on the respiratory health of children and implications for research. *Thorax* 1999; 54: 357–66.

120. Strachan DP, Cook DG. Health effects of passive smoking. 5. Parental smoking and allergic sensitisation in children. *Thorax* 1998; 53: 117–23.

121. Gergen PJ, Mullally DI, Evans R. National survey of prevalence of asthma in the United States. *Pediatrics* 1990; 81: 1–7.

122. Dybendal T, Hetland T, Vik H, Apold J, Elsayed S. Comparative measurements of antigenic and allergic proteins in dust vacuumed from carpeted and non-carpeted classrooms in Norwegian schools. *Clin Exp Allergy* 1989; 19: 217–24.

123. Cook DG, Whincup PH, Jarvis MJ, Strachan DP, Papacosta DP, Bryant A. Passive exposure to tobacco smoke in children aged 5–7 years: individual, family, and community factors. *BMJ* 1994; 308: 384–9.

124. Abramson MJ, Puy RM, Weiner JM. *Allergen immunotherapy for asthma (Cochrane Review)*. The Cochrane Library Issue 1. Oxford: Update Software, 1999.

125. Ostergaard PA, Kaad PN, Kristensen T. A prospective study on the safety of immunotherapy in children with severe asthma. *Allergy* 1986; 41: 588–93.

126. National Heart Lung and Blood Institute. *International consensus report on diagnosis and treatment of asthma*. Bethesda, MD: Department of Health and Human Services, 1992: 1–72.

127. Warner JO. The beta$_2$-agonist controversy and its relevance to the treatment of children. *Eur Respir Rev* 1994; 4: 21–6.

128. Spitzer WO, Suissa S, Ernst P *et al*. The use of β-agonists and the risk of death and near death from asthma. *N Engl J Med* 1992; 326: 501–506.

129. Ernst P, Habbick B, Suissa S *et al*. Is the association between inhaled beta-agonist use and life-threatening asthma because of confounding by severity? *Am Rev Respir Dis* 1993; 148: 75–9.

130. Sears MR, Taylor DR, Print CG *et al*. Regular inhaled beta-agonist treatment in bronchial asthma. *Lancet* 1990; 336: 1391–6.

131. Van Schayck CP, Dompeling E, Van Herwaarden CLA. Bronchodilator treatment in moderate asthma or chronic bronchitis: continuous or demand. A randomized control trial. *BMJ* 1991; 303: 1426–31.

132. O'Byrne PM, Kerstjens HAM. Inhaled β$_2$-agonists in the treatment of asthma. *N Engl J Med* 1996; 335: 888–9.

133. Verberne AA, Frost C, Roorda RJ, van der Laag H, Kerrebijn KF, and the Dutch Paediatric Asthma Study

134. Weinstein SF, Pearlman DS, Bronsky EA *et al*. Efficacy of salmeterol xinafoate powder in children with chronic persistent asthma. *Ann Allergy Asthma Immunol* 1998; 81: 51–8.

135. Russel G, Williams DAJ, Weller P, Price JF. Salmeterol xinafoate in children on high dose inhaled steroids. *Ann Allergy Asthma Immunol* 1995; 75: 423–8.

136. Greening AP, Ind PW, Northfield M, Shaw G, on behalf of Allen and Hanburys Limited UK Study Group. Added salmeterol versus higher-dose corticosteroid in asthma patients with symptoms on existing inhaled corticosteroid. *Lancet* 1994; 344: 219–24.

137. Pauwels RA, Lofdahl CG, Postma DS *et al*. Effect of inhaled formoterol and budesonide on exacerbations of asthma. Formoterol and Corticosteroids Establishing Therapy (FACET) International Study Group. *N Engl J Med* 1997; 337: 1405–11.

138. Verberne AA, Frost C, Duiverman EJ, Grol MH, Kerrebijn KF, and the Dutch Paediatric Asthma Study Group. Addition of salmeterol versus doubling the dose of beclomthethasone in children with asthma. *Am J Respir Crit Care Med* 1998; 158: 213–19.

139. Green CP, Price JF. Prevention of exercise induced asthma by inhaled salmeterol xinafoate. *Arch Dis Child* 1992; 67: 1014–17.

140. de Benedictis FM, Tuteri G, Pazzelli P, Niccoli A, Mezzetti D, Vaccaro R. Salmeterol in exercise-induced bronchoconstriction in asthmatic children: comparison of two doses. *Eur Respir J* 1996; 9: 2099–2103.

141. Verberne AAPH, Fuller R. An overview of nine clinical trials of salmeterol in an asthmatic population. *Respir Med* 1998; 92: 777–82.

142. Milgrom H, Bender B. Current issues in the use of theophylline. *Am Rev Respir Dis* 1993; 147: S33–S39.

143. Weinberger M. Theophylline: when should it be used? *J Pediatr* 1993; 122: 403–405.

144. Szefler SJ, Bender BG, Jusko WJ *et al*. Evolving role of theophylline for treatment of chronic childhood asthma. *J Pediatr* 1995; 127: 176–85.

Group. One year treatment with salmeterol compared with beclomethasone in children with asthma. *Am J Respir Crit Care Med* 1997; 156: 688–95.

145. Pauwels R, van Renterghem D, van der Straeten M, Johannesson N, Persson CGA. The effects of theophylline and enprophylline on allergen-induced bronchoconstriction. *J Allergy Clin Immunol* 1985; 76: 583–90.

146. Ward AJM, McKenniff M, Evans JM, Page CP, Costello JF. Theophylline-an immunmodulatory role in asthma? *Am Rev Respir Dis* 1993; 147: 518–23.

147. Sullivan P, Bekir S, Jaffar Z, Jeffery P, Costello J. Anti-inflammatory effects of low-dose oral theophylline in atopic asthma. *Lancet* 1994; 343: 1006–1008.

148. Reed CE, Offord KP, Nelson HS, Li JT, Tinkelman DG. Aerosol beclomethasone dipropionate spray compared with theophylline as primary treatment for chronic mild-to-moderate asthma. The American Academy of Allergy, Asthma and Immunology Beclomethasone Dipropionate-Theophylline Study Group. *J Allergy Clin Immunol* 1998; 101: 14–23.

149. Barnes PJ, Greening AP, Neville L, Timmers J, Poole GW. Single-dose slow-release aminophylline at night prevents nocturnal asthma. *Lancet* 1982; i: 299–301.

150. Brenner M, Berkowitz R, Marshall N, Strunk RC. Need for theophylline in severe steroid-requiring asthmatics. *Clin Allergy* 1988; 18: 143–50.

151. Schlieper A, Alcock D, Beaudry P, Feldman W, Leikin L. Effect of therapeutic plasma concentrations of theophylline on behavior, cognitive processing, and affect in children with asthma. *J Pediatr* 1991; 118: 449–55.

152. Bender BG, Ikle DN, DuHamel T, Tinkelman D. Neuropsychological and behavioral changes in asthmatic children treated with beclomethasone dipropionate versus theophylline. *Pediatrics* 1998; 101: 355–60.

153. Hendles L, Weinberger M, Szefler S, Ellis E. Safety and efficacy of theophylline in children with asthma. *J Pediatr* 1992; 120: 179–83.

154. Qureshi F, Pestian J, Davis P, Zaritsky A. Effect of nebulized ipratropium on the hospitalization rates of children with asthma. *N Engl J Med* 1998; 339: 1030–35.

155. Hodges IGC, Groggins RC, Milner AD, Stokes GM. Bronchodilator effects of inhaled ipratropium bromide in wheezy toddlers. *Arch Dis Child* 1981; 56: 729–32.

156. Everard ML, Kurian M. *Anti-cholinergic drugs for wheeze in children under the age of two years (Cochrane Review)*. The Cochrane Library Issue 1. 1999. Oxford: Update Software, 1999.

157. Beasley CRW, Rafferty P, Holgate ST. Bronchoconstrictor properties of preservatives in ipratropium bromide (Atrovent) nebuliser solution. *BMJ* 1987; 294: 1197–8.

158. ❂ Barnes PJ, Pedersen S, Busse WW. Efficacy and safety of inhaled corticosteroids. *Am J Respir Crit Care Med* 1998; 157: S1–S53.

159. Juniper EF, Kline PA, Vanzieleghem MA, Ramsdale EH, O'Byrne PM, Hargreave FE. Effect of long-term treatment with an inhaled corticosteroid (budesonide) on airway hyperresponsiveness and clinical asthma in nonsteroid-dependent asthmatics. *Am Rev Respir Dis* 1990; 142: 832–6.

160. Juniper EF, Kline PA, Vanzieleghem MA, Ramsdale EH, O'Byrne PM, Hargreave FE. Long-term effects of budesonide on airway responsiveness and clinical asthma severity in inhaled-steroid dependent asthmatics. *Eur Respir J* 1990; 3: 1122–7.

161. Haahtela T, Jarvinen M, Kava T *et al*. Comparison of a β$_2$-agonist, terbutaline, with an inhaled corticosteroid, budesonide, in newly detected asthma. *N Engl J Med* 1991; 325: 388–92.

162. van Essen-Zandvliet EE, Hughes MD, Waalkens HJ *et al*. Effects of 22 months treatment with inhaled corticosteroid and/or beta-2-agonist on lung function, airway responsiveness and symptoms in children with asthma. *Am Rev Respir Dis* 1992; 146: 547–54.

163. Pedersen S, Hansen OR. Budesonide treatment of moderate and severe asthma in children: a dose-response study. *J Allergy Clin Immunol* 1995; 95: 29–33.

164. van Essen-Zandvliet EE, Hughes MD, Waalkens HJ, Duiverman EJ, Kerrebijn KF, Dutch CNSLD study group. Remission of childhood asthma after long-term treatment with an inhaled corticosteroid (budesonide): Can it be achieved? *Eur Respir J* 1994; 7: 63–8.

165. Bisgaard H, Munck SL, Nielsen JP, Peterson W, Ohlsson SV. Inhaled budesonide for treatment of recurrent wheezing in early childhood. *Lancet* 1990; 336: 649–51.

166. Connett GJ, Warde C, Wooler E, Lenney W. Use of budesonide in severe asthmatics aged 1–3 years. *Arch Dis Child* 1993; 69: 351–5.

167. Gleeson JG, Price JF. Controlled trial of budesonide given by the nebuhaler in preschool children with asthma. *BMJ* 1988; 297: 163–6.

168. Greenough A, Pool J, Gleeson JGA, Price JF. Effect of budesonide on pulmonary hyperinflation in young asthmatic children. *Thorax* 1988; 43: 937–8.

169. Ilangovan P, Pedersen S, Godfrey S, Nikander K, Novisksi N, Warner JO. Treatment of severe steroid dependent preschool asthma with nebulised budesonide suspension. *Arch Dis Child* 1993; 68: 356–9.

170. Price JF, Weller PH. Comparison of fluticasone propionate and sodium cromoglycate for the treatment of childhood asthma (an open parallel group study). *Respir Med* 1995; 89: 363–8.

171. ✪ Waalkens HJ, van Essen-Zandvliet EE, Hughes MD *et al*. Cessation of long-term treatment with inhaled corticosteroid (Budesonide) in children with asthma results in detrioration. *Am Rev Respir Dis* 1993; 148: 1252–7.

172. Shapiro GG, Bronsky EA, LaForce CF *et al*. Dose-related efficacy of budesonide administered via a dry powder inhaler in the treatment of children with moderate to severe persistent asthma. *J Pediatr* 1998; 132: 976–82.

173. Geddes DM. Inhaled corticosteroids: benefits and risks. *Thorax* 1992; 47: 404–407.

174. Barnes PJ, Pedersen S. Efficacy and safety of inhaled corticosteroids in asthma. *Am Rev Respir Dis* 1993; 148: S1–S26.

175. Balfour-Lynn L. Growth and childhood asthma. *Arch Dis Child* 1986; 61: 1049–55.

176. Shohat M, Shohat T, Kedem R, Mimouni M, Danon YL. Childhood asthma and growth outcome. *Arch Dis Child* 1987; 62: 63–5.

177. Allen DB, Mullen M, Mullen B. A meta-analysis of the effect of oral and inhaled corticosteroids on growth. *J Allergy Clin Immunol* 1994; 93: 967–76.

178. Volovitz B, Amir J, Malik H, Kauschansky A, Varsano I. Growth and pituitary-adrenal function in children with severe asthma treated with inhaled budesonide. *N Engl J Med* 1993; 329: 1703–1708.

179. Ruiz RG, Price JF. Growth and adrenal responsiveness with budesonide in young asthmatics. *Respir Med* 1994; 88: 17–20.

180. Wolthers OD, Pedersen S. Measures of systemic activity of inhaled glucocorticosteroids in children: a comparison of urine cortisol excretion and knemometry. *Respir Med* 1995; 89: 347–9.

181. Agertoft L, Pedersen S. A randomized, double-blind dose reduction study to compare the minimal effective dose of budesonide Turbuhaler and fluticasone propionate Diskhaler. *J Allerg Clin Immunol* 1997; 99: 773–80.

182. Nicolaizik WH, Marchant JL, Preece MA, Warner JO. Endocrine and lung function in asthmatic children on inhaled corticosteroids. *Am J Respir Crit Care Med* 1994; 150: 624–8.

183. Doull IJ, Freezer NJ, Holgate ST. Growth of prepubertal children with mild asthma treated with inhaled beclomethasone dipropionate. *Am J Respir Crit Care Med* 1995; 151: 1715–19.

184. Law CM, Marchant JL, Honour JW, Preece MA, Warner JO. Nocturnal adrenal suppression in asthmatic children taking inhaled beclomethasone dipropionate. *Lancet* 1986; 1: 942–4.

185. Ninan TK, Reid IW, Carter PE, Smail PJ, Russell G. Effects of high doses of inhaled corticosteroids on adrenal function in children with severe persistent asthma. *Thorax* 1993; 48: 599–602.

186. Connett GJ, Lenney W. Inhaled budesonide and behavioural disturbances. *Lancet* 1991; 338: 634.

187. Simons FE, Persaud MP, Gillespie CA, Cheang M, Shuckett EP. Absence of posterior subcapsular cataracts in young patients treated with inhaled glucocorticoids. *Lancet* 1993; 342: 776–8.

188. Shaw NJ, Edmunds AT. Inhaled beclomethasone and oral candidiasis. *Arch Dis Child* 1986; 61: 788–90.

189. Deshpande A, McKenzie SA. Short course of steroids in home treatment of children with acute asthma. *Br Med J (Clin Res Ed)* 1986; 293: 169–71.

190. Harris JB, Weinberger MM, Nassif E, Smith G, Milavetz G. Stillerman A. Early intervention with short courses of prednisone to prevent progression of asthma in ambulatory patients incompletely responsive to bronchodilators. *J Pediatr* 1987; 110: 627–33.

191. Brunette MG, Lands L, Thibodeau LP. Childhood asthma: prevention of attacks with short-term corticosteroid treatment of upper respiratory tract infection. *Pediatrics* 1988; 81: 624–9.

192. Zora JA, Zimmerman D, Carey TL, O'Connell EJ, Yunginger JW. Hypothalamic-pituitary-adrenal axis suppression after short-term, high-dose glucocorticoid therapy in children with asthma. *J Allergy Clin Immunol* 1986; 77: 9–13.

193. Dolan LM, Kesarwala HH, Holroyde JC, Fischer TJ. Short-term, high-dose, systemic steroids in children with asthma: the effect on the hypothalamic–pituitary-adrenal axis. *J Allergy Clin Immunol* 1987; 80: 81–7.

194. Kamada AK, Spahn JD, Surs W, Brown E, Leung DYM, Szefler SJ. Coexistence of glucocorticoid receptor and pharmacokinetic abnormalities: factors that contribute to a poor response to treatment with glucocorticoids in children with asthma. *J Pediatr* 1994; 124: 984–6.

195. Gschwentner M, Susanna A, Schmarda A *et al*. ICIn: a chloride channel paramount for cell volume regulation. *J Allergy Clin Immunol* 1996; 98: S98–101.

196. Silverman M, Connolly NM, Balfour-Lynn L, Godfrey S. Long-term trial of disodium cromoglycate and isoprenaline in children with asthma. *Br Med J* 1972; 823: 378–81.

197. Godfrey S, Balfour-Lynn L, Konig P. The place of cromolyn sodium in the long-term management of childhood asthma based on a 3–5 year follow-up. *J Pediatr* 1975; 87: 465–73.

198. Furfaro S, Speir S, Drblik SP, Turgeon JP, Robert M. Efficacy of cromoglycate in persistently wheezing infants. *Arch Dis Child* 1994; 71: 331–4.

199. Yuksel B, Greenough A. The effect of sodium cromoglycate on upper and lower respiratory symptoms in children born prematurely. *Eur J Pediatr* 1993; 152: 615–18.

200. Tasche MJ, van der Wouden JC, Uijen JH *et al*. Randomised placebo-controlled trial of inhaled sodium cromoglycate in 1–4-year old children with moderate asthma. *Lancet* 1997; 350: 1060–1064.

201. Chudry N, Correa F, Silverman M. Nedocromil sodium and exercise induced asthma. *Arch Dis Child* 1987; 62: 412–14.

202. Comis A, Valletta EA, Sette L, Andreoli A, Boner AL. Comparison of nedocromil sodium and sodium cromoglycate administered by pressurized aerosol, with and without a spacer device in exercise-induced asthma in children. *Eur Respir J* 1993; 6: 523–6.

203. Armenio L, Baldini G, Bardare M *et al*. Double blind, placebo controlled study of nedocromil sodium in asthma. *Arch Dis Child* 1993; 68: 193–7.

204. Yuksel B, Greenough A. Inhaled nedocromil sodium in symptomatic young children born prematurely. *Respir Med* 1996; 90: 467–71.

205. de Benedictis FM, Tuteri G, Pazzelli P, Bertotto A, Bruni L, Vaccaro R. Cromolyn versus nedocromil: duration of action in exercise-induced asthma in children. *J Allergy Clin Immunol* 1995; 96: 510–14.

206. Sampson A, Holgate ST. Leukotriene modifiers in the treatment of asthma–look promising across the board of severity. *BMJ* 1998; 316: 1257–8.

207. Lipworth BJ. Leukotriene-receptor antagonists. *Lancet* 1999; 353: 57–62.

208. Kemp JP, Dockhorn RJ, Shapiro GG *et al*. Montelukast once daily inhibits exercise-induced bronchoconstriction in 6- to 14-year-old children with asthma. *J Pediatr* 1998; 133: 424–8.

209. Knorr B, Matz J, Bernstein JA *et al*. Montelukast for chronic asthma in 6- to 14-year-old children: a randomized, double-blind trial. Pediatric Montelukast Study Group. *JAMA* 1998; 279: 1181–6.

210. Leff JA, Busse WW, Pearlman D *et al*. Montelukast, a leukotriene-receptor antagonist, for the treatment of mild asthma and exercise-induced bronchoconstriction. *N Engl J Med* 1998; 339: 147–52.

211. Loftus BG, Price JF. Long-term, placebo-controlled trial of ketotifen in the management of pre-school children with asthma. *J Allergy Clin Immunol* 1987; 79: 350–55.

212. Kennedy JD, Hasham F, Clay MJD, Jones RS. Comparison of action of disodium cromoglycate and ketotifen on exercise-induced bronchoconstriction in childhood asthma. *BMJ* 1980; 281: 1458.

213. Iikura Y, Naspitz CK, Mikawa H *et al*. Prevention of asthma by ketotifen in infants with atopic dermatitis. *Ann Allergy* 1992; 68: 233–6.

214. Maclay WP, Crowder D, Spiro S, Turner P. Post-marketing surveillance: Practical experience with ketotifen. *BMJ* 1984; 288: 911–14.

215. Banner AS. Non-steroidal anti-inflammatory therapy for bronchial asthma. *Lancet* 1998; 351: 5–7.

216. Coren ME, Rosenthal M, Bush A. The use of cyclosporin in corticosteroid dependent asthma. *Arch Dis Child* 1999; 1997: 522–3.

217. Guss S, Portnoy J. Methotrexate treatment of severe asthma in children. *Pediatrics* 1992; 89: 635–9.

218. Niggemann B, Leupold W, Schuster A *et al*. Prospective, double-blind, placebo-controlled, multicentre study on the effect of high-dose, intravenous immunoglobulin in children and adolescents with severe bronchial asthma. *Clin Exp Allergy* 1998; 28: 205–210.

219. ♻ Balfour-Lynn I. Difficult asthma: beyond the guidelines. *Arch Dis Child* 1999; 80: 201–206.

220. Balon J, Aker PD, Crowther ER *et al*. A comparison of active and simulated chiropractic manipulation as adjunctive treatment for childhood asthma. *N Engl J Med* 1998; 339: 1013–1020.

221. Bowler SD, Green A, Mitchell CA. Buteyko breathing techniques in asthma: a blinded randomised controlled trial. *Med J Aust* 1998; 169: 575–8.

222. Reiser J, Warner JO. Inhalation treatment for asthma. *Arch Dis Child* 1986; 61: 88–94.

223. Pedersen S. Inhaler use in children with asthma. *Dan Med Bull* 1987; 34: 234–49.

224. ♻ Pedersen S. Inhalers and nebulizers: which to choose and why. *Respir Med* 1996; 90: 69–77.

225. Pedersen S, Frost L, Arnfred T. Errors in inhalation technique and efficiency in inhaler use in asthmatic children. *Allergy* 1986; 41: 118–24.

226. Pedersen S, Mortensen S. Use of different inhalation devices in children. *Lung* 1990; 168: S653–57.

227. Henry RL, Milner AD. Simple drug delivery system for use by young asthmatics. *BMJ* 1983; 286: 2021–22.

228. Everard ML, Clark AR, Milner AD. Drug delivery from holding chambers with attached facemask. *Arch Dis Child* 1992; 67: 580–85.

229. Bisgaard H. A metal aerosol holding chamber devised for young children with asthma. *Eur Respir J* 1995; 8: 856–60.

230. Barry PW, O'Callaghan C. Inhalational drug delivery from seven different spacer devices. *Thorax* 1996; 51: 835–40.

231. O'Callaghan C, Lynch J, Cant M, Robertson C. Improvement in sodium cromoglycate delivery from a spacer device by use of an antistatic lining, immediate inhalation, and avoiding multiple actuations of drug. *Thorax* 1993; 48: 603–606.

232. Rivlin J, Mindorff C, Reilly P, Levison H. Pulmonary response to a bronchodilator delivered from three inhalation devices. *J Pediatr* 1984; 104: 470–73.

233. Brown PH, Blundell G, Greening AP *et al*. Do large volume spacer devices reduce the systemic effects of high dose inhaled corticosteroids? *Thorax* 1990; 45: 736–9.

234. Prahl P, Jensen T. Decreased adreno-cortical suppression utilizing the Nebuhaler for inhalation of steroid aerosols. *Clin Allergy* 1987; 17: 393–8.

235. Freelander M, Van Asperen PP. Nebuhaler versus nebuliser in children with acute asthma. *BMJ* 1984; 288: 1873–4.

236. Sennhauser FM, Sly PD. Pressure flow characteristics of the valve in spacer devices. *Arch Dis Child* 1989; 64: 1305–1307.

237. O'Callaghan C, Milner AD, Swarbrick A. Spacer device with face mask attachment for giving bronchodilators to infants with asthma. *BMJ* 1989; 298: 160–61.

238. Gleeson JGA, Price JF. Nebuhaler technique. *Br J Dis Chest* 1988; 82: 172–4.

239. Wildhaber JH, Devadason SG, Eber E *et al*. Effect of electrostatic charge, flow, delay and multiple actuations on the *in vitro* delivery of salbutamol from different small volume spacers for infants. *Thorax* 1996; 51: 985–8.

240. Pedersen S. Aerosol treatment of bronchoconstriction in children, with or without a tube spacer. *N Engl J Med* 1983; 308: 1328–30.

241. Borgstrom L, Bondesson E, Moren F, Trofast E, Newman SP. Lung deposition of budesonide inhaled via Turbuhaler: a comparison with terbutaline sulphate in normal subjects. *Eur Respir J* 1994; 7: 69–73.

242. Pedersen S. How to use a rotahaler. *Arch Dis Child* 1986; 61: 11–14.

243. Pedersen S, Hansen OR, Fuglsang G. Influence of inspiratory flow rate upon the effect of a Turbuhaler. *Arch Dis Child* 1990; 65: 308–310.

244. Agertoft L, Pedersen S. Importance of training for correct Turbuhaler use in preschool children. *Acta Paediatr* 1998; 87: 842–7.

245. Agertoft L, Pedersen S. The importance of the inhalation device on the effects of budesonide. *Arch Dis Child* 1993; 69: 130–33.

246. The nebuliser project group of the British Thoracic Society Standards of Care Committee. Current best practice for nebuliser treatment: Guidelines. *Thorax* 1997; 52: S4–S16.

247. Bendefy IM. Home nebulisers in childhood asthma: survey of hospital supervised use. *BMJ* 1991; 302: 1180–81.

248. Everard ML, Clark AR, Milner AD. Drug delivery from jet nebulisers. *Arch Dis Child* 1992; 67: 586–92.

249. Barry PW, O'Callaghan C. Nebuliser therapy in childhood. *Thorax* 1997; 52: S79–S88.

250. Salmon B, Wilson NM, Silverman M. How much aerosol reaches the lungs of wheezy infants and toddlers. *Arch Dis Child* 1990; 65: 401–403.

251. Agertoft L, Andersen A, Weibull E, Pedersen S. Systemic availability and pharmacokinetics of nebulised budesonide in preschool children. *Arch Dis Child* 1999; 80: 241–7.

252. Agertoft L, Pedersen S. Effects of long-term treatment with an inhaled corticosteroid on growth and pulmonary function in asthmatic children. *Respir Med* 1994; 88: 373–81.

253. Wilson N, Sloper K, Silverman M. Effect of continuous treatment with topical corticosteroid on episodic viral wheeze in preschool children. *Arch Dis Child* 1995; 72: 317–20.

254. Doull IJ, Lampe FC, Smith S, Schreiber J, Freezer NJ, Holgate ST. Effect of inhaled corticosteroids on episodes of wheezing associated with viral infection in school age children: randomised double blind placebo controlled trial. *BMJ* 1997; 315: 858–62.

255. Wilson NM, Silverman M. Treatment of acute, episodic asthma in preschool children using intermittent high dose inhaled steroids at home. *Arch Dis Child* 1990; 65: 407–410.

256. Connett GJ, Lenney W. Prevention of viral induced asthma attacks using inhaled budesonide. *Arch Dis Child* 1993; 68: 85–7.

257. Anderson SD, duToit JI, Rodwell LT, Jenkins CR. Acute effect of sodium cromoglycate on airway narrowing induced by 4.5 percent saline aerosol. Outcome before and during treatment with aerosol corticosteroids in patients with asthma. *Chest* 1994; 105: 673–80.

258. Woolcock A, Lundback B, Ringdal N, Jacques LA. Comparison of addition of salmeterol to inhaled steroids with doubling of the dose of inhaled steroids. *Am J Respir Crit Care Med* 1996; 153: 1481–8.

259. Verberne AA, Frost C, Duiverman EJ, Grol MH, Kerrebijn KF. Addition of salmeterol versus doubling the dose of beclomethasone in children with asthma. The Dutch Asthma Study Group. *Am J Respir Crit Care Med* 1998; 158: 213–19.

260. Ukena D, Harnest U, Sakalauskas R *et al*. Comparison

of addition of theophylline to inhaled steroid with doubling of the dose of inhaled steroid in asthma. *Eur Respir J* 1997; 10: 2754–60.

261. Evans DJ, Taylor DA, Zetterstrom O, Chung KF, O'Connor BJ, Barnes PJ. A comparison of low-dose inhaled budesonide plus theophylline and high-dose inhaled budesonide for moderate asthma. *N Engl J Med* 1997; 337: 1412–18.

262. Paggiaro PL, Giannini D, Di Franco A, Testi R. Comparison of inhaled salmeterol and individually dose-titrated slow-release theophylline in patients with reversible airway obstruction. European Study Group. *Eur Respir J* 1996; 9: 1689–95.

263. Goldberg S, Algur N, Levi M *et al*. Adrenal suppression among asthmatic children receiving chronic therapy with inhaled corticosteroid with and without spacer device. *Ann Allergy Asthma Immunol* 1996; 76: 234–8.

264. Malo J-L, Cartier A, Merland N *et al*. Four-times-a-day dosing frequency is better than twice-a-day regimen in subjects requiring a high-dose inhaled steroid, budesonide, to control moderate to severe asthma. *Am Rev Respir Dis* 1989; 140: 624–48.

265. Sur S, Crotty TB, Kephart GM. *et al*. Sudden-onset fatal asthma–A distinct entity with few eosinophils and relatively more neutrophils in the airway submucosa. *Am J Respir Crit Care Med* 1993; 148: 713–19.

266. Beer S, Laver J, Karpuch J, Chabut S, Aladjem M. Prodromal features of asthma. *Arch Dis Child* 1987; 62: 345–8.

267. Young S, Arnott J, Le Soeuf PN, Landau LI. Flow limitation during tidal expiration in symptom-free infants and the subsequent development of asthma. *J Pediatr* 1994; 124: 681–8.

268. Bailey WC, Richards JN, Brooks N, Seng Jaw Soong, Windsor RA, Nanzelle BA. A randomised trial to improve the self management practices of adults with asthma. *Arch Intern Med* 1994; 150: 1664–8.

269. Hughes DM, McLeod M, Garner B, Goldbloom RB. Controlled trial of a home management and ambulatory programme for asthmatic children. *Pediatrics* 1991; 87: 54–61.

270. Zeiger RS, Heller S, Mellon MH, Wald J, Falkoff R,

Schatz M. Facilitated referral to asthma specialist reduces the relapses in asthma emergency room visits. *J Allergy Clin Immunol* 1991; 87: 1160–68.

271. Storr JE, Barrell E, Lenney W, Hatcher G. Effect of a single oral dose of prednisolone in acute childhood asthma. *Lancet* 1987; 1: 879–82.

272. Charlton I, Charlton G, Broomfield J, Mullee MA. Evaluation of peak flow and symptoms only self management plans for control of asthma in general practice. *BMJ* 1990; 301: 1355–9.

273. Garrett J, Williams S, Wong C, Holdaway D. Treatment of acute asthmatic exacerbations with an increased dose of inhaled steroid. *Arch Dis Child* 1998; 79: 12–17.

274. van Essen-Zandvliet EE, Lans C, Denteneer A, Van Stel H, Colland V. Can asthma exacerbations in children be reduced by using prodromal signs in a self-management plan? *Am J Respir Crit Care Med* 1999; 159: A757.

275. Svedmyr J, Nyberg E, Asbrink-Nilsson E, Hedlin G. Intermittent treatment with inhaled steroids for deterioration of asthma due to upper respiratory tract infections. *Acta Paediatr* 1995; 84: 884–8.

276. Svedmyr J, Nyberg E, Thunqvist P, Asbrink-Nilsson E, Hedlin G. Prophylactic intermittent treatment with inhaled corticosteroids of asthma exacerbations due to airway infections in toddlers. *Acta Paediatr* 1999; 88: 42–7.

277. Benton G, Thomas RC, Nickerson BG, McQuitty JC, Okikawa J. Experience with a metered dose inhaler with a spacer in the pediatric emergency department. *Am J Dis Child* 1989; 143: 678–81.

278. Marinker M. *Partnership in medicine taking: a consultative document*. Royal Pharmaceutical Society and Merck, Sharp and Dohme, 1996.

279. Williams JR, Bothner JP, Swanton RD. Delivery of albuterol in a pediatric emergency department. *Pediatr Emerg Care* 1996; 12: 263–7.

280. Batra V, Sethi GR, Sachdev HP. Comparative efficacy of jet nebulizer and metered dose inhaler with spacer device in the treatment of acute asthma. *Indian Pediatr* 1997; 34: 497–503.

281. Robertson CF, Norden MA, Fitzgerald DA *et al.* Treatment of acute asthma: salbutamol via jet nebuliser vs spacer and metered dose inhaler. *J Paediatr Child Health* 1998; 34: 142–6.

282. Dewar AL, Stewart A, Cogswell JJ, Connett GJ. A randomised controlled trial to assess the relative benefits of large volume spacers and nebulisers to treat acute asthma in hospital. *Arch Dis Child* 1999; 80: 421–3.

283. Clark NM, Northwehr F, Gong M *et al.* Physician–patient partnership in managing chronic illness. *Acad Med* 1995; 70: 957–9.

284. Guidelines on the management of asthma. *Thorax* 1993; 48: S1–S24.

285. McNicol KN, Williams HE. Spectrum of asthma in childhood. I. Clinical and physiological components. *BMJ* 1973; 4: 7–11.

286. Strachan DP. The prevalence and natural history of wheezing in early childhood. *J R Coll Gen Pract* 1985; 35: 182–4.

287. Wright AL, Taussig LM. Lessons from long-term cohort studies. Childhood asthma. *Eur Respir J* (suppl. 1) 1998; 27: 17s–22s.

288. Tattersfield AE. Asthma–where now? In: Lawson DH (ed). *Current Medicine*. Edinburgh: Churchill Livingstone, 1994; 29–49.

289. Williams HE, McNicol KN. Prevalence, natural history and relationship of wheezy bronchitis and asthma in children: an epidemiological study. *BMJ* 1969; 4: 321–5.

290. Clifford RD, Radford M, Howell JB, Holgate ST. Associations between respiratory symptoms, bronchial responsiveness to methacholine and atopy in two age groups of school children. *Arch Dis Child* 1989; 64: 1133–9.

291. ✪ Martinez FD, Morgan WJ, Wright AL, Holberg CJ, Taussig LM. Diminished lung function as a predisposing factor for wheezing respiratory illness in infants. *N Engl J Med* 1988; 319: 1112–17.

292. Taylor B, Wadsworth J. Maternal smoking during pregnancy and lower respiratory tract illness in early life. *Arch Dis Child* 1987; 62: 786–91.

293. Tager IB, Hanrahan JP, Tostesan TD *et al.* Lung function, pre- and post-natal smoke exposure, and wheezing in the first year of life. *Am Rev Respir Dis* 1993; 147: 811–17.

294. Chan KN, Wong YC, Silverman M. Relationship between infant lung mechanics and childhood lung function in children of very low birthweight. *Pediatr Pulmonol* 1990; 8: 74–81.

295. Horn MEC, Gregg I, Brain EA, Inglis JM, Yealland SJ, Taylor P. Respiratory viral infection and wheezy bronchitis in childhood. *Thorax* 1979; 34: 23–8.

296. Luyt DK, Burton P, Brooke AM, Simpson H. Wheeze in preschool children and its relation with doctor diagnosed asthma. *Arch Dis Child* 1994; 71: 24–30.

297. Selander P. Asthmatic symptoms in the first year of life. *Acta Paediatr Scand* 1960; 49: 265–9.

298. O'Callaghan C, Milner AD, Swarbrick A. Nebulised salbutamol does have a protective effect on airways in children under 1 year old. *Arch Dis Child* 1988; 63: 479–83.

299. Tepper RS. Airway reactivity in infants: a positive response to methacholine and metaproterenol. *J Appl Physiol* 1987; 62: 1155–9.

300. Henderson AJW, Young S, Stick S, Landau LI, Le Soeuf PN. Effect of salbutamol on histamine induced bronchoconstriction in healthy infants. *Thorax* 1993; 48: 317–23.

301. Prendiville A, Green S, Silverman M. Paradoxical response to salbutamol in wheezy infants. *Arch Dis Child* 1987; 42: 86–91.

302. Clough JB. Bronchodilators in infancy. *Thorax* 1993; 48: 308.

303. Tal A, Golan H, Grauer N, Aviram M, Albin D, Quastel MR. Deposition pattern of radiolabeled salbutamol inhaled from a metered-dose inhaler by means of a spacer with mask in young children with airway obstruction. *J Pediatr* 1996; 128: 479–84.

304. Loftus BG, Price JF. Treatment of asthma in preschool children with slow release theophylline. *Arch Dis Child* 1985; 60: 770–72.

305. Varsano I, Volovitz B, Malik H, Amir Y. Safety of

1 year of treatment with budesonide in young children with asthma. *J Allergy Clin Immunol* 1990; 85: 914–20.

306. Freigang B, Ashford DR. Adrenal cortical function after long-term beclomethasone aerosol therapy in early childhood. *Ann Allergy* 1990; 64: 342–4.

307. Webb MS, Milner AD, Hiller EJ, Henry RL. Nebulised beclomethasone dipropionate suspension. *Arch Dis Child* 1986; 61: 1108–10.

308. de Blic J, Delacourt C, Le Bourgeois M *et al.* Efficacy of nebulized budesonide in treatment of severe infantile asthma: a double-blind study. *J Allergy Clin Immunol* 1996; 98: 14–20.

309. Connett GJ, Warde C, Wooler E, Lenney W. Use of budesonide in severe asthmatics aged 1–3 years. *Arch Dis Child* 1993; 69: 351–5.

310. Connett G, Lenney W. Prevention of viral induced asthma attacks using inhaled budesonide. *Arch Dis Child* 1993; 68: 85–7.

311. Kaur B, Anderson HR, Austin J, Burr M, Harkins LS, Strachan DP. Prevalence of asthma symptoms, diagnosis, and treatment in 12–14 year old children across Great Britain (International Study of Asthma and Allergies in Childhood ISAAC UK). *BMJ* 1998; 316: 118–24.

312. Siersted HC, Boldsen J, Hansen HS, Mostgaard G, Hyldebrandt N. Population based study of risk factors for underdiagnosis of asthma in adolescence: Odense schoolchild study. *BMJ* 1998; 316: 651–5.

313. Martin AJ, McLennan LA, Landau LI, Phelan PD. The natural history of childhood asthma to adult life. *BMJ* 1980; 280: 1397–1400.

314. von Mutius E. Progression of allergy and asthma through childhood to adolescence. *Thorax* 1996; 51 (suppl. 1): S3–S6.

315. Proimos J. Confidentiality issues in the adolescent population. *Current Opinion in Pediatrics* 1997; 9: 325–8.

316. Viner R. Asthma in adolescence: communications is the key to effective management. *Asthma J* 1999; 4: 66–7.

317. ✪ McFadden ER Jr, Gilbert IA. Exercise-induced asthma. *N Engl J Med* 1994; 330: 1362–7.

318. Jones RS, Buston MH, Wharton MJ. The effect of exercise on ventilatory function in children with asthma. *Br J Dis Chest* 1962; 56: 78–86.

319. Hansen-Flaschen J, Schotland H. New treatments for exercise-induced asthma. *N Engl J Med* 1998; 339: 192–3.

320. McFadden ERJ, Zawadski DK. Vocal cord dysfunction masquerading as exercise-induced asthma, a physiologic cause for "choking" during athletic activities. *Am J Respir Crit Care Med* 1996; 153: 942–7.

321. Anderson SD, Silverman M, Konig P, Godfrey S. Exercise-induced asthma. *Br J Dis Chest* 1975; 69: 1–39.

322. Zawadski DK, Lenner KA, McFadden ER Jr. Effect of exercise on nonspecific airway reactivity in asthmatics. *J Appl Physiol* 1988; 64: 812–16.

323. Mussaffi H, Springer C, Godfrey S. Increased bronchial responsiveness to exercise and histamine after allergen challenge in children with asthma. *J Allergy Clin Immunol* 1986; 77: 48–52.

324. Edmunds AT, Tooley M, Godfrey S. The refractory period after exercise-induced asthma: its duration and relation to severity of exercise. *Am Rev Respir Dis* 1978; 117: 247–54.

325. Orenstein DM, Reed ME, Grogan FT, Crawford LV. Exercise conditioning in children with asthma. *J Pediatr* 1985; 106: 556–60.

326. Zanconato S, Baraldi E, Santuz P, Magagnin G, Zacchello F. Effect of inhaled disodium cromoglycate and albuterol on en energy cost of running in asthmatic children. *Pediatr Pulmonol* 1990; 8: 240–44.

327. Unnithan VB, Thomson KJ, Aitchison TC, Paton JY. β_2-agonists and running economy in prepubertal boys. *Pediatr Pulmonol* 1994; 17: 378–82.

328. Simons FE, Gerstner TV, Cheang MS. Tolerance to the bronchoprotective effect of salmeterol in adolescents with exercise-induced asthma using concurrent inhaled glucocorticoid treatment. *Pediatrics* 1997; 99: 655–9.

329. Leff JA, Busse WW, Pearlman D *et al.* Montelukast, a leukotriene-receptor antagonist, for the treatment of mild asthma and exercise-induced bronchoconstriction. *N Engl J Med* 1998; 339: 147–52.

330. Young S, Bitsaku H, Caric D, McHardy GJR. Coughing can relieve or exacerbate symptoms in asthmatic patients. *Respir Med* 1991; 85: 7–12.

331. Kelly YJ, Brabin BJ, Milligan PJ, Reid JA, Heaf D, Pearson MG. Clinical significance of cough and wheeze in the diagnosis of asthma. *Arch Dis Child* 1996; 75: 489–93.

332. Ninan TK, MacDonald L, Russell G. Persistent nocturnal cough in childhood: a population based study. *Arch Dis Child* 1995; 73: 403–407.

333. Wright AL, Holberg CJ, Morgan WJ, Taussig LM, Halonen M, Martinez FD. Recurrent cough in childhood and its relation to asthma. *Am J Respir Crit Care Med* 1996; 153: 1259–65.

334. Sheppard D, Rizk NW, Boushey HA, Bethel RA. Mechanism of cough and bronchoconstriction caused by distilled water. *Am Rev Respir Dis* 1983; 127: 691–4.

335. Thomson A, Pratt C, Simpson H. Nocturnal cough in asthma. *Arch Dis Child* 1987; 62: 1001–1004.

336. Chang AB. Isolated cough: probably not asthma. *Arch Dis Child* 1999; 1999: 211–13.

337. McKenzie S. Cough–but is it asthma? *Arch Dis Child* 1994; 70X: 3–4.

338. Chang AB, Phelan PD, Carlin JB, Sawyer SM, Robertson CF. A randomised, placebo controlled trial of inhaled salbutamol and beclomethasone for recurrent cough. *Arch Dis Child* 1998; 79: 6–11.

339. Stores G, Ellis AJ, Wiggs L, Crawford C, Thomson A. Sleep and psychological disturbance in nocturnal asthma. *Arch Dis Child* 1998; 78: 413–19.

340. Martin RJ, Cicutto LC, Ballard RD. Factors related to the nocturnal worsening of asthma. *Am Rev Respir Dis* 1990; 140: 33–8.

341. Meijer GG, Postma DS, Wempe JB, Gerritsen J, Knol K, van Aalderen WM. Frequency of nocturnal symptoms in asthmatic children attending a hospital out-patient clinic. *Eur Respir J* 1995; 8: 2076–80.

342. van Aalderen WM, Postma DS, Koeter GH, Knol K. The effect of reduction of maintenance treatment on circadian variation in peak expiratory flow rates in asthmatic children. *Acta Paediatr Scand* 1988; 77: 269–74.

343. Horn CR, Clark TJH, Cochrane GM. Inhaled therapy reduces morning dips in asthma. *Lancet* 1984; i: 1143–5.

344. Verberne A, Lenney W, Kerrebijn KF. A 3 way crossover study comparing twice daily dosing of salmeterol 25 mcg and 50 mcg with placebo in children with mild to moderate reversible airways disease. *Am Rev Respir Dis* 1991; 143: A20.

345. Zeitlin S, Rolles C, Antolainen I *et al*. An open, multicentre, cross-over comparison of albuterol controlled release tablets and individually titrated slow release theophylline in the treatment of childhood asthma. *Am Rev Respir Dis* 1988; 137: 33A.

346. Douglas NJ. Nocturnal asthma. *Thorax* 1993; 48: 100–102.

347. Hoskyns EW, Thomson AH, Decker E, Hutchins A, Simpson H. Effect of controlled release salbutamol on nocturnal cough in asthma. *Arch Dis Child* 1991; 66: 1209–12.

348. Wilson NM. Diet related asthma in children. *Paediatr Respir Med* 1993; 1: 14–20.

349. May CD. Objective clinical and laboratory studies of immediate reactions to foods in asthmatic children. *J Allergy Clin Immunol* 1976; 58: 500–515.

350. Matus I. Assessing the nature and clinical significance of psychological contributions to childhood asthma. *Am J Orthopsychiat* 1981; 51: 327–41.

351. Strunk RC. Identification of the fatality-prone subject with asthma. *J Allergy Clin Immunol* 1989; 83: 477–85.

352. Miller BD. Depression and asthma: a potentially lethal mixture. *J Allergy Clin Immunol* 1987; 80: 481–6.

353. Quinn CM. Children's asthma: new approaches, new understandings. *Ann Allergy* 1988; 60: 283–92.

354. Nocon A. Social and emotional impact of childhood asthma. *Arch Dis Child* 1991; 66: 458–60.

355. Barnes SD, Grob CS, Lachman BS, Marsh BR, Loughlin GM. Psychogenic upper airway obstruction presenting as refractory wheezing. *J Pediatr* 1986; 109: 1067–70.

356. Lask B, Matthew D. Childhood asthma. A controlled

trial of family psychotherapy. *Arch Dis Child* 1979; 54: 116–19.

357. Strunk RC, Fukuhara JT, LaBrecque JL, Mrazek DA. Outcome of long-term hospitalisation for asthma in children. *J Allergy Clin Immunol* 1989; 83: 17–25.

358. Brunekreef B, Dockery DW, Speizer FE, Ware JH, Spengler JD, Ferris BG. Home dampness and respiratory morbidity in children. *Am Rev Respir Dis* 1989; 140: 1363–7.

359. Dales RE, Zwanenburg H, Burnett R, Franklin CA. Respiratory effects of home dampness and molds among Canadian children. *Am J Epidemiol* 1991; 134: 196–203.

360. Nafstad P, Oie L, Mehl R *et al*. Residential dampness problems and symptoms and signs of bronchial obstruction in young Norwegian children. *Am J Respir Crit Care Med* 1998; 157: 410–414.

361. Honicky RE, Osborne III JS, Akpom CA. Symptoms of respiratory illness in young children and the use of wood-burning stoves for indoor heating. *Pediatrics* 1985; 75: 587–93.

362. Anderson HR, Bailey PA, Cooper JS, Palmer JC, West S. Morbidity and school absence caused by asthma and wheezing illness. *Arch Dis Child* 1983; 58: 777–84.

363. Bevis M, Taylor B. What do school teachers know about asthma? *Arch Dis Child* 1990; 65: 622–5.

364. Fillmore EJ, Jones N, Blankson JM. Achieving treatment goals for schoolchildren with asthma. *Arch Dis Child* 1997; 77: 420–22.

365. Jenkins MA, Hopper JL, Bowes G, Carlin JB, Flander LB, Giles GG. Factors in childhood as predictors of asthma in adult life. *BMJ* 1994; 309: 90–93.

366. Kelly WJW, Hudson I, Phelan PD, Pain MC, Olinsky A. Childhood asthma in adult life: a further study at 28 years of age. *BMJ* 1987; 294: 1059–62.

367. ✪ Godden DJ, Ross S, Abdalla MI *et al*. Outcome of wheeze in childhood: symptoms and pulmonary function 25 years later. *Am Rev Respir Dis* 1994; 149: 106–112.

368. Blair H. Natural history of childhood asthma. *Arch Dis Child* 1977; 52: 613–19.

369. Ross S, Godden DJ, McMurray D *et al*. Social effects of wheeze in childhood: a 25 year follow-up. *BMJ* 1992; 305: 545–8.

370. Sibbald B, Anderson HR, McGuigan S. Asthma and employment in young adults. *Thorax* 1992; 47: 19–24.

371. Strachan DP. Do chesty children become chesty adults? *Arch Dis Child* 1990; 65: 161–2.

372. Barnes PJ. General Pharmacologic Principles. In: Murray JF, Nadel JA (eds). *Textbook of Respiratory Medicine*. Philadelphia: W.B. Saunders, 1994; 1–2739.

373. Partridge MR. Problems with asthma care delivery. In: Mitchell DM (ed). *Recent Advances in Respiratory Medicine No. 5*. London: Churchill Livingstone, 1991: 61–78.

374. Paton JY. The safety of inhaled steroids in childhood asthma. *The Practitioner* 1994; 238: 322–6.

375. Robertson CF, Rubinfeld AR, Bowes G. Pediatric asthma deaths in Victoria: the mild are at risk. *Pediatr Pulmonol* 1992; 13: 95–100.

376. Weiss KB, Wagener DK. Changing patterns of asthma mortality–identifying target populations at high risk. *JAMA* 1990; 264: 1683–7.

377. Newcomb RW, Akhter J. Respiratory failure from asthma: a marker for children with high morbidity and mortality. *Am J Dis Child* 1988; 142: 1041–8.

Chapter 30

Management of Acute Asthma in Children

Søren Pedersen

The number of hospitalizations due to acute asthma has been increasing,[1,2] probably because of an increase in asthma prevalence or severity, but other factors including poor patient understanding, inadequate recognition and under-treatment also seem to have contributed substantially.[2–5] An acute severe asthma attack is a potentially life-threatening event, which should always be treated effectively without delay. The aims of the treatment are:

- to prevent death;
- to relieve hypoxaemia and normalize lung functions as quickly as possible;
- to avoid future relapses.

The principles and modalities of the treatment are the same as in adults. However, there are differences in dosages of medication and clinical assessment. A precondition for achieving the aims without unnecessary delay is a detailed knowledge about the optimal doses and mode of administration of the drugs used in the treatment of the condition and ability to recognize severe attacks.[6] Therefore, that will be discussed with special emphasis upon the results from controlled trials in the different age groups. This information will then form the basis for some suggestions of management strategies at home and in hospital.

β_2 AGONISTS

The value of inhaled β_2 agonists in the treatment of acute asthma in school and pre-school children has been demonstrated in several controlled trials.[7–27] Such treatment is superior to treatment with all other bronchodilators since it works effectively within minutes after the administration. Similarly, subcutaneous, intramuscular or intravenous administration is associated with a significant effect.[28–30]

Adrenaline has both α and β activity. Although it is an effective bronchodilator, the side-effects caused by its α and β_1 actions – anxiety, tremor, hypertension, tachycardia, palpitations and cardiac arrhythmias – are undesirable. It is sometimes suggested that adrenaline, with its α-adrenoceptor vasoconstricting activity would be better than other drugs at decreasing bronchial oedema because of its constrictor effects on arterioles. However, it also causes venous vasoconstriction and this effect could negate or even supersede any beneficial effect on arterial constriction. Controlled clinical trials do not demonstrate any advantages over the modern adrenoceptor agonists in relieving airway obstruction in children.[12,18,20,21,29,31–33] As a consequence its use in modern asthma treatment is obsolete. However, the α-stimulating action makes adrenaline the drug of choice for the treatment of anaphylactic shock.

Modes of Administration of β_2 Agonists

No direct comparisons between inhaled and systemic administration of β_2 agonist have been performed in children. However, in general the inhaled route provides a better clinical-effect to side-effect ratio than the systemic route in adults with severe acute symptoms.[34] Furthermore, the inhaled route appears to be less affected by the pre-treatment given prior to admission.[35] For these reasons inhalations are the best way to administer β_2 agonists to children with acute asthma.

Inhalation Systems

Nebulizers are simple to use and in the acute situation it is advantageous that oxygen can be administered through the nebulizer at the same time as the β_2 agonist. Therefore, nebulizers are still the delivery system of choice in the treatment of acute severe asthma in all age groups of hospitalized children even though most studies show that the same results can be obtained with other inhalation systems in schoolchildren.[7,8,16,17,26,27]

Simply varying the choice of compressor, jet-nebulizer and volume-fill has been shown to vary the mass of drug in respirable particles over a ten-fold range.[36] Therefore, conclusions from one nebulizer may not be transferred to other nebulizers or comparisons with other inhalers.

The inhalations should take place through tightly fitting face mask or a mouth-piece. Inhalation through a face mask 2–3 centimetres from the face, which is often seen, will reduce drug delivery to the patient by approximately 50% in schoolchildren, with a corresponding increase in release of aerosol to the environment. In agreement with this *in vitro* studies have reported an 85% reduction in the inhaled dose of respirable particles when the face mask was moved 2 cm from the inspiratory orifice.[37] The effect appears to be the same in schoolchildren whether the inhalation takes place through a mouth-piece or a face mask.[17]

Spacers are also easy to use[38] and virtually all schoolchildren can learn the use of these devices and also use them effectively during attacks of acute bronchoconstriction when they are as effective as nebulizers.[7,8,16,17,19,26,27,39] Because of the enormous variation in nebulizer output it is not possible to define exact equi-effective doses between nebulizers and spacers. However, normally lower doses are required from spacers to produce the same response as from a nebulizer.[19,26,27,39–41]

Normally actuation of more than one puff at a time into a spacer is not recommended[42,43] since the inhaled dose is reduced when several doses are fired into the spacer at a time because the fraction of airborne particles is reduced due to impaction and settling of particles on the inner wall of the spacer.

The output of respirable particles from some spacers may be markedly reduced if they are electrically charged due to static electricity. This may be a clinical problem with some new spacers or if the spacer is newly washed.[44,45] If such a spacer is used the patient may require higher doses than those normally recommended and therefore the attack may be assessed to be more severe than it is.

Fast inhalations are required to produce a maximum effect from *dry powder inhalers* (DPIs)[38,46–49] and therefore it sometimes suggested that dry powder inhalers are ineffective during acute attacks of wheeze. However, the majority of schoolchildren can generate a sufficient inspiratory flow rate also during episodes of acute wheeze.[47,50,51] Furthermore, the output and clinical effect of some dry powder inhalers are less dependent on the inspiratory flow rate generated by the patient.[52,53] Therefore dry powder inhalers can normally be used to treat even quite severe acute asthma attacks in schoolchildren.[50,54] However, many pre-school children may not be able to generate sufficiently high inspiratory flow rates during acute episodes of bronchoconstriction[38,47,55] and therefore DPIs should preferably be reserved for children older than 5 years. The same is true for *conventional metered dose inhalers*, which can normally only be used effectively in schoolchildren after careful tuition[38,56] but often not during episodes of acute wheeze.[57]

Dose Recommendations

It is always dangerous to recommend doses for acute severe asthma. This is because the dose required depends upon the response. The correct strategy is to administer enough drug for each individual patient under guidance of careful monitoring for adverse effects and measurement of the clinical response. Therefore, dose recommendations should be considered suggestions for an average patient. Furthermore, not all selective β_2 agonists have been extensively studied in children. When conclusions from studies with one drug are transferred to the others it must be remembered that some differences exist between the various agents.

Nebulized Therapy The optimal dose of nebulized β_2 agonists for acute asthma not only depends upon the nebulizer brand but also upon volume fill: more drug will be delivered if the same amount of drug is given in 4 ml than in 2 ml in the chamber. However, high doses of salbutamol (0.30 mg kg^{-1}) were better than low doses (0.15 mg kg^{-1}) when given at 3-hourly intervals.[14] No significant difference was observed in effect on heart rate or potassium levels between the two treatments. Furthermore, continuous nebulization of 0.3 mg salbutamol kg^{-1} h^{-1} produced better results than the same dose nebulized intermittently over 20 minutes every hour.[58] The value of continuous or frequent administration has also been emphasized by other investigators,[59–61] though several trials have failed to show any additional benefit of such strategy as compared with intermittent administration.[23,24]

A few years ago a study on less severe asthma attacks questioned the importance of dosing salbutamol per kilogram body weight (0.1 mg kg^{-1}), since a fixed dose of 2.5 mg to all children produced similar results.[62] This finding was recently supported by the results in other studies which have found a marked age-dependent lung deposition with various inhalation devices ,[63–66] lung deposition (in percentage of nominal or inhaled dose) being substantially lower in younger children than in older. So dosing inhaled therapy in mg kg^{-1} body weight in order to reduce the risk of unwanted systemic effects does not seem to be warranted with the inhalation devices presently available. Such strategy seems to involve a great risk of under-treating young children.

A dose–response study found that 5–10 mg nebulized metaproterenol seems to be the optimal bronchodilating dose for acute asthma in schoolchildren.[67]

Inhalation of high doses of β$_2$ agonists causes significant systemic absorption so that after some inhalations plasma drug levels are in the same range as after continuous systemic administration. As a consequence the same side-effects may be seen.[39,68,69] Therefore, this treatment combines the effects of local and systemic administration.

Spacers The optimal dose from a spacer is not known, but as for nebulizers dosing in mg kg^{-1} body weight does not seem to be warranted. Doses from 2 to 6 mg and doses around 0.1 mg kg^{-1} have been used without unacceptable side-effects.[7,8,16,17,19,39,40] In agreement with some nebulizer studies, frequent administration seems to be better than single high dose administration: a single dose of six puffs terbutaline (1500 µg) from a spacer was less effective than three puffs given twice at 15 minute intervals;[10] in addition one dose of 500 µg terbutaline was less effective than two doses of 250 µg given 5 minutes apart.[70]

Systemic Administration A significant correlation is seen between plasma drug levels and bronchodilating effect after systemic administration of a β agonist.[28,71] However, considerable inter-individual variations exist in plasma levels obtained after a given dose.[28,71] Therefore, standard doses are not feasible for effective therapy. Dosing should be individualized under the monitoring of the therapeutic response and the occurrence of side-effects.[72]

In a dose–response trial an intravenous loading dose of 2 µg kg^{-1} terbutaline followed by a continuous infusion of 5 µg kg^{-1} h^{-1} was optimal for the majority of children not receiving other therapy.[28] Furthermore, inhalation of 1 mg terbutaline from a Nebuhaler did

not further improve bronchodilation, indicating that maximum effect in these children could be achieved by systemic administration of drug. The same intravenous doses seem to apply when salbutamol is used.[73,75] In agreement with this addition of a 15 µg kg^{-1} infusion of salbutamol in the early treatment of children with acute severe asthma was recently found to curtail the clinical progression of asthma, reduce demand placed on hospital resources, and improve the quality of health care provided to the acutely sick child with asthma.[30] When systemic administration is combined with high-dose inhaled therapy the systemic doses should probably be reduced. Finally, doses around 10 µg kg^{-1} of terbutaline or salbutamol given subcutaneously or intramuscularly have produced significant clinical effect without unacceptable side-effects.[29,76] In one of these studies 12 µg kg^{-1} was better than 3 µg kg^{-1} and 6 µg kg^{-1}.

Special Considerations in Infants Several early studies failed to find any bronchodilator response to nebulized β$_2$ agonists in infants[77–80] and for many years it was believed that β agonists are ineffective in this age group though functioning β adrenoceptors are present. In agreement with these observations two recent studies assessing transcutaneous oxygen pressure and/or oxygen saturation found a fall in these parameters after treatment of acute wheeze in infants with nebulized salbutamol.[81,82] One of these studies suggested that some of the fall in Po_2 might be caused by the acidity of the aerosol.[81] In contrast, another study found an increase in tcPo_2 after nebulized salbutamol in children aged 11–30 months.[83] In accordance with this, recent placebo-controlled double-blind studies have demonstrated significant bronchodilator effects,[84–90] protective effects against broncoconstrictor agents[82,91–93] and clinical improvement in infants treated with β$_2$ agonists either alone or in combination with steroids.[80,94] The reason for this discrepancy is not clear. The various studies have differed with respect to dose, inhaler (spacer, nebulizer), baseline lung function, duration of symptoms and method of lung function measurement. The discrepancy is only seen in studies assessing bronchodilator effects. All studies find a significant protection against bronchoconstriction induced by various challenges. Thus, it seems that infants have functioning β$_2$ receptors from birth and that stimulation of these receptors can produce the same effects as in older children. However, often the response is rather small and marked inter-individual differences are seen. As a consequence further studies are needed to assess the optimal use during episodes of acute wheeze.

Side-Effects

Generally treatment of children with β_2 agonists is very safe. The occurrence of side-effects is directly proportional to the plasma concentrations of drug and therefore mainly depends on route of administration as well as on selectivity. Skeletal muscle tremor, headache, palpitations and some agitation are the most common complaints when high doses are used. After systemic administration the occurrence of side-effects can be used as an indication that the top of the bronchodilatory dose–response curve has been reached.[28] Tolerance to the side-effects seems to develop easily so that they will disappear with continued use of the drug.[95,96]

A small drop in blood pressure and a compensatory increase in pulse rate is seen after systemic use or administration of high doses of inhaled drug.[28] Furthermore, hyperglycaemia, hypokalaemia and an increase in free fatty acids are common under these conditions.[95,96] The hypokalaemia is more pronounced when concomitant high doses of steroids are used. The clinical importance of this remains to be elucidated since the changes seem to plateau even if the dose of β_2 agonists is increased and the measured changes are due to an increased transport of potassium into skeletal muscle. Thus there is no decrease in total body potassium level.

Asthma is associated with considerable ventilation-perfusion imbalance. This may result in low P_aO and hypoxaemia. β agonists have two pharmacological actions which may effect P_aO_2 in different directions. Firstly, they may decrease P_aO_2 by causing pulmonary vasodilatation, which increases perfusion of the poorly ventilated areas and thus increases the shunt effect. Secondly, β agonists will increase cardiac output, decrease peripheral resistance and cause bronchodilation, which will all increase P_aO_2. The net effect on P_aO_2 will be the balance of these effects. The significance of β agonist induced fall in P_aO_2 will depend on the initial oxygen tension of the patient, but normally it is without clinical importance and often occurs in patients with relatively high pretreatment P_aO_2. Concomitant use of theophylline seems to enhance most of the side-effects of β agonists.

STEROIDS

The beneficial effects of systemic steroids in the management of acute severe asthma has been shown in

several controlled trials in all age groups except infants[97–105] and the value of such therapy has only rarely been questioned, though some studies have found minimal or no benefit.[106,107] The optimal doses of steroid and route of administration have not been carefully evaluated, so the recommendations for this condition are rather empirical and based upon personal experience and the dose regimens used in studies evaluating the treatment. Undoubtedly, oral prednisolone is sufficient in the majority of children, especially when used early during the exacerbation.[100,108] Oral prednisolone is rapidly and reliably absorbed and therefore normally to be preferred. However, in some patients intravenous hydrocortisone or methylprednisolone may be necessary in case of gastrointestinal problems. Theoretically, methylprednisolone is preferable to hydrocortisone because of less mineralocorticoid effect and a better penetration into the lung tissue,[109] but no clinical differences in efficacy have been demonstrated. Very high doses of steroids are probably not necessary and may cause hypokalaemia, fluid retention and an acute myopathy.[110] Normally recommended steroid doses, which have produced significant effects in controlled trials are:

- *Prednisolone*: Loading dose 1–2 mg kg^{-1} (maximum 60 mg). This should be followed by 2 mg kg^{-1} every 24 hours, divided into two doses.
- *Methylprednisolone*: Loading dose 1–2 mg kg^{-1}. This should be followed by 1 mg kg^{-1} every 6 hours.
- *Hydrocortisone*: Loading dose 10 mg kg^{-1}, followed by 5 mg kg^{-1} every 6 hours.[61]

Systemic dexamethasone or oral prednisolone were of little benefit in infants with acute wheeze in two studies[111,112] but of significant benefit in another.[113] Therefore, further studies are needed in this age group.

Controlled trials have found that nebulized beclomethasone reduced the frequency (but not the severity) of respiratory symptoms and improved lung function in infants with post-bronchiolitis wheezing.[114,115]

High doses of inhaled corticosteroids are sometimes recommended for the treatment of exacerbations. However, at present there are an insufficient number of studies to support this. One study found a significant additional effect of nebulized budesonide in acute wheeze in children up to 18 months of age.[113] Another found that a short course of high-dose inhaled budesonide was at least as effective as oral prednisolone, without suppressing serum cortisol concentration in children who were treated in the emergency department.[116] Furthermore, if given early to young children with asthma provoked by viral upper respiratory tract infection such treatment can reduce the severity of asthma attacks though probably not the incidence of hospital admissions.[117,118] The studies assessing the value of increasing the dose of inhaled corticosteroid early during an exacerbation in older children have produced conflicting results.[119,120]

METHYLXANTHINES

Xanthine derivates (aminophylline or theophylline) have been used for many years in the treatment of acute severe asthma in children. The number of placebo-controlled studies assessing the acute effect is relatively sparse. It has been demonstrated that a bolus dose of theophylline causes significant increases in lung functions in schoolchildren with acute wheeze.[121–123] However, only two double-blind, controlled trials have supported its use in hospitalized children with severe asthma,[124,125] who were receiving other treatment including aggressive treatment with inhaled β_2 agonists.

No formal dose–response studies have been conducted in children with acute wheeze, but the bronchodilating effect seems to correlate with the plasma theophylline level.[123] Therefore it is normally recommended that the therapeutic strategy in such situations is to aim at plasma levels between 55 and 110 μmol l^{-1}. This can be achieved in all age groups by giving an intravenous bolus of 6 mg kg^{-1} lean body weight over 5 minutes to a child who has not received any theophylline for 12 hours prior to the treatment and then continue with theophylline infusion rates or oral therapy as shown in Table 30.1 Since the volume of distribution is around 0.5 l kg^{-1} such a bolus will result in a mean serum level of 12 μg ml^{-1} = 66 μmol l^{-1}. Gastrointestinal and rectal absorption of an aqueous solution is almost complete with peak serum theophylline levels being measured within one hour after the administration. Somewhat higher loading doses are required when these administration forms are used (8–9 mg kg^{-1}).[123,126] If the child is already receiving treatment with theophylline additional theophylline therapy should only be given under the guidance of plasma theophylline monitoring.

Though significant bronchodilating effects have been demonstrated in children the role of theophylline in the acute management of asthma has been questioned upon the basis of the findings in a recent study[127] which did not find any additional benefit of theophylline in children treated with steroids and frequent inhalations of β_2 agonist, probably because theophylline is a weaker bronchodilator than inhaled β_2 agonists.[128,129] In accordance with this is a recent meta-analysis of 13 double-blind controlled studies on the treatment of acute asthma in children and adults did not find any convincing evidence of any clinical benefit of adding theophylline to treatment with steroids and indeed β_2 agonists.

Theophylline has not been thoroughly studied in pre-school children and infants with wheeze.

Some knowledge about theophylline pharmacokinetics is important for effective, safe therapy. This has been thoroughly described in an excellent review.[130] Generally children metabolize theophylline much more rapidly than adults, and in the child population the elimination rate also varies with age so that young children have a much higher clearance than older children. The normally recommended theophylline doses for continuous therapy in different age groups are shown in Table 30.1.

These dose recommendations are based upon lean body weight and they aim at plasma theophylline levels between 55 and 110 μmol l^{-1}. Within each age group the inter-individual variations in theophylline half life may be up to 10-fold and in addition other drugs including β_2 agonists (increase clearance so that higher doses are required) and viral infections (reduce clearance) may also affect the metabolism. Therefore, theophylline dose must always be individualized and if high doses are used as in the treatment of acute asthma plasma theophylline levels must be measured. When dose adjustments are made upon the basis of serum theophylline determinations it is important to remember that theophylline often shows dose-dependent kinetics so that on average the percent change in serum concentration is about 50% greater than the percent change in dose.

Side-Effects

Theophylline has a narrow therapeutic window and potentially lethal side-effects when overdosed.[131–134] During the last decade, 63 deaths have been reported in studies with theophylline.[135] The most common side-effects are anorexia, nausea, vomiting and headache.[133,134,136] These symptoms are quite common. Mild central nervous stimulation, palpitations, tachycardia, arrhythmias, abdominal pain, diarrhoea and, rarely, gastric bleeding may also occur.

Table 30.1: Recommended average doses of the various drugs used to treat acute severe asthma in all age groups of children. Only the most commonly used drugs are mentioned. Individual dose adjustments should be made based upon the clinical response and occurrence of side-effects

β_2 *agonists*	
Nebulizer	2.5 mg salbutamol or 5 mg terbutaline Volume fill = 4 ml Mouth piece or tightly fitting face mask May be repeated at frequent intervals
Spacer device or other inhalers	One puff every minute until satisfactory response. If more than 10 puffs is required: consider admission
Subcutaneous or intramuscular	10 μg kg^{-1} salbutamol or terbutaline
Intravenous (salbutamol/terbutaline)	Loading dose: 2–5 μg kg^{-1} over 5 min Continuous: 5 μg kg^{-1} per hour
Ipratropium bromide	
Nebulizer	250 μg in a volume fill of 4 ml to all age groups May be repeated 4–6 hourly
Corticosteroids	
Prednisolone	Loading dose: 1–2 mg kg^{-1} (maximum 60 mg) Continuous: 2 mg kg^{-1} per day divided into two doses
Intravenous methylprednisolone	Loading dose: 1–2 mg kg^{-1} Continuous: 1 mg kg^{-1} 6 hourly
Intravenous hydrocortisone	Loading dose: 10 mg kg^{-1} Continuous: 5 mg kg^{-1} 6 hourly
Theophylline (for patients not receiving theophylline prior to treatment)	
Intravenous	Loading dose: 6 mg kg^{-1} lean body weight over 10 min
Oral or rectal administration	Loading dose: 8–9 mg kg^{-1} lean body weight
Continuous treatment (oral or intravenous)	<1 year: $(0.3) \times$ (age in weeks) + 8 mg kg^{-1} per 24 h
Measurement of serum levels required.	1–9 years: 24 mg kg^{-1} per 24 h 9–12 years: 20 mg kg^{-1} per 24 h 12–16 years: 18 mg kg^{-1} per 24 h Over 16 years: 14 mg kg^{-1} per 24 h

The most serious toxicity is the risk of seizures, which have been associated with a mortality rate as high as 50%. However, seizures appear to be rare at serum levels less than 220 μmol l^{-1}. In theophylline-induced seizures higher than normal doses of benzodiazepines should be used as theophylline antagonizes the effect of benzodiazepines on γ-aminobutyric acid (GABA) receptors in the brain.[137] If modern kinetic principles are used seizures should not occur.[130]

ANTI-MUSCASRINIC AGENTS

Virtually all pharmacodynamic data in children refer to one drug: ipratropium bromide. The dose-ranging studies in schoolchildren have all used a nebulizer for the delivery so the optimal dose is only known for this administration. It would be expected, however, to be lower if a metered dose inhaler with a spacer is used.[138] Normally, increasing the ipratropium bromide dose above 250 µg adds no extra benefit in protection against exercise-induced asthma,[139] cold air hyperventilation or in bronchodilation.[140] This dose (250 µg) has also been used in most studies on pre-school children. No formal dose–response studies have been performed in infants but a dose of 25 µg kg^{-1} has produced beneficial effects in one study.[141] The optimal dose frequency and optimal dose in acute severe wheeze remains unknown.

Generally, maximum bronchodilatation from these doses of ipratropium bromide seems to be slower and the duration of action similar to that of an inhaled β_2 agonist.

Anti-cholinergics result in less bronchodilatation than inhaled β_2 agonists[142] and administered alone these drugs have no role in the management of acute severe asthma in schoolchildren.[143] However, controlled studies have found that the combination of a β_2 agonist and an anti-cholinergic agent produces somewhat better results than either drug used alone[143–149] without an increase in side-effects. Though statistically highly significant, the advantages of the combination therapy were rather small in most studies. This may be the reason why other studies failed to find any benefit of such combined therapy.

It has been argued that the augmented effects elicited by the combination of adrenergic and anti-cholinergic agents might simply be a consequence of underdosing with the adrenergic drug. However, the additional effect has also been reported in studies using quite high doses of β_2 agonists. Furthermore, in one study frequent nebulized doses of salbutamol were administered to the children until a plateau in the response was seen. The children were then randomized to receive either ipratropium bromide or placebo. A significant additional increase in lung function of around 20% (placebo = 5%) was observed after 2 hours in the ipratropium bromide group compared with placebo.[147]

A clinical study in acute viral bronchiolitis in infants did not find any beneficial effects of ipratropium bromide[150] though other studies suggest some benefit in this conditions.[141,145]

So, although the findings have not been consistent the data do suggest that ipratropium bromide has a role as an adjunct to inhaled β_2 agonists in the treatment of acute asthma in children older than one year.

Side-Effects

Paradoxical bronchoconstriction after inhalation and dryness of the mouth may be a problem in some patients.[151,152] Some of these incidents seemed to be due to benzalkonium chloride which has now been removed from the nebulizer solution. Otherwise no important side-effects are associated with the use of anti-cholinergics.

ASSESSMENT OF SEVERITY

The asthma severity in children is often underestimated by physicians. The child may appear deceptively well and yet suffer from quite marked airway obstruction (PEF around 50–60% predicted normal or personal best value). Even in the presence of wheeze many children still want to participate in other children's activities. Therefore, objective measurements are important and necessary for a correct assessment. Even trained doctors may not be good at predicting a patient's lung function.[153] Table 30.2 provides some parameters, which are normally used in the assessment. Since these are guidelines only, all features in one category need not be present. When in doubt whether the condition should be categorized as moderate or severe it is normally severe.

Absolute criteria for admission or a particular treatment recommendation are difficult to formulate and depend upon several factors including past history, availability of treatment, social circumstances (parental understanding and capability of accurate monitoring) and geographic isolation. Unfortunately, there is no identifiable factor that can be used to predict which children will respond to the treatment.[153] In the lights of this the value of some of the parameters in Table 30.2 will be briefly discussed.

Special Considerations in Infants and Young Children

Differences in lung anatomy and physiology and a poorer response to treatment place infants at greater risk than older children. Marked hyperinflation is often prevalent in young children with wheeze.[154] As a consequence respiratory works is increased and these age groups are prone to develop hypercapnia (hypoventilation) and respiratory failure more readily than older

405

Table 30.2: Assessment of severity of asthma exacerbations in children

	Mild	Moderate	Severe
Treatment place	Home/out-patient	Home/out-patient	Hospitalization
Wheeze	Only end-expiratory	Loud	Loud or absent
Breathless			
Older child	Playing	Walking	Talks in single words
Infant	Crying	Difficult feeding	Stops feeding
Accessory muscle retractions	Usually not	Moderate	Marked
Respiratory rate			
<3 months	<60 min^{-1}	60–70 min^{-1}	>70 min^{-1}
3–12 months	<50 min^{-1}	50–60 min^{-1}	>60 min^{-1}
1–6 years	<40 min^{-1}	40–50 min^{-1}	>50 min^{-1}
>6 years	<30 min^{-1}	30–40 min^{-1}	>40 min^{-1}
Pulse rate			
<1 year	<150 min^{-1}	150–170 min^{-1}	>170 min^{-1}
1–2 years	<120 min^{-1}	120–140 min^{-1}	>140 min^{-1}
>2 years	<110 min^{-1}	110–130 min^{-1}	>130 min^{-1}
Pre-treatment PEFR	>70%	50–70%	<50%
Response to β_2 agonist	>3 hours	2–3 hours	<2 hours
P_aCO_2	<35 mmHg	<40 mmHg	>40 mmHg
S_aO_2 (on air)	>94%	92–94%	<92%

Life-threatening features

PEFR <40% of best
Cyanosis
Bradycardia
Fatigue/exhaustion/reduced consciousness
Silent chest
Paradoxical thoraco–abdominal movement
Disappearance of retractions without concomitant clinical
   improvement

High-risk patient:[180] low admission threshold

Recent withdrawal of oral steroids
Hospitalization for asthma in past year
Earlier catastrophic attacks
Psychiatric disease/psychosocial problems
Poor compliance
Young children (develop respiratory failure more readily and are more
   difficult to assess)

children. It is more common to underestimate severity in infants and generally young children are more severely obstructed and have higher P_{CO_2} than older children.[155] Therefore, measurement of time trends in P_{CO_2}, P_{O_2} or oxygen saturation is usually indicated in addition to the clinical observations in severe wheeze in these age groups.

History

History should always include likely triggers (infection, allergy, compliance), duration, treatment prior to admission (dose, drug, response) and other lung diseases. An acute asthma attack in a child assessed to suffer from mild asthma may be as dangerous as an attack in a child with moderate or severe asthma. Thus the majority of fatal asthma attacks are seen in patients with a history of mild asthma.[5]

Objective Findings

Symptom scores assessing degree of auscultatory findings, respiratory rate, patient distress, respiratory effort (retractions) and pallor have been used to assess severity and the efficacy of drugs in the treatment of acute asthma.[62,153,155–158] The various scores correlate weakly with oxygen saturation and lung function,[153] though not all studies have found this.[155] Furthermore, findings of a quiet chest on auscultation, inability to talk, and cyanosis or a high score strongly suggest hypercapnia and severe bronchoconstriction.[156,159] However, in the individual patient it cannot be used as a single criterion to predict outcome. It is important to remember that respiratory muscle fatigue may result in slowing of the respiration rate, disappearance of retractions and appearance of paradoxical thoraco-abdominal movement. *Remember that anxiety and confusion may be due to hypoxemia. Therefore, anxiety should never be treated with sedatives.*

Pulsus Paradoxus

The pulsus paradoxus of acute severe asthma is an exaggeration of the normal fall in systolic blood pressure during inspiration. Its size is thought to relate to the severity of the attack. However, pulsus paradoxus is difficult to measure in children and the association between worsening obstruction and increase in pulsus paradoxus is weak.[153] The sign is not present in one third of patients with severe obstruction and only a severe paradox (>20 mmHg) is a reliable indicator of a severe attack.[160]

Bronchodilator Response

It is normally suggested that the duration of effect following the administration of β_2 agonists is a useful guide to the severity. Those with a low or short effect (<2 hours) following inhalation of a β_2 agonist tend to be prone to a slower recovery.

Blood Gases

PCO_2 can be reliably measured on capillary blood which makes this parameter very useful particularly in young children. It may also be monitored transcutaneously together with PO_2. Normally, PCO_2 is low due to hyperventilation and a slight respiratory alkalosis is common.[161] When airway obstruction becomes excessive the low PCO_2 and high pH return to normal and severe respiratory failure may soon develop. Therefore, normal or elevated PCO_2 values should always be considered a sign of danger. High values, which increase in spite of aggressive treatment are one of the indications for assisted ventilation. One paper found that blood gases was the only satisfactory method to assess severity.

Oxygen Saturation

The initial arterial oxygen saturation has been evaluated as a criterion to decide to admit or discharge a child with acute asthmatic symptoms. An oxygen saturation level ≤ 91% was found predictive of a very severe condition requiring admission; saturation levels of 92–93% were borderline cases and ≥ 94% indicated moderate and mild attacks.[161] In that study post-bronchodilator saturation was not predictive of the outcome.[161] At variance with this other studies have found that a post-bronchodilator oxygen saturation <91% was the best predictor for a severe attack.[153,162] Whilst arterial oxygen saturation is a useful tool in the evaluation and surveillance of acute asthma, the correlation with lung function is weak and this parameter has not been shown to be sufficiently sensitive to be used as a single criterion for the admission to hospital of an acutely ill child.

Lung Functions

Most children ≥ 5 years can make reproducible measurements. Remember, however, that in the acute situation it is better to treat the child than to use the time training him/her in lung function measurements. Furthermore, forced expiratory manoeuvres may provoke/increase bronchoconstriction when the airways are very hyperreactive. The best way of assessing lung function is the measured value as a percentage of the child's personal best. If that is not known the percentage of predicted normal can be used. It is worthwhile remembering that normally the percentage predicted FEV_1 or $FEF_{25-75\%}$ is lower than the percentage predicted PEF. Though lung functions correlate to the various clinical signs and objective measurements the correlation is always weak and therefore these parameters are not good predictors in the individual patient. Lung functions are still the best measurement of the degree of airway obstruction and there is a highly significant association between low peak expiratory flow rate (<25% and <50%) as well as the percentage improvement after β_2 agonist treatment and need for intensive treatment.[163] Therefore, peak expiratory flow rates (or FEV_1 and FVC if the equipment is available) should be measured whenever it is possible. These measurements are the most valuable of all parameters for assessing the response to treatment and for decisions about stepping down treatment and discharging the patient. As for the other parameters, lung function may not be used as a single criterion for admission, though one study suggested that children with peak expiratory values >25% predicted normal or personal best could be managed outside hospital.[155] It is the author's personal opinion that 25% is a too low value. Therefore somewhat higher values are suggested in Table 30.2.

Chest X-rays

Chest X-rays are rarely helpful in acute asthma in children. It can be reserved for cases when the initial progression in clinical improvement is poor or objective findings or history suggest that complicating factors or differential diagnoses may be important.

Infections

Viral infections are frequent causes of exacerbations and nasopharyngeal swabs and sputum for viral and bacterial culture should be taken if infection is suspected as a precipitating cause.

TREATMENT AND MONITORING

There is more than one way to manage an acute asthma exacerbation in a child. No two patients or situations are alike and many excellent reviews have suggested various management plans.[164–171] The following is the author's suggestion of a protocol for treating acute asthma in various age groups of children. It is based upon the controlled studies mentioned earlier, personal experience, and the fact that the primary factors leading to obstruction are bronchoconstriction, inflamation, mucus plugging and oedema.

First of all it is important to ensure that the correct treatment has been applied and that it is improving the condition satisfactorily. Careful monitoring is therefore mandatory. It should include the assessment of the parameters in Table 30.2. It is recommended to do regular recordings of: respiration rate, pulse rate, peak expiratory flow rate, use of auxiliary muscles and retractions, colour, duration of effect of nebulized β_2 agonist, blood gases (especially PCO_2), oxygen saturation and the general clinical condition, including occurrence of side-effects (measurement of electrolytes (potassium) – see under β_2 agonists, p. 402). The frequency of assessment depends upon severity, but generally more frequent monitoring (every 30 minutes) is required in the beginning of the treatment and in the more severe cases.

GENERAL PRACTICE

The child should be seen without delay. It is important to assess the child both before, during and after treatment to get an accurate perception of the severity.

Immediate Treatment

All Children Independent of the initial assessment of severity of the acute attack a short-acting β_2 agonists should be given – preferably via an MDI and a spacer device. Use a face mask in pre-school children. If a spacer is not available other inhalers may be used (see inhalers). Give one puff every minute until satisfactory improvement occurs, i.e. the clinical condition is changed into mild severity (Table 30.2). Consider admission if this is not achieved after 10 puffs.

If inhaled treatment can not for some reason be given or taken by the child salbutamol or terbutaline $10 \, \mu g \, kg^{-1}$ can be administered subcutaneously or intramuscularly.

Subsequent Treatment

Mild Attacks Continue with regular inhaled β_2 agonist (every 3–6 hours) as long as it is required and consider doubling the normally taken dose or adding high-dose ($800 \, \mu g$ per day) inhaled corticosteroid until the conditions has been stable for 1 week. If 3–4 hourly treatments are still required after 24 hours, the attack should be considered as moderate and treated accordingly.

Moderate Attacks If the response to the initial treatment is good and the dose of β_2 agonist required to achieve the response is six puffs or less, continue with regular inhaled β_2 agonist (every 2–4 hours) as long as it is required and double the normally taken dose or add high-dose ($800 \, \mu g$ per day) inhaled corticosteroid until the condition has been stable for 1–2 weeks. If 3-hourly β_2 agonist is still required after 24 hours, add a short course of oral prednisolone.

If the response to the initial treatment is good but high doses of β_2 agonist doses are required to achieve the response, add a short course of oral prednisolone 2 mg kg^{-1} per day (maximum dose 60 mg) divided into two doses per day for 3–5 days to the suggested treatment.

If the response to the initial treatment is poor or of short duration (<2 hours), consider admission and give a 1–2 mg kg^{-1} dose of oral prednisolone (maximum dose 60 mg).

Severe Attacks Admission to hospital without delay after the initial treatment. Give a 1–2 mg kg^{-1} dose of oral prednisolone (maximum dose 60 mg).

The various treatments may be supplemented by continuous oral theophylline or oral β$_2$ agonist treatment for some days as suggested in Table 30.1.

All parents should be instructed in monitoring procedures and encouraged to call the doctor again if the resolution of the exacerbation is not progressing satisfactorily (individual criteria and a written action plan (see later) should be given according to the global assessment of the situation).

HOSPITAL MANAGEMENT

Immediate Treatment
All children

- Oxygen (8–10 l min^{-1}) via a face mask or nasal canula.
- Salbutamol or terbutaline 2.5 or 5 mg kg^{-1} in a volume fill of 4 ml via oxygen-driven nebulizer. If a face mask is used it should fit tightly to the child's face.
- Prednisolone 1–2 mg kg^{-1} body weight orally (maximum 60 mg).
- If the child is critically ill or vomits, oral prednisolone should be replaced by intravenous methylprednisolone 2 mg kg^{-1}

Subsequent Treatment
In many children the immediate treatment produces significant and marked improvement. Subsequent management in these cases may only require repeated nebulized β$_2$ agonist 2–4 hourly and continued treatment with oral prednisolone 2 mg kg^{-1} per day.[98]

In those with more severe asthma (the response to the initial treatment is poor or the duration less than 2 hours) the following should be tried in addition to continued prednisolone:

- Repeat nebulized β$_2$ agonist treatment and add 0.250 mg ipratropium bromide to the solution.
- This can be followed by frequent or continuous nebulized β$_2$ agonist in divided doses at 20–30 minute intervals or as continuous nebulization (if the equipment is available). 0.250 mg ipratropium bromide can be repeated.
- If the improvement is still not satisfactory consider intravenous β$_2$ agonists or theophylline as outlined in Table 30.1. These doses are average doses and should be adjusted upon the basis of the clinical effect, side-effects and (for theophylline) serum drug concentrations. If the child is already receiving oral theophyllines systemic β$_2$ agonists are preferred. In such patients serum theophylline concentration should be monitored before theophylline treatment is initiated. If the child is receiving systemic β$_2$ agonists the initial loading theophylline dose should be halved to minimize side-effects.

Additional Treatment

- Give supplemental oxygen to maintain saturation above 90%.
- Assess the need for intravenous fluids but do not overhydrate.
- Antibiotics should not be given routinely, but only to patients suspected of bacterial pneumonia or other bacterial infections.
- Acute asthma is a frightening condition and the child needs psychological support.

Useless or Dangerous Treatments Cough medicine is useless and never indicated in acute severe asthma. Sedatives are dangerous and may induce respiratory failure or apnoea. Therefore, these drugs should only be given at the intensive care unit when facilities for intubation and assisted ventilation are available and ready.

Indications for Intensive Care Children with acute severe asthma require intensive monitoring by experienced staff and all patients with life-threatening features (Table 30.2) not responding convincingly to treatment require intensive care.

Indications for Assisted Ventilation Not all children admitted to the intensive care unit need ventilation, but it may be necessary in a small number of patients as a life-saving procedure. In general, it is accepted that this procedure is necessary in those patients who fulfil the following criteria:

- P_aCO_2 of >8.6 kPa and rising
- P_aO_2 of <6.6 kPa and falling
- pH of 7.25 or less and falling
- Apnoea
- Respiratory arrest
- Cardiorespiratory arrest.

Stepping Down Treatment

- *Step 1*. When the condition has been stable for 12 hours the intensive treatment can be gradually reduced, starting with systemic β_2 agonists and theophylline. Some may want to continue with these treatments for some time. In that case the intravenous treatment can be stopped and oral maintenance treatment started with the doses given in Table 30.1.
- *Step 2*. The next step is less frequent β_2 agonists inhalations.
- *Step 3*. Finally, the patient is switched to inhaled therapy with corticosteroids and β_2 agonists with the inhaler that is going to be used at home. Oral prednisolone continues unchanged.

The duration of oral prednisolone treatment is individual depending upon severity of the attack and response. A rule of thumb is to continue after the condition is brought back to "mild" for twice as many days as it took to bring it there, but never less than 3 days. The dose may be gradually reduced or simply stopped based upon individual assessments.

Recovery and Discharge

An acute attack must always be considered a failure of prophylaxis and before discharge measures must be taken to prevent relapse, which has been reported to occur at a rate of 20–30% within the first 2 weeks after presentation.[158,161,172] Therefore, patients should not normally be discharged until:

- their symptoms have disappeared;
- lung function has stabilized (diurnal variability <25%); lung function has returned to its normal or best level (peak expiratory flow of >75% of the predicted or personal best);
- the child is stabilized on maintenance treatment, which should *always* include inhaled corticosteroids at a higher than pre-admission dosage;

- it has been ensured that the child is able to comply with the regimen.

The treatment with inhaled steroids should preferably be started 24–48 hours before discharge if the attack was severe. Nebulizers should be replaced by standard inhaler devices 24–48 hours before discharge unless the patient requires a nebulizer at home. Inhaled β_2 agonists should preferably be prescribed for use "as necessary". The inhalation technique should be checked and performance recorded. In patients requiring oral xanthines blood theophylline concentrations should be monitored.

Recovery after acute asthma is often very slow. Children can remain vulnerable despite appearing well. The airways can remain hyperreactive and smaller airways lung function compromised for many weeks after an acute asthmatic attack. Therefore, inhaled corticosteroids should continue throughout the recovery phase, which is often of 6–8 weeks duration.

Investigation of the Circumstances of Admission It is important to address the following questions, which relate to avoidable factors:

- Was there an avoidable precipitating cause? An allergy history should be taken.
- Was this a catastrophic sudden attack or was there a period of recognizable deterioration?
- Did the patient (or relatives) react appropriately when the asthma got worse?
- Was the patient complying with regular treatment, and, if not, can anything be done to help?
- Was medical management appropriate?

The admission to hospital provides an opportunity to educate patients about their asthma and train them to respond to changes in symptoms and peak flow. Children ≥ 5 years should have a peak expiratory flow meter and be taught how to use it. Peak expiratory flow rates should be recorded and brought at the first follow-up visit.

Self-Management Plan All patients should have a written self-management plan. The child and his or her parents:

- should know at what values of peak expiratory flow or level of symptoms to increase their treatment;
- how treatment should be increased and for how long;
- when to call their doctor, or readmit themselves to hospital.

In this respect it is important to remember that overuse of a β_2 agonist is a marker for uncontrolled asthma. Physicians should be alert for children who require frequent use (> twice daily) of a β_2 agonist. Such patients should be prescribed an inhaled steroid or have their inhaled steroid treatment modified to achieve symptom control. Furthermore, the patient should be instructed not to rely too much on the inhaled β_2 agonists during periods of worsening of symptoms.

Contact with a General Practitioner Good communication with the patient's general practitioner is essential. Discharge letters should include the peak expiratory flow on admission and at discharge (recorded on the patient's meter) and details of treatment to be continued at home and the self management plan.

Follow-Up Arrangements All children require follow-up. The initial outpatient appointment should be within a month. Clinical assessment including lung function and discussion of the home recordings with the child and his or her parents should be performed and a further management plan to enable the patient to lead normal life and to prevent further severe attacks should be made. It is also important to evaluate whether the patient has read and understood the information given at discharge, particularly the action plan.

Many of the measures suggested after the hospital treatment have not been thoroughly evaluated in controlled trials. However, several studies do suggest that use of steroids, good instructions, self-management plans and use of prophylactic medication markedly reduce morbidity and the occurrence of relapses.[173–178] Reduction of the total number of asthma exacerbations and hospital admissions in society requires an earlier diagnosis of asthma and an earlier and more widespread use of inhaled corticosteroids, especially in children with milder disease since this group contributes the largest number of exacerbations and admissions.[5] In areas where such strategies are adopted the number of asthma hospitalizations is reduced by 50–80%.[179,181]

KEY POINTS

1 Acute asthma in children can be managed in many different ways. No two patients or situations are alike and individualization is important.

2 Inhaled, β_2 agonists and systemic steroids are the cornerstone in the acute management. Other drugs are additional.

3 It may be difficult clinically to assess the severity of airway obstruction in children. Therefore objective measurements are important for a correct assessment and monitoring of response to treatment.

4 Young children and infants develop respiratory failure more readily than older children.

5 After initial treatment and stabilization, measures should be taken for preventing future attacks.

REFERENCES

1. Mitchell EA, Anderson HR, Freeling P, White PT. Why are hospital admission and mortality rates for childhood asthma higher in New Zealand than in the United Kingdom? *Thorax* 1990; 45: 176–82.

2. Anderson HR. Increase in hospital admissions for childhood asthma: Trends in referral, severity, and readmissions from 1970 to 1985 in a health region in the United Kingdom. *Thorax* 1989; 44: 614–19.

3. Fletcher HJ, Ibrahim SA, Speight N. Survey of asthma deaths in the Northern region, 1970–85.

Arch Dis Child 1990; 65: 163–7.

4. ✪ Pinnock H, Johnson A, Young P, Martin N. Are doctors still failing to assess and treat asthma attacks? An audit of the management of acute attacks in a health district. *Respir Med* 1999; 93: 397–401.

5. Robertson C, Rubinfeld A, Bowes G. Deaths from asthma in Victoria: a 12-month survey. *Med J Aust* 1990; 152: 511–17.

6. Webb LZ, Kuykendall DH, Zeiger RS *et al*. The impact of status asthmaticus practice guidelines on patient outcome and physician behaviour. *QRB Qual Rev Bull* 1992; 18: 471–6.

7. Pendergast J, Hopkins J, Timms B, Van Asperen PP. Comparative efficacy of terbutaline administered by Nebuhaler and by nebulizer in young children with acute asthma. *Med J Aust* 1989; 151: 406–408.

8. Fuglsang G, Pedersen S. Comparison of a new multidose powder inhaler with a pressurized aerosol in children with asthma. *Pediatr Pulmonol* 1989; 7: 112–15.

9. Watson WT, Becker AB, Simons FE. Comparison of ipratropium solution, fenoterol solution, and their combination administered by nebulizer and face mask to children with acute asthma. *J Allergy Clin Immunol* 1988; 82: 1012–18.

10. Phanichyakarn P, Kraisarin C, Sasisakulporn C, Kittikool J. A comparison of different intervals of administration of inhaled terbutaline in children with acute asthma. *Asian Pac J Allergy Immunol* 1992; 10: 89–94.

11. ✪ Kelly HW, McWilliams B, Katz R, Murphy S. Safety of frequent high dose nebulized terbutaline in children with acute severe asthma. *Ann Allergy* 1990; 64: 229–33.

12. Victoria MS, Battista CJ, Nangia BS. Comparison between epinephrine and terbutaline injections in the acute management of asthma. *J Asthma* 1989; 26: 287–90.

13. Portnoy J, Aggarwal J. Continuous terbutaline nebulization for the treatment of severe exacerbations of asthma in children. *Ann Allergy* 1988; 60: 368–71.

14. Schuh S, Reider MJ, Canny G *et al*. Nebulized albuterol in acute childhood asthma: comparison of two doses. *Pediatrics* 1990; 86: 509–513.

15. Pool J, Greenough A, Price J. Abnormalities of functional residual capacity in symptomatic and asymptomatic young asthmatics. *Acta Paediatr Scand* 1988; 77: 419–23.

16. Scalabrin DM, Naspitz CK. Efficacy and side effects of salbutamol in acute asthma in children: comparison of oral route and two different nebulizer systems. *J Asthma* 1993; 30: 51–9.

17. Lowenthal D, Kattan M. Facemasks versus mouthpieces for aerosol treatment of asthmatic children. *Pediatr Pulmonol* 1992; 14: 192–6.

18. Ben-Zvi Z, Lam C, Hoffman J, Teets-Grimm KC, Kattan M. An evaluation of the initial treatment of acute asthma. *Pediatrics* 1982; 70 (suppl 3): 348–53.

19. ✪ Kerem E, Levison H, Schuh S *et al*. Efficacy of albuterol administered by nebulizer versus spacer device in children with acute asthma. *J Pediatr* 1993; 123: 313–17.

20. Turpeinen M, Kuokkanen J, Backman A. Adrenaline and nebulized salbutamol in acute asthma. *Arch Dis Child* 1984; 59: 666–8.

21. Becker AB, Nelson NA, Simons FE. Inhaled salbutamol (albuterol) vs injected epinephrine in treatment of acute asthma in children. *J Pediatr* 1983; 102: 465–9.

22. Kelly HW, McWilliams B, Katz R, Murphy S. Safety of frequent high dose nebulized terbutaline in children with acute severe asthma. *Ann Allergy* 1990; 64: 229–33.

23. Ducharme FM, Davis GM. Randomized controlled trial of ipratropium bromide and frequent low doses of salbutamol in the management of mild and moderate acute pediatric asthma *J Pediatr* 1998; 133: 479–85.

24. Khine H, Fuchs SM, Saville AL. Continuous vs intermittent nebulized albuterol for emergency management of asthma. *Acad Emerg Med* 1996; 3: 1019–24.

25. Zar HJ, Brown G, Donson H, Brathwaite N, Mann MD, Weinberg EG. Home-made spacers for bronchodilator therapy in children with acute asthma: a randomised trial. *Lancet* 1999; 354: 979–82.

26. Robertson CF, Norden MA, Fitzerald DA *et al*. Treatment of acute asthma: salbutamol via jet nebuliser vs spacer and metered dose inhaler. *J Paediatr Child Health* 1998; 34: 142–6.

27. Williams JR, Bothner JP, Swanton RD. Delivery of albuterol in a pediatric emergency department. *Pediatr Emerg Care* 1996; 12: 263–7.

28. Fuglsang G, Pedersen S, Borgström L. Dose–response relationships of intravenously administered terbutaline in children with asthma. *J Pediatr* 1989; 114: 315–20.

29. Davis WJ, Pang LM, Chernack WJ, Mellins RB. Terbutaline in the treatment of acute asthma in childhood. *Chest* 1977; 72: 614–17.

30. ○ Browne GJ, Penna AS, Phung X, Soo M. Randomised trial of intravenous salbutamol in early management of acute severe asthma in children. *Lancet* 1997; 349: 301–305.

31. Ting CK, Liao MH. A comparative study of epinephrine injection and beta 2-agonist inhalation in the treatment of childhood asthma. *Acta Paediatr Sin* 1991; 32: 372–81.

32. Kornberg AE, Zuckerman S, Welliver JR, Mezzadri F, Aquino N. Effect of injected long-acting epinephrine in addition to aerosolized albuterol in the treatment of acute asthma in children. *Pediatr Emerg Care* 1991; 7: 1–3.

33. Uden DL, Goetz DR, Kohen DP, Fifield GC. Comparison of nebulized terbutaline and subcutaneous epinephrine in the treatment of acute asthma. *Ann Emerg Med* 1985; 14: 229–32.

34. Janson C. The role of adrenergics in the management of severe, acute asthma. *Res Clin Forums* 1993; 15: 9–14.

35. Swedish Society of Chest Medicine. High dose inhaled versus intravenous salbutamol combined with theophylline in acute severe asthma. *Eur Respir J* 1990; 3: 163–70.

36. Newman S, Pellow PGD, Clay M, Clarke SW. Evaluation of jet nebulizers for use with gentamycin solution. *Thorax* 1985; 40: 671–6.

37. Everard ML, Clark AR, Milner AD. Drug delivery from holding chambers with attached facemask. *Arch Dis Child* 1992; 67: 580–85.

38. Pedersen S. Inhaler use in children with asthma. *Danish Med Bull* 1987; 34: 234–49.

39. Fuglsang G, Pedersen S. Comparison of Nebuhaler and nebulizer treatment of acute severe asthma in children. *Eur J Respir Dis* 1986; 69: 109–113.

40. Blackhall M, O'Donnell SR. A dose-response study of inhaled terbutaline administered via nebuhaler or nebuliser to asthmatic children. *Eur J Respir Dis* 1987; 71: 96–101.

41. Freelander M, Van Asperen PP. Nebuhaler versus nebuliser in children with acute asthma. *BMJ* 1984; 288: 1873–4.

42. Clark AR, Rachelefsky G, Mason PL, Goldenhersh MJ, Hollingworth A. The use of reservoir devices for the simultaneous delivery of two metered-dose aerosols. *J Allergy Clin Immunol* 1990; 85: 75–9.

43. Newman S, Millar A, Lennard-Jones T, Moren F, Clarke SW. Improvement of pressurised aerosol deposition with nebuhaler spacer device. *Thorax* 1984; 39: 935–41.

44. O'Callaghan C, Lynch J, Cant M, Robertson C. Improvement in sodium cromoglycate delivery from a spacer device by use of an antistatic lining, immediate inhalation, and avoiding multiple actuations of drug. *Thorax* 1993; 48: 603–606.

45. Anhoj J, Bisgaard H, Lipworth BJ. Effect of electrostatic charge in plastic spacers on the lung delivery of HFA-salbutamol in children. *Br J Clin Pharmacol* 1999; 47: 333–6.

46. Pedersen S, Steffensen G. Fenoterol powder inhalator technique in children: Influence of inspiratory flow rate and breath-holding. *Eur J Respir Dis* 1986; 68: 207–14.

47. Pedersen S, Hansen OR, Fuglsang G. Influence of inspiratory flow rate upon the effect of a Turbuhaler. *Arch Dis Child* 1990; 65: 308–310.

48. Richards R, Dickson CR, Renwick AG, Lewis RA, Holgate S. Absorption and disposition kinetics of cromolyn sodium and the influence of inhalation technique. *J Pharmacol Exp Ther* 1987; 241: 1028–32.

49. Nielsen KG, Skov M, Klug B, Ifversen M, Bisgaard H. Flow-dependent effect of formoterol dry-powder inhaled from the Aerolizer. *Eur Respir J* 1997; 10: 2105–9.

50. Rufin P, Benoist MR, de Blic J, Braunstein G, Scheinmann P. Terbutaline powder in asthma exacerbations. *Arch Dis Child* 1991; 66: 1465–6.

51. Drblik SP, Spier S, Lapierre G et al. Peak inspiratory flow (PIF) measured with and without the Turbuhaler (Tb) dry powder inhaler (DPI) in 6–16 year olds during an acute asthmatic episode. *Am J Respir Crit Care Med* 1995; 151: A365.

413

52. Newhouse MT, Nantel NP, Chambers CB, Pratt B, Parry-Billings M. Clickhaler (a novel dry powder inhaler) provides similar bronchodilation to pressurized metered-dose inhaler, even at low flow rates. *Chest* 1999; 115: 952–6.

53. Nielsen KG, Ank IL, Bojsen K, Ifversen M, Klug B, Bisgaard H. Clinical effect of Diskus dry-powder inhaler at low and high inspiratory flow-rates in asthmatic children. *Eur Respir J* 1998; 11: 350–4.

54. Drblik S, Lapierre G, Thivierge R *et al.* Comparative efficacy of terbutaline sulfate delivered by Turbuhaler (TBH) dry powder inhaler or pressurized metered dose inhaler (pMDI) + Nebuhaler (Neb) spacer in children during an acute asthmatic episode. *Am J Respir Crit Care Med* 1998; 157: A709.

55. Agertoft L, Pedersen S. Importance of training for correct Turbuhaler use in preschool children. *Acta Paediatr Scand* 1998; 87: 842–7.

56. Pedersen S, Frost L, Arnfred T. Errors in inhalation technique and efficacy of inhaler use in asthmatic children. *Allergy* 1986; 41: 118–24.

57. Pedersen S. Aerosol treatment of bronchoconstriction in children, with or without a tube spacer. *New Engl J Med* 1983; 308: 1328–30.

58. ✪ Papo MC, Frank J, Thompson AE. A prospective, randomized study of continuous versus intermittent nebulized albuterol for severe status asthmaticus in children. *Crit Care Med* 1993; 21: 1479–86.

59. Robertson C, Smith F, Beck R, Levison H. Response to frequent low doses of nebulized salbutamol in acute asthma. *J Pediatr* 1985; 106: 672–4.

60. Portnoy J, Nadel G, Amado M, Willsie-Ediger S. Continuous nebulization for status asthmaticus. *Ann Allergy* 1992; 69: 71–9.

61. Singh M, Kumar L. Continuous nebulized salbutamol and oral once a day prednisolone in status asthmaticus. *Arch Dis Child* 1993; 69: 416–19.

62. Oberklaid F, Mellis C, Souef PN, Geelhoed G, Maccarrone AL. A comparison of a bodyweight dose versus a fixed dose of nebulised salbutamol in acute asthma in children. *Med J Aust* 1993; 158: 751–3.

63. Wildhaber JH, Devadason SG, Eber E, Hayden MJ, Summers QA, Le Souef P. Aerosol delivery to wheezy infants: a comparison between a nebulizer and two small volume spacers. *Pediatr Pulmonol* 1997; 23: 212–6.

64. Everard ML, Devadason SG, Macerlean C *et al.* Drug delivery from Turbuhaler to children with CF. *Am J Respir Crit Care Med* 1996; 153: A70.

65. Agertoft L, Andersen A, Weibull E, Pedersen S. Systemic availability and pharmacokinetics of nebulized budesonide in pre-school children with asthma. *Arch Dis Child* 1999; 80: 241–7.

66. Anhøj J, Thorsson L, Bisgaard H. The systemic exposure of budesonide inhaled from a metal spacer is similar in young children and adults. *Eur Respir J* 1998; 12: 378.

67. Shapiro G, Furukawa CT, Pierson W, Chapko MK, Sharpe M, Bierman C. Double-blind, dose-response study of metaproterenol inhalant solution in children with acute asthma. *J Allergy Clin Immunol* 1987; 79: 378–86.

68. Janson C, Herala M. Plasma terbutaline levels in nebulisation treatment of acute asthma. *Pulmonary Pharmacol* 1991; 4: 135–9.

69. Pedersen S. Treatment strategies for acute asthma in infants and children. *Res Clin Forums* 1993; 15. (no 4 part 2): 55–61.

70. Pedersen S. The importance of a pause between the inhalation of two puffs of terbutaline from a pressurized aerosol with a tube spacer. *J Allergy Clin Immunol* 1986; 77: 505–509.

71. Lonnerholm G, Foucard T, Lindstrom B. Oral terbutaline in chronic childhood asthma; effects related to plasma concentrations. *Eur J Respir Dis* 1984; 65: 205–210.

72. Morgan DJ. Clinical pharmacokinetics of beta-agonists. *Clin Pharmacokinet* 1990; 18: 270–94.

73. Bohn D, Kalloghlian A, Jenkins J, Edmunds J, Barker G. Intravenous salbutamol in the treatment of status asthmaticus in children. *Crit Care Med* 1984; 12: 892–6.

74. Ahlström H, Svenonius E, Svensson M. Treatment of asthma in children with inhalation of terbutaline

Turbuhaler compared with Nebuhaler. *Allergy* 1989; 44: 515–18.

75. Edmunds AT, Godfrey S. Cardiovascular response during severe acute asthma and its treatment in children. *Thorax* 1981; 36: 534–40.

76. Estelle F, Simons R, Gillies JD. Dose response of subcutaneous terbutaline and epinephrine in children with acute asthma. *Am J Dis Child* 1981; 135: 214–17.

77. Lenney W, Evans NAP. Nebulised salbutamol and ipratropium bromide in asthmatic children. *Br J Dis Chest* 1986; 80: 59–65.

78. Lenney W, Milner AD. At what age do bronchodilator drugs work? *Arch Dis Child* 1978; 53: 532–5.

79. O'Callaghan C, Milner AD, Swarbrick A. Paradoxical deterioration in lung function after nebulised salbutamol in wheezy infants. *Lancet* 1986; ii: 1424–5.

80. Tal A, Bavilski C, Yohai D, Bearman JE, Gorodischer R, Moses SW. Dexamethasone and salbutamol in the treatment of acute wheezing in infants. *Pediatrics* 1983; 71: 13–18.

81. Seidenberg J, Mir Y, Von der Hardt H. Hypoxaemia after nebulized salbutamol in wheezy infants: the importance of aerosol acidity. *Arch Dis Child* 1991; 66: 672–5.

82. Ho L, Collis G, Landau L, Le Souef P. Effect of salbutamol on oxygen saturation in bronchiolitis. *Arch Dis Child* 1981; 66: 1061–4.

83. ✪ Holmgren D, Bjure J, Engström I, Sixt R, Sten G, Wennergren G. Transcutaneous blood gas monitoring during salbutamol inhalations in young children with acute asthmatic symptoms. *Pediatr Pulmonol* 1992; 14: 75–9.

84. Yuksel B, Greenough A. Effect of nebulized salbutamol in preterm infants during the first year of life. *Eur Respir J* 1991; 4: 1088–92.

85. Wilkie RA, Bryan MH. Effect of bronchodilator on airway resistance in ventilator-dependent neonates with chronic lung disease. *J Pediatr* 1987; 111: 278–82.

86. Sosulski R, Abbasi S, Bhutani V, Fox W. Physiological effects of terbutaline on pulmonary function of infants with bronchopulmonary dysplasia. *Pediatr Pulmonol* 1986; 2: 269–73.

87. Kao LC, Durand DJ, Nickerson GB. Effects of inhaled metraproterenol and atropine on the pulmonary mechanics of infants with bronchopulmonary dysplasia. *Pediatr Pulmonol* 1989; 7: 74–80.

88. Cabal LA, Lanazabal C, Ramanathan R *et al.* Effects of metraproterenol on pulmonary mechanics, oxygenation and ventilation in infants with chronic lung disease. *J Pediatr* 1987; 110: 116–19.

89. Yuksel B, Greenough A. Effect of nebulized salbutamol in preterm infants during the first year of life. *Eur Respir J* 1991; 4: 1088–92.

90. Kraemer R, Frey U, Sommer CW, Russi E. Short term effect of albuterol, delivered via a new auxiliary device, in wheezy infants. *Am Rev Respir Dis* 1991; 144: 347–51.

91. Prendiville A, Green S, Silverman M. Airway responsiveness in wheezy infants. *Thorax* 1987; 42: 100–104.

92. ✪ O'Callaghan C, Milner AD, Swarbrick A. Nebulised salbutamol does have a protective effect on airways in children under one year old. *Arch Dis Child* 1988; 63: 479–83.

93. Prendiville A, Green S, Silverman M. Airway responsiveness in wheezy infants: evidence for functional beta adrenergic receptors. *Thorax* 1987; 42: 100–104.

94. Daugbjerg P, Brenoe E, Forchammer H *et al.* A comparison between nebulized terbutaline, nebulized corticosteroid and systemic corticosteroid for acute wheezing in children up to 18 months of age. *Acta Paediatr* 1993; 82: 547–51.

95. Larsson S, Svedmyr N, Thiringer G. Lack of bronchial beta adrenoceptor resistance in asthmatic patients during long term treatment with terbutaline. *J Allergy Clin Immunol* 1977; 59: 93–100.

96. Bengtsson B, Fagerström PO. Extrapulmonary effects of terbutaline during prolonged administration. *Clin Pharmacol Ther* 1982; 31: 726–32.

97. Deshpande A, McKenzie S. Short course of steroids in home treatment of children with acute asthma. *BMJ* 1986; 293: 169–71.

98. Connett G, Warde C, Wooler E, Lenney W. Prednisolone and salbutamol in the hospital treatment of acute asthma. *Arch Dis Child* 1994; 70: 170–73.

99. Shapiro G, Furukawa CT, Pierson EE, Gardinier R, Bierman C. Double blind evaluation of methylprednisolone versus placebo for acute asthma episodes. *Pediatrics* 1983; 71: 510–14.

100. ✪ Brunette MG, Lands L, Thibodeau LP. Childhood asthma: prevention of attacks with short-term corticosteroid treatment of upper respiratory tract infection. *Pediatrics* 1988; 81: 624–9.

101. ✪ Tal A, Levy N, Bearman JE. Methylprednisolone therapy for acute asthma in infants and toddlers: a controlled clinical trial. *Pediatrics* 1990; 86: 350–56.

102. Storr J, Barry W, Barrell E, Lenney W, Hatcher G. Effect of a single dose of prednisolone in acute childhood asthma. *Lancet* 1987; i: 879–82.

103. Younger RE, Gerber PS, Herrod HG, Cohen RM, Crawford LV. Intravenous methylprednisolone efficacy in status asthmaticus of childhood. *Pediatrics* 1987; 80: 225–30.

104. Gleeson JG, Loftus BG, Price J. Placebo controlled trial of systemic corticosteroids in acute childhood asthma. *Acta Paediatr Scand* 1990; 79: 1052–58.

105. FitzGerald JM, Kearon MC. Corticosteroids in acute asthma results of a meta-analysis. *Am Rev Respir Dis* 1991; 143: 624.

106. Kattan M, Gurwitz D, Levison H. Corticosteroids in status asthmaticus. *Pediatrics* 1980; 96: 596–9.

107. Pierson W, Bierman C, Kelly WC. A double blind trial of corticosteroid therapy in status asthmaticus. *Pediatrics* 1974; 54: 282–8.

108. Barnett PL, Caputo GL, Baskin M, Kuppermann N. Intravenous versus oral corticosteroids in the management of acute asthma in children. *Ann Emerg Med* 1997; 29: 212–17.

109. Vichyanond P, Irvin CG, Larsen G, Szefler S, Hill M. Penetration of corticosteroids into the lung: Evidence for a difference between methylprednisolone and prednisolone. *J Allergy Clin Immunol* 1989; 84: 867–73.

110. Shee CD. Risk factors for hydrocortisone myopathy in acute severe asthma. *Respir Med* 1990; 84: 229–33.

111. Tal A, Bavilski C, Yohai D, Bearman JE, Gorodisher R, Moses SW. Dexamethasone and salbutamol in the treatment of acute wheezing in infants. *Pediatrics* 1993; 71: 13–18.

112. Webb MS, Henry RL, Milner AD. Oral corticosteroids for wheezing attacks under 18 months. *Arch Dis Child* 1986; 61: 15–19.

113. Daugbjerg P, Brenøe E, Forchammer H *et al*. A comparison between nebulized terbutaline, nebulized corticosteroid and systemic corticosteroid for acute wheezing in children up to 18 months of age. *Acta Paediat* 1993; 82: 547–51.

114. Maayan C, Itzhaki T, Bar-Yishay E, Gross S, Tal A, Godfrey S. The functional response of infants with persistent wheezing to nebulized beclomethasone dipropionate. *Pediatr Pulmonol* 1986; 2: 9–14.

115. Carlsen KH, Leegard J, Larsen S, Orstravik I. Nebulised beclomethasone dipropionate in recurrent obstructive episodes after acute bronchiolitis. *Arch Dis Child* 1988; 63: 1428–33.

116. Volovitz B, Bentur L, Finkelstein Y *et al*. Effectiveness and safety of inhaled corticosteroids in controlling acute asthma attacks in children who were treated in the emergency department: a controlled comparative study with oral prednisolone. *J Allergy Clin Immunol* 1998; 102: 605–9.

117. Wilson N, Silverman M. Treatment of acute episodic asthma in preschool children using intermittent high dose inhaled steroids at home. *Arch Dis Child* 1990; 65: 407–410.

118. Connett G, Lenney W. Prevention of vira-induced asthma attacks using inhaled budesonide. *Arch Dis Child* 1993; 68: 85–7.

119. Svedmyr J, Nyberg E, Åsbrink-Nilsson E, Hedlin G. Intermittent treatment with inhaled steroids for deterioration of asthma due to upper respiratory tract infections. *Acta Paediatr Int J Paediatr* 1995; 84: 884–8.

120. Garrett J, Williams S, Wong C, Holdaway D. Treatment of acute asthmatic exacerbations with an increased dose of inhaled steroid. *Arch Dis Child* 1998; 79: 12–17.

121. Ishizaki T, Minegishi A, Morishita M *et al.* Plasma catecholamine concentrations during a 72-hours aminophylline infusion in children with acute asthma. *J Allergy Clin Immunol* 1988; 82: 146–54.

122. Roddick LG, South RT, Mellis C. Value of combining an oral sympathomimetic agent with oral theophylline in asthmatic children. *Med J Aust* 1979; 118: 153–4.

123. Pedersen S, Sommer B, Nissen P. Treatment of acute asthma in children with a solution of aminophylline given rectally. *Eur J Respir Dis* 1984; 65: 354–61.

124. Pierson W, Bierman C, Stamm S, Van Arsdel P. Double-blind trial of aminophylline in status asthmaticus. *Pediatrics* 1971; 48: 642–6.

125. Young M, South M. Randomised controlled trial of aminophylline for severe acute asthma. *Arch Dis Child* 1998; 79: 405–410.

126. Pedersen S, Sommer B. Rectal administration of theophylline in aqueous solution. *Acta Paed Scand* 1981; 70: 243–6.

127. ○ Carter E, Cruz M, Chesrown S, Shieh G, Reilly K, Hendeles L. Efficacy of intravenously administered theophylline in children hospitalized with severe asthma. *J Pediatr* 1993; 122: 470–76.

128. Barclay J, Whiting P, Mickey M, Addis G. Theophylline-salbutamol interaction: bronchodilator response to salbutamol at maximally effective plasma theophylline concentrations. *Br J Clin Pharmacol* 1981; 11: 203–208.

129. Fanta C, Rossing T, McFadden E. Treatment of acute asthma: is combination therapy with sympathomimetics and methylxanthines indicated? *Am J Med* 1986; 80: 5–10.

130. ○ Hendeles L, Iafrate R, Weinberger M. A clinical and pharmacokinetic basis for the selection and use of slow release theophylline products. *Clin Pharmacokinet* 1984; 9: 95–135.

131. Sarrazin E, Hendeles L, Weinberger M, Muir K, Riegelman S. Dose dependent kinetics for theophylline: Observations among ambulatory asthmatic children. *J Pediatr* 1980; 97: 825–8.

132. Hendeles L, Bighley L, Richardson RH, Hepler CD, Carmichael J. Frequent toxicity from IV aminophylline infusions in critically ill patients. *Drug Intell Clin Pharm* 1977; 11: 12–18.

133. Barker D. Theophylline toxicity in children. *J Pediatr* 1986; 109: 538–42.

134. Hendeles L, Weinberger M, Szefler S, Ellis E. Safety and efficacy of theophylline in children with asthma. *J Pediatr* 1992; 120: 177–83.

135. Tsiu SJ, Self TH, Burns R. Theophylline toxicity: update. *Ann Allergy* 1990; 64: 241–57.

136. Ellis E. Theophylline toxicity. *J Allergy Clin Immunol* 1985; 76: 297–301.

137. Niemand D, Martiness S, Arvidsson S *et al.* Adenosine in the inhibition of diazepamsedation by aminophylline. *Acta Anaesthet* 1986; 30: 493–5.

138. Gross NJ, Petty TL, Friedman M, Skorodin MS, Silvers GW, Donohue JF. Dose response to ipratropium as a nebulised solution in patients with chronic obstructive pulmonary disease. A three-center study. *Am Rev Respir Dis* 1989; 139: 1188–91.

139. Boner A, Vallone G, De Stefano G. Effect of inhaled ipratropium bromide on methacholine and exercise provocation in asthmatic children. *Pediatr Pulmonol* 1989; 6: 81–5.

140. Anonymous. Determination of dose–response relationship for nebulised ipratropium bromide in asthmatic children. *J Pediatr* 1984; 105: 1002–1005.

141. Wilkie RA, Bryan MH. Effect of bronchodilators on airway resistance in ventilator-dependent neonates with chronic lung disease. *J Pediatr* 1984; 11: 278–82.

142. Svenonius E, Arborelius M, Wiberg R, Ekberg P. Prevention of exercise-induced asthma by drugs inhaled from metered aerosols. *Allergy* 1988; 43: 252–7.

143. Watson WT, Becker AB, Simons FE. Comparison of ipratropium solution, fenoterol solution and their combination administered by nebuliser and face mask to children with acute asthma. *J Allergy Clin Immunol* 1988; 82: 1012–18.

144. Reisman J, Galdes-Sebaldt M, Kazim F, Canny G, Levison H. Frequent administration by inhalation of

salbutamol and ipratropium bromide in the initial management of severe acuta asthma in children. *J Allergy Clin Immunol* 1988; 81: 10–20.

145. Stokes GM, Milner AD, Hodges IGC, Elphick MC, Henry RI. Nebulised therapy in acute severe bronchitis in infancy. *Arch Dis Child* 1983; 58: 279–82.

146. Watson WT, Becker AB, Simons FE. Comparison of ipratropium solution, fenoterol solution, and their combination administered by nebulizer and face mask to children with acute asthma. *J Allergy Clin Immunol* 1988; 82: 1012–18.

147. Beck R, Robertson C, Galdes-Sebaldt M, Levison H. Combined salbutamol and ipratropium bromide by inhalation in the treatment of severe acute asthma. *J Pediatr* 1985; 107: 605–608.

148. Phanichyakarn P, Kraisarin C, Sasisakulporn C. Comparison of inhaled terbutaline and inhaled terbutaline plus ipratropium bromide in acute asthmatic children. *Asian Pac J Allergy Immunol* 1990; 8: 45–58.

149. Reisman J, Galdes-Sebaldt M, Kazim F, Canny G, Levison H. Frequent administration by inhalation of salbutamol and ipratropium bromide in the initial management of severe acute asthma in children. *J Allergy Clin Immunol* 1988; 81: 16–20.

150. Henry RC, Milner AD, Stokes GM. Ineffectiveness of ipratropium bromide in acute bronchiolitis. *Arch Dis Child* 1983; 58: 925–6.

151. Beasley CR, Rafferty P, Holgate S. Bronchoconstrictor properties of preservatives in ipratropium bromide (Atrovent) nebuliser solution. *BMJ* 1987; 294: 1197–8.

152. Mann JS, Howarth PH, Holgate S. Bronchoconstriction induced by ipratropium bromide in asthma: relation to hypotonicity. *BMJ* 1984; 289: 469.

153. Connett G, Lenney W. Use of pulse oximetry in the hospital management of acute asthma in childhood. *Pediatr Pulmonol* 1993; 15: 345–9.

154. Greenough A, Pool J, Gleeson JG, Price J. Effect of budesonide on pulmonary hyperinflation in young asthmatic children. *Thorax* 1988; 43: 937–8.

155. McKenzie S, Edmunds AT, Godfrey S. Status asthmaticus in children. *Arch Dis Child* 1979; 54: 581–6.

156. Moler FW, Hurwitz ME, Custer JR. Improvement in clinical asthma score and P_aCO_2 in children with severe asthma treated with continuously nebulized terbutaline. *J Allergy Clin Immunol* 1988; 81: 1101–1109.

157. Bentur L, Kerem E, Canny G, Reisman J, Schuh S, Stein R, Levison H. Response of acute asthma to a beta 2 agonist in children less than two years of age. *Ann Allergy* 1990; 65: 122–6.

158. Bishop J, Carlin J, Nolan T. Evaluation of the properties and reliability of clinical severity scale for acute asthma in children. *J Clin Epidemiol* 1992; 45: 71–6.

159. Mountain RD, Sahn SA. Clinical features and outcome in patients with acute asthma presenting with hypercapnia. *Am Rev Respir Dis* 1988; 138: 535–9.

160. Pearson MG, Spence DPS, Ryland I, Harrison BD. Value of pulsus paradoxus in assessing acute severe asthma. *BMJ* 1993; 307: 659.

161. Geelhoed G, Landau L, Le Souef P. Predictive value of oxygen saturation in emergency evaluation of asthmatic children. *BMJ* 1988; 297: 395–6.

162. Bishop J, Nolan T. Pulse oximetry in acute asthma. *Arch Dis Child* 1991; 66: 724–5.

163. Carson JWK, Taylor M. Relapse after single dose nebulized salbutamol in children with acute asthma. *Irish Med J* 1985; 78: 93–6.

164. Rachelefsky G, Warner J. International consensus on the management of pediatric asthma: a summary statement. *Pediatr Pulmonol* 1993; 15: 125–7.

165. Warner J, Gotz M, Landau L, Levison H, Milner AD, Pedersen S, Silverman M. Management of asthma: a consensus statement. *Arch Dis Child* 1989; 64: 1065–79.

166. Nelson DR, Sachs MI, O'Connell EJ. Approaches to acute asthma and status asthmaticus in children. *Mayo Clin Proc* 1989; 64: 1392–1402.

167. McWilliams B, Kelly HW, Murphy S. Management of acute severe asthma. *Pediatr Ann* 1989; 18: 774–5, 779.

168. Murphy S, Kelly HW. Management of acute asthma. *Pediatrician* 1991; 18: 287–300.

169. Press S, Lipkind RS. A treatment protocol of the acute asthma patient in a pediatric emergency department. *Clin Pediatr* 1991; 30(10): 573–7.

170. Henry RL, Robertson C, Asher I *et al.* Management of acute asthma. Respiratory paediatricians of Australia and New Zealand. *J Pediatr Child Health* 1993; 29: 101–103.

171. Niggemann B, Wahn U. Die Therapie des Status asthmaticus im Kindesalter. *Monatsschr Kinderheilkd* 1991; 139: 323–9.

172. Geelhoed G, Landau L, Le Souef P. Oximetry and peak expiratory flow in assessment of acute childhood asthma. *J Pediatr* 1990; 117: 907–909.

173. Zeiger RS, Heller S, Mellon M, Wald J, Falkoff R, Schatz M. Facilitated referral to asthma specialist reduces relapses in asthma emergency rooms visits. *J Allergy Clin Immunol* 1991; 87: 1160–68.

174. Chapman KR, Verbeek PR, White JG, Rebuck AS. Effect of short course of prednisone in the prevention of early relapse after the emergency room treatment of acute asthma. *New Engl J Med* 1991; 324: 788–94.

175. Akerman MJ, Sinert R. A successful effort to improve asthma care outcome in an inner-city emergency department. *J Asthma* 1999; 36: 295–303.

176. Wever-Hess J, Wever AM. Asthma statistics in The Netherlands 1980–94. *Respir Med* 1997; 91: 417–22.

177. Wesseldine LJ, McCarthy P, Silverman M. Structured discharge procedure for children admitted to hospital with acute asthma: a randomised controlled trial of nursing practice. *Arch Dis Child* 1999; 80: 110–14.

178. Madge P, McColl J, Paton J. Impact of a nurse-led home management training programme in children admitted to hospital with acute asthma: a randomised controlled study. *Thorax* 1997; 52: 223–8.

179. Bisgaard H, Moller H. Changes in risk of hospital readmission among asthmatic children in Denmark, 1978–93. *BMJ* 1999; 319: 229–30.

180. Wennergren G, Kristjansson S, Strannegard IL. Decrease in hospitalization for treatment of childhood asthma with increased use of antiinflammatory treatment, despite an increase in the prevalence of asthma. *J Allergy Clin Immunol* 1996; 97: 742–48.

181. Strunk RC. Identification of the fatality-prone subject with asthma. *J Allergy Clin Immunol* 1989; 83: 477–85.

Chapter 31

Management of Chronic Asthma in Adults

Romain Pauwels

INTRODUCTION

The most important objective of the management of chronic asthma for both patients and physicians would be to cure the disease. Cure is defined here as the absence of symptoms and physiological abnormalities even after stopping the treatment for a long time. Unfortunately, none of the currently available treatment options results in a significant cure rate of asthma. Only a minority of adult asthmatic patients develops a complete remission of the disease. A 25-year follow-up study in 181 adult patients, who had asthma as a child, showed that only 11% could be considered as no longer asthmatic.[1] The absence of asthma was defined as no bronchial hyperresponsiveness, a forced expiratory volume in 1 s (FEV_1) of more than 90% predicted, and the absence of pulmonary symptoms.

Although the mortality of asthma is relatively low, most of the asthma deaths are considered to be avoidable by appropriate management.[2-4] Prevention of mortality should therefore be an important objective of the management of chronic asthma. Another objective of the long-term treatment of asthma might be the prevention of the development of irreversible airflow limitation. There is an increasing body of evidence that patients with asthma have a faster decline in FEV_1 over time than non-asthmatics.[5-8] That prevention of irreversible airflow limitation is an achievable treatment objective is suggested by two studies on the role of early intervention in asthma.[9,10] Both studies showed that early treatment with inhaled steroids results in a better lung function than the delayed introduction of this treatment.

The main objectives for the treatment of chronic asthma are therefore to control the disease and to prevent irreversible airway damage and mortality from

asthma. Control of asthma is usually defined as absence of symptoms and exacerbations, no need for rescue medication, normal levels of activity including exercise and sports, a normal lung function and no adverse effects from the anti-asthma treatment (Table 31.1).[11]

Control of asthma, as defined in Table 31.1, can be achieved in the majority of asthma patients using currently available treatment. Complete control might not be possible in some patients, especially those with severe asthma, either because the risk of severe side-effects from the medications is too high, or because the patient is not prepared to follow completely the therapeutic recommendations. In both cases, a compromise will have to made in order to achieve the best achievable control. Reaching a normal lung function may also be unattainable in patients with long-standing asthma, due to the presence of irreversible changes of the airways. A normal lung function is usually defined as a peak expiratory flow (PEF) and/or a forced expiratory volume in 1 s (FEV_1) that is within the expected normal

Table 31.1: Control of asthma
No symptoms
No exacerbations
No emergency visits
No need for rescue medication
No limitation on activities, including exercise
Normal lung function or lung function at personal best level
No adverse effects from medication

range. An alternative approach, which encompasses the subjects with irreversible airway damage, is to use the personal best PEF or FEV_1 as reference value. This personal best value can be taken from historical recordings or can be measured after 2 weeks of maximal anti-asthma treatment. There is currently only indirect evidence that suboptimal treatment of asthma increases the risk of irreversible airway obstruction.[9,10,12] The recommendation that control of asthma should also involve reaching a normal lung function is therefore based rather on consensus than on hard evidence. The evidence that treatment of asthma should aim at normalization of the airway responsiveness to broncho-constrictor agonists such as histamine or methacholine is even scarcer[13] and most consensus documents do not include normal airway responsiveness as a goal of asthma management.

The limitation of the resources available for health care in almost all countries over the world has resulted in an increasing awareness about the cost-effectiveness of asthma management. Asthma is a disease with a substantial burden on the health-care budget. The cost-effectiveness of the different management options will therefore increasingly influence the choice and availability of therapy.

AVOIDANCE OF ASTHMA TRIGGERS

Secondary prevention of asthma symptoms and exacerbations is an important and often neglected part of asthma management. The avoidance of exposure to factors that worsen an existing asthma (triggers) should always be part of the approach to managing asthma in an individual patient. The type of triggers that cause a worsening of asthma varies from individual to individual. They include non-specific triggers such as cigarette smoke, cold air, exercise, air pollutants and specific triggers dependent of the individual's sensitivity to allergens, occupational sensitizers and medications. Avoidance measures will therefore need to be adapted to the patient's sensitivities, life-style and severity of asthma.

Avoidance of Non-Specific Triggers

Exposure to cold air and exercise are part of a normal life-style and should therefore not be avoided if the asthma can be controlled with treatment that does not carry the risk of severe long-term side-effects.

The avoidance of passive and active smoking is an important measure. Both active and passive smoking increase the frequency and severity of respiratory symptoms in patients with asthma.[14] All patients with asthma should therefore be advised to stop smoking and/or to avoid exposure to cigarette smoke. They should be firm in requesting the possibility to live and to work in a smoke-free environment.

The major air pollutants causing an increase in asthma symptoms are sulphur dioxide, nitric oxides, ozone and biologicals such as endotoxin. These pollutants can be present both indoor and outdoor. The major source of indoor pollutants is heating and cooking systems.[15] All furnaces should be vented to the outdoors and heating systems should be adequately maintained.

Some medications such as β-adrenergic blocking agents and muscarinic agonists cause airway narrowing in the majority of patients with asthma and should therefore in general be avoided by such patients except under very specific circumstances and specific control.

Specific Avoidance

The severity of asthma in subjects with documented allergy is related to the amount of allergen in the environment. Measures that reduce specific allergen exposure have proven to decrease the asthmatic symptoms and the need for anti-asthma medication in sensitized individuals. These measures should therefore be implemented whenever possible. The adherence to these measures is dependent on the socioeconomic status of the patient and his family.

Some subjects with asthma are hypersensitive to aspirin and other non-steroidal anti-inflammatory agents such as indomethacin, flurbiprofen, ibuprofen, diclofenac, and others. They usually have a rather severe form of asthma in combination with rhinitis and/or sinusitis. These sensitive subjects should strictly avoid aspirin and the other non-steroidal anti-inflammatory agents. Safe alternatives include salicylic acid and acetaminophen (paracetamol). Asthma induced by hypersensitivity to sulphite-containing foods or drinks is rather rare but these individuals should avoid such foods. However, sulphite use in foods and drinks has decreased so that this has become a rather rare cause of food-induced asthma symptoms.

PHARMACOLOGICAL TREATMENT AVAILABLE FOR ASTHMA MANAGEMENT

Although the avoidance of non-specific and specific triggers undoubtedly reduces the symptoms of asthma,

Table 31.2: Controller medication in asthma

Inhaled corticosteroids

Chronic oral glucocorticosteroids

Sodium cromoglycate

Nedocromil sodium

Long-acting β_2 agonists (inhaled or oral)

Sustained-release theophylline

Antileukotrienes

it is evident that the majority of patients with asthma require pharmacological treatment to attain control of asthma and/or to use as rescue medication when asthma worsens. Various classifications of anti-asthma drugs have been used but none of the classifications, based on mechanisms of action of the different drugs, has withstood the time, not at the least because our understanding of the mechanisms of action of anti-asthma medications is incomplete and evolving. The most accepted classification is based on outcome measures used in the evaluation of asthma therapy. Controller medication is medication that is used on a regular base in order to obtain long-term control of chronic asthma (Table 31.2).

Quick-relief medication is medication that is used to quickly relieve the symptoms of asthma but does not contribute substantially to the long-term control of asthma (Table 31.3). In fact, frequent or regular use of quick-relief medication might even decrease long-term control of asthma either by decreasing the compliance for the long-term-control medication or by mechanisms not yet fully understood.[16] In general,

Table 31.3: Quick-relief medication in asthma

Short-acting β_2 agonists (inhaled, oral, i.v.)

Anticholinergics

Short-acting theophylline

Short courses of glucocorticosteroids

patients with chronic asthma require both controller and quick-relief medication but optimal control is achieved when no or very little quick-relief medication is needed.

PHARMACOLOGICAL TREATMENT OF CHRONIC ASTHMA

The choice of the treatment should be guided by the severity of the disease, the availability and cost of different medications and the benefits and risks of each treatment. Cultural and patient preferences should be taken into account in establishing a chronic treatment plan. Such a plan is very often a compromise between what is considered to be optimal treatment and what the patient is prepared to take or can afford. Failure to take these considerations into account will result in bad compliance of the patient with the treatment regimen and suboptimal or bad control.

The establishment of a chronic treatment in asthma necessitates a thorough education of the patient with asthma. The objectives of the chronic treatment, the ways to avoid asthma triggers, the mode of action of medications and the use of inhalation devices should be clearly and repeatedly explained. If inhalation therapy is prescribed, then the physician should explain and demonstrate the use of the prescribed inhalation device. The patient should then be invited to use the device in the presence of the physician so that the necessary corrections can be made. If doubt persists about the appropriate use of the inhalation device even after repeated training efforts, then other devices or treatment options should be selected. The multiplication of different inhalation devices will undoubtedly enhance the confusion amongst physicians and patients and will necessitate that prescribing physicians limit their options to inhalation devices that they really know. They should also be aware about the large differences in efficacy of these inhalation devices and about the fact that the therapeutic effect of an inhaler not only depends on the medication that is contained in the inhaler but also on the amount of drug that is delivered to the appropriate site in the airways.[17]

All patients with asthma should receive a written treatment plan that clearly indicates and differentiates the maintenance treatment and the rescue medication. This action plan should also contain instructions on what the patient should do when she or he develops an exacerbation.

423

Initiation and Maintenance of Chronic Treatment for Asthma

The aim of the initial therapy is to achieve control of asthma as quickly as possible but there is still no good evidence on what is the most appropriate way to achieve this.[18] One can either start with a short course of potent anti-asthma therapy such as relatively high doses of inhaled glucocorticosteroids or even oral corticosteroids and then switch, once control is achieved, to the optimal medication necessary to maintain control or one can start immediately at the therapeutic level judged to be appropriate for the severity of the patient's asthma. The former approach has the advantage that control of asthma is achieved somewhat quicker and that the personal best values for lung function parameters can be established in a reliable way. It has also the theoretical advantage that an initial course of anti-inflammatory medication may bring the chronic asthmatic airway inflammation down to a level that is easily controlled with smaller doses of medication.[19] Once control of asthma is achieved, then every effort should be made to establish the minimal amount of medication necessary to maintain this control. This usually means an attempt to reduce progressively the amount of chronic medication. This reduction should be guided both by clinical parameters such as symptoms and signs but also by objective measurements of lung function such as peak flow or spirometry measurements. The occurrence of an acute severe exacerbation clearly indicates that control is insufficient and that the chronic treatment must be adapted. It is important to remember that asthma can be very variable and that therefore the patient should be observed for a sufficient length of time before the decision is taken to change the chronic treatment. An observation period of approximately 3 months seems to be appropriate to judge control of chronic asthma. There might be external circumstances that change the severity of asthma. Examples of this are the pollen season in pollen-allergic asthmatics, temporary changes in the living environment for patients allergic to house-dust mite, the introduction of a new pet or starting smoking. Whenever an unexpected worsening of chronic asthma occurs, appropriate investigations must be made to identify the cause and if possible eliminate it. If this is unachievable, then the chronic asthma treatment must be adapted to obtain control again.

Steps to Achieve and Maintain Control of Asthma

The severity of the chronic asthma is an important guide for the selection of the appropriate chronic treatment and therefore therapy appropriate for different levels of asthma severity is discussed using the stepwise approach as outlined in the recently adapted Global Strategy for Asthma Management and Prevention[11] (Table 31.4). The presence of one or more features of clinical severity places a patient at the respective therapeutic step.

In the stepwise approach to therapy, progression to the next step is indicated when control is not achieved or lost at the current step, and there is assurance the patient is using medication correctly. The frequent (e.g. more than three times a week) presence of such

Table 31.4: Classification of asthma by severity

	Symptoms	Night-time symptoms	PEF or FEV$_1$
Step 4 (Severe persistent)	Continuous; limited physical activity	Frequent	≤ 60% predicted
Step 3 (Moderate persistent)	Daily; use rescue medication daily	≥ ×1 a week	<80–>60% predicted
Step 2 (Mild persistent)	≥ ×1 a week but < × 1 a day	> ×2 a month but < ×1 a week	≥ 80% predicted
Step 1 (Intermittent)	< ×1 a week; asymptomatic in between	≤ ×2 a month	≥ 80% predicted

symptoms as cough, wheezing and dyspnoea, and the increased use of short-acting bronchodilators may indicate inadequate control of asthma. The presence of symptoms at night or early in the morning is an especially useful indicator. Increasing variability in PEF indicates inadequately controlled asthma. Measurement of PEF and its variability is helpful in the initial assessment of asthma severity and in monitoring the initial treatment, assessing changes in severity, and preparing step-down in therapy. Of course, specific medication plans should be tailored depending on the availability of anti-asthma medication, the conditions of the health-care system, and individual patient circumstances.

INTERMITTENT ASTHMA

Characteristics

A patient has intermittent asthma if the patient experiences episodes of asthma symptoms (cough, wheezing, or dyspnoea) less than once a week over a period of at least 3 months and the episodes are brief, generally lasting only a few hours to a few days. Nocturnal asthma symptoms do not occur more than twice a month. In between exacerbations the patient is asymptomatic and has a completely normal lung function, i.e. a pre-treatment baseline FEV_1 or PEF greater than 80% of predicted or personal best and PEF variability of less than 15%.

Intermittent asthma includes the patient with allergy who is occasionally exposed to the allergen (e.g. cat or dog) that is responsible for causing his or her asthma symptoms, but who is completely symptom-free and has normal lung function when not exposed to the allergen. Intermittent asthma also includes the patient who has occasional exercise-induced asthma (e.g. under bad weather circumstances). Intermittent asthma is not trivial. The severity of the asthma episode may vary from patient to patient and from time to time. Such an episode might even be life-threatening, although this is extremely rare in patients with intermittent asthma.

Treatment

The low frequency of the symptomatic episodes and the fact that in between exacerbations the patient has a completely normal lung function support the recommendations that no long-term treatment with a controller medication should be started. Furthermore, patient compliance with long-term therapy when the patient only experiences occasional symptoms could

be low. Rather, the exacerbations should be treated as such, depending on their severity. Treatment includes medication prior to exercise as needed (inhaled β_2 agonist, cromoglycate, nedocromil, or antileukotriene) or prior to allergen exposure (sodium cromoglycate or nedocromil). Treatment of exacerbation includes an inhaled short-acting β_2 agonist taken as needed to relieve the asthma symptoms. An inhaled anticholinergic, oral short-acting β_2 agonist or short-acting theophylline may be considered as alternatives to inhaled short-acting β_2 agonists, although these alternatives have a slower onset of action and/or a higher risk for side-effects. Occasionally, more severe or prolonged exacerbations may require a short course of oral glucocorticosteroids.

If medication is required more than once a week over a 3-month period, the patient should be moved to the next step of care, regardless of PEF measurements. The same applies if the lung function in between exacerbations becomes abnormal.

MILD PERSISTENT ASTHMA

Characteristics

A patient has mild persistent asthma if he or she experiences exacerbations, persistent symptoms, and/or declines in lung function with sufficient frequency to warrant daily long-term therapy with controller medication. Mild persistent asthma is present if the patient experiences exacerbations at least once a week but less than once a day over the last 3 months. Some of the exacerbations might affect sleep and activity levels; and/or if the patient has chronic symptoms that require symptomatic treatment almost daily and experiences nocturnal asthma symptoms more than twice a month. The patient with mild persistent asthma has a pre-treatment baseline PEF of more than 80% of predicted or personal best and PEF variability of 20–30%. Furthermore, cough-variant asthma should be treated as mild persistent asthma.

Treatment

Patients with mild persistent asthma require controller medication every day to achieve and maintain control of their asthma. The primary therapy for mild persistent asthma is regular use of anti-inflammatory medication taken on a daily basis. Treatment of mild persistent asthma can be started with inhaled corticosteroids, sodium cromoglycate, or nedocromil sodium, slow-release theophylline or an antileukotriene. In adults treatment should be started with inhaled glucocorticosteroids. The suggested introductory dose of inhaled corticosteroids is 200 to 500 µg per day of beclomethasone dipropionate (BDP) or budesonide or equivalent, divided over one dosing in the morning and one dosing in the evening. Budesonide can be used once daily. A spacer device and mouth washing after inhalation are recommended when using inhaled corticosteroids with a pressurized metered dose inhaler. Mouth rinsing is also advised when using powder inhalers. This is to reduce oropharyngeal side-effects. There is no doubt that treatment with a low dose of an inhaled glucocorticosteroid is more effective than regular treatment with cromoglycate or nedocromil or an antileukotriene.[20,21] The potential for systemic effects of low doses of inhaled glucocorticosteroids is extremely small.[22]

Long-term treatment with sustained-release theophylline may be considered, but the need for monitoring of serum concentration levels may make this treatment less feasible. The exact role of the antileukotrienes in the chronic treatment of mild persistent asthma is not clear.[23] The lack of comparative studies of sufficient duration with the recommended standard therapy of low dose of inhaled glucocorticosteroids precludes that they can be recommended as first-line therapy in mild persistent asthma. They should, until more data become available, be reserved for those patients who are unwilling or unable to take treatment with inhaled glucocorticosteroids.

Inhaled short-acting β_2 agonist should be available to take as needed to relieve symptoms, but should not be taken more than three to four times a day. An inhaled anticholinergic, oral short-acting β_2 agonist, or short-acting theophylline may be considered as an alternative to inhaled short-acting β_2 agonist, although they have a slower onset of action and/or a higher risk for side-effects. Because of the risk of serious side-effects, short-acting theophylline should not be used as rescue medication if the patient is already on long-term controller therapy with sustained-release theophylline. If the patient's long-term therapy was initiated with sustained-release theophylline, sodium cromoglycate or nedocromil sodium, and symptoms persist after 4 weeks of this initial treatment, then inhaled corticosteroids should be introduced. The inhaled corticosteroids may be initiated either instead of or together with the other medication to allow on overlap period.

If symptoms persist despite the initial dose of inhaled corticosteroids, and the health-care professional is satisfied that the patient is using the medications correctly, then the patient should be considered as having moderate persistent asthma.

MODERATE PERSISTENT ASTHMA

Characteristics

Moderate persistent asthma can be defined easily as persistent asthma that is insufficiently controlled by a low dose of inhaled glucocorticosteroids or as asthma that has one or more of the following characteristics. Moderate persistent asthma is characterized by daily symptoms over a prolonged time or nocturnal asthma more than once a week. The patient with moderate persistent asthma has a pre-treatment baseline PEF of more than 60% but less than 80% of predicted or personal best and PEF variability of 20–30%.

Treatment

Regular treatment with a long-acting bronchodilator should be added to a dose of at least 500 µg inhaled corticosteroids. The inhaled corticosteroids might be increased from 500 µg of beclomethasone equivalent to 1000 µg and 800 µg for beclomethasone and budesonide, respectively. The combination of a long-acting inhaled β_2 agonist with inhaled glucocorticosteroids is more effective in controlling asthma in patients with moderate persistent asthma than doubling the dose of inhaled glucocorticosteroids[19,24,25] in the majority of patients. High doses of inhaled glucocorticosteroids (>1 mg per day) should be reserved for patients with repeated severe asthma exacerbations despite treatment with the combination of low to moderate inhaled glucocorticosteroids and a long-acting inhaled β_2 agonist.

A long-acting inhaled β_2 agonist, sustained-release theophylline, an oral slow-release β_2 agonist or an antileukotriene might be used as add-on therapy to inhaled glucocorticosteroids. The preferred add-on therapy is the long-acting inhaled β_2 agonist. Add-on therapy with slow-release theophylline is less efficacious and more toxic than add-on therapy with a long-acting inhaled β_2 agonist.[26] Also treatment with an antileukotriene is less efficacious as add-on to inhaled glucocorticosteroids than therapy with a long-acting inhaled β_2 agonist.[27]

Inhaled short-acting β_2 agonists should be available to take as needed to relieve symptoms, but should not be taken more than three to four times a day.

SEVERE PERSISTENT ASTHMA

Characteristics

A patient has severe persistent asthma if the patient experiences highly variable, continuous symptoms, and frequent nocturnal symptoms; has limited activities; and experiences severe exacerbations in spite of medication. The patient with severe persistent asthma has a pre-treatment baseline PEF of less than 60% of predicted or personal best and PEF variability greater than 30%.

Treatment

Control of asthma as defined earlier may not be possible. In severe persistent asthma, the goal of therapy becomes achieving best possible results: the least symptoms, the least need for short-acting β_2 agonist, the best flow rates, the least circadian (night to day) variation, and the least side-effects from medication. Therapy usually requires multiple daily controller medications. Primary therapy includes inhaled glucocorticosteroids at higher doses (more than 800 to 2000 µg per day of beclomethasone dipropionate or equivalent). A long-acting bronchodilator is recommended in addition to the inhaled glucocorticosteroids, such as a long-acting inhaled β_2 agonist or oral sustained-release theophylline or oral β_2 agonist. A combination of different bronchodilators and/or an antileukotriene with high doses of inhaled glucocorticosteroids should be considered. A trial of the regular treatment with an inhaled anticholinergic (ipratropium) may be considered, particularly for those patients who experience adverse effects from β_2 agonist. Inhaled short-acting β_2 agonist should be available as needed up to three to four times a day to relieve symptoms.

Long-term oral glucocorticosteroids should be avoided when possible, but if needed be used in the lowest possible dose (alternate or single daily dose after a 3–7 day burst). Persistent trials of high doses of inhaled glucocorticosteroids administered with a spacer device in combination with therapy with long-acting bronchodilators should be made in an attempt to reduce oral corticosteroids. When patients are transferred from oral glucocorticosteroids to high-dose inhaled glucocorticosteroids combined with other therapy, they should be monitored closely for evidence of adrenal insufficiency and for the possible unmasking of an underlying Churg–Strauss syndrome.[28] Difficult-to-manage asthma may indeed herald a life-threatening underlying disorder such as Churg–Strauss syndrome or other forms of systemic vasculitis.

The complexity of a multiple daily medication regimen is often a factor in patient non-adherence, and this in turn complicates control of the asthma. Patients with severe persistent asthma may require particularly intensive patient education and referral to appropriate sources of support.

REDUCTION OF MAINTENANCE THERAPY

Asthma is a variable disorder, and spontaneous and therapy-induced variations in severity occur. Especially anti-inflammatory therapy has been shown to reduce asthma severity over the long term. Once control of asthma is achieved and maintained for at least 3 months, a gradual stepwise reduction of the maintenance therapy should be tried in order to identify the minimum therapy required to maintain control. This will help reduce the risk of side-effects and enhance patient adherence to the treatment plan. The therapy reduction should be done stepwise, following the reverse order of what has just been described with close monitoring of symptoms, clinical signs and, as much as possible, lung function.

IMMUNOTHERAPY

The role of immunotherapy in the management of asthma is not clearly defined.[29,30] There are large variations from country to country in its use for the treatment of asthma. These variations reflect the absence of controlled studies comparing a pure pharmacological approach versus an approach that combines immunotherapy and pharmacological treatment.

NON-CONVENTIONAL TREATMENTS

Alternative and complementary medicines (here called non-conventional treatments although some of the treatment modalities might be very conventional in their country or region of origin) are popular in many parts of the world. They include acupuncture, homeopathy, herbal medicine, Ayurvedic medicine, etc. Their efficacy has seldom been evaluated using the appropriate methods of clinical research and almost never compared with the long-term-control medication discussed in the preceding sections. The holistic approach used in many traditional methods of healing makes it very difficult to assess them in the standard randomized controlled clinical trials. One possibility would be to compare the non-conventional treatments with pharmacological management using outcome measures such as absence from work or school, emergency room visits and hospitalizations. Non-conventional therapies cannot be recommended for the management of asthma unless well-documented studies have proven their efficacy and compared them with the generally accepted long-term-control medications.

KEY POINTS

1. The main asthma guidelines are similar but the methods of assessment and treatment are chiefly based on expert opinion and require validation by clinical trials.

2. The treatment of asthma requires that the physician and patient understand the goals of treatment and how to achieve them.

3. Treatment is primarily directed to reverse and prevent airway inflammation.

4. An important component is avoidance of causes of airway inflammation and constriction.

REFERENCES

1. ✪ Panhuysen CIM, Vonk JM, Koeter GH *et al.* Adult patients may outgrow their asthma: A 25-year follow-up study. *Am J Respir Crit Care Med* 1997; 155: 1267–72.

2. Sears MR. Worldwide trends in asthma mortality. *Bull Int Union Tuberc Lung Dis* 1991; 66: 79–83.

3. Beasley R, Burgess C, Crane J, Pearce N, FitzGerald JM, Macklem P. Fatal asthma. *Allergy Proc* 1996; 47: 161–8.

4. Lange P, Ulrik CS, Vestbo J, The Copenhagen City Heart Study Group. Mortality in adults with self-reported asthma. *Lancet* 1996; 347: 1285–8.

5. Burrows B, Earle RH. Course and prognosis of chronic obstructive lung disease. The *N Engl J Med* 1969; 280: 397–404.

6. ✪ Peat JK, Woolcock AJ, Cullen K. Rate of decline of lung function in subjects with asthma. *Eur J Respir Dis* 1987; 70: 171–9.

7. Ulrik CS, Lange P. Decline of lung function in adults with bronchial asthma. *Am J Respir Crit Care Med* 1994; 150: 629–34.

8. ✪ Lange P, Parner J, Vestbo J, Schnohr P, Jensen G. A 15-year follow-up study of ventilatory function in adults with asthma. *N Engl J Med* 1998; 339: 1194–200.

9. ✪ Agertoft L, Pedersen S. Effects of long-term treatment with an inhaled corticosteroid on growth and pulmonary function in asthmatic children. *Respir Med* 1994; 88: 373–81.

10. ✪ Haahtela T, Jarvinen M, Kava T *et al.* Effects of reducing or discontinuing inhaled budesonide in patients with mild asthma. *N Engl J Med* 1994; 331: 700–705.

11. Global Initiative for Asthma. *Global Strategy for Asthma Management and Prevention*. 1995; Publ 95–3659, 1–176. Washington: National Heart, Lung and Blood Institute, National Institutes of Health.

12. Selroos O, Pietinalho A, Lofroos AB, Riska H. Effect of early vs late intervention with inhaled corticosteroids in asthma. *Chest* 1995; 108: 1228–34.

13. ✪ Sont JK, Willems LNA, Bel EH, van Krieken JHJM, Van der Broucke JP, Sterk PJ. Clinical control and histopathologic outcome of asthma when using airway hyperresponsiveness as an additional guide to long-term treatment. *Am J Respir Crit Care Med* 1999; 159: 1043–1051.

14. Strachan DP, Cook DG. Parental smoking and childhood asthma: longitudinal and case-control studies. *Thorax* 1998; 53: 204–212.

15. Jarvis D, Chinn S, Luczynska C, Burney P. Association of respiratory symptoms and lung function in young adults with use of domestic gas appliances. *Lancet* 1996; 347: 426–31.

16. Sears MR, Taylor DR, Print CG *et al*. Regular inhaled beta-agonist treatment in bronchial asthma. *Lancet* 1990; 336: 1391–6.

17. Pauwels R, Newman S, Borgstrom L. Airway deposition and airway effects of antiasthma drugs delivered from metered-dose inhalers. *Eur Respir J* 1997; 10: 2127–38.

18. van der Molen T, Meyboom de Jong B, Mulder HH, Postma DS. Starting with a higher dose of inhaled corticosteroids in primary care asthma treatment. *Am J Respir Crit Care Med* 1998; 158: 121–5.

19. ✪ Pauwels RA, Lofdahl CG, Postma DS *et al*. Effect of inhaled formoterol and budesonide on exacerbations of asthma. *N Engl J Med* 1997; 337: 1405–11.

20. Malmstrom K, Rodriguez Gomez G, Guerra J *et al*. Oral montelukast, inhaled beclomethasone, and placebo for chronic asthma–a randomized, controlled trial. *Ann Intern Med* 1999; 130: 487–95.

21. Laitinen LA, Naya IP, Binks S, Harris A. Comparative efficacy of zafirlukast and low dose steroids in asthmatics on prn β_2-agonists. *Eur Respir J* 1997; 10: 419s.

22. Derom E, van Schoor J, Verhaeghe W, Vincken W, Pauwels R. Systemic effects of inhaled fluticasone propionate and budesonide in adult patients with asthma. *Am J Respir Crit Care Med* 1999; 160: 157–161.

23. Drazen JM, Israel E, O'Byrne PM. Treatment of asthma with drugs modifying the leukotriene pathway. *N Engl J Med* 1999; 340: 197–206.

24. Greening AP, Ind PW, Northfield M, Shaw G. Added salmeterol versus higher dose corticosteroid in asthma patients with symptoms on existing inhaled corticosteroid. *Lancet* 1994; 344: 219–24.

25. Woolcock A, Lundback B, Ringdal N, Jacques LA. Comparison of addition of salmeterol to inhaled steroids with doubling of the dose of inhaled steroids. *Am J Respir Crit Care Med* 1996; 153: 1481–8.

26. Davies B, Brooks G, Devoy M. The efficacy and safety of salmeterol compared to theophylline: meta-analysis of nine controlled studies. *Respir Med* 1998; 92: 256–63.

27. ✪ Busse W, Nelson H, Wolfe J, Kalberg C, Yancey SW, Rickard KA. Comparison of inhaled salmeterol and oral zafirlukast in patients with asthma. *J Allergy Clin Immunol* 1999; 103: 1075–1080.

28. Wechsler ME, Garpestad E, Flier SR *et al*. Pulmonary infiltrates, eosinophilia, and cardiomyopathy following corticosteroid withdrawal in patients with asthma receiving zafirlukast. *JAMA* 1998; 279: 455–7.

29. Bousquet J, Hejjaoui A, Michel FB. Specific immunotherapy in asthma. *J Allergy Clin Immunol* 1990; 86: 292–305.

30. Bousquet J, Lockey R, Malling HJ. Allergen immunotherapy: therapeutic vaccines for allergic diseases. A WHO position paper. *J Allergy Clin Immunol* 1998; 102: 558–62.

Chapter 32

Management of Acute Asthma in Adults

Brian Harrison

INTRODUCTION

Pathology of Severe Asthma[1]

The lungs of patients who die from asthma are distended with trapped gas and the airways are frequently full of grey worm-like plugs of mucus and epithelial and inflammatory cellular debris. Histologically there is evidence of intense inflammation with infiltration of eosinophils, mast cells and T-lymphocytes, mucosal and sub-mucosal oedema, vasodilatation, smooth muscle hypertrophy and contraction and mucus gland hypertrophy, all reducing airway calibre. The airways are further obstructed by mucus and cellular debris in the lumen.

Some patients develop sudden severe attacks with rapid onset and rapid response to treatment.[2] The pathology in these attacks may be different and may be due to severe rapidly reversible bronchospasm, or even intense mucosal oedema. At autopsy these lungs are often "empty", i.e. contain little or no mucus plugging and the predominant inflammatory cells are neutrophils.[3]

The intense inflammation in acute severe asthma is why systemic steroid therapy as well as specific bronchodilator therapy is manadatory.

Physiology of Acute Severe Asthma[4–6]

The progressive airway narrowing caused by the inflammatory changes result in increased airflow resistance reflected in falling peak expiratory flow (PEF) and forced expired volume in 1 s (FEV$_1$). The lungs become hyperinflated with a marked increase in residual volume and total lung capacity. During recovery hyperinflation may resolve before there are major increases in PEF or FEV$_1$. As airway narrowing becomes progressively severe arterial carbon dioxide tension ($P_a CO_2$)

initially falls as a result of hyperventilation, then if the airway narrowing increases the $P_a CO_2$ returns to normal and may then rise steeply as alveolar ventilation falls. $P_a CO_2$ returns from low levels to the normal range when the FEV$_1$ falls to about 25% of predicted normal, corresponding to a PEF of about 30% predicted although there is much individual variation.[7,8] Alveolar hypoventilation can result from progressive airway narrowing, respiratory muscle exhaustion, or both. As the asthma becomes more severe arterial oxygen tension ($P_a O_2$) falls progressively due to falling ventilation–perfusion ratios and ultimately falling ventilation as well. Cyanosis occurs only when airflow obstruction is very severe. Patients who die from asthma die from hypoxaemia, which is the most serious and dangerous physiological consequence of severe asthma.

The dangers of severe hypoxia are why oxygen therapy should be given as soon as practicable in acute asthma.

Epidemiology of Severe Asthma

While asthma deaths steadily increased from the mid 1970s to the late 1980s in Britain and many other countries,[9,10] since 1988 asthma deaths have been declining in Britain.[9] Near-fatal asthma (NFA) or severe life-threatening asthma (SLTA) is defined as an attack of asthma with a raised $P_a CO_2$ or requiring intermittent positive pressure ventilation with raised inflation pressures. Statistics of NFA are more difficult to come by than those of asthma deaths, but where they have been collected NFA also seems to be becoming less common.[11] Studies of severe asthma or NFA have shown that most patients have had deteriorating asthma for days or even weeks and that very few patients have a severe attack from a state of demonstrably normal lung function over a period of hours. Studies of asthma deaths over the last

Table 32.1: Preventable factors identified in studies of asthma deaths

Underestimation of severity by doctor – usually because of failure to make objective measurements

Underestimation of severity by patient or relative

Under-treatment with systemic steroids

Adverse psychosocial factors

Inappropriate therapy

Failure to recognize and treat deterioration weeks or months before fatal attack

25 years have consistently shown potentially preventable factors associated with the majority of deaths. These factors are listed in Table 32.1. Studies in the 1970s[12-15] and 1980s[16-19] highlighted the first three factors: underestimation of severity by the doctor; underestimation of severity by the patient; and as a consequence under-treatment with systemic steroids. Studies during the 1990s[20-23] have shown that these "medical" factors, although they still occur, are occurring much less often. What these studies have highlighted is the importance of adverse psychosocial factors which are found in around three-quarters of the patients who have died. Similar adverse psychosocial factors have also been found in the majority of patients with near-fatal asthma (NFA).[11,21] Indeed, patients with NFA and those who die of asthma seem to come from the same population, the main differences being that patients with NFA are significantly younger, have fewer co-morbidities and reach medical help more quickly.[11,21] The implications of these studies include the importance of continuing to address, and improve where necessary, the medical assessment and treatment of acute severe asthma, but also developing strategies to help address the adverse psychosocial factors which are contributing to morbidity and mortality from asthma.

These were some of the reasons why, during the 1990s, groups in several countries have produced guidelines for managing acute severe asthma. Amongst the first of these were the British Guidelines published in 1990.[24] Since then the British group has revised the guidelines twice.[25,26] These guidelines have been amongst the most widely accepted, broadly based and specific and will form the basis of the next section.

MANAGEMENT OF ACUTE SEVERE ASTHMA[26]

Prevention of Acute Asthma

The implications of the studies reviewed above are that most attacks of acute severe asthma are preventable and that treatment should have begun at least a day before the presentation with acute severe asthma. Approaches to this are outlined in previous chapters and include symptoms and, where appropriate, peak flow monitoring. To emphasize the importance of this, when symptoms increase or peak flows fall below threshold levels, anti-inflammatory treatment and bronchodilator treatment should be increased by the patient, and when there is insufficient response should be increased further and medical help should be sought.

Recognition of Acute Asthma

Charts designed for use in primary care, accident and emergency departments and the acute hospital ward setting are reproduced in Fig 32.1–32.3.[26] Management of an acute exacerbation of asthma begins with the recognition of *uncontrolled asthma, acute severe asthma* or *life-threatening asthma* (Fig. 32.1). *Acute severe asthma* is reflected by the presence of one or more of the following: peak expiratory flow rate (PEF) of 50% or less of predicted or best; breathlessness that prevents the completion of a sentence in one breath; tachypnoea (≥ 25 min^{-1}); or tachycardia (≥ 110 min^{-1}). *Life-threatening* features are indicated by PEF $< 33\%$ predicted or best, a silent chest, cyanosis, feeble respiratory effort, bradycardia, hypotension, exhaustion, confusion or coma. Very severe attacks are also suggested by hypoxia indicated by oxygen saturation (S_aO_2) less than 92%. Arterial blood gases should be measured in any patient with any life-threatening features or $S_aO_2 < 92\%$. P_aO_2 below 8 kPa, a normal or elevated P_aCO_2 or a low pH, each confirms a very severe, life-threatening attack.

Treatment of Acute Asthma

Treatment of *uncontrolled asthma* is summarized in Fig. 32.1, which includes guidance for nebulized β_2-agonist therapy, use of systemic or increased inhaled

FIGURE 32.1: Acute severe asthma in adults in general practice. From The British Guidelines on Asthma Management. 1995 Review and Position Statement. *Thorax* 1997; 52: S1–S21. Inset from Greg & Nunn. *BMJ* 1989; 298: 1068–70 with permission from the BMJ Publishing Group.)

Acute severe asthma in adults in general practice

Many deaths from asthma are preventable: delay can be fatal

Factors include:

- Doctors failing to assess severity by objective measurement
- Patients or relatives failing to appreciate severity
- Underuse of corticosteroids

Regard each emergency consultation as for acute severe asthma until it is shown otherwise.

Assess and record:

- Symptoms and response to self treatment
- Heart and respiratory rates
- Peak expiratory flow (PEF)

Caution:
Patients with severe or life-threatening attacks may not be distressed and may not have all these abnormalities. The presence of any should alert the doctor.

Uncontrolled asthma

ASSESSMENT

- Speech normal
- Treat at home but response to treatment MUST be assessed before you leave

TREATMENT

Nebulized salbutamol 5 mg or terbutaline 10 mg

MONITOR RESPONSE 15–30 MIN AFTER NEBULIZER

If PEF >50–75% predicted/best
- Give prednisolone 30–60 mg
- Step up usual treatment

or

If PEF >75% predicted/best
- Step up usual treatment

FOLLOW-UP

- Monitor symptoms and PEF on PEF chart
- Self-management plan
- Surgery review ≤ 48 hours
- Modify treatment at review according to guidelines for chronic persistent asthma

CRITERIA FOR HOSPITAL ADMISSION

- Any life-threatening features
- Any features of acute severe asthma present after initial treatment, especially PEF <33%

LOWER THE THRESHOLD FOR ADMISSION IF:

Attack is in afternoon or evening, recent nocturnal symptoms etc, recent hospital admission, previous severe attacks, patient unable to assess own condition, concern over social circumstances.

Acute severe asthma

ASSESSMENT

- Can't complete sentences
- Pulse ≥110 beats min^{-1}
- Respiration ≥25 breaths min^{-1}
- PEF ≤50% predicted or best

MANAGEMENT

Seriously consider admission if more than one feature above present

TREATMENT

- Oxygen 40–60% if available
- Nebulized salbutamol 5 mg or terbutaline 10 mg
- Prednisolone 30–60 mg or intravenous hydrocortisone 200 mg

MONITOR RESPONSE 15–30 MIN AFTER NEBULIZER

If any signs of acute severe asthma persist
- Arrange admission
- Repeat nebulized β agonist plus ipratropium 0.5 mg
  or give subcutaneous terbutaline
  or give intravenous aminophylline (slowly) while awaiting ambulance

or

If good response to first nebulized treatment (symptoms improved, respiration and pulse settling, and PEF >50%):
- Step up usual treatment and continue prednisolone

FOLLOW-UP

- Monitor symptoms and PEF
- Self-management plan
- Surgery review ≤ 24 hours

Modify treatment at review according to guidelines for chronic persistent asthma

Life-threatening asthma

ASSESSMENT

- Silent chest
- Cyanosis
- Brachycardia or exhaustion
- PEF <33% of predicted or best

MANAGEMENT

Arrange immediate ADMISSION

TREATMENT

- Prednisolone 30–60 mg or intravenous hydrocortisone 200 mg immediately
- Oxygen driven nebulizer in ambulance
- Nebulized β agonist and ipratropium or subcutaneous terbutaline or intravenous aminophylline (250 mg slowly)

Stay with patient until ambulance arrives

NB If there is no nebulizer give 2 puffs of β agonist via a large volume spacer and repeat 10–20 times

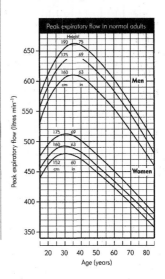

433

Acute severe asthma in adults

Recognition and assessment in hospital

Features of acute severe asthma

- Peak expiratory flow (PEF) †50% of predicted or best
- Can't complete sentences in one breath
- Respirations ‡25 breaths min^{-1}
- Pulse >110 beats min^{-1}

Life-threatening features

- PEF <33% of predicted or best
- Silent chest, cyanosis, or feeble respiratory effort
- Brachycardia or hypotension
- Exhaustion, confusion, or coma

If S_aO_2 <92% or a patient has **any life-threatening** features, measure arterial blood gases.

Blood gas markers of a very severe, life-threatening attack:

- Normal (5–6 kPa, 33–45 mmHg) or high P_aCO_2
- Severe hypoxia: P_aO_2 <8 kPa (60 mmHg) irrespective of treatment with oxygen
- A low pH (or high H$^+$)

No other investigations are needed for immediate management.

Caution:
Patients with severe or life-threatening attacks may not be distressed and may not have all these abnormalities. The presence of any should alert the doctor.

---

1 Immediate treatment

- Oxygen 40–60% (CO_2 retention is not usually aggravated by oxygen therapy in asthma)
- Salbutamol 5 mg or terbutaline 10 mg via an oxygen driven nebulizer
- Prednisolone tablets 30–60 mg or intravenous hydrocortisone 200 mg or both if very ill
- No sedatives of any kind
- Chest radiograph to exclude pneumothorax

IF LIFE-THREATENING FEATURES ARE PRESENT:

- Add ipratropium 0.5 mg to the nebulized β agonist
- Give intravenous aminophylline 250 mg over 20 mins or salbutamol or terbutaline 250 μg over 10 mins. Do not give bolus aminophylline to patients already taking oral theophyllines

2 Subsequent management

IF PATIENT IS IMPROVING CONTINUE:

- 40–60% Oxygen
- Prednisolone 30–60 mg daily or intravenous hydrocortisone 200 mg 6-hourly
- Nebulized β agonist 4-hourly

IF PATIENT IS NOT IMPROVING AFTER 15—30 MINUTES:

- Continue oxygen and steroids
- Give nebulized β agonist more frequently up to every 15-30mins
- Add ipratropium 0.5 mg to nebulizer and repeat 6-hourly until patient is improving

IF PATIENT IS STILL NOT IMPROVING GIVE:

- Aminophylline infusion (small patient 750 mg every 24 hours, large patient 1500 mg every 24 hours); monitor blood concentrations if it is continued for over 24 hours
- Salbutamol or terbutamine infusion as an alternative to aminophylline

3 Monitoring treatment

- Repeat measurement of PEF 15–30 mins after starting treatment
- Oximetry: maintain S_aO_2 >92%
- Repeat blood gas measurements within 2 hours of starting treatment if

– initial P_aO_2 <8 kPa (60 mmHg) unless subsequent S_aO_2 >92%
– P_aO_2 normal or raised
- Chart PEF before and after giving nebulized and inhaled β agonists and at least 4 times daily throughout hospital stay

Transfer patient to the intensive care unit accompanied by a doctor prepared to intubate if there is:

- Deteriorating PEF, worsening or persisting hypoxia, or hypercapnia
- Exhaustion, feeble respirations, confusion or drowsiness
- Coma or respiratory arrest

4 When discharged from hospital, patients should have:

- Been on discharge medication for 24 hours and *have had inhaler* technique checked and recorded
- PEF >75% of predicted or best and PEF diurnal variability <25% unless discharge is agreed with respiratory physician
- Treatment with oral and inhaled steroids in addition to bronchodilators
- Own PEF meter and written self-management plan
- GP follow-up arranged within 1 week
- Follow-up appointment in respiratory clinic within 4 weeks

Also

- Determine reason(s) for exacerbation and admission
- Send details of admission, discharge and potential best PEF to GP.

Peak expiratory flow in normal adults

FIGURE 32.2: Acute severe asthma in adults. From The British Guidelines on Asthma Management. 1995 Review and Position Statement. *Thorax* 1997; 52: S1–S21. Inset from Greg & Nunn. *BMJ* 1989; 298: 1068–70 with permission from the BMJ Publishing Group.

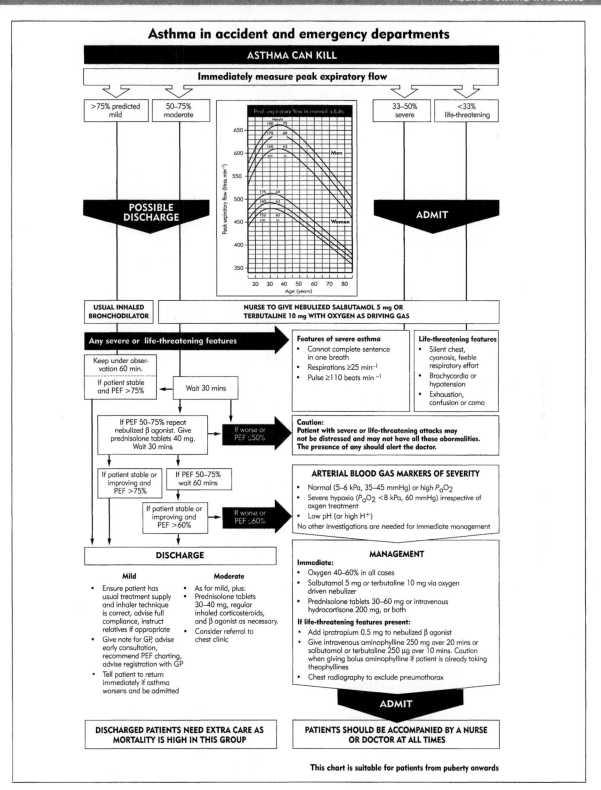

FIGURE 32.3: Asthma in accident and emergency departments. From The British Guidelines on Asthma Management. 1995 Review and Position Statement. *Thorax* 1997; 52 (Suppl. 1): S1–S21 with permission from the BMJ Publishing Group.

steroid medication and criteria for hospital admission. Immediate treatment of *acute severe asthma* consists of high-flow oxygen, high doses of inhaled β agonists and systemic corticosteroids. In addition there is now convincing evidence to support the addition of ipratropium 0.5 mg to the initial nebulization of β agonists with repeated doses 6-hourly.[27,28] If *life-threatening* features are present in addition to nebulized β agonist and ipratropium, intravenous bronchodilators are added. Subsequent management (Fig. 32.2) is determined by progress and response to treatment monitored by repeated PEF measurements, repeated oximetry aiming for an oxygen saturation above 92% and, if necessary, repeated blood gas measurements.

Indications for Intensive Care and Intermittent Positive Pressure Ventilation (IPPV)

Indications for transfer to the intensive care unit are given in Fig. 32.2. Not all such patients will require ventilation, but those with worsening hypoxia or hypercapnia, drowsiness or unconsciousness and those who have had a respiratory arrest require IPPV.[5] Intubation in such patients is very difficult and should ideally be performed by an experienced anaesthetist.[5]

Management Just Before and After Discharge from Hospital

Recommendations are outlined in Fig. 32.2. In particular, patients should have had their inhaler technique checked and should be comfortable with the inhaler system prescribed. Their peak flow should generally be above 75% of predicted or best with diurnal variability less than 25%. Almost all patients should be on oral steroid therapy in addition to their inhaled steroid therapy and bronchodilator therapy. It is wise for the dose of inhaled steroid to be at least a BTS step higher than the dose the patient was taking before the severe episode. Since they have been ill enough to be admitted to hospital they should be given a written self-management plan and their own peak flow meter with peak flow thresholds upon which to base their treatment.

It is important at this stage to look into the circumstances preceding their admission (Table 32.2). Physicians can then determine whether there were preventable factors that can be addressed to try to avoid a recurrence.

Ideally, follow-up would be arranged with the patient's general practitioner or primary care physician within one week of discharge and follow-up in the specialist respiratory clinic within 4 weeks. There are many studies which show that the care of patients admitted to hospital with acute severe asthma is superior when provided by a respiratory specialist as compared with a general physician with another sub-specialist interest.[29–33] This is why, ideally, patients should be transferred to the care of a respiratory specialist during their admission and why all patients admitted with asthma should be followed up by the respiratory specialist.

At-Risk Register[23,34,35]

Features associated with patients who are at risk of developing severe or fatal attacks of asthma are listed in Table 32.3.[23,34,35] It is wise for physicians in primary and secondary care to develop a register of such at-risk asthmatics. Such patients need special vigilance from their physicians and asthma nurses. Doctors running out of hours, deputizing or co-op covering services need to be aware of patients on the at-risk asthma register. In particular, if these patients do not attend us in our surgeries and clinics then we should make attempts to attend them since the major problems with such patients are not pharmacotherapeutic but behavioural.

COMPARISON BETWEEN THE 1997 BRITISH GUIDELINES[26] AND THE 1997 AMERICAN GUIDELINES[36]

The similarities between the most recent versions of the British (Figs 32.1–32.3) and the American and

Table 32.2: Circumstances preceding admission		
Was there an avoidable precipitating cause?	(YES)	(NO)
Was this a catastrophic sudden attack? (i.e. no period of recognizable deterioration before the acute attack)	(YES)	(NO)
Did the patient (or relatives) react appropriately when the asthma deteriorated?	(YES)	(NO)
Was the patient complying with regular therapy?	(YES)	(NO)
Can we do anything to help? If so, what?	(YES)	(NO)
Was medical management appropriate?	(YES)	(NO)

Table 32.3: Patients at risk of developing severe or fatal asthma

Previous *life-threatening attacks*

Severe disease reflected by:
(a) *three or more categories* of anti-asthmatic drug prescribed
(b) ever admitted with their asthma *especially in the previous year*
(c) requiring *emergency* steroids and or nebulized bronchodilators

With *psychiatric morbidity, behavioural difficulties, especially denial, and socioeconomic deprivation.* (Recognize denial or anger by non-attendance, unwillingness to comply with therapy or monitoring, unwillingness to accept the diagnosis or the need to take regular medication)

Calling for GP, or attending surgery, or A & E Department with *emergency deterioration*

Patient's *non-compliance*

Discontinuity of medical care

Peak flow falling below 50% of their best or predicted value

Requiring *two or more* bronchodilator inhalers *monthly*

Discuss these issues frankly with the patient and their relative

indeed the Canadian[23,37] and International guidelines[38] are more impressive and more important than their differences. Indeed the overall agreement is extremely reassuring.

IMPORTANT DIFFERENCES

The important differences between the two Guidelines reflect different practice in Britain and the USA and relate to the doses and frequency of administration of nebulized bronchodilators and the doses of systemic steroids.

β-Agonist Therapy

For patients with acute severe asthma the British Guidelines recommend nebulized salbutamol 5 mg or terbutaline 10 mg initially. If the patient is improving

this dose is repeated 4-hourly. If the patient is not improving after 15–30 minutes, the dose is repeated more frequently up to every 15–30 minutes. The US Guidelines recommend nebulized albuterol (salbutamol) 2.5 to 5 mg every 20 minutes for three doses, and then 2.5 to 10 mg every 1–4 hours, as needed, or 10 to 15 mg per hour continuously. There is no evidence to favour one or other of these different approaches.

Ipratropium
There is now good evidence for the addition of ipratropium bromide 0.5 mg to the nebulized β agonist in the initial treatment of acute severe or life-threatening asthma. Ipratropium is a long-acting bronchodilator and British studies have recommended 4–6 hourly doses. In the US Guidelines, the recommendation is for 0.5 mg every 30 minutes for three doses and then every 2–4 hours, as needed. Again, there is no evidence to favour either of these approaches.

Systemic Steroids
The British Guidelines recommend 30–60 mg of prednisolone orally immediately and then the same dose repeated daily. In the US the recommendation is for 120–180 mg daily in three or four divided doses for 48 hours, then 60–80 mg daily. Again, there is no evidence to favour one of these dosage regimens over the other.

AREAS OF CONTROVERSY AND UNCERTAINTY (Table 32.4)

Peak Flow Thresholds
The view that a PEF of less than 33% of predicted or best reflects a very severe life-threatening attack of

Table 32.4: Some areas of uncertainty

PEF thresholds for recognizing acute severe asthma, life threatening asthma and for recommending hospital admission

Role of intravenous aminophylline

Role of oxygen saturation measurements in reducing need for arterial gas measurement

PEF diurnal variability criterion for appropriateness for discharge from hospital asthma is supported by several studies.[4–8,39] The use of a PEF of 50% or less of predicted normal or best to define a severe attack, though included in the British,[26] US[36] and Canadian[37] Guidelines, is not supported by any clinical scientific study. However, the British audit of 766 patients admitted to hospital with acute severe asthma provides some empirical support for this figure, since the median PEF on admission was 40% of the best achieved by the patient whilst still in hospital.[32] Clearly, using PEF thresholds expressed as a percentage of predicted normal or best is only valid for patients whose best PEF approaches their predicted normal when they are well and in remission. These thresholds, therefore, do not apply to the many patients who have a combination of smoking-induced and asthmatic airways obstruction, or to that group of usually elderly patients with asthma who develop a greater or lesser degree of fixed airways narrowing.

Role of Intravenous Aminophylline

Some[40] but not all[41] studies seem to show an advantage when intravenous aminophylline is added to subcutaneous or nebulized β_2 agonists in the management of asthma in patients seen in the emergency room. These were both short-term studies and included patients whose pre-treatment function and rapid response to treatment indicates that their asthma was not particularly severe. Some[41] but not all[40,42] studies have shown more adverse effects when aminophylline is added. On the basis of experience and published evidence it seems reasonable to include intravenous aminophylline in the initial treatment of very severe life-threatening asthma and in the patient who has not responded to initial treatment with oxygen, nebulized β_2 agonist plus ipratropium and systemic steroid therapy.[26]

Role of Oxygen Saturation Measurements

The potential for using oxygen saturation measurements to reduce the need for arterial puncture and blood gas measurement has been reported in one study of 89 patients admitted to hospital with acute severe asthma. The authors concluded that blood gases are not required if the patient's arterial saturation measured by pulse oximetry is 92% or higher, since only 5% of patients with saturations in this range had P_aO_2 or P_aCO_2 in the respiratory failure range, and none of these patients was either severely hypoxaemic or hypercapnic.[43]

Diurnal Variability of PEF

Guidelines recommend that patients should not be discharged from hospital until their PEF is above 75% of their predicted or best and their diurnal variability, i.e.

$$\frac{\text{highest PEF} - \text{lowest PEF}}{\text{highest PEF}} \times 100$$

in each 24 hours is less than 25%.[26] This is based on one published report, which concluded that patients should not be discharged until their PEF variability was less than 20%.[44] It is hoped that such guidance will result in fewer re-admissions, but the importance of hospitalization as opposed to therapy in such patients has not been established.

AUDIT

One of the original intentions of the British Guidelines was to use them as a basis for audit. Using the guidelines as a standard against which to measure practice, audit of all patients admitted with acute severe asthma to 36 hospitals in August and September 1990, and in the same 2 months a year later, was undertaken and the results of these two audits have been published.[32,33] One of the most striking results of this first audit was the difference in care of patients admitted under respiratory physicians compared with those admitted under general physicians (see Table 51.6). Several studies had shown this difference before.[29–31] They had also shown that practice can be improved but that the quality of care provided by respiratory physicians remains at a higher level than that provided by general physicians.[31,33] This should not be surprising, since it would appear to be unreasonable to expect general physicians whose main subspecialty interest is in a different field to remain abreast of all the literature and advances in the field of asthma care. As a consequence of these observations, the following suggestions have been made.[45]

(1) All patients admitted to hospital with acute severe asthma should be admitted under the care of a respiratory physician or managed according to guidelines agreed by the local respiratory physician and transferred to the care of the respiratory physician on the next full working day.

(2) All patients requiring hospital follow-up as outpatients should be attending respiratory medical

clinics and not the clinics of general physicians whose specialty interest is not respiratory medicine.[26,38]

A further result of the audit concerns systolic paradox. This was measured in fewer than half the 766 patients in the first audit and was found to be abnormal (10 mmHg or greater) in less than half of those. It was the only abnormal sign of those signs used to define a severe attack in under 5% of the patients.[46] Consequently systolic paradox is not included as a useful sign in recognizing severe asthma in the revised guidelines.[25,26]

KEY POINTS

1 Studies of asthma deaths have consistently found potentially preventable factors in over three-quarters of patients. Before 1990 the three factors mainly highlighted were underestimation of severity by the doctor, underestimation of severity by the patient, and as a consequence undertreatment with systemic steroids. In the 1990s studies have highlighted the importance of adverse psychosocial factors.

2 Patients at risk of developing severe or fatal asthma can usually be identified by features listed in Table 32.3. Doctors in primary and secondary care should develop a register of such "at-risk" patients and make it available to all doctors and nurses to whom such patients might present.

3 Management of acute severe asthma requires recognition and assessment of the severity based on objective clinical measurements; treatment with prednisolone tablets, (or rarely intravenous hydrocortisone), nebulized β_2 agonists and oxygen (augmented if necessary by intravenous bronchodilators); monitoring with repeated PEF and oxygen saturation measurements; and appropriate discharge planning.

4 Recommendations
Inpatients with asthma should be cared for by respiratory physicians or managed according to their local protocols and transferred to the care of the respiratory team on the next full working day.

REFERENCES

1. Dunnill MS. The pathology of asthma. In: Porter R and Birch J (eds). *Identification of Asthma*. Ciba Foundation Study Group No. 38. Edinburgh: Churchill Livingstone, 1971: 35.

2. Wasserfallen JB, Schaller MD, Perret CH. Life threatening asthma with dramatic resolution. *Chest* 1993; 104: 616.

3. Sur S, Crotty T, Kephart G et al. Sudden-onset fatal asthma. A district entity with few eosinophils and relatively more neutrophils in the airway submucosa? *Am Rev Respir Dis* 1993; 148: 713–19.

4. McFadden ER, Lyons HA. Arterial blood gas tension in asthma. *N Engl J Med* 1968; 78: 1027–32.

5. Rebuck AS, Read J. Assessment and management of severe asthma. *Am J Med* 1971; 51: 788–98.

6. McFadden ER, Kiser R, deGroot WJ. Acute bronchial asthma. *N Engl J Med* 1973; 288: 211.

7. Harrison BDW, Swarbrick ET. Peak flow percentage in asthma. *Lancet* 1971; ii: 494.

8. Nowak RM, Tomlanovich MC, Sarkar DD, Kvale PA, Anderson JJ. Arterial blood gases and pulmonary function testing in acute bronchial asthma. *JAMA* 1983; 249: 2043–6.

9. Lung and Asthma Infromation Agency. *Trends in asthma mortality in Great Britain*. Factsheet 97/3.

10. Sears MR. Descriptive epidemiology of asthma. *Lancet* 1997; 350 (suppl. II): 1–4.

11. Innes NJ, Reid A, Halstead et al. Psychosocial factors in near-fatal asthma and in asthma deaths. *J R Coll Physicians Lond* 1998; 32: 430–34.

12. Cochrane GM, Clark TJH. A survey of asthma mortality in patients between ages 35 and 64 in the Greater London hospitals. *Thorax* 1975; 30: 300–5.

13. MacDonald JB, Seaton A, Williams JA. Asthma deaths in Cardiff 1963–74: 90 deaths outside hospital. *BMJ* 1976; 1: 1493–5.

14. MacDonald JB, MacDonald ET, Seaton A, Williams DA. Asthma deaths in Cardiff 1963–74: 53 deaths in hospital. *BMJ* 1976; 2: 721–3.

15. Bateman JRM, Clarke SW. Sudden death in asthma. *Thorax* 1979; 34: 40–4.

16. Ormerod LP, Stableforth DE. Asthma mortality in Birmingham 1975–7: 53 deaths. *BMJ* 1980; 280: 687–90.

17. British Thoracic Association. Death from asthma in two regions of England. *BMJ* 1982; 285: 1251–5.

18. Sears MR, Rea HH, Beaglehoe RG *et al*. Asthma mortality in New Zealand: a two year national study. *N Z Med J* 1985; 98: 271–5.

19. Eason J, Markowe HLJ. Controlled investigation of deaths from asthma in hospitals in the North East Thames Region. *BMJ* 1987; 294: 1255–8.

20. Wareham NJ, Harrison BDW, Jenkins PF, Nicholls J, Stableforth DE. A district confidential enquiry into death due to asthma. *Thorax* 1993; 48: 1117–40.

21. ✪ Campbell DA, McLennan G, Coates JR *et al*. A comparison of asthma deaths and near-fatal asthma attacks in South Australia. *Eur Respir J* 1994; 7: 490–7.

22. Somerville M, Williams EMI, Pearson MG. Asthma deaths in Mersey region 1989–90. *J Publ Health Med* 1995; 17: 397–403.

23. ✪ Mohan G, Harrison BDW, Badminton RM *et al*. A confidential enquiry into deaths caused by asthma in an English health region: implictions for general practice. *Br J Gen Pract* 1996; 46: 529–32.

24. Statement by the British Thoracic Society, Research Unit of the Royal College of Physicians of London, King's Fund Centre, National Asthma Campaign. Guidelines for management of asthma in adults: II–acute severe asthma. *BMJ* 1990; 301: 767–800.

25. Statement by the British Thoracic Society and others. Guidelines on the Management of Asthma. *Thorax* 1993; 48: S1–S24.

26. ✪ The British Guidelines on Asthma Management. 1995 Review and Position Statement. *Thorax* 1997; 52: S1–21.

27. Beveridge RC, Grunfeld AF, Hodder RV, Verbeek R. Guidelines for the emergency management of asthma in adults. *Can Med Assoc J* 1996; 155: 25–7.

28. Brophy C, Ahmed B, Bayston S *et al*. How long should Atrovent be given in acute asthma? *Thorax* 1998; 53: 363–7.

29. Osman J, Ormerod LP, Stableforth DE. Management of acute asthma: a survey of hospital practice and comparison between thoracic and general physicians in Birmingham and Manchester. *Br J Dis Chest* 1987; 81: 232–41.

30. Bucknall CE, Robertson C, Moran F, Sevenson RD. Differences in hospital asthma management. *Lancet* 1988; i: 748–50.

31. Baldwin DR, Ormerod LP, Mackay AD, Stableforth DE. Changes in hospital management of acute severe asthma by thoracic and general physicians in Birmingham and Manchester during 1978 and 1985. *Thorax* 1990; 4: 130–4.

32. ✪ Pearson MG, Ryland I, Harrison BDW. A national audit of acute severe asthma in adults admitted to hospital. *Quality in Health Care* 1995; 4: 24–31.

33. Pearson MG, Ryland I, Harrison BDW. Comparison of the process of care of acute severe asthma in adults admitted to hospital before and 1 year after the publication of national guidelines. *Respir Med* 1996; 90: 539–45.

34. Sears MR, Rea HH. Patients at risk of dying of asthma: New Zealand experience. *J Allergy Clin Immunol* 1987; 80: 477–81.

35. ✪ Strunk RC. Identification of the fatility-prone subject with asthma. *Allergy Clin Immunol* 1989; 83: 477–85.

36. NHLBI Expert Panel Report II. *Guidelines for the Diagnosis and Management of Asthma*. NIH publication No. 97-Bethesda MD, 1997.

37. Hargreaves FE, Dolovich J, Newhouse MT (eds). The Assessment and Treatment of Asthma: A Conference Report. *J Allergy Clin Immunol* 1990; 85: 1098–111.

38. International Consensus Report on the Diagnosis and Management of Asthma. *Clin Exp Allergy* 1992; 22 (suppl.): 1–72.

39. Arnold AG, Lane DJ, Zapata E. The speed of onset and severity of acute severe asthma. *Br J Dis Chest* 1982; 76: 157–63.

40. Rossing TH, Fanta CH, McFadden ER. A controlled trial of the use of single versus combined drug therapy in the treatment of acute episodes of asthma. *Am Rev Respir Dis* 1981; 123: 190–4.

41. Siegel D, Sheppard D, Gelb A, Weinberg PF. Aminophylline increases the toxicity but not the efficacy of an inhaled beta-adrenergic agonist in the treatment of acute exacerbations of asthma. *Am Rev Respir Dis* 1985; 132: 283–6.

42. Fanta CJ, Rossing TH, McFadden ER. Emergency room treatment of asthma. Relationships among therapeutic combinations, severity of obstruction and time course of response. *Am J Med* 1982; 72: 416–22.

43. Carruthers D, Harrison BDW. Arterial blood gas analysis or oxgyen saturation in the assessment of acute asthma. *Thorax* 1995; 50: 186–8.

44. Udwadia ZF, Harrison BDW. An attempt to determine the optimal duration of hospital stay following a severe attack of asthma. *J Coll Physicians Lond* 1990; 24: 112–4.

45. Harrison BDW, Pearson MG. Audit in acute severe asthma–who benefits. *J R Coll Physicians Lond* 1993; 27: 387–90.

46. Pearson MG, Spence DPS, Ryland I, Harrison BDW. Value of pulsus paradoxus in assessing acute severe asthma. *BMJ* 1993; 307: 659.

Chapter 33

Specific Problems: Occupational Asthma

Jean-Luc Malo and Moira Chan-Yeung

INTRODUCTION AND DEFINITION

Although interest in occupational diseases has focused primarily on conditions that affect the lung parenchyma, referred to as pneumoconiosis (asbestosis and silicosis being the most common), there is now growing interest in conditions that involve the airways. These include bronchial cancer, chronic bronchitis and fixed airway obstruction, and asthma. Occupational asthma (OA) is now the most common occupational respiratory ailment in developed countries.[1,2] In epidemiological surveys, it has been estimated that approximately 5% of adult-onset asthma is attributable to the workplace.[3] Occupational asthma can be defined as "a disease characterized by variable airflow limitation and/or airway hyperresponsiveness due to causes and conditions attributable to a particular occupational environment and not to stimuli encountered outside the workplace".[4,5] Two types of OA are distinguishable by whether or not they appear after a latency period. The usual form develops after a latency period that is necessary for "sensitization", although, in many instances of OA due to low molecular weight agents, the mechanism for sensitization is unknown. Some of the agents causing OA with a latency period can be classified as high or low molecular weight (greater or less than 1000–5000). The principal differences between OA caused by high and low molecular weight agents are listed in Table 33.1. The other form of OA occurs without a latency period and follows exposure(s) to high concentrations of an irritant product.

HOW TO DIAGNOSE OCCUPATIONAL ASTHMA

It is important to remove subjects from exposure to an occupational agent that causes their asthma as OA can lead to permanent impairment/disability.[6] Several retrospective studies have shown that the earlier affected workers are removed from exposure to a causal agent present at work, the more likely it is they will recover, if this is going to occur.[6] Not diagnosing OA can therefore have a significant impact on respiratory health. A diagnosis of OA carries serious social consequences. Workers have to leave their job, which implies a diminished quality of life and financial loss.[2,7–9] For these reasons, objective evidence in confirming the diagnosis is very important. The various means of diagnosing OA have been reviewed in different guidelines and statements.[10,11] They include the following.

Medical Questionnaire

All asthmatic subjects should be questioned as to possible exposure to causal agents at their current or previous workplaces. As asthmatic subjects could be left with permanent asthma after removal from the workplace, their current asthma symptoms could result from previous exposure to occupational causal agents. Physicians should be aware that certain workplaces are at high risk of exposing subjects to agents that can cause asthma. They should also have ready access to a databank of causal agents. There are national agencies that offer these services. The most successful one is the French MINITEL system, which gives physicians access to a databank listing causes according to workplaces and agents.[4] This databank is also available from the American Academy of Asthma, Allergy and Immunology. Safety data sheets on all products used in the workplace should be obtained from employers and/or from local safety committees. Table 33.2 lists the most frequent causes of OA and the most commonly implicated workplaces.

Clinical questionnaires should be sensitive although, in general, they are not very specific tools.[12] Exposure

443

Table 33.1: Characteristics of high and low molecular weight agents

	High molecular weight	Low molecular weight
Physical size	<1000–5000	>1000–5000
Examples of agents	Proteins, enzymes gums, flour	Isocyanates, white and red cedar
Immunological mechanism		
Humoral mechanism	IgE	Non-IgE
Clinical		
Predisposition	Atopy, smoking (?)	Unknown
Interval between onset of exposure and symptoms	Longer	Shorter
Functional		
Temporal patterns of reaction on specific inhalation challenges	Isolated immediate, dual	Late, atypical
Epidemiological		
Prevalence in high-risk populations	<5%	>5%
Model	"Extrinsic asthma"	"Intrinsic asthma"

Table 33.2: Common agents causing occupational asthma and frequently implicated workplaces

Agent	Workplace
High molecular weight agents	
Cereals	Bakers, millers
Animal-derived allergens	Animal handlers
Enzymes	Detergent, pharmaceutical, bakers
Gums	Carpet, pharmaceutical
Latex	Health professional
Seafoods	Seafoods processors
Low molecular weight agents	
Isocyanates	Spray painters, insulation, plastics and rubbers, foam
Wood-dusts	Forest workers, carpenters, cabinet makers
Anhydrides	Plastics, epoxy resins users
Amines	Shellac and lacquer handlers, solderers
Fluxes	Electronic workers
Chloramine T	Janitor–cleaners
Dyes	Textile industries
Persulphate	Hairdressers
Formaldehyde, glutaraldehyde	Hospital staff
Acrylate	Adhesive handlers, painters
Drugs	Pharmaceutical companies, health professionals
Metals	Solderers, refiners

to a known causal agent at work and the presence of asthma should be sufficient to alert the physician to the possibility of OA, even though the temporal relationship between exposure at work and symptoms may seem discordant. Subjects with OA may experience improvement in their symptoms at weekends and on vacations, but it is our experience that this occurs at the beginning of the illness only. Once OA is well-established, it is sometimes difficult for subjects to notice any significant improvement on these occasions. The possibility of the presence of nasal or conjunctival symptoms should be addressed. Ocular and nasal symptoms often accompany or even precede, in the case of high molecular weight agents, the occurrence of OA.[13]

Immunological Testing

Atopy, defined as the presence of immediate cutaneous reactivity to at least one of a battery of common inhalant allergens (pollens, house dust, moulds, etc.) is a predisposing factor for OA due to high molecular weight agents, but its positive predictive value is weak.[14,15] Allergy skin tests should not be used to exclude atopic subjects from high-risk workplaces. Skin-prick tests can be done with extracts derived from specific high molecular weight agents. However, the presence of immediate skin sensitivity only indicates the presence of sensitization and does not confirm the diagnosis of OA. The target organ, the bronchial tubes in this instance, should be shown to be hyperresponsive. This can be done through the assessment of non-allergic airway responsiveness (see below). The combination of positive skin test reaction to a relevant occupational allergen and non-allergic airway hyperresponsiveness means that there is a ~80% likelihood that the patient has OA.[16]

Assessment of Non-Allergic Airway Responsiveness

In order to make a diagnosis of OA, it is important to demonstrate the presence of asthma. Non-allergic airway hyperresponsiveness can be shown either by assessing the response to bronchodilators, if there is airway obstruction, or by estimating the degree of bronchoconstrictive response to a pharmacological agent. If the worker is still employed, non-allergic airway responsiveness should be evaluated on a working day after a minimum period of 2 weeks at work, as it may be normal when the subject has not been exposed for a period of time[17] although this is not always the rule.[6] The absence of non-allergic airway hyperresponsive-

ness in a subject when still working and exposed to the agent(s) suspected of causing OA virtually excludes OA.

Assessment of Airway Calibre and Its Fluctuations

As in the diagnosis of non-occupational asthma, it is important to assess the degree of airway obstruction serially over time. Serial measurement of peak expiratory flow rates (PEF) in the diagnosis and management of asthma[18,19] has been used since the late 1970s.[20] In the investigation of OA, workers are asked to measure and register their PEFR at least four times a day and to record their medication, symptoms and whether they are at work or away from work (Fig. 33.1). Although monitoring of PEF has been found to have satisfactory sensitivity and specificity in the diagnosis of OA,[21,22] several aspects of this method of monitoring have yet to be explored as reviewed elsewhere:[23] (a) compliance which is far from being satisfactory in most instances[24] but can be verified with portable instruments that store results; (b) comparison with a more suitable functional index

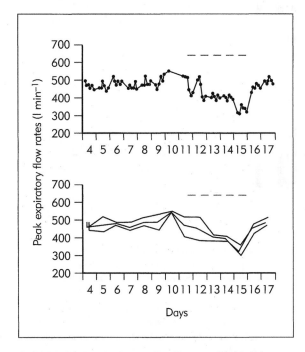

FIGURE 33.1: Peak expiratory flow rates for periods away from work and at work (horizontal bars). Individual results plotted in the upper section and maximum, mean and minimum daily values in the lower graph according to the method proposed by Burge and co-workers.[20] Progressive weekly pattern of falls in PEFR during a week spent at work.

such as forced expiratory volume in 1 s (FEV_1) which seems to favour PEF according to recent findings;[25] (c) tracing, analysis and interpretation of results for which computerized methods have been suggested.[26]

Specific Inhalation Challenges

Exposing individuals to the potential causal agent(s) in a hospital laboratory or at the workplace under careful supervision is a good method to confirm OA. This method was first proposed in the 1970s by Professor Jack Pepys at the Brompton Hospital in London, UK.[27] However, these tests require the expertise of highly trained personnel and can only be done in specialized centres. They should be performed in a dose–response manner, exposing subjects to increasing concentrations but non-irritant levels of the agent with serial monitoring of FEV_1 following exposure for at least 8 hours.[28] Several patterns of reaction have been described. Isolated immediate and dual reactions occur more commonly after exposure to high molecular weight agents while isolated late reactions or atypical reactions occur as a rule after exposure to low molecular weight agents.[29] These tests have furthered our understanding of the mechanism of asthma.

The investigation of OA is a step-wise procedure as shown in Table 33.3 and further illustrated in Fig. 33.2. It can be seen that several methods have to be used together to confirm the diagnosis of OA.

Table 33.3: Step-wise approach to the assessment of occupational asthma. (Modified from Bernstein DI. Clinical assessment and management of occupational asthma. In: Bernstein IL, Chan-Yeung M, Malo JL, Bernstein DI (eds). Asthma in the Workplace. New York: Marcel Dekker, 1993: 103–23.

(1) Suspect an occupational aetiology

(2) Obtain a medical and occupational history

(3) Research all suspect agents in the medical literature and databank

(4) Obtain information on the nature of the exposure

(5) Instruct the worker (if the asthma is not severe) not to leave his or her job until a diagnosis is confirmed or excluded

(6) Follow specific steps using guidelines to confirm or exclude a diagnosis as shown in Fig. 33.2. Referral to or consultation with a specialist may be necessary

(7) Once the diagnosis is confirmed, institute measures to eliminate exposure to causative agent(s)

Screening Programmes in High-Risk Groups

Physicians may be asked to screen for OA in subjects exposed to known causal agents or in a workplace where cases of OA have been identified.[30] These programmes may include pre-employment testing and periodic assessment. Pre-employment testing should include a questionnaire, spirometry and assessment of non-allergic airway responsiveness to document the baseline status. Workers with pre-existing asthma should not be excluded as there is no reason to believe that asthmatic subjects are more likely to develop OA than anyone else. It is important to measure baseline lung function and the degree of airway responsiveness so that any change can be detected. Figure 33.3 illustrates the steps in the assessment of workers according to the nature of the agent. It is difficult to recommend a frequency for screening assessments. It has been estimated that 40% of subjects with OA due to low molecular weight agents develop their symptoms during the first year of exposure, while the corresponding figure for high molecular weight agents is 20%.[31] After that, there is a progressive reduction in the rate of development of OA. From these findings, it seems advisable to assess subjects in the workplace 1 year after exposure begins and every 2 years thereafter.

HOW TO MANAGE OCCUPATIONAL ASTHMA ONCE THE DIAGNOSIS IS MADE

Once the diagnosis of OA is confirmed, subjects should be advised to avoid exposure to the causal agent. Wearing a mask does not reduce symptomatology or functional abnormalities.[32] It is unknown whether treatment with inhaled steroids while keeping the subject at work is justified. On the other hand, in subjects who are unable to leave their job, this measure should be considered. For some, treatment with inhaled steroids coupled with removal from exposure has accelerated recovery.[33] Subjects with OA whose symptoms persist after removal from exposure should be treated in the same way as patients with non-occupational asthma.

Patients with OA should be offered suitable help in finding another job, either with the same employer or another one, provided there is no further exposure to the causal agent (Table 33.4). Subjects aged 55 or over should be offered early retirement, and young subjects should be retrained for a new job, all with financial compensation. Compensation boards or similar medicolegal agencies should offer these programmes to workers and

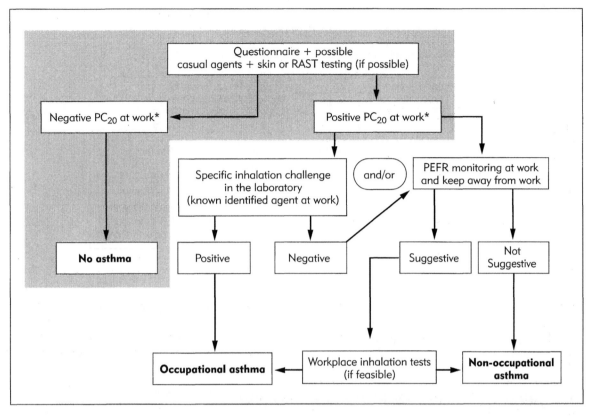

FIGURE 33.2: Step-wise scheme for investigating occupational asthma. The white zone corresponds to the investigation that should be carried out in specialized centres whereas the grey zone represents the steps that should be followed by allergologists, pneumologists and internists implicated in the initial step of the investigation. *, Assessed at the end of a working day and after a minimal period of 2 weeks at work. †, The choice depends on the facilities of the investigation centre. (From Ref. 4 by courtesy of Marcel Dekker Inc.)

assess the cost-effectiveness of them. The time needed to make a diagnosis of OA and to implement a programme is very long, causing hardship to the subjects.[2,34]

Because OA can lead to permanent impairment/disability, subjects should be re-assessed periodically. The first assessment should take place 2 years after removal from exposure, when a plateau of improvement can occur, as in the case of a high molecular weight agent such as snow-crab.[35] Impairment/disability should be assessed using different tools from those proposed for pneumoconiosis. Impairment is the functional abnormality resulting from a medical condition; disability is the total effect of impairment on a patient's life. The three main criteria for assessing impairment/disability for asthma are: (1) airway calibre; (2) airway responsiveness either to a bronchodilator if airway obstruction is present or a bronchoconstrictor if this is not the case;

(3) the need for medication, which is a reflection of the clinical severity of asthma.

A SPECIFIC ENTITY: IRRITANT-INDUCED OA OR REACTIVE AIRWAYS DYSFUNCTION SYNDROME (RADS)

A type of irritant-induced asthma was labelled "RADS" by Brooks et al.[36] It involves the onset of asthma symptoms and the presence of non-allergic airway hyperresponsiveness in subjects exposed in an acute manner to high concentrations of an occupational irritant product. This can be a single exposure, as proposed by Brooks and co-workers[36] or multiple exposures, provided that respiratory symptoms occur on each occasion. There seems to be a dose-dependent relationship between exposure and the likelihood of permanent disability/impairment.[37–39]

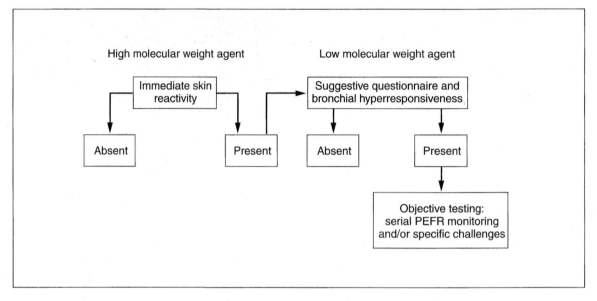

FIGURE 33.3: Suggested surveillance programme for occupational asthma, distinguishing between high and low molecular weight agents. In the first instance, skin reactivity is the cornerstone whereas for low molecular weight agents, questionnaires and airway hyperresponsiveness are the key factors.

Table 33.4: How to manage occupational asthma once the diagnosis is confirmed*
Removal from exposure
Assess for temporary disability

Refer to a rehabilitation programme
    Finding a job with the same employer without exposure to the causal agent
    Finding a job with a different employer without exposure to the causal agent
    Retraining for a new job
    Early retirement
    When a subject cannot change jobs, minimize exposure and treat asthma with anti-inflammatory preparations

Treat asthma
For those who are unable to change jobs, ensure minimal exposure to the causal agent

Assess for permanent disability 2 years after cessation of exposure
    Ensure that asthma is in a stable clinical condition
    Set disability/impairment using the following criteria:
    (a) airway calibre;
    (b) responsiveness to a bronchodilator or a bronchoconstrictive agent;
    (c) need for medication to treat asthma

Re-assess periodically if necessary
*Refer to a medicolegal agency (if not done) or a private insurance programme. The diagnosis should be confirmed as rapidly as possible.

Chlorine and ammonia are common causal agents. Prevention is mandatory in high-risk workplaces where such inhalational accidents can occur. Assessment of methacholine airway responsiveness should also be considered as a pre-employment test so that, if an accident occurs, comparisons are possible.[40]

CONCLUSION

Occupational asthma is the most common occupational respiratory condition in developed countries. It is important to diagnose the condition with precision so that proper medical and medicolegal advice can be given. Moreover, screening programmes should be available to workers in high-risk industries. If a worker develops OA, proper compensation, including temporary and permanent impairment/disability, through a medicolegal agency or access to private insurance, should be offered.

KEY POINTS

1 Occupational asthma is a disease characterized by variable airflow limitation and/or airway hyperresponsiveness due to causes and conditions attributable to a particular occupational environment and not to stimuli encountered outside the workplace.

2 Occupational asthma is the most common occupational respiratory condition in developed countries. It is important to diagnose the condition with precision so that proper medical and medicolegal advice can be given.

3 Screening programmes for occupational asthma should be available to workers in high-risk industries.

REFERENCES

1. Ross DJ, Keynes HL, McDonald JC. SWORD '97: Surveillance of work-related and occupational respiratory disease in the UK. *Occup Med* 1998; 48: 481–5.

2. Dewitte JD, Chan-Yeung M, Malo JL. Medicolegal and compensation aspects of occupational asthma. *Eur Respir J* 1994; 7: 969–80.

3. Kogevinas M, Anto JM, Soriano JB, Tobias A, Burney P. The risk of asthma attributable to occupational exposures. *Am J Respir Crit Care Med* 1996; 154: 137–43.

4. ✪ Bernstein IL, Chan-Yeung M, Malo JL, Bernstein D. *Asthma in the Workplace*, second edition. New York: Marcel Dekker, 1999.

5. ✪ Chan-Yeung M, Malo JL. Occupational asthma. *N Engl J Med* 1995; 333: 107–112.

6. Chan-Yeung M, Malo JL. Natural history of occupational asthma. In: Bernstein IL, Chan-Yeung M, Malo JL, Bernstein DI (eds). *Asthma in the Workplace*. New York: Marcel Dekker, 1993; 299–322.

7. Malo JL, Dewitte JD, Cartier A, *et al.* Quality of life of subjects with occupational asthma. *J Allergy Clin Immunol* 1993; 91: 1121–7.

8. Marabini A, Ward H, Kwan S, Kennedy S, Wexler-Morrison N, Chan-Yeung M. Clinical and socioeconomical features of subjects with red cedar asthma–a follow up study. *Chest* 1993; 104: 821–4.

9. Gannon PFG, Weir DC, Robertson AS, Burge PS. Health, employment, and financial outcomes in workers with occupational asthma. *Br J Ind Med* 1993; 50: 491–6.

10. Bernstein DI, Cohn JR. Guidelines for the diagnosis and evaluation of occupational immunologic lung disease: preface. *J Allergy Clin Immunol* 1989; 84: 791–3.

11. ✪ Chan-Yeung M. Assessment of asthma in the workplace. *Chest* 1995; 108: 1084–1117.

12. ✪ Malo JL, Ghezzo H, L'Archevêque J, Lagier F, Perrin B, Cartier A. Is the clinical history a satisfactory means of diagnosing occupational asthma? *Am Rev Respir Dis* 1991; 143: 528–32.

13. Malo JL, Lemière C, Desjardins A, Cartier A. Prevalence and intensity of rhinoconjunctivitis in subjects with occupational asthma. *Eur Respir J* 1997; 10: 1513–15.

14. Slovak AJM, Hill RN. Does atopy have any predictive value for laboratory animal allergy? A comparison of

different concepts of atopy. *Br J Ind Med* 1987;
44: 129–32.

15. Venables KM. Epidemiology and the prevention of occupational asthma. (editorial). *Br J Ind Med* 1987; 44: 73–5.

16. Malo JL, Cartier A, L'Archevêque J, Ghezzo H, Lagier F, Trudeau C, Dolovich J. Prevalence of occupational asthma and immunologic sensitization to psyllium among health personnel in chronic care hospitals. *Am Rev Respir Dis* 1990; 142: 1359–66.

17. Hargreave FE, Ramsdale EH, Pugsley SO. Occupational asthma without bronchial hyperresponsiveness. *Am Rev Respir Dis* 1984; 130: 513–5.

18. Epstein SW, Fletcher CM, Oppenheimer EA. Daily peak flow measurements in the assessment of steroid therapy for airway obstruction. *BMJ* 1969; 1: 223–5.

19. Turner-Warwick M. On observing patterns of airflow obstruction in chronic asthma. *Br J Dis Chest* 1977; 71: 73–86.

20. Burge PS, O'Brien IM, Harries MG. Peak flow rate records in the diagnosis of occupational asthma due to colophony. *Thorax* 1979; 34: 308–16.

21. Côté J, Kennedy S, Chan-Yeung M. Sensitivity and specificity of PC 20 and peak expiratory flow rate in cedar asthma. *J Allergy Clin Immunol* 1990; 85: 592–8.

22. Perrin B, Lagier F, L'Archevêque J, Cartier A, Boulet LP, Côté J, Malo JL. Occupational asthma: validity of monitoring of peak expiratory flow rates and non-allergic bronchial responsiveness as compared to specific inhalation challenge. *Eur Respir J* 1992; 5: 40–48.

23. ✪ Moscato G, Godnic-Cvar J, Maestrelli P, Malo JL, Burge PS, Coifman R. Statement on self-monitoring of peak expiratory flows in the investigation of occupational asthma. *J Allergy Clin Immunol* 1995; 96: 295–301.

24. Malo JL, Trudeau C, Ghezzo H, L'Archevêque J, Cartier A. Do subjects investigated for occupational asthma through serial PEF measurements falsify their results? *J Allergy Clin Immunol* 1995; 96: 601–607.

25. Leroyer C, Perfetti L, Trudeau C, L'Archevêque J, Chan-Yeung M, Malo JL. Comparison of serial monitoring of peak expiratory flow and FEV$_1$ in the diagnosis of occupational asthma. *Am J Respir Crit Care Med* 1998; 158: 827–32.

26. Gannon PFG, Newton DT, Belcher J, Pantin CFA, Burge PS. Development of OASYS-2: a system for the analysis of serial measurement of peak expiratory flow in workers with suspected occupational asthma. *Thorax* 1996; 51: 484–9.

27. Pepys J, Hutchcroft BJ. Bronchial provocation tests in etiologic diagnosis and analysis of asthma. *Am Rev Respir Dis* 1975; 112: 829–59.

28. ✪ Vandenplas O, Malo JL. Inhalation challenges with agents causing occupational asthma. *Eur Respir J* 1997; 10: 2612–29.

29. Perrin B, Cartier A, Ghezzo H *et al*. Reassessment of the temporal patterns of bronchial obstruction after exposure to occupational sensitizing agents. *J Allergy Clin Immunol* 1991; 87: 630–9.

30. Malo JL. Occupational asthma. In: Hirsch A, Goldberg M, Martin JP, Masse M (eds). *Prevention of Respiratory Diseases*. Lung Biology in Health and Disease Series, vol 68. New York: Marcel Dekker, 1993: 117–31.

31. Malo JL, Ghezzo H, D'Aquino C, L'Archevêque J, Cartier A, Chan-Yeung M. Natural history of occupational asthma: relevance of type of agent and other factors in the rate of development of symptoms in affected subjects. *J Allergy Clin Immunol* 1992; 90: 937–44.

32. Côté J, Kennedy S, Chan-Yeung M. Outcome of patients with cedar asthma with continuous exposure. *Am Rev Respir Dis* 1990; 141: 373–6.

33. Malo JL, Cartier A, Côté J *et al*. Influence of inhaled steroids on the recovery of occupational asthma after cessation of exposure: an 18-month double-blind cross-over study. *Am J Crit Care Respir Med* 1996; 153: 953–60.

34. Ameille J, Pairon JC, Bayeux MC *et al*. Consequences of occupational asthma on employment and financial status: a follow-up study. *Eur Respir J* 1997: 10: 55–8.

35. Malo JL, Cartier A, Ghezzo H, Lafrance M, McCants M, Lehrer SB. Patterns of improvement of spirometry, bronchial hyperresponsiveness, and specific IgE antibody levels after cessation of exposure in occupational asthma caused by snow-crab processing. *Am Rev Respir Dis* 1988; 138: 807–12.

36. Brooks SM, Weiss MA, Bernstein IL. Reactive airways dysfunction syndrome (RADS). Persistent asthma syndrome after high level irritant exposures. *Chest* 1985; 88: 376–84.

37. Kennedy SM, Enarson DA, Janssen RG, Chan-Yeung M. Lung health consequences of reported accidental chlorine gas exposures among pulpmill workers. *Am Rev Respir Dis* 1991; 143: 74–9.

38. Kern DG. Outbreak of the reactive airways dysfunction syndrome after a spill of glacial acetic acid. *Am Rev Respir Dis* 1991; 144: 1058–64.

39. Bhérer L, Cushman R, Courteau JP *et al.* Survey of construction workers repeatedly exposed to chlorine over a three to six month period in a pulpmill: II. Follow up of affected workers by questionnaire, spirometry and assessment of bronchial responsiveness 18 to 24 months after exposure. *Occup Environ Med* 1994; 51: 225–8.

40. Leroyer C, Malo JL, Infante-Rivard C, Dufour JG, Gautrin D. Changes in airway function and bronchial responsiveness after acute occupational exposure to chlorine leading to treatment in a first-aid unit. *Occup Med* 1998; 55: 356–9.

Chapter 34

Specific Problems: Asthma Induced by Aspirin and Other Non-Steroidal Anti-Inflammatory Drugs

Barbro Dahlén, Olle Zetterström and Sven-Erik Dahlén

INTRODUCTION

Aspirin (acetylsalicylic acid) was introduced with considerable success for the treatment of fever and inflammatory disorders in 1899, but a few years later severe intolerance reactions, including life-threatening asthma, were reported among subjects taking therapeutic doses of aspirin.[1–3] Aspirin and other non-steroidal anti-inflammatory drugs (NSAIDs) are today widely used for a number of different indications, from alleviation of common ailments to prevention of cardiovascular fatalities. Therefore, it is important for every physician to be aware of the syndrome of aspirin intolerance. In particular, it is unacceptable that deaths are reported every year to the drug regulatory authorities around the world because of failure to recognize that most NSAIDs may trigger adverse reactions in aspirin-intolerant asthmatic subjects.

CLINICAL MANIFESTATIONS

A typical intolerance reaction occurs within 30 minutes to 2 hours after intake of an NSAID. Ocular injection, rhinorrhoea and nasal congestion is very common. There may be a heat rash, increased perspiration and flushing on the chest and face. The symptoms from the lower respiratory tract include dry cough and feeling of tightness in the chest. Although auscultation may reveal relatively few rhonchi, the pulmonary function test will generally demonstrate a severe airway obstruction. In addition to the symptoms from the eyes, nose and lungs, the patients often experience fatigue and a general feeling of malaise. The reaction may progress to shock, unconsciousness and respiratory arrest. Sometimes gastrointestinal symptoms including vomiting and diarrhoea occur, and occasionally urticaria

or angio-oedema develops. Subjects with chronic urticaria may in addition display isolated intolerance reactions in the skin to ingested NSAIDs, whereas asthmatic subjects preferentially display the more severe respiratory manifestations. However, there is no given sequence of events during an episode of NSAID intolerance; the described symptoms may occur in isolation or combination, and in any order.[4–6]

The first episode of an NSAID intolerance reaction in the airways is often unexpected. However, there is a strong preponderance of rhinitis with recurrent nasal polyposis among those subjects who develop NSAID intolerance, providing the clinical triad Samter's triad of nasal polyposis, asthma and aspirin intolerance.[4,7] Eosinophilia in blood and tissues is often prominent,[8–11] but it can obviously not be considered a specific sign. NSAID intolerance is rare among children, more common among women and usually presents during the second or third decade of life. Typically, intermittent watery rhinitis develops, eventually followed by chronic nasal congestion, recurrent nasal polyposis, sinusitis, loss of ability to smell and finally the appearance of asthma and aspirin intolerance. This course of events may progress during a couple of months or take one or two decades. However, there are also cases where the first intolerance reaction appears to precipitate the onset of asthma and rhinitis. As a further example of the unpredictable nature of this syndrome, there are several patients with an identical clinical picture who apparently never develop aspirin intolerance and, at the opposite end of the spectrum, a few rare patients whose asthma is relieved by aspirin.[12–14]

The prevalence of atopy in aspirin-intolerant patients has been reported to be low[4,15,16] and there are no strong indications of family aggregations of aspirin intoler ance,[17] which together with the observation that aspiri intolerance often develops after viral infections[6,18] suggests an acquired disease. Due to the variable clinical picture and the difficulties relating to diagnosis of aspirin intolerance, estimations of the prevalence of aspirin intolerance very considerably, but most authors have concluded that around 10% of adult asthmatic subjects may belong to this group (reviewed in Ref. 6). The information on the epidemiology and natural course of aspirin-induced asthma is incomplete. It is generally agreed that NSAID-intolerant asthmatic subjects display a particularly severe variety of asthma, which often requires chronic treatment with high doses of oral or inhaled glucocorticosteroids (GCS).[5,6,8] However, the association between aspirin intolerance and asthma may not be causal, since desensitization to aspirin appears to have little influence on the clinical course of the airway disease[19] and chronic asthma persists despite careful avoidance of NSAIDs.[4]

DIAGNOSIS

Although NSAID intolerance may be the first presenting symptom, an asthmatic subject with chronic rhinitis and/or recurrent nasal polyposis should always be considered as an individual at risk for development of aspirin intolerance. In the absence of a predictable *in vitro* test, the diagnosis depends upon provocations to demonstrate intolerance towards aspirin and other NSAIDs. Skin tests with aspirin have not been successful[3,15] and may in fact be dangerous if accidental systemic injection occurs.[20] Nasal provocations with lysine-aspirin (a more water-soluble derivative of aspirin) have rather low sensitivity,[21,22] but would be of interest to develop further as an initial screening test. Oral provocations with aspirin have been used for many years to diagnose aspirin-induced asthma,[6,23,24] although the procedure is fairly time-consuming and always associated with significant risk of provoking severe bronchial and/or systemic reactions. In the most cautious protocols, the patient is challenged with increasing doses of aspirin over the course of 3 days,[6] but it has been concluded that oral challenges generally are unsuitable for routine clinical practice. Bronchial provocation with lysine-aspirin was introduced by Bianco *et al.*[25] in 1977 and has been documented to be simpler to perform, less time-consuming and considerably safer than the oral challenge test,[26] presumably because the inhalation challenge produces a reaction limited to the airways.[26] By inhalation of

increasing doses of lysine-aspirin, the provocative dose for a 20% decrease (PD_{20}) in forced expiratory volume is 1 s (FEV_1) can be determined in protocols similar to those used for conventional bronchial reactivity testing with histamine or methacholine,[26–28] and the repeatability of the challenge is excellent.[28] Although the reaction to inhaled lysine-aspirin in intolerant individuals in some respects resembles the early reaction to inhaled allergen in atopic asthmatic subjects, it should be noted that the response to aspirin is not followed by a late phase reaction.[27,28]

After a positive provocation response to inhaled or oral aspirin, a state of refractoriness to further doses of aspirin or other NSAIDs follows.[7,25,29,30] The refractory period lasts between 2 and 5 days. As a corollary, desensitization as well as cross-desensitization may be retained provided aspirin is ingested with a maximum interval of 48 hours. Complete sensitivity to aspirin and other NSAIDs reappears about 7 days after the last exposure to these drugs.[29] Therefore, repeated challenges for diagnosis or research purpose should be separated by at least 1 week. Another pitfall that may produce false-negative aspirin provocations is that high doses of GCS may mask aspirin intolerance.[31]

To summarize the diagnostic tests, the inhalation challenge test with lysine-aspirin should be the preferred method to demonstrate aspirin intolerance in the airways. Oral challenge with aspirin should only be used if negative inhalation challenges have been performed but suspicion of extra-pulmonary NSAID intolerance remains. Due to the ability of aspirin intolerance to wax and wane,[5,32,33] it should be remembered that a negative history or challenge test in an asthmatic subject with nasal polyposis never excludes the possibility that the patient in the future will acquire intolerance to NSAIDs.

PATHOPHYSIOLOGY

The mechanisms that create the state of aspirin intolerance in certain individuals remain completely unknown. It is well documented (reviewed in Refs 6 and 24) that the common denominator among the NSAIDs that precipitate intolerance reactions is their ability to inhibit the cyclooxygenase enzyme that catalyses the initial step in the formation of prostaglandins (PG) and thromboxane from arachidonic acid (Fig. 34.1). There is no evidence of immunological hypersensitivity reactions towards this large family of structurally unrelated compounds,[15,16]

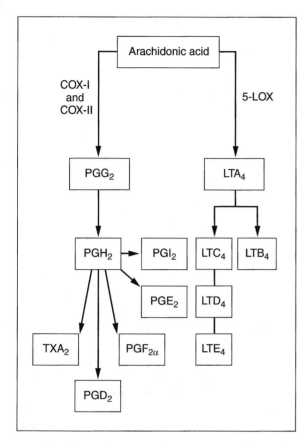

FIGURE 34.1: Schematic drawing of the cyclooxygenase (COX) and 5-lipoxygenase (5-LOX) pathways for cellular oxygenation of arachidonic acid. PG, prostaglandin; LT, leukotriene. COX-I and COX-II denote the constitutive and inducible COX-isoenzymes, respectively. They catalyse the same reactions, but differ in structure and with respect to kinetics and susceptibility to pharmacologic antagonism (see text and Refs 34–36). However, the currently available NSAIDs inhibit both isoenzymes with little practical difference in affinity.

and other alternative hypotheses[7–9] all suffer from a lack of critical experimental support. A great number of findings have firmly established the cyclooxygenase theory originally proposed by Szczeklik et al.[40] Thus, there is a positive correlation between the potency of NSAIDs to induce airway obstruction and the potency of the same drugs as cyclooxygenase inhibitors in vitro.[40,41] In further support of the cyclooxygenase theory, NSAIDs with cyclooxygenase-inhibiting properties always elicit airway obstruction in intolerant subjects, whereas those NSAIDs

that do not inhibit cyclooxygenases in therapeutic doses usually are well-tolerated.[5,42,43] It was recently shown that the plasma level of acetylsalicylic acid during the development of aspirin-induced bronchoconstriction is in the concentration range known to be required for in vivo inhibition of the cyclooxygenase enzyme.[44] Moreover, after aspirin desensitization, cross-tolerance to other cyclooxygenase inhibitors is also achieved.[29,45]

Although it is clear that cyclooxygenase inhibition is central in the pathogenesis of NSAID intolerance, it is not known which cells are activated during the intolerance reaction to aspirin. In vitro investigations have generally failed to show specific and reproducible metabolic or functional abnormalities in any single population of the great number of different cells that have been collected from aspirin-intolerant asthmatic subjects. In vivo, it has been shown that aspirin challenge is associated with release of histamine,[46] leukotrienes[22,46–50] and, at least during systemic reactions to aspirin, tryptase,[51] together suggesting that the mast cell may be a key effector cell. In this context, it is of considerable interest that a marked overproduction of the mast cell metabolite PGD$_2$, increased histamine excretion and elevated serum tryptase levels were reported in a subset of patients with systemic mastocytosis who had attacks provoked by low doses of aspirin and aspirin-like drugs.[52] The almost anaphylactic nature of the intolerance reactions makes it natural to assume that the mast cell is involved, but its obligatory role has yet to be proved conclusively.

Despite the acknowledged uncertainties concerning several critical steps and the role of different cells in the intolerance reactions to NSAIDs, a number of recent investigations have firmly established that leukotrienes are important mediators of the airway obstruction, and perhaps leukotrienes mediate also some of the extra-pulmonary manifestations. First, the cysteinyl-leukotrines (LTC$_4$, LTD$_4$ and LTE$_4$), previously known as the presumed mediator of asthma and hypersensitivity, slow reacting substance of anaphylaxis (SRS-A) (for reviews of biological activities and biochemistry see Refs 53–55), are potent inducers of bronchconstruction in aspirin-intolerant asthmatic subjects.[56] In fact, there are interesting observations suggesting that aspirin-intolerant asthmatic subjects display a specific and unique airway hyperresponsiveness to LTE$_4$ when compared with other asthmatic subjects.[57] Second, aspirin provocation is associated with increased excretion of cysteinly-leukotrienes in nasal washings,[22,46] in the urine[47–49] and in bronchoalveolar lavages (BAL).[58] The third, and most definite piece of evidence, is provided by recent investigations which document that pre-treatment with anti-leukotriene drugs provide partial or complete prevention[28,59,60] of the airway obstruction induced by aspirin challenge. Since the leukotriene biosynthesis inhibitor zileuton also attenuated nasal, gastrointestinal and dermal symptoms induced by oral challenge with aspirin,[60] it is possible that leukotrienes also mediate significant components of the extra-pulmonary symptoms in the aspirin-intolerance syndrome.

There are also indications that leukotrienes may be important regulators of baseline bronchomotor tone in aspirin-intolerant asthmatic subjects. First, several independent observations have documented that aspirin-intolerant asthmatic subjects have an over-production of cysteinyl-leukotrienes, expressed as an increased basal (i.e. prior to aspirin challenge) excretion of urinary LTE_4 compared with other asthmatic subjects.[47,48,61] It is known that the basal levels of urinary LTE_4 generally overlap considerably between asthmatic and non-asthmatic subjects,[62] whereas aspirin-sensitive asthmatic subjects have been reported to have basal values of urinary LTE_4 that are significantly (two to five times) higher than those of other asthmatic subjects. Second, the leukotriene receptor antagonist MK-0679 was found to produce a long-lasting baseline bronchodilation in a group of aspirin-intolerant asthmatic subjects[63] (Fig. 34.2). The response varied among the studied individuals, but interestingly correlated directly both with general disease severity and the sensitivity to aspirin in the subjects.

The contribution of leukotrienes is supported by evidence that in a placebo-controlled clinical trial, treatment with zileuton improved asthma management when added to usual asthma therapy in patients with sensitivity to aspirin.[64]

Lastly, studies have demonstrated over-expression of the enzyme leukotriene C_4 synthase, necessary for cysteinyl leukotriene production, in airway biopsies from aspirin-intolerant asthmatics.[65]

The mechanism by which aspirin and other cyclo-oxygenase inhibitors trigger enhanced dependence upon the leukotriene system remains elusive. It has been speculated that arrested formation of prostaglandin endo-peroxides after inhibition of the cyclooxygenase enzyme by NSAIDs would result in shunting of the common substrate arachidonic acid into the

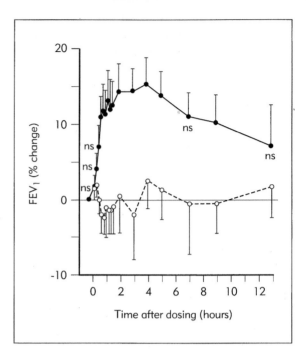

FIGURE 34.2: Basal pulmonary function was followed as FEV_1 in eight ASA-sensitive asthmatic subjects for 12 hours after ingestion of placebo (○) or the leukotriene receptor antagonist MK-0679 (825 μg) (●) on two different occasions in a double-blind cross-over design. Each point represents mean ± SE in the group. The mean maximal improvement in FEV_1 was 18 ± 3.5%, calculated from the peak effect in each individual. For comparison, inhalation of a nebulized solution of salbutamol (2500 μg) produced a 22.8 ± 4.3% improvement of FEV_1 in this group of subjects. Data are expressed as percentage change from baseline FEV_1 (mean of first two recordings upon arrival to clinic) during each study day. The difference between placebo and MK-0679 is significant (P ≤ 0.05) at all time points except when indicated (ns, not significant, P > 0.05). (Modified from Dahlén B, Margolskee DJ, Zetterström O, et al. Effect of the leukotriene-antagonist MK-0679 on baseline pulmonary function in aspirin-sensitive asthmatics. *Tharax* 1993; 48: 1205–16.

leukotriene pathway (Fig. 34.1), but there is no experimental proof of this "shunting hypothesis" and there are theoretical arguments against it. Further, the "shunting hypothesis" does not seem to explain why aspirin-tolerant asthmatic subjects fail to produce more leukotrienes after inhibition of the cyclooxygenase system. One, perhaps more likely, hypothesis assumes that aspirin-intolerant asthmatic subjects are particularly dependent upon one or several continuously produced cyclooxygenase products, which tonically act to inhibit release of mediators from different inflammatory cells. Incidentally, the concentration of PGE_2, which has several anti-inflammatory effects including *in vivo* inhibition of mast cell mediator release,[66] was recently found to be elevated in the airways of aspirin-intolerant asthmatic subjects.[58] The "PGE_2-hypothesis" would thus explain the almost anaphylactic reaction to cyclooxygenase inhibitors as a consequence of removal of a brake (PGE_2) that certain individuals (aspirin intolerant) need to control their mediator-producing cells. One could speculate that the induction of the aspirin-intolerant state through viral infections or other factors has altered some key regulatory cell resulting in enhanced production of PGE_2 or increased expression of its receptors. Inhalation of PGE_2 has recently been found to inhibit airway obstruction induced by allergen[67] and exercise,[68] suggesting that the general function of PGE_2 in the airways is to act as a modulator that protects against bronchoconstriction and inflammatory mediators. For unknown reasons, NSAID-intolerant subjects may be especially dependent upon this protection.

Finally in this context, it has recently been discovered[34–36] that there exist at least two cyclooxygenase (COX) isoenzymes, one constitutive (COX-I) that may mediate the physiological functions of the prostaglandins and one (COX-II) that is induced at inflammatory sites and may be the desired target of anti-inflammatory drugs. The present generation of NSAIDs are generally unselective and inhibit both isoenzymes. The findings have created the hypothesis that NSAIDs which are selective for COX-II may have lesser side-effects by preserving gastrointestinal mucosal integrity, platelet and renal function, to mention some of the tissues associated with severe side-effects of NSAIDs in individuals without aspirin idiosyncrasy. It will be of great interest to find out which isoenzyme is involved in aspirin intolerance.

CURRENT TREATMENT STRATEGIES

Treatment of the asthma in NSAID-intolerant individuals follows the general guidelines for treatment of asthma outlined in other chapters. The nasal affliction and in particular the recurrent nasal polyposis requires continuous treatment with topical GCS, and frequently also repeated surgical interventions.

Asthmatic subjects with a history of an episode of unequivocal NSAID intolerance or a previous positive aspirin-provocation test should for the future refrain from using NSAIDs (Table 34.1). It has previously been

Table 34.1: Effects of some NSAIDs in aspirin-intolerant subjects.

Precipitate intolerance reactions	Well-tolerated
Salicylates	Sodium salicylate[a]
Aspirin (acetylsalicylic acid)	Choline salicylate
Diflunisal	Choline magnesium
Salsalate (salicylsalicylic acid)	trisalicylate[a]
Polycyclic acids	Salicylamide
Acetic acids	Dextropropoxyphene
Indomethacin	Benzydamine
Sulindac	Chloroquine
Diclofenac	Paracetamol
Tolmetin	(acetaminophen)[b]
Aryl aliphatic acids	
Naproxen	
Fenoprofen	
Ibuprofen	
Ketoprofen	
Tiaprofenic acid	
Flurbiprofen	
Enolic acids	
Piroxicam	
Tenoxicam	
Fenemates	
Mefenamic acid	
Flufenamic acid	
Cyclofenamic acid	
Pyrazolones	
Aminopyrine	
Noramidopyrine	
Sulphinpyrazone	
Phenylbutazone	
Azapropazone	
Phenazone	
Ketorolac	

[a] Well tolerated in controlled studies, but two cases of bronchoconstriction after sodium salicylate[69,70] and one after choline magnesium trisalicylate[71] have been reported.
[b] Adverse reactions occur in no more than 5% of aspirin-sensitive asthmatic subjects.[5,72] It is recommended that when beginning therapy, half a tablet should be given under observation for 2–3 hours.

457

suggested that there is an association between hypersensitivity to tartrazine and related dyes among aspirin-intolerant subjects, but a large multicentre study showed that this was not the case.[73] Hydrocortisone and in particular its succinate salts have also been reported to elicit adverse reactions among individual aspirin-intolerant asthmatic subjects,[74–77] but a general cross-reactivity between hydrocortisone and NSAIDs could not be confirmed in a recent large population study.[78] Very recently, adverse reactions to biphosphonate were reported among a few aspirin-intolerant asthmatic subjects,[79] but the general importance of this finding remains to be evaluated. As evident from Table 34.1, when NSAID-intolerant asthmatic subjects need to instil anti-pyretic or analgesic treatment for milder afflictions, paracetamol (acetaminophen), dextropropoxyphene or salicylic acid may be used. (Interestingly, salicylic acid, the immediate metabolite of acetylsalicylic acid is a weak cyclooxygenase inhibitor[80] and is tolerated by NSAID-intolerant subjects.) It has been reported[5,71] that some 5% of NSAID-intolerant asthmatic subjects also react to paracetamol (acetaminophen), but this appears to be a question of dosing, and the likelihood of an intolerance reaction appears insignificant when the dose is less than 1000 mg. In ambiguous cases, it may be advised to give the first doses of paracetamol (acetaminophen) under supervision and to start with a lower than usual dose, e.g. 250 mg. In cases of more severe inflammation, e.g. osteoarthritis or rheumatic diseases, desensitization with aspirin is an alternative that will allow for use of regular NSAIDs. However, this should be performed at specialist centres with considerable experience, and the selected individuals must understand that only a few days of withdrawal of the NSAID may result in a dangerous intolerance reaction if the regular dose is taken again. In severe GCS-resistant inflammation, other alternatives may be treatment with chloroquine, cyclosporin A or methotrexate.

CONCLUSIONS AND PROSPECTS FOR THE FUTURE

By more widespread use of the lysine-aspirin inhalation test, it is hoped that more definite information about the prevalence and clinical course of NSAID intolerance will be obtained in the future. The discovery of cyclooxygenase isoenzymes has the potential to provide further insight into the molecular defects behind the abnormal reaction to NSAIDs in aspirin-intolerant asthmatic subjects and, on a speculative note, perhaps even produce a group of isoenzyme-selective NSAIDs that are tolerated among these patients. The recent indications that cysteinyl-leukotrienes are important and perhaps even the predominant mediators both of spontaneous and aspirin-induced airway obstruction in aspirin-intolerant asthmatic subjects has both diagnostic and therapeutic implications. First, the findings of elevated urinary LTE_4 among NSAID-intolerant asthmatic subjects should be evaluated as a marker to use when screening for NSAID intolerance. Second, since aspirin-sensitive asthmatic subjects as discussed above may display both an over-production and a hyper-responsiveness to cysteinyl-leukotrienes compared with other asthmatic subjects, one could speculate that this subgroup of asthmatic subjects should respond espe-

KEY POINTS

1 An asthmatic with chronic rhinits and/or nasal polyposis should always be suspected of being of risk of intolerance to aspirin and other non-steroidal anti-inflammatory drugs.

2 Inhibition of the cyclooxygenase enzyme is the common feature, of all drugs that elicit this syndrome and these patients must thus always refrain from using common non-steroidal anti-inflammatory drugs.

3 For treatment of pain acetaminophen (paracetamol) or dexfropropoxyphen, or these in combination should be used.

4 Inhalation challenge with lysine-aspirin, or other non-steroidal anti-inflammatory drugs is the preferred method of confirming a diagnosis of aspirin intolerance. Oral challenge with aspirin is always associated with a risk of severe reactions.

5 Apart from avoidance of NSAIDs, the treatment of subjects with aspirin-induced asthma currently follows the same principles as in aspirin tolerant subjects.

cially well to recently developed anti-leukotriene drugs. It is therefore possible that anti-leukotrienes may provide a new approach in the treatment of aspirin-induced asthma. Irrespective of the outcome of the new exciting basic discoveries relating to NSAID intolerance, it remains important for the practising physician to always remember the clinical triad of rhinitis with nasal polyposis, asthma and aspirin intolerance, and the fact that virtually all NSAIDs produce the sometimes fatal intolerance reactions in the predisposed individuals.

ACKNOWLEDGEMENTS

Barbro Dahlén is supported by grants from the Swedish Heart Lung Foundation and the Swedish Association Against Asthma and Allergy, and Sven-Erik Dahlén's research position is funded by the Swedish Heart Lung Foundation. The research projects from the authors' laboratories have been supported by grants from the Swedish Medical Research Council (project 14X-09071), the Swedish Association Against Chest and Heart Diseases, the Swedish Association Against Asthma and Allergy (RmA), the Swedish National Board for Laboratory Animals (CFN), the Scientific Council of the Swedish Association Against Use of Experimental Animals in Research, the Institute of Environmental Medicine, the Swedish Environment Protection Board (5324069–3), the Swedish Public Health Institute, and Karolinska Institutet.

REFERENCES

1. Hirschberg VGS. Mitteilung über ein Fall von Nebenwirkung des Aspirin. *Deutsch Med Wochenschr* 1902; 28: 416.

2. Gilbert GB. Unusual idiosyncrasy to aspirin. *JAMA* 1911; 56: 1262.

3. Cooke RA. Allergy in drug idiosyncrasy. *JAMA* 1919; 73: 759–60.

4. Samter M, Beers RF. Intolerance to aspirin. Clinical studies and considerations of its pathogenesis. *Ann Intern Med* 1968; 68: 975–83.

5. Szczeklik A, Gryglewski RJ, Czerniawska-Mysik G. Clinical patterns of hyper-sensitivity to nonsteroidal anti-inflammatory drugs and their pathogenesis. *J Allergy Clin Immunol* 1977; 60: 276–84.

6. ✪ Stevenson DD, Simon RA. Aspirin sensitivity: Respiratory and cutaneous manifestations. In: Middleton E Jr, Reed CE, Ellis EF, Adkinson NF, Yunginger JW (eds) *Allergy, Principles and Practice*. St Louis: CV Mosby, 1988: 1537–54.

7. Widal F, Abrami P, Lermoyez J. Anaphylaxie et idiosyncrasie. *Presse Med* 1922; 30: 189–93.

8. Friedlaender S, Feinberg S. Aspirin allergy: Its relationship to chronic intractable asthma. *Ann Intern Med* 1947; 26: 734–40.

9. Salén EB, Arner B. Some views on the aspirin-hypersensitive allergy group. *Acta Allergol* 1948; 1: 47–84.

10. Godard P, Chaitreull J, Damon M *et al.* Functional assessment of alveolar macrophages: comparison of cells from asthmatics and normal subjects. *J Allergy Clin Immunol* 1982; 70: 88–93.

11. Lumry WR, Curd JG, Zeiger RS, Pleskow WW, Stevenson DD. Aspirin-sensitive rhinosinusitis: the clinical syndrome and effects of aspirin administration. *J Allergy Clin Immunol* 1983; 71: 580–7.

12. Cooke RA, *Allergy in Theory and Practice*. Philadelphia: W.B. Saunders, 1947.

13. Kordansky D, Adkinson F, Norman PS, Rosenthal RR. Asthma improved by non steroidal anti-inflammatory drugs. *Ann Intern Med* 1978; 88: 508–11.

14. Szczeklik A, Nizankowska E. Asthma improved by aspirin-like drugs. *Br J Dis Chest* 1983; 77: 153–8.

15. Schlumberger HD, Löbbecke EA, Kallós P. Acetylsalicylic acid intolerance. Lack of N-acetylsalicylic acid specific, skin-sensitizing antibodies in the serum of intolerant individuals. *Acta Med Scand* 1974; 196: 451–8.

16. Delaney JC, Kay AB. Complement components and IgE in patients with asthma and aspirin idiosyncrasy. *Thorax* 1976; 31: 425–7.

17. Lockey RF, Rucknagel DL, Vanselow NA. Familial occurrence of asthma, nasal polyps and aspirin intolerance. *Ann Intern Med* 1973; 78: 57–63.

18. Szczeklik A. Aspirin-induced asthma as a viral disease. *Clin Allergy* 1988; 18: 15–20.

19. Stevenson DD, Pleskow WW, Simon RA. Aspirin-sensitive rhinosinusitis asthma: a double blind crossover study of treatment with aspirin. *J Allergy Clin Immunol* 1984; 73: 500–7.

20. Storm van Leeuwen W. Pathognomonische Bedeutung der Ueber-empfindlichkeit gegen Aspirin bei Asthmatikern. *Münch Med Wschr* 1928; 37: 1588–90.

21. Patriarca G, Nucera E, DiRienzo V, Schiavino D, Pellegrino S, Fais G. Nasal provocation test with lysine acetylsalicylate in aspirin-sensitive patients. *Ann Allergy* 1991; 67: 60–2.

22. Picado C, Ramis I, Rosellò J et al. Release of peptide leukotriene into nasal secretions after local instillation of aspirin in aspirin-sensitive asthmatic patients. *Am Rev Respir Dis* 1992; 145: 65–9.

23. Rosenhall L. Evaluation of intolerance to analgesics, preservatives and food colorants with challenge tests. *Eur Respir Dis* 1982; 63: 410–9.

24. ✪ Szczeklik A, Virchow C, Schmitz-Schumann M. Pathophysiology and pharmacology of aspirin-induced asthma. In: Page CP, Barnes PJ (eds). *Handbook of Experimental Pharmacology: Pharmacology of Asthma*. Berlin: Springer-Verlog, 1991: 291–314.

25. Bianco S, Robuschi M, Petrini G. Aspirin-induced tolerance in aspirin-asthma detected by a new challenge test. *IRCS J Med Sci* 1977; 5: 129.

26. ✪ Dahlén B, Zetterström O. Comparison of bronchial and per oral provocation with aspirin in aspirin-sensitive asthmatics. *Eur Respir J* 1990; 3: 527–34.

27. ✪ Phillips GD, Foord R, Holgate ST. Inhaled lysine-aspirin as a bronchoprovocation procedure in aspirin-sensitive asthma: Its repeatability, absence of late-phase reaction, and the role of histamine. *J Allergy Clin Immunol* 1989; 84: 232–41.

28. ✪ Dahlén B, Kumlin M, Margolskee DJ et al. The leukotriene-receptor antagonist MK-0679 blocks airway obstruction induced by inhaled lysine-aspirin in aspirin-sensitive asthmatics. *Eur Respir J* 1993; 6: 1018–26.

29. Pleskow WW, Stevenson DD, Mathison DA, Simon RA, Schatz M, Zeiger RS. Aspirin desensitization in aspirin-sensitive asthmatic patients: clinical manifestations and characterization of the refractory period. *J Allergy Clin Immunol* 1982; 69: 11–9.

30. Zeiss CR, Lockey RF. Refractory period to aspirin in a patient with aspirin-induced asthma. *J Allergy Clin Immunol* 1976; 57: 440–8.

31. Nizankowska E, Szczeklik A. Glucocorticosteroids attenuate aspirin-precipitated adverse reactions in aspirin-intolerant patients with asthma. *Ann Allergy* 1989; 63: 159–62.

32. Pleskow WW, Stevenson DD, Mathison DA, Simon RA, Schatz M, Zeiger RS. Aspirin-sensitive rhinosinusitis/asthma: spectrum of adverse reactions to aspirin. *J Allergy Clin Immunol* 1983; 71: 574–9.

33. Prieto L, Palop J, Castro J, Basomba A. Aspirin-induced asthma in a patient with asthma previously improved by non-steroidal anti-inflammatory drugs. *Clin Allergy* 1988; 18: 629–32.

34. Meade EA, Smith WL, DeWitt DL. Differential inhibition of prostaglandin endoperoxide synthase (cyclooxygenase) isoenzymes by aspirin and other non-steroidal anti-inflammatory drugs. *J Biol Chem* 1993; 268: 6610–4.

35. Masferrer JL, Seibert K, Zweifel B, Needleman P. Endogenous glucocorticoids regulate an inducible cyclooxygenase enzyme. *Proc Natl Acad Sci USA* 1992; 89: 3917–21.

36. O'Neill GP, Ford-Hutchinson AW. Expression of mRNA for cyclooxygenase-I and cyclooxygenase-2 in human tissues. *FEBS Lett* 1993; 330: 156–60.

37. Capron A, Ameisen JC, Joseph M, Auriault C, Tonnel AB, Caen J. New function for platelets and their pathological implications. *Int Arch Allergy Appl Immunol* 1985; 77: 107–14.

38. Pearson DJ, Suarez-Mendez VJ. Abnormal platelet hydrogen peroxide metabolism in aspirin hypersensitivity. *Clin Exp Allergy* 1990; 20: 157–63.

39. Williams WR, Pawlowicz A, Davies BH. *In vitro* tests for the diagnosis of aspirin-sensitive asthma. *J Allergy Clin Immunol* 1990; 86: 445–51.

40. Szczeklik A, Gryglewski RJ, Czerniawska-Mysik G. Relationship of inhibition of prostaglandin biosynthesis by analgesics to asthma attacks in aspirin-sensitive patients. *BMJ* 1975; 1: 67–9.

41. Stevenson DD, Hougham AJ, Schrank PJ, Goldlust MB, Wilson RR. Salsalate cross-sensitivity in aspirin-sensitive patients with asthma. *J Allergy Clin Immunol* 1990; 86: 749–58.

42. Bianco S, Petrigni G, Felisi E, Robuschi M. Tolerance of guaiacolic ester of acetylsalicylic acid by patients with aspirin-asthma. *Scand J Respir Dis* 1979; 60: 350–4.

43. Szczeklik A, Nizankowska E, Dworski R. Choline magnesium trisalicylate in patients with aspirin-induced asthma. *Eur Respir J* 1990; 3: 535–9.

44. Dahlén B, Boréus LO, Anderson P, Andersson R. Plasma acetylsalicylic acid and salicylic acid levels during aspirin provocation in aspirin-sensitive subjects. *Allergy* 1994; 49: 43–9.

45. Kowalski ML, Grzelewska-Rzymowska I, Rozniecki J, Szmidt M. Aspirin tolerance induced in aspirin-sensitive asthmatics. *Allergy* 1984; 39: 171–8.

46. Ferreri NR, Howland WC, Stevenson DD, Spiegelberg HL. Release of leukotrienes, prostaglandins, and histamine into nasal secretions of aspirin-sensitive asthmatics during reaction to aspirin. *Am Rev Respir Dis* 1988; 137: 847–54.

47. Christie PE, Tagari P, Ford-Hutchinson AW *et al.* Urinary leukotriene E_4 concentrations increase after ASA challenge in ASA-sensitive asthmatic subjects. *Am Rev Respir Dis* 1991; 143: 10s5–9.

48. ✪ Kumlin M, Dahlén B, Björck T, Zetterström O, Granström E, Dahlén S-E. Urinary excretion of leukotriene E_4 and 11-dehydro-thromboxane B_2 in response to bronchial provocations with allergen, aspirin, leukotriene D_4 and histamine in asthmatics. *Am Rev Respir Dis* 1992; 146: 96–103.

49. Knapp HR, Sladek K, FitzGerald GA. Increased excretion of leukotriene E_4 during aspirin-induced asthma. *J Lab Clin Med* 1992; 119: 48–51.

50. Sladek K, Szczeklik A. Cysteinyl leukotrienes overproduction and mast cell activation in aspirin-provoked bronchospams in asthma. *Eur Respir J* 1993; 6: 391–9.

51. Bosso JV, Schwartz LB, Stevenson DD. Tryptase and histamine release during aspirin-induced respiratory reactions. *J Allergy Clin Immunol* 1991; 88: 830–7.

52. Roberts LJ II, Sweetman BJ, Lewis RA, Austen KF, Oates JA. Increased production of prostaglandin D_2 in patients with systemic mastocytosis. *N Engl J Med* 1980; 303: 1400–4.

53. Samuelsson B, Dahlén S-E, Lindgren JÅ, Rouzer CA, Serhan CN. Leukotrienes and lipoxins: structures, biosynthesis, and biological effects. *Science* 1987; 237: 1171–6.

54. Lewis RA, Austen KF, Soberman RJ. Leukotrienes and other products of the 5-lipoxygenase pathway. Biochemistry and relation to pathobiology in human diseases. *N Engl J Med* 1990; 323: 645–55.

55. Dahlén S-E. Leukotrienes as mediators of airway obstruction and bronchial hyperresponsiveness. In: Page C, Gardiner PJ (eds). *Airway Hyperresponsiveness: Is it Really Important for Asthma?* Oxford: Blackwell Scientific Publications, 1993: 188–205.

56. Arm JP, O'Hickey SP, Spur BW, Lee TH. Airway responsiveness to histamine and leukotriene E_4 in subjects with ASA-induced asthma. *Am Rev Respir Dis* 1989; 140: 148–53.

57. Christie PE, Schmitz-Schumann M, Spur BW, Lee TH. Airway responsiveness to leukotriene C_4 (LTC_4), leukotriene E_4 (LTE_4) and histamine in aspirin-sensitive asthmatic subjects. *Eur Respir J* 1993; 6: 1468–73.

58. Sladek K, Dworski R, Soja J *et al.* Eicosanoids in broncheoalveolar lavage fluid of aspirin-intolerant patients with asthma after aspirin challenge. *Am J Respir Crit Care Med* 1994; 149: 940–6.

59. Christie PE, Smith CM, Lee TH. The potent and selective sulfidopeptide leukotriene antagonist, SK&F 104353, inhibits aspirin-induced asthma. *Am Rev Respir Dis* 1991; 144: 957–8.

60. ✪ Israel E, Fischer AR, Rosenberg MA *et al.* The pivotal role of 5-lipoxygenase products in the reaction

of aspirin-sensitive asthmatics to aspirin. *Am Rev Respir Dis* 1993; 148: 1447–51.

61. Smith CM, Hawksworth RJ, Thien FCK, Christie PE, Lee TH. Urinary leukotriene E$_4$ in bronchial asthma. *Eur Respir J* 1992; 5: 693–9.

62. Kumlin M, Stensvad F, Larsson L, Dahlén B, Dahlén S-E. Validation and application of a new simple strategy for measurements of urinary leukotriene E$_4$ in humans. *Clin Exp Allergy* 1995; 25: 467–79.

63. ✪ Dahlén B, Margolskee DJ, Zetterström O, Dahlén S-E. Effect of the leukotriene-antagonist MK-0679 on baseline pulmonary function in aspirin-sensitive asthmatics. *Thorax* 1993; 48: 1205–10.

64. Dahlén B, Nizankowska E, Szczeklik A *et al.* Benefits from adding the 5-lipoxygenase inhibitor zileuton to conventional therapy in aspirin-intolerant asthmatics. *Am J Respir Crit Care Med* 1998; 157: 1187–94.

65. Cowburn AS, Sladek K, Soja J *et al.* Overexpression of leukotriene C4 synthase in bronchial biopsies from patients with aspirin-intolerant asthma. *J Clin Invest* 1998; 101: 834–46.

66. Raud J, Dahlén SE, Sydbom A, Lindbom L, Hedqvist P. Enhancement of acute allergic inflammation by indomethacin is reversed by prostaglandin E2: Apparent correlation with in vivo modulation of mediator release. Proc Natl Acad Sci USA 1988; 85: 2315–9.

67. Pavord ID, Wong CS, Williams J, Tattersfield AE. Effect of inhaled prostaglandin E$_2$ on allergen-induced asthma. *Am Rev Respir Dis* 1993; 148: 87–90.

68. Melillo E, Wooley KL, Manning PJ, Watson RM, O'Byrne PM. Effect of inhaled prostaglandin E$_2$ on exercise-induced bronchoconstriction in asthmatic subjects. *Am J Respir Crit Care Med* 1994; 149: 1138–41.

69. Park HS, Lim YS, Suh JE, Rhu NS, Cho D III, Kim JW. Sodium salicylate sensitivity in an asthmatic patient with aspirin sensitivity. *J Korean Med Sci* 1991; 6: 113–7.

70. Schäufele A, Schmitz-Schumann M, Virchow JChr Jr, Menz G, Virchow Chr Sr. Eignet sich Natriumsalizylat (NaS) als Protektivum beim Analgetika-asthma-syndrom (AIA)? *Pneumologie* 1990; 44: 371–2.

71. Shudwin DS, Strub M, Golden RE, Frey CDO, Richmond GW, Luskin T. Sensitivity to non acetylated salicylates in a patient with asthma, nasal polyps and rheumatoid arthritis. *Ann Allergy* 1986; 57: 133–4.

72. Settipane RA, Stevenson DD. Cross sensitivity with acetaminophen in aspirin-sensitive subjects with asthma. *J Allergy Clin Immunol* 1989; 84: 26–33.

73. Virchow Ch, Szczeklik A, Bianco S *et al.* Intolerance to tartrazine in aspirin-induced asthma: results of a multicenter study. *Respiration* 1988; 53: 20–3.

74. Partridge MR, Gibson GJ. Adverse bronchial reactions to intravenous hydrocortisone in two aspirin sensitive patients. *BMJ* 1978; 1: 1521–2.

75. Dajani BM, Sliman NA, Shubair KS, Hamzeh YS. Bronchospasm caused by intravenous hydrocortisone sodium succinate (Solu-Cortef) in aspirin-sensitive asthmatics. *J Allergy Clin Immunol* 1981; 68: 201–4.

76. Szczeklik A, Nizankowska E, Czerniawska-Mysik G, Sek S. Hydrocortisone and airflow impairment in aspirin-induced asthma. *J Allergy Clin Immunol* 1985; 76: 530–6.

77. Tanaguchi M, Sato A. Aspirin-induced asthmatics (AIA) have cross-sensitivity with the steroid succinate esters *N Engl Reg Allergy Proc* 1988; 9: 338(A 358).

78. Feigenbaum BA, Stevenson DD, Simon RA. Lack of cross-sensitivity to iv hydrocortisone in subjects with aspirin-sensitive asthma. *ACI News* 1994; suppl 2: 156 (A 563).

79. Rolla G, Bucca C, Brussino L. Biphosphonate-induced bronchoconstriction in aspirin-sensitive asthma. *Lancet* 1994; 343: 426–7.

80. Vane JR. Inhibition of prostaglandin synthesis as a mechanism of action for aspirin-like drugs. *Nature New Biol* 1971; 231: 232–5.

Chapter 35

Specific Problems: Allergic Bronchopulmonary Aspergillosis

Rachel Limbrey and Peter Howarth

INTRODUCTION

Allergic bronchopulmonary aspergillosis (ABPA) is an immunologically mediated response within the airways to inhaled *Aspergillus* spores in an *Aspergillus*-sensitive patient which results in a chronic inflammatory response associated with altered tissue architecture. This typically arises in the proximal bronchi but may extend into the small airways and alveoli. Although it is classically described in asthmatics, it may also occur in patients with cystic fibrosis and there are a number of reports in the literature of ABPA in atopic non-asthmatics. The diagnosis is based on a combination of clinical, serological and radiological criteria. At present there is no single diagnostic test. The importance of early diagnosis in this condition is that intervention may prevent progression to endstage lung fibrosis. Corticosteroids remain the mainstay of treatment, although there are case reports of good response to anti-fungals emerging in the literature.

ASPERGILLUS

The fungus *Aspergillus* derives its name from its microscopic resemblance to a brush used for sprinkling holy water called an aspergillum.[1] It is a common fungus, with over 150 species described.[2] In the UK *Aspergillus fumigatus* and *Aspergillus niger* are the most prevalent and of these, *Aspergillus fumigatus* is the commonest cause of ABPA. It is appreciated, however, that other *Aspergillus* species and indeed other fungi can cause an identical disease.

Aspergillus fumigatus (AF) is ubiquitous. It is commonly found in decaying matter such as in compost heaps, old hay and fallen leaves. Peak spore counts are encountered in the autumn and winter months, which is the likely explanation for the increase in exacerbations of ABPA in these seasons.[3,4]

The spores are 2–3.5 µm in diameter. Their small size allows them to deposit throughout the airways after inhalation, penetrating down to the respiratory bronchioles. *Aspergillus* species are thermotolerant and thus grow well at body temperature. While the upper limit for growth for most fungi is 35°C, *Aspergillus* species have been demonstrated to grow at temperatures between 15 to 55°C. The germinated spores grow into a meshwork of hyphae which measure 7–10 µm in diameter. It is the hyphae that are expectorated, or recovered at bronchoscopy.

Aspergillus can be identified in tissue by routine haematoxylin and eosin staining, although periodic acid–Schiff and silver staining are better.[5]

CLINICAL DIAGNOSIS

ABPA was first described in 1952 by Hinson *et al.*[6] This publication reported details of three patients who experienced recurrent episodes of wheeze, fever, eosinophilia and sputum production associated with fleeting shadows on their chest X-ray. They were identified as having bronchial plugging with secretions containing *Aspergillus fumigatus* hyphae. Since then ABPA has become widely recognized with cases reported worldwide.

ABPA is reported to affect between 1–6% of all asthmatics[7,8] rising to 10% in those who are steroid-dependent.[9] The diagnosis of ABPA is based on the presence of a number of criteria. An initial seven were suggested by Rosenberg *et al.* in 1977[41] with one further criterion added by Wang and Patterson in 1978[18]. The criteria are:

(1) Asthma.

(2) Immediate cutaneous reactivity to *Aspergillus fumigatus* (i.e. skin-prick positive).

(3) Elevated total serum IgE >1000 iu ml^{-1}.

(4) Peripheral blood eosinophilia >0.5 × 10^9 l^{-1}.

(5) Precipitating serum IgG to *Aspergillus fumigatus*.

(6) Elevated, specific IgG and IgE to *Aspergillus fumigatus* in serum.

(7) Fleeting chest X-ray infiltrates.

(8) Central bronchiectasis.

None of the above criteria are considered essential for the diagnosis of ABPA, but clearly the more criteria satisfied the more certain the diagnosis. Although the diagnosis would be difficult in the absence of evidence for elevated IgE and IgG for an *Aspergillus* or an alternative fungal species, the criterion alone is insufficient as some diagnostic difficulty may be encountered in asthmatics sensitized to *Aspergillus fumigatus* due to the overlap of a number of the clinical and laboratory findings. Skin-prick tests to *Aspergillus fumigatus* can be positive in 13–38% of asthmatic subjects without ABPA.[10–13] Serum precipitating antibodies to *Aspergillus fumigatus* are present in 69–90% of cases of ABPA[3,14,15] but are also present in 25% of atopic asthmatics[13] and 3% of non-atopic asthmatics who do not have clinical evidence of ABPA.

It has recently been shown that it is possible to differentiate between ABPA and *Aspergillus fumigatus* sensitization by the difference in IgE-mediated immune responses to single, recombinant *Aspergillus fumigatus* allergens.[16,17] This may be of assistance in difficult diagnostic cases.

Despite the overlap of laboratory findings described above, measurement in the serum of elevated IgG-Af and IgE-Af relative to control sera is considered necessary for a diagnosis of ABPA[18–20] and possibly essential.[8] It is important to use age-appropriate control serum when performing serological tests for ABPA in children, as adults with asthma can have increased serum IgE-Af concentrations when compared with children with asthma, despite having three- to ten-fold lower concentrations of serum IgE.[21]

The total serum IgE is usually greater than 1000 iu ml^{-1} and may be as high as 20 000 iu ml^{-1} in acute cases.[8] Although most of the serum IgE is not *Aspergillus fumigatus* specific this increase in total IgE can be used as a marker to monitor the response to therapy, with falls in total IgE of 35–50% being consistent with adequate treatment. Effective therapy does not, however, restore total IgE levels to normal.[22]

The peripheral blood eosinophilia may be muted in those treated with steroids and thus not available as a diagnostic criterion.

The presence of central bronchiectasis in the absence of cystic fibrosis and other congenital ciliary disorders is virtually pathognomonic for ABPA.[23] However it is recognized that there are a group of asthmatic subjects who satisfy all the criteria for ABPA but do not have central bronchiectasis.[24,25] It appears that this group of seropositive ABPA (ABPAs) as opposed to ABPA with central bronchiectasis (ABPAcb) has a milder form of the disease or is presenting at an earlier stage in the disease's natural history. Patients with ABPAs have significantly lower IgG-Af than those with ABPAcb.[24] In a small series of 11 patients with ABPAs followed for a total of 63 patient years while receiving appropriate treatment no patient progressed to end-stage lung disease.[24]

CHEST RADIOLOGY

The radiological changes seen on ABPA may be fixed or transient[23] and need not be present at diagnosis. Fleeting chest X-ray infiltrates are, however, inevitable at some stage of the disease. Transient changes that resolve with corticosteroid treatment appear to be the result of parenchymal infiltrates, mucoid impaction or secretions in damaged bronchi. The appearances on plain chest radiography of these pathological processes include pulmonary infiltrates, perihilar infiltrates resembling lymphoedema, homogenous consolidation that may be unilateral or bilateral, "toothpaste" shadows from mucoid impaction in damaged bronchi, or "gloved finger" shadows from distally occluded bronchi filled with secretions. The changes occur more frequently in the upper than the lower lobes, but shrinkage occurs almost exclusively in the upper lobes.[26]

The radiological appearances are typically confined to one or two segments during an exacerbation, with the shadowing occurring in either the same area or elsewhere within the lung with recurrent episodes. When central bronchiectasis is present then ring shadows, 1–2 cm diameter circular markings on the chest X-ray produced by dilated bronchi viewed *en face*, or parallel hair-line shadows extending from the hilum may be seen.

High-resolution computerized tomography (HRCT) is the gold standard for demonstrating bronchiectasis.[27]

Previously bronchography was considered the gold standard, but this is a procedure now considered unsafe in asthma. HRCT compared with bronchography has a sensitivity of 83% and a specificity of 92% in detecting central bronchiectasis in patients with ABPA.[28] Central bronchiectasis with normal peripheral bronchi is pathognomonic for ABPA. Panchal et al. in 1997 evaluated the CT appearances of 23 patients with ABPA. Central bronchiectasis was identified in all patients, involving 114 (85%) of the 134 lobes and 210 (52%) of the 406 segments studied. Bronchial, parenchymal and pleural abnormalities were also documented. The pleura was involved in 10 (43%) patients. The occurrence of central bronchiectasis in this group of patients is slightly higher than in similar studies and is thought to be due to the delay in diagnosis caused by the radiological similarity to pulmonary tuberculosis.[29]

Angus et al. in 1994 looked at the CT changes in asthmatics with ABPA (17 patients) and asthmatics without ABPA, but with a positive skin-prick test to Aspergillus fumigatus (nine patients). Evidence of bronchiectasis was found in 43 of a possible 102 lobes of patients with ABPA, compared with three of a possible 66 in the non-ABPA group. Bronchial wall thickening was common to both groups, but pleural thickening was noted in 14 of those with ABPA but in only three of the non-ABPA group.[30]

Late radiological findings in ABPA include cavitation, local emphysema, contracted upper lobes and honeycomb fibrosis.[31] Spontaneous pneumothorax may be a complication in very advanced ABPA especially when bullous changes are present.[32]

PATHOLOGY

Histology is not routinely examined in patients with ABPA. Bronchoscopy with biopsy and washings may help to establish the diagnosis in atypical cases either where the disease is unsuspected or where the "criteria" are not met. Mucoid impaction and the histological finding of "allergic" mucin containing fungal hyphae are diagnostic of ABPA.[33] "Allergic" mucin is defined as pale staining, eosinophilic-to-basophilic mucus containing Charcot–Leyden crystals, Curshmann's spirals, fibrin and abundant eosinophils arranged in parallel layers.[34,35]

A granulomatous disease (bronchocentric granulomatosis) has also been described with aspergillosis. Whether this is related to ABPA is, at present, unclear.

PATHOGENESIS

As ABPA is rare in non-asthmatics it is presumed that asthmatic airways provide favourable conditions for Aspergillus. It is suggested that the tenacious mucus traps the Aspergillus spores. The thermotolerance of the species enables them to germinate at body temperature and produce hyphae. As a result antigenic material is produced and an immunological response is generated. In addition to IgE-mediated tissue effects, Aspergillus species, including Aspergillus fumigatus in culture, have been shown to generate proteolytic enzymes which may contribute to the inflammation and bronchial wall destruction that occurs in ABPA.[36]

IMMUNOLOGY

The precise nature of the immunological response is not fully understood at present. Aspergillus fumigatus generates a vigorous polyclonal antibody response leading to elevated total IgE as well as specific IgE, IgG and IgA.[37,38] The presence of IgE has been shown in animal models to enhance the tissue damaging effect of IgG precipitating antibodies.[39] The cellular infiltrate in ABPA is rich in eosinophils and mononuclear cells with evidence of T-cell activation. In vitro, populations of Aspergillus fumigatus antigen-specific T-cells proliferate on exposure to Aspergillus fumigatus and are able to stimulate B-cell IgE production, while T-cell clones to Aspergillus fumigatus have been shown to recognize Aspergillus fumigatus antigen. It is thus probable that the activated T-cells release TH_2-like cytokines such as IL-4, IL-5 and IL13. T-cells in asthmatics have increased gene expression for IL-4 and IL-5[40] and these cells are also capable of synthesizing IL-3 and granulocyte macrophage colony stimulating factor (GM-CSF). IL-4 and IL13 promote IgE synthesis from B-cells and can account for the substantial increase in IgE. The generation of IL-5 can be considered responsible for eosinophil differentiation as this cytokine along with IL-3 and GM-CSF will stimulate the production of eosinophil progenators in the bone marrow as well as increase eosinophil differentiation and tissue recruitment and survival. T-cell activation can thus explain the eosinophilia found in ABPA.

The tissue fibrosis is likely to be a consequence of the local airway inflammation secondary to the persistently high IgE levels and presence of antigen. Both activated eosinophils and mononuclear cells are able to synthesize and release fibrogenic factors such as transforming growth factor B (TGF-B), platelet-derived growth factor (PDGF), and basic fibroblast growth factor (bFGF). These factors will stimulate fibroblast proliferation and increase collagen synthesis, particularly for collagen types III and V, and promote the deposition of extracellular matrix protiens such as fibronectin and tenascin.

NATURAL HISTORY

ABPA may occur at any age and has been described in children as young as 14 months, but is rare at the extremes of age.

Patterson and Greenberger identified five stages of ABPA: (I) Acute; (II) Remission; (III) Exacerbation; (IV) Corticosteroid-dependent asthma; (V) Fibrotic.

Patients with stage I disease present with symptoms of fever, malaise, deteriorating or poorly controlled asthma and cough, classically productive of golden brown plugs of sputum. On examination there may be signs of consolidation in the chest. With treatment most patients will progress to remission (stage II).

During remission the patient's asthma is easily managed with bronchodilators and regular inhaled steroids. Exacerbations can be recognized by a change in asthma severity and the recurrence of symptoms and signs as in stage I. However, in up to 35% of exacerbations of ABPA the patient may be asymptomatic,[41] the exacerbation only becoming apparent through a rise in serum IgE. A doubling of the serum IgE is significant. A prolonged remission does not imply cure as exacerbations have been reported after remission of periods as long as 7.5 years.[42]

Patients are said to have stage IV disease when in the presence of ABPA oral corticosteroids are required to control their symptoms of asthma and it is no longer possible to wean them from their oral therapy once disease control is achieved.

The fibrotic stage is an advanced stage of radiographic abnormalities with asthma, irreversible and partially reversible obstructive pulmonary function changes, and poor prognosis.

The natural history of the disease is varied. In a review of 17 patients with stage V disease the interval between diagnosis and stage V varied from 5 months to 35 years.[43] The prognosis for patients with a forced expiratory volume in 1 s (FEV_1) of less than 0.81 at the time of diagnosis is poor with death occurring within 7 years.[43]

TREATMENT

Oral corticosteroids are the cornerstone of treatment of ABPA. After the initial treatment phase, the corticosteroid dose is adjusted according to serial measurements of total serum IgE along with identification of radiological resolution. The original guidelines for treatment were suggested by Wang et al. in 1979 and remain sensible advice.[44] After diagnosis oral prednisolone 0.5 mg kg^{-1} as a single daily dose should be given for the first 2 weeks and then continued as an alternate daily dose for 3 months. After this the dose can be gradually tapered over a further 3 months. The speed at which the corticosteroids can be reduced is dictated by the clinical and objective response to treatment.

Recognition of ABPA early in the disease process and effective treatment with corticosteroids and prolonged follow-up appears to prevent progression to lung damage and stage V disease.[8,24] It is not clear whether all patients with ABPA are at risk of progressing to chronic lung damage or whether exacerbations could be managed with shorter courses of steroids tailed over a period of 1 month.[38]

Inhaled steroids are useful to control the symptoms of asthma during remissions but have not been helpful during exacerbations of ABPA.[44,45]

Follow-Up

During the initial treatment period an improvement in symptoms accompanied by resolution of pulmonary infiltrates and a fall in IgE should be seen. It is important to perform regular chest X-rays to confirm the resolution of changes and then at 4-monthly intervals for the first 2 years of follow-up, extending eventually to an annual chest X-ray. Serum total IgE levels should be determined at presentation and then monthly for the following year. After this the interval between IgE measurements can be gradually extended. A fall in total serum IgE of approximately 35% is expected after 4–6 weeks of treatment[8] and a plateau level should be seen by 6 months treatment. Failure to achieve these criteria suggests under-treatment and a more prolonged initial course of corticosteroid prior to reduction is required. Prolonged follow-up of ABPA patients is essential, as exacerbations have been described as long as 7.5 years after remission.[42]

Anti-Fungals

Anti-fungal agents are very attractive in theory to reduce the antigenic load in patients with ABPA, but have not been clearly established as routine therapy by clinical trials. A randomized, placebo-controlled trial of nebulized natamycin in ABPA showed no benefit of treatment over placebo in terms of steroid sparing or markers of disease activity after 1 year of treatment.[46] Trials of newer oral anti-fungal agents such as itraconazole suggest beneficial effects as an adjuvant therapy. The open introduction of itraconazole in the treatment of ABPA led to a reduction in oral corticosteroid dose, a fall in total serum IgE and an improvement in spirometeric values when treatment was continued for up to 6 months.[47,48] These were non-controlled, non-randomized studies with small patient numbers. There has also been a recent case report of good response to itraconazole alone.[49] There is a need for carefully conducted, controlled clinical trials of this anti-fungal agent in patients with ABPA.

KEY POINTS

1 Diagnosis

Maintain a high index of suspicion in susceptible patients (i.e. with asthma, cystic fibrosis) look for:

(a) Skin-prick positive *Aspergillus fumigatus*,
(b) Elevated total serum IgE
(c) Eosinophilia
(d) *Aspergillus fumigatus* precipitins
(e) Specific IgE-Af and IgG-Af
(f) Fleeting shadows on chest X-ray
(g) Central bronchiectasis

2 Treatment

Oral corticosteroids tailored to clinical response, radiological resolution and reduction in total serum IgE. An adequate response produces a fall in total IgE of 35–50%

3 Follow-up

Long term, as prolonged remissions reported. Exacerbations may be a symptomatic. Suggest annual chest X-ray and monitor total serum IgE.

REFERENCES

1. Raper K, Fennel D. *The Genus Aspergillus*. Huntington, NY: Robert E Krieger, 1973.

2. Richeson R, Stander P. Allergic bronchopulmonary aspergillosis. *Postgrad Med* 1990; 88: 217–22.

3. McCarthy D, Pepys J. Allergic bronchopulmonary aspergillosis. Clinical immunology: (1) clinical features. *Clin Allergy* 1971; 1: 261–86.

4. Safirstein B, D'Souza M, Simon G, Tai E, Pepys J. Five year follow-up of bronchopulmonary aspergillosis. *Am Rev Respir Dis* 1973; 108: 450–9.

5. Ricketti AJ, Greenberger PA, Patterson R. Varying presentations of allergic bronchopulmonary aspergillosis. *Int Arch Allergy Appl Immunol* 1984; 73(3): 283–5.

6. ✪ Hinson K, Moon A, Plummer N. Bronchopulmonary aspergillosis: a review and a report of eight new cases. *Thorax* 1952; 7: 317–33.

7. Greenberger P, Patterson R. Allergic bronchopulmonary aspergillosis and the evaluation of the patient with asthma. *J Allergy Clin Immunol* 1988; 81: 646–50.

8. Ganz M, Greenberger P, Patterson R (eds). *Hypersensitivity Pneumonitis and Allergic Bronchopulmonary Aspergillosis*, 3rd edn. Boston: Little, Brown and Co, 1993.

9. Basich JE, Graves TS, Baz MN *et al*. Allergic bronchopulmonary aspergillosis in corticosteroid-dependent asthmatics. *J Allergy Clin Immunol* 1981; 68(2): 98–102.

10. Henderson A, English M, Vecht R. Pulmonary aspergillosis: A survey of its occurrence in patients with chronic lung disease and discussion of the significance of diagnostic tests. *Thorax* 1968; 23: 513–23.

11. Bardana E, Gerber J, Craig S, Cianciulla F. The general and specific humoral immune response to pulmonary aspergillosis. *Am Rev Respir Dis* 1975; 112: 799–805.

12. Hendrick D, Davis R, D'Souza M, Pepys J. An analysis of skin prick test reaction in 656 asthmatic patients. *Thorax* 1975; 30 (suppl.): 2.

13. Longbottom J, Pepys J. Pulmonary aspergillosis: Diagnosis and immunological significance of antigens and C-substance in *Aspergillus fumigatus*. *J Pathol Bacteriol* 1964; 88: 141–51.

14. Campbell M, Clayton Y. Bronchopulmonary aspergillosis. *Am Rev Respir Dis* 1964; 89: 186–96.

15. Faux J, Shale D, Lane D. Precipitans and specific IgG antibody to *Aspergillus furnigatus* in a chest unit population. *Thorax* 1992; 47: 48–52.

16. Crameri R, Hemmann S, Ismail C, Menz G, Blaser K. Disease-specific recombinant allergens for the diagnosis of allergic bronchopulmonary aspergillosis. *Internat Immunol* 1998; 10(8): 1211–16.

17. Banerjee B, Greenberger P, Fink J, Kurup V. Immunological characterization of *Asp f 2*, a major allergen from *Aspergillus fumigatus* associated with allergic bronchopulmonary aspergillosis. *Infect Immun* 1998; 66(11): 5175–82.

18. Wang J, Patterson R, Rosenberg M, Roberts M, Cooper B. Serum IgE and IgG antibody activity against *Aspergillus fumigatus* as a diagnostic aid in allergic bronchopulmonary aspergillosis. *Am Rev Resp Dis* 1978; 117: 917–27.

19. Greenberger P, Patterson R. Application of enzyme linked immunosorbent assay (ELISA) in diagnosis of allergic bronchopulmonary aspergillosis. *J Lab Clin Med* 1982; 99: 288–93.

20. Kurup V, Resnick A, Kalbfleish J, Fink J. Antibody isotype responses in *Aspergillus*-induced disease. *J Lab Clin Med* 1990; 115: 298–303.

21. Greenberger P, Liotta J, Roberts M. The effects of age on isotypic antibody responses to *Aspergillus fumigatus*: implications regarding *in-vitro* measurements. *J Lab Clin Med* 1989; 114: 278–84.

22. Patterson R, Greenberger PA, Lee TM *et al*. Prolonged evaluation of patients with corticosteroid-dependent asthma stage of allergic bronchopulmonary aspergillosis. *J Allergy Clin Immunol* 1987; 80(5): 663–8.

23. ✪ Mintzer R, Rogers L, Kriglik G. The spectrum of radiological findings in allergic bronchopulmonary aspergillosis. *Radiology* 1978; 127: 301–7.

24. Greenberger P, Miller T, Roberts M, Smith L. Allergic bronchopulmonary aspergillosis in patients with and without evidence of bronchiectasis. *Ann Allergy* 1993; 70: 333–8.

25. Patterson R, Greenberger PA, Halwig JM, Liotta JL, Roberts M. Allergic bronchopulmonary aspergillosis. Natural history and classification of early disease by serologic and roentgenographic studies. *Arch Intern Med* 1986; 146(5): 916–8.

26. Phelan MS, Kerr IH. Allergic broncho-pulmonary aspergillosis: the radiological appearance during long-term follow-up. *Clin Radiol* 1984; 35(5): 385–92.

27. Neeld DA, Goodman LR, Gurney JW, Greenberger PA, Fink JN. Computerized tomography in the evaluation of allergic bronchopulmonary aspergillosis. *Am Rev Respir Dis* 1990; 142(5): 1200–5.

28. Panchal N, Pant C, Bhagat R, Shah A. Central bronchiectasis in allergic bronchopulmonary aspergillosis: comparative evaluation of computed tomography of the thorax with bronchography. *Eur Respir J* 1994; 7(7): 1290–3.

29. Panchal N, Bhagat R, Pant C, Shah A. Allergic bronchopulmonary aspergillosis: the spectrum of computed tomography appearances. *Respir Med* 1997; 91(4): 213–9.

30. Angus RM, Davies ML, Cowan MD, McSharry C, Thomson NC. Computed tomographic scanning of the lung in patients with allergic bronchopulmonary aspergillosis and in asthmatic patients with a positive skin test to *Aspergillus fumigatus*. *Thorax* 1994; 49(6): 586–9.

31. McCarthy DS, Simon G, Hargreave FE. The radiological appearances in allergic broncho-pulmonary aspergillosis. *Clin Radiol* 1970; 21(4): 366–75.

32. Ricketti AJ, Greenberger PA, Mintzer RA, Patterson R. Allergic bronchopulmonary aspergillosis. *Chest* 1984; 86(5): 773–8.

33. Aubry M, Fraser R. The role of bronchial biopsy and washing in the diagnosis of allergic bronchopulmonary aspergillosis. *Mod Pathol* 1998; 11(7): 607–611.

34. Jelihovsky T. The structure of bronchial plugs in mucoid impaction, bronchocentric granulomatosis and asthma. *Histopathology* 1983; 7(2): 153–67.

35. Bosken CH, Myers JL, Greenberger PA, Katzenstein AL. Pathologic features of allergic bronchopulmonary aspergillosis. *Am J Surg Pathol* 1988; 12(3): 216–22.

36. Greenberger P. Diagnosis and management of allergic bronchopulmonary aspergillosis. *Allergy Proc* 1994; 15(6): 335–9.

37. Patterson R, Rosenberg M, Roberts M. Evidence that *Aspergillus fumigatus* growing in the airway of man can be a potent stimulus of specific and nonspecific IgE Formation. *Am J Med* 1977; 63: 257–62.

38. Wardlaw A, Geddes D. Allergic bronchopulmonary aspergillosis: a review. *J Royal Soc Med* 1992; 85: 747–51.

39. Slavin R. Allergic bronchopulmonary aspergillosis. *Clin Rev Allergy* 1985; 3: 167.

40. Robinson D, Hamid Q, Ying Sea. Predominant TH_2 like bronchoalveolar T-lymphocyte population in atopic asthma. *N Engl J Med* 1992; 326: 298–304.

41. ○ Rosenberg M, Patterson R, Mintzer R, Cooper B, Roberts M, Harris K. Clinical and immunological criteria for the diagnosis of allergic bronchopulmonary aspergillosis. *Ann Int Med* 1977; 86: 405–414.

42. Halwing M, Greenberger P, Patterson R, Levine M. Recurrence of allergic bronchopulmonary aspergillosis after seven years remission. *J Allergy Clin Immunol* 1984; 74: 319–23.

43. ○ Lee T, Greenberger P, Patterson R, Roberts M, Liotta J. Stage V (fibrotic) allergic bronchopulmonary aspergillosis. A review of 17 cases followed from diagnosis. *Arch Intern Med* 1987; 147: 319–23.

44. Wang JL, Patterson R, Roberts M, Ghory AC. The management of allergic bronchopulmonary aspergillosis. *Am Rev Respir Dis* 1979; 120(1): 87–92.

45. Vaughan LM. Allergic bronchopulmonary aspergillosis. *Clin Pharm* 1993; 12(1): 24–33.

46. Currie DC, Lueck C, Milburn HJ *et al*. Controlled trial of natamycin in the treatment of allergic bronchopulmonary aspergillosis. *Thorax* 1990; 45(6): 447–50.

47. Denning D, Van Wye J, Lewiston N, Stevens D. Adjunctive therapy of allergic bronchopulmonary aspergillosis with itraconazole. *Chest* 1991; 3: 813–19.

48. Germaud P, Tuchais E. Allergic bronchopulmonary aspergillosis treated with itraconazole [letter; comment]. *Chest* 1995; 107(3): 883.

49. Nikaido K, Nagata N, Yamamoto T, Yoshii C, Ohmori H, Kido M. A case of allergic bronchopulmonary aspergillosis successfully treated with itraconazole. *Resp Med* 1998; 92: 118–24.

Chapter 36

Specific Problems: Exercise-Induced Asthma

Sandra Anderson and John Brannan

DEFINITION AND MECHANISM

"Exercise-induced asthma (EIA) and exercise-induced bronchoconstriction (EIB) are the terms used to describe the transitory increase in airways resistance which follows vigorous exercise".[1] While EIA/EIB most commonly occurs in people with clinically recognized asthma, there are many reports of EIA/EIB in asymptomatic healthy subjects, e.g. schoolchildren, defence force recruits, elite athletes, and skaters.[2–6] It has recently been suggested that the term EIA be reserved to describe the changes in lung function and response to drugs in those with known asthma.[7]

It has long been recognized that the intensity, duration, and type of exercise are important in determining severity of EIA.[8] However, it is the ventilation rate reached and sustained during exercise,[9] and the water content of the air inspired during exercise[10] that are the primary determinants of severity of EIA. Exercise, *per se*, is not necessary to provoke airway narrowing and isocapnic hyperventilation with dry air at high-flow rates is used as a laboratory challenge to substitute for exercise.[11–13]

The stimulus to EIA is the loss of water from the airways by bringing large volumes of inspired air to alveolar conditions in a short time.[10,14,15] The precise mechanism whereby water lost by evaporation leads to airway narrowing is unknown, but it appears that thermal[16,17] and osmotic[18] effects of dehydration are important.[19] One hypothesis suggests that it is the thermal effects of water loss acting to increase permeability of the bronchial microcirculation, with consequent vascular engorgement and airway oedema causing the airways to narrow independently of contraction of bronchial smooth muscle.[16,17] However thermal factors, such as airway cooling followed by re-warming, are not

pre-requisites for EIA to occur,[20,21] and may simply be epiphenomena that occur during breathing of cold air. Exercise-induced asthma is provoked by breathing hot dry air when abnormal cooling and re-warming are absent but water loss is still significant.[22–25] The osmotic hypothesis suggests that EIA is a result of the dehydrating effects of water loss causing a transient increase in osmolarity of the airway surface liquid and epithelium with subsequent release of mediators.[18,20,26–30] Mast cell mediators and sensory neuropeptides are thought to cause the airways to narrow by contraction of bronchial smooth muscle, with or without airway oedema. While technical issues have made it difficult to obtain direct evidence for mediator release some investigators have been successful.[31–34] However the most convincing evidence for mediator release comes from the inhibitory effects on EIA by specific antagonists of histamine and leukotrienes.[35–40]

DIAGNOSIS OF EIA BY HISTORY

A diagnosis of EIA can frequently be made on history and the response to inhaled drug therapy. A patient who complains of shortness of breath that is worse after rather than during exercise, and who reports that the symptoms are relieved by inhaling a β_2-adrenoceptor agonist (β agonist), has a history consistent with EIA. If the shortness of breath after exercise is prevented by taking either a β_2-adrenoceptor agonist, nedocromil sodium or sodium cromoglycate immediately before exercise, the diagnosis of EIA is confirmed. Obtaining a clear history of EIA suggests that the FEV_1 and PEFR have fallen at least 20% as symptoms are rare with mild EIA. It is difficult however to assess the severity of EIA by history alone or by resting lung function. Severe EIA can occur in patients with good lung function and lung function cannot be used to predict the amount of therapy required to control EIA.

It should be noted that the diagnosis of EIA cannot be simply made on a history of post-exercise cough. While it is important to recognize cough as a symptom consistent with EIA, not all those with post-exercise cough have EIA.[41–43]

DIAGNOSIS BY LABORATORY TESTING

When there is doubt about the diagnosis, severity, or the amount of medication required to control EIA, the patient should be referred to a laboratory for a standardized exercise test. Such patients should be screened carefully before referral to exclude cardiovascular disease. Although many physicians may use a "run up the stairs" to confirm a diagnosis of EIA, it should be kept in mind that a standardized stimulus is required to document severity and to evaluate the effect of therapy. The conditions for evaluating the presence and severity of EIA/EIB modified from those of Folgering et al.[44] are given in Table 36.1.

It is also important to confirm that the protocol used in the laboratory will be sufficient to provoke EIA in a trained athlete. Nowadays we choose isocapnic hyperventilation with dry air[11–13,45] for most subjects referred for EIA testing, but we always use it to assess trained athletes. Cold air[46] can be used but is not necessary and inhaling compressed air at room temperature is usually an adequate stimulus, providing the appropriate ventilation rate is reached and sustained.[47]

Exercise-induced asthma is quantified by expressing the reduction in PEFR or FEV_1 that occurs in the 20 minutes after exercise as a percentage of the pre-exercise value (percentage fall index). (Table 36.1). Historically EIA has been classified as mild when the FEV_1 falls 10–24%, moderate when it falls 25–50% and severe when the fall in FEV_1 is greater than 50.1%. However these values for defining severity were assigned before the widespread use of inhaled steroids to treat asthma. Because inhaled steroids are now being prescribed more frequently, in higher doses and earlier in the treatment of asthma, it seems appropriate to modify the original classification. Thus for those patients, otherwise well-controlled on steroids, but who still get EIA, the following classification is suggested. Mild EIA <20% fall in FEV_1, moderate EIA 20–30%, and severe EIA greater than 30% fall in FEV_1.

The value of 10% as the cut-off point for diagnosis of EIA is based on the responses measured in healthy subjects exercising in both temperate and cold environments.[8,13,48] If two tests are performed within one month, the percentage fall index will usually vary less than 20%, providing the two exercise tests are performed under standardized conditions.[47,49] In addition to the percentage fall index, it is useful for a physician to have the pre-exercise level of FEV_1 and the lowest value for FEV_1 measured after exercise reported as a percentage of the predicted normal value. These values may reveal the benefit of treatment with aerosol steroids on pre-and post-exercise lung function and symptoms, even though the percentage fall index may remain the same. The reason for this is that FEV_1 improves within days of starting steroids, whereas the severity of EIA may not necessarily be reduced for weeks or even months.[50,51] When assessing the acute affect of a drug it is useful to know what the response is after a placebo medication. The protection afforded by a drug is taken as the difference in the percentage fall after the placebo and the active drug expressed as a percentage of the percentage fall on the placebo. A value for protection greater than 50% is regarded as a significant drug effect as it takes into account the repeatability of the test.[47]

DIAGNOSIS IN THE FIELD

Many health-care professionals are now involved in assessing EIA/EIB. Providing they have been properly trained in the safety of these procedures and emergency equipment is available if required, it would seem appropriate that the recognized athlete with asthma can be followed up outside the laboratory. For children in schools with the appropriate equipment, the physical educationists could also be encouraged to make measurements of flow rates after exercise in children suspected of having EIA. This has been made easier with hand-held spirometers for measuring FEV_1 now being more readily available (Micromedical Ltd, Kent, UK).

Various protocols for use in the field have been described,[52–54] and one that has adapted many of the requirements for the standardized procedure in a laboratory is presented in Fig. 36.1.[54] The subject exercises, by running for 6 to 8 minutes, at a speed sufficient to raise the oxygen consumption to >35 ml kg^{-1} per min (Fig. 36.2).[55–57] This intensity of exercise should be sufficient to provoke EIA and can be confirmed by the

Table 36.1: Conditions for evaluating the presence and severity of exercise-induced bronchoconstriction. (Modified from Folgering H, Palange P, Anderson S. Clinical exercise testing with reference to lung diseases: indications and protocols. *Eur Respir Mon* 1997; 6: 51–71.)

Safety	Risk factors or contraindications for exercise should be assessed when considering patients with EIB. Arterial oxygen saturation (S_aO_2) at rest should be >94% and pulse oximetry should be monitored continuously during the test, in addition to adherence to general guidelines for safety
Measurement	FEV_1 measurement is recommended, pre-exercise and 1, 3, 5, 7, 10, 15, and 20 min post-exercise. In elite athletes, FEF_{25-75} should also be measured to assess EIB.
FEV_1 at rest	>75% predicted or 80% of patient's usual value (if known) and reproducible, i.e. <10% variation
Medications withheld	8 h for short-acting bronchodilators, sodium cromoglycate, nedocromil sodium; 48 h for long-acting bronchodilators, theophylline, leukotriene antagonists and antihistamines; and no steroids or caffeine on the study day
Control for time of last	(a) EIB > 3 h; (b) infection >6 weeks; and (c) exposure to pollen (note if test performed in/out of season for pollen sensitive subjects)
Type of exercise	Cycling or running. Cycling is recommended as safest and easiest. Workload set at 60% 1st min, 75% 2nd min and 90% 3rd min and 100% thereafter and may be back-titrated for VE to be sustained for 4 min
Intensity of exercise	V_{O_2} sufficient to raise exercise VE to 18.5 ± 3.5 times predicted FEV_1 for at least 4 min; Target work load in watts = $(53.76 \times FEV_1) - 11.07$. For treadmill, V_{O_2} target will need to be greater than 35 ml kg^{-1} to achieve the required VE (Fig. 36.2)[56,57] For most subjects this will be achieved by running at 4–6 kph up a 15% or greater slope
Duration of exercise	6–8 min to allow target VE to be achieved and sustained for at least 4 min
Inspired air	Compressed dry air is recommended. Room air containing <10 mg H_2O l^{-1} T°C <25°C, <50% relative humidity is adequate. Cold air only needed if it represents environmental conditions.
Index of severity	If patient not taking inhaled or oral steroids: (a) 10% <ΔFEV_1 <25%, mild;(b) 25% <ΔFEV_1 <50%, moderate; (c) ΔFEV_1 >50%, severe
Recovery	Spontaneous or with administration of a β_2 agonist. Supplemental O_2 should be provided if needed at any time during the test

FEV_1: forced expiratory volume in 1 s; FEF_{25-75}: forced mid-expiratory flow; V_{O_2}: oxygen consumption; VE: minute ventilation; ΔFEV_1: fall in FEV_1

measurement of heart rate at the radial or carotid pulse or by using a heart rate meter. The values for oxygen consumption can be estimated by knowing the weight of the subject, the distance run, and the time over which the distance was run.[56,57] To ensure adequate water loss from the airways,[23] the exercise is performed while breathing through the mouth and when the inspired air has a water content less than 10 mg l^{-1} (23°C, 50% RH). Having established the diagnosis of EIA the management of its severity can begin. A value of 15% fall in

FEV_1 is taken as the cut-off point as the diagnosis for EIA in field studies.[2]

MANAGEMENT OF EIA

Treatment of EIA

The usual approach to the management of EIA is prevention; however it is important to know how to treat EIA when it occurs. The reason EIA should not be ignored is that it is associated with arterial hypoxaemia

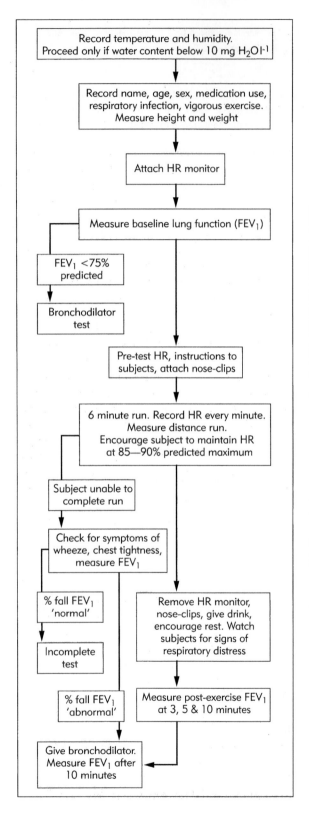

FIGURE 36.1: Field procedure for identifying exercise-induced bronchoconstriction. After Haby et al.[54]

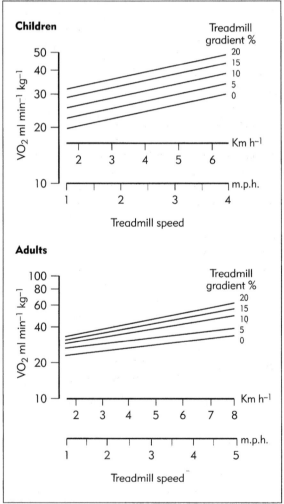

FIGURE 36.2: Predicted oxygen consumption in ml min⁻¹ kg⁻¹ during running in children and adults in relation to treadmill speed and slope. The illustration for children is taken from Silverman, and Anderson[56] and for adults is constructed from the data given by Givoni and Goldman.[57]

and hyperinflation of the lungs.[58,59] It is the hypoxaemia associated with exercise that makes it dangerous for a person to continue or resume exercise at a time when the FEV_1 or PEFR is falling. If a person feels an attack of asthma coming on during exercise, he should be advised to stop immediately. It can be predicted that the attack will worsen on the cessation of exercise, usually within the first 5 minutes, but often as late as 10 minutes. For most asthmatic subjects, the attack of asthma can be reversed quickly by inhaling a β_2-adrenoceptor agonist. For mild to moderate EIA, two or three inhalations of a bronchodilator with 1–2 minutes separating each inhalation is usually all that is required. Spacing devices such as the Nebuhaler and Volumatic can aid in the delivery of drug as co-ordination between delivery and inspiration is not required and the drug can be given over two or three tidal breaths. In severe cases of EIA up to 10 inhalations of a β_2-adrenoceptor agonist can be given.[60] Ideally, in severe cases of EIA, a bronchodilator should be delivered by a nebulizer with oxygen. There have been deaths after exercise, both in children and adults, who have competed successfully without apparent compromised exercise performance. As the severity of the attack is usually at its greatest 10 minutes after ceasing exercise, it is advisable to monitor lung function and watch closely individuals with EIA within this time.

About 50% of people with EIA become refractory to exercise if it is repeated within 30 to 90 minutes. In order to identify refractoriness, a person needs to recover spontaneously from an attack of EIA with lung function returning to within 5% of the pre-challenge value.[61] If an identical exercise test is performed and results in less than 50% of the fall observed on the first test, the person is said to be refractory.[61] The ingestion of non-steroidal anti-inflammatory drugs such as indomethacin can prevent refractoriness[62] and athletes taking these drugs should be advised accordingly.

PREVENTION OF EIA

For most patients who have normal lung function, EIA will be prevented by any of the short-acting β_2-adrenoceptor agonists or sodium cromoglycate or nedocromil sodium taken immediately before exercise.[47,63,64] For patients with reduced lung function before exercise, the use of β_2-adrenoceptor agonist is recommended if maximal exercise performance is to be achieved. If patients have less than 75% of the normal predicted lung function or less than 80% of their normal lung function, after medication, they should be advised not to exercise and their treatment should be reviewed.

β_2-Adrenoceptor Agonists

The short-acting β agonists taken in the standard dose 10–15 minutes before exercise have been shown to be effective in most patients with EIA. They usually provide 60–75% protection against EIA when exercise is performed within 30 minutes of taking the drug.[47,49]

While β agonists are the most effective treatment for prevention of EIA there is current concern about their regular use. Daily use of short-acting β_2-adrenoceptor agonists can affect airway responsiveness[65] and daily use of long-acting β agonists can cause tolerance to their protective effects. Both these problems are relevant to the management of EIA. Thus severity of untreated EIA can be made worse with daily use of 800 μg of salbutamol for one week even though the effectiveness of an acute dose of 200 μg of salbutamol to prevent the EIA, in the same subjects, was still evident[66] (Fig. 36.3). Further, it has been shown that when bronchoconstriction is provoked in people taking β agonists daily, they have a reduced rate of recovery in response to the acute administration of a β agonist.[67,68] This slower rate of recovery to baseline lung function in those taking β agonists regularly occurs whether the subjects are taking inhaled steroids daily or not.[68] Given that most short-acting β_2-adrenoceptor agonists in use have a protective effect against EIA of 2 hours or less (Fig. 36.4) they are likely to be used many times in a day by some asthmatics! For these people, alternative strategies to using multiple doses of β agonists, should be considered for controlling EIA.

The longer acting β agonists salmeterol,[47,69,70] and formoterol[71–73] also provide good protection against EIA. Salmeterol has a slower onset of its protective effect compared with formoterol, however, some patients are well-protected from EIA 30 minutes after administration of salmeterol.[47] The optimal benefit of salmeterol is observed 2.5 hours after administration (Fig. 36.4). For those with mild EIA, protection from these long-acting agents may be afforded for 8–12 hours;[70,73] however some patients with moderate to severe EIA may be protected only for 4–6 hours.[47]

The major disadvantage in using these long-acting drugs for the prevention of EIA is that, when taken on a twice daily basis for one month, tolerance develops to

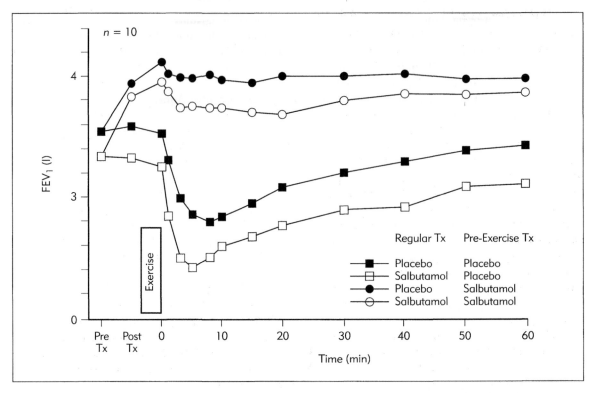

FIGURE 36.3: Mean values for FEV₁ before during and after steady-state exercise for 5 minutes breathing dry air at approximately 60% predicted maximum work load on four occasions. The symbols denote the regular treatment in which case the subject had taken no medication for 8 hours prior to exercise and pre-exercise treatment where subject took the medication 5 minutes before exercise. (Data redrawn From Inman et al[66]).

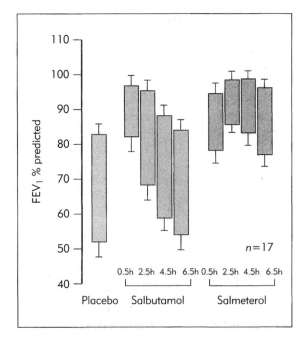

FIGURE 36.4: Mean values ±1 SEM for FEV₁ before (top of the column) and lowest value after exercise (bottom of column) expressed as a percentage of the predicted normal value in 17 asthmatic subjects. Exercise was by cycling for 8 minutes while breathing compressed dry air between 22°C and 26°C. The target workload [(53.76 × FEV₁) − 11.07] in watts was set to give a ventilation of FEV₁ predicted × 18.5 (see Table 36.1). During the first 3 minutes of exercise the workload was increased from 60% to 75% to 90% and, in the 4th minute to 100% of the workload calculated to produce the target ventilation. Exercise tests were performed at 0.5 hours after placebo and 0.5, 2.5, 4.5 and 6.5 hours after 200 μg of salbutamol and 50 μg of salmeterol on two separate days. (Data taken from Anderson et al[47]).

their protective effect against exercise. This tolerance is evidenced by a reduction in the duration of the protective effect against EIA.[74–76] This tolerance which has been demonstrated in adults and children is also evident in those taking inhaled steroids.[75] Thus the relative advantage of using a long-acting agent such as salmeterol may be offset by its slower onset of action and reduced period of protection. The optimal use of salmeterol for EIA would seem to be for those subjects not taking the drug daily and willing to wait 30 minutes before exercising. While it is not yet known if tolerance develops to the protective effect of formoterol there is no reason to expect otherwise.

It would seem advisable that β_2-adrenoceptor agonists be used with more caution than in the past and other therapy, such as using nedocromil sodium, be considered as an alternative for controlling EIA. However a β_2-adrenoceptor agonist must be available for those who develop EIA unexpectedly and who are in need of rescue medication.

Oral bronchodilators such as terbutaline, salbutamol and theophylline are not useful in the prevention of EIA.[77–79] Patients may feel better on their oral bronchodilator, compared with no drugs, because their flow rates before and after exercise will be higher, however the percentage fall in FEV_1 after exercise is usually unaffected by the active drug.

Nedocromil Sodium and Sodium Cromoglycate

Exercise-induced asthma may be prevented simply by inhaling 10 to 20 mg of sodium cromoglycate,[80–82] or 4 to 8 mg of nedocromil sodium immediately before exercise.[64,82,83] In a recent meta-analysis reported by Spooner in the Cochrane Library for evidence-based medicine,[64] nedocromil sodium was shown to have a 50% protection from EIA and to be equally effective in adults and children, and in those with severe (>30% fall in lung function) or mild EIA (Fig. 36.5). Both sodium cromoglycate and nedocromil sodium have an immediate onset of action and only the few seconds it takes for the inhaled particles to settle in the airways are required for onset of action. These drugs can be effective at first dosing so that no pre-treatment time is required for efficacy. Their duration of action is 1.5–2.5 hours. There are no reports of tolerance developing to the protective effects of these agents and they can be taken many times in a day. They are not bronchodilators and are thought to prevent airway narrowing by a number of mechanisms.[84,85] They are most likely to be

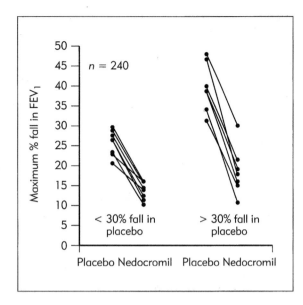

FIGURE 36.5: Mean values for the maximum percentage fall in FEV_1 after placebo and after acute prophylactic treatment with nedocromil sodium (4–8 mg) in studies of subjects who had a fall in FEV_1 less than 30% and greater than 30% of baseline after exercise. (Taken from the data of Spooner et al[64]).

effective in persons with normal lung function before exercise.

Inhaled Corticosteroids

The recognition that asthma is an inflammatory disease of the airways[86] and that EIA is a manifestation of this has led to early introduction of inhaled corticosteroids in the treatment of EIA. Treatment with inhaled steroids usually reduces the severity of EIA within days or weeks.[50,51,87–91] Further, the type and amount of additional medication, e.g. a β agonist to control EIA, can be reduced markedly by daily use of inhaled steroids.[50] The decrease in severity of EIA within hours or days[88,90] is probably due to the reduction in airway oedema by steroids, the reduction of severity over weeks is likely due to a reduction in number of mast cells in the airways.[86]

It is important to know that EIA can still occur when the daily dose of aerosol steroid is sufficient to achieve normal lung function, eliminate symptoms, and reduce diurnal airflow variability.[91] The dose of steroids may need to be titrated to inhibit EIA (Fig. 36.6). In a study of asthmatic children, 800 μg per day of budesonide

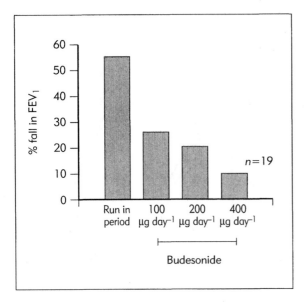

FIGURE 36.6: Mean values for the fall in FEV$_1$ expressed as a percentage of baseline during the run in period and 4 weeks after treatment with 100, 200 and 400 µg per day of budesonide given via a Turbuhaler to children. The values after treatment were significantly different to the run in period. (Data taken from Pedersen and Hansen[91]).

The advantage to the patient for using this type of drug is that it may only require once or twice day dosing. Further tolerance does not develop to their protective effect after weeks of use[96] and the inhibitory effect on EIA is still evident at the end of a dosing period.[40] The disadvantage is that several days of treatment is likely to be needed before the protective effect against EIA is evident. In view of other effective inhaled therapy and on the basis of the studies so far, at this time it is hard to recommend this orally administered drug solely on the basis of managing EIA. However a patient prescribed a leukotriene antagonist for treatment of asthma is likely to benefit from a reduction in symptoms and severity of EIA, a situation similar to that which occurs with inhaled steroids.

For some asthmatics, exercise is the only factor provoking an attack. Whether such patients should be treated with inhaled steroids or leukotriene antagonists remains an unanswered question. If the severity of EIA is a reflection of airway inflammation, this may be an important question to be answered. EIA is highly specific to asthma[97] yet not all persons with documented EIA give symptoms of asthma.[2,98] When exercise and hyperpnoea with dry air are used in epidemiological studies, persons falling into this category are being recognized in increasing numbers.[2,98,99] For this reason, a decision should be made as to whether EIA without symptoms should be prevented and the underlying pathology treated with anti-inflammatory agents.

halved the severity of EIA, but EIA still occurred in 55% of the children.[51] It is those patients who will still need prophylactic medication to prevent EIA.

Leukotriene Antagonists

There are now a number of leukotriene receptor antagonists[37–40,92,93] and 5-lipoxygenase inhibitors[94,95] that have been investigated in asthmatic subjects and their acute and chronic effects on EIA documented. The traditional analysis of comparing the maximum percentage fall in FEV$_1$ from baseline on the active and placebo has, in some studies, been replaced with an analysis of the area under the post-exercise FEV$_1$ time curve.[40,92] This is probably justified, given that the fall in lung function after exercise may be mediated by histamine initially but sustained by the release of leukotrienes some 5–10 minutes later. The likelihood is that, for the patient taking a leukotriene antagonist, EIA may still occur but for a shorter time o, it may be reduced to less than a 20% fall in FEV$_1$, a situation when symptoms are less readily perceived. The protective effect of these drugs against EIA is reported to be about 38%.

Non-Pharmacological Methods to Prevent EIA

Changing Inspired Air Conditions When it was realized that EIA could be prevented, or markedly reduced, by having the patient inhale air of alveolar conditions, i.e. 34–37°C and 100% humidity,[10,14,15,26] attention was given to techniques and devices that could reduce respiratory water loss and thus the severity of EIA. A number of masks and re-breathing devices were designed and shown to reduce the severity of EIA.[100–102] These devices simply allow some of the heat and water lost during expiration to be re-breathed during inspiration. However we have found that patients are unwilling to use them regularly or in public. A similar beneficial effect on EIA can be had by nose,[103] however the nasal mucosa can also respond to evaporative water loss with an increase in nasal resistance.[104]

Physical Training Because exercise is a potent stimulus for provoking an attack of asthma it is often avoided by asthmatics.[105] However there are many physical and social benefits in exercising regularly and asthmatics should be encouraged to be physically active. This can be achieved easily by using the appropriate medication before exercise. Asthmatics should also be encouraged to improve their cardiovascular fitness in order to reduce the ventilation rate required for a particular exercise intensity.[106,107]

Programs have been designed to evaluate the effects of physical training on EIA. The investigators have all concluded that there are definite social benefits to be had from physical training[108] but the results in terms of effect on EIA have been inconsistent. For example, some investigators[109–111] found exercise tolerance improved after training when exercise intensity was increased after training, but there was no reduction in severity of EIA. By contrast other investigators[112–114] found both an improvement in exercise tolerance and a reduction in EIA. No change in lung function was found[112] and medication was used to prevent EIA during training.

Physical training has the potential to benefit those who are unfit by raising the intensity of exercise at which EIA occurs. However training in those who are already fit is likely to have little or no effect. It should also be kept in mind that ventilating large volumes of dry and cool air may have a detrimental effect on resting airway calibre[114–115] as a result of dehydration.[28,29] This may be the reason that there is a high prevalence of bronchial responsiveness to exercise in trained athletes.[5,116]

Warm-Up and EIA

This is also an area of research that has not brought consistent results. The work of Morton and colleagues in the 1970s[117–118] demonstrated that warm-up of various duration was without effect in preventing EIA. However in 1980 Schnall and Landau[119] reported that multiple sprints of 30 seconds duration, 30 minutes before exercise, did reduce the severity of EIA. This has been confirmed for suboptimal exercise performed for 20 minutes, some half an hour before exercise challenge[120] or for 15 minutes immediately before exercise.[121] It may be that findings on the effect of warm-up were variable because of differences in its intensity and duration used by different investigators. The mechanism whereby warm-up can lead to a reduction in EIA is not clear. It may relate to an increase in bronchial blood flow, and thus an increase in delivery of water to the airways, thus reducing the rate of dehydration.

Air Pollution and EIA

It has been reported that the severity of EIA is enhanced when the inspired air contains sulphur dioxide or other air pollutants.[122] The reason for this may relate to the interactive effects between airway drying and sulphur dioxide, particularly on sensory nerves. It does not appear to relate to the higher doses of sulphur dioxide given as a result of the hyperpnoea of exercise.[122] Pre-exposure to low levels of ozone (0.025 ppm) prior to exercise does not enhance responsiveness to exercise.[123,124] It would seem however sensible to advise asthmatics not to exercise heavily during high pollution days.

Vocal Cord Dysfunction and EIA

There have been several recent reports on vocal cord dysfunction occurring in patients, usually elite athletes, who present with a "history" of EIA.[125,126] The failure to demonstrate EIA in the laboratory or have the patient's symptoms relieved by medication taken in the field should alert the physician to the possibility that symptoms are due to extra-thoracic airway obstruction such as vocal cord dysfunction. This obstruction can be identified by measuring a reduction in inspiratory flow at the time of symptoms. If the symptoms are not provoked by exercise, eucapnic hyperventilation with dry air for 6 minutes at maximum ventilation can be tried.

Hyperosmolar Challenge to Identify EIA

Since the evaporative water loss may increase airway osmolarity and lead to EIA[18] many investigators have compared the responses to hyperosmolar challenge and exercise in the same subjects.[12,127–130] These studies demonstrate that persons with EIA can be identified using hyperosmolar challenge (Fig. 36.7) and that sensitivity to the two challenges is similar. There are other similarities between challenge with hyperosmolar agents and exercise including the profile of mediators released and cross refractoriness.[130] These findings suggest that this relatively inexpensive technique to identify EIA may become more widely used.

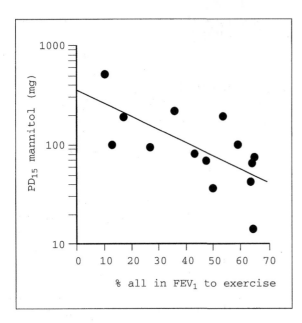

FIGURE 36.7: Individual values for percentage fall in FEV_1 after exercise in relation to the dose of mannitol required to provoke a 15% fall in FEV_1 in asthmatic subjects not taking steroids. (Brannan et al.[12], Official Jounal of the American Thoracic Association. ©American Lung Association.)

REFERENCES

1. Anderson SD. Exercise-induced asthma. In: Kay AB (ed). *Allergy and Allergic Diseases.* 692–711. Oxford: Blackwell Scientific Publications, 1997: 692–711.

2. ✪ Haby MM, Peat JK, Mellis CM, Anderson SD, Woolcock AJ. An exercise challenge for epidemiological studies of childhood asthma: validity and repeatability. *Eur Respir J* 1995; 8: 729–36.

3. Nish WA, Schwietz LA. Underdiagnosis of asthma in young adults presenting for USAF basis training. *Ann Allergy* 1992; 69: 239–42.

4. O'Donnell AE, Fling J. Exercise-induced airflow obstruction in a healthy military population. *Chest* 1993; 103: 742–4.

5. Rupp NT, Brudno S, Guill MF. The value of screening for risk of exercise-induced asthma in high school athletes. *Ann Allergy* 1993; 70: 332–339.

6. Mannix ET, Farber MO, Palange P, Galassetti P, Manfredi F. Exercise-induced asthma in figure skaters. *Chest* 1996; 109: 312–15.

7. Anderson SD, Henriksen J. Management of exercise-induced asthma. In: Carlsen K-H, Ibsen TB (eds). *Exercise-Induced Asthma and Sports in Asthma.* Copenhagen: Munksgaard Press, 1999: 99–108.

8. Anderson SD, Silverman M, Konig P, GodFrey S. Exercise-induced asthma. A Review. *Br J Dis Chest* 1975; 69: 1–39.

9. Deal EC, McFadden ER, Ingram RH, Jaeger JJ. Hyperpnea and heat flux: initial reaction sequence in exercise-induced asthma. *J Appl Physiol: Respirat Environ Exercise Physiol* 1979; 46: 476–83.

10. Strauss RH, McFadden ER, Ingram RH, Deal EC, Jaegar JJ, Stearns D. Influence of heat and humidity on the airway obstruction induced by exercise in asthma. *J Clin Invest* 1978; 61: 433–40.

11. ✪ Argyros GJ, Roach JM, Hurwitz KM, Eliasson AH, Phillips YY. Eucapnic voluntary hyperventilation as a bronchoprovocation technique. Development of a standardized dosing schedule in asthmatics. *Chest* 1996; 109: 1520–24.

12. ✪ Brannan JD, Koskela H, Anderson SD, Chew N. Responsiveness to mannitol in asthmatic subjects with exercise- and hyperventilation-induced asthma. *Am J Respir Crit Care Med* 1998; 158: 1120–26.

13. Hurwitz KM, Roach JM, Eliasson AH, Phillips YY. Interpretation of eucapnic voluntary hyperventilation in the diagnosis of asthma. *Chest* 1995; 108: 1240–45.

14. Chen WY, Horton DJ. Heat and water loss from the airways and exercise-induced asthma. *Respiration* 1977; 34: 305–13.

15. Bar-Or O, Neuman I, Dotan R. Effects of dry and humid climates on exercise-induced asthma in children and preadolescents. *J Allergy Clin Immunol* 1977; 60: 163–8.

16. McFadden ER, Lenner KA, Strohl KP. Postexertional airway rewarming and thermally induced asthma. *J Clin Invest* 1986; 78: 18–25.

17. Gilbert IA, McFadden ER. Airway cooling and rewarming. The second reaction sequence in exercise-induced asthma. *J Clin Invest* 1992; 90: 699–704.

18. Anderson SD. Is there a unifying hypothesis for exercise-induced asthma? *J Allergy Clin Immunol* 1984; 73: 660–65.

19. Godfrey S. Exercise-induced asthma. In: Barnes PJ, Grunstein MM, Leff AR, Woolcock AJ (eds). *Asthma*. Philadelphia: Lippencott-Raven, 1997: 1105–1120.

20. Anderson SD, Daviskas E. The airway microvasculature and exercise-induced asthma. *Thorax* 1992; 47: 748–52.

21. Anderson SD, Daviskas E. An evaluation of the airway cooling and rewarming hypothesis as the mechanism for exercise induced asthma. In: Holgate S, Kay AB, Lichtenstein L, Austen F (eds). *Asthma: Physiology, Immunopharmacology, and Treatment. 4th International Symposium*. London: Academic Press, 1993: 323–35.

22. Deal EC, McFadden ER, Ingram RH, Strauss RH, Jaeger JJ. Role of respiratory heat exchange in production of exercise-induced asthma. *J Appl Physiol Respir Environ Exercise Physiol* 1979; 46: 467–75.

23. Hahn A, Anderson SD, Morton AR, Black JL, Fitch KD. A re-interpretation of the effect of temperature and water content of the inspired air in exercise-induced asthma. *Am Rev Respir Dis* 1984; 130: 575–9.

24. Anderson SD, Schoeffel RE, Black JL, Daviskas E. Airway cooling as the stimulus to exercise-induced asthma–a re-evaluation. *Eur J Respir Dis* 1985; 67: 20–30.

25. Argyros GJ, Phillips YY, Rayburn DB, Rosenthal RR, Jaeger JJ. Water loss without heat flux in exercise-induced bronchospasm. *Am Rev Respir Dis* 1993; 147: 1419–24.

26. Anderson SD, Schoeffel RE, Follet R, Perry CP, Daviskas E, Kendall M. Sensitivity to heat and water loss at rest and during exercise in asthmatic patients. *Eur J Respir Dis* 1982; 63: 459–71.

27. Anderson SD, Daviskas E, Smith CM. Exercise-induced asthma: a difference in opinion regarding the stimulus. *Allergy Proc* 1989; 10: 215–26.

28. Anderson SD, Daviskas E. Pathophysiology of exercise-induced asthma: role of respiratory water loss. In: Weiler J (ed). *Allergic and Respiratory Disease in Sports Medicine*. New York: Marcel Dekker, 1997: 87–114.

29. Anderson SD, Daviskas E. Airway drying and exercise induced asthma. In: McFadden ER (ed). *Exercise Induced Asthma*. New York: Marcel Dekker, 1999: 77–113.

30. Anderson SD. Inflammatory mediators and exercise-induced asthma Chapter 37. In: Holgate ST, Busse WW (eds). *Inflammatory Mechanisms in Asthma*. New York: Marcel Dekker, 1998.

31. Anderson SD, Bye PTP, Schoeffel RE, Seale JP, Taylor KM, Ferris L. Arterial plasma histamine levels at rest, during and after exercise in patients with asthma: Effects of terbutaline aerosol. *Thorax* 1981; 36: 259–67.

32. Pliss LB, Ingenito EP, Ingram RH, Pichurko B. Assessment of bronchoalveolar cell and mediator response to isocapnic hyperpnea in asthma. *Am Rev Respir Dis* 1990; 142: 73–8.

33. ✪ O'Sullivan S, Roquet A, Dahlen B *et al*. Evidence for mast cell activation during exercise-induced bronchoconstriction. *Eur Respir J* 1998; 12: 345–50.

34. Nagakura T, Obata T, Shichijo K *et al*. GC/MS analysis of urinary excretion of 9alpha, 11beta-PGF2 in acute and exercise-induced asthma in children. *Clin Exp Allergy* 1998; 28 (2): 181–6.

35. Patel KR. Terfenadine in exercise-induced asthma. *BMJ* 1984; 85: 1496–7.

36. Finnerty JP, Holgate ST. Evidence for the roles of histamine and prostaglandins as mediators in exercise-induced asthma: the inhibitory effect of terfenadine and flurbiprofen alone and in combination. *Eur Respir J* 1990; 3: 540–47.

37. ✪ Manning PJ, Watson RM, Margolskee DJ, Williams VC, Schwartz JI, O'Byrne PM. Inhibition of exercise-induced bronchoconstriction by MK-571, a potent

leukiotriene D4-receptor antagonist. *N Engl J Med* 1990; 323: 1736–9.

38. Robuschi M, Riva E, Fuccella LM *et al*. Prevention of exercise-induced bronchoconstriction by a new leukotriene antagonist (SK & F 104353): a double-blind study versus disodium cromoglycate and placebo. *Am Rev Respir Dis* 1992; 45: 1285–8.

39. Finnerty JP, Wood-Baker R, Thomson H, Holgate S. Role of leukotrienes in exercise-induced asthma. Inhibitory effect of ICI 204219, a potent leukotriene D$_4$ receptor antagonist. *Am Rev Respir Dis* 1992; 145: 746–9.

40. ❂ Leff JA, Busse WW, Pearlman D *et al*. Montelukast, a leukotriene-receptor antagonist, for the treatment of mild asthma and exercise-induced bronchoconstriction. *N Engl J Med* 1998; 339 (3): 147–52.

41. Banner AS, Green J, O'Connor M. Relation of respiratory water loss to coughing after exercise. *N Engl J Med* 1984; 311: 883–6.

42. Katz RM, Siegel SC, Rachelefsky GS. Chronic cough in athletes. *Clin Rev Allergy* 1988; 6: 431–41.

43. Drobnic F, Casan P, Banquells M, Miralda R, Sanchis J. Cough after exercise in the elite athlete. *Sports Med Training Rehab* 1996; 6: 309–315.

44. Folgering H, Palange P, Anderson S. Clinical exercise testing with reference to lung diseases: indications and protocols. *Eur Respir Mon* 1997; 6: 51–71.

45. Argyros GJ, Roach JM, Hurwitz KM, Eliasson AH, Phillips YY. The refractory period after eucapnic voluntary hyperventilation challenge and its effect on challenge technique. *Chest* 1995; 108: 419–24.

46. Koskela HO, Räsänen SH, Tukiainen HO. The diagnostic value of cold air hyperventilation in adults with suspected asthma. *Respir Med* 1997; 91 (8): 470–78.

47. Anderson SD, Rodwell LT, Du Toit J, Young IH. Duration of protection of inhaled salmeterol in exercise-induced asthma. *Chest* 1991; 100: 1254–60.

48. O'Cain CF, Dowling NB, Slutsky AS *et al*. Airway effects of respiratory heat loss in normal subjects. *J Appl Physiol Respir Environ Exercise Physiol* 1980; 49: 875–80.

49. Anderson SD, Morton AR, Lambert S, Brannan JD, Briggs M. Comparison of the bronchoprotective effect of single doses of Albuterol administered by Diskus dry powder inhaler and by metered dose inhaler against exercise-induced bronchoconstriction. *Am J Respir Crit Care Med* 1999; 153: A879.

50. Henriksen JM, Dahl R. Effects of inhaled budesonide alone and in combination with low-dose terbutaline in children with exercise-induced asthma. *Am Rev Respir Dis* 1983; 128: 993–7.

51. ❂ Waalkans HJ, van Essen-Zandvliet EEM, Gerritsen J *et al*. The effect of an inhaled corticosteroid (budesonide) on exercise-induced asthma in children. *Eur Respir J* 1993; 6: 652–6.

52. Rundell KW, Wilbur RL, Szmedra L, Jenkinson DM, Mayers LB, Im J. Excercise-induced asthma screening of elite athletes: field versus laboratory exercise challenge. *Medicine and Science in Sports and Exercise* 2000; 32: 309–316.

53. Freeman W, Weir DC, Sapiano SB, Whitehead JE, Burge PS, Cayton RM. The twenty-metre shuttle-running test: a combined test for maximal oxygen uptake and exercise-induced asthma? *Respir Med* 1990; 84: 31–5.

54. Haby MM, Anderson SD, Peat JK, Mellis CM, Toelle BG, Woolcock AJ. An exercise challenge protocol for epidemiological studies of asthma in children: comparison with histamine challenge. *Eur Respir J* 1994; 7: 43–9.

55. Anderson SD, Mellis CM. Clinical presentation and ongoing clinical and physiological assessment of asthma in children. Taussig L, Landau LI (eds). *Pediatric Respiratory Medicine*. New York: Mosby 1998: 938–60.

56. Silverman M, Anderson SD. Metabolic cost of treadmill exercise in children. *J Appl Physiol* 1972; 33: 696–8.

57. Givoni B, Goldman RF. Predicting metabolic energy cost. *J Appl Physiol* 1971; 30: 429–33.

58. Anderson SD, Silverman M, Walker SR. Metabolic and ventilatory changes in asthmatic patients during and after exercise. *Thorax* 1972; 27: 718–25.

59. Anderson SD, McEvoy JDS, Bianco S. Changes in lung volumes and airway resistance after exercise in asthmatic subjects. *Am Rev Respir Dis* 1972; 106: 30–37.

60. Freelander M, Van Asperen PP. Nebuhaler versus nebuliser in children with acute asthma. *BMJ* 1984; 288: 873–4.

61. Anderson SD. Exercise-induced asthma. The state of the art. *Chest* 1985; 87S: 191S–195S.

62. O'Byrne PM, Jones GL. The effect of indomethacin on exercise-induced bronchoconstriction and refractoriness after exercise. *Am Rev Respir Dis* 1986; 134: 69–72.

63. Comis A, Valletta EA, Sette L, Andreoli A, Boner AL. Comparison of nedocromil sodium and sodium cromoglycate administered by pressurized aerosol, with and without a spacer device in exercise-induced asthma in children. *Eur Respir J* 1993; 6: 523–6.

64. Spooner CH, Saunders LD, Rowe BH. Nedocromil sodium as single dose prophylactic treatment of exercise-induced bronchoconstriction. Oxford: Update Software, 1998. The Cochrane Library; vol 3.

65. Sears M. Asthma treatment: inhaled beta-agonists. *Can Respir J* 1998; Jul–Aug; 5 (suppl. A): 54A–59A.

66. Inman MD, O'Byrne PM. The effect of regular inhaled albuterol on exercise-induced bronchoconstriction. *Am J Respir Crit Care Med* 1996; 153: 65–9.

67. Grove A, Lipworth BJ. Bronchodilator subsenstivity to salbutamol after twice daily salmeterol in asthmatic patients. *Lancet* 1995; 346: 201–206.

68. Hancox RJ, Aldridge RE, Cowan JO *et al.* Tolerance to beta-agonists during acute bronchoconstriction. *Eur Respir J* 1999; 14: 283–7.

69. Newnham DM, Ingram CG, Earnshaw J, Palmer JBD, Dhillon DP. Salmeterol provides prolonged protection against exercise-induced bronchoconstriction in a majority of subjects with mild, stable asthma. *Respir Med* 1993; 87: 439–44.

70. Kemp JP, Dockhorn RJ, Busse WW, Bleecker ER. Prolonged effect of inhaled salmeterol against exercise-induced bronchospasm. *Am J Respir Crit Care Med* 1994; 150: 1612–15.

71. Patessio A, Podda A, Carone M, Trombetta N, Donner CF. Protective effect and duration of action of formoterol aerosol on exercise-induced asthma. *Eur Respir J* 1991; 4: 296–300.

72. Henriksen JM, Agertoft L, Pedersen S. Protective effect and duration of action of inhaled formoterol and salbutamol on exercise-induced asthma in children. *J Allergy Clin Immunol* 1992; 89: 1176–82.

73. Bronsky E, Yegen U, Yeh CM, Cioppa GD, Larsen L. Foradil provides rapid and long acting protection against exercise-induced bronchospasm. *Am J Respir Crit Care Med* 1997; 155: A964.

74. ✪ Ramage L, Lipworth BJ, Ingram CG, Cree IA, Dhillion DP. Reduced protection against exercise induced bronchoconstriction after chronic dosing with salmeterol. *Respir Med* 1994; 88: 363–8.

75. Simons FE, Gerstner TV, Cheang MS. Tolerance to the bronchoprotective effect of salmeterol in adolescents with exercise-induced asthma using concurrent inhaled glucocorticoid treatment. *Pediatrics* 1997; 99 (5): 655–9.

76. ✪ Nelson JA, Strauss L, Skowronshi M, Ciufo R, Novak R, McFadden ER. Effect of long-term salmeterol treatment on exercise-induced asthma. *N Engl J Med* 1998; 339 (3): 141–6.

77. Anderson SD, Seale JP, Rozea P, Bandler L, Theobald G, Lindsay DA. Inhaled and oral salbutamol in exercise-induced asthma. *Am Rev Respir Dis* 1976; 114: 493–500.

78. Laursen LC, Johannesson N, Weeke B. Effects of enprophylline and theophylline on exercise-induced asthma. *Allergy* 1985; 40: 506–509.

79. Fuglsang G, Hertz B, Holm E-B. No protection by oral terbutaline against exercise-induced asthma in children: a dose-response study. *Eur Respir J* 1993; 6: 527–30.

80. Tullett WM, Tan KM, Wall RT, Patel KR. Dose-response effect of sodium cromoglycate pressurised aerosol in exercise induced asthma. *Thorax* 1985; 40: 41–4.

81. Patel KR, Wall RT. Dose-duration effect of sodium cromoglycate aerosol in exercise-induced asthma. *Eur J Respir Dis* 1986; 69: 256–60.

82. Koenig P, Hordvik NL, Kreutz C. The preventative effect and duration of action of nedocromil sodium and cromolyn sodium on exercise-induced asthma (EIA) in adults. *J Allergy Clin Immunol* 1987; 79: 64–8.

83. Albbazzaz MK, Neale MG, Patel KR. Dose-response study of nebulised nedocromil sodium in exercise induced asthma. *Thorax* 1989; 44: 816–19.

84. Bernstein JA, Bernstein IL. Cromones. In: Barnes PJ, Grunstein MM, Leff AR, Woolcock AJ (eds). *Asthma*. Philadelphia: Lippincott-Raven, 1997: Vol. 2, 1647–65.

85. Anderson SD, Rodwell LT, Daviskas E, Spring JF, du Toit J. The protective effect of nedocromil sodium and other drugs on airway narrowing provoked by hyperosmolar stimuli: A role for the airway epithelium. *J Allergy Clin Immunol* 1996; 98 (5 Part 2 suppl. S): S124–134S.

86. Laitinen LA, Laitinen A, Haahtela T. Airway mucosal inflammation even in patients with newly diagnosed asthma. *Am Rev Respir Dis* 1993; 147: 697–704.

87. Henriksen JM. Effect of inhalation of corticosteroids on exercise induced asthma: randomised double blind crossover study of budesonide in asthmatic children. *BMJ* 1985; 291: 248–9.

88. Thio BJ, Slingerland GLM, Nagelkerke AF, Dankert-Roelse JE. Single high dose inhaled fluticasone propionate (FP) reduces exercise induced bronchial obstruction. *Am J Respir Crit Care Med* 1998; 157: A710.

89. Vathenen AS, Knox AJ, Wisniewski A, Tattersfield AE. Effect of inhaled budesonide on bronchial reactivity to histamine, exercise, and eucapnic dry air hyperventilation in patients with asthma. *Thorax* 1991; 46: 811–16.

90. Papalia SM. *Aspects of inhaled budesonide use in asthma and exercise*. PhD Thesis. Perth: University of Western Australia, 1997: 1–185.

91. ✪ Pedersen S, Hansen OR. Budesonide treatment of moderate and severe asthma in children: a dose-response study. *J Allergy Clin Immunol* 1995; 95 (1 Pt 1): 29–33.

92. Adelroth E, Inman MD, Summers E, Pace D, Modi M, O'Byrne PM. Prolonged protection against exercise-induced bronchoconstriction by the leukotriene D4-receptor antagonist cinalukast. *J Allergy Clin Immunol* 1997; 99 (2): 210–215.

93. Reiss TF, Hill JB, Harman E *et al*. Increased urinary excretion of LTE4 after exercise and attenuation of exercise-induced bronchospasm by montelukast, a cysteinyl leukotriene receptor antagonist. *Thorax* 1997; 52 (12): 1030–35.

94. Meltzer SS, Hasday JD, Cohn J, Bleecker ER. Inhibition of exercise-induced bronchospasm by zileuton: a 5-lipoxygenase inhibitor. *Am J Respir Crit Care Med* 1996; 153 (3): 931–5.

95. Lehnigk B, Rabe KF, Dent G, Herst RS, Carpentier PJ, Magnussen H. Effects of a 5-lipoxygenase inhibitor, ABT-761, on exercise-induced bronchoconstriction and urinary LTE$_4$ in asthmatic patients. *Eur Respir J* 1998; 11: 617–23.

96. Villarin C, O'Neill S, Helbing A *et al*. Montelukast versus salmeterol in patients with asthma and exercise-induced bronchoconstriction. *J. Allergy Clin Immunol* 1999; 104: 547–53.

97. Godfrey S, Springer C, Noviski N, Maayan C, Avital A. Exercise but not methacholine differentiates asthma from chronic lung disease in children. *Thorax* 1991; 46: 488–92.

98. Backer V, Ulrik CS. Bronchial responsiveness to exercise in a random sample of 494 children and adolescents from Copenhagen. *Clin Exp Allergy* 1992; 22: 741–7.

99. Weiss JW, Rossing TH, McFadden ER, Ingram RH. Relationship between bronchial responsiveness to hyperventilation with cold air and methacholine in asthma. *J Allergy Clin Immunol* 1983; 72: 140–44.

100. Gravelyn TR, Capper M, Eschenbacher WL. Effectiveness of a heat and moisture exchanger in preventing hyperpnoea induced bronchoconstriction in subjects with asthma. *Thorax* 1987; 42: 877–80.

101. Millqvist E, Bake B, Bengtsson U, Lowhagen O. A breathing filter exchanging heat and moisture prevents asthma induced by cold air. *Allergy* 1995; 50: 225–8.

102. Nisar M, Spence DPS, West D *et al*. A mask to modify inspired air temperature and humidity and its effect on exercise induced asthma. *Thorax* 1992; 47: 446–50.

103. Mangla PK, Menon MPS. Effect of nasal and oral breathing on exercise-induced asthma. *Clin Allergy* 1981; 11: 433–9.

104. Anderson SD, Togias A. Dry air and hyperosmolar challenge in asthma and rhinitis. In: Busse WW, Holgate ST (eds). *Asthma and Rhinitis*. Boston: Blackwell Scientific Publications, 1994: 1178–95.

105. Carlsen K-H, Boe J. Exercise-induced asthma in children. *Eur Respir J* 1993; 6: 614–16.

106. Cochrane LM, Clark CJ. Benefits and problems of a physical training programme for asthmatic patients. *Thorax* 1990; 45: 345–51.

107. Varray A, Mercier J, Savy-Pacaux A-M, Préfaut C. Cardiac role in exercise limitation in asthmatic subjects with special reference to disease severity. *Eur Respir J* 1993; 6: 1011–17.

108. Emtner M, Herala M, Stålenheim G. High-intensity physical training in adults with asthma. *Chest* 1996; 109: 323–30.

109. Fitch KD, Blitvich JD, Morton AR. The effect of running training on exercise-induced asthma. *Ann Allergy* 1986; 7: 90–94.

110. Nickerson BG, Bautista DB, Naney MA, Richards W, Keens TG. Distance running improves fitness in asthmatic children without pulmonary complications of changes in exercise-induced bronchospasm. *Pediatrics* 1983; 71: 147–52.

111. Bundgaard A, Ingemann-Hansen T, Schmidt A, Halkjaer-Kristensen J. Effect of physical training on peak oxygen consumption rate and exercise-induced asthma in adult asthmatics. *Scand J Clin Lab Invest* 1982; 42: 9–13.

112. Henriksen JM, Nielsen TT. Effect of physical training on exercise-induced bronchoconstriction. *Acta Paediatr Scand* 1983; 72: 31–6.

113. Svenonius E, Kautto R, Arborelius M. Improvement after training of children with exercise-induced asthma. *Acta Paediatr Scand* 1983; 72: 23–30.

114. Haas F, Pasierski S, Levine N *et al.* Effect of aerobic training on forced expiratory airflow in exercising asthmatic humans. *J Appl Physiol* 1987; 63: 1230–35.

115. Schaefer O, Eaton RDP, Timmermans FJW, Hildes JA. Respiratory function impairment and cardiopulmonary consequences in long-term residents of the Canadian Arctic. *Canadian Med Assoc J* 1980; 123: 997–1004.

116. Tikkanen HO, Helenius I, Haahtela T. Prevalence of asthma and allergy in track and field athletes and swimmers in Finland. In: Carlsen K-H, Ibsen TB (eds). *Exercise-Induced Asthma and Sports in Asthma*. Copenhagen: Munksgaards, 1999: 57–60.

117. Morton AR, Fitch KD, Davis T. The effect of "warm-up" on exercise-induced asthma. *Ann Allergy* 1979; 42: 257–60.

118. Morton AR, Hahn AG, Fitch KD. Continuous and intermittent running in the provocation of asthma. *Ann Allergy* 1982; 48: 123–9.

119. Schnall RP, Landau LI. Protective effects of repeated short sprints in exercise-induced asthma. *Thorax* 1980; 35: 828–32.

120. Reiff DB, Choudry NB, Pride NB, Ind PW. The effect of prolonged submaximal warm-up exercise on exercise-induced asthma. *Am Rev Respir Dis* 1989; 139: 479–84.

121. McKenzie DC, McLuckie SL, Stirling DR. The protective effects of continuous and interval exercise in athletes with exercise-induced asthma. *Med Sci Sports Exerc* 1994; 26(8): 951–6.

122. Lin WS, Shamoo DA, Anderson KR, Whynot SD, Avol EL, Hackney JD. Effects of heat and humidity on the responses of exercising asthmatics to sulphur dioxide exposure. *Am Rev Respir Dis* 1985; 131: 221–5.

123. Weymer AR, Gong J, Lyness A, Linn WS. Pre-exposure to ozone does not enhance or produce exercise-induced asthma. *Am J Respir Crit Care Med* 1994; 149: 1413–19.

124. Fernandes AL, Molfino NA, McClean PA *et al.* The effect of pre-exposure to 0.12 ppm of ozone on exercise-induced asthma. *Chest* 1994; 106(4): 1077–82.

125. McFadden ER, Zawadski DK. Vocal cord dysfunction masquerading as exercise-induced asthma. A physiologic cause for "choking" during athletic activities. *Am J Respir Crit Care Med* 1996; 153: 942–7.

126. Landwehr LP, Wood RP, Blager FB, Milgrom H. Vocal cord dysfunction mimicking exercise-induced bronchospasm in adolescents. *Pediatrics* 1996; 98 (5): 971–4.

127. Smith CM, Anderson SD. Inhalational challenge using hypertonic saline in asthmatic subjects: a

comparison with responses to hyperpnoea, methacholine, and water. *Eur Respir J* 1990; 3: 144–51.

128. Belcher NG, Lee TH, Rees PJ. Airway responses to hypertonic saline, exercise and histamine challenges in bronchial asthma. *Eur Respir J* 1989; 2: 44–8.

129. Boulet LP. Comparative effects of hyperosmolar saline inhalation and exercise in asthma. *Immunol Allergy Practice* 1989; 11: 93–100.

130. Anderson SD. Asthma provoked by exercise, hyperventilation, and the inhalation of non-isotonic aerosols. In: Barnes P, Rodger I, Thomson NC (eds). *Asthma: Basic Mechanisms and Clinical Management*, 3rd *edn*. London: Academic Press, 1998; 569–88.

Chapter 37

Specific Problems: Nocturnal Asthma

Richard Martin

INTRODUCTION

To fully understand asthma, it is important for the clinician to know about alterations which occur on a circadian (24-hour cycle) basis. There are several important reasons for this concept. Symptoms of obstructive lung disease, independent of medication, occur more commonly during the sleep-related time interval with the peak at approximately 4.00 a.m.[1] Additionally, Turner-Warwick has shown in a large population study that "stable" asthmatic outpatients, when specifically asked, have frequent problems with their asthma at night.[2] Thirty-nine percent of these patients are symptomatic every night of the week, 64% three nights per week, and 74% have difficulty at least one night a week.

Does this high frequency of nocturnal problems translate into anything more than a simple nuisance? Fitzpatrick and colleagues have shown that these patients have poorer daytime cognitive function than a matched control population.[3] Thus, asthmatic children with nocturnal worsening of their disease would tend to perform at a lower level in school, and similarly adults may not function up to their capacity at work. Furthermore, asthma morbidity (respiratory arrests) and mortality have the greatest occurrence during the sleeping hours.[4,5] Recent statistics show a worldwide trend for increased asthma mortality, and those studies which analyse time of death have shown the majority of cases to occur at night.[6,7] This figure is probably low as the death may occur during the day, but the process begins or accelerates during the night. Thus to understand and control the nocturnal worsening of asthma, in reality, will improve asthma over the 24-hour cycle.

ASSESSMENT

Assessment of an asthmatic patient for nocturnal asthma is, fortunately, relatively easy. However, one must always keep in mind other diseases that can mimic asthma. As an example, with the increasing prevalence of asthma in the geriatric population, cardiac problems must be differentiated in this specific asthmatic population. In fact, cardiac function normally decreases at night which in a patient with compromised cardiac function can lead to nocturnal heart failure. This cardiac decompensation can present as nocturnal "wheezing" which can be confused with asthma. Additionally, intermittent recurrent small pulmonary emboli can present with nocturnal problems in the older population. Other types of obstructive lung diseases, e.g. chronic obstructive pulmonary disease (COPD), all have the potential to worsen during the night and give symptoms similar to asthma. One must keep in mind that most if not all disease processes have the potential for circadian alterations with symptoms and signs worse at night. This would be true for all age groups. If that particular disease process affects the upper (such as allergic rhinitis) or lower airways, symptoms may mistakenly be confused with nocturnal asthma.

Objectively measuring lung function is important in determining the severity of nocturnal asthma. The peak flow meter is relatively inexpensive and gives the patient and physician an accurate objective assessment of alterations in lung function that may occur overnight. This objectivity has an added benefit in that it allows the patient to become more "aware" of changes in lung function and thus more "in tune" with his/her asthma. This subject awareness of asthma, particularly at night, is important. Turner-Warwick's study[2] showed that less than 50% of asthmatic patients with problems every night of the week considered their asthma to be severe. The majority considered their asthma to be mild or moderate. Many patients become "used to" the bronchoconstriction and incorporate this into their "normal" routine. Another group of asthmatic patients have a blunted perception of the degree of bronchoconstriction. Thus, objectivity (using peak flow measurements) is extremely helpful in evaluating nocturnal asthma. This has also been stressed in multiple, recent national and in an international asthma guidelines report.[8]

In a very small segment of the asthma population (exact percentage unknown), the patient only has asthma during sleep. Thus, daytime spirometry, response to inhaled bronchodilators, and even airway responsiveness (response to agents that produce bronchoconstriction) may be relatively normal and cast the diagnosis of asthma into doubt. Here the use of a peak flow meter at home will show the overnight changes in lung function if they are present. If further information about asthma in this situation is needed, methacholine challenge testing can be set up (with difficulty in most institutions) to be performed at 4.00 a.m. Airway responsiveness is much greater in nearly all asthmatics during the night[9] even if nocturnal worsening of expiratory flow rates is absent.

Thus, it is important for the physician to evaluate the asthmatic patient not only during the day but also during the night. In doing so the physician truly understands the patient's asthma and does not erroneously make assumptions of the clinical status on daytime measurements in the office. The effectiveness of any medical intervention can then also be determined in the home setting. In addition, the patient has an objective parameter to follow. This not only educates the patient to his/her disease, but also gradual impending problems can be noted earlier and more easily dealt with compared with delaying intervention to where the patient is eventually seen in the emergency room.

MANAGEMENT (Fig. 37.1)

To understand the management of nocturnal asthma, the clinician must realize that nocturnal asthma is a multifaceted process. Figure 37.2 shows the multiple factors which can interact in producing nocturnal asthma. The nocturnal decrement in cortisol, adrenaline, and body temperature and the increase in vagal

tone are actually normally occurring circadian rhythms. The increase in inflammation is specifically related to worsening of asthma at night. This indeed may occur due to the decrement in cortisol and adrenaline allowing the "brakes" to be released and nocturnal inflammation to develop in those individuals primed for this event.

Reversible Factors

Although most patients will not have easily identifiable extrinsic factors, these still should be considered. Even if the patient is asymptomatic during the daytime, causative agents at work or home may produce delayed effects and nocturnal asthma. Examples of work place factors are western red cedar[10] and grain dust exposure.[11] At home be certain the patient is not sleeping with the family dog or cat, a not uncommon occurrence in those households with pets.

Asthma is a disease of both intra- and extra-thoracic airways and sinusitis occurs in about 40–60% of all asthmatics. If aspiration of the sinus secretions occurs, this can worsen asthma. Correcting the sinusitis with nasal saline irrigation, oral decongestants and nasal steroids can improve nocturnal asthma in this subset of patients. Oral steroids and 3–4 weeks of antibiotics may be needed in severe cases of sinusitis. A sinus surgical procedure is rarely needed for control of sinusitis in asthma.

Gastroesophageal (GE) reflux in and of itself has not been proven to be an aetiologic factor in nocturnal asthma.[12] However, aspiration of reflux material may play an important and potentially correctable role in nocturnal asthma. The patient who complains of a bitter or sour taste upon arising may be the subset of reflux patients that aspirate during sleep. In this situation a trial of 4-inch wood or brick blocks under the head of the bed (raising the head with pillows will not work) and medication to increase gastric emptying (metaclopramide) would be indicated. Surgery to solidify the GE junction is rarely indicated, but should be considered if aspiration is documented and the above therapy is not of benefit.

Those asthmatic patients that have daytime hypersomnolence, loud snoring, increased irritability, restless sleep, hypertension, erythrocytosis or any of the other signs and symptoms of sleep apnoea should be evaluated for this possibility. Both adults and children with asthma and associated sleep apnoea can have significant worsening of their asthma at night.[13,14] Of inter-

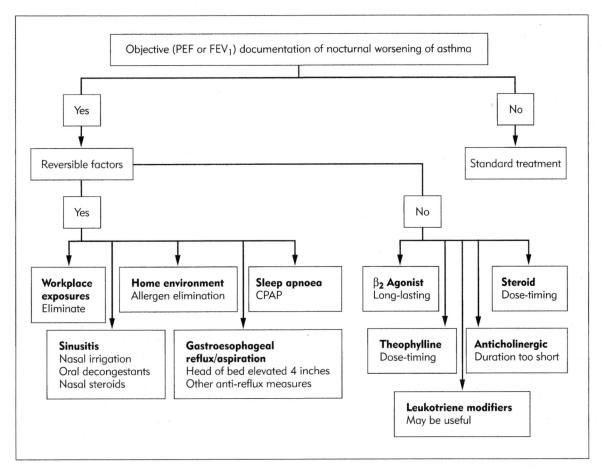

FIGURE 37.1: Algorithm for treatment of nocturnal asthma. (See the text for specific treatment.)

est, when the sleep apnoea is corrected, not only is the nocturnal asthma component improved but also the daytime asthma controlled. This suggests what many investigators have seen with asthma, i.e. control the night and the day will follow suit. There are many modes of therapy for sleep apnoea,[15] but nasal CPAP usually is the most successful.

β₂-Adrenergic Agonists

As longer acting β_2 agonists become available, particularly inhaled, the use of these agents may be of benefit in nocturnal asthma. Salmeterol, a long-acting β_2 agonist, has been shown to be of use in nocturnal asthma.[16] Doses of 50 and 100 μg inhaled twice daily overall improved the morning peak flow rates compared with placebo. Of interest, only the 50 μg dose objectively improved sleep quality. It appears that the higher dose of salmeterol produced a stimulating central nervous system effect. A study in more severe nocturnal asthma demonstrated that the bedtime and awakening lung function values were both increased, but the overnight fall remained the same.[17]

Theophyllines

Zwillich *et al.*[18] showed the superiority of a sustained release (12-hour) theophylline preparation (Theo-Dur) in treating asthmatic patients with mild-to-moderate nocturnal asthma compared with a shorter acting (8-hour duration) inhaled β_2 agonist (bitolterol, Tornalate). Not only was the FEV_1 improved in the morning, but there was less nocturnal oxygen desaturation while on theophylline. Importantly, sleep quality and architecture were unchanged between the different preparations, demonstrating that the presence of theophylline did not alter sleep compared with the β_2 agonist.

489

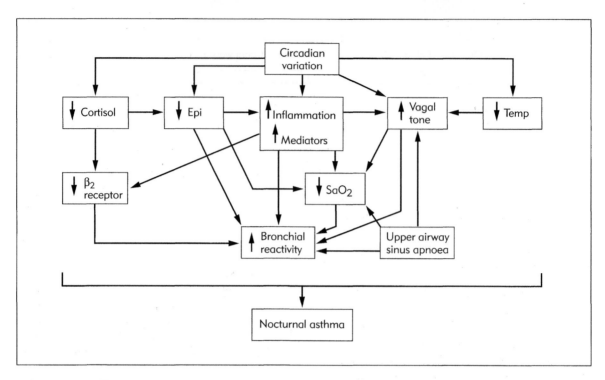

FIGURE 37.2: There are multiple and interactive factors which produce nocturnal worsening of asthma. (From Martin RJ. Nocturnal asthma: an overview. In: Martin RJ (ed). *Nocturnal Asthma: Mechanisms and Treatment*. New York: Futura Publishing, 1993: 101, with permission.)

In subjects with more significant nocturnal asthma, a chronotherapeutic approach is indicated. That is, obtaining higher serum theophylline concentrations (STC) during the night where the disease is the worst and lower STC during the daytime where it is easier to control the bronchoconstriction. Comparing two theophylline preparations with different pharmacokinetics, Martin et al.[19] showed that higher STC (about 15 µg ml^{-1}) from 3 to 5.00 a.m. produced a marked improvement in the overnight worsening of lung function versus lower therapeutic levels (about 11.5 µg ml^{-1}). During the daytime the agent that gave a higher nocturnal STC (Uniphyl, given once daily at 7.00 p.m.) will have a progressive decrease in the STC with a nadir of about 8 µg ml^{-1} before the next dose. The other agent (Theo-Dur) given twice a day had higher daytime STC levels compared with night-time. The FEV$_1$ levels measured every 2 hours during the daytime were not significantly different between the agents even though the STCs were different. This reinforces the importance of delivering higher concentrations of medica-

tion when most needed, i.e. at night. Furthermore, sleep quality and architecture were not altered between the higher and lower therapeutic STC, but there was less nocturnal oxygen desaturation with the higher levels. Many other studies using theophylline in a chronotherapeutic method have shown similar beneficial results.

It is of interest that many recent studies strongly suggest that theophylline has anti-inflammatory properties.[20–22] Inflammation is increased at night and the improvement in nocturnal asthma by theophylline has been linked to the decrease in leukotriene B$_4$ and granulocytes in the lung.[23]

Corticosteroids
Another example of chronotherapy is in the use of oral corticosteroids. If an asthma patient needs steroids, then every effort should be made to use inhaled steroids. However, inhaled steroids improve nocturnal asthma in only about 50% of patients if individual data and not group means are analysed. There are many

oral steroid-dependent asthmatic patients with nocturnal asthma. Commonly, increasing the morning steroid dosing in these individuals usually leads to more steroid complications without improvement in nighttime asthma control. Reinberg and colleagues[24,25] have suggested that the time of corticosteroid administration during the day may be relevant in attenuating the nocturnal worsening of asthma.

Beam *et al.*[26] have begun to clarify the contribution of timing of corticosteroids to their ability to block the circadian recruitment of inflammatory cells into the lung. The results of their data highlight the relevance of prednisone dose-timing in attenuating the nocturnal worsening of asthmatic lung function and decrement in airways inflammation. A 3.00 p.m. dose produced significant improvement in overnight FEV_1 (placebo control, $-28\% \pm 7\%$; steroid, $-10\% \pm 4\%$). Additionally, the 3.00 p.m. dose of prednisone produced a pancellular reduction in the 4.00 a.m. bronchoalveolar lavage cytology. Neither an 8.00 a.m. or 8.00 p.m. dose phase produced an improvement in overnight spirometry or reduction in any bronchoalveolar lavage cellular profile. It is noteworthy that Martin and colleagues[27] demonstrated elevations in total white cell number, neutrophil, eosinophil, and lymphocyte counts in the bronchoalveolar lavage fluid at 4.00 a.m. in nocturnal asthma subjects compared with 4.00 p.m. These observations support a collaborative cellular mechanism of inflammation at night that is corticosteroid sensitive, but dependent on timing in addition to dosage.

The use of inhaled steroids is of interest in patients with nocturnal asthma. One would think that these agents would be ideal for this problem. However, studies have given mixed results. Horn *et al.*[28] showed that in 14 asthmatic patients with nocturnal symptoms and morning decrease in peak flow, only eight patients resolved the nocturnal component using inhaled beclomethasone (also taking inhaled salbutamol). The dose of beclomethasone was higher than standard, 400 µg four times per day. Although the other six patients had improved daytime lung function, the overnight decrements in lung function did not improve. The question arises if there is also a dose-time for inhaled steroids that would work better in the treatment of nocturnal asthma.

Pincus and colleagues[29,30] clearly demonstrated in a general asthma population that 3.00 p.m. dosing of the entire daily dosage of an inhaled steroid is equiva-

lent in multiple outcome variables to a four times a day dosing schedule. Although total dosing at 8.00 a.m. does improve asthma, it is not as good as the four times a day schedule. Finally, 5.30 p.m. total dosage is better than 8.00 a.m., but it is not as good as the 3.00 p.m. or four times a day schedule. Thus even for inhaled steroids, timing is important.

Anticholinergics

Vagal tone is increased at night in everyone. This would suggest that a vagalytic would be of benefit in treating nocturnal asthma. Morrison and colleagues[31] have shown that atropine produces marked bronchodilatation at 4.00 a.m. compared with 4.00 p.m. Presently, an anticholinergic of long enough durations is not available for this form of therapy to work. Higher bedtime dosing compared with the usual daytime dosing is needed to lengthen the duration of effective action of the drug, but side-effects are then increased. If the patient wakes during the night, then inhalation of atropine or ipratropium bromide may be of benefit.

Leukotriene Modifiers

These new agents need extensive evaluation in regard to dose-timing and if the inflammatory response is truly altered during the night. However, in patients who are not responding well to the above described interventions, these agents can be tried. Following objective measurements such as peak flow rates and objective symptoms will allow the caregiver to determine the efficacy in individual patients.

CONCLUSION

As Eugene Robin stated 40 years ago, "the sleeping patient is still a patient. His disease not only goes on while he sleeps, but indeed may progress in an entirely different fashion from its progression during the waking state".[32] Today we can see how accurate that notion was, because any disease process of any organ system has the potential to worsen during sleep. To neglect this area of medicine hinders the care of the patient and accelerates the disease process. The future will bring tremendous advances to our understanding and ability to treat the nocturnal aspect of asthma and thus the disease itself.

REFERENCES

1. Dethlefsen U, Repgas R. Ein neues Therapieprinzip bei nachtlichen Asthma. *Klin Med* 1985; 80: 44–7.

2. Turner-Warwick M. Epidemiology of nocturnal asthma. *Am J Med* 1988; 85 (suppl. 1B): 6–8.

3. ✪ Fitzpatrick MF, Engelman H, Whyte KF, Deary IJ, Shapiro CM, Douglas NJ. Morbidity in nocturnal asthma: sleep quality and daytime cognitive performance. *Thorax* 1991; 46: 569–73.

4. Cochrane GM, Clark TJH. A survey of asthma mortality in patients between ages 35 and 65 in the greater London hospitals in 1971. *Thorax* 1975; 30: 300–315.

5. Hetzel MR, Clark TJH, Branthwaite MA. Asthma: analysis of sudden deaths and ventilatory arrest in hospital. *BMJ* 1977; 1: 808–811.

6. Jackson RT, Sears MR, Beaglehole R, Reatt H. International trends in asthma mortality; 1970–1985. *Chest* 1988; 94: 914–18.

7. Robertson CE, Rubinfeld AR, Bowej G. Deaths from asthma in Victoria: a 12-month study. *Med J Aust* 152: 511–17.

8. NHLBI-NIH. *International Consensus Report on Diagnosis and Treatment of Asthma*. Publication No. 91–3091, 1992.

9. Martin RJ, Cicutto LC, Ballard RD. Factors related to the nocturnal worsening of asthma. *Am Rev Respir Dis* 1990; 141: 33–8.

10. Gandevia B, Milne J. Occupational asthma and rhinitis due to western red cedar (*Thuja plicata*), with special reference to bronchial reactivity. *Br J Ind Med* 27: 235–44.

11. Davies RJ, Green M, Schofield N. Recurrent nocturnal asthma after exposure to grain dust. *Am Rev Respir Dis* 1976; 114: 1011–19.

12. Tan WC, Martin RJ, Pandey R *et al*. Effects of spontaneous and simulated gastroesophageal reflux on sleeping asthmatics. *Am Rev Respir Dis* 1990; 141: 1394–9.

13. Chan CS, Woolcock AJ, Sullivan CE. Nocturnal asthma: role of snoring and obstructive sleep apnea. *Am Rev Respir Dis* 1988; 137: 1502–1504.

14. Guilleminault C, Quera-Salva MA, Powell N *et al*. Nocturnal asthma: snoring, small pharynx and nasal CPAP. *Eur Respir J* 1988; 1: 902–907.

15. Sanders MH. The management of sleep-disordered breathing. In: Martin RJ (ed). *Cardiorespiratory Disorders During Sleep*. New York: Futura Publishing, 1990: 141–88.

16. Fitzpatrick MF, Mackay T, Driver H, Douglas NJ. Salmeterol in nocturnal asthma: a double blind, placebo controlled trial of a long acting inhaled β_2 agonist. *BMJ* 1990; 301: 1365–8.

17. ✪ Kraft M, Wenzel SE, Bettinger CM, Martin RJ. The effect of salmeterol on nocturnal symptoms, airway function, and inflammation in asthma. *Chest* 1997; 111: 1249–54.

18. Zwillich CW, Neagley SR, Cicutto L, White DP, Martin RJ. Nocturnal asthma therapy. *Am Rev Respir Dis* 1989; 139: 470–74.

19. Martin RJ, Cicutto LC, Ballard RD, Goldenheim PD, Cherniack RM. Circadian variations in theophylline concentrations and the treatment of nocturnal asthma. *Am Rev Respir Dis* 1989; 139: 475–8.

20. Ward AJ, McKenniff M, Evans JM, Page CP, Costello JF. Theophylline–an immunomodulatory role in asthma? *Am Rev Respir Dis* 147: 518–23.

21. Sullivan P, Bekir S, Jaffar Z, Page C, Jeffer P, Costello J. Antiinflammatory effects of low-dose oral theophylline in atopic asthma. *Lancet* 1994; 343: 1006–1008.

22. Kidney J, Dominguez M, Taylor PM, Rose M, Chung KF, Barnes PJ. Immunomodulation by theophylline in asthma. Demonstration by withdrawal of therapy. *Am J Respir Crit Care Med* 1995; 151: 1907–1914.

23. Kraft M, Torvik JA, Trudeau JB, Wenzel SE, Martin RJ. Theophylline: potential antiinflammatory effects in nocturnal asthma. *J Allergy Clin Immunol* 1996; 97: 1242–6.

24. Reinberg AE. Circadian timing of methylprednisolone effects in asthmatic boys. *Chronobiologia* 1974; 1: 333–47.

25. Reinberg A, Gervais P, Chaussade M, Fraboulet G, Duburque B. Circadian changes in effectiveness of corticosteroids in eight patients with allergic asthma. *J Allergy Clin Immunol* 1983; 71: 425–33.

26. ✪ Beam WR, Weiner DE, Martin RJ. Timing of prednisone and alterations of airways inflammation in nocturnal asthma. *Am Rev Respir Dis* 1992; 146: 1524–30.

27. Martin RJ, Cicutto LC, Ballard RD, Smith HR, Szefler SJ. Airways inflammation in nocturnal asthma. *Am Rev Respir Dis* 1991; 143: 351–7.

28. Horn CR, Clark TJH, Cochrance GM. Inhaled therapy reduces morning dips in asthma. *Lancet* 1984; 1: 1143–5.

29. ✪ Pincus DJ, Szefler SJ, Ackerson LM, Martin RJ. Chronotherapy of asthma with inhaled steroids: the effect of dosage timing on drug efficacy. *J Allergy Clin Immunol* 1995; 95: 1172–8.

30. ✪ Pincus DJ, Humeston TR, Martin RJ. Further studies on the chronotherapy of asthma with inhaled steroids: the effect of dosage timing on drug efficacy. *J Allergy Clin Immunol* 1997; 100: 771–4.

31. Morrison JFJ, Pearson SB, Dean HG. Parasympathetic nervous system in nocturnal asthma. *BMJ* 1988; 296: 1427–9.

32. Robin ED. Some interrelations between sleep and disease. *Arch Int Med* 1958; 102: 669–75.

Chapter 38

Specific Problems: Asthma in Pregnancy and Pre-Menses

Amjad Tuffaha and William Busse

INTRODUCTION

The prevalence of asthma has increased. Consequently, most physicians who care for asthma patients are likely to face the clinical problems of the asthma patient during pregnancy, and further more, asthma complicates approximately 1% of all pregnancies.[1] To more fully appreciate the effects of asthma on the pregnant patient, it is necessary to first understand the changes in respiratory physiology that occur during pregnancy and how these effects can produce symptoms in normal gravidas as well as in patients with asthma. The following discussion will focus on the effects of pregnancy on asthma, the perinatal outcome in the patient with asthma, and options for effective and appropriate medical management with an emphasis on medications frequently used in pregnancy. Finally, we will briefly discuss the effects of the menstrual cycle on asthma with attention on the possibility of pre-menstrual exacerbations of airflow obstruction in asthma.

PULMONARY FUNCTION DURING PREGNANCY

Pregnancy causes changes in physiology to meet the requirments of the fetus, including increased blood flow to the uterus and the placenta, oxygen consumption secondary to fetal demands, and blood volume in addition to a reduction in oncotic pressure which promotes formation of tissue oedema. Despite these changes, it is remarkable how little the normal lung function is altered during a normal pregnancy.

Upper Respiratory Tract

Hormonal changes in pregnancy affect the upper respiratory tract and the airway mucosa, leading to hyper-aemia, mucosal oedema, hypersecretion, and increased friability. Thirty percent of pregnant women have rhinitis symptoms[2] which peak in the third trimester and cause nasal obstruction, epistaxis, and voice changes.[3] Oestrogen is likely responsible for many of these effects through the development of tissue oedema, capillary congestion, and mucus gland hyperplasia.

Chest Wall and Abdominal Mechanics

As the uterus enlarges during pregnancy, there is an elevation of the diaphragm (up to 4 cm) and an increase in the anterior–posterior and transverse diameter of the lower thorax (by 2 cm).[4,5] Diaphragmatic function is not impaired. On the contrary, an elevation of the diaphragm increase the area of opposition between the diaphragm and the lateral wall of the thoracic cage, allowing further expansion of the thoracic cage with diaphragmatic muscle contraction.[6] This efficient coupling of the diaphragm and thoracic cage is responsible for the increase in tidal volume (TV) during pregnancy.

Pregnancy causes a progressive increase in chest wall compliance with an enlargement of the substernal angle from 68° to 103°. The chest wall changes in elastic property are thought to be secondary to the effects of the hormone relaxin.[7,8] Given these effects on the diaphragm and chest wall, there are associated changes in pulmonary function.

Pulmonary Function

Lung Volumes There is little change in static lung volumes during pregnancy (Fig. 38.1). Total lung capacity (TLC) remains normal or is minimally reduced; residual volume (RV) is slightly decreased; and small or no changes in vital capacity (VC) occur during pregnancy.[9-11] The most consistent change in static lung volumes found with pregnancy is a reduction in

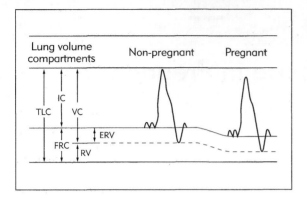

FIGURE 38.1: Changes in lung volumes with pregnancy. (From Elkus R, Popovich J. Respiratory physiology in pregnancy *Clin Chest Med* 1992; 13: 555–65, with permission.)

functional residual capacity (FRC) and expiratory reserve volume (ERV).[12] A reduction in ERV is accompanied with a compensatory increase in the inspiratory capacity (IC) to preserve VC. FRC falls progressively by 10–25% during pregnancy, beginning during the second trimester.[9] The reduction in FRC correlates with an increase in end-expiratory gastric pressure, but not with end-expiratory oesophageal pressure, suggesting that the fall in FRC is caused by the mechanical effects of the enlarged uterus.[4] The causes for the reduction in RV are not yet well-established, though it is thought that the diminished RV may reflect improved expiratory muscle function during pregnancy. The improvement in expiratory muscle function will help in generating effective intra-abdominal pressures, which are advantageous to the pregnant woman at delivery.

Spirometry and Airflow Mechanics Pregnancy has no significant effects on FEV_1 or FEV_1/FVC ratio.[13,14] Consequently, non-pregnant baseline measures and references for evaluation of lung function can be used during pregnancy. Slight reductions have been found in peak expiratory flow rates (PEFR), and are felt to be effort-dependent. The ratio of the maximum expiratory airflow at 50% and 25% of FVC (MEF_{50}/MEF_{25}) is normal throughout pregnancy, indicating small airway dysfunction does not occur in non-smoking pregnant women.

Ventilation and Gas Exchange A significant increase in resting minute ventilation occurs during pregnancy, begins in the first trimester, and reaches 20–40% over

baseline at term.[9,15] The increase in minute ventilation is both due to an increase in metabolic CO_2 production as well as a heightened respiratory drive due to elevated serum progesterone level.[4] Progesterone is considered a direct respiratory stimulant and also changes the respiratory centre's sensitivity to CO_2.[4,16] Minute ventilation increases as a result of an increase in tidal volume, which is elevated by about 30–35%.[15] The respiratory rate remains relatively constant or increases slightly.[9,15] These normal changes of the respiratory physiology during pregnancy may contribute to the perception of dyspnoea, which is often an isolated symptom and does not reflect cardiopulmonary dysfunction.

With an increase in minute ventilation, CO_2 falls to 32–34 mmHg;[17] these changes are compensated by renal excretion of bicarbonate thereby reducing serum bicarbonate to 15–20 meq l^{-1}.[18] The resulting respiratory alkalosis increases levels of erythrocyte 2,3-diphosphoglycerate (2,3-DPG) to cause a rightward shift of the oxyhaemoglobin dissociation curve and greater oxygen transfer across the placenta.[19]

Increases in alveolar ventilation during pregnancy produce arterial Po_2 levels of 100–105 mmHg.[20] The alveolar–arterial oxygen difference remains normal in the upright position.[21] Table 38.1 summarizes the changes in lung functions with pregnancy.

EFFECTS OF PREGNANCY ON ASTHMA

The course of asthma during pregnancy is generally unpredictable.[22] Gluck and Gluck[23] reviewed ten retrospective studies of 1087 pregnancies with asthma between 1930 and 1964, and found 36% of the pregnant asthmatics improved, 23% worsened, and 41% remained unchanged. However, when these studies were evaluated separately, the results differed significantly due to the fact that the asthma severity assessment methods differed between these studies. Juniper and Newhouse[24] performed a systematic review and meta-analysis of 14 studies beginning 1953; they concluded that one-third of pregnant women with asthma experience improvement, one-third worsen, and one-third remain the same. The variable effect of pregnancy on the course of asthma, however, appears to be more than random fluctuation in the natural history of asthma since changes in asthma during pregnancy revert toward the pre-pregnancy status within 3 months of delivery.[25]

There have been some general observations on the effect of pregnancy on asthma. Severe asthma is more

Table 38.1: Changes in lung functions with pregnancy. (Adapted from Wise R. Pulmonary function during pregnancy. In: Schatz M, Zeiger RS, Calman HN (eds). Asthma and Immunologic Disease in Pregnancy and Early Infancy. New York: Marcel Dekker, 1998)

Measure	Change with pregnancy
TLC	Decreased or no change
VC	Increased or no change
FRC	Decreased
RV	No change or decreased
Lung compliance	No change
Chest wall compliance	Decrease
Total respiratory compliance	Decrease
P_aO_2	Increased
P_aCO_2	Decreased
pH	No change
Minute ventilation	Increased
Tidal volume	Increased
Breathing rate	No change
Airway conductance	Increased
FEV_1	No change
MEF_{50}/MEF_{25}	No change
PEFR	No change or decreased
CO lung diffusing capacity (DL_{CO}) rest upright	No change
DL_{CO} rest supine	Decreased
DL_{CO} exercise	No change

the last 4 weeks of pregnancy, asthma symptoms lessen in comparison to any other gestational period.[25] Moreover, increased asthma severity during labour is rare if asthma control is maintained during pregnancy.[25] Interestingly, the changes in asthma severity generally repeat in subsequent pregnancies.[25]

Studies to evaluate pulmonary function parameters during pregnancy have shown variable responses. When spirometry was compared in 27 asthma vs 11 non-asthma subjects, no significant effects of pregnancy on airflow obstruction were found.[22] However, Juniper *et al.* evaluated methacholine sensitivity in 16 pregnant women and found a two-fold improvement in airway responsiveness during pregnancy.[27] The same investigators showed the improvement in airway responsiveness during pregnancy paralleled a reduction in asthma severity.

The mechanisms which determine the pattern of asthma during pregnancy have not been defined. The potential physiologic changes which occur during pregnancy, to either improve or worsen disease severity, are summarized in Table 38.2.

EFFECTS OF ASTHMA ON PREGNANCY

Analysis of controlled studies to compare pregnancy outcomes between asthma and non-asthma subjects indicate that poorly controlled asthma increases the risk for perinatal complications including pre-term births, low birth weight infants, and perinatal mortality.[28] Maternal mortality,[29] pre-eclampsia, and the need for emergency caesarean section[30] are also linked to severe uncontrolled asthma. Gordon *et al.* reported the perinatal outcomes in 16 women with severe asthma.[29] This group of women experienced two abortions, three fetal deaths, and one neonatal death. Three of the 11 live births had low birth weight; two of the ten surviving infants manifested neurological abnormality at one year of age. Moreover, there is an association between perinatal deaths and status asthmaticus during pregnancy.[30,31] Greenberg and Patterson found significantly lower birth weights in the infants of mothers hospitalized for asthma during pregnancy compared with infants of mothers who did not require any emergency or rescue treatment for gestational asthma.[32] Schatz *et al.* prospectively evaluated the relationship between FEV_1 and the incidence of intrauterine growth retardation, and found it to be independent from maternal smoking or medication use.[33] Similar findings were

likely to worsen during pregnancy.[23,26] In addition, the peak increase in asthma symptoms during pregnancy occurs between 24 and 36 weeks of gestation.[23,25] In

Table 38.2: Potential mechanisms of the change in asthma course during pregnancy. From Schatz M. Journal of Allergy and Clinical Immunology 1999; 103 (2 pt 2): 330–36. Mosby, Inc, with permission).

Factors that may improve asthma

Progesterone-mediated bronchodilation
Oestrogen or progesterone-mediated potentiation of β-adrenergic bronchodilation
Decreased plasma histamine-mediated bronchoconstriction
Pulmonary effects of increased serum-free cortisol
Glucocorticoid-mediated increased β-adrenergic responsiveness
Prostaglandin E-mediated bronchodilation
Prostaglandin I_2-mediated bronchial stabilization
Atrial natriuretic factor-induced bronchodilation
Increased half-life or decreased protein-binding of endogenous bronchodilators

Factors that may worsen asthma

Pulmonary refractoriness to cortisol effects because of competitive binding to glucocorticoid receptors by progesterone, aldosterone, or deoxycorticosterone
Prostaglandin $F_{2\alpha}$-mediated bronchoconstriction
Decreased functional residual capacity with resultant airway closure during tidal breathing and altered ventilation–perfusion ratios
Increased placental major basic protein reaching the lungs
Increased viral or bacterial respiratory tract infection-triggered asthma
Increased gastroesophageal reflux-induced asthma
Increased stress

described by Mabie *et al.* who reported an increase in the incidence of intrauterine growth retardation in infants of mothers with moderate to severe asthma compared with infants whose mother's asthma was mild.[34] Perlow *et al.* found that patients with corticosteroid-dependent asthma were more likely to have low birth weight and pre-term infants at delivery.[35]

Maternal complications associated with asthma include chronic hypertension[36,37] and increased incidence of caesarean section.[38,39] None of the studies that evaluated for congenital malformations noted an increased incidence of this outcome in the infants of asthmatic versus control mothers.

To further emphasize the importance of asthma control during pregnancy, Schatz *et al.* compared nearly 500 pregnant women with asthma with a non-asthmatic control group and found the perinatal outcomes for women with well-controlled asthma during pregnancy did not differ significantly from the non-asthmatic population.[37] Data such as these indicate the importance of good asthma control to a desired outcome during pregnancy.

ASTHMA MANAGEMENT DURING PREGNANCY

The goals of asthma therapy during pregnancy are directed towards optimizing airway function and the preventing an acute asthma exacerbation, which can cause an anoxic insult. By identifying and avoiding those factors which trigger asthma, it is possible to improve asthma control. This process can be aided by selective use of immunoassays like radioallergosorbent test (RAST). Routine skin testing for allergens during pregnancy is not recommended since a small risk of anaphylaxis exists in some patients.[40] Immunotherapy appears to be safe during pregnancy[41,42] and can be continued if pregnant women are deriving benefit, do not have systemic reactions, and are at a maintenance dose.[40] Initiation if immunotherapy during pregnancy is not recommended due to the possibility of systemic reactions. Sinusitis is a frequent cause of deterioration of asthma and needs to be treated adequately during pregnancy. Careful selection of antibiotics is necessary. Special attention to smoking cessation and controlling gastroesophageal reflux also improves the asthma control during pregnancy.

Pharmacological Management

When choosing a medication in pregnancy, the potential therapeutic benefits must be weighed against possible risks to both mother and fetus. Most drugs used to treat asthma and allergic rhinitis have not been shown to have harmful effects. However, some medications have been more extensively evaluated and have a more extensive safety and efficacy record; these medications are the "drugs of choice" during pregnancy (Table 38.3). In this regard, the Food and Drug Administration (FDA) in the USA has published guidelines for prescribing medications to pregnant women. Drugs are categorized into four groups (Table 38.4) depending on their adverse effects in human or animal studies. This information can be useful in establishing a safe therapeutic program for asthma during pregnancy.

Bronchodilators

β-ADRENERGIC AGONISTS β$_2$-adrenergic agents are the most frequently used bronchodilators for asthma. All β$_2$-adrenergic agonists are FDA category C with the exception of terbutaline (FDA category B) (Table 38.5). Schatz *et al.* followed 259 pregnant women who used inhaled β-agonist bronchodilators (primarily metaproterenol) and found no significant increase in perinatal mortality, congenital malformations, pre-term births, low birth weight, or labour and delivery complications of bleeding.[43] Long-term adverse effects in the offspring have not been noted with β$_2$ sympathomimetics as a group.[44]

Intravenous β-adrenergic agents have been used as tocolytic agents in premature labour. β agonists relax

Table 38.3: Suggested medications for use in asthma during pregnancy

Bronchodilators
  Terbutaline by inhalation
  Theophylline

Anti-inflammatory agents
  Cromolyn sodium
  Beclomethasone dipropionate
  Prednisone

Antibiotics
  Penicillins
  Cephalosporins

Allergy medication
  Chlorpheniramine
  Tripelennamine
  Nasal beclomethasone (for allergic rhinitis)

Table 38.4: Food and Drug Administration pregnancy categories (From Federal Register, Index publication 44, FR 37462, 26 June 1979)

Category	Animal studies	Human data	Benefit outweighs risk
A	Negative	Studies negative[a]	Yes
B	Negative	Studies not done	Yes
B	Positive	Studies negative	Yes
C	Positive	Studies not done	Yes
C	Not done	Studies not done	Yes
D	Positive or negative	Studies or reports positive	Yes
X	Positive	Studies or reports positive	No

[a] Adequate and well-controlled studies in pregnant women

Table 38.5: Bronchodilators used for asthma during pregnancy

Drug	Animal teratogenicity studies	Malformation or other effect	Class
Inhaled β agonists			
Metaproterenol	Positive	May inhibit labour	C
Albuterol/salbutamol	Positive	May inhibit labour	C
Pirbuterol	Negative Positive		C
Terbutaline	Negative	May inhibit labour Preserves or increases utero–placental blood flow	B
Adrenaline	Positive	Possible malformation Associated with reduced utero-placental blood flow in animals	C
Isoproterenol/isoprenaline	Positive		C
Ephedrine	Positive	Reduction in uterine blood flow (animals)	C
Theophylline	Positive	Newborn theophylline intoxication May inhibit labour, may reduce risk of pre-eclampsia	C

uterine smooth muscle and cause uterine atony. Terbutaline is the most frequently used such agent. As a result, β-adrenergic agonists may have the theoretical potential to inhibit labour. Inhaled β agonists have minimal systemic effects so the likelihood of significant prolongation of labour is small. Systemic β agonists, however, should be avoided in the late-term interval.

Salmeterol is a long-acting β$_2$-adrenergic agonist. Currently there are not sufficient data on human fetal effects to evaluate the safety of salmeterol. Nevertheless, it is not recommended to use salmeterol instead of the older β$_2$ agonists; however, benefit-to-risk consideration may favour salmeterol continuation during pregnancy for some subjects.

The use of adrenaline, a non-selective β agonist, in the pregnant asthmatic patient should be limited to subcutaneous dosing in severe asthma episodes when selective β$_2$-adrenergic agonists are not available or have not been effective. Gatling reported limb defects in chick embryo with adrenaline use,[45] and Heinonen was the only one to find an association between first trimester exposure to epinephrine and an increased risk of major and minor malformations.[46] The same association could not be found with the use of isoproterenol.

ANTICHOLINERGICS Ipratropium bromide appears to be safe to use in pregnancy (FDA category B). It can be helpful in acute asthma exacerbations when given in conjunction with β$_2$ agonists and can be also used in patients intolerant to β agonists. Ipratropium bromide is poorly absorbed systemically, and no increased risk of congenital malformations has been observed although rigorous safety studies are not available.

Methylxanthines Theophylline is a commonly used medicine for asthma and does not have teratogenic effects when used at therapeutic dosages[47] (Table 38.5). Pharmacokinetics of theophylline may change during pregnancy and require the dosing schedule to be adjusted accordingly. In a small number of patients, theophylline clearance was reduced by 25–30% in the third trimester;[48] this has not been adequately confirmed by others.[49] Because fetal theophylline levels are similar to those of the mother,[50] it is advantageous to follow maternal theophylline levels closely, particularly in the third trimester. Xanthines also have the potential to decrease uterine contractility by inhibiting phosphodiesterase. This effect could prolong or even complicate labour. Alternatively, lower rates of perinatal death and respiratory distress syndrome,[51] as well as lowered rates of pre-eclampsia,[36] have been reported with theophylline use.

Theophylline rapidly crosses the placenta and appears in the breast milk with milk to plasma ratio of 0.7.[52] Breast-feeding just before drug administration limits neonatal exposure and minimizes the transient tachycardia, jitteriness and irritability observed with maternal theophylline use during pregnancy.

Anti-Inflammatory Agents

CROMOLYN SODIUM AND NEDOCROMIL SODIUM Cromolyn has little systemic absorption, and is devoid of side-effects (FDA category B). Wilson reported 296 pregnancies with cromolyn use. There was no increase in fetal abnormalities or perinatal mortality.[53] Nedocromil sodium (FDA category B) showed no adverse reproductive effects in rats and rabbits when significantly high doses were used.[54] However, there are no published human data (Table 38.6).

CORTICOSTEROIDS In animals, high doses of systemic corticosteroids cause congenital malformations such as cleft palate.[55] Neonatal adrenal insufficiency has also been a concern with corticosteroid use.[56] Initial studies reported an increase in stillbirth and fetal mortality in mothers who received corticosteroids during pregnancy; however, these studies did not control for the severity of underlying disease as a factor affecting the outcome of pregnancy. Moreover, recent clinical studies have not demonstrated an increase in the risk for congenital malformations, stillbirths or fetal mor-

tality with the use of inhaled or systemic corticosteroids during pregnancy.[57,8]

Dexamethsone and betamethasone cross the placenta rapidly and in high concentrations.[58] In contrast, methylprednisolone appears to cross the placenta poorly.[59] Prednisone also crosses the placenta poorly, as exhibited by the low incidence of adrenal suppression of infants of mothers treated with this drug.[60] Although data are limited, prednisone and methylprednisolone are the preferred systemic corticosteroids in treatment of acute asthma during pregnancy.

All inhaled corticosteroids are FDA category C. Beclomethasone dipropionate is suggested as the inhaled corticosteroid of choice for gestational use because of the published experience with its use during pregnancy compared with other inhaled corticosteroids.[61] Inhaled triamcinolone and flunisolide (FDA category C) have been associated with teratogenicity in animals and fetal growth retardation in humans (triamcinolone).[62] There are no published data on inhaled fluticasone propionate and budesonide (FDA category C) during human pregnancy (Table 38.6).

LEUKOTRIENE INHIBITORS AND ANTAGONISTS Three oral leukotriene modifying drugs have been available for use in the United States, zafirlukast (FDA category B), zileuton (FDA category C), and montelukast (FDA category B). No human data have been reported for these medications; therefore they cannot be recommended for use during pregnancy at this time.

Table 38.6: Anti-inflammatory therapy

Drug	Animal studies	Human studies	Class
Cromolyn sodium	Negative	No congenital malformation or increase in perinatal mortality	B
Nedocromil sodium	Not well-studied in pregnancy		
Corticosteroids			
Beclomethasone	Negative (inhalation)	No congenital malformation Increased LBW infants	C
Triamcinolone	Positive (inhalation)	Fetal growth retardation in patients using 40 mg daily topically	D
Flunisolide	Positive		C
Fluticasone	Positive	No human studies	C
Budesonide	Positive	No human studies	C

501

Management of Asthma During Pregnancy

Asthma management during pregnancy should consider the following goals: maintain normal to near-normal lung function, maintain normal activity levels, control symptoms, prevent acute exacerbations, avoid medication side-effects, and deliver a healthy infant. It should be emphasized that early intervention during acute exacerbations is a key factor to the prevention of impaired maternal–fetal oxygenation.

Patient education also is critical to successful asthma management and should be initiated prior to pregnancy. Education should include methods to monitor pulmonary function at home using PEFR and avoidance of specific asthma provokers.

The fetus is most susceptible to the teratogenic effects of asthma medications early in the first trimester. Avoiding medications that have possible teratogenic effects is important at this critical time. Fetal monitoring with sonography at 12–20 weeks should be performed to assess fetal growth.[63] In addition, continuous fetal heart monitoring is indicated both during asthma exacerbations and labour.

Asthma control during pregnancy is similar to that for non-pregnant adults. Patients with symptoms limited to brief intermittent flares, without symptoms between these exacerbations and PEFR $\geq$ 80% of baseline, can be managed on an as needed inhaled β_2 agonists (preferably terbutaline). Patients who experience symptoms more than 1–2 times per week, have exacerbations lasting for few days, and register PEFR about 60–80% of baseline during symptoms, need inhaled anti-inflammatory therapy with either cromolyn sodium or beclomethasone (the preferred treatment) in addition to as needed inhaled β_2 agonists. Theophylline may be used in this category of patients. Patients with continuous symptoms, frequent asthma exacerbations, and PEFR <60% of baseline should be treated with short bursts of systemic corticosteroids in addition to continuous dosing with inhaled corticosteroids. In this situation, oral prednisone is generally used and has not shown teratogenic effects in humans.[64]

For an acute asthma exacerbation during pregnancy, the principal goal of treatment should be control of hypoxia. Supplemental oxygen is essential with continuous maternal and fetal electronic monitoring. Terbutaline or albuterol can be delivered by nebulizer every 20 minutes for the first hour. If parenteral β_2 agonists are needed, terbutaline is preferred over adrenaline, as adrenaline may decrease utero–placental blood flow and possibly cause congenital malformations as shown in animal studies.[65] Intravenous corticosteroids should be added early in therapy.

Labour and Delivery

The majority of asthma patients, especially those who are well controlled, do not require specific intervention during labour. Nonetheless, specific concerns exist during labour and delivery, and should be kept in mind. First, intravenous β agonists, if given in a substantial dose, could cause uterine relaxation, inhibit labour and alter utero–placental blood flow. Theophylline also has the potential to inhibit myometrial contractility; intravenous aminophylline should probably be avoided during labour and delivery. If the patient received systemic corticosteroids within 4 weeks prior to delivery, hydrocortisone (100 mg i.v. q 8 hours) should be administered during labour and for the 24 hours following delivery to control an adrenal insufficiency.[66]

Oxytocin and PGE_2 can be safely used, whereas 15-methyl $PGF_{2\alpha}$ and methylergonovine should be avoided as they can induce bronchospasm. Magnesium sulphate is the drug of choice for treating pre-term labour in pregnant asthmatics; this product has shown some bronchodilator properties in very selective situations.

Epidural anaesthesia is preferred because it reduces oxygen consumption and minute ventilation during labour.[67] Fentanyl is a better choice than meperdine which may cause histamine release. Regional anaesthesia is optimal for non-emergency caesarean delivery; ketamine induction of general anaesthesia has the potential advantage that it may prevent bronchospasm.[68]

The Post-Partum Period

Altered control of asthma during pregnancy usually reverts back to a pre-pregnancy state within 3 months of delivery. Breast-feeding should be encouraged and medications that are considered safe during pregnancy can be administered during lactation. Although it has been reported to cause irritability and jitteriness, theopylline is generally well-tolerated. Very little of administered prednisone enters into breast milk; consequently, low to moderate dosages of prednisone are unlikely to cause effects on the infant. As a rule, inhaled medications have a low systemic absorption and are well-tolerated.

ASTHMA AND MENSES

The association between asthma exacerbations and the pre-menstrual period has long been of interest. In

1931, Frank described increased asthma symptoms in one patient prior to the onset of her menses.[69] Rees[70] studied 81 female patients with asthma and found 27 (33%) to have an increased tendency for asthma attacks in the 10 days prior to the onset of menses with a peak incidence during 2 to 3 days before menses. Gibbs et al.[71] reported 36/91 women with asthma who answered "yes" when asked if their asthma worsened before their menstrual period. These and similar studies rely on patient impression and recollection. Hanley[72] reported a statistically significant drop in peak flow rate at the time of menstruation in women whose asthma flared at this time compared with subjects who were unaffected. Pauli et al.[73] examined the relationship between pulmonary function and the menstrual cycle and found that asthmatic subjects develop both increased asthma symptoms and decreased morning peak flow when compared with non-asthma controls.

The mechanisms proposed to explain pre-menstrual worsening of asthma include hormonal, immunological and psychological processes. For example, there is a cyclic elevation of both oestrogen and progesterone, and a fall of progesterone immediately prior to menses. Progesterone induces uterine smooth muscle relaxation and may have a similar effect on bronchial smooth muscle. However, recent studies have failed to associate changes in pulmonary function or airway hyper-responsiveness with progesterone.[74] Oestrogen and progesterone, similar to other steroid hormones, may act to potentiate the effects of catecholamines;[75] whether or not this has clinical relevance has yet to be established.

Other hormonal influences associated with the menstrual cycle include prostaglandins and catecholamines. As noted previously, $PGF_{2\alpha}$ is a potent bronchoconstrictor and its levels vary during different phases of the menstrual cycle. In addition, investigators have found an association between asthma and pre-menstrual symptoms. It has been proposed that pre-menstrual peaks of $PGF_{2\alpha}$ are responsible for these symptoms. However, Eliasson et al. was unable to confirm a pre-menstrual rise in prostaglandin metabolites.[76] Also, meclofenamate, a prostaglandin synthesis inhibitor, had no effect on pre-menstrual asthma although it did have some effect on other menstrual symptoms.

There are many additional factors that may influence pre-menstrual asthma, including increased autonomic tone and autonomic lability, higher emotional lability and increased oedema of the bronchial wall.[70]

Many other aetiological agents may be involved, as the hormonal changes involved in menstruation are very complex.

Management of pre-menstrual asthma, primarily exacerbations, should be treated like any other acute or worsening asthma episode. Other treatments that have been considered include diuretics and non-steroidal anti-inflammatory agents. Benyon et al. used intra-muscular injections of progesterone to prevent severe pre-menstrual attacks in three patients.[77] These therapies, however, must still be considered experimental.

SUMMARY

Asthma in women can present a special and unique situation. During menstruation, some women will notice an increase in disease severity. Although the mechanisms underlying these changes are not established, escalation in therapy can be helpful. Pregnancy can also pose special problems; pregnancy is complicated by inherent changes in pulmonary physiology which occur in all subjects. Moreover, the presence of a developing fetus requires special considerations and attention for medication use. Understanding how pregnancy may affect asthma is critical to optimal asthma care during the gestational period. The physician who manages asthma during pregnancy must keep in mind that the goals of therapy during pregnancy are the general overall goals of asthma therapy: minimize symptoms, normalize pulmonary functions and prevent acute exacerbations. With noted exceptions, the available medications should allow the physician to achieve these goals.

KEY POINTS

The influences of pregnancy on asthma can include:
* alteration in lung physiology;
* exacerbations of asthma;
* need to modify medication in use because of potential adverse effects on the fetus.

REFERENCES

1. Gordon M, Niswander KR, Berendes H, Kantor AG. Fetal morbidity following potentially anoxiogenic conditions. VII. Bronchial asthma. *Am J Obstet Gynecol* 1970; 106: 421–9.

2. Mabry RL. Rhinitis of pregnancy. Southern *Med J* 1986; 79: 965–71.

3. Elkus R, Popovich J. Respiratory physiology in pregnancy. *Clin Chest Med* 1992; 13: 555–65.

4. Contreras G, Gutierrez M, Berozia T *et al.* Ventilatory drive and respiratory muscle function in pregnancy. *Am Rev Respir Dis* 1991; 144: 837–41.

5. Bonica JJ. Maternal respiratory changes during pregnancy and parturition. In: Marx GF (ed). *Parturition and Perinatology.* Philadelphia: FA Davis, 1973; 2–19.

6. Mead J. Functional significance of the area of apposition of diaphragm to ribcage. *Am Rev Resp Dis* 1979; 119 (2 pt 2): 31–2.

7. Sherwood OD, Downing SJ, Guico-Lamm ML *et al.* The physiological effects of relaxin during pregnancy: studies in rats and pigs. *Oxford Rev Reprod Biol* 1993; 15: 143–89.

8. Greenberger PA, Patterson R. Beclomethasone dipropionate for severe asthma during pregnancy. *Ann Int Med* 1983; 98: 478–80.

9. Cugell DW, Frank NR, Gaensler EA, Badger TL. Pulmonary function in pregnancy: I. Serial observations in normal women. *Am Rev Tuberc* 1953; 67: 568–89.

10. Gazioglu K, Kaltreider NL, Rosen M, Yu PN. Pulmonary function during pregnancy in normal women and in patients with cardiopulmonary disease. *Thorax* 1970; 25: 445–50.

11. Gee JBL, Packer BS, Millen JE, Robin ED. Pulmonary mechanics during pregnancy. *J Clin Invest* 1967; 46: 945–52.

12. Russell IF, Chambers WA. Closing volume in normal pregnancy. *Br J Anaesthesia* 1981; 53: 1043–7.

13. Milne JA. The respiratory response to pregnancy. *Postgrad Med J* 1979; 55: 318–24.

14. Mokkapatti R, Prasad EC, Venkatraman, Fatima K. Ventilatory functions in pregnancy. *Ind J Physiol Pharmacol* 1991; 35: 237–40.

15. Rees GB, Pipkin FB, Symonds EM, Patrick JM. A longitudinal study of respiratory changes in normal human pregnancy with cross-sectional data on subjects with pregnancy induced hypertension. *Am J Obstet Gynecol* 1990; 162: 826–30.

16. Bayliss DA, Millhorn DE. Central neural mechanisms of progesterone action: Application to the respiratory system. *J Appl Physiol* 1992; 73: 393–404.

17. Prowse CM, Gaensler EA. Respiratory acid–base changes during pregnancy. *Anesthesiology* 1965; 26: 381–92.

18. Lucius H, Gablenbeck H, Kleine HO, Fabel H, Bartels H. Respiratory function, buffer system and electrolyte concentrations of blood during human pregnancy. *Respir Physiol* 1970; 9: 311–15.

19. Sherman HF, Scott LM, Rosemurgy AS. Changes affecting the initial evaluation and care of the pregnant trauma victim. *J Emerg Med* 1990; 8: 575–82.

20. Templeton A, Kelman GR. Maternal blood gas, PAO_2–PaO_2, physiological shunt and V_dV_t in normal pregnancy. *Br J Anaesthesia* 1967; 48: 1001–1008.

21. Liberatore SM, Pistelli R, Patalano F, Moneta E, Incalzi RA, Ciappi G. Respiratory function during pregnancy. *Respiration* 1984; 46: 145–50.

22. Sims CD, Chamberlain CVP, deSwiet M. Lung function tests in bronchial asthma during and after pregnancy. *Br J Obstet Gynaecol* 1976; 83: 434–7.

23. ✪ Gluck JC, Gluck PA. The effects of pregnancy on asthma: A prospective study. *Ann Allergy* 1976; 37: 164–8.

24. ✪ Juniper EF, Newhouse MT. Effect of pregnancy on asthma: A systematic review and meta-analysis. In: Schatz M, Zeiger RS, Calman HN (eds). *Asthma and Immunologic Disease in Pregnancy and Early Infancy.* New York: Marcel Dekker, 1988.

25. Schatz M, Harden K, Forsythe A *et al.* The course of asthma during pregnancy, postpartum and with successive pregnancies: A prospective analysis. *J Allergy Clin Immunol* 1988; 81: 509–17.

26. Williams DA. Asthma and pregnancy. *Acta Allergol* 1967; 22: 311–23.

27. ✪ Juniper EF, Daniel EF, Roberts RS, Kline PA, Hargreave FE, Newhouse MT. Improvement in airway responsiveness and asthma severity during pregnancy. *Am Rev Respir Dis* 1989; 140: 924–31.

28. ✪ Schatz M. Asthma and pregnancy. *Immunol Allergy Clin N Am* 1996; 16: 893–916.

29. Gordon M, Niswander KR, Berendes H, Kantor AG. Fetal morbidity following potentially anoxigenic obstetric conditions: VII. Bronchial Asthma. *Am J Obstet Gynecol* 1970; 106: 421–9.

30. Gelber M, Sidi Y, Gassner L *et al.* Uncontrollable life threatening status asthmaticus – an indicator for termination of pregnancy by cesarean section. *Respiration* 1984; 46: 320–22.

31. Warrell DW, Taylor R Outcome for the foetus of mothers receiving prednisolone during pregnancy. *Lancet* 1968; 1: 117–18.

32. Greenberger PA, Patterson R. The outcome of pregnancy complicated by severe asthma. *Allergy Proc* 1988; 9: 539–43.

33. Schatz M, Zeiger RS, Hoffman CP, and the Kaiser-Permanente Asthma and Pregnancy Study Group. Intrauterine growth is related to gestational pulmonary function in pregnant asthmatic women. *Chest* 1990; 98: 389–92.

34. Mabie WC, Barton JR, Wasserstrum N, Sibal BM. Clinical observations on asthma in pregnancy. *J Maternal-fetal Med* 1992; 1: 45–50.

35. Perlow JH, Montgomery D, Morgan MA *et al.* Severity of asthma and perinatal outcome. *Am J Obstet Gynecol* 1992; 167: 963–7.

36. Dombrowski MP, Bottoms SF, Boike GM, Wald J. Incidence of preeclampsia among asthmatic patients lower with theophylline. *Am J Obstet Gynecol* 1986; 155: 265–7.

37. ✪ Schatz M, Zeiger RS, Hoffman CP *et al.* Perinatal outcomes in the pregnancies of asthmatic women: A prospective controlled analysis. *Am J Respir Crit Care Med* 1995; 151: 1170–74.

38. Lao TT, Huengsburg M. Labour and delivery in mothers with asthma. *Eur J Obstet Gynecol Reprod Biol* 1990; 35: 183–90.

39. Stenius-Aarniala B, Piirila P, Teramo K. Asthma and pregnancy: A prospective study of 198 pregnancies. *Thorax* 1988; 43: 12–18.

40. Schatz M, Zeiger RS. Asthma and allergy in pregnancy. *Clin Perinatol* 1997; 24: 407–431.

41. Metzger WJ, Turner E, Patterson R. The safety of immunotherapy during pregnancy. *J Allergy Clin Immunol* 1978; 61: 268–72.

42. Shaikh WA. A retrospective study on the safety of immunotherapy in pregnancy. *Clin Exp Allergy* 1993; 23: 857–60.

43. Shatz M, Zeiger RS, Harden KM *et al.* The safety of inhaled beta-agonist bronchodilators during pregnancy. *J Allergy Clin Immunol* 1988; 82: 686–95.

44. ✪ Ravenscraft SA, Lupo VR. Asthma: Management during pregnancy. *Sem Respir Crit Care Medici* 1998; 19: 221–30.

45. Gatling RR. The effect of sympathomimetic agents on the chick embryo. *Am J Pathol* 1962; 40: 113–27.

46. Heinonen OP, Slone D, Shapiro S. *Birth Defects in Pregnancy.* Littleton, MA: Publishing Sciences Group, 1977.

47. Greenberger P, Patterson R. Safety of therapy for allergic symptoms during pregnancy. *Ann Intern Med* 1978; 89: 234–7.

48. Carter BL, Driscoll CF, Smith GD. Theophylline clearance during pregnancy. *Obstet Gynecol* 1986; 68: 555–9.

49. Gardner MJ, Schatz M, Cousins L, Zeiger R, Middleton E, Jusko WJ. Longitudinal effects of pregnancy on the pharmacokinetics of theophylline. *Eur J Clin Pharmacol* 1987; 31: 289–95.

50. Labovitz E, Spector S. Placental theophylline transfer in pregnant asthmatics. JAMA 1982; 247: 786–8.

51. Hadjigeorgiou E, Kitsiou S, Psaroudakis A, Sagos C, Nicolopoulos D, Kaskarelis D. Antepartum aminophylline treatment for prevention of respiratory

distress syndrome in premature infants. *Am J Obstet Gynecol* 1979; 135: 257–60.

52. Wood M, Wood ATJ. Changes in plasma drug binding and α_1-acid glycoprotein in mother and newborn infant. *Clin Pharmacol Therapeut* 1981; 29: 522–6.

53. Wilson J. Use of sodium cromoglycate during pregnancy. *J Pharmacol Med* 1982; 8: 45–51.

54. Clark B, Clarke AJ, Bamford DG, Greenwood B. Nedocromil sodium preclinical safety evaluation studies: A preliminary report. European *J Respir Dis* 1986; 69 (147 suppl.): 248–51.

55. Fainstat T. Cortisol induced congenital cleft palate in rabbits. *Endocrinology* 1964; 55: 502–511.

56. Walsh SD, Clark FR. Pregnancy in patients on long term corticosteriod therapy. *Scottish Med J* 1967; 12: 302–306.

57. Fitzimmons R, Greenberger PA, Patterson R. Outcomes of pregnancy in women requiring corticosteroids for severe asthma. *J Allergy Clin Immunol* 1986; 78: 349–53.

58. Ballard PL, Granberg P, Ballard RA. Glucocorticoid levels in maternal and cord serum after prenatal betamethasone therapy to prevent respiratory distress syndrome. *J Clin Invest* 1975; 56: 1548–54.

59. Taeusch HW Jr, Frigoletto R, Kitzmiller J. Risk of respiratory distress syndrome after prenatal dexamethasone treatment. *Pediatrics* 1979; 63: 64–72.

60. Block MF, Kling OR, Corsby WM. Antenatal glucocorticoid therapy for prevention of respiratory distress syndrome in the premature infant. *Am J Obstet Gynecol* 1978; 131: 538.

61. ✪ Schatz M. Asthma treatment during pregnancy: What can be safely taken? *Drug Safety* 1997; 16: 342–50.

62. Romero R, Lockwood C. The use of anti-asthmatic drugs in pregnancy. In: Neibyl JR (ed). *Drug Use in Pregnancy*, 2nd edn. Philadelphia: Lea and Febiger, 1988; 67–82.

63. Venkataraman MT, Harvey MS. Pregnancy and asthma. *J Asthma* 1997; 34: 265–71.

64. Stablein JJ, Lockey RF. Managing asthma during pregnancy. *Comp Therapeut* 1984; 10: 45–52.

65. Schardein JL. *Drugs as Teratogens*. Cleveland: CRC Press, 1976.

66. ✪ National Asthma Education Program. Management of asthma during pregnancy. Report of the working group on asthma and pregnancy. Publication # NIH 93–3279, 1993.

67. Hagerdal M, Morgan CW, Sumner AE *et al.* Minute ventilation and oxygen consumption during labor with epidural analgesia. *Anesthesiology* 1983; 59: 425–7.

68. Hirshman CA, Downes H, Farbood A *et al.* Ketamine block of bronchospasm in experimental canine asthma. *Br J Anaesthesia* 1979; 518: 713–18.

69. Frank RT. The hormonal cause of premenstrual tension. *Arch Neurol Psychiatry* 1931; 26: 1053.

70. Rees L. An aetiological study of premenstrual asthma. *J Psychosomat Res* 1963; 7: 191–7.

71. Gibbs CJ, Coutts H, Lock R *et al.* Premenstrual exacerbation of asthma. *Thorax* 1984; 39: 833–6.

72. Hanley SP. Asthma variation with menstruation. *Br J Dis Chest* 1981; 74: 87–94.

73. Pauli BD, Reid RL, Mont PW, Wingle RD, Forkert L. Influence of the menstrual cycle on airway function in asthmatic and normal subjects. *Am Rev Resp Dis* 1989; 140: 358–62.

74. Juniper EF, Kline PA, Roberts S, Hargreave EF, Daniel EE. Airway responsiveness to methacholine during the natural menstrual cycle and the effect of oral contraceptives. *Am Rev Respir Dis* 1987; 135: 1039–42.

75. Foster PS, Goldie RG, Paterson JW. Effect of steroids on beta-adrenoreceptor mediated relaxation of pig bronchus. *Br J Pharmacol* 1983; 78: 441–5.

76. Eliasson O, Densmore MJ, Scherzer HH, DeGraff AC. The effect of sodium meclofenamate in premenstrual asthma. A controlled trial. *J Allergy Clin Immunol* 1987; 79: 909–18.

77. Benyon HL, Garbett ND, Barnes PJ. Severe premenstrual exacerbations of asthma: Effects of intramuscular progesterone. *Lancet* 1988; 2: 370–72.

Chapter 39

Specific Problems: Glucocorticoid-Resistant Asthma

Stephen Lane, Gordon Cochrane and Tak Lee

INTRODUCTION

Glucocorticoids are the mainstay of treatment for bronchial asthma and inhaled glucocorticoids are now the appropriate first-line treatment for patients who require inhalation with β_2 agonists more than once daily as recommended in national and international guidelines.[1] Short-term treatment with high-dose oral prednisolone dramatically improves the clinical, physiological and pathological changes of asthma in most cases.[2] Both low- and high-dose inhaled glucocorticoids improve symptoms and lung function in newly diagnosed asthmatic children and adults to a greater degree than that provided by β_2 agonists alone in studies up to 2 years.[3] In addition, inhaled glucocorticoids attenuate the accelerated decline in lung function seen in asthmatic subjects and recent evidence suggests that a delay in the initiation of glucocorticoid therapy lessens the subsequent glucocorticoid response and so may contribute to an eventual suboptimal response to glucocorticoids.[4]

In recent years there has been increasing recognition of a group of asthmatic patients who do not appear to benefit from glucocorticoid therapy, i.e. the glucocorticoid-resistant (GR) asthmatic.[5] If the mechanisms for GR asthma are understood, it may in turn provide insight into the key mechanism of glucocorticoid action and allow a rational way to treat these individuals whose disease tends to be severe. Glucocorticoid resistance is not limited to asthma and is a feature of other inflammatory diseases, such as rheumatoid arthritis and renal transplant rejection.[6,7] Thus, the cause for the relative lack of glucocorticoid response in this sub-group of asthmatic individuals has important implications for biology and medicine in the wider sense. Glucocorticoid responsiveness is probably a continuous spectrum with individuals who demonstrate glucocorticoid resistance falling at one end of a unimodal distribution. For clinical purposes, the failure of an asthmatic patient to improve forced expiratory volume in 1 s (FEV_1) by 15% from a baseline of $\leq 75\%$ predicted after an adequate dose (e.g. 40 mg prednisolone) for an adequate duration of time (e.g. 1–2 weeks) would satisfy the definition for glucocorticoid resistance, despite demonstrating greater than 15% reversibility to an inhaled β_2 agonist and provided compliance was ensured.[8] Glucocorticoid-sensitive (GS) asthma is defined in this context as patients whose FEV_1 increases by $\geq 15\%$ from a baseline of $\leq 75\%$ predicted after a similar course of prednisolone while demonstrating greater than 15% reversibility to an inhaled β_2 agonist. This is a pragmatic definition, which nevertheless is useful because it defines a sufficiently high dose of glucocorticoid and a duration of usage after which physicians would feel uncomfortable in maintaining patients on continuous systemic glucocorticoids. Furthermore, irrespective of whether glucocorticoid resistance is part of a continuum of glucocorticoid responsiveness or whether it is a distinct population, the definition stated above allows research to be conducted on patients at polar extremes of the clinical spectrum of asthma.

In 1981 Carmichael described 58 subjects with chronic asthma who were clinically resistant to prednisolone therapy.[9] Compared with GS subjects, these patients had a longer duration of asthma, a more frequent family history of asthma, poorer morning lung function, and a greater degree of bronchial reactivity. These early clinical studies suggested that both genetic (family history of asthma) and environmental (longer duration of asthma) factors may play a role in the pathogenesis of this condition (Table 39.1).

Table 39.1: Characteristics of GR asthmatics

Chronic asthma

Family history of asthma

Susceptible to steroid-induced side-effects

In vitro and *in vivo* defects in mononuclear cell function

Excess mononuclear cell AP-1 activity

DIFFERENTIAL DIAGNOSIS OF GR ASTHMA

Before a diagnosis of GR asthma can be entertained certain conditions need to be ruled out which may lead to apparent glucocorticoid resistance. These conditions fall broadly into four categories and deal with issues relating to a suboptimal therapeutic response in an otherwise GS patient, inappropriate diagnoses, failure to recognize primary diseases of which asthma is a manifestation, i.e. secondary asthma and asthma induced by drug therapy (Table 39.2).

Table 39.2: Differential diagnosis of GR asthma

Sub-optimal response
    Compliance
    Adequate dose for adequate time
    Suitable delivery system
    Control exposure to precipitating factor

Inappropriate diagnosis
    Gastroesophageal reflux disease
    Post-nasal drip
    C_1 inhibitor deficiency
    Vocal cord dysfunction

Secondary asthma
    Aspirin-sensitive syndrome
    Allergic bronchopulmonary aspergillosis
    Churg–Strauss syndrome
    HIV infection

Drug related asthma
    β-Adrenergic agents
    NSAIDs
    ACE inhibitors

The main factor contributing to a suboptimal response to glucocorticoids is that of compliance and indeed some institutions, including our own, admit patients for a trial of supervised therapy including measurements of urinary cortisol and suppression of the hypothalamic–pituitary–adrenal (HPA) axis.[10] The recent launch of inhaled β_2-agonist and glucocorticoid combination therapy in the same delivery system may help address this difficult issue.[11] Other important issues relating to optimizing the response to glucocorticoids include ensuring that the patient is on an adequate dose of glucocorticoids for a sufficient time. There is wide variability in the responsiveness of patients with asthma to the therapeutic effects of glucocorticoids and it is therefore important to be aware that the patient may be under-treated.[12,13] It is important that each patient uses an appropriate delivery system, is not taking drugs that can non-specifically increase bronchoconstriction and is removed, if possible, from the site of continual allergen exposure. The latter factor is particularly important in patients with asthma provoked by occupational agents as early removal from the site of exposure may result in a marked clinical improvement.[14]

Some diseases may mimic the clinical presentation of asthma and lead to an inappropriate diagnosis. Upper airway obstruction secondary to vocal cord dysfunction is a rare condition, which may mimic asthma.[15] This condition can be ruled out by a combination of flow-volume loops and direct endoscopy when paradoxical adduction of the vocal cords is seen on inspiration. There is accumulating evidence that chronic gastro-esophageal reflux disease (GERD) may play an important role in difficult-to-control asthma either by microaspiration or more probably by vagal hyperreactivity provoked by the presence of acid in the oeso-phagus.[16] Studies have indicated that it is present in between 34–89% of asthmatics and may be clinically silent. There is evidence that a large proportion of asthmatics with GERD have abnormalities of oesophageal tone, increased inflammation on biopsy, and increased number of reflux episodes per hour and time that the oesophageal pH is below 4. If this condition is suspected clinically, patients should undergo 24-hour oesophageal pH monitoring, which has a 95% sensitivity and 93% specificity, and if positive should undergo a 3-month trial of a proton pump inhibitor such as omeprazole.[17] Recurrent angioedema may present as intermittent upper airway obstruction mimicking asthma.[18] Stridor, rather than wheeze are often the main symptom and there may be associated facial swelling, skin urticarial eruptions and a known provoking factor. If this diagnosis is suspected functional and quantitative complement studies should be undertaken to rule out deficiencies in the C_1 inhibitor. Post-nasal drip is very common in asthmatics and usually occurs secondary to disease in the sinuses.[19] It usually presents as recurrent cough and its treatment has been shown to improve asthma control. Hysterical conversion presenting as asthma can often be an extremely difficult, and indeed dangerous, positive diagnosis to make in the absence of a suitably accurate non-invasive marker of asthma.

Asthma may occur as a manifestation of administration of asthma-inducing/unmasking drugs or as part of a multisystem disease. β-blocking drugs can precipitate novel asthma or render established asthma more difficult to control.[20] Aspirin (or, more accurately non-steroidal anti-inflammatory drug (NSAID)) sensitive syndrome is thought to affect between 5 and 30% of asthmatics, presenting in the third decade in patients without a previous exposure history.[21] Characteristically symptoms of facial flushing, asthma and rhinitis appear 30 minutes to 2 hours after ingestion of aspirin or other non-steroidal anti-inflammatory drugs. It is important to recognize this condition as it is responsive to specific therapies in the form of desensitization and, in addition, is acutely sensitive to the newly available leukotriene inhibitor class of drugs.[22] Asthma can occur as a manifestation of the Churg–Strauss syndrome and should be suspected in the older asthmatic with co-existing rhinitis, skin lesions and constitutional symptoms such as weight loss.[23] Laboratory abnormalities include an increase blood and tissue eosinophils, erythrocyte sedimentation rate (ESR) and a positive p-anti-neutropil cytoplasmic antibody (p-ANCA). Allergic bronchopulmonary aspergillosis (ABPA) is thought to occur secondary to a hypersensitivity to *Aspergillus* species.[24] Patients characteristically expectorate sputum plugs and mucus suggestive of intrapulmonary infection. ABPA is associated with an eosinophilia, very high IgE, positive precipitating IgG antibodies to *Aspergillus* and a chest CT scan appearance of central airway bronchiectasis. Finally, it is becoming more evident that the CD_4 T-lymphocyte depletion characteristic of infection with HIV can lead to an acquired atopic state presenting with difficult-to-control asthma. This becomes particularly apparent when the CD_4 count falls below 200 CD_4 T-cells per μl.[25] The mechanisms underlying this acquired atopic state are, at present, poorly understood.

In addition to aspirin, it has been described widely that β-blocking drugs can precipitate an asthma attack or render asthma more difficult to control secondary to loss of sympathomimetic bronchdilator tone. This effect can be significant in patients on even the highly cardioselective β-blocking or upon exposure to β blockers in the form of topical eye medication. Once recognized this is rarely a problem as there are many alternatives to their usage. A more recent problem is that of angiotensin converting enzyme (ACE) inhibitor-induced cough and in these situations again a substitute drug should be sought.[26]

CELLULAR AND MOLECULAR ABNORMALITIES IN GR ASTHMA

Clinically relevant glucocorticoid resistance cannot be linked to either disorders of bioavailability or defects in glucocorticoid receptor function.[27,28] Many studies have now demonstrated that GR asthma is associated with impaired *in vitro* and *in vivo* responsiveness of monocytes and T-lymphocytes to the suppressive effects of glucocorticoids.[29] Molecular studies on these cells have demonstrated specific increased activity of the transcription factor activating peptide-1 (AP-1).[30,31,32] Overproduction of AP-1 can result in glucocorticoid resistance by two mechanisms. Excess AP-1 can result in decreased anti-inflammatory activity of the glucocorticoid receptor (GR) by direct protein–protein sequestration. In addition, it can perpetuate asthmatic inflammation by leading to enhanced production of the pro-inflammatory cytokines IL-5 and GM-CSF that are central to asthmatic inflammation. Experiments using antisense oligonucleotides to AP-1 have demonstrated that overproduction of the c-fos component of AP-1 accounts for 63% of the resistant activity as detected in a GR binding assay. This indicates that increased c-fos synthesis is a major component of glucocorticoid resistance in bronchial asthma.

ASSESSMENT AND MANAGEMENT

Patients with true glucocorticoid-resistant asthma provide a difficult management problem. All patients should have a thorough clinical evaluation, chest X-ray, skin-prick allergy tests and full biochemical and haematological screen. Before a diagnosis of GR asthma can be entertained it is essential to rule out suboptimal therapeutic response in an otherwise GS patient, inappropriate diagnoses and failure to recognize primary diseases of which asthma is a manifestation, i.e. secondary asthma as indicated above. A $\geq 15\%$ improvement in FEV_1 or PEFR must be demonstrated either spontaneously or in response to a bronchodilating agent (Fig. 39.1). Patients with suspected GR asthma should be given 40 mg prednisolone orally (corrected for body surface area) for 14 days and FEV_1 measured at the beginning and at the end of the trial period. This trial should be repeated on at least two separate occasions. It is also important to monitor PEFR continuously throughout the trial period on at least a twice-daily

basis. The vast majority of patients will demonstrate a $\geq 15\%$ improvement in FEV_1 in response to this dose of prednisolone. GR asthmatic subjects will show a $\leq 15\%$ improvement in FEV_1 after a similar dose for a similar time period, although in our experience this improvement amounts generally to about 5%.

General management measures applicable to all asthmatic subjects should be applied rigorously to patients with GR asthma (Fig. 39.2). It is essential to detect and improve upon poor compliance and to optimize a delivery system for inhaled medication that the patient finds effective and easy to use. The patient

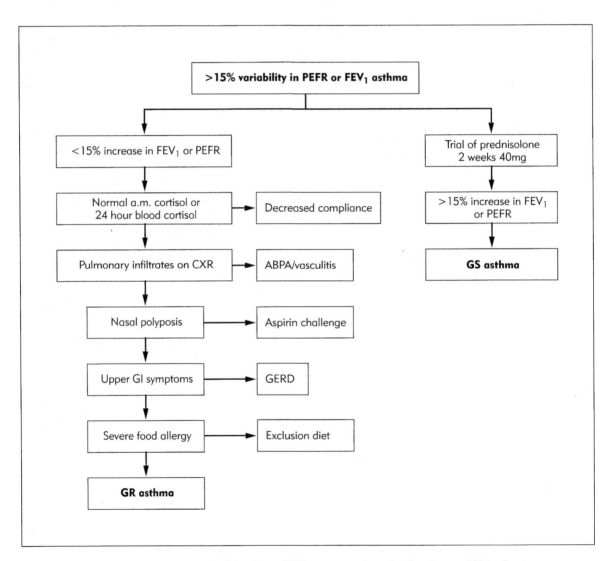

FIGURE 39.1: Assessment algorithm for GR asthma. GERD: gastroesophageal reflux disease; ABPA: allergic bronchopulmonary aspergillosis.

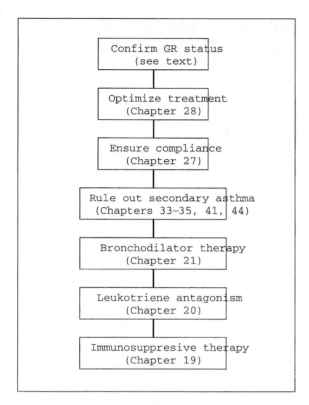

FIGURE 39.2: Outline of management for GR asthma.

should be educated concerning the nature of the underlying condition and given an easily understood customized self-management plan. Specific triggers such as allergens, irritants, drugs, GERD, and uncontrolled rhinosinusitis should be neutralized as much as possible. Specific pharmacotherapy in GR asthma, as in GS asthma, is incremental depending upon severity.

BRONCHODILATOR THERAPY IS FIRST-LINE TREATMENT

This treatment includes β_2 agonists via the inhaled, oral, subcutaneous or intravenous routes as indicated. The newer long-acting β_2 agents are very potent bronchodilators and should be used in combination with other non-steroidal anti-allergic drugs. Inhaled anticholinergics have an additional bronchodilating role and are very effective in a minority of GR subjects. Oral and intravenous theophyllines afford additional bronchodilatation in this difficult group of patients, but is important to bear in mind their narrow toxic/therapeutic ratio and their many drug interactions. Leukotriene antago-

nists (LTAs) may be particularly effective in a subgroup of patients particularly in those with co-existing upper and lower airways disease and in those patients with aspirin sensitivity.[33]

IMMUNOSUPPRESSIVE DRUGS

The efficacy of most of these drugs has been investigated as steroid-sparing agents in glucocorticoid-dependent asthma. The most striking results have been with methotrexate and cyclosporin A. Mullarkey *et al.* have demonstrated a mean daily reduction from 26.9 to 6.3 mg prednisolone which was sustained over an 18-month period in 25 patients with very little associated toxicity.[34] This implies an anti-inflammatory mechanism independent of glucocorticoids and thus a 6–12 month trial is justified in the more severely afflicted patient. Alexander *et al.* have shown that in a group of 33 steroid-dependent asthmatic subjects a 12-week course of cyclosporin reduced the frequency of disease exacerbations by 48%, improved the baseline FEV_1 by 17% and reduced the diurnal variation of PEFR by 27%.[35] In view of its additional role in suppressing glucocorticoid resistant interferon-γ (IFN-γ) and interleukin 2 (IL-2) generation from mitogen-stimulated T-lymphocytes *in vitro*, a trial of cyclosporin is therefore indicated in any severe GR asthmatic subject.

ROLE OF GLUCOCORTICOIDS

Glucocorticoid-resistant asthmatics show a disappointing response even to large and prolonged doses of oral or intravenous glucocorticoids and they therefore have a very limited role to play. Dose and time studies have indicated that 40 mg prednisolone for 14 days effectively selects for the majority of GS subjects.[12,13] However, there may be the very rare patient who will respond at much higher doses and thus a more aggressive therapeutic trial is indicated in any severely ill non-responsive GR patient. It is important to note that these patients are at equal risk of developing the "Cushingoid" steroid-induced side-effects, as resistance appears to be selective to the anti-inflammatory component of steroid action.[36,37]

SUMMARY

Glucocorticoid-resistant asthma is associated with disease chronicity, positive family history for asthma and an *in vitro* and *in vivo* defect in mononuclear cell function. At a molecular level GR asthma is associated with excess AP-1 activity which can perpetuate enhanced asthmatic-type inflammation and render the action of glucocorticoids less effective. Glucocorticoid resistance is specific to the anti-inflammatory component of glucocorticoid action and these patients are therefore susceptible to the side-effects of these drugs. Management of this difficult condition includes ruling out suboptimal therapeutic response in an otherwise GS patient, inappropriate diagnoses and failure to recognize primary diseases of which asthma is a manifestation, i.e. secondary asthma. Bronchodilatation is the mainstay of therapy; however, immunosuppression and the use of the new LTA class of drugs may be effective is certain individuals.

KEY POINTS

- GR asthma is defined as failure of FEV_1 to improve by $\geq$ 15% after 2 weeks of 40 mg prednisolone on two separate occasions.

- GR asthmatics are susceptible to steroid-induced side-effects

- Suboptimal treatment, inappropriate diagnoses and secondary asthma need to be ruled out.

- GR asthma is associated with defects in mononuclear cell function.

- GR asthma is associated with excess AP-1 activity.

REFERENCES

1. Guidelines for the management of asthma: a summary. British Thoracic Society and others [published erratum appears in *BMJ* 1993; 307(6911): 1054]. *BMJ* 1993; 306 (6880): 776–82.

2. Barnes PJ. Efficacy of inhaled corticosteroids in asthma. *J Allergy Clin Immunol* 1998; 102 (4 Pt 1): 531–8.

3. Laitinen LA, Laitinen A, Haahtela T. A comparative study of the effects of an inhaled corticosteroid, budesonide, and a beta 2-agonist, terbutaline, on airway inflammation in newly diagnosed asthma: a randomized, double-blind, parallel-group controlled trial. *J Allergy Clin Immunol* 1992; 90 (1): 32–42.

4. ❂ Haahtela T, Jarvinen M, Kava T *et al.* Effects of reducing or discontinuing inhaled budesonide in patients with mild asthma. *N Engl J Med* 1994; 331 (11): 700–5.

5. ❂ Lane SJ. Pathogenesis of steroid-resistant asthma. *Br J Hosp Med* 1997; 57 (8): 394–8.

6. Langhoff E, Ladefoged J, Jakobsen BK *et al.* Recipient lymphocyte sensitivity to methylprednisolone affects cadaver kidney graft survival. *Lancet* 1986; 1 (8493): 1296–7.

7. Kirkham BW, Corkill MM, Davison SC, Panayi GS. Response to glucocorticoid treatment in rheumatoid arthritis: *in vitro* cell mediated immune assay predicts *in vivo* responses. *J Rheumatol* 1991; 18 (6): 821–5.

8. Lane SJ, Lee TH. Mechanisms of corticosteroid resistance in asthmatic patients. *Int Arch Allergy Immunol* 1997; 113 (1–3): 193–5.

9. Carmichael J, Paterson IC, Diaz P, Crompton GK, Kay AB, Grant IW. Corticosteroid resistance in chronic asthma. *BMJ (Clin Res Ed)* 1981; 282 (6274): 1419–22.

10. ❂ Cochrane GM. Therapeutic compliance in asthma; its magnitude and implications. *Eur Respir J* 1992; 5 (1): 122–4.

11. Chapman KR, Ringdal N, Backer V, Palmqvist M, Saarelainen S, Briggs M. Salmeterol and fluticasone propionate (50/250 mg) administered via combination Diskus inhaler: As effective as when given via separate Diskus inhalers. *Can Respir J* 1999; 6 (1): 45–51.

12. Webb J, Clark TJ, Chilvers C. Time course of response to predinisolone in chronic airflow obstruction. *Thorax* 1981; 36 (1): 18–21.

13. Webb JR. Dose response of patients to oral corticosteroid treatment during exacerbations of asthma. *BMJ (Clin Res Ed)* 1986; 292 (6527): 1045–7.

14. Guidelines for the evaluation of impairment/disability in patients with asthma. American Thoracic Society. Medical Section of the American Lung Association. *Am Rev Respir Dis* 1993; 147 (4): 1056–61.

15. Newman KB, Mason UG 3rd, Schmaling KB. Clinical features of vocal cord dysfunction. *Am J Respir Crit Care Med* 1995; 152 (4 Pt 1): 1382–6.

16. Simpson WG. Gastroesophageal reflux disease and asthma. Diagnosis and management. *Arch Intern Med* 1995; 155 (8): 798–803.

17. ◐ Harding SM, Richter JE, Guzzo MR, Schan CA, Alexander RW, Bradley LA. Asthma and gastroesophageal reflux: acid suppressive therapy improves asthma outcome. *Am J Med* 1996; 100 (4): 395–405.

18. Frank MM. The C1 esterase inhibitor and hereditary angioedema. *J Clin Immunol* 1982; 2 (2): 65–8.

19. Irwin RS, Corrao WM, Pratter MR. Chronic persistent cough in the adult: the spectrum and frequency of causes and successful outcome of specific therapy. *Am Rev Respir Dis* 1981; 123 (4 Pt 1): 413–7.

20. Lewis RV, Lofthouse C. Adverse reactions with beta-adrenoceptor blocking drugs. An update. *Drug Safety* 1993; 9 (4): 272–9.

21. Lee TH. Mechanism of aspirin sensitivity. *Am Rev Respir Dis* 1992; 145 (2 Pt 2): S34–6.

22. Dahlen B, Nizankowska E, Szczeklik A *et al.* Benefits from adding the 5-lipoxygenase inhibitor zileuton to conventional therapy in aspirin-intolerant asthmatics. *Am J Respir Crit Care Med* 1998; 157 (4 Pt 1): 1187–94.

23. Churg J, Strauss SL. Allergic angiitis and periarteritis nodosa. *Am J Pathol* 1951; 27: 2777.

24. Greenberger PA, Patterson R. Diagnosis and management of allergic bronchopulmonary aspergillosis. *Ann Allergy* 1986; 56 (6): 444–8.

25. Lin RY, Lazarus TS. Asthma and related atopic disorders in outpatients attending an urban HIV clinic. *Ann Allergy Asthma Immunol* 1995; 74 (6): 510–5.

26. Pylypchuk GB. ACE inhibitor-versus angiotensin II blocker-induced cough and angioedema. *Ann Pharmacother* 1998; 32 (10): 1060–6.

27. Lane SJ, Palmer JB, Skidmore IF, Lee TH. Corticosteroid pharmacokinetics in asthma [letter]. *Lancet* 1990; 336 (8725): 1265.

28. Lane SJ, Lee TH. Glucocorticoid receptor characteristics in monocytes of patients with corticosteroid-resistant bronchial asthma. *Am Rev Respir Dis* 1991; 143 (5 Pt 1): 1020–4.

29. Lane SJ, Lee TH. Mononuclear cells in corticosteroid-resistant asthma. *Am J Respir Crit Care Med* 1996; 154 (2 Pt 2): S49–51; discussion S52.

30. ◐ Lane SJ, Adcock IM, Richards D, Hawrylowicz C, Barnes PJ, Lee TH. Corticosteroid-resistant bronchial asthma is associated with increased c-fos expression in monocytes and T lymphocytes. *J Clin Invest* 1998; 102 (12): 2156–64.

31. ◐ Hamid QA, Wenzel SE, Hauk PJ *et al.* Increased glucocorticoid receptor beta in airway cells of glucocorticoid-insensitive asthma. *Am J Respir Crit Care Med* 1999; 159 (5): 1600–1604.

32. Corrigan CJ, Brown PH, Barnes NC, Tsai JJ, Frew AJ, Kay AB. Glucocorticoid resistance in chronic asthma. Peripheral blood T lymphocyte activation and comparison of the T lymphocyte inhibitory effects of glucocorticoids and cyclosporin A. *Am Rev Respir Dis* 1991; 144 (5): 1026–32.

33. Lane SJ. Leukotriene antagonism in asthma and rhinitis. *Respir Med* 1998; 92 (6): 795–809.

34.. Mullarkey MF, Blumenstein BA, Andrade WP, Bailey GA, Olason I, Wetzel CE. Methotrexate in the treatment of corticosteroid-dependent asthma. A double-blind crossover study. *N Engl J Med* 1988; 318 (10): 603–7.

35. Alexander AG, Barnes NC, Kay AB. Trial of cyclosporin in corticosteroid-dependent chronic severe asthma. *Lancet* 1992; 339 (8789): 324–8.

36. ◐ Lane SJ, Atkinson BA, Swaminathan R, Lee TH. Hypothalamic–pituitary–adrenal axis in corticosteroid-resistant bronchial asthma. *Am J Respir Crit Care Med* 1996; 153 (2): 557–60.

37. ◐ Lane SJ, Vaja S, Swaminathan R, Lee TH. Effects of prednisolone on bone turnover in patients with corticosteroid resistant asthma. *Clin Exp Allergy* 1996; 26 (10): 1197–201.

Chapter 40

Specific Problems: Psychological Factors

Richard Ruffin, Anne Marie Southcott and Robert Adams

The focus of this chapter will be on adults with asthma, but it is important to recognize that asthma in children can impact on a family and that a greater impact is seen in caretaking parents with high levels of emotional distress and low levels of perceived support.[1] A recent review of psychosocial aspects of severe paediatric asthma provides a reasonable starting point for those wishing to review the paediatric aspects.[2]

WHAT IS THE EVIDENCE FOR PSYCHOLOGICAL FACTORS IN ADULT ASTHMA?

The literature is adorned with anecdotal reports of asthma and emotions being related. Some reports imply that there is a causal effect of emotions, and the aggravation or development of asthma; and others imply that there are emotional responses or consequences to having significant asthma.

Case–control studies of asthma deaths and near fatal asthma attacks, and case series of patients with near-fatal asthma attacks and brittle asthma have provided most evidence of an association between psychological factors and more severe asthma. From the case control studies the following statements can be made:

(1) Medications prescribed for psychosocial problems in people with asthma are associated with a higher risk of asthma death.[3–5]
(2) Non-compliance in people with asthma is associated with a higher risk of asthma deaths.[6,7]
(3) Depression, conflict and psychiatric illness are associated with a higher risk of asthma death.[6]

Case series of patients with near-fatal asthma attacks (defined as respiratory failure, respiratory arrest or an episode of unconsciousness related to asthma) have shown associations with the following factors:

(1) Depression or other psychiatric illness, which may be current or previous.[8,9]
(2) Denial.[8–10]
(3) Psychiatric caseness defined using the general health questionnaire.[9]

The specific psychiatric diagnoses in the follow-up of near-fatal asthmatics in one study were anxiety state 9/25, panic disorder 7/25, post-traumatic stress disorder 2/25, and depression 1/25.[8]

A similar pattern has been observed in a reported series of brittle asthmatics with large peak expiratory flow variability where psychiatric caseness was present in 21/29 compared with 3/29 with non-brittle asthma.[11] Also in the same series brittle asthmatics had significant denial present in 14/29.[11] The information described above has been derived after the critical event, that is death, ventilation, hospital admission etc. Thus it is difficult to describe these psychological factors in a causal relation with poor asthma outcomes. The psychological factors may result as sequelae to previous asthma events or be consequences of the inherent severity of asthma.

HOW DOES THE EVIDENCE IMPACT ON ASTHMA MANAGEMENT?

There is a need to have a broad framework to develop an assessment and management approach in the patient population with severe or difficult to control asthma. The framework needs to be able to integrate the areas for which there is evidence for the association of psychological factors. A conceptual framework is useful to develop the issues, but a clinical approach (Fig. 40.1) is most likely to be useful in patient–doctor interaction.

Conceptually, psychological factors can influence the broad areas of symptom perception, the level of

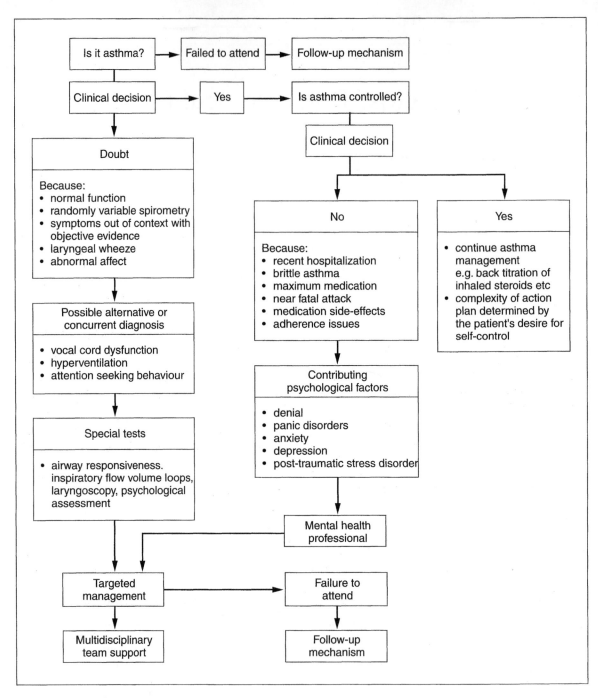

FIGURE 40.1: The asthma review.

bother caused by asthma, the emotional impact of the bother from asthma, and compliance with treatment strategies.[12,13]

For the individual asthmatic the level of symptom perception and symptom anticipation is influenced by psychological factors[12] and hence anxious depressive personalities perceive symptoms more readily. This view is supported by Rushford *et al.* who recently described exaggerated perceivers in an asthma population attending a hospital respiratory function laboratory.[14] Exaggerated perceivers had a higher frequency of anxiety and depression than asthmatics with normal perception.

In contrast, an effective coping style allows someone to minimize the bother from asthma and undertake normal activity despite the presence of airways obstruction. Hence it is important to distinguish the effective coping person from a poor perceiver of airway obstruction. This is why the practice of checking on symptom perception correlated with spirometry change to bronchodilator in the laboratory or clinic is important. This practice assists in the appropriate targeting of peak flow meter use for the poor perceiver. The emotional impact of asthma is a complex interaction of personality traits, coping skills and attitudes so that a severe episode of asthma may lead to a positive approach to life in some individuals, but have the opposite effect in others. Intentional non-compliance may be influenced by a range of issues from low self-esteem and depression to desire for self-control and coping styles.[13]

It should also be recognized that there can be interaction between psychological factors and social factors. There is growing evidence to support the association between a range of social factors and poor asthma outcomes, e.g. unemployment, low income and social isolation. Determination of adverse social factors should form part of the asthma assessment process. This knowledge may allow appropriate resources to be mobilized to minimize the impact of adverse social conditions on an individual with asthma and their family.

The clinical message from the asthma death and near-fatal attack case control studies and case series is that patients assessed as having severe asthma or difficult to control asthma need to have the potential for psychiatric disorders considered as part of their management. Harrison describes the practice of holding multi-disciplinary clinics with psychiatrists and respiratory physicians in the same clinic to facilitate management of patients with significant asthma.[15] So how do we place this knowledge in our day-to-day management of the patient with asthma? In the clinical situation of the review of the apparently difficult to control asthmatic, it is helpful to consider the knowledge about psychological factors under the broad headings of asthma diagnosis and long-term asthma management.

ASTHMA DIAGNOSIS

Asthma diagnosis is most often straight forward with reversible airflow obstruction being readily identified by spirometry. The diagnosis of asthma may be doubted by a clinician in the settings of: normal spirometry; wide random variation in spirometry results at the one sitting; failed conventional therapy; inappropriate affect for the level of symptoms; or a wheeze that is localized to the throat in the presence of high medication usage. The presence of these events should signal the possibility of psychological factors being operational. At this time conditions such as vocal cord dysfunction, hyperventilation, or attention-seeking behaviour need to be considered. Vocal cord dysfunction can be diagnosed at laryngoscopy by the findings of adducted cords with a posterior chink sign, or with inspiratory flow volume loops showing a pattern of upper airway obstruction. Vocal cord dysfunction can sometimes be associated with asthma but can also mimic asthma. A recent controlled study on vocal cord dysfunction in adolescents showed that those with vocal cord dysfunction and asthma had more anxiety than adolescents with moderate to severe chronic asthma.[16] The management of vocal cord dysfunction can be difficult and generally requires a multi-disciplinary approach with the respiratory physician, speech therapist, otolaryngologist, and mental health professional. Speech exercises may help control anxiety in vocal cord dysfunction. The potential role of antidepressants in the treatment of vocal cord dysfunction has not been determined.

Hyperventilation and attention-seeking behaviour become apparent to the more experienced clinician when symptoms and actions are occurring when the patient is under direct health professional observation, or when there is wide random variability in spirometry readings within an assessment visit. In this setting discussion with a mental health professional is important so that an understanding of the circumstances leading to the behaviour can be determined and then strategies developed to best manage the situation.

LONG-TERM ASTHMA MANAGEMENT

Psychological factors are most likely to be present in patients who appear to have severe chronic asthma or difficult to control asthma. There are many factors to consider. One may be that the patient is an exaggerated perceiver and has more symptoms than can be correlated with physiological measurements. Identification of these patients should result in involvement of a mental health professional because of the high associated psychiatric morbidity. Other modalities that need to be explored by further research are the potential for behavioural desensitization of a patient with exaggerated perception, and considering psychotropic medication. This group of patients are potentially at risk of being over-treated with medications and developing substantial medication side-effects. In the same category we must include patients who have the combination of vocal cord dysfunction and asthma because they are also at risk of being over-treated.

Patients with a high level of denial will delay seeking treatment and probably not accept that they have a significant problem requiring regular treatment. A mental health professional needs to be involved with the clinician in the management of these patients and explore associations with specific psychiatric diagnoses. Frequent review of these patients with defined short-term achievable goals may improve outcomes in these patients.

Each of the specific psychological factors or diagnoses ranging from anxiety, depression, panic disorders to post-traumatic stress disorder require a similar approach: the clinician must think of the possibility of the factor or diagnosis, and then involve a mental health professional in a team approach with or without the use of psychotropic medications.

The identification of psychological factors can be facilitated by questionnaires to assess denial[17] and bother[18] which can be used as a pre-interview screening tool. Another marker for the presence of psychological factors is non-attendance for review. A follow-up mechanism (e.g. phone call) should be undertaken for such asthmatics.[19]

GENERAL ASTHMA MANAGEMENT PERSPECTIVES

Knowledge of an individual patient's need or desire for control is important to the clinician, as this factor has an important role in determining the patient's behaviour. Those patients who are enquiring and demanding to know a lot about their asthma and are desirous of high control are the ones most likely to follow complex treatment regimes and self-monitor asthma carefully. On the other hand those patients with a low need for control require a very simple regime and probably need to have support in the form of a family member or other persons providing encouragement for them to use regular medication and to react appropriately to an action plan. Therefore in the day-to-day management of patients with any level of asthma it is appropriate to identify the level of desire for self-control. Those wishing for that control may manage a sophisticated individualized action plan. However those who do not wish to take control need to be supplied with a fail-safe mechanism (e.g. attend a hospital emergency department) to facilitate activation of an action plan. Such a mechanism needs to be communicated to all services involved and preferably a register developed.[19]

CONCLUSION

In the severe or difficult to control asthmatic patient think about the presence of psychological factors; involve a mental health professional and develop an appropriate management strategy with a multi-disciplinary team. For all asthmatics assess their desire for self-control: if it is low, use a simple asthma action plan.

KEY POINTS

1 Think about the possibility of psychological factors in severe or difficult to control asthma.

2 Exaggerated perceivers of symptoms exist.

3 Distinguish between poor perceivers of airflow obstruction and those people with an effective coping style.

4 Intentional non-compliance suggests the possibility of psychological factors.

5 Clinical factors such as normal spirometry or a laryngeal wheeze may suggest the presence of vocal cord dysfunction or hyperventilation.

6 In difficult to control asthma get support from a mental health professional.

7 Organize follow-up for non-attenders.

8 Assess the desire for self-control in all asthmatic patients; if low use a simple action plan.

REFERENCES

1. Frankel K, Wamboldt M Z. Chronic childhood illness and maternal medical health–why should we care? *J Asthma* 1998; 35: 621–30.

2. ✪ Wamboldt MZ, Wamboldt FS. Psychosocial aspects of severe asthma in children. In: Szefler SJ, Leung DYM (eds). *Severe Asthma Pathogenesis and Clinical Management. Lung Biology in Health and Disease*, Vol 86. New York: Marcel Dekker, 1996: 465–95.

3. Ryan G, Musk AW, Perera DM, Stock H, Knight JL, Hobbs MS. Risk factors for death in patients admitted to hospital with asthma; a follow-up study. *Aust NZ J Med* 1991; 21: 681–5.

4. Crane J, Pearce N, Burgess C, Woodman K, Robson B, Beasley R. Markers of risk of asthma death or readmission in the 12 months following a hospital admission for asthma. *Internat J Epidemiol.* 1992; 21: 737–44.

5. Joseph KS, Blais L, Ernst P, Suissa S. Increased morbidity and mortality related to asthma among asthmatic patients who use major tranquillisers. *BMJ* 1996; 312: 79–82.

6. Ernst P, Habbick B, Suissa S *et al.* Is the association between inhaled beta-agonist use and life-threatening asthma because of confounding by severity? *Am Rev Respir Dis* 1993; 148: 75–9.

7. Rea HH, Scragg R, Jackson R, Beaglehole R, Fenwick J, Sutherland DC. A case–control study of deaths from asthma. *Thorax* 1986; 41: 833–9.

8. ✪ Yellowlees PM, Ruffin RE. Psychological defences and coping styles in patients following a life-threatening attack of asthma. *Chest* 1989; 95: 1298–1303.

9. Campbell DA, Yellowlees PM, McLennan G *et al.* Psychiatric and medical features of near fatal asthma. *Thorax* 1995; 50: 254–9.

10. Innes NJ, Reid A, Halstead J, Watkin SW, Harrison BDW. Psychosocial risk factors in near-fatal asthma and in asthma deaths. *J R Coll Physicians* 1998; 32: 430–34.

11. ✪ Miles JF, Garden GM, Tunnicliffe WS, Cayton RM, Ayres JG. Psychological morbidity and coping skills in patients with brittle and non-brittle asthma: a case control study. *Clin Exp Allergy* 1997; 27: 1151–7.

12. Hyland ME. A Reformation of quality of life for medical science. *Qual Life Res* 1992; 1: 267–72.

13 Hyland ME. Types of non compliance. *Eur Respir Rev* 1998; 8: 255–9.

14. Rushford N, Tiller JWG, Pain MCF. Perception of natural fluctuations in peak flow in asthma: clinical severity and psychological correlates. *J Asthma* 1998; 25: 251–9.

15. ✪ Harrison BDW. Psychosocial aspects of asthma in adults. *Thorax* 1998; 53: 519–25.

16. Gavin LA, Wamboldt M, Brugman S, Roesler TA, Wamboldt F. Psychological and family characteristics of adolescents with vocal cord dysfunction. *J Asthma* 1998; 35: 409–17.

17. Pilowsky I, Spence ND. *Manual for the Illness Behaviour Questionnaire (IBQ)*, 2nd edn. Adelaide, Australia: University of Adelaide, 1983.

18. ✪ Hyland ME, Ley A, Fisher DW, Woodward V. Measurement of psychological distress in asthma and asthma management programmes. *Br J Clin Psychol* 1995; 34: 601–11.

19. Mohan G, Harrison BDW, Badminton RM, Mildenhall S, Wareham NJ. A confidential enquiry into deaths caused by asthma in an English health region: implications for general practice. *Br J Gen Pract* 1996; 46: 529–32.

Chapter 41

Specific Problems: Gastroesophageal Reflux and Asthma

Christopher Allen and Michael Newhouse

INTRODUCTION

Gastroesophageal reflux (GOR) occurs when gastric contents regurgitate through the lower oesophageal sphincter (LOS) into the oesophagus. Reflux is typically associated with heartburn, a retrosternal burning sensation that tends to occur after meals or when lying down, and acid regurgitation, a sour or bitter taste in the mouth often, but not invariably, associated with heartburn. Other symptoms may include dysphagia and choking, chest pain often due to oesophageal spasm and flatulent dyspepsia. More severely affected patients may have episodes of acid or food regurgitation in the recumbent position. Normal individuals who undergo oesophageal pH monitoring demonstrate short episodes of reflux into the lower oesophagus that most frequently occur after meals. Conversely patients with pathological reflux experience more frequent reflux episodes which last longer, occur in the recumbent position and at night.

Population surveys have shown that symptomatic reflux is common. Among the US population 37% experienced heartburn and regurgitation in the previous month.[1] In Sweden 26% of the population experienced heartburn and acid regurgitation in the previous 6 months.[2] In the UK 34% of the population complained of heartburn in the preceding 12 months and 58% had experienced heartburn at some time in their life.[3] Symptoms of reflux are more common in asthmatic patients than the general population with an average incidence of 57%.[4–8] A recent survey of asthmatic patients showed that at some time 77% had experienced heartburn and 55% acid regurgitation.[9] In the preceding 6 weeks 62% of patients complained of heartburn and 37% complained of acid regurgitation.

Objective studies of reflux in asthmatic patients similarly show a high incidence of reflux. When studies were pooled, oesophagitis was found in 43%,[5,10] reduction in LOS tone in 35%,[5,8,11] and 24-hour oesophageal pH monitoring was abnormal in 58%.[11–16] This association between asthma and reflux cannot be attributed to bronchodilator medication.[13,17] Not all patients with proven asthma and GOR complain of typical reflux symptoms – there was objective evidence of reflux without typical symptoms ("silent reflux") in 23% of asthmatics.[6,18]

Two mechanisms are proposed to explain the association of asthma and GOR: vagally mediated oesophago-bronchial reflexes and microaspiration. Both the oesophagus and the proximal airways develop from the foregut resulting in cross innervation through the vagus between the oesophagus and the airway. Many studies (cited by Harding[19,20]) have shown a statistically significant 5–10% fall in either FEV_1 or peak flow rate during the instillation of acid into the mid-oesophagus. This response is inhibited by pretreatment with atropine and is not due to aspiration.[19] Reflux may enhance the bronchoconstriction induced by methacholine or isocapnic hyperventilation in asthmatics.[12] If provocative testing with hyperventilation under eucapnic conditions is undertaken while acid is infused into the mid-oesophagus, the induced bronchoconstriction is more than doubled. Similarly, if acid is instilled during methacholine inhalation there is a 30% drop in the provocative dose of methacholine that causes a 20% fall in FEV_1.[12]

Aspiration of gastric contents may be suspected but is hard to prove. The patient may give a history of choking episodes, laryngitis, and cough in association with acid reflux. If aspiration is suspected, two-channel pH monitoring with the upper electrode in the upper oesophagus or oropharynx should be considered. In children, lipid-laden alveolar macrophages have been reported in patients with reflux and chronic respiratory disease suggesting aspiration,[21] but this observation awaits confirmation in adults.

While it is evident that GOR is very common in patients with bronchial asthma and reflux may amplify the bronchoconstriction to external stimuli, the evidence from randomized controlled trials that control of reflux improves asthma is still controversial. The consensus from systematic overviews is that treatment of GOR may improve the symptoms of asthma, but there is no change in spirometry or peak flow.[20,22,23] Where perhaps reflux is most important is in the difficult to control asthmatic.[18] For example the "asthmatic" who is unresponsive to high-dose corticosteroids therapy, may not have asthma and may in reality have GOR, masquerading as asthma. When reviewing patients with asthma that is not responding, reflux should be considered, even if there are no typical symptoms of GOR, and if present the GOR should be treated. We do not recommend routine use of anti-reflux measures in patients presenting with asthma that is controlled and responding to standard therapy.

RECOMMENDATIONS

Enquiry for GOR should be part of any respiratory history. Pay particular attention to reflux-associated respiratory symptoms which occur in patients who develop cough or wheeze or chest pain at the same time as they experience dyspepsia, heartburn or acid regurgitation. Reflux-associated respiratory symptoms may occur in 45% of asthmatics[9,24] and when present may predict an improvement in respiratory symptoms with anti-reflux therapy.[24]

A history of choking, or globus-like symptoms localizing to the upper oesophagus or crico-pharyngeus may be obtained in 30% of asthmatics with GOR.[8] Nocturnal symptoms, particularly cough, or respiratory symptoms after meals, likewise may be suggestive of reflux-related respiratory disease. An asthmatic patient with a prominent cough, recurrent pulmonary infiltrates, or acute bronchitis without obvious cause should also be assessed for reflux.

MANAGEMENT

In general, the management of GOR in patients with asthma should proceed in three stages.

Stage 1

In a person under 40 with a history with typical reflux symptoms, it may be enough to give a trial of diet and life-style measures supplemented by antacid, alginic antacid combination and/or an H_2 antagonist. In patients over 40, particularly if there are persistent or unexplained symptoms such as weight loss or anaemia, careful clinical examination and appropriate additional investigation is mandatory. Too often the focus of anti-reflux therapy in patients with asthma is on drugs and antacids. Diet and life-style measures (including weight reduction) are essential and elevation of the head of the bed may be the single most effective measure. If an H_2 antagonist is used the dosage should be adequate and the literature suggests using ranitidine 300 mg twice daily (famotidine 40 mg, cimetidine 600–800 mg) and it is best absorbed if taken about 60 minutes before breakfast and the evening meal. These agents should not be taken at the same time as antacids.

Stage 2

If first line measures do not control the reflux, or if asthma continues to deteriorate, specific investigations are necessary. There needs to be objective evidence for both asthma and GOR. Specific respiratory investigations such as methacholine inhalation testing will support a diagnosis of asthma. To diagnose reflux, endoscopy would be considered the first line by many physicians. Oesophageal pH monitoring can be very helpful because it will document GOR in the ambulatory setting and permit correlation of respiratory symptoms with oesophageal acid reflux. If GOR is confirmed, most gastroenterologists at this point would place the patient on 3 months treatment with a proton pump inhibitor (e.g. omeprazole, lansoprazole or pantoprazole). The dose of proton pump inhibitor is important. Harding[25] showed that 30% of asthmatics did not have control of gastric acid secretion with the usual recommended dose of omeprazole 20 mg daily. If the dose of omeprazole was optimized, 75% of patients experienced improvement in their asthma symptoms. Based on our experience we would recommend starting with a twice daily regimen of a proton pump inhibitor.

Stage 3

At the end of a 3-month trial with a proton pump inhibitor, if symptoms persist the patient will need to be re-evaluated and if reflux is refractory to medical therapy anti-reflux surgery could be considered. In carefully selected respiratory patients operated on by an experience oesophageal surgeon, one should expect a 90% long-term success in controlling heartburn and acid regurgitation,[26] and about a 75% long-term success in controlling or eliminating the respiratory complaints, particularly cough, after anti-reflux surgery.[27–29]

KEY POINTS

1 Gastroesophageal reflux is very common in patients with bronchial asthma – in some patients reflux may exacerbate respiratory symptoms, and enhance the bronchoconstriction resulting from natural stimuli.

2 Twenty-five percent of asthmatic subjects with proven gastroesophageal reflux do not have the typical reflux symptoms of heartburn and acid regurgitation.

3 It is particularly important to consider reflux in the "asthmatic" who appears not to respond to standard treatment for asthma.

4 A carefully monitored trial of anti-reflux therapy in addition to optimal asthma therapy may be the best way to assess the contribution of reflux.

5 Patients in whom reflux is suspected but who do not respond to anti-reflux therapy should be referred for further investigations such as endoscopy and 24-hour oesophageal pH monitoring.

REFERENCES

1. Nebel OT, Fornes MF, Castell DO. Symptomatic gastroesophaeal reflux: incidence and precipating factors. *Am J Dig Dis* 1976; 21: 953–6.

2. Ruth M, Mansson I, Sandberg N. The prevalence of symptoms suggestive of esophageal disorders. *Scand J Gastroenterol* 1991; 26: 73–81.

3. Corder AP, Jones RH, Sadler GH, Daniels P, Johnson CD. Heartburn, oesophagitis and Barrett's oesophagus in self-medicating patients in general practice. *Br J Clin Pract* 1996; 50: 245–8.

4. Perrin Fayolle M. Gastroesophageal reflux and chronic respiratory disease in adults. Influence and results of surgical therapy. *Clin Rev Allergy* 1990; 8: 457–69.

5. Perrin-Fayolle M, Bel A, Kofman J. Asthma and gastro-esophageal reflux. Results of a survey over 150 cases. *Poumon Coeur* 1980; 36: 225–30.

6. Mays EE. Intrinsic asthma in adults. Association with gastroesophageal reflux. *JAMA* 1976; 236: 2626–8.

7. Clemencon GH, Ihre B, Plengier LH. Hiatal hernia in bronchial asthma. *Gastroenterologia* 1960; 93: 337–56.

8. Kjellen B, Brundin A, Tibbling L, Wranne B. Oesophageal function in asthmatics. *Eur J Resp Dis* 1981; 62: 87–94.

9. ✪ Field SK, Underwood M, Brant R, Cowie RL. Prevalence of gastroesophageal reflux symptoms in asthma. *Chest* 1996; 109: 316–22.

10. Sontag SJ, Schnell TG, Miller TQ *et al*. Prevalence of oesophagitis in asthmatics. *Gut* 1992; 33: 872–6.

11. Peters O, Smekens L, Schandevyl W, Devis G. Prevalence of asymptomatic gastroesophageal reflux in bronchial asthma. *Gastroenterology* 1986; 90 (5 pt 2): 1584.

12. ✪ Herve P, Denjean A, Jian R, Simonneau G, Duroux P. Intraesophageal perfusion of acid increases the bronchomotor response to methacholine and to isocapnic hyperventilation in asthmatic subjects. *Am Rev Respir Dis* 1986; 134: 986–9.

13. Sontag SJ, O'Connell S, Khandelwal S *et al*. Most asthmatics have gastroesophageal reflux with or without bronchodilator therapy. *Gastroenterology* 1990; 99: 613–20.

14. ✪ Vincent D, Cohen-Jonathan AM, Leport J *et al*. Gastro-oesophageal reflux prevalence and relationship

with bronchial reactivity in asthma. *Eur Respir J* 1997; 10: 2255–9.

15. Campo S, Morini S, Re MA *et al*. Esophageal dysmotility and gastroesophageal reflux in intrinsic asthma. *Dig Dis Sci* 1997; 42: 1184–8.

16. Schnatz PF, Castell JA, Castell DO. Pulmonary symptoms associated with gastroesophageal reflux: use of ambulatory pH monitoring to diagnose and to direct therapy. *Am J Gastroenterol* 1996; 91: 1715–8.

17. Schindlbeck NE, Muller LS. Asthmatics' gastroesophageal reflux with or without bronchodilator therapy [letter]. *Gastroenterology* 1991; 101: 876–7.

18. ❂ Irwin RS, Curley FJ, French CL. Difficult-to-control asthma. Contributing factors and outcome of a systematic management protocol. *Chest* 1993; 103: 1662–9.

19. Harding SM, Schan CA, Guzzo MR, Alexander RW, Bradley LA, Richter JE. Gastroesophageal reflux-induced bronchoconstriction. Is microaspiration a factor? *Chest* 1995; 108: 1220–7.

20. Harding SM, Richter JE. The role of gastroesophageal reflux in chronic cough and asthma. *Chest* 1997; 111: 1389–402.

21. Nussbaum E, Maggi JC, Mathis R, Galant SP. Association of lipid-laden alveolar macrophages and gastroesophageal reflux in children. *J Pediatr* 1987; 110: 190–4.

22. Field SK, Sutherland LR. Does medical antireflux therapy improve asthma in asthmatics with gastroesophageal reflux?: a critical review of the literature. *Chest* 1998; 114: 275–83.

23. Sontag SJ. Gastroesophageal reflux and asthma. *Am J Med* 1997; 103: 84S–90S.

24. Ekstrom T, Lindgren BR, Tibbling L. Effects of ranitidine treatment on patients with asthma and a history of gastro-oesophageal reflux: a double blind crossover study. *Thorax* 1989; 44: 19–23.

25. Harding SM, Richter JE, Guzzo MR, Schan CA, Alexander RW, Bradley LA. Asthma and gastroesophageal reflux: acid suppressive therapy improves asthma outcome. *Am J Med* 1996; 100: 395–405.

26. ❂ Anvari M, Allen CJ. Laparoscopic Nissen fundoplication. Two year comprehensive follow-up of a technique of minimal paraesophageal dissection. *Ann Surg* 1998; 227: 25–32.

27. ❂ Allen CJ, Anvari MA. Gastroesophageal reflux related cough and its response to laparoscopic fundoplication. *Thorax* 1998; 53: 963–8.

28. Perrin Fayolle M, Gormand F, Braillon G *et al*. Long-term results of surgical treatment for gastroesophageal reflux in asthmatic patients. *Chest* 1989; 96: 40–5.

29. Larrain A, Carrasco E, Galleguillos F, Sepulveda R, Pope CD. Medical and surgical treatment of nonallergic asthma associated with gastroesophageal reflux. *Chest* 1991; 99: 1330–5.

Chapter 42

Specific Problems: Cough

Philip Ind

Cough is probably the commonest of all human symptoms with up to 30% of the general population reporting recurrent cough.[1] Cough, with or without sputum, is a cardinal symptom of asthma and can occur in the absence of wheeze or breathlessness.

IMPORTANCE OF COUGH IN ASTHMA

In addition to its prevalence as a common symptom cough has additional importance in asthma (Table 42.1). Cough may reflect uncontrolled asthma acutely, as an early feature of an exacerbation of asthma indicating the need to increase therapy, or it may reflect

Table 42.1: Factors affecting cough in asthma	
Uncontolled asthma	Acutely (developing exacerbation) Chronic under-treatment
Irritant triggers	Smoking Occupational exposure Pollution
Associated conditions	Rhinosinusitis (particularly post-nasal drip) Gastroesophageal reflux Extrathoracic airway hyperresponsiveness
Iatrogenic factors	MDIs (inhaled steroids $>\beta_2$ agonists) Non-steroidal anti-inflammatory drugs ACE-inhibitors
Psychological factors	

chronically uncontrolled asthma. It may represent the sole presentation ("cough-variant asthma") or it may present a difficult problem in differential diagnosis. In addition to chronic cough occurring as a feature of asthma it may occur coincidentally due to another cause. Cough may lead to over-diagnosis or over-treatment of asthma. Associated factors may include smoking, upper airway or oesophageal problems, and other iatrogenic or psychological factors. Cough and wheeze can occur independently in asthma and have different pathophysiological mechanisms. Anti-asthma therapy is of variable efficacy probably depending on what the cough implies (Table 42.1). Cough monitoring is in its infancy and treatment is difficult and may be unsuccessful adversely affecting quality of life.

EPIDEMIOLOGY OF COUGH

Cough prevalence rates vary between 5 to 40%.[2] Cough is more common in younger age groups and rates fall in late childhood.[3,4] In 7-year-olds, in the absence of wheeze, cough is reported by 15% while by the age of 11[5] this has fallen to about 6%. Unlike wheeze, cough is not more common in male children.[6] In the elderly chronic cough is usually associated with airflow obstruction;[7] 26% of over 65-year-olds in the general population reported chronic cough compared with wheeze in 15% and self-reported asthma in 8%.[8] As with wheeze the prevalence of cough varies throughout the world,[5] but it is not clear whether its prevalence is increasing.

COUGH IN CHILDREN

The natural history of cough differs from that of wheeze in children. In a cohort of Tasmanian children followed from birth,[9] children who wheezed at age 7, were two and a half times more likely to develop persistent symptoms than those with cough alone. At 12 years of age 57% of children had wheeze, compared with 33% of children who had cough alone. 11% of coughers later developed wheeze.[9] Conversely in young adults persistence of childhood asthma was a common cause of chronic cough.[10] In the Tucson Children's Respiratory Study, 27% of nearly 1000 children reported two or more episodes of cough from 5–6 years.[11] The more frequent the episodes of cough, the more likely wheeze was to be present. Nearly 12% of children had recurrent cough without wheeze. By age 11 the prevalence of cough had fallen to 18%. About 65% of children with recurrent cough and wheeze at age 6 still had recurrent cough at age 11, compared with 35% of those who had only recurrent cough at age 6. Markers of allergy at age 6 were associated with recurrent cough at age 11. Recurrent coughers without wheeze had normal serum IgE, skin test responses, lung function and bronchial responsiveness to cold air in contrast to those who wheezed. Recurrent cough in the absence of wheeze also differs from classic asthma in terms of the risk factors including male gender, maternal allergy, high IgE, and wheezing lower respiratory infection in early life. Others have found that wheeze as opposed to cough is associated with lower lung function, greater bronchial responsiveness and peak flow variation.[12]

In children with asthma, cough is more likely in association with indoor and outdoor air pollution,[13] parental smoking,[14] pets, respiratory infections, familial crowding and maternal and paternal allergy.[15]

It is not clear whether asthma is currently overdiagnosed in children who present to their GPs with cough. Two years after presentation with chronic cough in general practice,[16] 34 out of 106 children had been diagnosed with chronic asthma, 16 with typical intermittent asthma symptoms. Studying the antecedent features of asthma[17] in 36 children at age 10–20 years, cough at age 5–9 was associated with a four-fold increased risk of developing asthma (equivalent to the risk of atopy). The combination of atopy and cough had an odds ratio of 9.5 for the development of asthma.[17]

COUGH VARIANT ASTHMA

Cough as a sole or predominant feature of asthma has been appreciated only relatively recently. A patient with exercise-induced asthma with episodes caused by cough, spontaneous or induced, or respiratory manoeuvres associated with high flow rates was described in 1970 by Stanescu and Teculescu.[18] He responded to an inhaled β agonist and prednisolone. Five patients with paroxysmal non-productive cough, without wheezing or breathlessness, were described as "variant asthma" in 1972.[19] McFadden contrasted a group of eight adult asthmatics who complained of cough or exertional breathlessness[20] rather than wheezing with another group of patients with intermittent asthma. The patients with predominant cough demonstrated marked change in airway resistance as opposed to a marked increase in residual volume in the other group of patients suggesting that the cough patients had more localized central airway narrowing. Bronchial responsiveness to histamine[21] or methacholine[22] was shown to be common in patients presenting with chronic cough. Similar results were described in children.[23,24] Monitoring response to a β agonist is now suggested as diagnostic.[25]

PATHOPHYSIOLOGY OF COUGH

Cough is usually seen as a defence mechanism with dual functions of protecting the lungs from aspiration of noxious materials, and clearing the respiratory tract of secretions. In humans cough is a voluntary act as well as a defensive reflex.

The mechanisms involved in cough have been well reviewed recently.[2,26] The cough reflex is initiated in response to a wide range of stimuli, affecting epithelial and subepithelial sensory nerve endings of the larynx and tracheobronchial tree. No specific cough receptor has yet been anatomically identified. It is thought likely that rapidly adapting (irritant) receptors are activated by chemical and mechanical stimuli with fast conducting myelinated fibres subserving the response. Slowly adapting stretch receptors facilitate cough, airway relaxation and the Hering Breuer reflex, mediated by myelinated fibres. Laryngeal, bronchial and pulmonary C-fibre nerve endings and unmyelinated fibres also mediate cough and airway contraction.

Sensory afferent nerves, predominantly from the vagus, but also from supralaryngeal nerves, synapse with second order neurones in the medullary nucleus tractus solitarius, closely related to the "cough centre". The afferent output via the vagus, superior laryngeal and phrenic nerves closely integrates activation of upper airway, intercostal muscles, diaphragm and facial muscles. The cough motor response is divided into four phases: exaggerated inspiration; compression (with glottic closure and increase in intrathoracic pressure); expulsive expiration (after rapid glottis opening); and relaxation of expiratory muscles and resumption of normal ventilation.

AIRWAY INFLAMMATION AND COUGH

Airway inflammation is a cardinal feature of asthma. Its characteristics are now well-established; involving activated eosinophils, mast cells and T-lymphocytes producing TH_2 predominant cytokines. The role of airway inflammation in other forms of cough is less clear. Bronchial biopsy and bronchoalveolar lavage (BAL) fluid findings suggested inflammation in a mixed group of patients with non-asthmatic cough,[27] whereas 16 patients with idiopathic persistent non-productive cough (IPNPC) showed no obvious inflammation on bronchial biopsy[28] or in BAL.[29] Heino found evidence of epithelial injury, increased eosinophils and mast cells in children with chronic cough after lower respiratory tract illness.[30] Increased neutrophil numbers and neutrophil associated cytokines have recently been reported in induced sputum from patients with chronic cough including IPNPC.[31] A recent report contrasts airway inflammation in 14 patients with cough variant asthma and 21 classic asthmatics.[32] Eosinophilic inflammation on bronchial biopsy and in BAL and serum did not differ between the two groups of asthmatics though both differed from controls.

EOSINOPHILIC BRONCHITIS

Eosinophilic bronchitis is a term coined by Gibson et al.[33] to describe initially seven patients with chronic cough with no evidence of variable airflow obstruction or bronchial hyperresponsiveness, but with a response to oral or inhaled steroid therapy. Subsequently, a further eight patients were examined.[34] BAL findings were compared in a third group of nine patients with corticosteroid responsive chronic cough to 12 asthmatics.[35] BAL eosinophils were elevated in both groups and gene expression, using reverse transcriptase polymerase chain reaction, for cytokines IL5 and GMCSF was detected in two-thirds to three-quarters of each group, suggesting a similar pattern of inflammation. Eosinophilic bronchitis without asthma has been reported as a drug reaction.[36] More recently an abstract

from Nottingham[37] suggests that this may be a much more common cause of chronic cough than previously appreciated.

ASSESSMENT OF COUGH

Quantification and Measurement of Cough

Methods of quantification used clinically, and in research, are surprisingly inconsistent and poorly validated. In clinical practice cough is not formally quantified. Patients are asked directly about severity, or information about indirect effects, e.g. sleep disturbance, social embarrassment, stress incontinence, effect on quality of life etc is sought. More precise quantification has been attempted using:

- patient or observer administered subjective scores;
- indirect measurement of the sensitivity of the cough reflex;
- direct objective measurement of cough.

Subjective Methods of Cough Measurement

A variety of different subjective cough scores have been used. In many studies cough is simply recorded as present, resolved, or substantially improved. Cough diaries, visual analogue scales (VAS), or specifically designed verbal category descriptive scoring (VCDS) systems, using a series of cross-over questions, have been employed. VCDS are based on a series of graded statements which are assigned specific scores and probably work by reiterating and constraining patients responses. Cough diaries were found to correlate poorly with recorded cough.[38] VAS reflected daytime cough reasonably well but was less reliable for nocturnal cough.[38,39] The crossover was found to be more consistent and to correlate best with objective 24-hour recording.[39,40]

COUGH REFLEX SENSITIVITY IN ASTHMA

Much of the available information regarding the sensory and motor physiology of the cough reflex has been obtained from experimental animals. However, challenge studies in humans, using a variety of tussive agents (Table 42.2), have produced much relevant information. In general capsaicin is thought to be relatively selective for C-fibres[26,41] though effects on laryngeal or tracheobronchial irritant receptors and myelinated fibres are not excluded. Solutions lacking

Table 42.2: Inhaled tussive agents used to investigate cough

Vanilloids	Capsaicin
Organic acids	Citric acid Tartaric acid Acetic acid Sulphur dioxide Sodium metabisulphite
Altered electrolyte solutions	Distilled water Isotonic (1.26%) sodium bicarbonate Isotonic (5%) dextrose Urea Hypertonic (4.5%) saline
"Mediators"	Acetylcholine Nicotine Histamine Prostaglandins Bradykinin
Other	Cigarette smoke Lactose Dust

permeant anions (e.g. low chloride) may involve rapidly adapting irritant receptors, particularly in the larynx.[26] Citric acid, like other organic acids probably exerts its effects through change in pH. It shows differences from capsaicin in humans and is characterized by rapid tachyphylaxis, but in guinea pigs it involves capsaicin sensitive nerves.[41]

Cough challenge methodology has recently been reviewed.[42,43] A large amount of information is summarized in Table 42.3. In general cough responsiveness to citric acid,[44] prostaglandins,[45] low chloride,[46] capsaicin[46,47,49,51] and tartaric acid[48] appears to be normal in mild to moderate asthmatic patients in stable clinical state. However, cough responsiveness is increased in asthmatics who complain of cough[47,49,50] and acute exacerbations of asthma.[51] Patients with severe asthma have not been reported.

COUGH RECORDING

Direct recording of cough sounds has been attempted since the 1950s.[52] Spectral analysis or tussiphonography unequivocally identifies cough but the necessary high sampling rates make this impractical for prolonged ambulatory recording. Digital and audiotape recording

Table 42.3: Cough reflex afferent sensitivity in asthma

Author	Ref.	Patients	Tussive agent	Sensitivity
Pounsford (1985)	44	Stable asthma	Citric acid	Normal
Costello (1985)	45	Stable asthma	$PGF_{2\alpha}$	Normal
Stone (1991)	46	Stable asthma Cough variant	Low Cl⁻/capsaicin Low Cl⁻/capsaicin	Normal Increased
Choudry (1992)	47	Asthma–cough Asthma+cough	Capsaicin Capsaicin	Normal Increased
Fujimura (1992)	48	Stable asthma	Tartaric acid	Normal
O'Connell (1994)	49	Cough variant	Capsaicin	Increased
Fujimura (1995)	50	Stable asthma	Capsaicin	Increased
Chang (1997)	51	Stable asthma[a] Acute asthma[a]	Capsaicin	Increased in "coughers" Increased acutely in "coughers"

[a] Children mean age 8 years.

allows cough sounds to be analysed by computer or played back for human analysis.[53] These systems are well-validated, but too labour-intensive for routine 24-hour recording. An alternative approach relies on recording of the audio signal together with another synchronous measurement to accurately identify cough. The Digitrapper device (Medtronic) uses an oesophageal balloon to record oesophageal pressure (reflecting intrathoracic pressure swings). The Logan Sinclair system relies on surface abdominal electromyographic recording. This has been well-validated.[40,54] Other devices[55,56] have been described. Arguably 24-hour cough recording should become the gold standard for pharmacological studies. However, much more work is required to compare the different methods, to assess repeatability and reliability, and to validate other measures against them. They are unlikely to be widely used until they are less expensive and analysis is more automated.

Few studies compare the severity of cough symptoms and cough reflex sensitivity. Weak or non-existent correlations have been published.[57,58] Using an ambulatory monitor we found no relationship between cough reflex sensitivity and cough frequency though we included few patients with asthma (Myers, personal communication). Any relationship between the sensitivity of the cough reflex and cough severity would necessarily be very indirect.

The importance of hyperresponsiveness of the upper airways in asthmatic cough is unclear.[59,60]

PATIENTS REFERRED WITH CHRONIC COUGH

The anatomic–diagnostic approach originally described by Irwin[61] is now widely used in the diagnosis and treatment of chronic cough. Despite incorporating more intensive investigation and therapy, the initially reported success rates are rarely duplicated, probably due to variations in local practice and referral patterns. Idiopathic chronic persistent non-productive cough (ICPNPC) was not initially recognized though this is reported in 18–31% patients in more recent series.[31,49,60] However, the observation that asthma, alone or in combination with other conditions, particularly post-nasal drip (with or without allergic rhinosinusitis) or oesophageal reflux accounts for an important number (11–35%) of these patients holds generally true[31,49,60] (Table 42.4).

MANAGEMENT OF COUGH IN ASTHMA

Cough quite commonly occurs as a result of inhaled asthma therapy, particularly corticosteroids and long-acting β_2 agonists by metered dose inhaler. It may result

Table 42.4: Asthma in adult patients referred with chronic cough					Diagnosis established			
Authors	Ref.	n	Age (years)	Cough duration (months)	Asthma alone	Asthma + others	Asthma total	Idiopathic
Irwin (1981)	61	49	50	40	25%	18%	43%	0
Poe (1989)	63	139	45	–	27%	6%	33%	12%
Irwin (1990)	64	102	51	53	24%	21%	45%	1%
Pratter (1993)	65	45	47	35	7%	24%	31%	0%
O'Connell (1994)	49	87	49	53	6%	5%	11%	31%
Carney (1997)	60	30	56	57	3%	20%	23%	23%
McGarvey (1998)	29	43	48	67	23%	12%	35%	18%

529

from aerosol propellants or other incipients or from associated deep inspiration. This cause should be obvious from the history and direct observation. Management consists of changing to a dry powder device and addition of a large volume spacer. Pretreatment with a short-acting β_2 agonist may help.

Otherwise management of cough in the context of established asthma requires some modification of Irwin's approach.[61] The aim is to ascertain whether cough is a residual symptom of asthma or due to a coincident cause. Both possibilities commonly occur since cough may be more resistant to therapy than bronchoconstriction (relieved by bronchodilators) while other causes of cough, allergic or non-allergic rhinosinusitis and oesophageal reflux occur commonly in association with asthma. The mechanism(s) by which oesophageal reflux causes cough are unclear.[62] However, oesophageal reflux may occur commonly in severe asthma and may even be exacerbated by theophylline or other therapy (see Chapter 41). Conventional management is usually successful,[49] but it may be important to confirm resolution of reflux if cough persists in case there are multiple causes.

Suggested Approach

An approach which we have adopted, but not prospectively assessed, is to utilize a steroid trial (usually with prednisolone 30–40 mg daily but occasionally, in the presence of contraindications, e.g. severe obesity or borderline diabetes, with high-dose inhaled steroids (2000 µg BDP, or equivalent, daily) for 2–4 weeks. It is important to ensure compliance as far as possible. If cough responds then it is likely to be due to uncontrolled asthma and/or associated upper airway allergy, or coincident eosinophilic bronchitis. Attention to administering adequate high-dose inhaled steroids (correct device with or without spacer, encouraging compliance and monitoring response) and perhaps nasal steroids, with or without decongestants initially, should then resolve or improve the problem.

Cough which does not respond, at least partially, is presumed to be unlikely to be due to uncontrolled allergy or asthma (steroid non-responsive asthma may remain a possibility). In this case the anatomic–diagnostic approach is adopted focusing on chest X-ray (with or without other imaging) for a coincident airway or parenchymal problem (e.g. associated bronchiectasis or complicated ABPA or a tumour or foreign body). Sputum (spontaneous or induced) cytology may be useful to confirm few eosinophils (large numbers suggest possible non-compliance). Large numbers of neutrophils may suggest infection or bronchiectasis or asthma exacerbation. Oesophageal pH monitoring (preferred to barium or endoscopic examination) would also then be indicated. Assessment of capsaicin responsiveness is contributory in a negative sense. If it is not markedly enhanced it suggests a lower airway abnormality or psychological component. Objective 24-hour cough monitoring may be helpful. The importance of thoroughness in conducting these investigations cannot be over emphasised. Although some patients appear psychologically abnormal, we should be reluctant to ascribe cough as a result (rather than a cause) of this.

Anti-Tussive Therapy

The actions of a variety of anti-asthma drugs in cough suppression are summarized in Table 42.5. These effects relate mainly to relief of associated bronchoconstriction[22,24,25,71,72] or airway inflammation[70,75] including antagonizing specific mediators.[65,67,76–79] Actions on neuronal mechanisms may be relevant.[66,68,69,74,75] In many asthma controlled trials specific information on cough is not available in the literature; cough data are included in the total symptom score. For example as regards the leukotriene modifiers[76–79] a single report refers to use in cough variant asthma.[80]

The effectiveness of various drugs, e.g. bronchodilators[81–83] differs with respect to different cough challenges and non-specific[2,66] and asthmatic cough.[2,22,24,25,71,72] It is not clear to what extent contradictory evidence represents differences between the different challenges[2,81–86] nor what this implies with respect to their use in predicting anti-tussive effects in symptomatic cough.

Unfortunately treatment of cough can be difficult. No specific agents apart from opiates[2,26,82] and local anaesthetics[2,26,89] are available. Both are relatively contraindicated in asthma. Anti-histamine preparations[2,65,67,84] and demulcents[2] and aromatics, e.g. menthol[90] show small benefits.

No matter how thorough the investigation a number of patients will have persistent cough whether due to their asthma or not. Chronic cough can be very disabling. Cough may trigger bronchoconstriction. Morbidity includes: impairment of social functioning; sleep loss; exhaustion; depression; irritability; stress incontinence; cough syncope; conjunctival haemor-

Table 42.5: Pharmacological treatment of cough (reference numbers in brackets)

	β₂ Agonist	Anti-cholinergic	Anti-histamines	Theophylline	Long-acting β₂	Cromones	Inhaled steroid	LT mod
Non-specific cough	–(2)	–(2, 66)	±(2, 65, 67)	?	?	+(2, 68, 69)	–(70)	?
Asthmatic cough	+(22, 24, 25)	?(2)	±(2)	±(24,71)	+(72)	+(2, 73, 74)	++(75)	+(76–79)
Citric acid/ other challenge	+(2,81–83)	+(2, 81)	+(84)	?	?	–(2, 85)	?	?
Capsaicin	–(2, 82)	–(2)	–(2)	?	?	+(86)	?	–(87)

Response of various forms of cough to anti-asthma therapy: – no effect; + inhibitory effect; ± uncertain; ? unknown.

rhage; muscle strain; rib fractures, occasionally leading to pneumothorax; pneumomediastinum; or subcutaneous emphysema.

Future Possible Pharmacological Approaches

Research into more effective, more specific cough suppressants is ongoing. There is considerable experimental evidence for the involvement of sensory nerves and tachykinins in cough and in asthma.[91] The initial promise of FK-224 in inhibiting bradykinin-induced cough[92] (in three asthmatics) has not been fulfilled by other studies of neurokinin 1 and 2 blockers.[91,93,95] Potential future anti-tussive agents include novel anti-inflammatory agents[94], neuropeptide inhibitors, e.g. bradykinin antagonists,[96] centrally acting drugs, e.g. non-sedative opiates,[97] and agents which modify central[98] or peripheral neurotransmission, e.g. baclofen.[99] In the context of asthma the priority in treating cough is to ensure that the other facets of the asthmatic process are well-controlled.

KEY POINTS

1 Cough is common in asthma and may reflect chronic poor control, an exacerbation, irritant triggers, associated conditions, iatrogenic or psychosocial factors.

2 Assessment of cough is in its infancy; VCDS may be superior to VAS. Twenty-four hour cough recording is a gold standard for research, but equipment is expensive and analysis is time-consuming.

3 Cough reflex responsiveness to a variety of stimuli is normal in stable asthma, in adults and in children, but is increased in asthma exacerbations.

4 Management of cough in asthma involves a trial of steroids. Responders have their anti-asthma and rhinosinusitis therapy (particularly inhaled steroids) optimized. In non-responders another (additional) cause is sought with investigation according to a modified anatomic–diagnostic approach.

5 Treatment can be difficult as there are no suitable, effective specific anti-tussives currently available but there are potentially promising pharmacological approaches.

REFERENCES

1. Wynder EL, Lenon FR, Mantel N. Epidemiology of persistent cough. *Am Rev Respir Dis* 1965; 91: 679–700.

2. Fuller RW, Jackson DM. Physiology and treatment of cough. *Thorax* 1990; 45: 425–30.

3. Luyt DK, Burton PR, Simpson H. Epidemiological study of wheeze, doctor diagnosed asthma, and cough in preschool children in Leicestershire. *BMJ* 1998; 306: 1386–90.

4. Robertson CE, Bishop J, Sennhauser FH, Mallol J. International comparison of asthma prevalence in children: Australia, Switzerland, Chile. *Pediatr Pulmonol* 1993; 16: 219–26.

5. Clifford RD, Radford M, Howel J, Holgate ST. Prevalence of respiratory symptoms among 7 and 11 year old schoolchildren and association with asthma. *Arch Dis Child* 1989; 64: 1118–25.

6. Robertson CE, Heycock E, Bishop J, Nolan T, Olinsky A, Phelan PD. Prevalence of asthma in Melbourne schoolchildren: changes over 26 years. *BMJ* 1991; 302: 1116–18.

7. Enright PL, Kronmal RA, Higgins MW, Schenker MB, Haponik EF. Prevalence and correlates of respiratory symptoms and disease in the elderly. *Chest* 1994; 106: 827–34.

8. Burrows B, Barber RA, Cline MG, Knudson RJ, Leibowitz MD. Characteristics of asthma among elderly adults in a sample of the general population. *Chest* 1991; 100: 935–42.

9. Giles GG, Gibson HB, Lickless N, Shaw K. Respiratory symptoms in Tasmanian adolescents: a follow up of the 1961 birth cohort. *Aust NZ J Med* 1984; 14: 631–7.

10. Strachan DP, Anderson HR, Bland JM, Peckham C. Asthma as a link between chest illness in childhood and chronic cough and phlegm in young adults. *BMJ* 1988; 296: 890–93.

11. Wright AL, Holberg CJ, Morgan WJ, Taussing LM, Halonen M, Martinez FD. Recurrent cough in childhood and its relation to asthma. *Am J Respir Crit Care Med* 1996; 153: 1259–65.

12. Clough JB, Holgate ST. Episodes of respiratory morbidity in children with cough and wheeze. *Am J Respir Crit Care Med* 1994; 150: 48–53.

13. Ostro BD, Lipsett MJ, Mann JK, Weiner MB, Selner J. Indoor air pollution and asthma. Results from a panel study. *Am J Resp Crit Care Med* 1994; 149: 1400–1406.

14. Charlton A. Children's coughs related to parental smoking. *BMJ* 1984; 288: 1647–49.

15. Duffy DL, Mitchell CA. Lower respiratory tract symptoms in Queensland schoolchildren: risk factors for wheeze, cough and diminished ventilatory function *Thorax* 1993; 48: 1021–24.

16. Spelman R. Two-year follow up of the management of chronic or recurrent cough in children according to an asthma protocol. *Br J Gen Pract* 1991; 41: 406–409.

17. Dodge R, Burrows B, Lebowitz MD, Cline MG. Antecedent features of children in whom asthma develops during the second decade of life. *J Allergy Clin Immunol* 1993; 92: 744–9.

18. Stanescu DC, Teculescu DB. Exercise and cough-induced asthma. *Respiration* 1970; 27: 377–83.

19. Glauser E. Variant asthma. *Ann Allergy* 1972; 30: 457–9.

20. McFadden ER. Exertional dyspnea and cough as preludes to acute attacks of asthma. *N Engl J Med* 1975; 292: 555–9.

21. Cockcroft DW, Killian DN, Mellon JJ, Hargreave FE. Bronchial reactivity to inhaled histamine: a method and clinical survey. *Clin Allergy* 1977; 7: 235–43.

22. Corrao WM, Braman SS, Irwin RS. Chronic cough as the sole presenting manifestation of bronchial asthma. *N Engl J Med* 1979; 300: 633–7.

23. Hanaway PJ, Hopper DK. Cough variant asthma in children. *JAMA* 1982; 247: 206–208.

24. Cloutier MM, Loughlin GM. Chronic cough in children: a manifestation of airway hyperactivity. *Pediatrics* 1981; 67: 6–12.

25. Irwin RS, French CT, Smyrnios NA, Carley FJ. Interpretation of positive results of a methacholine inhalation challenge and 1 week of inhaled

bronchodilator use in diagnosing and treating cough variant asthma. *Arch Intern Med* 1997; 157: 1981–7.

26. Stone RA, Fuller RW. Mechanisms of cough. In: Busse WW, Holgate ST (eds). *Asthma and Rhinitis* Boston: Blackwell, 1995: Chapter 82 1075–83.

27. Boulet L-P, Milot J, Boutet M, St Georges F, Laviolette M. Airway inflammation in nonasthmatic subjects with chronic cough. *Am J Respir Crit Care Med* 1994; 149: 482–9.

28. O'Connell F, Springall DR, Moradoghli-Haftvani A *et al*. Abnormal intraepithelial airway nerves in persistent unexplained cough? *Am J Respir Crit Care Med* 1995; 152: 2068–75.

29. McGarvey LPA, Heaney LG, Lawson JT *et al*. Evaluation and outcome of patients with chronic non-productive cough using a comprehensive diagnostic protocol. *Thorax* 1998; 53: 738–43.

30. Heino M, Juntunen-Backman K, Leijala M, Rapola J, Laitenen LA. Bronchial epithelial inflammation in children with chronic cough after early lower respiratory tract illness. *Am Rev Respir Dis* 1990; 141: 428–32.

31. Jatakanon A, Lalloo UG, Lim S, Chung KF, Barnes PJ. Increased neutrophils and cytokines, TNF-α and IL-8, in induced sputum of non-asthmatic patients with chronic dry cough. *Thorax* 1999; 54: 234–7.

32. Niimi A, Amitani R, Suzuki K, Tanaka E, Murayama T, Kuze F. Eosinophilic inflammation in cough variant asthma. *Eur Respir J* 1998; 11: 1064–9.

33. Gibson PG, Dolovich J, Denburg JA, Ramsdale EH, Hargreave FE. Chronic cough eosinophilic bronchitis without asthma. *Lancet* 1989; 1: 1346–8.

34. Gibson PG, Hargreave FE, Girgis-Gabardo A, Morris M, Denburg JA, Dolovich J. Chronic cough with eosinophilic bronchitis: examination for variable airflow obstruction and response to corticosteroid. *Clin Exp Allergy* 1995; 25: 127–32.

35. Gibson PG, Zlatic K, Scott J, Sewell W, Woolley K, Saltos N. Chronic cough resembles asthma with IL-5 and granulocyte-macrophage colony-stimulating factor gene expression in bronchoalveolar cells. *J Allergy Clin Immunol* 1998; 101: 320–26.

36. Ogawa H, Fujimara M, Heki U, Kitagawa M, Matsuda T. Eosinophilic bronchitis presenting with only severe dry cough due to bucillamine. *Respir Med* 1995; 89: 210–21.

37. Brightling CE, Ward R, Goh K-L, Wardlaw AJ, Pavord ID. Eosinophilic bronchitis is an important cause of cough. *Thorax* 1998; 53:(suppl. 4) A39.

38. Hsu JY, Stone RA, Logan-Sinclair RB, Worsdell M, Busst CM, Chung KF. Coughing frequency in patients with persistent cough: assessment using a 24 hour ambulatory recorder. *Eur Respir J* 1994; 7: 1246–53.

39. Chang AB, Newman RG, Carlin JB, Phelan PD, Robertson CF. Subjective scoring of cough in children: parent-completed vs child-completed diary cards vs an objective method. *Eur Respir J* 1998; 11: 462–6.

40. Myers JD, Shakur BHK, Ind PW, Pride NB. Use of ambulatory cough recording to validate other measures of cough. *Eur Resp J* 1997; 10: 422s.

41. Morice AH. Inhalation cough challenge in the investigation of the cough reflex and antitussives. *Pulm Pharmacol* 1996; 9: 281–4.

42. Ind PW, Pride NB. Assessment of airway responses and the cough reflex. In: Hughes JM, Pride NB (eds). *Lung Function Tests: Physiological Principles and Clinical Applications* London: WB Saunders, 1999; Chapter 14, 223–36.

43. Szallasi A, Blumberg PM. Vanilloid (capsaicin) receptors and mechanisms. *Pharmacol Rev* 1999; 51: 159–211.

44. Pounsford JC, Saunders KB. Effect of bronchodilators on the cough response to inhaled citric acid in normal and asthmatic subjects. *Thorax* 1985; 40: 662–7.

45. Costello JF, Dunlop LS, Gardiner PJ. Characteristics of prostaglandin induced cough in man. *Br J Clin Pharmacol* 1985; 20: 355–9.

46. Stone RA, Barnes PJ. Patients with cough are sensitised to low chloride solution and capsaicin compared to normal volunteers and patients with asthma. *Respir Med* 1991; 86: 78-abs.

47. Choudry NB, Fuller RW. Sensitivity of the cough reflex in patients with chronic cough. *Eur Respir J* 1992; 5: 296–300.

48. Fujimura M, Sakamoto S, Kamio Y, Matsuda T. Cough receptor sensitivity and bronchial responsiveness in normal and asthmatic subjects. *Eur Respir J* 1992; 5: 291–5.

49. O'Connell F, Thomas VE, Pride NB, Fuller RW. Capsaicin cough sensitivity decreases with successful treatment of chronic cough. *Am J Respir Crit Care Med* 1994; 150: 374–80.

50. Fujimura M, Kamio Y, Kasahara K, Bando T, Hashimoto T, Matsuda T. Prostanoids and cough response to capsaicin in asthma and chronic bronchitis. *Eur Respir J* 1995; 8: 1499–1505.

51. Chang AB, Phelan PD, Robertson CF. Cough receptor sensitivity in children with acute and non-acute asthma. *Thorax* 1997; 52: 770–74.

52. Piirila P, Sovijarvi AR. Objective assessment of cough. *Eur Respir J* 1995; 8: 1949–56.

53. Subburaj S, Parvez L, Rajagopalan TG. Methods of recording and analysing cough sounds. *Pulm Pharmacol* 1996; 9: 269–79.

54. Munyard P, Busst C, Logan-Sinclair R, Bush A. A new device for ambulatory cough recording. *Pediatr Pulmonol* 1994; 18: 178–86.

55. Chang AB, Newman R, Phelan PD, Robertson CF. A new use for an old Holter monitor: an ambulatory cough meter. *Eur Respir J* 1997; 10: 1637–9.

56. Kohler D, Klauke M, Schonhofer B. A new portable monitor for long-term cough recording. *Pneumologie* 1997; 51: 555–9.

57. Riordan MF, Beardsmore CS, Brooke AM, Simpson H. Relationship between respiratory symptoms and cough receptor sensitivity. *Arch Dis Child* 1994; 70: 299–304.

58. Yeo WW, Chadwick IG, Kraskiewicz M, Jackson PR, Ramsay LE. Resolution of ACE inhibitor cough: changes in subjective cough and responses to inhaled capsaicin, intradermal bradykinin and substance-P. *Br J Clin Pharmacol* 1995; 40: 423–9.

59. Bucca C, Rolla G, Brussino L, De Rose L, Bugiani M. Are asthma-like symptoms due to bronchial or extrathoracic airway dysfunction? *Lancet* 1995; 346: 791–5.

60. Carney AK, Gibson PG, Muree-Allen K, Saltos N, Olson LG, Hensley MJ. A systematic evaluation of mechanisms in chronic cough. *Am J Respir Crit Care Med* 1997; 156: 211–16.

61. Irwin RS, Corrao WM, Pratter MR. Chronic persistent cough in the adult: the spectrum and frequency of causes and successful outcome of specific therapy. *Am Rev Respir Dis* 1981; 123: 413–17.

62. Ing AI, Nigu MC, Bueslin ABX. Pathogenesis of chronic persistent cough associated with gastroesophageal reflux. *Am J Respir Crit Care Med* 1994; 149: 160–67.

63. Poe HR, Harder RV, Israel RH *et al*. Chronic persistent cough: experience in diagnosis and outcome using an anatomic diagnostic protocol. *Chest* 1989; 95: 723–7.

64. Irwin RS, Curley FJ, French CL. Chronic cough: the spectrum and frequency of causes, key components of the diagnostic evaluation and outcome of specific therapy. *Am Rev Resp Dis* 1990; 141: 640–47.

65. Pratter R, Bartter T, Akers S, DuBois J. An algorithmic approach to chronic cough. *Ann Intern Med* 1993; 119: 977–83.

66. Lowry R, Wood A, Higenbottam T. The effect of anticholinergic bronchodilator therapy on cough during upper respiratory tract infection. *Br J Clin Pharmacol* 1994; 37: 182–91.

67. Ciprandi G, Buscaglia S, Catrullo A, Marchesi E, Bianchi B, Canonica W. Loratadine in the treatment of cough associated with allergic rhinoconjuntivitis. *Ann Allergy Asthma Immunol* 1995; 75: 115–20.

68. Hargreaves MR, Benson MK. Inhaled sodium cromoglycate in angiotensin-converting enzyme inhibitor cough. *Lancet* 1995; 345: 13–16.

69. Moroni M, Porta C, Gualtieri G, Nastasi G, Tinelli C. Inhaled sodium cromoglycate to treat cough in advanced lung cancer patients. *Br J Cancer* 1996; 74: 309–11.

70. Evald T, Munch EP, Kok-Jensen A. Chronic non-asthmatic cough is not affected by inhaled beclomethasone dipropionate. *Allergy* 1989; 44: 510–14.

71. Furukawa CT, Shapiro G, Bierman CW, Kraemer MJ, Ward DJ, Pierson WE. A double-blind study comparing

the effectiveness of cromolyn sodium and sustained-release theophylline in childhood asthma. *Pediatrics* 1984; 74: 453–9.

72. Tattersfield AE. Clinical pharmacology of long acting beta-receptor agonists. *Life Sci* 1993; 52: 2161–9.

73. Edwards A. Sodium cromoglycate (Intal) as an anti-inflammatory agent for the treatment of chronic asthma. *Clin Exp Allergy* 1994; 24: 612–23.

74. Fink NJ, Forman S, Silvers WS, Soifer MM, Tashkin DP, Wilson AF. A double-blind study of the efficacy of nedocromil sodium in the management of asthma in patients using high doses of bronchodilators. *J Allergy Clin Immunol* 1994; 94: 473–81.

75. Barnes PJ, Pedersen S. Efficacy and safety of inhaled steroids in asthma. *Am Rev Respir Dis* 1993; 148: S1–S26.

76. Spector SL, Smith LJ, Glass M. Accolate Asthma Trialists Group. Effects of 6 weeks of therapy with oral doses of ICI 204, 219, a leukotriene D_4 receptor antagonist, in subjects with bronchial asthma. *Am J Respir Crit Care Med* 1994; 150: 618–23.

77. Israel E, Cohn J, Dube L, Drazen JM. Effect of treatment with zileuton, a 5-lipoxygenase inhibitor, in patients with asthma: a randomized controlled trial. *JAMA* 1996; 275: 931–6.

78. Barnes NC, Pujet JC. Pranlukast, a novel leukotriene receptor antagonist: results of the first European, placebo controlled, multicentre clinical study in asthma. *Thorax* 1997; 52: 523–7.

79. Reiss TF, Chervinsky P, Dockhorn RJ, Shingo S, Seidenberg B, Edwards TB. Montelukast, a once-daily leukotriene receptor antagonist, in the treatment of chronic asthma: a multicenter, randomized, double-blind trial. *Arch Intern Med* 1998; 158: 1213–20.

80. Nishi K, Watanabe K, Ooka T, Fujimura M, Matsuda T. Cough variant asthma successfully treated with a peptide leukotriene receptor antagonist. *Nihon Kyobu Shikkan Gakkai Zasshi* 1997; 35: 117–23.

81. Lowry R, Wood A, Johnson T, Higenbottam T. Antitussive properties of inhaled bronchodilators on induced cough. *Chest* 1988; 6: 1186–9.

82. Fujimura M, Sakamoto S, Kamio Y, Matsuda T. Effect of methacholine induced bronchoconstriction and procaterol induced bronchodilation on cough receptor sensitivity to inhaled capsaicin and tartaric acid. *Thorax* 1992; 47: 441–5.

83. Shimizu T, Mochizuki H, Tokuyama K, Morikawa A. Relationship between the acid-induced cough response and airway responsiveness and obstruction in children with asthma. *Thorax* 1996; 51: 281–7.

84. Tanaka S, Hirata K, Kurihara N, Yoshikawa J, Takeda T. Effect of loratadine, an H_1 antihistamine, on induced cough in non-asthmatic patients with chronic cough. *Thorax* 1996; 51: 810–14.

85. Fuller RW, Collier JG. Sodium cromoglycate and atropine block the fall in FEV_1 but not the cough induced by hypotonic mist. *Thorax* 1984; 39: 766–70.

86. Collier JG, Fuller RW. Capsaicin inhalation in man and the effects of sodium cromoglycate. *Br J Pharmacol* 1984; 81: 113–17.

87. Dicpinigaitis PV, Dobkin JB. Effect of zafirlukast on cough reflex sensitivity in asthmatics. *J Asthma* 1999; 36: 265–70.

88. Fuller RW, Karlsson J-A, Choudry NB, Pride NB. Effect of inhaled and systemic opiates on responses to inhaled capsaicin in humans. *J Appl Physiol* 1988; 65: 1125–30.

89. Choudry NB, Fuller RW, Anderson N, Karlsson J-A. Separation of cough and reflex bronchoconstriction by inhaled local anaesthetics. *Eur Respir J* 1990; 3: 579–83.

90. Morice AH, Marshall AE, Higgins KS, Grattan TJ. Effect of inhaled menthol on citric acid induced cough in normal subjects. *Thorax* 1994; 49: 1024–6.

91. Advenier C, Lagenta V, Boichot E. The role of tachykinin receptor antagonists in the prevention of bronchial hyperresponsiveness, airway inflammation and cough. *Eur Respir J* 1997; 10: 1892–1906.

92. Ichinose M, Nakajima N, Takahashi T, Yamauchi H, Inoue H, Takashima T. Protection against bradykinin-induced bronchoconstriction in asthmatic patients by neurokinin receptor antagonist. *Lancet* 1992; 340: 1248–51.

92. Joos GF, Pauwels R, Van der Straeten M. Effect of inhaled substance P and neurokinin A on the airways of normal and asthmatic subjects. *Thorax* 1987; 42: 779–83.

93. Joos GF, Van Schoor J, Kips JC, Pauwels RA. The effect of inhaled FK224, a tachykinin NK-1 and NK-2 receptor antagonist, on neurokinin A-induced bronchoconstriction in asthmatics. *Am J Respir Crit Care Med* 1996; 153: 1781–4.

94. Sharara AM, Hijazi M, Tarawneh M, Ind PW. Nebulized glyceryl trinitrate exerts acute bronchodilator effects in patients with acute bronchial asthma. *Pulm Pharmacol Therapeut* 1998; 11: 65–70.

95. Fahy JV, Wong HH, Geppetti P *et al*. Effect of an NK$_1$ receptor antagonist (CP-99,994) on hypertonic saline-induced bronchoconstriction and cough in male asthmatic subjects. *Am J Respir Crit Care Med* 1995; 152: 879–84.

96. Akbary AM, Wirth KJ, Schölkens BA. Efficacy and tolerability of Icatibant (Hoe 140) in patients with moderately severe chronic bronchial asthma. *Immunopharmacology* 1996; 33: 238–42.

97. O'Connell F, Thomas VE, Fuller RW, Pride NB. Effect of pizotifen on the antitussive action of morphine in healthy humans using the capsaicin model. *Eur Respir J* 1995; 8: 347s.

98. O'Connell F, Thomas VE, Fuller RW, Pride NB. Effect of dopaminergic and cholinergic agonists and antagonists on capsaicin-induced cough and reflex bronchoconstriction. *Thorax* 1993; 48: 1084P.

99. Dicpinigaitis PV, Dobkin JB, Rauf K, Adrich TK. Inhibition of capsaicin-induced cough by the gamma-aminobutyric acid agonist baclofen. *J Clin Pharmacol* 1998; 38: 364–7.

Chapter 43

Specific Problems: Chronic Rhinosinusitis and Asthma

Paraya Assanasen and Robert Naclerio

INTRODUCTION

Sinusitis has manifestations ranging from an acute illness following an upper respiratory tract infection to an unremitting illness associated with a genetic abnormality in the epithelium of patients with cystic fibrosis. It is a major health-care problem that is increasing in prevalence.[1] It currently afflicts about 15% of the US population.[2] Asthma affects approximately 5% of the general population.[3] Forty to seventy-five percent of patients with asthma have chronic sinusitis,[4] and 35% with chronic sinusitis have asthma.[5]

Patients with asthma and sinusitis have been shown to have diminished social function and low perception of their functioning in work and in daily activity.[6] Between 1990 and 1992, approximately 73 million restricted activity days per year were reported by persons who had sinusitis, a 50% increase from the figures reported between 1986 and 1988.[7] In 1992, 13 million antibiotic prescriptions were given for acute and chronic sinusitis, more than a two-fold increase from 5.8 million prescriptions in 1985.[8] Direct medical costs of sinusitis, not including the cost of surgery, were approximately $2.4 billion in 1992,[8] establishing sinusitis as one of the most costly disorders experienced by the US population.

Acute sinusitis typically follows a viral respiratory infection and can trigger an asthmatic attack. Although most cases of sinusitis are acute and self-limited, a significant number of individuals develop chronic sinusitis. The underlying cause of chronic sinusitis is poorly defined. Some conditions associated with the development of this malady are listed in Table 43.1.[9] In a recent series of 200 consecutive cases of chronic sinusitis, allergic rhinitis was found in 56% of the patients and non-allergic rhinitis in another 26%.[10]

It is hypothesized that certain individuals have a predisposition to develop chronic sinusitis. In these persons, environmental factors, such as allergens, viruses, and air pollutants, trigger epithelial alterations that induce inflammation and subsequently decrease mucociliary transport, causing sinus ostial obstruction. Stasis of mucus in the sinuses then leads to bacterial infections that may further adversely influence the epithelium. If this cycle is not interrupted, the epithelium develops metaplastic changes, and the underlying mucosa proliferates, leading to a self-perpetuating cycle. This cycle manifests itself clinically as chronic sinusitis and is no longer dependent upon either the bacteria or the anatomy that initiated the process.

DEFINITION

Sinusitis implies inflammation of the paranasal sinuses. Uncomplicated colds in healthy patients are associated with radiographic evidence of sinusitis.[11,12] Because the mucosa of the nasal and sinus tissue are contiguous and the inflammatory process that causes sinusitis is frequently associated with inflammation of the nasal passages, the term *rhinosinusitis* describes this disease state more precisely.[13] Rhinosinusitis may be classified as acute fulminant, subacute, recurrent acute, chronic, or acute exacerbation of chronic, based on clinical picture[14] (Table 43.2). Chronic rhinosinusitis is defined as signs and symptoms of inflammation of the sinuses persisting for more than 12 weeks and documented by positive imaging study at least 4 weeks after appropriate medical treatment in the absence of an intervening acute episode.[15] Signs and symptoms of chronic sinusitis are non-specific and overlap with other nasal disorders that should be considered in the differential diagnosis of rhinosinusitis.

Table 43.1: Conditions that predispose to chronic rhinosinusitis

Rhinitis
Allergic rhinitis
Non-allergic rhinitis
Nasal polyps

Nasal anatomic abnormalities
Septal deviation
Concha bullosa
Paradoxical middle turbinate
Haller cell
Prominent ethmoid bulla
Atelectatic uncinate process

Lower respiratory disease
Asthma
Cystic fibrosis
Bronchiectasis

Immune deficiencies
Panhypogammaglobulinaemia
Deficiencies of selective antibody response; e.g. IgA
    deficiency, IgG-subclass deficiency

Miscellaneous
Cigarette smoke
Pollution
Dental caries, dental extraction/injections (second
    premolar or first molar teeth)
Foreign bodies (transnasal tubes)
Ciliary dyskinesia, Kartagener's syndrome, Young's
    syndrome
Aspirin sensitivity
Acquired immunodeficiency syndrome
Rhinitis medicamentosa
Cocaine abuse
Wegener's granulomatosis
Facial trauma, barotrauma, iatrogenic surgical causes
Viral infections
Swimming and diving

RELATIONSHIP BETWEEN SINUSITIS AND ASTHMA

An association between the presence of chronic sinusitis and asthma has been known for more than a century. It has been reported that 20–70% of a large number of adult asthmatics had coexistent sinusitis.[16–18] A frequent occurrence in patients with asthma is a worsening of lower airway disease with sinusitis.[19] There was radiographic evidence of sinusitis in 50–70% of children and adults with asthma.[20,21] De Cleyn et al.[22] found that 54% of 270 asthmatic patients had abnormal plain sinus films, and children had more opacifications than did adults. Zimmerman et al.[23] found that plain sinus films of 138 asthmatic patients showed abnormalities in 31%, compared with none of 50 patients who had dental complaints. Schwartz et al.[24] reported that 47% of asthmatic flare-ups were associated with abnormal sinus radiographs, a significantly greater percentage than that for rhinitic patients with flare-ups (29%). Rossi et al.[25] noted that 87% of patients with exacerbation of asthma had abnormal sinus radiographs. In another study, the prevalence of sinusitis in 558 children 3–6 years old who had bronchial asthma was 37.3%, which was far greater than that among patients with other non-atopic pulmonary diseases (5.9%). A correlation between the severity of asthma and the prevalence of sinusitis was found.[26] In a study of 80 patients with chronic sinusitis, asthma was noted to be associated with extensive disease as determined by the computed tomography (CT) score of the paranasal sinuses.[5] In contrast, Ferrante et al.[27] studied the prevalence of sinusitis and its relationship to bronchial asthma in 120 young male asthmatics. There were no statistical differences between asthmatics with and those without sinusitis with regard to the severity of asthma, basal lung function, and bronchial hyperresponsiveness.

These studies do not imply a cause-and-effect relationship. Both conditions may merely coexist and represent the same inflammatory process occurring in different organ systems. Several mechanisms, however, have been proposed for the way in which sinusitis could initiate or worsen asthma. These include aspiration of infected sinus secretions into the lungs, enhanced vagal stimulation producing reflex bronchospasm, excessive airway drying of the tracheobronchial tree from mouth breathing, and production of cytokines and bronchoconstrictive mediators in an infected sinus that affects the lungs directly or indirectly via their influence on circulating cells.[28]

The postulated neuroanatomic pathways that could connect the paranasal sinuses to the lungs are as follows: receptors in the nose, pharynx, and presumably in the paranasal sinuses give rise to afferent fibres that pass to the brain stem, where it can connect via the reticular formation with the dorsal vagal nucleus. From the vagal nucleus, parasympathetic efferent fibres travel in the

Table 43.2: Classification of rhinosinusitis

Classification	Duration	Characteristics
Acute fulminant	Occurs within hours to days	Severe symptoms Often indicates intraorbital or intracranial complications Requires urgent attention
Subacute	1–12 weeks	Persistent symptoms following upper respiratory tract infection Usually complete resolution after effective medical therapy
Recurrent acute	≥ Four episodes per year, with each episode lasting ≥ 7–10 days and absence of intervening signs and symptoms of chronic rhinosinusitis	Suspect anatomic abnormalities or immune deficiency
Chronic	≥ 12 weeks	Requires imaging study after adequate medical treatment Poor response to therapy
Acute exacerbations of chronic	–	Treat acute episodes like subacute sinusitis and manage like chronic sinusitis

vagus nerve to the bronchi. The cholinergic parasympathetic nervous system plays a role in maintaining resting bronchial muscle tone as well as in mediating an acute bronchospastic response.[29]

Stimulation of receptors in the nose or nasopharynx either via chemical or mechanical methods has been shown to cause reflex bronchoconstriction in both animals and man. Kratchmer demonstrated that a variety of irritants applied to the nasal mucous membranes of cats and rabbits provoked bronchoconstriction.[30] Dixon and Brodie found that, after vagus nerve resection, bronchoconstriction caused by mechanical or electric stimulation of the nasal mucosa was abolished.[31] Evidence for such a connection in man has been shown by Kaufman and Wright.[32] The nasal and nasopharyngeal mucosa of healthy subjects was exposed to silica particles. Lower airway resistance increased significantly, and the effect was abolished by atropine administration. They also demonstrated that, after trigeminal nerve resection, reflex bronchospasm induced by nasal and nasopharyngeal irritation was abolished.[33] Bucca et al.[34] performed a histamine challenge to the lower airway of 106 patients with chronic sinusitis before and after medical treatment of sinusitis. During sinusitis exacerbation, 76 patients had extrathoracic airway hyperresponsiveness, which was associated in 46 with bronchial hyperresponsiveness. The changes in bronchial and extrathoracic airway hyperresponsiveness were strongly associated with pharyngitis as determined by history, physical examination, and nasal lavage. They proposed that airway hyperresponsiveness in sinusitis might depend on pharyngobronchial reflexes triggered by seeding of the inflammatory process into the pharynx via post-nasal drip of mediators and infected material from affected sinuses. These observations seem to support the existence of a nasobronchial reflex in man, as Sluder originally proposed.[35] In an attempt to prove the existence of a reflex from the sinus, Baroody et al.[36] studied the response of the maxillary sinus to histamine provocation in non-allergic subjects and found that no sinonasal reflex was demonstrated because there was no contralateral nasal-reflex secretory response. In their view, based on these findings, the presence of a sino-pulmonary reflex is probably unlikely.

In patients with chronic sinusitis, increases in the number of eosinophils[37] and CD4+ lymphocytes[38] have been found in tissue biopsies. In a recent study, nasal turbinate tissues from 16 individuals with allergic or non-allergic chronic sinusitis and 10 normal controls were examined for eotaxin mRNA. Eotaxin is a relatively specific eosinophil chemokine. The numbers of cells expressing eotaxin mRNA and protein were increased significantly in patients with both allergic and non-allergic chronic sinusitis when compared with normal controls.[39] This suggests a potential role of this chemokine in the recruitment of eosinophils in patients with chronic sinusitis.

Harlin et al.[40] found a significant association between sinus tissue eosinophilia and asthma in adults with chronic sinusitis. In contrast, sinus tissue from patients with chronic sinusitis alone had no eosinophils. Immunofluorescence studies demonstrated an association between the presence of extracellular deposition of major basic protein and damage to the sinus mucosa. The histopathology of the paranasal respiratory epithelium was similar to that described in bronchial asthma. Eosinophils seem to act as effector cells in chronic inflammatory disease in the paranasal epithelium. Sinus disease in patients with asthma may be caused by the same mechanism that causes damage to the bronchial epithelium.

Newman et al.[41] found a strong relationship among allergy, peripheral blood eosinophilia, and sinusitis in asthmatic patients. Extensive paransal sinus disease (as assessed by computed tomography) correlated well with asthma, specific IgE antibodies, and peripheral blood eosinophilia. Moreover, the correlation with eosinophilia was noted in patients without a history of wheezing or allergy. Newman et al. suggested that inflammation in the sinus mucosa could lead to release of chemotactic cytokines (IL-5), which could recruit inflammatory cells (e.g. eosinophils) into the circulation. It may facilitate their recruitment into the bronchial mucosa, leading to exacerbation of asthmatic inflammation.

Other possible mechanisms by which sinusitis may initiate bronchospasm are aspiration of infected material or local stimulation of irritant receptors by inflammatory mediators, with resultant reflex bronchospasm. Bardin et al.[42] performed a study attempting to mimic the aspiration postulate in asthmatics who had sinusitis. When they used a radionuclide technique, pulmonary aspiration of upper airway secretions could not be demonstrated in neurologically intact individuals. This suggests that aspiration of mucopurulent or even locally produced inflammatory mediators is unlikely to cause pulmonary symptoms in asthmatics.

Rolla et al.[43] performed a histamine inhalation challenge and nasopharyngeal biopsies in 24 non-asthmatic patients who had exacerbation of chronic sinusitis. They found that pharyngeal damage as indicated by epithelial thinning might contribute to airway dysfunction by favouring the access of irritants to submucosal nerve endings, with activation of constrictive reflexes to the extrathoracic airway. Proliferation of sensory neurons as indicated by increased submucosal nerve density, consequent to long-lasting pharyngeal inflammation, may cause more severe extrathoracic airway narrowing and activate pharyngobronchial reflex.

Moreover, Brugman et al.[44] studied the association between abnormal lower airway function and sinusitis in rabbits. Sterile sinusitis was induced by instillation of the active complement component C5a into the maxillary sinuses. After the C5a injection, the rabbits had a marked increase in bronchial responsiveness. When the rabbits were positioned head down or intubated for blocking of the passage of cells or mediators from the nose to the lower airways, they failed to show lower airway hyperresponsiveness. However, this aspiration may reflect the effect of the anaesthetic agent and may not be relevant to non-anaesthetized human subjects. These studies suggest that drainage of material to the pharynx or lower airway may contribute to changes in airway function.

An example of an association between disorders of the upper and lower respiratory tract is "the aspirin triad". This syndrome includes ASA (acetylsalicylic acid) intolerance, nasal polyps, and asthma and usually indicates chronic intractable rhinosinusitis, persistent asthma of greater than average severity, and higher than ordinary medication requirements. The majority of ASA-sensitive asthmatics, if challenged with aspirin, demonstrate, in addition to bronchospasm, nasal responses heralded by rhinorrhoea, sneezing, and nasal obstruction.[45] The nasal responses to ASA challenge, however, are superimposed on existing pathology of the upper respiratory tract including chronic rhinitis, sinusitis, and nasal polyposis. The incidence of sinusitis by roentgenogram in ASA-sensitive asthmatics is as high as 95%, and the frequency of nasal polyps may be as high as 70–90%, compared with about 5% in the general asthmatic population.[45] There is a high recurrence of nasal polyps and a frequent need for endoscopic sinus surgery in this group of patients. This disorder probably represents the coexistence of changes in both the lower and upper airways rather than a cause-and-effect relationship.

Additional evidence suggesting a sino-bronchial relationship comes from observations that appropriate and effective treatment of sinusitis has resulted in improvement or stabilization of a patient's lower airway disease. Rachelefsky et al.[46] studied 48 children with asthma. All had symptoms and were under active treatment. Sinus radiographs showed abnormalities in all 48 children. After receiving treatment for sinusitis, they had significant alleviation of their asthmatic symptoms, and nearly 80% had normal sinus radiographs. Of the children tested, 67% had normal pulmonary function. Finally, at the completion of treatment, only 21% required bronchodilator treatment. Similar results were reported in another group of children with asthma and sinusitis.[47] Treatment of sinusitis in asthmatic children has been shown to improve their bronchial hyper-responsiveness to methacholine and to decrease their symptoms, with appropriate response of their sinuses to clinical therapy.[48] The caveat is that medical treatment of sinusitis does not affect only the sinuses, but also the lungs.

Furthermore, patients with asthma may be unresponsive to therapy until co-existing sinus disease is successfully treated. Weille[49] examined 500 patients with asthma, 72% of whom had concomitant chronic sinus disease. Of 100 patients who underwent sinus surgery, 56 subsequently experienced improvements in chest symptoms, and complete resolution of asthma occurred in 10. In another study, 23 of 24 patients with simultaneous chronic sinusitis and asthma experienced a 75% or greater improvement in asthma symptoms after surgical drainage.[50] Mings and colleagues[51] showed that 62% of 16 patients who underwent bilateral intranasal sphenoethmoidectomy after not responding to aggressive medical management of sinusitis had subjective improvement of their asthma. Eighty-eight percent of the patients reported a significantly reduced prednisolone requirement. Functional endoscopic sinus surgery (FESS) has provided equally good results. One report presented results for 205 steroid-dependent patients with the aspirin triad. After FESS, 40% of the patients were able to discontinue steroids; another 44% had their illness controlled with alternate-day steroid therapy or bursts.[52] Manning et al.[53] studied 14 children with severe asthma requiring at least intermittent systemic steroid therapy. Eleven of 14 patients who underwent FESS demonstrated a significant reduction in hospitalization and schooldays missed. Twelve of the 14 patients experienced a reduc-

tion in glucocorticoid requirements. Eleven of 14 and 13 of 14 patients experienced a significant improvement in asthma and sinusitis symptoms scores, respectively. Similar results in 52 children were addressed by Parsons and Philips.[54] After FESS, there was a reduction of 89% in chronic cough and a 96% decrease in asthmatic symptoms. There was also a significant reduction of the number of exacerbations per month and of emergency department visits. Another study investigated 20 asthma patients aged 16 to 72 years who underwent FESS for chronic sinusitis. Eighty-five percent reported that their asthma was less severe after FESS. There was a reduction of 75% in hospitalizations and of 81% in emergency department/urgent physician office visits after FESS.[55] In contrast, another recent study showed that, although asthma was a critical factor negatively affecting the outcome of sinus surgery, sinus disease extension did not correlate with asthma severity at any stage. FESS failed to produce any significant change in lung function scores or any post-operative improvement of asthmatic symptoms.[56]

Unfortunately, the majority of the above-cited studies are retrospective and poorly controlled, and thus the evidence for a causal relationship between sinusitis and asthma is not clear-cut. Well-designed prospective studies are needed for establishment of a definite causal relationship between sinusitis and asthma.

MICROBIOLOGY

The microbiology of chronic sinusitis is less well-understood than that of acute sinusitis. One reason is that microbiologic testing is often performed on patients who have received multiple courses of antibiotics during the course of their illness.[57] The bacteriology of community-acquired acute sinusitis has been studied by antral punctures of maxillary sinuses in adults and children (Table 43.3). In both age groups, *Streptococcus pneumoniae* and *Haemophilus influenzae* are the predominant organisms.[58] In children, *Moraxella catarrhalis* is another important organism.[59] Gwaltney[60] compiled the results of a number of studies and showed the prevalence of infective organisms in acute rhinosinusitis to be as follows: *S. pneumoniae*, 31%, unencapsulated *H. influenzae*, 21%, anaerobes, 6%, *S. aureus*, 4%, *S. pyogenes*, 2% and *M. catarrhalis*, 2%. Viruses were also found in the cultures, often in conjunction with bacteria.

Table 43.3: Organisms associated with rhinosinusitis

Acute sinusitis
Bacteria
    Streptococcus pneumoniae
    Haemophilus influenzae
    Moraxella catarrhalis
    Streptococcus pyogenes
Viruses
    Rhinovirus
    Influenza virus
    Parainfluenza virus

Chronic sinusitis
Coagulase-negative *Staphylococcus*
Staphylococcus aureus
Anaerobes
Streptococcus pneumoniae
Fungi

Nosocomial sinusitis
Gram-negative organisms
Fungi
Methicillin-resistant *Staphylococcus aureus*

Although the organisms have remained fairly constant, the pattern of antibiotic resistance has changed. The bacteria that predominate in sinusitis can resist penicillin through the production of the enzyme β-lactamase (*Haemophilus influenzae* and *Moraxella catarrhalis*) or through changes in penicillin-binding sites (*Streptococcus pneumoniae*).[61] Twenty to 30% of *Streptococcus pneumoniae* strains have been reported to be penicillin-resistant in the USA,[62] whereas 30–40% of *Haemophilus influenzae* and 75–95% of *Moraxella catarrhalis* are β-lactamase producers.[63] In nosocomial sinusitis (particularly in patients with tubes transversing the nasal cavity) and sinusitis in impaired hosts, a greater spectrum of organisms, including Gram-negative organisms, fungi, and methicillin-resistant *Staphylococcus aureus*, has been cultured. Pathogens in patients with cystic fibrosis and sinusitis include *Pseudomonas aeruginosa*, *Escherichia coli*, *Staphylococcus aureus*, and *Aspergillus fumigatus*, in addition to the common organisms.

The bacteriology of chronic sinusitis has been studied by tissue or secretion culture during surgery. Chronic sinusitis has been associated with a mixed flora of anaerobic and aerobic organisms. In adults, one study showed anaerobic bacteria in only 17% and aerobic bacteria in only 53% of their 30 subjects. Mixed aerobic and anaerobic isolates were recovered from 30% of patients.[64] Another study demonstrated that anaerobes and viridans *streptococci* predominated in chronic maxillary sinusitis, whereas coagulase-negative *staphylococci* (70%) and *streptococci* (33%) predominated in chronic ethmoid sinusitis.[65] In children, Muntz and Lusk[66] cultured ethmoid mucosal specimens obtained at surgery and found mainly alpha-haemolytic *Streptococcus* (23%) and *S. aureus* (19%) as single organisms. Thirty percent of specimens grew multiple organisms. Another study of surgical specimens from the ethmoid in children showed that *Staphylococcus epidermidis* and viridans *streptococci* predominated.[67]

Goldenhersh *et al.*[68] studied 12 children between 3 and 11 years of age who had asthma. All subjects had documented respiratory allergy and chronic respiratory symptoms of at least 30 days' duration, consistent with chronic sinusitis. When maxillary sinus aspiration was performed, *M. catarrhalis* was recovered from six patients, and mixed cultures of *streptococci* were recovered from three patients. Only one patient had anaerobic *streptococci* mixed with aerobic *streptococci*. Ramadan[69] obtained tissue for cultures from endoscopic sinus surgery in 76 patients to study the microbiology of chronic sinusitis. Of the positive cultures, 80% grew coagulase-negative *Staphylococcus* species, 21% grew *S. aureus*, 8% grew anaerobes, and 4% grew *S. pneumoniae*.

In chronic sinusitis, there is some evidence based on experience that antibiotic treatment alone does not cure the disease in most cases.[57,70] Thus, it is not clear whether the cultures reflect causative organisms or colonization of functionally impaired sinus cavities. It also indicates that the ongoing pathologic process in chronic sinusitis is not due solely to bacterial infection.

EVALUATION OF THE PATIENT

Although the causal relationship between chronic sinusitis and asthma is still being debated, physicians treating asthma should be prepared to evaluate and manage chronic sinusitis.

History

The evaluation of chronic sinusitis begins with a history of symptoms, with particular emphasis on risks and exacerbating factors, starting by defining the onset and duration of the illness and its temporal relationship to seasonal or life events (e.g. change in school or house, acquiring a pet, trauma). Diseases with known associations between the upper and lower airways, such as allergy, immotile cilia syndrome, cystic fibrosis, immunodeficiency syndrome, and aspirin intolerance should be addressed. Both a personal and a family history of atopic diseases (allergic rhinitis, asthma, atopic dermatitis) and environmental history (type of home heating, chemical exposure, employment, presence of humidification) are helpful. Acute sinusitis typically is manifested as a persistent upper respiratory infection. Symptoms that suggest sinusitis should be asked about. A history of these nasal symptoms preceding an exacerbation of asthma should alert the physician to the possibility of co-existing active sinus disease. Inquiry into the sense of smell aids in determining the degree of airflow obstruction. In children, paroxysmal nocturnal cough, bad breath, and sleep disturbance are more prominent than in adults. The history should detail previous medical and surgical treatments such as use of prescribed and over-the-counter drugs (aspirin, topical decongestants), antibiotics, and steroids.

Physical Examination

A complete ear, nose, and throat examination should be performed with special focus on the nasal cavity. Ear examination may show unilateral or bilateral otitis media with effusion, suggesting nasopharyngeal pathology or eustachian tube dysfunction. Patients with chronic rhinosinusitis usually have no facial swelling or oedema. Facial swelling as well as abnormal eye or neurological examination findings should alert the physician to a potential complication. Chronic nasal obstruction as in allergic rhinitis may have special clues such as an allergic shiner (discolouration beneath the eyelids), allergic salute (pushing the nasal tip upward with the palm of the hand to relieve nasal itching and obstruction), and adenoid facies (under-development of the zygoma, nasal processes, and maxillary sinuses).

After examination of the external nares for obvious structural abnormalities such as signs of old trauma, a rhinophyma, or a collapsed nasal valve, a nasal speculum is used for examining the anterior third of the nasal cavity under good illumination. The examination should include visualization of the nasal septum to assess for anterior septal deviation that could cause airflow obstruction. Structural deviations or asymmetry should raise the suspicion of trauma or congenital deformities. Examination of the nasal cavity with the otoscope is helpful in small children, in whom endoscopy cannot be performed. Unilateral signs should raise the suspicion of foreign bodies in children or of tumour in adults.

Applying a topical decongestant permits improved visualization of the nasal cavity. A slow or absent response to a decongestant indicates a hyperplastic mucosa. A well-decongested nasal cavity can provide better visualization of the anterior aspect of the middle turbinate. The openings to the frontal, maxillary, and anterior ethmoidal sinuses are located lateral to the anterior portion of the middle turbinate in the middle meatus. Occasionally, polyps or polypoid changes may be seen in this area. Nasal polyposis causes chronic symptoms and may predispose patients to recurrent infections. Polyps appear as a glistening pedunculated mass, sometimes with a bluish or yellowish hue that differentiates them from the normal pink-coloured nasal mucosa. Nasal polyps are uncommon in children, and their presence should prompt evaluation for possible cystic fibrosis. A unilateral nasal polyp should raise the suspicion of an inverted papilloma or carcinoma in adults, or of dermoid cysts, encephaloceles, and gliomas in children.

Persistent purulent nasal secretions usually seen coming from inside the middle meatus are characteristic of sinusitis. Nasal cultures obtained without endoscopy are not specific for the identification of bacteria responsible for chronic sinusitis. Examination of the oral cavity may show post-nasal drip or a high arched palate with poor dental occlusion that is related to chronic mouth breathing. The physical examination should also include signs of diseases that predispose to sinusitis (Table 43.1).

Nasal Endoscopy

Nasal endoscopy has advanced the diagnosis and treatment of rhinosinusitis. It provides excellent visualization of the entire nasal cavity, and pus draining from the sinus ostium can be cultured. Cultures from the middle meatus or ostio-meatal complex area have been shown to correlate with cultures obtained from within the sinuses in patients undergoing sinus surgery.[67,71] Nasal endoscopy was demonstrated to identify more disease than did anterior rhinoscopy (85% vs 74%), and to have a sensitivity of 84% and a specificity of 92%.[72] Although flexible endoscopy does not provide as good an illumination and breadth of examination as does rigid endoscopy, it provides a more thorough, less painful examination, particularly in children, because more of the examination can be performed. It is also useful for getting into the sinus cavity in post-operative patients. Anatomical abnormalities, purulence, septal deformities, masses, mucosal changes, and naso-pharyngeal pathology can be identified. Endoscopic examinations need not to be performed in every patient who has nasal complaints. However, any patient whose diagnosis remains questionable or who does not respond to treatment should be considered for endoscopic evaluation.

Other Diagnostic Tests

Skin tests or *in vitro* IgE measurements help to confirm the diagnosis of allergic rhinitis. Nasal cytology can identify eosinophils, pointing to an allergic problem or non-allergic rhinitis with eosinophilia syndrome (NARES). The presence of bacteria and neutrophils suggests infectious disease. Quantitative sweat chloride tests for the diagnosis of cystic fibrosis should be considered in children with nasal polyps and/or colonization of the nose and sinuses with *Pseudomonas* sp. A complete blood count with differential, CH50 levels, measurement of complement components, quantitative immunoglobulins, and the response to protein and polysaccharide antigens may indicate confounding immunological defects in cases of chronic or recurrent sinusitis. Nasal/paranasal sinus biopsy may be required for diagnosis in suspected cases of tumour, granulomatous disease, fungal infection, or immotile cilia syndrome.

Plain sinus radiographs serve reasonably well for diagnosing maxillary, frontal, and sphenoid sinusitis. However, they are less reliable in depicting abnormalities in the ethmoid sinuses, the area most commonly affected by inflammatory disease. For example, CT scans of the paranasal sinuses demonstrated ethmoid sinusitis in 45 patients in whom plain films were negative.[73] Compared to sinus CT, plain films prove to be less specific and sensitive in depicting the extent and specific location of sinus abnormalities.[74] Coronal sinus CT scans are presently considered the best imaging mode for patients suspected of having chronic sinusitis.[75] Although nasal endoscopy was moderately sensitive and highly specific in predicting the results of CT scans,[75] a normal-appearing nasal cavity on endoscopy does not rule out chronic sinusitis, and a patient with suggestive symptoms should undergo CT scanning for definitive diagnosis. The CT scan is the most sensitive

and non-invasive means of diagnosing disease in the sinus cavity, although patient-based reports of paranasal sinus symptoms failed to be correlated with findings on CT scan.[76]

Importantly, individuals with no complaints may have changes within the sinus. Sinus abnormalities may be seen in asymptomatic patients because of previous colds or other undetermined causes and do not require treatment.[11,77,78] This points to the necessity of relating patient complaints, endoscopic findings, and CT findings when a diagnosis is made. Besides determining the degree of mucosal involvement, a CT scan can define anatomical abnormalities that interfere with sinus drainage.[79] These abnormalities are risk factors, and their correction is the object of surgical intervention.

Unilateral symptomatic chronic sinusitis that is unresponsive to appropriate medical treatment should raise the suspicion of fungal sinusitis or neoplasms. Fungal sinusitis often causes a non-homogeneous appearance of the enlarged mucous membrane, especially in the maxillary sinus. Patients should receive antibiotic and other indicated medical treatment before obtaining CT scans. The rationale for the duration of pre-medication is obscure, but it is known that mucosal abnormalities after acute sinusitis can persist for weeks. The CT examination is usually performed with the patient prone on the scanner bed with the chin in hyperextension. In patients who cannot tolerate being placed on their chin, scans are performed in hyperextension. In young children, coronal scans cannot always be obtained. In these individuals, axial scans with coronal reconstruction should be obtained.

Magnetic resonance imaging (MRI) is more costly than CT scans and does not show air–bone interfaces as well as does CT.[80] MRI is excellent for demonstrating the presence of inflammatory disease in the paranasal sinuses. Its main benefit is in distinguishing sinusitis from tumour or to help in the diagnosis of fungal sinusitis and mucocoeles.[81]

TREATMENT

Medical

Antibiotics The key to medical therapy is accurate diagnosis. In acute rhinosinusitis or a flare-up of chronic sinusitis, antibiotic therapy should be directed to *S. pneumoniae* and *H. influenzae* (Table 43.4). The appropriate duration of antibiotic therapy for acute sinusitis

Table 43.4: Antibiotic treatment of rhinosinusitis

	Dosage	
	Adult	**Children**
First-line antibiotics		
Amoxicillin	250–500 mg t.i.d.	30–40 mg kg^{-1} day^{-1} divided t.i.d
(In penicillin-allergic patients: trimethoprim-sulphamethoxazole)		
Trimethoprim-sulphamethoxazole	1 DS b.i.d. (DS: TMP 160 mg/SMX 800 mg)	8–12 mg TMP/40–60 mg SMX kg^{-1} day^{-1} divided b.i.d.
Second-line antibiotics		
Amoxicillin-clavulanate	500–875 mg b.i.d.	30–40 mg kg^{-1} day^{-1} divided b.i.d. or t.i.d
Clarithromycin	250–500 mg b.i.d.	15 mg kg^{-1} day^{-1} divided b.i.d.
Loracarbef	400 mg b.i.d.	30 mg kg^{-1} day^{-1} divided b.i.d.
Cefpodoxime proxetil	100 mg b.i.d.	10 mg kg^{-1} day^{-1} divided b.i.d.
Cefprozil	500 mg q.d.	30 mg kg^{-1} day^{-1} divided b.i.d.
Cefuroxime axetil	250–500 mg b.i.d.	20–30 mg kg^{-1} day^{-1} divided b.i.d.
Cefixime	400 mg q.d.	8 mg kg^{-1} day^{-1} divided q.d. or b.i.d.
Ceftibuten	400 mg q.d. or 200 mg b.i.d.	9 mg kg^{-1} day^{-1} divided q.d. or b.i.d.
Ciprofloxacin	500–750 mg b.i.d.	Not approved for age <18 years
Levofloxacin	500 mg q.d.	Not approved for age <18 years

is not well defined, but a 10-day course is probably adequate for most patients with acute sinusitis. Amoxicillin (amoxycillin) or trimethoprim-sulphamethoxazole as a first order of therapy is generally effective, inexpensive, and well-tolerated. If the patient fails to respond after 3 days, antibiotics should be switched. The choice of second-line antibiotic therapy should be based on factors that include previous antibiotic therapy, information about the resistance patterns of the pathogenic organisms within the community, dosing schedules, cost, side-effects, and the patient's drug allergy history. In chronic rhinosinusitis, data as to which antibiotic is most effective are not available for either children or adults, nor has the optimal treatment duration been established. Antibiotic therapy should be directed toward *Staphylococcus* species, *Streptococcus* species, and anaerobes (Table 43.4).

The currently recommended duration of antibiotic therapy for chronic rhinosinusitis is usually listed as 4–6 weeks, although there are no data to support this recommendation. On the basis of clinical experience, antimicrobial treatment should be continued for at least 1 week after the patient appears to be symptom-free.

Prior use of broad-spectrum antibiotics, presence of foul breath from the nasal cavity, or the results of a culture of sinus secretions should raise the suspicion of an anaerobic infection. It may then be appropriate to add metronidazole or clindamycin to the antibiotic regimen. Low-dose macrolide has been suggested for use in long-term therapy for chronic sinusitis. It was shown to reduce IL-8 in inflammatory sites[82] and to decrease subjective and objective symptoms in 80% or more of the patients.[83] *Pseudomonas aeruginosa* may colonize in patients who have cystic fibrosis and those who had prior surgery. This group of patients requires oral quinolones or intravenous tobramycin or ceftazidime for control of an acute exacerbation. In the clinical setting of persistent or aggravated asthma symptoms and radiographic evidence of sinusitis, with or without sinusitis symptoms, a medical trial of sinusitis therapy seems warranted.[20,21,29,46]

Adjuvants Besides administration of antibiotics, multiple other therapies have been used in the treatment of sinus disease. These include topical and systemic corticosteroid, topical and systemic decongestants and antihistamine, mucolytics, steam inhalations, and saline irrigations. Each adjuvant has a rationale that ranges form increasing ostial patency and thinning mucus to providing symptomatic relief. Although adjunctive treatments are widely recommended, few prospective studies have been directed toward evaluating their effectiveness.

CORTICOSTEROID There appears to be evidence that a topical steroid spray, alone or in conjunction with topical antibiotic therapy, may have some benefit for the treatment of chronic sinusitis, especially in patients with polyps.[84,85] Adding topical flunisolide to antibiotic treatments of 50 acute sinusitis patients was demonstrated to improve global evaluations slightly, possibly reduce exacerbation, and aid regression of radiographic abnormalities compared with placebo spray in a double-blind, randomized evaluation.[86] Budesonide administration in addition to antibiotic treatment for chronic rhinosinusitis was also shown to yield a slight reduction of nasal symptoms more effectively than did placebo, and mucosal thickening as evaluated radiologically was decreased more clearly in the budesonide group than in the placebo group.[87] Moreover, in one recent study, treatment of acute sinusitis in children with antibiotic and intranasal budesonide spray significantly reduced coughing and nasal discharge earlier in the course of acute sinusitis than did placebo spray.[88] The benefit in acute sinusitis seems small, and whether the additional cost and issues of compliance in taking multiple medication justify its use remains unknown.

Topical steroids help to reduce mucosal oedema and inflammation and may improve drainage. They have been shown to reduce nasal symptoms, polyp size,[89,90] and the number of recurrences after polypectomy[91] especially in patients who have previously been subjected to frequent polypectomies.[91] Consequently, topical corticosteroid should be used both before and after surgical removal of polyps. Additionally, nasal steroids have favourable effects on lower airway disease, thus allowing for concomitant reduction of airway hyperresponsiveness.[92,93] Systemic steroids are also of great benefit in allergic patients with chronic rhinosinusitis. A short course of systemic steroids may help even in patients who fail intranasal steroids because of drug distribution issues.

DECONGESTANTS AND ANTIHISTAMINE Decongestants stimulate α-adrenergic receptors on blood vessels,

resulting in vasoconstriction with subsequent shrinking of a swollen or oedematous mucosa. They are expected to decrease nasal swelling, to restore patency of ostia, and to improve ventilation. Minimal data are available to confirm the benefit of decongestants for the treatment of sinusitis. Systemic side-effects frequently occur with the use of systemic decongestants. Topical decongestants are helpful on a short-term basis, but continued use causes rhinitis medicamentosa.

Anti-histamines are traditionally used in the treatment of chronic sinusitis in patients with concomitant allergic rhinitis. There is one study showing that the addition of loratadine to antibiotics and oral corticosteroid reduced sneezing and nasal obstruction in patients with acute exacerbation of rhinosinusitis more than did placebo.[94]

MUCOLYTICS AND HUMIDITY There appears to be some evidence that mucolytics and nasal irrigations may be helpful for the treatment of chronic sinusitis.[95–98] A mucolytic drug was shown to accelerate the healing process and proper regeneration of the epithelium, and to lead to reduction of the period of antibiotic administration in the treatment of inflammatory changes in the paranasal sinuses.[99] The efficacy of guaifenesin was studied in a double-blind, placebo-controlled manner in 23 HIV-infected patients with rhinosinusitis. The guaifenesin group reported significantly less nasal congestion and thinner post-nasal drainage compared with the placebo group.[100] Shoseyov and co-workers[101] found that hypertonic saline irrigation improved two clinical scores (cough and nasal secretion/post-nasal drip) and the radiology score significantly in paediatric patients with chronic sinusitis compared with the use of normal saline.

OTHER AGENTS Intravenous immune serum globulin is useful in selected patients who have chronic sinusitis and proven impairment of humoral immunity. It was also demonstrated to decrease the duration of the course of antibiotics and episodes of sinusitis, and to improve the sinus CT findings in children whose sinus disease was recalcitrant to the usual therapeutic modalities.[102] Leukotriene inhibitors may play some role in patients with sinusitis and aspirin sensitivity. This syndrome is believed to be caused by increased production of leukotrienes.[103] Medications which interfere with leukotrienes, either by inhibiting leukotriene synthesis (zileuton) or by blocking leukotriene receptors (zifirlukast and monteleukast), appear to provide subjective improvement in nasal congestion and sense of smell.[104] Zileuton significantly reduced the decrease in FEV_1, angioedema, nasal congestion, and gastrointestinal symptoms that occurred after aspirin ingestion in triad patients.[105] These products are not licensed for use in sinusitis, but may be worth trying for difficult-to-manage patients.

Surgical

Surgical intervention for asthmatic patients with sinusitis is reserved for those in whom attempts at appropriate medical therapy fail to clear sinus disease or for those with recurrent acute problems in whom clear-cut anatomical abnormalities are present. Patients with asthma and sinusitis need to understand that their disease requires chronic management. Surgery assists patients to live more comfortably with their disease, but rarely eliminates it. Patients usually require chronic medications for their asthma and sinusitis. They need to have their asthma well-controlled before surgery. Short bursts of oral steroids are often prescribed for 2–3 days prior to surgery, particularly when intubation is planned.

The aim of surgery is to reduce the patient's need for medication, possibly turning the steroid-dependent patient into a steroid-independent patient, and to reduce the number of exacerbations of asthma caused by sinusitis.

Before a surgical approach to the management of refractory sinus disease is undertaken, a CT scan of the paranasal sinuses in mandatory. It not only helps to establish the extent of the disease, but also provides an indispensable view of the individual patient's anatomy. FESS, as initially described by Messerklinger and expanded upon by Kennedy and Stammberger, is a limited approach directed to the sinus involved, as assessed by pre-operative endoscopic evaluation and CT scan.[106] This surgery has become the most commonly used technique because of the reduced morbidity in comparison with that after traditional procedures. The major principle is that anatomical anomalies in the areas of mucociliary transport from the sinuses compromise drainage. Correction of outflow obstruction promotes drainage and leads to reversal of mucosal changes within the paranasal sinuses. Recent advances in endoscopic surgery involve computer-assisted navigation within the naris and power instrumentation.[107–109] With the new imaging technique, patients with extensive sinus disease and those undergoing revision surgery can benefit from image-guided surgery. It helps to localize areas of the sinuses within 2 mm, improve the thoroughness of the surgery, and limit complications. After surgery, post-operative care, adequate medical treatment, and follow-up are still necessary. Subjective improvement after FESS was reported by Kennedy.[110] Eighty-five percent of 120 patients followed up for an average of 18 months after surgery have had a very good subjective outcome, 12% a good outcome, and 3% a poor outcome. Recently, excellent subjective results (98.4% improvement in overall symptoms compared with the status before surgery) after FESS were demonstrated in a long-term follow-up (average, 7.8 years).[111] In an objective evaluation, endoscopic sinus surgery has also been shown to lead to significant improvement in ciliary beat frequency[112,113] or mucociliary clearance as measured by saccharin test,[113,114] and in olfactory ability.[112,115–117]

CONCLUSION

Experimental and clinical observations suggest that sinonasal infection can worsen asthma; however, the exact nature of this relationship is still unknown.

KEY POINTS

1. The prevalence of chronic sinusitis in patients with asthma is high.

2. History of an upper respiratory tract infection preceding the worsening of asthma should raise the suspicion of sinusitis.

3. Nasal endoscopy provides excellent visualization of the nasal cavity and sinus ostial area that helps in diagnosing sinusitis.

4. Coronal sinus CT scan after medical management is the preferred radiographic diagnostic method for evaluating sinus disease.

5. Appropriate and effective treatment of co-existing sinusitis may result in improvement of asthma.

Identification of chronic sinusitis in asthmatic patients by use of nasal endoscopy and imaging techniques has enhanced patient care and leads to better treatment of sinusitis. Physicians should consider the diagnosis of chronic sinusitis in difficult-to-control asthmatic patients. It is now clear that some individuals with chronic sinusitis, in particular, patients with co-existing pulmonary disease, have problems that extend beyond anatomy and microbiology. More investigation is needed to elucidate the pathophysiology of chronic sinus disease and the interrelationship between the upper and lower airways.

REFERENCES

1. National Disease and Therapeutic Index. Plymouth Meeting, PA: IMS Inc, 1994: 963–7.

2. Benson V, Marano MA. Current estimates from the 1993 National Health Interview Survey. National Center for Health Statistics. *Vital Health Stat* 1994; 10: 190.

3. Weiss KB, Gergen PH, Hodgson TA. An economic evaluation of asthma in the United States. *N Engl J Med* 1992; 326: 862–6.

4. ○ Spector SL, Bernstein IL, Li JT *et al*. Complete guidelines and references. In: Parameters for the diagnosis and management of sinusitis. *J Allergy Clin Immunol* 1998; 102: S132.

5. ○ Hoover G, Newman LJ, Platts-Mills TAE *et al*. Chronic sinusitis: risk factors for extensive disease. *J Allergy Clin Immunol* 1997; 100: 185–91.

6. Gliklich R, Metson R. The health impact of chronic sinusitis in patients seeking otolaryngologic care. *Otolaryngol Head Neck Surg* 1995; 113: 104–9.

7. Collins JG. Prevalence of selected chronic conditions: United States, 1986–88. National Center for Health Statistics. *Vital Health Stat* 1993; 10: 1–87.

8. McCaig LF, Hughes JM. Trends in antimicrobial drug prescription among office-based physicians in the United States. *JAMA* 1995; 273: 214–9.

9. Chaen T, Watanabe N, Mogi G, Mori K, Takeyama M. Substance P and vasoactive intestinal peptide in nasal secretions and plasma from patients with nasal allergy. *Ann Otol Rhinol Laryngol* 1993; 102: 16–21.

10. McNally PA, White MV, Kaliner MA. Sinusitis in an allergist's office: analysis of 200 consecutive cases. *Allergy Asthma Proc* 1997; 18: 169–76.

11. Gwaltney JM Jr, Phillis CD, Miller RD, Riker DK. Computed tomographic study of the common cold. *N Engl J Med* 1994; 330: 25–30.

12. Puhakka T, Makela MJ, Alanen A *et al*. Sinusitis in the common cold. *J Allergy Clin Immunol* 1998; 102: 403–8.

13. ○ Kaliner MA, Osguthorpe JD, Fireman P *et al*. Sinusitis: bench to bedside. *J Allergy Clin Immunol* 1997; 99: S829–48.

14. Lanza DC, Kennedy DW. Adult rhinosinusitis defined. In: Anon JB (eds). Report of the Rhinosinusitis Task Force Committee meeting. *Otolaryngol Head Neck Surg* 1997; 117: S1–7.

15. Kennedy DW. International conference on sinus disease: terminology, staging, therapy. *Ann Otol Rhinol Laryngol* 1995; 104: 10.

16. Gottlieb MJ. Relation of intranasal disease in the production of bronchial asthma. *JAMA* 1925; 85: 105–7.

17. Bullen SS. Incidence of asthma in 400 cases of chronic sinusitis. *J Allergy* 1932; 4: 402–7.

18. Weille FL. Studies in asthma: nose and throat in 500 cases of asthma. *N Engl J Med* 1936; 215: 235–9.

19. Druce HM, Slavin RG. Sinusitis: a critical need for further study. *J Allergy Clin Immunol* 1991; 88: 675–7.

20. Rachelefsky GS, Goldberg M, Katz RM. Sinus disease in children with respiratory allergy. *J Allergy Clin Immunol* 1978; 61: 310–4.

21. Friedman R, Ackerman M, Wald E *et al*. Asthma and bacterial sinusitis in children. *J Allergy Clin Immunol* 1984; 74: 185–9.

22. De Cleyn KM, Kersschot EA, De Clerck LS *et al*. Paranasal sinus pathology in allergic and non-allergic respiratory tract disease. *Allergy* 1986; 41: 313–8.

23. Zimmerman B, Stringer D, Feanny S *et al*. Prevalence of abnormalities found by sinus X-rays in childhood asthma: Lack of relation to severity of asthma. *J Allergy Clin Immunol* 1987; 80: 268–73.

24. Schwartz HJ, Thompson JS, Sher TH, Ross RJ. Occult sinus abnormalities in the asthmatic patient. *Arch Intern Med* 1987; 147: 2194–6.

25. Rossi OVJ, Pireila T, Laitinen J *et al*. Sinus aspirates and radiographic abnormalities in severe attacks of asthma. *Int Arch Allergy Immunol* 1994; 103: 209–16.

26. Krajewski Z, Makuch B, Latos T. Prevalence of nasal sinusitis in children with bronchial asthma. *Pneumonol Allergol Pol* 1997; 65: (suppl. 1): 40–3.

27. Ferrante ME, Quatela MM, Corbo GM *et al*. Prevalence of sinusitis in young asthmatics and its relation to bronchial asthma. *Mil Med* 1998; 163: 180–3.

28. Marney SR Jr. Pathophysiology of reactive airways disease and sinusitis. *Ann Otol Rhinol Laryngol* 1996; 105: 98–100.

29. ✪ Slavin RG. Complications of allergic rhinitis: Implications for sinusitis and asthma. *J Allergy Clin Immunol* 1998; 101: S357–60.

30. Kratchmer I. Physiologic relationships between nasal breathing and pulmonary function. *Laryngoscope* 1996; 76: 30–5.

31. Dixon WE, Brodie TG. The bronchial muscles. Their innervation, and the action of drugs upon them. *J Physiol* 1903; 29: 93–7.

32. Kaufman J, Wright GW. The effect of nasal and nasopharyngeal irritation on airway resistance in man. *Am Rev Respir Dis* 1969; 100: 626–30.

33. Kaufman J, Chen J, Wright GW. The effect of trigeminal resection on reflex bronchoconstriction after nasal and nasopharyngeal irritation in man. *Am Rev Respir Dis* 1970; 101: 768–9.

34. Bucca C, Rolla G, Scappaticci E *et al*. Extrathoracic and intrathoracic airway responsiveness in sinusitis. *J Allergy Clin Immunol* 1995; 95: 52–9.

35. Sluder G. Asthma as a nasal reflex. *JAMA* 1919; 73: 589–91.

36. Baroody F, Gungor A, de Tineo M, Haney L, Blair C, Naclerio RM. A comparison of the response to histamine challenge of the nose and the maxillary sinus: effect of loratadine. *J Appl Physiol* (In Review).

37. Baroody FM, Hughes CA, McDowell P, Hruban R, Zinreich SJ, Naclerio RM. Eosinophilia in chronic childhood sinusitis. *Arch Otolaryngol Head Neck Surg* 1995; 12: 1396–1402.

38. Driscoll PV, Naclerio RM, Baroody FM. CD4+ lymphocytes are increased in the sinus mucosa of children with chronic sinusitis. *Arch Otolaryngol Head Neck Surg* 1996; 122: 1071–6.

39. Minshall EM, Cameron L, Lavigne F *et al*. Eotaxin mRNA and protein expression in chronic sinusitis and allergen-induced nasal responses in seasonal allergic rhinitis. *Am J Respir Cell Mol Biol* 1997; 17: 683–90.

40. Harlin SL, Ansel DG, Lane SR, Myers J, Kephart GM, Gleich GJ. A clinical and pathologic study of chronic sinusitis: the role of the eosinophil. *J Allergy Clin Immunol* 1988; 81: 867–75.

41. Newman LJ, Platts-Mills TA, Phillips CD *et al*. Chronic sinusitis. Relationship of computed tomographic findings to allergy, asthma, and eosinophilia. *JAMA* 1994; 271: 363–7.

42. Bardin PG, Van Heerden BB, Joubert JR. Absence of pulmonary aspiration of sinus contents in patients with asthma and sinusitis. *J Allergy Clin Immunol* 1990; 86: 82–8.

43. Rolla G, Colagrande P, Scappaticci E *et al*. Damage of the pharyngeal mucosa and hyperresponsiveness of airway in sinusitis. *J Allergy Clin Immunol* 1997; 100: 52–7.

44. Brugman SM, Larsen GC, Henson PM, Honor S, Irvin CG. Increased lower airways responsiveness associated with sinusitis in a rabbit-model. *Am Rev Respir Dis* 1993; 147: 314–20.

45. Kowalski ML. Aspirin sensitive rhinosinusitis and asthma. *Allergy Proc* 1995; 16: 77–80.

46. Rachelefsky GS, Katz RM, Siegel SC. Chronic sinus disease with associated reactive airway disease in children. *Pediatrics* 1984; 783: 526–9.

47. Friedman R, Ackeman M, Wald E. Asthma and bacterial sinusitis in children. *J Allergy Clin Immunol* 1984; 74: 185–9.

48. ❂ Oliveira CA, Sole D, Naspitz CK, Rachelefsky GS. Improvement of bronchial hyperresponsiveness in asthmatic children treated for concomitant sinusitis. *Ann Allergy Asthma Immunol* 1997; 79: 70–4.

49. Weille F. Studies in asthma: nose and throat in 500 cases of asthma. *N Engl J Med* 1936; 215: 235–6.

50. Davison F. Chronic sinusitis and infectious asthma. *Arch Otolaryngol* 1969; 90: 292–307.

51. Mings R, Friedman WH, Linford P *et al*. Five year follow-up of the effects of bilateral intranasal sphenoethmoidectomy in patients with sinusitis and asthma. *Am J Rhinol* 1988; 71: 123–32.

52. English GM. Nasal polypectomy and sinus surgery in patients with asthma and aspirin idiosyncrasy. *Laryngoscope* 1986; 96: 374–80.

53. Manning SC, Wasserman RL, Silver R, Phillips DL. Results of endoscopic sinus surgery in pediatric patients with chronic sinusitis and asthma. *Arch Otolaryngol Head Neck Surg* 1994; 120: 1142–5.

54. Parsons DS, Phillips SE. Functional endoscopic sinus surgery in children. *Laryngoscope* 1993; 103: 899–903.

55. Nishioka GJ, Cook PR, Davis WE, Mckinsy JP. Functional endoscopic sinus surgery in patients with chronic sinusitis and asthma. *Otolaryngol Head Neck Surg* 1994; 110: 494–500.

56. Dinis PB, Gomes A. Sinusitis and asthma: how do they interrelate in sinus surgery? *Am J Rhinol* 1997; 11: 421–8.

57. Sykes DA, Wilson R, Chan KL *et al*. Relative importance of antibiotic and improved clearance in topical treatment of chronic mucopurulent rhinosinusitis. *Lancet* 1986; 16: 359–60.

58. Gwaltney J. Microbiology of sinusitis. In: Druce H (ed). *Sinusitis Pathophysiology and Treatment*. New York: Marcel Dekker 1994: 41–56.

59. Wald E, Milmoe G, Bowen A, Ledosma-Modina J, Salamon N, Bluestone CD. Acute maxillary sinusitis in children. *New Engl J Med* 1981; 304: 749–54.

60. Gwaltney JM. Acute community-acquired sinusitis. *Clin Infect Dis* 1996; 25: 1209–25.

61. Brook I. Microbiology of common infections in the upper respiratory tract. *Prim Care* 1998; 25: 633–48.

62. Doern GV, Brueggemann A, Holley HP, Rauch AM. Antimicrobial resistance of *Streptococcus pneumoniae* recovered from outpatients in the United States during the winter months of 1994 to 1995; results of a 30-center national surveillance study. *Antimicrob Agents Chemother* 1996; 40: 1208–13.

63. Wald ER, Reilly JS, Casselbrant M *et al*. Treatment of acute maxillary sinusitis in childhood: a comparative study of amoxicillin and cefaclor. *J Pediatr* 1984; 104: 297–302.

64. Radosz-Komoniewska H, Kapp-Burzynska Z, Klaptocz B, Wilk I, Ekiel A. Aerobic and anaerobic bacterial flora in chronic sinusitis in adults. *Med Dosw Mikrobiol* 1997; 49: 89–94.

65. Doyle PW, Woodham JD. Bacterial flora in acute and chronic sinusitis. *J Clin Neurol* 1991; 29: 2396–9.

66. Muntz HR, Lusk RP. Bacteriology of the ethmoid bulla in children with chronic sinusitis. *Otolaryngol Head Neck Surg* 1991; 117: 179–81.

67. Orobello PW, Park RI, Belcher LJ *et al*. The microbiology of chronic sinusitis in children. *Arch Otolaryngol Head Neck Surg* 1991; 117: 980–92.

68. Goldenhersh MJ, Rachelefsky GS, Dudley J *et al*. The bacteriology of chronic maxillary sinusitis in children with respiratory allergy. *J Allergy Clin Immunol* 1990; 85: 1030–9.

69. Ramadan HH. What is the bacteriology of chronic sinusitis in adults? *Am J Otolaryngol* 1995; 16: 303–6.

70. Evans FO, Sydnor JB, Moore WE *et al*. Sinusitis of the maxillary antrum. *N Engl J Med* 1975; 293: 735–9.

71. Gold SM, Tami TA. Role of middle meatus aspiration culture in the diagnosis of chronic sinusitis. *Laryngoscope* 1997; 107: 1586–9.

72. Hughes RG, Jones NS. The role of nasal endoscopy in outpatient management. *Clin Otolarygol* 1998; 23: 224–6.

73. Gonzalez Morales JE, Leal de Hernandez L, Gonzalez Spencer D. Usefulness of simple paranasal sinus radiographs and axial computed tomography in the diagnosis of chronic sinusitis. *Rev Alerg Mex* 1998; 45: 17–21.

74. Goldstein JH, Phillips CD. Current indications and techniques in evaluating inflammatory disease and neoplasia of the sinonasal cavities. *Curr Probl Diagn Radiol* 1998; 27: 41–71.

75. Rosbe KW, Jones KR. Usefulness of patient symptoms and nasal endoscopy in the diagnosis of chronic sinusitis. *Am J Rhinol* 1998; 12: 167–71.

76. Bhattacharyya T, Piccirillo J, Wippold FJ. Relationship between patient-based descriptions of sinusitis and paranasal sinus computed tomographic findings. *Arch Otolaryngol Head Neck Surg* 1997; 123: 1189–92.

77. Havas TE, Motbey JA, Guillane DJ. Prevalence of incidental abnormalities on computerized tomography of the paranasal sinuses. *Arch Otolaryngol Head Neck Surg* 1988; 114: 856–9.

78. McAlister WA, Lusk RP, Muntz HR. Comparison of plain radiographs and coronal CT scans in infants and children with recurrent sinusitis. *Am J Roentgenol* 1989; 153: 1259–64.

79. Zinreich SJ, Kennedy DW, Rosenbaum AE *et al*. Paranasal sinuses: CT imaging requirements for endoscopic surgery. *Radiology* 1987; 163: 769–75.

80. Kennedy DW, Zinreich SJ. Physiological mucosal changes within the nose and ethmoid sinus: imaging of the nasal cycle by MRI. *Laryngoscope* 1988; 98: 928–33.

81. Som PM, Shapiro MD, Biller HF *et al*. Sinonasal tumors and inflammatory tissues: Differentiation with MRI imaging. *Radiology* 1991; 167: 803–8.

82. Suzuki H, Shimomura A, Ikeda K *et al*. Inhibitory effect of macrolides on interleukin-8 secretion from cultured human nasal epithelial cells. *Laryngoscope* 1997; 107: 1661–6.

83. Kimura N, Nishioka K, Nishizaki K *et al*. Clinical effect of low-dose, long-term roxithromycin chemotherapy in patients with chronic sinusitis. *Acta Med Okayama* 1997; 51: 33–7.

84. Krouse HA, Phung ND, Klaustermeyer WB. Intranasal beçlomethasone in severe rhinosinusitis and nasal polyps. *Ann Allergy* 1983; 50: 385–8.

85. Rebhun J. Effectiveness of antibiotic nasal sprays on the treatment of severe chronic bacterial sinusitis. *Immunol Allergy Pract* 1993; 40: 164–9.

86. ✪ Meltzer EO, Orgel HA, Backhaus JW *et al*. Intranasal flunisolide spray as an adjunct to oral antibiotic therapy for sinusitis. *J Allergy Clin Immunol* 1993; 92: 812–23.

87. Qvarnberg Y, Kantola O, Salo J *et al*. Influence of topical steroid treatment on maxillary sinusitis. *Rhinology* 1992; 30: 103–12.

88. Barlan IB, Erkan E, Bakir M, Berrak S, Basaran MM. Intranasal budesonide spray as an adjunct to oral antibiotic therapy for acute sinusitis in children. *Ann Allergy Asthma Immunol* 1997; 78: 598–601.

89. Lildholdt T, Rundcrantz H, Lindqvist N. Effect of topical corticosteroid powder for nasal polyps: a double-blind, placebo-controlled study of budesonide. *Clin Otolaryngol* 1995; 20: 26–30.

90. Johansen LV, Illum P, Kristensen S *et al*. The effect of budesonide in the treatment of small and medium-sized nasal polyps. *Clin Otolaryngol* 1993; 18: 524–7.

91. Lildholdt T, Mygind N. Corticosteroids: locally and systemically. In: Mygind N, Lildholdt T (eds). *Nasal Polyposis: An Inflammatory Disease and Its Treatment*. Copenhagen: Munksgaard 1997: 160–9.

92. Pederson D, Dahl R, Lindqvist N, Mygind N. Nasal inhalation of the glucocorticoid budesonide from a spacer for the treatment of patients with pollen rhinitis and asthma. *Allergy* 1990; 45: 451–6.

93. Aubier M, Levy J, Clerici C, Neukirch F, Herman D. Different effects of nasal and bronchial glucocorticosteroid administration on bronchial hyperresponsiveness in patients with allergic rhinitis. *Am Rev Respir Dis* 1992; 146: 122–6.

94. ✪ Braun JJ, Alabert JP, Michel FB *et al*. Adjunct effect of loratadine in the treatment of acute sinusitis in patients with allergic rhinitis. *Allergy* 1997; 52: 650–5.

95. Ziment I. Acetylcysteine. A drug that is much more than a mucokinetic. *Biomed Pharmacother* 1988; 42: 513–20.

96. Saketkoo K, Januszkiewicz A, Sackner MA *et al.* Effects of drinking hot water, cold water, and chicken soup on nasal mucosis velocity and nasal airflow resistance. *Chest* 1978; 74: 408–10.

97. Van Bever HPS, Bosmans J, Stevens NJ. Nebulization treatment with saline compared to bromhexine in treating chronic sinusitis in asthmatic children. *Allergy* 1987; 42: 33–6.

98. Grossan M. A device for nasal irrigation. *Trans Am Acad Ophthalmol Otol* 1974; 47: 279–81.

99. Szmeja Z, Golusinski W, Mielcarek-Kuchta D, Laczkowska-Przybylska J. Use of mucolytic preparations (Mucosolvan) in selected diseases of the upper respiratory tract. *Otolaryngol Pol* 1997; 51: 480–6.

100. Wawrose SF, Tami TA, Amoils CP. The role of guaifenesin in the treatment of sinonasal disease in patients infected with the human immunodeficiency virus. *Laryngoscope* 1992; 102: 1225–8.

101. Shoseyov D, Bibi H, Shai P, Shoseyov N *et al.* Treatment with hypertonic saline versus normal saline nasal wash of pediatric chronic sinusitis. *J Allergy Clin Immunol* 1998; 101: 602–5.

102. Ramesh S, Brodsky L, Afshani E *et al.* Open trial of intravenous immune serum globulin for chronic sinusitis in children. *Ann Allergy Asthma Immunol* 1997; 79: 119–24.

103. Kowalski ML. Pathophysiology of rhinosinusitis in aspirin sensitive patients. In: Oehling AK, Huerta Lopez JG (eds). *Progress in Allergy and Clinical Immunology.* Volume 4. Seattle: Hogrefe and Huber, 1997: 174–8.

104. Wooding LG, Incaudo GA. The effect of zileuton on anosmia in aspirin-sensitive asthmatics. *Am J Rhinol* 1996; 10: 101–3.

105. Israel E, Fischer AR, Rosenberg MA *et al.* The pivotal role of 5-lopoxygenase products in the reaction of aspirin-sensitive asthmatics to aspirin. *Am Rev Respir Dis* 1993; 148: 1441–51.

106. Stammberger H. *Functional Endoscopic Sinus Surgery.* Philadelphia: BC Decker, 1991.

107. Freysinger W, Gunkel AR, Thumfart WF. Image-guided endoscopic ENT surgery. *Eur Arch Otorhinolaryngol* 1997; 254: 343–6.

108. Gunkel AR, Freysinger W, Thumfart WF. Computer-assisted surgery in the frontal and maxillary sinus. *Laryngoscope* 1997; 107: 631–3.

109. Mendelson MG, Gross CW. Soft-tissue shavers in pediatric sinus surgery. *Otolaryngol Clin North Am* 1997; 30: 443–9.

110. Kennedy D. Prognostic factors, outcomes and staging in ethmoid sinus surgery. *Laryngoscope* 1992; 102: 1–18.

111. ❂ Senior BA, Kennedy DW, Tanabodee J *et al.* Long-term results of functional endoscopic sinus surgery. *Laryngoscope* 1998; 108: 151–7.

112. Abdel-Hak B, Gunkel A, Kanonier G *et al.* Ciliary beat frequency, olfaction and endoscopic sinus surgery. *ORL J Otorhinolaryngol Relat Spec* 1998; 60: 202–5.

113. Hafner B, Davris S, Riechelmann H, Mann WJ, Amedee RG. Endonasal sinus surgery improves mucociliary transport in severe chronic sinusitis. *Am J Rhinol* 1997; 11: 271–4.

114. Kaluskar SK. Pre- and postoperative mucociliary clearance in functional endoscopic sinus surgery. *Ear Nose Throat J* 1997; 76: 884–6.

115. Delak KW, Stoll W. Olfactory function after functional endoscopic sinus surgery for chronic sinusitis. *Rhinology* 1998; 36: 15–9.

116. Rowe-Jones JM, Mackay IS. A prospective study of olfaction following endoscopic sinus surgery with adjuvant medical treatment. *Clin Otolaryngol* 1997; 22 (4): 377–81.

117. Hosemann W, Goertzen W, Wohlleben R. Olfaction after endoscopic endonasal ethmoidectomy. *Am J Rhinol* 1993; 7: 11–5.

Chapter 44

Specific Problems: Food Allergy in Asthma

Jean Bousquet, Dany Jaffuel, Pascal Chanez and François-B. Michel

Adverse reactions to foods can be classified on the basis of the mechanisms of the reaction. Allergic reactions are immunologically mediated. The best known example of such a reaction is IgE-mediated food anaphylaxis, but other types of hypersensitivity reactions have been associated with food allergy. Although IgG or IgG_4 might be involved, there is no definite proof that these immunoglobulin isotypes are important in food allergy. Other reactions involve immune-complex reactions and lymphocyte activation. All other non-immunological adverse reactions such as sulphite or aspirin-induced asthma should be classified as food intolerance.[1,2] Besides allergen-specific mechanims, there are many non-specific mechanisms which may aggravate respiratory symptoms due to food allergy such as exercise, cold drinks, aspirin or concomitant intake of alcohol. Alcohol-induced asthma,[3] a phenomenon characteristic of Asians, is due to differences in alcohol metabolism, particularly acetaldehyde metabolism due to a defect in acetylaldehyde dehydrogenase 2.[4] Wine can also induce symptoms, but wine-induced asthma appears to be a complex phenomenon and may involve several mechanisms that are codependent[5] including sulphite sensitivity and elevated histamine levels.[6]

Food allergy has always been a difficult problem to assess, especially in asthma, where some investigators deny its existence whilst others tend to over-estimate its importance. Moreover, the diagnosis of food allergy is always difficult and double-blind food challenges should often be performed to confirm the diagnosis of food-induced asthma. Food allergy only rarely induces asthma[7,8] except possibly in young children.[9]

CLINICAL PRESENTATION

There are several cases which demonstrate that asthma can be triggered by foods, and that this reaction can be controlled by an alteration in diet. However, many reports are only speculative and, when the delay between the ingestion and symptoms exceeds 24 hours, it is extremely difficult to ascribe an asthma attack to food allergy owing to the great variability of the airways obstruction in chronic asthmatics. The best demonstration is given by double-blind food challenges (Fig. 44.1) but in some highly allergic individuals or in ocupational allergy (e.g. bakers) inhalation challenges with foods can lead to an immediate bronchial response. Elimination diets can also be demonstrative,

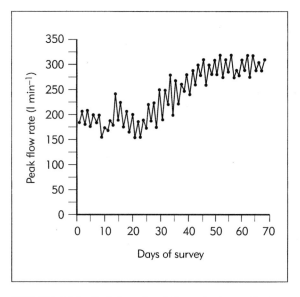

FIGURE 44.1: Evolution of peak flow rates in a patient allergic to eggs after an egg-free diet. (From Bousquet J, Metcalfe D, Warner J. Food allergy. Report of the Codex Alimentarius. ACI International 1997; 9: 10–21, with permission.)

but their interpretation may be difficult when patients are allergic both to foods and inhaled allergens.

Respiratory symptoms due to an IgE-mediated food allergic reaction can suddenly occur if the food is not routinely ingested and may be associated with other symptoms of generalized anaphylaxis. These acute outbreaks of asthma may be extremely severe and fatalities have been reported.[10–12] However, if the food is ingested routinely, the patient may present chronic asthma which is often associated with atopic dermatitis. Often, such patients present with severe asthma which is difficult to control. The severity of chronic asthma varies widely and may in mild cases only present as a persistent cough or as exercise-induced asthma.[13] It has also been observed that foods only increase the non-specific bronchial hyperreactivity without causing frank wheezing[14] or acute asthma.[15]

In infants, symptoms may take the form of classical asthma, but there may also be intermittent attacks of dyspnoea, tachypnoea and occasionally fever. Other symptoms of food allergy are often present concommitantly.[16]

DIAGNOSIS OF FOOD ALLERGY-INDUCED ASTHMA

Suspicion of Food Allergy in Asthma

Food allergy may be suspected (1) when asthma started early in life, especially if the patient has had or currently presents atopic dermatitis;[7] (2) in patients who have suffered from anaphylactic symptoms or acute urticaria due to food allergy; and (3) in any patient, even in adults, with poorly controlled asthma and elevated total serum IgE levels. However, it must be pointed out that suspicion of food allergy alone cannot be used as the basis for diagnosis.[17]

Diagnosis of Food Allergy in Asthma

The diagnosis of food allergy in asthma is difficult because of the quality of the tests available, but also because it should be demonstrated that the suspected food causes asthma. Such diagnoses are based on a suggestive clinical history, the demonstration of an IgE-mediated allergic reaction to food allergens and, at best, a food challenge.

Skin Tests and Allergen-Specific IgE Antibodies

The value of skin tests and serum specific IgE is dependent upon a number of variables amongst which the quality of the allergen extract used is of major importance. Allergen extracts currently available are not standardized, and their stability often remains poorly established.[2] For allergen extracts which are rapidly degraded such as those from fruits and vegetables, skin tests may be falsely negative in food allergic individuals. When available, recombinant allergens may be of great importance for the diagnosis of food allergy.[18] Allergen extracts from egg, milk, fish, shellfish, nuts, peanuts and cereals are usually of better quality.

The diagnosis should be started using skin-prick tests with foods. For fruits and vegetables, skin-prick tests with raw fresh foods are required (prick–prick test).[19] Intradermal skin tests are more sensitive than prick tests, but they are less specific. They may be used when prick tests are negative. The titration of serum food-specific IgE is available for many foods, but, in contrast with better characterized inhalant allergens, the sensitivity of the test is not yet fully known for most unpurified food allergens, Moreover, even more than in inhalant allergy, the presence of food-IgE in serum or positive skin tests to foods do not necessarily correlate with food allergy since many patients outgrow their allergy with age[20,21] and not all patients with food-specific IgE have a clinical sensitivity. The presence of positive skin-prick test and/or serum specific IgE does not preclude a positive result for food challenge since only one-third of patients presenting with positive skin-prick tests and/or serum specific IgE have asthma during food challenge,[22] so that a diet should not be started before food challenges have been performed.[23]

Patients who developed acute urticaria or anaphylaxis often make the diagnosis of "food intolerance" by themselves, and the presence of positive skin tests and/or serum specific IgE correlating with the claims of the patient make possible a diagnosis without performing a food challenge. This test may cause severe untoward reactions in patients with anaphylaxis and should be performed with extreme care. However, in asthma, patients rarely identify a food as a cause of wheezing, so it is necessary to confirm the diagnosis by double-blind food challenge.[23]

Food Challenge

Food challenges should be performed in a manner similar to that reported by Bock,[24] or Sampson and Albergo.[25] The food suspected as causing symptoms should be eliminated from the diet for a minimum of 2 weeks before testing. The selection of foods for administration is based upon positive skin tests and/or specific IgE or on a clear anecdotal history despite negative skin-prick tests and/or RAST. Patients should stop anti-asthma medications that might modify the performance of the test for an appropriate delay. However, medication withdrawal may induce a deterioration of lung function making evaluation difficult. Moreover, in patients with severe asthma it is not possible to discontinue all medications and occasionally the challenge has to be done in a patient receiving β agonists and/or theophylline and/or inhaled corticosteroids. In this case, the medications should be identical on placebo and test days. When possible, lyophilized foods should be placed in size 0 dye-free opaque capsules, or if administered as a liquid, they should be mixed in a broth or in a juice to disguise the taste. Although patients who have presented anaphylactic symptoms should not be tested, it is advisable to increase the dose slowly from 100 mg to 10 g. Challenges should ideally be conducted in a double-blind manner, but if several foods are implicated, a screening with single-blind challenges may be done first. In case of food-induced asthma, serial pulmonary function tests should be carried out for up to 8 hours since late reactions can occur.[7] During all challenges, a physician should follow up the patient since some untoward systemic reaction might occur. The challenge is only considered to be positive if PD_{20} FEV_1 is reached on a test day without any such drop in FEV_1 during a placebo day (Fig. 44.2). For asthma, the test with placebo is critical owing to the great variability of pulmonary function which is a characteristic of the disease. In young children, pulmonary function tests are not easy to do and to interpret without sophisticated equipment (which is rarely available) and so the diagnosis of asthma may be based on clinical examination alone. Some patients develop gastrointestinal symptoms, acute urticaria or atopic dermatitis without any airways response. If the challenge is inconclusive, it has been suggested that the patient be asked to eat the amount of food ingested during a usual meal and to measure the pulmonary function serially.

Food challenge data may be augmented by assessing non-specific bronchial hyperreactivity[15] or by measuring the release of mediators in peripheral blood or the increased gut permeability.

A positive food challenge does not necessarily imply that the patient presents an IgE-mediated allergy, but suggests that he or she is intolerant to certain foods. If

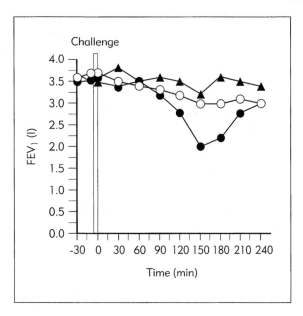

FIGURE 44.2: Evolution of FEV_1 during food challenge. ▲, placebo; ●, fish; ○, fish + disodium cromoglycate. (From Onorato J, Merland N, Terral C et al. Placebo-controlled double-blind food challenge in asthma. *J Allergy Clin Immunol* 1986; 78: 1139–46, with permission.)

specific IgE and/or prick tests to a specific food-stuff are positive, an IgE-mediated mechanism is likely to be involved. In situations where oral cromoglycate is commercially available, a further food challenge is advisable in order to test the efficacy of this drug prior to prescribing such a treatment. The results of double-blind food challenge in asthma are similar to those observed with other food-induced symptoms and only one-quarter to one-third of patients with positive skin tests and/or specific IgE have a positive oral challenge.[7,24–26]

Elimination Diets

Elimination diets are used primarily for the diagnosis of diseases such as eczema and rhinitis. In the case of asthma, it is often difficult to make the diagnosis of food allergy by elimination diets for many reasons.[7,26] (1) food allergy is almost constantly associated with inhalant allergy and possibly with other triggers, and variations in the airways obstruction may be due to factors unrelated to foods; (2) food allergens as well as inhalant allergens aggravate the non-specific bronchial hyperreactivity and it may take days or even weeks to observe an improvement of asthma; and (3) the great variability of the airways obstruction in chronic asthmatics may shadow the benefits of dietary manipulations. However, when a patient is highly allergic to a given food, significant improvement or even complete remission of asthma can be observed.

Unproven Techniques

As for other forms of food allergy, unproven and controversial techniques such as cytotoxic tests or sublingual provocation tests have absolutely no value. The titration of serum food specific IgG or IgG_4 has no value in clinical practice.

PREVALENCE OF FOOD ALLERGY IN ASTHMA

Asthma due to foods may be caused by immunological and non-immunological mechanisms. IgE-mediated allergy appears to be much less common than food intolerance as a trigger of asthma and reports of high incidence of food allergy in asthma did not differentiate between the mechanisms of food-induced asthma. Methodological problems limit the evaluation of the prevalence of food allergy in asthma. Methods commonly used in epidemiology of allergic diseases (e.g. skin tests and eventually serum specific IgE) are not completely reliable. Only double-blind food challenges combined with skin tests or IgE can screen asthmatics allergic to foods, but this method cannot be used in epidemiologic studies. Thus either epidemiological studies are performed in a random population with inappropriate methods, or they are performed in selected populations with appropriate techniques.

Most cases of food-induced asthma are observed in early infancy and are then often related to cow's milk hypersensitivity in which asthma has been noted in 7–29% of cases,[27–29] but there appears to be an increasing number of infants allergic to egg, flour and peanuts. The incidence of food allergy decreases with age, and although some investigators have proposed that many intrinsic adult asthmatics may in fact be allergic to foods,[30] the few controlled studies performed by food challenges[7,8] do not substantiate this assertion. In areas where mugwort and birch pollens are rare, food allergy only represents a minor cause of perennial asthma, being present in 4–6% of asthmatic children[31,32] and in 1–4% of asthmatic adults.[7,8,33] However, when these pollen species are prevalent, allergy due to cross-reactive food epitopes, such as celery, nuts or fruits, may be more important, but anaphylactic or gastro-intestinal and dermatologic symptoms are likely to be more frequent than asthma. In non-Caucasian populations the incidence of food allergy may be greater and these figures may also be increased. Finally, according to the regular diet of a given country, differences may be observed, such as dye-allergy that was reported to be relatively frequent in the UK.

TREATMENT OF ASTHMA INDUCED BY FOOD ALLERGY

The presence of a positive skin-prick test or serum IgE test to a given food should not lead to an elimination diet because only 30–40% of patients have asthma when they are challenged orally with the offending food. A positive food challenge favours dietary avoidance,[34] but nutritional balance must always be maintained especially in infants and young children since many infants are now being placed on dangerously inadequate diets.[35] Also, the reintroduction of a food, accidental or intentional, may be associated with anaphylaxis or severe respiratory obstruction since individual patients tend to continue to react with the same symptoms as they had before.

KEY POINTS

1. Food allergy is a rare event in asthma. Its prevalence ranges from 4 to 6% in children but is less than 1% in adult asthmatic subjects.

2. In areas where birch and mugwort pollen are common sensitizers food allergy is more common due to cross-reactive allergens.

3. Except in infancy, most patients with food allergy are also sensitized to inhalant allergens.

4. Current or previous atopic dermatitis is frequently associated with asthma in patients with food allergy.

5. Although food allergy is infrequent, it should be recognized since patients often present severe symptoms that are improved by a diet.

6. An elimination diet should be based on food challenge.

The efficacy of oral sodium cromoglycate is not completely established, but this drug was found in some studies to prevent asthma due to food allergy.[10,30] It is clear that only a fraction of patients benefits from this treatment but, when available and effective, it may be used (1) to decrease the reactivity of the gastrointestinal tract to dietary allergens and (2) to allow a less restrictive diet. Ketotifene was also used and seemed to have a greater value in the treatment of skin symptoms.

There is at present no evidence to support specific immunotherapy by either the oral or the parenteral route. If such a treatment is administered it must be done for research purposes, in an intensive care setting by specialized doctors, since deaths have been reported.

The prevention of food allergy may be attempted in the high-allergic risk newborn, but at present there is not clear demonstration that breast-feeding, even prolonged over a long period of time, may prevent the onset of allergy.[31]

REFERENCES

1. ✪ Bruinzeel-Koomen C, Ortolani C, Aas K et al. Adverse reactions to foods. Position Paper of the European Academy of Allergy and Clinical Immunology. *Allergy* 1995; 50: 623–35.

2. Bousquet J, Metcalfe D, Warner J. Food allergy. Report of the Codex Alimentarius. *ACI International* 1997; 9: 10–21.

3. Myou S, Fujimura M, Nishi K et al. Effect of ethanol on airway caliber and nonspecific bronchial responsiveness in patients with alcohol-induced asthma. *Allergy* 1996; 51: 52–5.

4. Takao A, Shimoda T, Kohno S, Asai S, Harda S. Correlation between alcohol-induced asthma and acetaldehyde dehydrogenase-2 genotype. *J Allergy Clin Immunol* 1998; 101: 576–80.

5. Vally H, Carr A, El-Saleh J, Thompson P. Wine-induced asthma: a placebo-controlled assessment of its pathogenesis. *J Allergy Clin Immunol* 1999; 103: 41–6.

6. Wantke F, Hemmer W, Haglmuller T, Gotz M, Jarisch R. Histamine in wine. Bronchoconstriction after a double-blind placebo-controlled red wine provocation test. *Int Arch Allergy Immunol* 1996; 110: 397–400.

7. ✪ Onorato J, Merland N, Terral C, Michel FB, Bousquet J. Placebo-controlled double-blind food challenge in asthma. *J Allergy Clin Immunol* 1986; 78: 1139–46.

8. Woods RK, Weiner JM, Abramson M, Thien F, Walters EH. Do dairy products induce bronchoconstriction in adults with asthma? *J Allergy Clin Immunol* 1998; 101: 45–50.

9. ✪ Rance F, Kanny G, Dutau G, Moneret-Vautrin DA. Food hypersensitivity in children: clinical aspects and distribution of allergens. *Pediatr Allergy Immunol* 1999; 10: 33–8.

10. Yunginger JW, Sweeney KG, Sturner WQ et al. Fatal food-induced anaphylaxis. *JAMA* 1988; 260: 1450–2.

11. ✪ Sampson HA, Mendelson L, Rosen JP. Fatal and near-fatal anaphylactic reactions to food in children and adolescents. *N Engl J Med* 1992; 327: 380–4.

12. Foucard T, Malmheden Yman I. A study on severe food reactions in Sweden–is soy protein an underestimated cause of food anaphylaxis? *Allergy* 1999; 54: 261–5.

13. Kidd JD, Cohen SH, Sosman AJ, Fink JN. Food-dependent exercise-induced anaphylaxis. *J Allergy Clin Immunol* 1983; 71: 407–11.

14. Wilson N, Vickers H, Taylor G, Silverman M. Objective test for food sensitivity in asthmatic children: increased bronchial reactivity after cola drinks. *Br Med J Clin Res* 1982; 284: 1226–8.

15. ✪ James JM, Eigenmann PA, Eggleston PA, Sampson HA. Airway reactivity changes in asthmatic patients undergoing blinded food challenges. *Am J Respir Crit Care Med* 1996; 153: 597–603.

16. Hill DJ, Firer MA, Shelton MJ, Hosking CS. Manifestations of milk allergy in infancy: clinical and immunologic findings. *J Pediatr* 1986; 109: 270–6.

17. Woods RK, Abramson M, Raven JM, Bailey M, Weiner JM, Walters EH. Reported food intolerance and respiratory symptoms in young adults. *Eur Respir J* 1998; 11: 151–5.

18. Hoffmann-Sommergruber K, Demoly P, Crameri R et al. IgE reactivity to *Api g* 1, a major celery allergen,

in a Central European population is based on primary sensitization by *Bet v* 1. *J Allergy Clin Immunol* 1999; 104: 478–84.

19. Dreborg S, Foucard T. Allergy to apple, carrot and potato in children with birch pollen allergy. *Allergy* 1983; 38: 167–72.

20. Dannaeus A, Inganas M. A follow-up study of children with food allergy. Clinical course in relation to serum IgE- and IgG-antibody levels to milk, egg and fish. *Clin Allergy* 1981; 11: 533–9.

21. Kulig M, Bergmann R, Klettke U, Wahn V, Tacke U, Wahn U. Natural course of sensitization to food and inhalant allergens during the first 6 years of life. *J Allergy Clin Immunol* 1999; 103: 1173–9.

22. Metcalfe DD. Food hypersensitivity. *J Allergy Clin Immunol* 1984; 73: 749–62.

23. Yunginger JW. Proper application of available laboratory tests for adverse reactions to foods and food additives. *J Allergy Clin Immunol* 1986; 78: 220–3.

24. Bock SA. A critical evaluation of clinical trials in adverse reactions to foods in children. *J Allergy Clin Immunol* 1986; 78: 165–74.

25. Sampson HA, Albergo R. Comparison of results of skin tests, RAST, and double-blind, placebo-controlled food challenges in children with atopic dermatitis. *J Allergy Clin Immunol* 1984; 74: 26–33.

26. Atkins FM, Steinberg SS, Metcalfe DD. Evaluation of immediate adverse reactions to foods in adult patients. I. Correlation of demographic, laboratory, and prick skin test data with response to controlled oral food challenge. *J Allergy Clin Immunol* 1985; 75: 348–55.

27. Hill MR, Gotz VP, Harman E, McLeod I, Hendeles L. Evaluation of the asthmogenicity of propafenone, a new antiarrhythmic drug. Comparison of spirometry with methacholine challenge. *Chest* 1986; 90: 698–702.

28. Nichaman MZ, McPherson RS. Estimating prevalence of adverse reactions to foods: principles and constraints. *J Allergy Clin Immunol* 1986; 78: 148–54.

29. Host A, Halken S. Epidemiology and prevention of cow's milk allergy. *Allergy* 1998; 53: 111–3.

30. Oehling A, Baena-Cagnani CE. Food allergy and child asthma. *Allergol Immunopathol Madr* 1980; 8: 7–14.

31. Novembre E, Veneruso G, Sabatini C et al. Incidence of asthma caused by food allergy in childhood. *Pediatr Med Chir* 1987; 9: 399–404.

32. Senechal H, Geny S, Desvaux FX et al. Genetics and specific immune response in allergy to birch pollen and food: evidence of a strong, positive association between atopy and the HLA class II allele HLA-DR7. *J Allergy Clin Immunol* 1999; 104: 395–401.

33. Burr ML, Fehily AM, Stott NC, Merrett TG. Food-allergic asthma in general practice. *Hum Nutr Appl Nutr* 1985; 39: 349–55.

34. Hoj L, Osterballe O, Bundgaard A, Weeke B, Weiss M. A double-blind controlled trial of elemental diet in severe, perennial asthma. *Allergy* 1981; 36: 257–62.

35. Isolauri E, Sutas Y, Salo MK, Isosomppi R, Kaila M. Elimination diet in cow's milk allergy: risk for impaired growth in young children. *J Pediatr* 1998; 132: 1004–9.

Chapter 45

Specific Problems: Difficult, Therapy-resistant Asthma

Kian Chung

INTRODUCTION

Asthma is a chronic inflammatory disorder of the airways which is increasing in prevalence and which can pose significant morbidity and mortality. Current treatment options involve the use of inhaled inflammatory agents such as corticosteroids to control airway inflammation, and the use of bronchodilators such as β_2 agonists to relieve airways obstruction.[1] Such treatment is usually effective in the majority of patients with asthma, resulting in adequate control of symptoms. Not uncommonly, however, practitioners are faced with patients who fail to respond to these therapies. The introduction of national and international guidelines for the management of asthma has allowed a consensus to develop regarding the use of effective treatments for asthma. This has made it possible to achieve a definition of "difficult-to-treat" or "therapy-resistant" asthma as poorly controlled asthma in terms of chronic symptoms, episodic exacerbations, persistent and variable airways obstruction and a continued requirement for short-acting β_2 agonists despite the use of high doses of inhaled corticosteroids, i.e. daily doses of 2000 µg of beclomethasone, or 1600 µg of budesonide or 1000 µg of fluticasone in adults.[2] Some patients may also require pulses or continuous doses of oral corticosteroids to maintain reasonable control of asthma. Therefore, difficult asthma may manifest with chronic symptoms but also with recurrent exacerbations in a patient who in between is well-controlled; it may also encompass a patient who remains well-controlled but needs regular doses of oral corticosteroids to achieve this control.

EPIDEMIOLOGY AND ECONOMIC COSTS

Accurate figures on the prevalence of difficult asthma are not available mainly because of a lack of precise figures for the prevalence of asthma itself, and partly because of a lack of a uniform definition. However, there are pointers to the increasing burden of asthma worldwide, not only from the point of view of increasing numbers of asthma, but from more patients using health care resources, and, in some countries, to the increasing asthma deaths. In a survey of 3373 asthmatic patients in the community in England, 1% of patients were on continuous oral corticosteroid therapy, with 14.6% on inhaled corticosteroids with or without a long-acting bronchodilator (Step 3 or above).[3] These patients most frequently needed at least one course of oral corticosteroids during the past year. From the pharmacoeconomic point of view, patients with severe asthma which form a minority contribute the most to asthma costs through hospitalization, attendances at emergency departments, absence from work or school and the use of medication. For example, in Canada, 10% of asthmatics were deemed to have severe asthma, but they accounted for 54% of costs,[4] while in Australia, 6% of patients with severe asthma used 47% of costs.[5]

DIAGNOSIS OF DIFFICULT ASTHMA

Before a diagnosis of difficult asthma is reached, one asks whether the patient has asthma, and other diagnoses that can masquerade as asthma should be excluded as deemed necessary (Table 45.1). Vocal cord dysfunction presenting as laryngeal or upper airway wheeze may masquerade as asthma or accompany severe asthma as an expression of stress of anxiety.[6,7] Such paroxysms of wheezing and dyspnoea may occur and are not responding to usual treatment, and therefore fall in the category of difficult-to-treat asthma.[8] Localized obstruction of the large airways by an intraluminal tumour or by extrinsic compression may also mimic

Table 45.1: Diagnoses that may masquerade as difficult therapy-resistant asthma

Children:
  Obliterative bronchiolitis
  Vocal cord dysfunction
  Bronchomalacia
  Inhaled foreign bodies
  Cystic fibrosis
  Recent aspiration (particularly in handicapped children)
  Developmental abnormalities of upper airway
  Immunoglobumin deficiencies
  Primary ciliary dyskinesia

Adults:
  Cystic fibrosis
  Bronchiectasis
  Inhaled foreign body
  Tracheobronchomalacia
  Recurrent aspiration
  Chronic obstructive pulmonary disease
  Congestive cardiac failure
  Tumours in or impinging on central airways
  Obstructive bronchiolitis
  Vocal cord dysfunction
  Bronchial amyloidosis

As part of the asthmatic diathesis:
  Allergic bronchopulmonary aspergillosis
  Pulmonary eosinophilic syndromes (e.g. Churg–Strauss)

asthma. Asthma is sometimes incorrectly diagnosed in patients with chronic obstructive pulmonary disease (COPD), although these two conditions may co-exist, particularly in an asthmatic patient who has been a long-standing smoker. Other conditions include congestive cardiac failure, particularly with nocturnal dyspnoeic episodes.[9] A significant bronchodilator response to an inhaled β agonist such as salbutamol, or an improvement of airways obstruction with a course of oral prednisolone (e.g. 40 mg per day for 2 weeks), or evidence of peak flow variability are useful in supporting a diagnosis of asthma. The diagnosis of asthma very much rests on the clinical history and physiological evidence of variable and reversible airways obstruction and on the exclusion of alternative diagnoses.

Vocal Cord Dysfunction

Vocal cord dysfunction is a term used to indicate the presence of upper laryngeal airway obstruction caused by adduction of the anterior two-thirds of the vocal cords, that can present with a wheeze and feeling of breathlessness which can be mistaken for asthma ("pseudoasthma").[6,7] This can present in patients with or without asthma and some consider this to be a hysterical conversion syndrome with secondary gain. However, it may also be observed in asthmatic patients with an on-going attack of asthma. Many patients may be admitted regularly to hospital as cases of acute severe asthma and may be treated with maximal asthma therapy including oral corticosteroid therapy, since they often report symptoms of acute wheeze, cough and dyspnoea. Other symptoms may include chest pain, stridor, hoarseness of voice and the lack of effect of bronchodilators. Often, there is evidence of suboptimal effort with variable forced expiratory tracings, and of flow-volume loops showing reduced inspiratory effort or truncation of the inspiratory loop. Plethysmographic measurements of airways resistance or conductance may be normal. Direct examination of the vocal cords is diagnostic and shows the characteristic adduction of the vocal cords in association with wheezing,[7,10] but this may occur only intermittently. Management of the condition is reassurance but is difficult, particularly when it co-exists with asthma. However, it should be possible to withdraw any excessive therapies such as oral corticosteroids/ high-dose oral steroids. Psychiatric assessment is necessary and speech therapy may be useful. Hypnotherapy and neuro-feedback training have been reported to be of benefit, but some patients may continue to have such episodes for many years.[11]

Treatment: Adequacy and Adherence

It is important to establish that the asthmatic has been given an adequate dose of inhaled corticosteroid therapy; sometimes a trial of maximal inhaled corticosteroids is needed. Institution of other therapy should be considered as appropriate to the level of asthma severity. Under-treatment may lead to a patient with continuing symptoms being labelled as suffering from difficult asthma.[12] In addition to making sure that inhaler techniques are satisfactory, adherence to the treatment must be ensured because poor control of asthma can result from poor compliance to therapy.[13] Patients with the highest levels of compliance had significantly fewer exacerbations than those with a confirmed record of poor compliance.[14] Reported levels of compliance to treatment with inhaled corticosteroid therapy has ranged from as low as 30% in adolescents to 55% in adults.[15] In one study, although mean compliance with inhaled therapy was satisfactory at 60–70%, treatment was only taken as prescribed on 30–40% of days.[16] Even compliance to taking corticosteroid tablets in a corticosteroid trial was only 26%.[17] Poor adherence to asthma treatment appears be related to the inhaled route since better compliance with oral theophylline than with inhaled corticosteroids has been found.[15] This also indicates that for patients prescribed theophylline, persistently low serum theophylline level may identify the patient with general poor adherence to treatment. Poor compliance to inhaled corticosteroids may also be related to the lack of immediate effect of this treatment, to an undue fear of unwanted effects, or to psychosocial factors, and poor patient education and comprehension.

The degree of adherence to prescribed therapy in a particular asthmatic patient remains difficult to estimate, but this should always be attempted by checking prescriptions and direct questioning. The best objective measures are made by using a computerized monitor attached to the inhaler, but these are not widely available. Compliance can be improved by regular medical consultations and by instituting an asthma educational programme that explains to the patient the rationale of treatment together with a self-management plan.

EXACERBATING FACTORS

A number of medical factors can contribute to poor control of asthma and these need to be addressed in each patient (Table 45.2).

Gastroesophageal Reflux
Gastroesophageal reflux is commonly noted in asthmatics, with a reported incidence of up to 60% in children with moderate to severe asthma.[18,19] It has been implicated as causing asthma exacerbations and increasing asthma symptoms, by mechanisms involving vagally-mediated oesophago-bronchial reflex or direct effects of microaspiration into the upper airways. Studies of the effects of spontaneous reflux or distal acid perfusion of the oesophagus have revealed only small responses in terms of pulmonary function changes,[20–22] but it is not known whether the effects of oesophageal reflux would be amplified in patients with difficult asthma. A precise mechanistic link between gastroesophageal reflux and a decline in asthma control is not established and only varying degrees of improve-

Table 45.2: Factors that may contribute to loss of control of asthma
Poor compliance/adherence to therapy
Psychosocial and emotional factors
Inadequate medical facilities
Poor access to medical facilities
Inadequate treatment
Exposure to allergens
Viral respiratory tract infections
Indoor/outdoor pollution
Gastroesophageal reflux
Sinorhinitis
Genetic factors

ment in asthma has been observed when concomitant gastroesophageal reflux have been treated.[23–25] Some studies demonstrate little beneficial effect of treating gastroesophageal reflux on asthma symptoms and control.[26,27] However, it would make sense to treat any concomitant gastroesophageal reflux in patients with difficult severe asthma. Future trials are needed to establish the value of this treatment in the difficult asthma patient.

Sinusitis/Rhinitis
Strong co-existence of rhinosinusitis with asthma suggests that there is a relationship between nasal and sinus disease, and the airways. Several mechanisms have been proposed by which disease of the sinuses could exacerbate asthma. These include rhinobronchial reflexes, enhancement of systemic airway inflammatory responses, or direct deposition of inflammatory mediators and cytokines from the upper airways in the lower airways. Significant improvement in asthma control may be obtained with targeted treatment for sinusitis/rhinitis[28–30] in children and adults with severe or refractory asthma. Treatment of rhinosinusitis includes topical nasal steroids, short courses of topical vasoconstrictors, antibiotics and sometimes, surgical interventions.

Allergen Exposure

Other factors may include exposure to allergens, indoor and outdoor air pollution and endotoxin.[31–34] The most common domestic allergens are house-dust mite, cats and moulds, but often exposure to other allergens including cockroaches[35] and other domestic pets may contribute to difficult asthma. Severe exacerbations of asthma leading to respiratory arrest has been attributed to aeroallergen mould spores.[36] Sensitization to a fungus, *Trichophyton*, has been described as causing severe asthma in non-atopic asthmatics, which was controlled once anti-fungal therapy was given.[37] Reversal of bronchial hyperresponsiveness with reduction in oral steroid requirement during prolonged hospitalization in a low house-dust mite environment has been reported in mild to moderately severe asthmatics.[38] Sensitization and seasonal exposure to *Alternaria* has been proposed as a risk factor for sudden death from asthma.[39,40] The degree of exposure of patients with severe brittle asthma to relevant aeroallergens in their home is not known, but this may be relevant to their rapid episodes of deterioration. Related to allergen exposure is the possibility of being exposed to allergens or chemical sensitizers at the work-place; an occupational history is an essential part of the evaluation of the severe asthmatic patient.

Drugs

Aspirin and non-steroidal anti-inflammatory drugs may cause exacerbation of asthma, but the condition of aspirin-sensitive asthma may present with particularly difficult asthma even in the absence of ingestion of such drugs. Aspirin-sensitive asthma usually presents as non-atopic late-onset asthma with the presence of rhinosinusitis and nasal polyps. There is increased production of cysteinyl-leukotrienes, particularly if the attack is precipitated by ingestion of aspirin. Over-expression of leukotriene (LT) C_4 synthase enzyme has been shown in bronchial biopsies, particularly in eosinophils, when compared with patients with non-aspirin-sensitive asthma.[41] Aspirin-sensitive asthma is more frequently associated with a genetic polymorphism in the promoter sequence of LTC_4 synthase leading to increased enzyme expression.[42] Aspirin-induced asthmatic attacks are blocked by leukotriene inhibitors, and aspirin-induced asthma is also improved by these agents.[43–46]

β blockers precipitate acute exacerbations of asthma, and must be avoided in patients with asthma. Even β blockers such as timolol delivered as eye-drops may precipitate asthma. Selective $β_1$-receptor blockers are not necessarily devoid of this adverse effect. All β-adrenergic receptor blockers should be avoided in asthmatic patients. Alternative therapies should be used as indicated such as in the treatment of ischaemic heart disease or hypertension. Angiotensin converting enzyme (ACE) inhibitors are well-known to be associated with the induction of a non-productive cough, but are not recognized as precipitating asthma.

Respiratory Tract Infections

Virus infections of the upper respiratory tract are important precipitants of acute severe exacerbations of asthma,[31] but their mechanisms are unknown. No specific preventive measures are available. *Mycoplasma pneumoniae* has been found in patients with chronic stable asthma and has been proposed as a contributory factor for asthma severity.[47] In children, persistent infection with *Chlamydia pneumoniae* has been associated with more frequent exacerbations of asthma.[48] In patients with severe corticosteroid-dependent asthma, treatment of *Chlamydia* with antibiotics such as clarithromycin or azithromycin may lead to an improvement in asthma.[49] The role of these infections in asthma severity needs further investigation.

Psychosocial Factors

Psychosocial factors are present in fatal, near-fatal and severe asthma. In a retrospective analysis of asthma deaths, these factors have been linked with or compounded by poor patient compliance and to lack of appropriate medical care.[50] High scores of psychiatric morbidity have been correlated with severe asthma and in the families of children who die of asthma. Although there is no causal relationship between psychosocial factors and asthma severity, it is clear that many psychosocial factors such as denial, panic, fear, depression, low socioeconomic class, minority status, alcoholism, marital problems and avoidance coping are linked to poor asthma outcomes.[50,51] An association between psychiatric disturbances and asthma morbidity has been reported in near-fatal asthma attacks and, in particular, the importance of denial has been emphasized as a barrier to the use of appropriate self-management plans. Bad experience at the time of a severe attack will predispose to post-traumatic stress disorder.[52] It is often difficult to clarify how psychosocial factors and pathophysiological determinants of the disease interrelate in determining the severity of asthma. However, patients commonly cite emotional factors or stress as an exacerbating factor.

PATTERNS OF DIFFICULT-TO-TREAT ASTHMA

A number of terms are used by clinicians to describe "difficult-to-treat" asthma patients such as difficult acute, difficult chronic, chronic severe, acute severe, therapy-resistant, difficult-to-control, corticosteroid-resistant or corticosteroid-dependent, life-threatening and fatal asthma, illustrating the heterogeneity of the clinical presentation of difficult asthma. Distinct subgroups of patients with severe asthma have been described usually on the basis of anecdotal reports. These have been characterized by the temporal sequence of exacerbations and of symptoms, the chronicity and rapidity of onset of symptoms and the response to treatment,[53] and include: (1) patients experiencing a fatal or near-fatal episode of asthma that is associated with hypercapnia and/or needing mechanical ventilation; (2) recurrent episodes of severe airway obstruction that occur rapidly over minutes to hours, which may occur at any time of the day ("brittle" asthma); (3) persistent falls in lung function at night or in the morning on waking, with marked diurnal peak flow measurements; (4) persistent airway obstruction with or without episodes of deterioration; the terms "fixed" obstruction or "corticosteroid-dependence" is often used for such patients.

Brittle Asthma

Brittle asthma was a term first used to describe patients with asthma who had a wide and chaotic variation in peak expiratory flow (PEF) despite high doses of inhaled steroids,[53] distinct from the more regular patterns of PEF seen in patients with less-well controlled asthma. It was implied that these patients had more life-threatening disease from the rapidity of onset of the severe bronchoconstriction. Two types of brittle asthma have been proposed: Type 1, with persistent and chaotic variability in peak flow despite considerable medical therapy, and Type 2, with sporadic sudden falls in PEF rate on a background of normal or near-normal lung function and well-controlled asthma.[54] Type 1 brittle asthma often fails to respond to inhaled β_2 agonists administered by nebuliser or long-acting β_2 agonists. Many of these patients have psychological problems.[55] The attacks of Type 2 brittle asthma appear

not to be controlled or prevented by steroids, and often do not respond sufficiently to inhaled β_2 agonists. Patients with Type 2 brittle asthma have a high incidence of food allergy, which appears to be a risk factor in death and near-death from asthma.[56] Since the attacks are unpredictable, they are difficult to pre-empt. In addition, there is an impaired perception of airway narrowing and a reduced ventilatory response to hypoxia in patients with sudden onset near-fatal attacks of asthma,[57,58] leading to reduced awareness of the severity of attacks and subsequent delay in taking appropriate therapy.

Chronic Difficult Asthma

This term is often used for patients affected by chronic symptoms interfering with sleep, exercise tolerance, ability to go to work or attending school or classes. There may be frequent exacerbations of these symptoms which persist despite the use of maximal asthma therapy. Such patients have evidence of airflow limitation, and may or may not demonstrate significant variability. They may already be established on chronic oral corticosteroid therapy. Higher doses of corticosteroids may lead to further improvement of airflow obstruction, and they may experience worsening of asthma when corticosteroids are reduced or discontinued. Therefore, the term "corticosteroid-dependent" asthma is often used for these patients. Rarely, some patients show no airway response to prednisolone (40 mg per day) administered for 2 weeks, despite a bronchodilator response to inhaled β_2 agonists[59] and, according to this definition, are labelled as corticosteroid-resistant asthma.[60] However, it is possible that they may respond to higher doses of corticosteroids. Some patients may have developed asthma in later years rather than in childhood, and some may not demonstrate evidence of atopy as measured by skin-prick tests to common aeroallergens ("intrinsic" asthma). However, recent immunohistopathological evidence indicates that the inflammatory airway mucosal infiltrate is not different between the atopic ("extrinsic") and non-atopic ("intrinsic") asthmatic patient.[61] Some patients with difficult atopic asthma have high levels of serum IgE, but the role of IgE is not known.

Fatal Asthma

Difficult asthma also includes patients that have an increased risk of severe attacks or asthma deaths. Patients with brittle asthma are particularly at risk, but asthma deaths are not confined only to this group.[62] The characteristics of the fatality-prone asthmatic have been described from retrospective analyses of case–control studies of asthma deaths and include patients who have had an episode of respiratory failure needing intubation, respiratory acidosis associated with an attack of asthma not requiring intubation, two or more hospitalizations for asthma despite the chronic use of oral corticosteroid therapy, and two episodes of acute pneumomediastinum or pneumothorax associated with an attack of asthma.[63,64] The risk of asthma deaths is also greater in patients with previous attacks that occurred suddenly or were associated with hypoxic seizures, hypercapnia, very low peak flows, and the use of medication from three or more classes of therapy for asthma.[65]

Pre-Menstrual Worsening of Asthma

Exacerbations of asthma during the premenstrual and the menstrual periods have been recognized from as far back as 1938, later confirmed by recordings of significant falls in peak expiratory flow rate occurring 7–10 days before the onset of menses.[66] This cyclical worsening of the airways obstruction occurring during the late luteal phase at a time when the circulating progesterone and oestrogen levels fall to their nadir remains largely unexplained. Its prevalence amongst ovulating asthmatic female patients is also unclear with reports of up to one-third of female patients surveyed in a hospital asthma clinic.[67,68] Some patients experience very severe episodes of pre-menstrual worsening, often resistant to high doses of corticosteroids.[69,70] Use of intramuscular synthetic progestin, medroxyprogesterone acetate, has been reported to control premenstrual exacerbations in three patients,[69] but this compound also displays potent corticosteroid activity. Gonadotrophin-releasing hormone agonist analogues may be used to suppress the menstrual cycle by creating a "pseudo menopause", but there are long-term risks of osteoporosis and atherosclerotic cardiovascular disease.

PATHOPHYSIOLOGY OF DIFFICULT THERAPY-RESISTANT ASTHMA

Lung Mechanics and Airway Responsiveness

Lung mechanics and airway responsiveness are major determinants of the clinical severity and expression of difficult therapy-resistant asthma. One of the patho-physiological features of severe asthma is excessive airway narrowing, as demonstrated by the loss of a maximal plateau response following inhalation of bronchoconstrictor stimuli.[71] This unlimited airway narrowing may be related to an increased amount of airway smooth muscle,[72,73] exudative swelling of the airway wall,[74,75] and to airway–parenchymal interactions.[76] One particular feature of severe asthma is the loss of bronchodilatation with a deep inspiration, which may be associated with airways inflammation[77] and with excessive narrowing during bronchoconstriction.[78] The loss of deep-breath induced bronchodilatation may contribute to increased perception of breathlessness in patients with asthma.[79] Loss of mechanical load may also affect the behaviour of airway smooth muscle by favouring the development of force-maintenance.[80] These observations may be the basis for the rapidity of development of severe airway narrowing in certain patients and also for the chronic shortness of breath observed in some patients with difficult asthma. It is not known whether the difficult therapy-resistant asthma patient demonstrates more pronounced abnormalities of airway smooth muscle mass and contractility, or of loss of airway–parenchymal interdependence.

Airway Inflammation

In patients with mild asthma, patchy loss of the surface epithelium, thickening of the reticular basement membrane, and an increased cellular infiltrate in the bronchial mucosa consisting mainly of eosinophils, often mast cells and T-lymphocytes are observed in bronchial biopsy sections.[81–83] The severity of asthma as measured by the expression of symptoms and degree of airflow limitation has been associated with the presence of activated eosinophils and expression of certain cytokines in the mucosa (e.g. Il-5, GM-CSF).[84–86] T-cell activation and eosinophilia in bronchoalveclar lavage fluid correlated with asthma severity.[87] In more severe asthmatics on chronic oral steroid therapy, a marked neutrophilia in bronchoalveolar lavage fluid and in endo- and trans-bronchial biopsies has been observed, while moderately severe asthmatics not on oral steroids demonstrated eosinophilia.[88] Analysis of induced sputum shows the presence of eosinophils, with greater release of the eosinophil product, eosinophil cationic protein (ECP), in the more difficult therapy-resistant asthmatics, together with increased numbers of neutrophils, together with increased IL-8 levels in the supernatants.[89] In addition, some patients with difficult severe asthma have excessive levels of nitric oxide in their exhaled breath despite high dose glucocorticoid therapy.[90]

Studies in patients with nocturnal asthma have revealed differences in the inflammatory components during the night compared with the day. Thus, increased airway eosinophils, superoxide levels and histamine levels in bronchoalveolar lavage fluid at 4.00 a.m. in subjects with nocturnal asthma, when compared with 4.00 p.m.[91,92] Significant inflammation is present in both proximal airways and alveolar tissues in subjects with asthma, but it is the alveolar tissue inflammation that increases significantly during the night, compared with the proximal airways of patients in whom there is no significant diurnal change.[93] A significant elevation of LTB_4, cysteinyl leukotrienes and thromboxane in bronchoalveolar lavage fluid has been reported.[94] Therefore, severe asthmatics may demonstrate both higher levels of activated eosinophils, and also neutrophilia, although the potential contribution of corticosteroid therapy to the neutrophilia is unknown.

Immunohistochemical studies of fatal asthma, compared with mild non-fatal asthma, have not provided any clear indications as to possible contributing factors to the severe obstruction. The eosinophilic inflammatory response is worse in the proximal airways with a redistribution of T-lymphocytes away from the airway epithelium while others emphasize the even distribution of inflammation in both small and large airways.[95,96] Neutrophilic inflammation has also been reported during acute exacerbations of asthma, and in cases of fatal asthma attacks of sudden onset.[97] Submucosal vascular congestion may also be an important feature.

Airway Wall Remodelling

A proportion of patients with asthma experience an accelerated decline in lung function,[98,99] which may be partially resistant to corticosteroid therapy. What underlies this decline in lung function is unclear but it may reflect chronic progressive airway wall "remodelling". In addition, airway wall remodelling may cause a loss of airway dynamic distensibility and persistent bronchial hyperresponsiveness. Airway remodelling has been defined as structural changes with the appearance of subepithelial fibrosis with collagen deposition ("basement membrane thickening"), an increase in the number of submucosal blood vessels and airway smooth muscle mass, and changes to the airway epithelium with an increase in goblet cells and submucosal glands.[100,72,101–103] These will contribute to an increase in airway wall thickness, which also includes the inflammatory cellular influx, the extravasation of plasma and the increased vascularity.[104] Subepithelial fibrosis is found in even mild episodic asthma, and has been reported to be increased in severe asthma in one study,[105] but not in another study.[106] Although there has been description of both airway smooth muscle hypertrophy and hyperplasia in the airways of patients who have died from asthma,[72] there are no data on chronic severe asthma. In cases of fatal and non-fatal asthma, the total and outer airway wall areas are greater than in control cases. However, in cartilaginous airways, cases with fatal asthma show greater total wall, inner wall, outer wall, smooth muscle and mucus gland areas than non-fatal and control cases.[107]

High resolution computed tomography (HRCT) of the lungs has been used as a non-invasive method of assessing the intrapulmonary airways in asthma. The clinical severity of asthma was related to the degree of airway thickening and airway dilatation,[108] while another study related it to the degree of air trapping measured on inspiratory and expiratory lung computed tomograms.[109] Whether these airway wall changes are a reflection of thickening of the muscle or submucosa, or of oedema is not known. The value of HRCT in assessing airway wall remodelling is unclear and the significance of radiological evidence of airway wall thickening and dilatation in a patient with asthma remains speculative in the absence of pathological correlation.

The pathogenesis of airway wall remodelling as well as its physiological consequences may involve the expression of growth factors and pro-inflammatory cytokines influencing the deposition and breakdown of collagen matrix, the increase in airway smooth muscle mass, the increase in submucosal blood vessels, and the augmentation of mucus production by an excess of mucus goblet cells, and submucosal glands. A greater number of airway mucosal eosinophils expressing transforming-growth factor (TGF) β_1 mRNA and protein has been reported to correlate with the severity of asthma and the degree of subepithelial fibrosis,[105] but this is not confirmed in other studies.[106] Although insulin-growth factor (IGF) expression was not increased in the airways of patients with asthma with a thickened reticularis lamina of their basement membrane, inhaled corticosteroid treatment is associated with a reduction in the expression of IGF in the airways, associated with a reduced lamina reticularis.[110] Epidermal growth factor (EGF) expression is increased in the epithelium of patients with asthma.[111] Established airway wall remodelling is assumed to be irreversible by inhaled corticosteroid treatment, but the early use of inhaled corticosteroids may prevent irreversible changes in lung function.[112,113] This may prevent the establishment of airway wall remodelling.

Corticosteroid Responsiveness

The proposed definition of difficult therapy-resistant asthma rests on the therapeutic response of asthmatic patients to inhaled or oral corticosteroid therapy. Difficult asthma may be viewed as a disease that responds suboptimally to inhaled or oral corticosteroids, thus necessitating high doses of these treatments at the risk of side-effects. Much of the work has focused on "steroid-resistant" asthma, but the response to corticosteroids is relative to the doses of corticosteroids used.[114] In the "steroid-resistant" asthmatic, the inflammatory infiltrate of eosinophils in the airways submucosa is similar to that of the steroid-sensitive patient; in addition, there is similar expression of the T-helper type 2 cytokines IL-4 and IL-5.[115] However, corticosteroid treatment does not cause a reduction in eosinophils, or suppression of expression of IL-4 and IL-5 mRNA in the airways submucosa of steroid-resistant asthmatics.[115] Levels of IL-12 mRNA did not change with corticosteroid therapy in steroid-resistant asthma, although they were increased in corticosteroid-sensitive asthmatics. Corticosteroids also do not inhibit the *ex vivo* proliferation of peripheral blood T-cells of steroid-resistant asthmatics.[116] A reduction in the number of glucocorticoid receptors available for binding to DNA in steroid-resistant asthmatics may be attributed to an increased activation of the transcription factor, activating-protein-1 (AP-1).[117] The mechanisms underlying steroid-resistant asthma may shed light on those underlying difficult asthma.[118] Circulating mononuclear cells of patients with deteriorating asthma on exposure to allergen show decreased binding affinity of corticosteroid receptors, which recovers on treatment with oral corticosteroids.[119] A decreased binding affinity of circulating mononuclear cells is also observed in severe patients on long-term oral corticosteroids, but this is not secondary to the effect of long-term treatment with oral corticosteroids.[120] Drugs that may

reverse the partial lack of response of corticosteroids in severe asthma may be beneficial. There are, however, very little data regarding the state of the corticosteroid receptors in the airways, and their properties. Corticosteroid receptors are particularly well-expressed in the airway epithelial cells of non-asthmatics and mild asthmatics,[121] and these may well reflect the responsiveness of the airways to corticosteroid therapy, as the epithelium is exposed to the highest concentrations of topical corticosteroids.

MANAGEMENT

It is best to manage difficult asthma in a specialized asthma centre where the patient can be seen regularly over a period of 6–12 months for confirmation of the diagnosis, features of the difficulty in asthma ascertained, treatment maximized and its effects observed, and adherence to treatment and delivery of care optimized. Table 45.3 shows the range of investigations that may be necessary in the patient with difficult, therapy-resistant asthma. Referral to specialized asthma centres is also important because it would allow for the collection of databases for such patients for clinical and cellular characterization. Many aspects of diagnosis, exacerbating factors, optimization of treatment and improving adherence to treatment have already been addressed and attention to these factors may improve the control of difficult asthma to a considerable extent.[25] However, newer effective therapies are needed for the difficult, therapy-resistant asthma patient,[122] and clinical trials of newer agents are needed in this group. This is another reason for having specialized asthma centres for such patients. Specific points will be made regarding the use of currently-available asthma drugs.

Inhaled Corticosteroids

By definition, the difficult asthmatic will be receiving high doses of inhaled corticosteroid therapy, often together with oral corticosteroids. Studies of dose–response relationships of inhaled corticosteroids indicate that, in terms of symptoms and peak expiratory flows, there appears to be a progressively diminishing response above 800 µg per day of budesonide or 400 µg per day of fluticasone propionate.[123,124] A twice-daily dosing is advised, although a four-times daily regime may be more efficacious.[125] Individual patients may however respond well to higher doses and it would be

Table 45.3: Investigation of difficult therapy-resistant asthma

Assessment of severity
Symptom score chart and use of β₂-agonist reliever therapy
Measurement of spirometry, lung volumes and gas transfer
Bronchial responsiveness to methacholine/histamine
Diurnal variation of peak expiratory flow
Quality of life assessment

Pharmacological responsiveness
Assessment of compliance to therapy and inhaler technique
Bronchodilator response to β₂-adrenergic agonists
Response to prednisolone (corticosteroid responsiveness)

Radiology
Chest radiograph
Barium swallow
Computed tomography of sinuses
High-resolution computed tomograms of the lungs

Blood tests
Full blood count including eosinophil count
Serum immunoglobulins G, A, M and IgG subclasses
Serum total immunoglobulin E (IgE)
Specific IgE to selected allergens
Thyroid function tests

Others
Biomarkers of inflammation (exhaled nitric oxide, eosinophils
    in induced sputum)
Sweat test and genetic assessment of cystic fibrosis
    transmembrane conductance regulator mutations
    (if indicated)
24-hour oesophageal pH monitoring
Examination of nasopharyngeal airways
Tests of ciliary function
Skin prick test to common aeroallergens
Fibreoptic bronchoscopy with bronchial biopsy and
    bronchoalveolar lavage
Psychological assessment

advisable to perform a trial of higher doses of inhaled steroids for a limited period. Reversal to the lower doses is important if there is no substantial benefit from using the higher doses. The use of high-dose topical corticosteroids delivered from a nebulizer has been advocated, but more data demonstrating their efficacy is required. The search for even more potent topical corticosteroids continues despite the apparent limited therapeutic gains of higher doses; however, this would

be an advance if these were devoid of potential systemic side-effects.

Oral Corticosteroids

Addition of maintenance oral corticosteroids may occur in a number of clinical situations: (1) patients with chronic symptoms and exacerbations may be started on a trial of prednisolone, followed by a step-down strategy to find the minimum effective dose; (2) patients with frequent severe exacerbations of asthma despite high-dose inhaled corticosteroid therapy may be treated intermittently for these episodes, but subsequently maintained on a chronic dose in an attempt to reduce these exacerbations; (3) patients already on a chronic daily dose of prednisolone needing further increases in the dose with worsening asthma or with an exacerbation of asthma.[114,126] Prednisone or prednisolone is the best characterized corticosteroid to use, usually administered once daily in the mornings to minimize adrenal suppression. Administration of a single dose of oral prednisone at 3.00 p.m. resulted in better overnight spirometric values and greater effect on cellular inflammation than a similar dose administered at 8.00 a.m. or 8.00 p.m.[127] This has not been investigated in larger studies. There is a suggestion that a twice daily regime of prednisone or prednisolone may be more beneficial, but there has been no formal proof of this in the treatment of asthma. Alternate-day regimes are also not entirely satisfactory in the control of severe asthma.

Of the many potential side-effects of chronic oral steroid therapy, the development of osteoporosis can now be clinically addressed. In patients with severe asthma embarking on a potentially long duration of oral corticosteroid therapy, it is now mandatory to assess and correct any dietary calcium and/or vitamin D deficiencies. Advice should be given concerning lifestyle where appropriate (regular exercise, a calcium-rich diet, or calcium supplements), and bone mass must be assessed using bone densitometry as early as possible. Consideration should be given to the need for primary or secondary prevention with oestrogen replacement therapy in perimenopausal women, or with bone-sparing agents such as bisphosphonates which are effective in the primary and secondary prevention of corticosteroid-induced bone loss.[128–130] The doses of corticosteroids should be reviewed frequently and adjusted to the minimal doses necessary to control asthma.

567

Short-Acting β-Adrenergic Agonists

Short-acting (SA) inhaled β_2-adrenergic agonists are used for the immediate relief of asthma symptoms and should be used on demand only. Their use in asthma is one measure of the severity of the disease. Excessive reliance on these agents is not advisable because of the following issues which remain controversial: (1) regular use of high-dose SA β_2 agonist may cause a partial loss of effectiveness, which in turn may lead to the use of even higher doses; (2) high doses of SA β_2 agonists may be detrimental to the control of asthma perhaps by interfering with corticosteroid action.[131] What constitutes an optimal and "safe" level of SA β_2 agonists has not been determined. Reducing excessive use of SA β_2 agonists (such as more than 24 puffs of salbutamol per day) nevertheless appears to be a reasonable step to take. Studies of β_2-receptor polymorphisms may be helpful in determining patients who will be relatively unresponsive to SA β_2-agonist therapy or may show severe tolerance to the effects of these drugs. One study showed that a mutation from arginine to glycine at position 16 is associated with increased down-regulation compared with the wild-type β_2 receptor.[132] The use of SA β_2 agonists delivered at high doses from a nebulizer should be reserved for the treatment of exacerbations. Continuous subcutaneous administration of terbutaline may be helpful in controlling the rapid attacks of brittle asthma.[133] How a beneficial effect is achieved from a subcutaneous infusion of terbutaline is unclear. Patients with a Type 2 brittle asthma should be given a self-administered syringe pre-loaded with adrenaline to be used in extreme situations.

Long-Acting β-Adrenergic Agonists

A complementary action of long-acting β_2 agonists with middle or high doses of inhaled corticosteroid therapy has been reported in moderately severe asthma both in terms of improvement in lung function and in the prevention of asthma exacerbations.[134,135] Such benefits persist for up to one year. Therefore, the addition of long-acting β_2 agonists to corticosteroid therapy in difficult asthma is a reasonable step. This may also help to reduce any excessive use of SA β_2 agonists. Such an addition does not worsen asthma control or accelerates the decline in lung function when administered in conjunction with inhaled corticosteroids. However, markers of airway inflammation such as eosinophils in induced sputum persist and may increase with the combination therapy of inhaled corticosteroids and long-acting β agonists.[136]

Theophylline

Theophylline, in addition to its bronchodilator properties, has immunomodulatory properties in asthma.[137,138] Its potential value in difficult asthma is unclear. Addition of slow-release theophylline to moderate doses of inhaled corticosteroids in moderately severe asthma provided similar or better control of asthma when compared with high-dose inhaled corticosteroid therapy.[139] Beneficial effects of theophylline have been reported in five cases of severe difficult asthma already on established high-dose inhaled and oral corticosteroids.[140]

Leukotriene Inhibitors

Leukotriene inhibitors, particularly leukotriene receptor antagonists, have been added in patients already taking inhaled corticosteroids, with or without oral corticosteroid therapy and with consequent improvement in lung function and a reduction in SA β_2 agonist use.[141,142] An inhaled steroid-sparing effect of one leukotriene receptor antagonist has been demonstrated in moderate-to-severe asthma,[143] while other preliminary studies show equivocal effects. Leukotriene inhibitors have been shown to be of particular benefit in patients with aspirin-induced asthma.[44] Corticosteroids do not reduce leukotriene biosynthesis as measured by urinary leukotriene E_4 excretion,[144,145] and therefore the combination of leukotriene inhibitors with corticosteroids may provide additional benefit for some patients with difficult asthma already taking high-dose inhaled or oral corticosteroid therapy.[146] Such data indicate that in certain patients with difficult asthma, the severity of the asthma may result from increased sulphidopeptide leukotriene production.

Immunosuppressants and Antimetabolities

Methotrexate, gold salts and cyclosporin A have been examined in oral corticosteroid-dependent asthmatics in double-blind placebo-controlled studies and significant oral corticosteroid-sparing effects have been found.[147-150] On average, a halving of the dose of corticosteroids has been reported after 4–5 months of continuous therapy. These medications are potentially toxic and should be instituted in specialized centres. Other treatments that have been reported include intravenous immunoglobulins (particularly in children), lignocaine aerosols, dapsone, colchicine and hydroxychloroquine but these trials have been open and small.[151-153] Patients with difficult, therapy-resistant asthma need newer effective asthma therapies.

KEY POINTS

KEY POINTS

1 In patients presenting with difficult-to-control asthma, it is necessary to confirm the diagnosis of asthma, to exclude alternative diagnoses, and to make sure that adequate asthma treatment is given and being adhered to.

2 Exacerbating factors such as gastroesophageal reflux, sinorhinitis, allergen exposure, drugs, respiratory tract infections and psychosocial factors must be addressed and treated, if possible.

3 Difficult therapy-resistant asthma may be defined as poorly controlled asthma in terms of chronic symptoms, episodic exacerbations, persistent and variable airways obstruction despite a continued requirement for short-acting β_2 agonists despite the use of high doses of inhaled steroids.

4 Difficult, therapy-resistant asthma is likely to consist of several clinical sub-groups characterized by the temporal sequence of exacerbations and symptoms, the chronicity and rapidity of symptoms and response to treatment, such as brittle asthma, chronic difficult asthma and fatal asthma.

5 The pathophysiological mechanisms of difficult asthma include excessive airway narrowing, excessive cellular inflammation and activation, increased airway wall remodelling and loss of responsiveness to the anti-inflammatory effects of corticosteroids.

6 Management of difficult asthma is best carried out in an asthma centre with attention to aspects of diagnosis, exacerbating factors, optimization of treatment and improving adherence to treatment and with regular follow-up of patients.

7 Specific asthma therapies in difficult asthma include short-acting and long-acting β_2-adrenergic agonists, slow-release theophylline, and inhaled and oral corticosteroids. Addition of leukotriene inhibitors may provide additional benefit.

8 For patients needing regular oral corticosteroids for satisfactory control, immunosuppressants such as methotrexate, cyclosporin A and gold salts may be used as corticosteroid-sparing agents. Bone-sparing measures should also be considered.

REFERENCES

1. British Thoracic Society. Guidelines for management of asthma in adults: I–chronic persistent asthma. *Br Med J* 1990; 301: 651–3.

2. ✪ Chung KF, Godard P. ERS Task force: Difficult therapy-resistant asthma. *Eur Respir J* 1999; 13: 1198–208.

3. Walsh LJ, Wong CA, Cooper S, Guhan AR, Pringle M, Tattersfield AE. Morbidity from asthma in relation to regular treatment: a community based study. *Thorax* 1999; 54: 296–300.

4. Glaxo Canada (Boston Consulting Group). *The Cost of Adult Asthma in Canada*. Princeton, NJ: Communications Media for Education, 1993.

5. National Asthma Campaign. *Report on the cost of asthma in Australia.* Melbourne: NAC, 1992.

6. Christopher KL, Wood RP, Eckert RC, Blager FB, Raney RA, Souhrada JF. Vocal-cord dysfunction presenting as asthma. *N Engl J Med* 1983; 308: 1566–70.

7. Newman KB, Mason UG, Schmaling KB. Clinical features of vocal cord dysfunction. *Am J Respir Crit Care Med* 1995; 152: 1382–6.

8. O'Connell MA, Sklarew PR, Goodman DL. Spectrum of presentation of paradoxical vocal cord motion in ambulatory patients. *Ann Allergy Asthma Immunol* 1995; 74: 341–4.

9. Snashall PD, Chung KF. Airway obstruction and bronchial hyperresponsiveness in left ventricular

failure and mitral stenosis. *Am Rev Respir Dis* 1991; 144: 945–56.

10. Nahmias J, Tansey M, Karetzky MS. Asthmatic extrathoracic upper airway obstruction: laryngeal dyskinesis. *N Engl J Med* 1994; 91: 616–20.

11. Hayes JP, Nolan MT, Brennan N, FitzGerald MX. Three cases of paradoxical vocal cord adduction followed up over a 10-year period. *Chest* 1993; 104: 678–80.

12. Bousquet J, Knani J, Henry C *et al*. Undertreatment in a nonselected population of adult patients with asthma. *J Allergy Clin Immunol* 1996; 98: 514–21.

13. Cochrane GM. Therapeutic compliance in asthma; its magnitude and implications. *Eur Respir J* 1992; 5: 122–4.

14. Milgrom H, Bender B, Ackerson L, Bowry P, Smith B, Rand C. Noncompliance and treatment failure in children with asthma. *J Allergy Clin Immunol* 1996; 98: 1051–7.

15. Kelloway JS, Wyatt RA, Adlis SA. Comparison of patients' compliance with prescribed oral and inhaled asthma medications. *Arch Intern Med* 1994; 154: 1349–52.

16. Bosley CM, Parry DT, Cochrane GM. Patient compliance with inhaled medication: does combining beta-agonists with corticosteroids improve compliance?. *Eur Respir J* 1994; 7: 504–9.

17. Hatton MQ, Allen MB, Vathenen SV, Feely MP, Cooke NJ. Compliance with oral corticosteroids during steroid trials in chronic airways obstruction. *Thorax* 1996; 51: 323–4.

18. Gustafsson PM, Kjellman NI, Tibbling L. Oesophageal function and symptoms in moderate and severe asthma. *Acta Paediatr Scand* 1986; 75: 729–36.

19. Martin ME, Grunstein MM, Larsen GL. The relationship of gastroesophageal reflux to nocturnal wheezing in children with asthma. *Ann Allergy* 1982; 49: 318–22.

20. Goodall RJ, Earis JE, Cooper DN, Bernstein A, Temple JG. Relationship between asthma and gastro-oesophageal reflux. *Thorax* 1981; 36: 116–21.

21. Herve P, Denjean A, Jian R, Simonneau G, Duroux P. Intraesophageal perfusion of acid increases the bronchomotor response to methacholine and to isocapnic hyperventilation in asthmatic subjects. *Am Rev Respir Dis* 1986; 134: 986–9.

22. Tan WC, Martin RJ, Pandey R, Ballard RD. Effects of spontaneous and simulated gastroesophageal reflux on sleeping asthmatics. *Am Rev Respir Dis* 1990; 141: 1394–9.

23. Harper PC, Bergner A, Kaye MD. Antireflux treatment for asthma. Improvement in patients with associated gastroesophageal reflux. *Arch Intern Med* 1987; 147: 56–60.

24. Spaulding HS Jr, Mansfield LE, Stein MR, Sellner JC, Gremillion DE. Further investigation of the association between gastroesophageal reflux and bronchoconstriction. *J Allergy Clin Immunol* 1982; 69: 516–21.

25. ❂ Irwin RS, Curley FJ, French CL. Difficult-to-control asthma. Contributing factors and outcome of a systematic management protocol. *Chest* 1993; 103: 1662–9.

26. Ford GA, Oliver PS, Prior JS, Butland RJ, Wilkinson SP. Omeprazole in the treatment of asthmatics with nocturnal symptoms and gastro-oesophageal reflux: a placebo-controlled cross-over study. *Postgrad Med J* 1994; 70: 350–54.

27. Larrain A, Carrasco E, Galleguillos F, Sepulveda R, Pope CE. Medical and surgical treatment of nonallergic asthma associated with gastroesophageal reflux. *Chest* 1991; 99: 1330–35.

28. Rachelefsky GS, Katz RM, Siegel SC. Chronic sinus disease with associated reactive airway disease in children. *Pediatrics* 1984; 73: 526–9.

29. Friedman R, Ackerman M, Wald E, Casselbrant M, Friday G, Fireman P. Asthma and bacterial sinusitis in children. *J Allergy Clin Immunol* 1984; 74: 185–9.

30. Adinoff AD, Cummings NP. Sinusitis and its relationship to asthma. *Pediatr Ann* 1989; 18: 785–90.

31. Pattemore PK, Johnston SL, Bardin PG. Viruses as precipitants of asthma symptoms. I. Epidemiology. *Clin Exp Allergy* 1992; 22: 325–36.

32. Delfino RJ, Coate BD, Zeiger RS, Seltzer JM, Street DH, Koutrakis P. Daily asthma severity in relation to personal ozone exposure and outdoor fungal spores. *Am J Respir Crit Care Med* 1996; 154: 633–41.

33. Michel O, Kips J, Duchateau J *et al*. Severity of asthma is related to endotoxin in house dust. *Am J Respir Crit Care Med* 1996; 154: 1641–6.

34. Strachan DP, Carey IM. Home environment and severe asthma in adolescence: a population based case-control study. *BMJ* 1995; 311: 1053–6.

35. Rosenstreich DL, Eggleston P, Kattan M *et al*. The role of cockroach allergy and exposure to cockroach allergen in causing morbidity among inner-city children with asthma. *N Engl J Med* 1997; 336: 1356–63.

36. O'Hollaren MT, Yunginger JW, Offord KP *et al*. Exposure to an aeroallergen as a possible precipitating factor in respiratory arrest in young patients with asthma. *N Engl J Med* 1991; 324: 359–63.

37. Ward GW Jr, Karlsson G, Rose G, Platts Mills TA. Trichophyton asthma: sensitisation of bronchi and upper airways to dermatophyte antigen. *Lancet* 1989; 1: 859–62.

38. Platts-Mills TA, Mitchell EB, Nock P, Tovey ER, Moszar H, Wilkins S. Reduction of bronchial hyperreactivity during prolonged allergen avoidance. *Lancet* 1982; ii: 675–8.

39. ✪ Neukirch C, Henry C, Leynaert B, Liard R, Bousquet J, Neukirch F. Is sensitisation to *Alternaria alternata* a risk factor for severe asthma? A population-based study. *J Allergy Clin Immunol* 1999; 103: 709–11.

40. Call RS, Ward G, Jackson S, Platts Mills TA. Investigating severe and fatal asthma. *J Allergy Clin Immunol* 1994; 94: 1065–72.

41. Cowburn AS, Sladek K, Soja J *et al*. Overexpression of leukotriene C4 synthase in bronchial biopsies from patients with aspirin-intolerant asthma. *J Clin Invest* 1998; 101: 834–46.

42. Sanak M, Simon HU, Szczeklik A. Leukotriene C4 synthase promoter polymorphism and risk of aspirin-induced asthma. *Lancet* 1997; 350: 1599–1600.

43. Dahlen B, Margolskee DJ, Zetterstrom O, Dahlen SE. Effect of leukotriene receptor antagonist MK-0679 on baseline pulmonary function in aspirin-sensitive asthmatic subjects. *Thorax* 1993; 48: 1205–10.

44. Dahlen B, Nizankowska E, Szczeklik A *et al*. Benefits from adding the 5-lipoxygenase inhibitor zileuton to conventional therapy in aspirin-intolerant asthmatics. *Am J Respir Crit Care Med* 1998; 157: 1187–94.

45. Dahlen B, Kumlin M, Margolskee DJ *et al*. The leukotriene-receptor antagonist MK-0679 blocks airway obstruction induced by bronchial provocation with lysine-aspirin in aspirin-sensitive asthmatics. *Eur Respir J* 1993; 6: 1018–26.

46. Israel E, Fischer AR, Rosenberg MA *et al*. The pivotal role of 5-lipoxygenase products in the reaction of aspirin-sensitive asthmatics to aspirin. *Am Rev Respir Dis* 1993; 148: 1447–51.

47. Kraft M, Cassell GH, Henson JE *et al*. Detection of *Mycoplasma pneumoniae* in the airways of adults with chronic asthma [published erratum appears in *Am J Respir Crit Care Med* 1998 Nov; 158 (5 Pt 1): 1692]. *Am J Respir Crit Care Med* 1998; 158: 998–1001.

48. Cunningham AF, Johnston SL, Julious SA, Lampe FC, Ward ME. Chronic *Chlamydia pneumoniae* infection and asthma exacerbations in children. *Eur Respir J* 1998; 11: 345–9.

49. Hahn DL, Bukstein D, Luskin A, Zeitz H. Evidence for *Chlamydia pneumoniae* infection in steroid-dependent asthma. *Ann Allergy Asthma Immunol* 1998; 80: 45–9.

50. Miller BD, Strunk RC. Circumstances surrounding the deaths of children due to asthma. A case–control study. *Am J Dis Child* 1989; 143: 1294–9.

51. Wareham NJ, Harrison BD, Jenkins PF, Nicholls J, Stableforth DE. A district confidential enquiry into deaths due to asthma. *Thorax* 1993; 48: 1117–20.

52. Yellowlees PM, Ruffin RE. Psychological defenses and coping styles in patients following a life-threatening attack of asthma. *Chest* 1989; 95: 1298–1303.

53. Turner-Warwick M. Observing patterns of airflow obstruction in chronic asthma. *Br J Dis Chest* 1971; 71: 73–86.

54. Ayres JG, Miles JF, Barnes PJ. Brittle asthma. *Thorax* 1998; 53: 315–21.

55. Miles JF, Garden GM, Tunnicliffe WS, Cayton RM, Ayres JG. Psychological morbidity and coping skills in patients with brittle and non-brittle asthma: a case–control study. *Clin Exp Allergy* 1997; 27: 1151–9.

56. Ernst P, Habbick B, Suissa S *et al*. Is the association between inhaled beta-agonist use and life-threatening asthma because of confounding by severity? *Am Rev Respir Dis* 1993; 148: 75–9.

57. Town GI, Allan C. Ventilatory responses to hypoxia and hypercapnia in asthmatics with previous respiratory failure. *Aust NZ J Med* 1989; 19: 426–30.

58. Kikuchi Y, Okabe S, Tamura G *et al*. Chemosensitivity and perception of dyspnea in patients with a history of near-fatal asthma. *N Engl J Med* 1994; 330: 1329–34.

59. Woolcock AJ. Corticosteroid-resistant asthma. Definitions. *Am J Respir Crit Care Med* 1996; 154: S45–8.

60. Chan MT, Leung DY, Szefler SJ, Spahn JD. Difficult-to-control asthma: clinical characteristics of steroid-insensitive asthma. *J Allergy Clin Immunol* 1998; 101: 594–601.

61. Humbert M, Durham SR, Ying S *et al*. IL-4 and IL-5 mRNA and protein in bronchial biopsies from patients with atopic and nonatopic asthma: evidence against "intrinsic" asthma being a distinct immunopathologic entity. *Am J Respir Crit Care Med* 1996; 154: 1497–1504.

62. ✪ Benatar SR. Fatal asthma. *N Engl J Med* 1986; 314: 423–9.

63. Walker CL, Greenberger PA, Patterson R. Potentially fatal asthma. *Ann Allergy* 1990; 64: 487–93.

64. Miller TP, Greenberger PA, Patterson R. The diagnosis of potentially fatal asthma in hospitalized adults. Patient characteristics and increased severity of asthma. *Chest* 1992; 102: 515–18.

65. Crane J, Pearce N, Burgess C, Woodman K, Robson B, Beasley R. Markers of risk of asthma death or readmission in the 12 months following a hospital admission for asthma. *Int J Epidemiol* 1992; 21: 737–44.

66. Hanley SP. Asthma variation with menstruation. *Br J Dis Chest* 1981; 75: 306–308.

67. Eliasson O, Scherzer HH, De Graft AC. Morbidity in asthma in relation to the menstrual cycle. *J Allergy Clin Immunol* 1986; 77: 87–94.

68. Gibbs CJ, Coutts II, Lock R, Finnegan OC, White RJ. Premenstrual exacerbation of asthma. *Thorax* 1984; 39: 833–6.

69. Beynon HLC, Garbett ND, Barnes PJ. Severe premenstrual exacerbations of asthma: effect of intramuscular progesterone. *Lancet* 1988; ii: 370–72.

70. Barkman RP. Sudden death in asthma. *Med J Aust* 1981; 1: 316–7.

71. Woolcock AJ, Salome CM, Yan K. The shape of the dose–response curve to histamine in asthmatic and normal subjects. *Am Rev Respir Dis* 1984; 130: 71–5.

72. Ebina M, Takahashi T, Chiba T, and Motomiya M. Cellular hypertrophy and hyperplasia of airway smooth muscle underlying bronchial asthma. *Am Rev Resp Dis* 1993; 148: 720–26.

73. Lambert RK, Wiggs BR, Kuwano K, Hogg JC, Pare PD. Functional significance of increased airway smooth muscle in asthma and COPD. *J Appl Physiol* 1993; 74: 2771–81.

74. Bel EH, Van der Veen H, Kramps JA, Dijkman JH, Sterk PJ. Maximal airway narrowing to inhaled leukotriene D4 in normal subjects. Comparison and interaction with methacholine. *Am Rev Respir Dis* 1987; 136: 979–84.

75. Kimura K, Inoue H, Ichinose M *et al*. Bradykinin causes airway hyperresponsiveness and enhances maximal airway narrowing. Role of microvascular leakage and airway edema. *Am Rev Respir Dis* 1992; 146: 1301–1305.

76. Macklem PT. A theoretical analysis of the effect of airway smooth muscle load on airway narrowing. *Am J Respir Crit Care Med* 1996; 153: 83–9.

77. Pliss LB, Ingenito EP, Ingram RHJC, Ingram RH Jr. Responsiveness, inflammation, and effect of deep breaths on obstruction in mild asthma. *J Appl Physiol* 1989; 66: 2298–2304.

78. Brusasco V, Pellegrino R, Violante B, Crimi E. Relationship between quasi-static pulmonary

hysteresis and maximal airway narrowing in humans. *J Appl Physiol* 1992; 72: 2075–80.

79. Sont JK, Booms P, Bel EH, Vandenbroucke JP, Sterk PJ. The severity of breathlessness during challenges with inhaled methacholine and hypertonic saline in atopic asthmatic subjects. The relationship with deep breath-induced bronchodilation. *Am J Respir Crit Care Med* 1995; 152: 38–44.

80. Fredberg JJ, Jones KA, Nathan M *et al.* Friction in airway smooth muscle: mechanism, latch, and implications in asthma. *J Appl Physiol* 1996; 81: 2703–12.

81. Azzawi M, Bradley B, Jeffery PK *et al.* Identification of activated T lymphocytes and eosinophils in bronchial biopsies in stable atopic asthma. *Am Rev Respir Dis* 1990; 142: 1407–13.

82. Djukanovic R, Roche WR, Wilson JW *et al.* Mucosal inflammation in asthma. *Am Rev Respir Dis* 1990; 142: 434–57.

83. Laitinen LA, Laitinen A, Haahtela T. Airway mucosal inflammation even in patients with newly diagnosed asthma. *Am Rev Respir Dis* 1993; 147: 697–704.

84. Bousquet J, Chanez P, Lacoste JY *et al.* Eosinophilic inflammation in asthma. *N Engl J Med* 1990; 323: 1033–9.

85. Hamid Q, Azzawi M, Ying S *et al.* Expression of mRNA for interleukins in mucosal bronchial biopsies from asthma. *J Clin Invest* 1991; 87: 1541–6.

86. Broide DH, Lotz M, Cuomo AJ. Cytokines in symptomatic asthma. *J Allergy Clin Immunol* 1992; 89: 958–67.

87. Walker C, Virchow JC, Bruijnzeel PLB, Blaser K. T Cell subsets and their soluble products regulate eosinophilia in allergic and non allergic asthma. *J Immunol* 1991; 146: 1829–35.

88. ✪ Wenzel SE, Szefler SJ, Leung DYM, Sloan SI, Rex MD, Martin RJ. Bronchoscopic evaluation of severe asthma: persistent inflammation associated with high dose glucocorticoids. *Am J Respir Crit Care Med* 1997; 156: 737–43.

89. Jatakanon A, Uasuf C, Maziak W, Lim S, Chung KF, Barnes PJ. Neutrophilic inflammation in severe persistent asthma. *Am J Respir Crit Care Med* 1999; 160: 1532–9.

90. Stirling RG, Kharitonov S, Campbell D, Durham SR, Chung KF, Barnes PJ. Exhaled NO is elevated in difficult asthma and correlates with symptoms and disease severity despite treatment with oral and inhaled corticosteroids. *Thorax* 1998; 53: 1030–34.

91. Martin RJ, Cicutto LC, Smith HR *et al.* Airway inflammation in nocturnal asthma. *Am Rev Respir Dis* 1991; 143: 351–7.

92. Jarjour NN, Busse WW, Calhoun WJ. Enhanced production of oxygen radicals in nocturnal asthma. *Am Rev Respir Dis* 1992; 146: 905–911.

93. Kraft M, Djukanovic R, Wilson S, Holgate ST, Martin RJ. Alveolar tissue inflammation in asthma. *Am J Respir Crit Care Med* 1996; 154: 1505–1510.

94. Wenzel SE, Trudeau JB, Kaminsky DA, Cohn J, Martin RJ, Westcott JY. Effect of 5-lipoxygenase inhibition on bronchoconstriction and airway inflammation in nocturnal asthma. *Am J Respir Crit Care Med* 1995; 152: 897–905.

95. Synek M, Beasley R, Frew AJ *et al.* Cellular infiltration of the airways in asthma of varying severity. *Am J Respir Crit Care Med* 1996; 154: 224–30.

96. Carroll N, Cooke C, James A. The distribution of eosinophils and lymphocytes in the large and small airways of asthmatics. *Eur Respir J* 1997; 10: 292–300.

97. Sur S, Crotty TB, Kephart GM *et al.* Sudden-onset fatal asthma: A distinct entity with few eosinophils and relatively more neutrophils in the airway submucosa? *Am Rev Resp Dis* 1993; 148: 713–19.

98. Peat JK, Woolcock AJ, Cullen K. Rate of decline of lung function in subjects with asthma. *Eur J Respir Dis* 1987; 70: 171–9.

99. Lange P, Parner J, Vestbo J, Schnohr P, Jensen G. A 15-year follow-up study of ventilatory function in adults with asthma. *N Engl J Med* 1998; 339: 1194–2000.

100. Roche WR, Beasley R, Williams JH, Holgate ST. Subepithelial fibrosis in the airways of asthmatics. *Lancet* 1989; 520–22.

101. Dunnill MS. The pathology of asthma with special reference to changes in the bronchial mucosa. *J Clin Path* 1960; 13: 27–33.

102. Laitinen LA, Heino M, Laitinen A, Kava T, Haahtela T. Damage of the airway epithelium in patients with asthma. *J Allergy Clin Immunol* 1992; 90: 32–42.

103. Li X, Wilson JW. Increased vascularity of the bronchial mucosa in mild asthma. *Am J Respir Crit Care Med* 1997; 156: 229–33.

104. Redington AE, Howarth PH. Airway wall remodelling in asthma. *Thorax* 1997; 52: 310–312.

105. Minshall EM, Leung DYM, Martin RJ *et al*. Eosinophil-associated TGFβ1 mRNA expression and airways fibrosis in asthma. *Am J Respir Cell Mol Biol* 1997; 17: 326–33.

106. Chu HW, Halliday JL, Martin RJ, Leung DYM, Szefler SJ, Wenzel SE. Collagen deposition in large airways may not differentiate severe asthma from milder forms of the disease. *Am J Respir Crit Care Med* 1998; 158: 1936–44.

107. Carroll N, Elliott J, Morton A, James A. The structure of large and small airways in nonfatal and fatal asthma. *Am Rev Resp Dis* 1993; 147: 405–410.

108. Paganin F, Trussard V, Seneterre E *et al*. Chest radiography and high resolution computed tomography of the lungs in asthma. *Am Rev Respir Dis* 1992; 146: 1084–7.

109. Carr DH, Hibon S, Rubens M, Chung KF. Peripheral airways obstruction on high-resolution computed tomography in chronic severe asthma. *Respir Med* 1998; 92: 448–53.

110. Hoshino M, Nakamura Y, Sim JJ *et al*. Inhaled corticosteroid reduced lamina reticularis of the basement membrane by modulation of insulin-like growth factor (IGF)-I expression in bronchial asthma. *Clin Exp Allergy* 1998; 28: 568–77.

111. Vignola AM, Chanez P, Chiappara G *et al*. Transforming growth factor-beta expression in mucosal biopsies in asthma and chronic bronchitis. *Am J Respir Crit Care Med* 1997; 156: 591–9.

112. Haahtela T, Jarvinen M, Kava T. Comparison of a β$_2$

113. Haahtela T, Jarvinen M, Kava T *et al*. Effects of reducing or discontinuing inhaled budesonide in patients with mild asthma. *N Engl J Med* 1994; 331: 700–705.

114. Ogirala RG, Aldrich TK, Prezant DJ, Sinnett MJ, Enden JB, Williams MH Jr. High-dose intramuscular triamcinolone in severe, chronic, life-threatening asthma [published erratum appears in *N Engl J Med* 1991 May 9; 324 (19): 1380]. *N Engl J Med* 1991; 324: 585–9.

115. Leung DY, Martin RJ, Szefler SJ *et al*. Dysregulation of interleukin 4, interleukin 5, and interferon gamma gene expression in steroid-resistant asthma. *J Exp Med* 1995; 181: 33–40.

116. Adcock IM, Lane SJ, Brown CR, Peters MJ, Lee TH, Barnes PJ. Differences in binding of glucocorticoid receptor to DNA in steroid-resistant asthma. *J Immunol* 1995; 154: 3500–3505.

117. Adcock IM, Lane SJ, Brown CR, Lee TH, Barnes PJ. Abnormal glucocorticoid receptor-activator protein I interaction in steroid-resistant asthma. *J Exp Med* 1995; 182: 1951–8.

118. ○ Barnes PJ, Adcock IM. Steroid resistance in asthma. *Q J Med* 1995; 88: 455–68.

119. Nimmagadda SR, Szefler SJ, Spahn JD, Surs W, Leung DY. Allergen exposure decreases glucocorticoid receptor binding affinity and steroid responsiveness in atopic asthmatics. *Am J Respir Crit Care Med* 1997; 155: 87–93.

120. Irusen E, Barnes PJ, Adcock IM, Chung KF. Altered affinity of dexamethasone for the glucocorticoid receptor (GR) in oral steroid-dependent asthmatics. *Eur Respir J* 1998; 13 (suppl.): 2822.

121. Adcock IM, Gilbey T, Gelder CM, Chung KF, Barnes PJ. Glucocorticoid receptor localization in normal and asthmatic lung. *Am J Respir Crit Care Med* 1996; 154: 771–82.

122. Chung KF. The role of new asthma treatments. *Allergol Internat* 1998; 47: 237–46.

123. Dahl R, Lundback B, Malo JL *et al*. A dose-ranging study of fluticasone propionate in adult patients with

agonist terbutaline with an inhaled steroid in newly detected asthma. *N Engl J Med* 1991; 325: 388–92.

moderate asthma. International Study Group. *Chest* 1993; 104: 1352–8.

124. Busse WW, Chervinsky P, Condemi J *et al.* Budesonide delivered by Turbuhaler is effective in a dose-dependent fashion when used in the treatment of adult patients with chronic asthma. *J Allergy Clin Immunol* 1998; 101: 457–63.

125. Toogood JH, Baskervill JC, Jennings B, Lefcoe NM, Johanson SA. Influence of dosing frequency and schedule on the response of chronic asthmatics to the aerosol steroid, budesonide. *J Allergy Clin Immunol* 1982; 70: 288–98.

126. Grandordy B, Belmatong N, Morelle A, De Lauture D, Marsac J. Effect of betamethasone on airway obstruction and bronchial response to salbutamol in prednisolone resistant asthma. *Thorax* 1986; 42: 65–71.

127. Beam WR, Weiner DE, Martin RJ. Timing of prednisone and alterations of airways inflammation in nocturnal asthma. *Am Rev Respir Dis* 1992; 146: 1524–30.

128. Mulder H, Struys A. Intermittent cyclical etidronate in the prevention of corticosteroid-induced bone loss. *Br J Rheumatol* 1994; 33: 348–50.

129. Struys A, Snelder AA, Mulder H. Cyclical etidronate reverses bone loss of the spine and proximal femur in patients with established corticosteroid-induced osteoporosis. *Am J Med* 1995; 99: 235–42.

130. Adachi JD, Bensen WG, Brown J *et al.* Intermittent etidronate therapy to prevent corticosteroid-induced osteoporosis. *N Engl J Med* 1997; 337: 382–7.

131. Adcock IM, Stevens DA, Barnes PJ. Interactions of glucocorticoids and beta 2-agonists. *Eur Respir J* 1996; 9: 160–68.

132. Tan S, Hall IP, Dewar J, Dow E, Lipworth B. Association between β_2-adrenoceptor polymorphism and susceptibility to bronchodilator desensitisation in moderately severe stable asthmatics. *Lancet* 1997; 350: 995–9.

133. Ayres J, Fish DR, Wheeler DC, Wiggins J, Cochrane GM, Skinner C. Subcutaneous terbutaline and control of brittle asthma or appreciable morning dipping. *Br Med J Clin Res Ed* 1984; 288: 1715–16.

134. Greening AP, Ind PW, Northfield M, Shaw G. Added salmeterol versus higher-dose corticosteroid in asthma patients with symptoms on existing inhaled corticosteroid. *Lancet* 1994; 344: 219–24.

135. Pauwels RA, Lofdahl C, Postma D *et al.* Effect of inhaled formoterol and budesonide on exacerbations of asthma. *New Engl J Med* 1997; 337: 1405–11.

136. McIvor RA, Pizzichini E, Turner MO, Hussack P, Hargreave FE, Sears MR. Potential masking effects of salmeterol on airway inflammation in asthma. *Am J Respir Crit Care Med* 1998; 158: 924–30.

137. Kidney J, Dominguez M, Taylor PM, Rose M, Chung KF, Barnes PJ. Immunomodulation by theophylline in asthma. Demonstration by withdrawal of therapy. *Am J Respir Crit Care Med* 1995; 151: 1907–14.

138. Sullivan P, Bekir S, Jaffar Z, Page C, Jeffery P, Costello J. Anti-inflammatory effects of low-dose oral theophylline in atopic asthma [published erratum appears in *Lancet* 1994 Jun 11; 343 (8911): 1512]. *Lancet* 1994; 343: 1006–1008.

139. Evans DJ, Taylor DA, Zetterstrom O, Chung KF, O'Connor BJ, Barnes PJ. Theophylline plus low dose inhaled steroid is as effective as high dose inhaled steroid in the control of asthma. *New Engl J Med* 1997; 337: 1412–18.

140. Brenner M, Berkowitz R, Marshall N, Strunk RC. Need for theophylline in severe steroid-requiring asthmatics. *Clin Allergy* 1988; 18: 143–50.

141. Spector SL, Smith LJ, Glass M. Effects of six weeks of therapy with oral doses of ICI 204,219, a leukotriene D4 receptor antagonist, in subjects with bronchial asthma. *Am J Respir Crit Care Med* 1994; 150: 618–23.

142. Reiss TF, Chervinsky P, Dockhorn RJ, Shingo S, Seidenberg B. Montelukast, a once-daily leukotriene receptor antagonist, in the treatment of chronic asthma: a multicenter, randomized, double-blind trial. Montelukast Clinical Research Study Group. *Arch Int Med* 1998; 158: 1213–20.

143. Tamaoki J, Kondo M, Sakai N *et al.* Leukotriene antagonist prevents exacerbation of asthma during reduction of high-dose inhaled corticosteroid. The Tokyo Joshi-Idai Asthma Research Group. *Am J Respir Crit Care Med* 1997; 155: 1235–40.

144. Dworski R, Fitzgerald GA, Oates JA, Sheller JR. Effect of oral prednisone on airway inflammatory mediators in atopic asthma. *Am J Respir Crit Care Med* 1994; 149: 953–9.

145. O'Shaughnessy KM, Wellings R, Gillies B, Fuller RW. Differential effects of fluticasone propionate on allergen-evoked bronchoconstriction and increased urinary leukotriene E4 excretion. *Am Rev Respir Dis* 1993; 147: 1472–6.

146. Virchow J, Hassall SM, Summerton L. Improved asthma control over 6 weeks with Accolate (zafirlukast) in patients on high dose corticosteroids. *Allergy* 1997; 52: 183.

147. Nierop G, Gijzel WP, Bel EH, Zwinderman AH, Dijkman JH. Auranofin in the treatment of steroid dependent asthma: a double blind study. *Thorax* 1992; 47: 349–54.

148. Shiner RJ, Nunn A, Chung KF, Geddes DM. Steroid-sparing effect of methotrexate in the treatment of chronic severe asthma: a double-blind controlled study. *Lancet* 1990; 336: 137–40.

149. Alexander AG, Barnes NC, Kay AB. Cyclosporin A in corticosteroid-dependent chronic severe asthma. *Lancet* 1992; 339: 324–7.

150. Lock SH, Kay AB, Barnes NC. Double-blind, placebo-controlled study of cyclosporin A as a corticosteroid-sparing agent in corticosteroid-dependent asthma. *Am J Respir Crit Care Med* 1996; 153: 509–514.

151. Mazer BD, Gelfand EW. An open-label study of high-dose intravenous immunoglobulin in severe childhood asthma. *J Allergy Clin Immunol* 1991; 87: 976–83.

152. Landwehr LP, Jeppson JD, Katlan MG *et al.* Benefits of high-dose i.v. immunoglobulin in patients with severe steroid-dependent asthma. *Chest* 1998; 114: 1349–56.

153. Hunt LW, Swedlund HA, Gleich GJ. Effect of nebulized lidocaine on severe glucocorticoid-dependent asthma. *Mayo Clin Proc* 1996; 71: 361–8.

Chapter 46

Specific Problems: Steroid-Induced Side-Effects

Neil Barnes

Systemic corticosteroids were first used in the management of asthma in the 1930s when crude extracts of adrenocorticotrophic hormone (ACTH) were administered. The first properly conducted trials of oral corticosteroids were performed in the 1950s in two MRC-sponsored studies.[1,2] The trial in chronic asthma[1] used a low and variable dose of cortisone and showed a benefit over part of the treatment period in the steroid-treated group. The second study[2] in acute severe asthma showed compelling evidence of benefit. In the absence of other effective anti-inflammatory agents, oral corticosteroids became widely used in asthma and in other inflammatory diseases such as rheumatoid arthritis. Within a few years the serious long-term side-effects of treatment with oral corticosteroids became apparent. Since then the goal in treating asthma has been to effectively control the disease without the long-term use of oral corticosteroids. This goal has been clearly set out in various guidelines:[3,4] the objective is control of the disease with best possible lung function, minimizing the chance of a severe attack and with the least possible side-effects from drugs.

Effective anti-asthma therapy has decreased the percentage of patients who require long-term oral steroids. There remain three broad patterns of use of systemic steroids in the treatment of asthma. The first and most common is the use of short courses of oral steroids for the treatment of acute exacerbations of asthma. The second is the long-term maintenance treatment and the third pattern is repeated short courses of steroids with only short gaps between them. Although side-effects are potentially the same, the principal concern differs. For instance, with a short course of oral steroids the principal concerns may be over dyspepsia, bleeding ulcers, electrolyte disturbances and impairment of glucose tolerance, whereas with long-term oral steroids the principal concerns will be over disturbances of protein metabolism, osteoporosis, skin thinning, easy bruising and cataract formation. The frequent use of short courses of oral steroids may lead to concern over both patterns of side-effects. The side-effects of oral steroids (Table 46.1) are dependent upon the dose of steroids and the duration of treatment. However, there is evidence particularly for effects on bone[5] that the most rapid bone loss is seen early in treatment with the rate of bone loss becoming less rapid as treatment progresses. When attempting to minimize the side-effects of oral steroids two considerations are necessary: first, how can the dose or duration of treatment be minimized and, second, how can other measures be taken to counteract the side-effects?

MINIMIZING THE USE OF ORAL STEROIDS

Allergen Avoidance

While the routine use of allergen avoidance in the proven control of asthma is controversial, it seems clear that in occupational asthma removal from offending allergen or improved work practices can lead to a very significant improvement in asthma. Therefore, treatment of any occupational component that can be identified is of importance.

Smoking

Advising patients to stop smoking is a routine part of the management of asthma. There is some evidence that patients with asthma who smoke are more resistant to treatment.[6] There is no specific proof that stopping smoking can prevent or decrease the use of oral steroids. However, smoking is known to increase the risk of osteoporosis, peptic ulceration,

Table 46.1: Complications of using systemic corticosteroids

	Problems occurring with both acute and chronic usage	Problems mainly related to chronic usage
Metabolic	Hypokalaemia Diabetes mellitus Hypothalamic–pituitary–adrenal axis suppression	Hyperlipidaemia Cushingoid appearance Secondary amenorrhoea Impotence
Cardiovascular	Hypertension Exacerbation of congestive cardiac failure Oedema	
Gastrointestinal tract	Peptic ulceration Oesophagitis Pancreatitis Intestinal perforation	
Infective complications	Increased susceptibility to infection Reactivation of infection Dissemination of live vaccine	
Skin		Skin thinning and fragility Easy bruising Hirsuitism
CNS	Psychological changes Convulsions	
Musculoskeletal	Myopathy Aseptic necrosis of head of femur	Osteoporosis Loss of muscle mass
Ocular	Glaucoma	Cataracts

the cardiovascular complications of hypertension and to worsen the complications of diabetes and therefore it is important that patients are strongly advised to stop smoking.

Immunotherapy

Immunotherapy is a treatment that remains controversial and there is no proof that it decreases the requirements for oral steroids.

β₂ Agonists

The possible benefits and side-effects of regular treatment with β_2 agonists for asthma have been controversial. A recent study of decreasing the dose of β_2 agonists has shown no evidence of improved control.[7] There is no proof that regular β_2 agonists either increase or decrease requirement for oral steroids.

Theophyllines

Some authorities consider oral theophyllines to have an anti-inflammatory role in asthma, although this role is not clearly defined. There are a number of studies suggesting that theophyllines may decrease requirement for oral steroids.[8–10] A trial of oral controlled-release theophyllines is worth while in patients with steroid-dependent asthma.

Anti-Cholinergics

There is no well-documented proof that anti-cholinergic drugs decrease requirement for oral corticosteroids.

Disodium Cromoglycate (DSCG) and Nedocromil Sodium

There are conflicting results of studies of DSCG and nedocromil sodium for their ability to decrease requirement for oral corticosteroids. In an early study DSCG led to an improvement in patients on oral steroids but steroid reduction was not attempted.[11] Other studies have investigated the ability to control asthma without steroids but not steroid reduction directly.[12] With nedocromil sodium both positive[13] and negative[14] trials have been reported. In practice, any oral steroid-sparing effect they have is small or non-existent in the presence of adequate doses of inhaled corticosteroids. Furthermore, as compliance with inhaled therapy is a significant problem, it is likely that any small beneficial effect obtained may well be outweighed by the fact that these drugs have to be taken three or four times a day and may increase compliance with the more important inhaled corticosteroids.

Inhaled Corticosteroids

These are undoubtedly the most effective way of decreasing the requirement for long-term oral steroids. Early trials with beclomethasone dipropionate (BDP) were performed in patients who were dependent on oral steroids and demonstrated the ability of these drugs to decrease requirement for oral steroids.[15] Open studies have suggested that high-dose inhaled steroids can further reduce the number of patients dependent on long-term oral steroids.[16] However, these studies are open to criticism and controversy remains about the beneficial effects of increasing doses of inhaled steroids above 800–1000 µg daily.[17,18] The recent introduction of the new, more potent, inhaled steroid fluticasone propionate has allowed further research into the role of inhaled steroids in decreasing requirement for oral steroids. In a study comparing 1.5 and 2 mg daily of inhaled fluticasone with placebo for the ability to decrease the requirement for oral steroids, 88% of patients on the highest dose of inhaled steroids managed to stop their oral steroids with an increase in pulmonary function compared with only 3% of patients stopping oral steroids on placebo.[19] There was also evidence in this study of a dose-related effect. Open uncontrolled[20] and anecdotal evidence suggests that in some patients increasing the dose of BDP or budesonide above 2 mg daily may further decrease requirement for oral steroids, but as these patients provide a harder and more difficult core of oral steroid-dependent asthmatic patients the return from increasing the dose becomes smaller. Both budesonide and fluticasone propionate are available as nebulizer solutions; however, there is no evidence that they have any advantage over the same dose given by either metered dose inhaler or dry powder inhaler.

Although concern has been expressed about the side-effects of inhaled steroids when used at high dose for a long time, any effects they have are far less than those that occur with the regular use of oral steroids. However it is important that any systemic effects are minimized. This can be achieved by using the lowest effective dose of inhaled steroids, by using a large-volume spacer with a metered dose inhaler and further decreasing the gastrointestinal deposition by gargling and spitting out. Evidence suggests that at high dose fluticasone propionate may have an improved safety-to-efficacy ratio compared with the established inhaled steroids BDP and budesonide;[21] if further studies confirm this fluticasone should be considered particularly in patients requiring oral steroids.

Immunosuppressants

A number of trials have demonstrated that immunosuppressants can decrease the requirement for oral steroids. However, their use remains controversial. Although several immunosuppressants have been shown to decrease the requirement for oral corticosteroids in trials of several months' duration, all of these drugs have serious side-effects and it is not yet clear whether the benefit from reduction of oral steroid requirement outweighs the side-effects of these immunosuppressant drugs. At present the use of these drugs should be in clinical trials or on an individual patient basis with the clinician attempting to weigh-up the benefits and risks of the treatment for the particular patient. They should only be used once other avenues of treatment, particularly the use of high-dose inhaled corticosteroids, has been found to be inadequate.

Methotrexate

The most widely used immunosuppressant in asthma is methotrexate. This acts on all dividing cells and has an established role as a steroid-sparing agent and anti-inflammatory drug in rheumatoid arthritis. The initial observation by Mullarkey *et al* that methotrexate decreased oral steroid requirement in a patient with asthma was followed by a clinical trial demonstrating an impressive decrease in oral steroid requirement.[22]

However, the group of patients studied had a very high requirement for oral steroids and the use of other anti-asthma drugs in this group was ill-defined. A well-performed study by Shiner et al.[23] investigated the steroid-sparing effect of methotrexate at a dose of 15 mg orally per week over a 24-week period in a randomized, placebo-controlled, parallel group study. The study demonstrated that methotrexate caused a 50% decrease in oral steroid requirement compared with a 14% decrease on placebo; however the effect had not maximized by the end of the study. There was also a decrease in exacerbations of asthma without any change in pulmonary function. Other studies have not shown such a marked beneficial effect of methotrexate.[24,25] A recent systematic review has confirmed that methotrexate has a steroid-sparing effect in steroid-dependent asthma.[26] There have been reports of side-effects, notably *Pneumocystis carinii* pneumonia[27] and methotrexate-induced pneumonitis.[28] Apart from an increase in opportunistic infections, the other specific side-effect of methotrexate is liver fibrosis and it is recommended by some that a liver biopsy should be performed every 2 years in patients on long-term methotrexate.[29] At present if methotrexate is to be used it should probably only be in patients on long-term oral steroids, despite high-dose inhaled steroids. A trial of treatment of at least 3 months is needed to see if there is any beneficial effect. If no decrease in steroid requirement is seen at this time then it is probably best to stop. If a beneficial effect is seen it may be worth continuing until the lowest possible dose of oral steroids is reached. Regular monitoring of liver function tests and full blood count are necessary and prompt treatment of any intercurrent infection will be needed.

Azathioprine

Azathioprine was the subject of two small-scale, short-term studies.[30,31] These were most certainly of inadequate length to determine if azathioprine had a steroid-sparing role. Although it is likely that azathioprine would have a steroid-sparing role in asthma its use cannot be advocated in the absence of any controlled trials.

Cyclosporin A

With the increased understanding of the role of T-lymphocytes in asthma[32] and evidence that cyclosporin A (CsA) is active in other steroid-responsive diseases, such as psoriasis and atopic dermatitis,[33,34] an investigation into the role of CsA in steroid-dependent asthma became attractive.

Three controlled trials have now been performed and there has been a report of the use of CsA on an open basis. Alexander et al.[35] showed an increase in pulmonary function with a decrease in exacerbations of asthma that required rescue courses of prednisolone in a group of steroid-depending asthmatic subjects on high-dose inhaled steroids. Two further controlled trials have been performed specifically searching for a steroid-sparing effect. Lock et al.[36] have shown a significant steroid-sparing effect of CsA over a 36-week period with a small rise in pulmonary function. Nizanowska et al.[37] have shown a decrease in oral steroid requirement without an increase in pulmonary function in a group of steroid-dependent asthmatic subjects. In these studies and in experience with the open use of CsA[38] it seems that only 50% or so of patients respond at the dose used (5 mg kg^{-1} daily). CsA should only be used in patients dependent on oral steroids or high-dose inhaled steroids. There should be no contraindications to use, particularly previous malignancy or significant renal disease, and regular monitoring of renal function is necessary during treatment. Treatment should be given for 3 months to see if there is any beneficial effect. Anecdotal experience suggests that in patients who respond doses lower than 5 mg kg^{-1} daily can be used, and if a response is achieved then it is worth trying to wean down the dose of CsA. On stopping treatment there seems to be no long-term beneficial effect, although there is no evidence of any rebound or worsening of asthma.[35–37]

Oral Gold

Oral gold is well established as a steroid-sparing agent in rheumatoid arthritis and has been used for a number of years in Japan in the treatment of asthma. An open, uncontrolled study in asthma suggested benefit.[39] Recently, a well-conducted placebo-controlled study has been performed in patients with difficult asthma most of whom were on oral steroids.[40] This study suggested a small but statistically significant oral steroid-sparing effect with a slight improvement in lung function. Side-effects were mild and included rashes and slight proteinuria. In common with other steroid-sparing treatments the effect was slow in onset and a 3- or 4-month trial of therapy would be necessary to determine if oral gold was effective in an individual patient.

Intravenous Immunoglobulins (IVIG)

There have been anecdotal reports and small, uncontrolled studies of the use of intravenous immunoglobulins, particularly in adolescents with difficult asthma.[41] Reports of two trials have shown no evidence of benefit[42,43] and cases of aseptic meningitis have been reported.[44] It is not possible to advocate the use of IVIG at present.

Hydroxychloroquine

Hydroxychloroquine is established as a steroid-sparing agent in rheumatoid arthritis. There has been an uncontrolled study in steroid-dependent asthmatic subjects that indicated benefit.[45] In the absence of controlled studies it is difficult to advocate the use of this treatment.

Troleandomycin

Troleandomycin (TAO) is a macrolide antibiotic that has the odd property of slowing the metabolism of methylprednisolone.[46] Thus if methylprednisolone is the oral steroid being used in a patient, the use of TAO can decrease the number of milligrams of treatment taken while the therapeutic effect remains unaltered.[47] In addition it has been claimed that TAO has other vaguely specified immunosuppressant activity. The theoretical benefit from decreasing the number of milligrams of methylprednisolone used while steroid side-effects remain unchanged is difficult to justify. TAO also interferes with theophylline metabolism and has hepatic side-effects. A well-performed study of TAO in steroid-dependent asthma has shown no benefit and considerable side-effects.[48] Its use cannot be recommended.

Alternative Therapies

A number of alternative therapies[49] such as homeopathy and acupuncture[50] have been suggested. In the absence of any properly conducted, controlled trials showing benefit it is difficult to justify the use of these treatments in steroid-dependent asthma.

New Therapies

A large number of novel therapies are currently being investigated in asthma. These have mostly been studied in mild asthma. The first to be introduced will probably be the leukotriene antagonists and 5-lipoxygenase inhibitors. The leukotriene receptor antagonist Accolate (ICI204,219) has been shown to be effective in patients taking inhaled corticosteroids,[51] but no trials of oral steroid reduction have been reported. In clinical practice some patients do seem to be able to decrease their oral steroid requirement. However, in some patients the eosinophilic vasculitis, Churg–Strauss syndrome has been reported particularly in patients on oral steroids. It seems most likely that this is due to unmasking of pre-existing CSS.[52] A recent study with a specific anti-IgE monoclonal antibody has suggested that it may decrease oral steroid requirement in atopic asthma patients.[62]

Preventing and Minimizing Side-Effects of Oral Steroids

The side-effects during both the acute and chronic administration of oral steroids are listed in Table 46.1. Some side-effects such as osteoporosis are mainly a problem during chronic usage, whereas others such as stomach ulceration can occur during both acute and chronic administration.

For many of the side-effects no specific preventative treatment is available. As there is a relationship between the dose of steroid and the incidence and severity of adverse events, keeping the dose of steroid to a minimum is essential. It is also important to be aware that steroids can cause this range of problems so that prompt treatment is given and needless tests for other causes are avoided. This section will concentrate on these steroid-induced problems for which specific measures need to be taken.

Metabolic

Electrolyte imbalance, particularly hypokalaemia, can be a problem as patients may be receiving high-dose inhaled β_2 agonists and theophyllines that lower plasma potassium. Plasma potassium should be monitored and appropriate replacement therapy given as necessary.

Diabetes mellitus may be unmasked or exacerbated in patients receiving high-dose oral steroids. Plasma glucose should be monitored with either blood tests or Dextrastix and treatment with oral hypoglycaemic agents or insulin administered as required. Usually when the steroid is stopped the diabetes will resolve.

The Cushingoid appearance and weight gain is a side-effect that causes patients considerable concern. Steroids cause weight gain mainly by an increase in appetite with a minor contribution from fluid retention. Furthermore there is redistribution of body mass from the peripheries to the centre. As it is always easier to prevent weight gain rather than to treat established obesity, it is important that patients are warned of this so that dietary advice can be given.

Cardiovascular

Exacerbations of existing hypertension or mild to moderate hypertension are relatively common complications of the long-term use of oral steroids. As other cardiovascular risk factors, particularly glucose intolerance, obesity and lack of exercise, may also be present it is important to detect and control any hypertension. β blockers are obviously completely contraindicated in asthma, so other alternative treatment anti-hypertensive agents must be used. Thiazide diuretics are best avoided unless there is co-existing fluid retention, as they will tend to exacerbate any hypokalaemia and may theoretically increase plasma viscosity, thus worsening cardiovascular risk profile. Calcium antagonists such as nifedipine or amlodipine are a good choice in hypertensive patients with asthma. Angiotensin-converting enzyme (ACE) inhibitors may be used but can precipitate cough in some patients; they may be of particular use in patients with co-existing diabetes.

Fluid retention and peripheral oedema are a particular problem in older patients who may have co-existing heart disease. A small dose of diuretic is usually sufficient to control this; however a potassium-sparing diuretic is preferable in view of the problems with hypokalaemia detailed above.

Gastrointestinal Tract

Many patients suffer from dyspepsia when taking oral steroids and these effects can be minimised by the use of enteric-coated prednisolone. The association of oral steroids with peptic ulceration and gastrointestinal haemorrhage is controversial, with conflicting results from meta-analysis of studies.[53,54] With doubt over the role of steroids in peptic ulceration the benefit of prophylactic anti-ulcer drugs is also the subject of some debate. However, H_2 agonists or proton pump inhibitors are often given to cover courses of high-dose oral steroids.

Infective Complications

Oral steroids may suppress the overt signs of infection so that a patients with, for instance, pneumonia may present with an insidious illness rather than obvious fever, dyspnoea and malaise. The clinician needs to be alert to the masking of signs by steroids.

Controversy exists over the risk of reactivation of tuberculosis in patients with oral steriods.[55] Patients with evidence of previous tuberculosis, who have not received adequate anti-tuberculosis therapy, should be considered for isoniazid prophylaxis, particularly if doses of prednisolone above 10 mg per day are used.

The danger of the dissemination of live viral vaccinations means that they are contraindicated.[56]

Musculoskeletal

Osteoporosis, particularly in post-menopausal women, is one of the most serious and worrying side-effects for both patients and doctors and is undoubtedly a common side-effect in patients on long-term oral steroids. Minimizing the risk of osteoporosis can be divided into non-pharmacological and pharmacological means. Many of these therapies have been directly tested in osteoporosis induced by steroids. There is evidence that the bone architecture in steroid-induced osteoporosis is different from age-related osteoporosis and that it is at least potentially reversible.[57]

Non-Pharmacological Treatments

There are a number of factors that have been clearly identified as increasing the risk of osteoporosis. Smoking increases the risk of osteoporosis and patients should be strongly advised to give up smoking[58] and be given any help with smoking cessation clinics and nicotine replacement therapy. Excess alcohol consumption is associated with an increased risk of osteoporosis and a patient should be advised about sensible alcohol consumption. Physical exercise helps to maintain bone mass and, within the limits of their asthma, patients should be advised to take regular exercise.

Pharmacological Treatments

There is little evidence that calcium supplementation in patients on a normal diet is of benefit in preventing osteoporosis; however, if there are any concerns about dietary insufficiency then calcium and vitamin D supplementation should be provided.[57] In peri-menopausal women hormone replacement therapy has been shown to help to maintain bone mass;[59] however greater benefit is seen when treatment is started within 5 years of the menopause. With the risks of long-term hormone replacement therapy, particularly with regard to endometrial carcinoma, careful follow-up is necessary. In men, hypogonadism may also be present and can accelerate osteoporosis; if there is evidence of testosterone insufficiency this should be investigated and treated. There is now evidence that bisphosphonates such as etidronate or alendronate may be helpful in maintaining bone mass and preventing fractures in patients with osteoporosis.[60] A trial of intranasal calcitonin has shown benefit in maintaining bone mass in patients on long-term oral steroids, but this cannot yet be considered part of routine treatment.[61]

Sodium fluoride can increase bone mass, but may not alter fracture rate. It has significant side-effects and is difficult to use. At present treatment or prevention of osteoporosis is not universally used in patients on oral steroids. With new treatments available more attention should now be paid to prevention and treatment (Table 46.2).

Muscle wasting and a degree of myopathy occurs in many patients on long-term steroids. A particular problem occurs in patients ventilated for acute severe asthma and treated with intravenous hydrocortisone. Whether the problem occurs to a greater extent with hydrocortisone than other steroids is not known. It has been suggested that other factors such as virally induced myopathy may also play a part.

Ocular

Glaucoma is common in the elderly and preventable. Old people on long-term steroids, particularly with a family history, should have intra-ocular pressure measured.

Table 46.2: Prevention of osteoporosis in patients on long-term oral steroids

1. Stop smoking
   Reduce alcohol intake
   Correct dietary calcium or vitamin D deficiency

2. Measure bone density if low
   Hormone replacement therapy in peri- or
      post-menopausal women
   Detect and treat hypogonadism in men
   Cyclical etidronate (2 weeks every 13 weeks) or
      alendronate

3. If still unsatisfactory consider:
   Nasal calcitonin
   Sodium fluoride

CONCLUSION

Although only a minority of patients now need treatment with long-term oral corticosteroids they are a group who suffer significant problems both from their disease and its treatment. Effective strategies exist to minimize or eliminate the need for oral steroids and to minimize the risk of systemic side-effects (Table 46.3).

KEY POINTS

1 The most important method of preventing steroid side-effects is to minimize the dose of oral steroids and the most effective way of doing this is with inhaled steroids.

2 Poor compliance with inhaled steroids or poor inhaler technique is a common cause of treatment failure.

3 It is important to minimize side-effects and the following need to be considered.
   (a) Monitor and treat hypertension.
   (b) Check for hypokalaemia.
   (c) Check for diabetes mellitus.
   (d) Warn about weight gain.
   (e) Avoid live vaccines.

4 Osteoporosis is a serious side-effect. It can be minimized by:
   (a) hormone replacement therapy;
   (b) bisphosphonates;
   (c) correcting calcium or vitamin D deficiency.

5 A trial of immunosuppressants may be justified in some patients. Proven agents are:
   (a) methotrexate;
   (b) oral gold;
   (c) cyclosporin A.

6 Avoiding smoking is very important as it worsens asthma and increases the risk of cardiovascular, gastrointestinal and bone side-effects.

Table 46.3: A checklist to consider when treating a patient with asthma on long-term oral steroids

Minimize allergen exposure
Stop smoking
Optimize inhaled corticosteroid therapy using doses of BDP or budesonide up to 2 mg per day
Trial of theophyllines
Gradually wean down oral steroids

If this fails
Consider higher doses of inhaled steroids or fluticasone propionate 2 mg per day

If this fails
Consider immunosuppressant trial of 3 months' duration if:
    Sufficient concern over steroid dose
    No contraindications after screening
Options:
    Low-dose methotrexate 15 mg per week initial dose
    Cyclosporin A 5 mg kg^{-1} daily initial dose
    Oral gold
Patients will need to be fully informed of risks and benefits and closely monitored

If still on oral steroids
Regular measurement of blood pressure
Regular testing of glucose
Minimize the risk of osteoporosis (see Table 46.2)
Remember the immunosuppressant effect of steroids if intercurrent illness occurs
Remember infections may be masked and present insidiously

REFERENCES:

1. Medical Research Council. Controlled effects of cortisone acetate in chronic asthma. *Lancet* 1956; ii: 798–803.

2. Medical Research Council. Controlled trial of cortisone acetate in status asthmaticus. *Lancet* 1956; ii: 803–6.

3. British Thoracic Society, Research Unit of the Royal College of Physicians, King's Fund Centre, National Asthma Campaign. Guidelines for the management of asthma in adults. I: Chronic persistent asthma. *BMJ* 1990; 301: 651–3.

4. International Consensus Report on Diagnosis and Management of Asthma. *Clin Exp Allergy* 1992; 22 (suppl. 1).

5. Smith R. Corticosteroids and osteoporosis. *Thorax* 1990; 45: 573–8.

6. ✪ Smoking and asthma study in *Am J Respir Crit Care Med.*

7. Harrison TW, Oborne J, Wilding PJ, Tattersfield AE. Randomised placebo controlled trial of β agonist dose reduction in asthma. *Thorax* 1999; 54: 98–102.

8. Scher MS, Scherr LB, Morton JL. Use of inhaled beclomethasone diproprionate and optimized theophylline doses in asthmatic children at Camp Bronco Junction, 1977–1978. *Ann Allergy* 1980; 44: 82–8.

9. Nassif EG, Weinberger M, Thompson R, Huntley W. The value of maintenance theophyllines in steroid dependent asthma. *N Engl J Med* 1981; 304: 71–5.

10. Brenner M, Berkowitz R, Marshall N, Strunk RC. Need for theophylline in severe steroid requiring asthmatics. *Clin Allergy* 1988; 18: 143–50.

11. Howell JBL, Altounyon REC. A double-blind trial of disodium cromoglycate in the treatment of allergic bronchial asthma. *Lancet* 1967; ii: 539–42.

12. Brompton Hospital/Medical Research Council Collaborative Trial. Long-term study of disodium cromoglycate in treatment of severe extrinsic or intrinsic bronchial asthma in adults. *BMJ* 1972; 4: 383–8.

13. Boulet LP, Cartier A, Cockroft DW *et al*. Tolerance to reduction of oral steroid dosage in severely asthmatic patients receiving nedocromil sodium. *Respir Med* 1990; 84: 317–23.

14. Golden JB, Bateman EA. Does nedocromil sodium have a steroid sparing effect in adult asthmatic patients requiring maintenance oral corticosteroids. *Thorax* 1988; 43: 982–6.

15. Morrow-Brown H, Storey G, George WMS. Beclomethasone dipropionate: a new steroid aerosol for the treatment of allergic asthma. *BMJ* 1971; 1: 585–90.

16. Smith MJ, Hodson ME. High dose beclomethasone inhaler in the treatment of asthma. *Lancet* 1983; i: 265–9.

17. Hummel S, Lehtonen L. Comparison of oral steroid sparing by high and low dose inhaled steroid in maintenance treatment of severe asthma. *Lancet* 1992; 340: 1483–7.

18. Geddes DM. Inhaled corticosteroids: benefits and risks. *Thorax* 1992; 47: 404–7.

19. Noonan MJ, Chervinsky P, Weisberg SC *et al*. Fluticasone proprionate aerosol therapy permits reductions of prednisolone while improving pulmonary function and asthma symptoms (abstract). *Am J Respir Crit Care Med* 1994; 149 (suppl.): A214.

20. Otulana BA, Varna N, Bullock A, Higenbotham T. High dose nebulised steroid in the treatment of chronic steroid-dependent asthma. *Respir Med* 1992; 86: 105–8.

21. Barnes NC, Hallett C, Harris TA. Clinical experience with fluticasone propionate in asthma: a meta-analysis of efficacy and systemic activity compared with budesonide and beclomethasone dipropionate at half the microgram dose or less. *Respir Med* 1998; 92: 95–104.

22. Mullarkey MF, Blumenstein BA, Andrade WP, Bailey GA, Ulason I, Wetzel CE. Methotrexate in the treatment of corticosteroid-dependent asthma. *N Engl J Med* 1988; 318: 603–7.

23. Shiner RJ, Nunn AJ, Chung KF, Geddes DM. Randomised, double-blind, placebo-controlled trial of methotrexate in steroid-dependent asthma. *Lancet* 1990; 336: 137–40.

24. Erzurum SC, Leff JA, Cochran JE *et al*. Lack of benefit of methotrexate in severe steroid-dependent asthma: a double-blind, placebo-controlled study. *Ann Intern Med* 1991; 114: 353–60.

25. Trigg CJ, Davies RJ. Comparison of methotrexate 30 mg per week with placebo in chronic steroid-dependent asthma: a 12-week double-blind, cross-over study. *Respir Med* 1993; 87: 211–6.

26. Marin GM. Low-dose methotrexate spares steroid usage in steroid-dependent asthmatic patients. *Chest* 1997; 112: 29–33.

27. Kuitert LM, Harrison AC. *Pneumocystis carinii* pneumonia as a complication of methotrexate treatment of asthma. *Thorax* 1991; 46: 936–7.

28. White DA, Rankin JA, Storer PE, Gellene RA, Gupta S. Methotrexate pneumonitis. Bronchoalveolar lavage findings suggest an immunologic disorder. *Am Rev Respir Dis* 1989; 139: 19–21.

29. Health and Public Policy Committee, American College of Physicians. Methotrexate in rheumatoid arthritis. *Ann Intern Med* 1987; 107: 418–9.

30. Hodges NG, Brewis RAL, Howell JBL. An evaluation of azathioprine in severe chronic asthma. *Thorax* 1971; 26: 734.

31. Asmundsson T, Kilburn KH, Lazzlo J, Krock CJ. Immunosuppressive therapy of asthma. *J Allergy* 1971; 47: 136–47.

32. Corrigan CJ, Kay AB. T-Lymphocytes. In: Barnes PJ, Rodger IW, Thomson NC (eds). *Asthma Basic Mechanisms and Clinical Management*, 2nd edn. London: Academic Press, 1992: 125–41.

33. Ellis CN, Fradin MS, Messona JM *et al*. Cyclosporine for plaque-type psoriasis. Results of a multidose, double-blind trial. *N Engl J Med* 1991; 324: 277–84.

34. Sourden JM, Berth-Jones J, Ross JS *et al*. Double-blind controlled cross-over study of cyclosporin in adults with

severe refractory atopic dermatitis. *Lancet* 1991; 338: 137–40.

35. Alexander AG, Barnes NC, Kay AB. Trial of cyclosporin A in corticosteroid-dependent chronic severe asthma. *Lancet* 1992; 339: 324–8.

36. Lock SH, Barnes NC, Kay AB. Cyclosporin A (CsA) as a corticosteroid sparing agent in corticosteroid dependent asthma. *Thorax* 1994; 49: 1051P (Abstract).

37. Nizanowska E, Soja J, Pinis G. Treatment of steroid-dependent asthma with cyclosporin (abstract). *Am Rev Respir Dis* 1993; 147 (suppl.): A294.

38. Szczeklik A, Nizanowska E, Dworski R, Danagalen B, Pinis G. Cyclosporin for steroid-dependent asthma. *Allergy* 1992; 47: 349–54.

39. Bernstein DI, Bernstein L, Bodenheimer SS, Pietrusko RG. An open study of Auranofin in the treatment of steroid-dependent asthma. *J Clin Immunol* 1988; 81: 6–16.

40. Nierop G, Gijzel WP, Bel EM, Zwinderman AM, Dijkman JM. Auranofin in the treatment of steroid-dependent asthma: a double-blind study. *Thorax* 1992; 47: 349–54.

41. Mazer BD, Gelfand EW. An open-label study of high dose intravenous immunoglobulin in severe childhood asthma. *J Allergy Clin Immunol* 1991; 87: 976–83.

42. Jakobsson T, Croner S, Kjellman N, Pettersson A, Vassella C, Bjorksten B. Slight steroid sparing effect of intravenous immunoglobulin in children and adolescents with moderately severe bronchial asthma. *Allergy* 1994; 49: 413–20.

43. Valacer DJ, Kishiyama JL, Com B *et al.* A multi-center, randomized, placebo-controlled trial of high dose intravenous gammaglobulin (IVIG) for oral corticosteroid dependent asthma. *Am J Respir Crit Care Med* 1997; 155: A659.

44. Pallares DE, Marshall GS. Acute aseptic meningitis associated with administration of intravenous immunoglobulin. *Am J Paediatr Hematol Oncol* 1992; 14: 279–81.

45. Charous BL. Open study of hydroxychloroquine in the treatment of severe symptomatic or corticosteroid-dependent asthma. *Ann Allergy* 1990; 65: 53–8.

46. Szefler SJ, Rose JQ, Ellis EF, Spector SL, Green AW, Jusko WJ. The effect of troleandomycin on methylprednisolone elimination. *J Allergy Clin Immunol* 1980; 66: 447–51.

47. Zeiger RS, Schatz M, Sperling W, Simon RA, Stevenson DD. Efficacy of troleandomycin in out-patients with severe corticosteroid-dependent asthma. *J Allergy Clin Immunol* 1980; 66: 438–66.

48. Nelson HS, Hamilos DL, Corsello PR, Levesque NV, Buchmeier AD, Bucher BL. A double-blind study of troleandomycin and methylprednisolone in asthmatic subjects who require daily corticosteroids. *Am Rev Respir Dis* 1993; 147: 398–404.

49. Alternative and complementary medicine for asthma. *Thorax* 1991; 46: 787–97.

50. Kleijnen J, ter Reit G, Knipschild P. Acupuncture and asthma: a review of controlled trials. *Thorax* 1991; 46: 799–802.

51. Hui KP, Barnes NC. Lung function improvement in asthma with a cysteinyl leukotriene receptor antagonist. *Lancet* 1991; 337: 1062–3.

52. D'Cruz DP, Barnes NC, Lockwood CM. Difficult asthma or Churg–Strauss syndrome. *BMJ* 1999; 318: 475–6.

53. Conn HU, Blitzer BL. Non-association of adrenocorticosteroid therapy and peptic ulcer. *N Engl J Med* 1976; 294: 473–9.

54. Messer J, Reitman D, Sacks HS, Smith H, Chalmers TC. Association of adrenocorticosteroid therapy and peptic ulcer disease. *N Engl J Med* 1983; 309: 21–4.

55. Bateman ED. Is tuberculosis chemoprophylaxis necessary for patients receiving corticosteroids for respiratory disease? *Respir Med* 1983; 87: 485–7.

56. ✪ CSM viral evidence.

57. Hosking DJ. Effects of corticosteroids on bone turnover. *Respir Med* 1993; 87 (suppl. A): 15–21.

58. Hopper JL, Seeman E. The bone density of female twins discordant for tobacco use. *N Engl J Med* 1994; 330: 387–92.

59. Lindsay R, Aitken JM, Anderson JB, Hart DM; MacDonald EB, Clarke AC. Long-term prevention of osteoporosis by oestrogen. *Lancet* 1976; i: 1038–41.

60. Storm T, Thamsburg G, Stenicke T, Genart HK, Sorensen OM. Effect of intermittent cyclical etidronate therapy on bone mass in women with post-menopausal osteoporosis. *N Engl J Med* 1990; 322: 1265–71.

61. Luengo M, Pons F, de Osaba MJM, Picado C. Prevention of further bone mass loss by nasal calcitonin in patients on long-term gluco-corticoid therapy for asthma a two year follow-up. *Thorax* 1994; 49: 1099–102.

62. Milgrom H, Fick RB, Su JQ *et al*. Treatment of allergic asthma with monoclonal anti-IgE antibody. rhuMAb-E25 Study Group. *N Engl J Med* 1999; 341: 1966–73.

Chapter 47

Acute Complications of Asthma

Bernadette Hickey and Haydn Walters

Despite better understanding of the pathophysiology of acute asthma attacks, both the incidence of and mortality from acute asthma may be rising.[1] Asthma can be a life-threatening disease, particularly in patients who are either poorly responsive to, or compliant with, anti-inflammatory treatment. The difficulties in treating acute asthma requiring hospitalization are well-recognized. Unfortunately little attention has been paid to documenting the morbidity of these exacerbations. One might infer from the current medical literature that acute severe asthma is a condition from which one either dies or makes a predictable recovery. This is not the case; there are a number of complications associated with both the disease process and its treatment.

COMPLICATIONS OF THE DISEASE

Air Flow Obstruction

Air flow obstruction, the hallmark of acute asthma, produces major changes in respiratory mechanics. The inspiratory muscles must generate an increased negative thoracic pressure to overcome the rise in airway resistance. Expiratory flow is limited by both the increased airway resistance and inspiratory muscle activity continuing through expiration. Airway closure occurs before expiration is complete and "gas trapping" results. These changes produce increases in both functional residual capacity (FRC) and residual volume (RV) as an acute attack progresses. This so-called *dynamic hyperinflation*, and the resulting positive alveolar pressure at the completion of expiration, has been described as auto PEEP (positive end-expiratory pressure) or intrinsic PEEP.[2] This positive pressure may have a protective role, opposing early airway closure and atelectasis during acute asthma. However as the attack continues, increased negative pressure must be generated during inspiration to "overcome" this intrinsic PEEP thus increasing the work of breathing.[2,3]

Work of breathing describes the energy cost of breathing. It is a function of the pressure the respiratory muscles are required to generate and the volume of gas displaced per unit time. This energy is used to overcome the pulmonary resistance due to air flow obstruction, intrinsic PEEP and elastic resistance. During acute asthma attacks all these components of lung resistance are increased and the recruitment of the expiratory muscles further increases energy demand and oxygen consumption. At the same time inspiratory muscle power is compromised, because over-inflation stretches the inspiratory muscles beyond their optimal length. If asthma remains unresponsive to therapy, these factors may lead to respiratory muscle fatigue and contribute to ventilatory failure. Fatigue is identified by a combination of patient characteristics and changes in the arterial blood gases (Table 47.1).

The expanding lungs may compress the heart, increase the pericardial pressure, limit venous return and diastolic filling and essentially tamponade right and left ventricular stoke volume. As the acute asthmatic attack develops the thoracic and adjacent structures are

Table 47.1: Markers of fatigue
Subjective difficulty: "the asthmatic knows best"!
Falling oxygenation despite increasing PEF
No longer able to speak
Floppy, lethargic, unable to cough
Rising P_aCO_2

Table 47.2: Extra-thoracic effects of increased intra-thoracic pressure

Gastroesophageal reflux[4]

Rectal or urethral incontinence or prolapse

Diaphragmatic, inguinal and abdominal hernias

Vaginal prolapse

Rupture viscus, e.g. hydrocele, stomach, spleen[5,6]

subjected to substantial swings in pressure. This elevated intrathoracic pressure may have adverse effects on visceral function (Table 47.2)

Coughing is a consequence of airway inflammation. It produces transient massive rises in intrathoracic pressure. These increases are superimposed on the already increased intrathoracic pressure and may cause further tissue damage (Table 47.3)

Air leaks from alveolar rupture may occur. These are caused by a rise in intra-alveolar pressure and radial wall tension, especially distal to airways that are "slow" to empty during expiration. When gas escapes from the pulmonary tree it will follow the pathway of least resistance finding its way to pleural space (pneumothorax), mediastinum, peritoneum, subcutaneous tissue and even the epidural space. Air flow obstruction ensures high airways pressures are maintained during expiration which assists gas leakage out of a ruptured alveolus. The gas itself is of little consequence, but it may exert considerable pressure if localized in a confined space, causing compression of surrounding structures. The most serious situation is "tension" in the

Table 47.3: Cough complications

Musculo-skeletal chest pain

Rib fractures

Sub-conjunctival haemorrhage

Syncope

Ruptured viscus

Nausea and vomiting

pleura or mediastinum causing impairment of myocardial function. This requires emergency drainage.

In the setting of acute asthma, most pneumothoraces should be drained to protect against large volumes of gas escaping under the elevated airway pressure. Even in the absence of classic tension, accumulation of gas in the pleural space will decrease ventilation to the affected side and contribute to hyperventilation of the opposite lung so predisposing to the disastrous situation of bilateral pneumothoraces. Very small uncomplicated air leaks may be managed conservatively, without drainage, except in mechanically ventilated patients when all air leaks should be drained to minimize the morbidity from rapidly evolving tamponade.

Consequences of Altered Gas Exchange: Hypoxia, Hypercapnia, Acidosis

Hypoxaemia (usually defined as a $P_aO_2 < 80$ mmHg) is the initial manifestation of the gas exchange defect which occurs during an acute asthma attack. Obstructed lung units participate in gas transfer roughly proportional to the degree of obstruction. This varies between different lung units, from complete obstruction with mucus plugs to minimal obstruction. Ventilation varies across the lung as different lung units develop different time constants. Hypoxia is initially associated with hypocapnia due to an increase in total minute ventilation. As the asthma attack continues hypoxia may worsen, with increases in ventilation/perfusion mismatch and oxygen consumption, as well as falling alveolar ventilation.

Severe, prolonged or inadequately treated attacks may progress to ventilatory failure. As the minute ventilation falls, hypoxia worsens and is accompanied by hypercapnia and acidosis. Compromised tissue oxygen delivery contributes a metabolic component to the evolving acidosis. These changes affect most organ systems producing severe physiological impairment as hypercapnia and acidosis progress. (Table 47.4)

Normal circulatory responses to hypoxia, hypercapnia and acidosis are potentially impaired in the severe asthmatic. Right and left ventricular filling may be limited by the rise in intra-thoracic pressure. Cardiac output is maintained by increasing heart rate, but this may be at the expense of decreasing myocardial oxygen delivery. Myocardial ischaemia is of concern, especially for the right ventricle, because the raised pulmonary pressure increases the right ventricular after-load and therefore

Table 47.4: Complications of hypercapnia and effects of acidosis

Complications of hypercapnia
Circulatory
   Hypotension
   Vasodilatation
   Decreased myocardial contractility
Respiratory
   Dyspnoea
   Impaired respiratory muscle function
   Increased V/Q mismatch
CNS
   Cerebral vasodilation and oedema
   Confusion, coma, seizures

Effects of acidosis
Decreased intracellular enzyme activity
Altered drug absorption
Decreased plasma protein binding, e.g. muscle relaxants
Decreased drug-receptor binding, e.g. β agonists
Impaired pathways for drug elimination

the stroke work and oxygen consumption. Although ECG abnormalities consistent with right ventricular strain have been reported[4] there is limited published data describing the haemodynamic changes during acute asthma using direct measurements. This may be due to difficulties in both inserting, and interpreting the data from, pulmonary artery catheters in patients with severe airflow obstruction. The risk of myocardial ischaemia in the setting of an acute asthma attack is probably only of clinical significance in patients who have underlying structural heart disease.

Right and left ventricular failure have both been described during acute asthma, but remain uncommon. It is worth remembering that "capillary leak" is a component of airway inflammation which, when combined with pulmonary venous congestion produces a predisposition to oedema formation.[5] Accurate clinical assessment of volume status may be difficult during an acute asthma attack and the potential for volume depletion from poor oral intake and increased insensible losses should be considered. Volume replacement therapy should be administered with these conditions in mind. Tissue hypoxaemia is an important sequela of this combination of hypoxaemia and hypotension during an acute asthmatic attack. The cerebral circulation may be the most sensitive to inadequate oxygen

delivery. A proportion of patients who die from acute asthma despite arriving at hospital, have irreversible cerebral hypoxia.

Mucus, Secretions, Infection

Increased mucus production, alteration in its viscosity and impaired mucociliary clearance are typical of the inflammation of asthma.[6] They combine to exacerbate airway narrowing and cause airway plugging and atelectasis. Although this most commonly occurs in sub-segmental bronchi, lobar obstruction with resultant collapse is well-described. This usually resolves with appropriate bronchodilator and physical therapy, but fibreoptic bronchoscopy to remove plugs may be required if airway obstruction persists, or lung collapse is associated with major physiological impairment. Prolonged collapse of lung tissue should be avoided as it predisposes to infection and possibly permanent airway damage with bronchectasis and fibrosis.

Patients who require intubation and assisted ventilation have an increased risk of developing nosocomial lower respiratory tract infection.

COMPLICATIONS OF TREATMENT

Pharmacological

Much has been written about the relationship between use of pharmacological agents and morbidity in acute asthma (Table 47.5).

Mechanical

Mechanical ventilation is necessary in a small number of asthmatics with respiratory failure. The mortality in ventilated asthmatics during the 1980s was reported as being between 10 and 38%.[7] Recently, methods of controlled hypoventilation designed to limit pulmonary hyperinflation have been implemented with significant decrease in mortality.[8,9]

The majority of morbidity in acute asthma occurs in mechanically ventilated patients. Therefore it is preferable to avoid assisted ventilation if possible.[10] Unfortunately a number of patients are unable to maintain adequate gas exchange and require mechanical assistance despite optimal treatment. Status asthmaticus has been managed with non-invasive positive pressure ventilation (NPPV).[11] Although in this study the patients treated with NPPV had less severe airflow obstruction, they required substantially less mechanical assistance and sedation and were both out of the intensive care

591

Table 47.5: Complications of pharmacological treatment

Class of drug	Complication
β Agonist	Common: tremor, restlessness, anxiety, dreams, tachycardia
	Rare: arrhythmias, myocardial ischaemia, dilated cardiomyopathy, lactic acidosis, hypokalaemia, hyperglycaemia
Theophylline	Gastrointestinal disturbances, seizures, arrhythmias
Corticosteroid	Psychosis, metabolic alkalosis, hypokalaemia, glucose intolerance, myopathy
Sedative	Decreased cough, impaired mucociliary clearance, ventilatory failure
Muscle relaxant	Skeletal muscle dysfunction rhabdomyolysis, anaphylaxis, malignant hyperpyrexia

unit and hospital much sooner than the intubated patients. The development of ultrasensitive flow triggered inspiratory valves should improve the application of NPPV. Although it remains to be fully evaluated in acute asthma, the potential for NPPV to limit the morbidity associated with intubation is exciting. It is possible that NPPV could be used to provide mechanical support early in an acute asthma attack to prevent severe acidosis and fatigue.

Intubation and positive pressure ventilation (IPPV) is currently the recommended method of mechanical ventilation in acute asthma. Intubation and initiation of assisted ventilation pose special problems in asthmatic patients. Asthmatics are more liable to laryngospasm and to allergic reactions to induction agents or muscle relaxants. Drugs associated with histamine release may exacerbate bronchospasm. The asthmatic may be hypovolaemic in the setting of impaired venous return due to rising intra-thoracic pressure and peripheral vasodilatation due to hypoxia and hypercapnia. Hypovolaemia, hypoxia and sympathetic activation, followed by sedatives and relaxants for intubation, and then the application of positive pressure to the thorax, can pre-cipitate circulatory collapse and cardiac arrest.[7] Awake nasal intubation may avoid some of this instability; however oropharangeal intubation with a larger sized endotracheal tube is recommended to minimize the intrinsic PEEP and facilitate weaning.

Because of the difficulty of evaluating over-inflation during "hand" ventilation, asthmatics should be promptly connected to a volume-cycled, preferably pressure-limited ventilator with, initially slow breath rates, high inspiratory flow rates and a low inspiration to expiration ratio. The objective at this stage should be to achieve adequate oxygenation, without circulatory compromise, if necessary permitting hypercapnia. When it is necessary to use a transport ventilator for an asthmatic patient, extra vigilance is required to monitor for hyperinflation.

Pulmonary hyperinflation, which we have already described occurring in spontaneously breathing acute asthma, may be exacerbated during positive pressure ventilation because the tidal volume is no longer limited by the patient's ability to generate a high inspiratory pressure gradient. Large increases in intra-thoracic volume may occur during artificial ventilation as modern ventilators are able to generate high "working pressures" and deliver large tidal volumes despite increased airway resistance. The sequelae of hyperinflation are limited in the spontaneously breathing asthmatic by fatigue of the inspiratory muscles due to the increased work of breathing. In the mechanically ventilated patient this protection is lost and hyperinflation and circulatory compromise may occur rapidly. It has been suggested that dynamic hyperinflation is the variable that best correlates with significant asthma morbidity.[12]

A range of strategies have been described to avoid over-ventilating acute asthmatics, but the optimal method is still debated. The aim of mechanical ventilation should be to ensure oxygenation, relieve the mechanical load and clear secretions. This usually requires a ventilatory pattern that permits hypercapnia, so as to prevent the complications of over-inflation. Normalization of ventilation is achieved when the airway obstruction resolves. If necessary acidosis may be controlled with intravenous sodium bicarbonate.

Evaluation of controlled hypoventilation has been troubled by the absence of an accepted objective measurement of "over-inflation". Tuxen *et al.* have described a method for grading pulmonary hyperinflation by measuring the volume at end inspiration

(VEI) and report that it predicts the incidence of complications.[13] They use this measurement to control the mechanical ventilation of all asthmatics and report a resulting fall in the incidence of hypotension.

Sedation and often paralysis is necessary during controlled hypoventilation. Sedation alone is preferable and often sufficient to allow adequate mechanical ventilation. However non-depolarizing muscle relaxant may be necessary for periods of severe bronchoconstriction where respiratory muscle resistance may prevent acceptable ventilation. Both these drugs may be additive to hypoxia, acidosis and hypercapnia as insults to intracellular metabolism. This concern is highlighted by the growing evidence for acute neuromyopathy occurring in ventilated patients.[13]

The application of positive pressure may cause mechanical damage to the lung. This can be attributed to a "stretch" damage from the change in volume (volutrauma) or from "pressure" damage (barotrauma). Mechanical damage to the lung has traditionally been defined in physiological terms; however recently the cellular and molecular effects have been investigated. Clinically there are three recognized variants:

(1) Escape of gas from the alveolar space follows rupture of the alveolar membrane as discussed above for spontaneously breathing patients. This is of greater concern during positive pressure ventilation because the intra-thoracic pressure may rise rapidly producing tamponade of the circulation. One must have a high level of suspicion to detect air leaks in the intensive care unit setting. A lateral decubitus X-ray of the chest may be more sensitive at confirming a pneumothorax than the traditional supine anterior–posterior views.

(2) Systemic gas embolism occurs when alveolar gas enters the systemic circulation. This is uncommon, but recorded in ventilated patients with the very high airway pressures that may be seen in severe acute asthma.

(3) Diffuse lung injury, with plasma extravasation and hyaline membrane formation, is proposed in patients ventilated for pulmonary oedema or acute respiratory distress syndrome, where high pressures and oxygen concentrations are applied to the lung for extended periods. It is unusual for these conditions to be required for prolonged periods in acute asthma, and therefore the risk

and incidence of this type of diffuse lung injury in ventilated asthmatics is uncertain.

Weakness syndromes are a well-described sequela of mechanical ventilation especially in asthmatics.[13] Muscle weakness is associated with increased duration of assisted ventilation and difficulty with weaning.[13] The initial reports of weakens following a severe asthma attack described changes consistent with myopathy which was attributed to drug toxicity in particular the effect of high-dose corticosteroids.[14] However, it is now clear that muscle weakness following mechanical ventilation may be due to disuse atrophy, acute myopathy, neuromuscular junction abnormalities, or acute neuropathy. The use of high-dose glucocorticoids, neuromuscular blocking drugs (probably all types) and β-adrenergic agonists as well as metabolic abnormalities such as acidosis, hypoxia, fever or hypophosphataemia may combine to produce neuromuscular damage. In cases of severe weakness nerve conduction studies, serum creatine kinase, CSF examination and possibly muscle biopsy may be helpful in determining the predominant pathology. A moderately aggressive approach to diagnosis is warranted because it is possible for plasmaphoresis or hyperimmuneglobulin to be beneficial in Guillain-Barré syndrome. Hopkin's syndrome, an acute poliomyelitis-like condition, was described in paediatric asthmatic patients and may be a separate clinical entity.[15] The potential for weakness to impair

KEY POINTS

1. Acute asthma is a potentially lethal condition.

2. Beware of not only airflow obstruction but also gas trapping and over-inflation.

3. Be patient, airflow obstruction may take many days to improve.

4. Consider the possibility of mucus and airway plugs causing gas exchange defects.

3. The side-effects of therapy are a major cause of asthma complications.

4. Prevention remains the best approach to acute asthma complications.

the recovery of asthmatic patients after a period of mechanical ventilation suggests muscle strength should be routinely assessed. For the present time it would seem that the benefits of paralysis in patients with severe airflow obstruction and pulmonary hyperinflation outweigh the concerns about muscle damage. However, the routine use of muscle relaxants in less severe asthmatics should be discouraged.

REFERENCES

1   Beasley R, Pearce N, Crane J. International trends in asthma mortality. *Ciba Found Symp* 1997; 206: 140–50.

2   Smith TC, Marini JJ. Impact of PEEP on lung mechanics and work of breathing in severe airflow obstruction. *J Appl Physiol* 1988; 65: 1488–99.

3   Fleury B, Murciano D, Talamo C *et al.* Work of breathing in patients with chronic obstructive pulmonary disease in acute respiratory failure. *Am Rev Resp Dis* 1985; 131: 822–7.

4   Quint HJ, Miller JI, Drach GW. Rupture of a hydrocele: an unusual event. *J Urol* 1992; 147: 1375–7.

5   McQueen M, Gollock RJ, Fergusson RJ. Spontaneous gastric rupture complicating acute asthma. *Br Med J* 1982; 285: 692–3.

6   Rebuck AS, Read J. Assessment and management of severe asthma. *Am Med J* 1971; 51: 788–98.

7   O'Riordan TG, Zwang J, Smaldone GC. Mucociliary clearance in adult asthma. *Am Rev Resp Dis* 1992; 146: 598–603.

8   Webb AK, Bilton AH, Hanson GC. Severe bronchial asthma requiring ventilation. A review of 20 cases and advice on management. *Post Grad Med J* 1979; 55: 161–70.

9   Mansel JK, Stogner SW, Petrini MF, Norman JR. Mechanical ventilation in patients with acute severe asthma. *Am J Med* 1990; 89: 42–8.

10   Tuxen DV. Detrimental effects of positive end-expiratory pressure during controlled mechanical ventilation of patients with severe airflow obstruction. *Am Rev Resp Dis* 1989; 140: 5–9.

11   Williams TJ, Tuxen DV, Scheinkestel CD, Czarny D, Bowes G. Risk factors for morbidity in mechanically ventilated patients with acute severe asthma. *Am Rev Resp Dis* 1992; 146: 607–15.

12   Meduri GU, Cook TR, Turner RE, Cohen M, Leeper KV. Noninvasive positive pressure ventilation in status asthmaticus. *Chest* 1996; 110: 767–74.

13   Tuxen DV, Williams TJ, Scheinkestel CD, Czarny D, Bowes G. Use of a measurement of pulmonary hyperinflation to control the level of mechanical ventilation in patients with acute severe asthma. *Am Rev Resp Dis* 1992; 146: 1136–42.

14   Nates JI, Cooper DJ, Day B, Tuxen DV. Acute weakness syndromes in critically ill patients-a reappraisal. *Anaesth Intens Care* 1997; 25: 502–13.

15   Cohen HA, Ashkenasi A, Ring H *et al.* Polimyelitis-like syndrome following asthmatic attack (Hopkins' syndrome)–recovery associated with i.v. gamma globulin treatment. *Infection* 1998; 26: 247–9.

Chapter 48

Chronic Complications of Asthma

Nick ten Hacken, Huib Kerstjens and Dirkje Postma

INTRODUCTION

In this chapter the chronic complications of asthma are discussed. Inevitably there will be some overlap with the former chapter on acute complications, because there is a continuum between acute and chronic complications. We have chosen to group complications in four categories (Table 48.1): (1) pulmonary complications; (2) extra-pulmonary complications; (3) psychosocial complications; and (4) complications related to the management of asthma. First, we will discuss briefly the first three categories; thereafter we will pay special attention to decline in lung function and airway remodelling. Group 4 complications will be dealt with in other chapters of this book.

Patients often adapt to their chronic impairments and disabilities. Yet, some chronic complications can be reduced, cured or even prevented. Therefore, awareness by the physician for the development of chronic complications can be important for the individual patient.

PULMONARY COMPLICATIONS

Chronicity of Airway Obstruction and Asthma Symptoms

Chronic airway inflammation is a characteristic feature of asthma and is associated with increased hyper-responsiveness. In contrast, airway obstruction and symptoms like wheeze, cough, sputum production, chest tightness and dyspnoea come and go. Some patients may develop continuous symptoms and airway obstruction, which is referred to as chronic asthma. Both endogenous and exogenous factors may contribute to the chronic nature of asthma. Endogeneous factors are, for example, the degree of airway inflammation, serum

Table 48.1: Chronic complications of asthma

1. Pulmonary complications directly related to asthma
   Chronicity of airway obstruction and symptoms
   Irreversible airway obstruction, decline in lung function, airway remodelling
   Development of hyperinflation, emphysema, bronchiectasis
   Infections with *Aspergillus fumigatus* (ABPA)[a], *Chlamydia pneumoniae*, *Mycoplasma pneumoniae*

2. Extra-pulmonary complications
   Worsening of gastroesophageal reflux (see also Ch. 41)
   Ischaemic heart disease, cor pulmonale
   Inactivity, deconditioning

3. Psychosocial complication
   Decreased quality of life
   Psychological/psychiatric disturbances (see also Ch. 40)
   Decreased sleep quality (see also Ch. 37)
   Work disability

4. Complications related to the management of severe asthma due to:
   Corticosteroids: growth retardation, delayed puberty, osteoporosis (see Ch. 46)
   Immunosuppressive agents (see also Chs 19 and 45)

[a]ABPA: allergic bronchopulmonary aspergillosis. (see also Ch. 35)

adrenaline and cortisol, thyroid status, and the menstrual cyclus. Examples of exogenous factors are environmental temperature and humidity, inhalation of aeroallergens, use of bronchodilators or corticosteroids. According to international guidelines, the continuous presence of symptoms and airway obstruction with adequate treatment has to be classified as "severe" and this ultimately leads to the administration of high doses of oral or inhaled corticosteroids.[1,2]

Chronic symptoms rather frequently occur in asthmatic patients of various ages. Five percent of the 2.7 million US children with active asthma reported continuous asthma symptoms.[3] Wheezing on most days was reported in 10% of the adults with asthma, and in 32% of the astmatics older than 65 years.[4] Two-thirds of the asthmatic children had symptoms over a longer period of time. Persistence of disease is associated with early age of asthma onset, severity of asthma symptoms, lower lung function, associated atopic conditions, female gender, and lower levels of lung function.[5–7] Roorda and co-workers followed a cohort of 406 ten-year-old asthmatic children for approximately 15 years.[8] Respiratory symptoms persisted or recurred during young adulthood in the majority (76%) of subjects, with a less favourable prognosis for children with more symptoms, more severe bronchial responsiveness and low FEV_1. Despite the persistence of symptoms, only 19% of the adult subjects was still under a physician's supervision; the incidence of cigarette smoking was high (33%); and only 32% of the subjects used maintenance medication.

Thus, only a small number of children with asthma may become asymptomatic and actually seem to be in remission. Even asymptomatic patients have persistently increased airway responsiveness, irrespective of the presence of airway obstruction.[9]

Panhuysen et al. demonstrated in a 25-year follow-up study that 20 out of 181 adult patients (11%) may outgrow their asthma.[10] Absence of asthma was defined in this study as no hyperresponsiveness, $FEV_1 > 90\%$ predicted, and absence of symptoms. The authors suggested that milder disease and earlier intervention are important for a beneficial outcome of adult asthma.

The above studies indicate that asthma generally is a chronic disease that requires persistent vigilance by the physician in order to prevent or reduce chronic complications.

Irreversible Airway Obstruction, Decline in Lung Function, Airway Remodelling

Irreversible airway obstruction is known to be a late complication of asthma. Brown et al. showed that the persistent airway obstruction in asthmatics was more closely related to duration of asthma than to age.[11] He, therefore, suggested that its development was associated with previous poor control of wheeze.[11] Connolly et al. confirmed that persistent airway obstruction was directly related to duration of asthma, whereas age was an additional factor in males, but not in females.[12] Finally, Braman et al. showed in older asthmatics that those who developed asthma at advanced age (>65 years) had a lower degree of airway obstruction than those with early onset asthma.[13] These cross-sectional data suggest that the longer duration of asthma leads to more severe airway obstruction. Whether this is related to treatment needs to be elucidated. Longitudinal studies are needed to clarify the contributing factors for the relatively rapid decline in lung function of subjects with asthma. These studies are discussed separately in a later section of this chapter.

Development of Hyperinflation, Signs of Emphysema, Bronchiectasis

Chronic airway obstruction may lead to airtrapping and hyperinflation in a number of subjects. This is reflected by an elevated functional residual capacity,[14] and by hyperinflation of the ribs on common chest radiographs.[15] Hyperinflation may be caused by active contraction of the inspiratory muscles, which often show an increased muscle endurance.[16] Some asthmatic subjects may develop "passive" hyperinflation, compatible with other signs of emphysema, e.g. the absence of "normal" reversibility of airway obstruction after inhaling high doses of β agonists as generally seen in asthma. A deficiency of α_1-antitrypsin has to be ruled out in these patients in the first place. There is a suggestion that smoking in asthma induces emphysema. A significant correlation has been demonstrated between the emphysema score on a CT scan and the number of pack years of cigarette smoking and CO diffusion in asthmatics who smoke.[17] Not withstanding this, non-smoking asthmatics frequently show features of a low degree of emphysema on high-resolution CT-scans.[18,19] Whether this is the consequence of asthma itself has not been established. Theoretically, emphysema might occur in asthma patients since a recent study showed that inflammation is not only present inside the large airways, but also outside the airways, in the alveolar attachments.[20] So far, several reports have reported changes of emphysema in asthma as assessed by CT scans. However, in clinical practice emphysema is not a common feature in asthma. Bronchiectases are another regular finding on CT scans of patients with even mild asthma.[18,21]

Respiratory Infections

The importance attributed to respiratory infections in asthma has changed somewhat in recent years. In the past, upper and lower respiratory infections were mainly seen as triggers which led to a temporary worsening of established asthma. Nowadays, there are indications that pulmonary infections in early childhood may play a role in the induction of asthma.[22] Furthermore, it is recognized that certain pulmonary infections do not tend to subside, but persist and even contribute to chronic airway obstruction in asthma. For example, *Aspergillus* is a common fungus in the community that may colonize the central airways in 1–2% of the asthmatics. Allergic bronchopulmonary aspergillosis (ABPA) may lead in a number of these patients to corticosteroid-dependent asthma, central bronchiectasis and pulmonary fibrosis.[23,24] Remarkable improvements have been documented after administration of oral itraconazole over a period of 6 months.[25] Less well-known microorganisms that may contribute to chronic asthma are *Mycoplasma pneumoniae* and *Chlamydia pneumoniae*. *M. pneumoniae* was detected with PCR techniques in 10 of 18 patients with chronic asthma versus 1 of 11 controls.[26] Treatment with clarithromycin resulted in an improvement in asthma symptoms and airway wall inflammation. Chronic infection with *C. pneumoniae* has been reported in severe corticosteroid-dependent asthmatics with improvement after treatment with clarithromycin or azithromycin.[27] It is not clear whether severe asthma, or intensive treatment of severe asthma, leads to colonization with such pathogens, or vice versa.

Several studies have suggested that impaired humoral immunity plays a role in chronic asthma. For example, Hamilos *et al.* demonstrated in 12 subjects out of 101 unselected asthmatics the presence of IgG hypogammaglobulinaemia.[28] This hypogammaglobulinaemia was strongly associated with the use of systemic corticosteroids. However, the clinical relevance of hypogammaglobulinaemia seemed not very large. Only three patients showed an impaired response to pneumococcal vaccination and they were not clinically distinguishable on the basis of sinus disease or pneumonia. In addition, two other studies showed a normal antibody response to pneumococcal or influenza vaccination in glucocorticoid-treated pulmonary patients.[29,30]

On the other hand, there are also two studies indicating that humoral abnormalities in asthmatic patients occur and even may be clinically important. In the first study of Oehling *et al.*, immunoglobulin G levels in steroid-dependent asthmatics with fewer or more than three respiratory infections per year were respectively 17% and 34% lower than in non-steroid-dependent asthmatics.[31] In this retrospective study, weak negative correlations were found between blood CD4/CD8 ratios, IgG levels, and the daily glucocorticoid dose. In the second study, Ayres *et al.* compared serum total immunoglobulins and IgG subclass levels in three groups of asthmatic patients: those with brittle asthma, those with infective exacerbations, and those with mild and stable asthma.[32] The group with brittle asthma showed lower total IgG, IgG_1, IgG_2, IgG_3 and IgA levels, whereas the asthmatics with infective exacerbations showed lower total IgG, IgG_1 and IgG_2 levels compared with mild asthmatics. In this study there was no significant relationship with the use of corticosteroids. So far the exact role of impaired humoral immunity and the relationship of this impaired immunity with corticosteroid use is not clear in patients with chronic asthma.

EXTRA-PULMONARY COMPLICATIONS

Worsening of Gastroesophageal Reflux

Gastroesophageal reflux and asthma often occur together. In a questionnaire-based cross-sectional study in Canada, 77% of the asthmatic subjects frequently reported heartburn, 55% regurgitation, and 24% swallowing difficulties.[33] These figures are in line with the findings of Sontag *et al.* who demonstrated that 40% of the asthmatics who attended the out-patient and in-patient clinic have endoscopic evidence of erosive oesophagitis.[34] The reasons for the strong association between asthma and gastroesophageal reflux are not fully understood, but several factors can be pointed out. In the presence of asthma attacks the abdominal pressure may rise during (forced) expiration and it may exceed the gastroesophagal sphincter tone. Moreover, most bronchodilators used for control of asthma theoretically are able to reduce this tone. Once gastroesophageal reflux occurs, asthmatic airway obstruction may be augmented because of vagal stimulation or microaspiration.[35] Nocturnal asthma is especially often associated with gastroesophageal reflux.[36] However, the use of anti-reflux medication did not improve asthma symptoms in most reports,[37] nor did it improve the severity of airway hyperresponsiveness.[38] In addition to worsening of asthma, gastroesophageal reflux can lead to bacterial tracheitis and bronchitis, aspiration pneumonia, atelectasis and ultimately to pulmonary fibrosis.[39] In patients with difficult asthma the presence of latent gastroesophageal reflux should always be considered as a contributing factor.[35,40]

Ischaemic Heart Disease, Cor Pulmonale

Cardiovascular complications are not frequently reported in asthma literature. Myocardial ischaemia may occur in elderly asthmatics and may be masked by severe dyspnoea. Factors predisposing to myocardial ischaemia are hypoxia, vasospasm related to anxiety and mediator release, electrolyte disturbances and dysrhythmias associated with asthma medications.[41] Toren et al. described in a Swedish study a relative risk of 2.1 for dying from ischaemic heart disease in patients with severe asthma.[42] However, such results may be confounded by physical inactivity and smoking habits. A statistically significant, independent association has been described between idiopathic dilated cardiomyopathy and a history of asthma, in individuals less than 55 years of age.[43] In a later study, the use of β agonists was suggested to play an aetiologic role in idiopathic dilated cardiomyopathy.[44] However, a large population-based study indicated that asthma was not an independent risk factor for survival in patients with idiopathic dilated cardiomyopathy.[45]

Eosinophilic pericarditis has also been described in relation with asthma, and in such cases one should always be alert for alternative explanations, e.g. Churg–Strauss disease.[46,47] With increasing age, some asthmatic patients may develop an important irreversible airway obstruction, only seldomly resulting in pulmonary hypertension and cor pulmonale.[48] Nevertheless, cor pulmonale has also been described in asthmatic children dying from fatal asthma.[49] It can be concluded that asthma is, although not frequently, complicated or associated with cardiac diseases.

Inactivity, Deconditioning

Theoretically, subjects with severe asthma may suffer from limited exercise capacity and become inactive. Large epidemiological studies in children and adults did not show a significant difference in the level of physical activities between asthmatic and non-asthmatic subjects.[50] However, in adults significant correlations were demonstrated between spirometric values and intensities of physical activity at work and during leisure time in male asthmatics. Furthermore, in aging subjects, asthma has shown to be one of the independent risk factors for physical disability.[51]

Moving from epidemiological studies to studies performed in the lung function lab, it is obvious that most asthmatics have normal aerobic capacities. Nevertheless, stable asthmatic children with a sedentary lifestyle were demonstrated to be less fit than asthmatic children who participated in organized sports or engaged in free-play.[52] The poor cardiovascular fitness of these asthmatic children was not related to ventilatory limitations during incremental exercise testing. Young adults with mild to moderate asthma did show a normal incremental exercise capacity, which was not related to the severity of hyperresponsiveness or airway obstruction.[53] On the other hand, a significant correlation was demonstrated between habitual leisure-time activity and aerobic capacity. In addition, with an exercise questionnaire, it was suggested that asthmatics perceive their disease as a limiting factor to improve aerobic fitness. Thus, most asthmatic subjects af all age groups have a normal exercise capacity if they avoid a sedentary life-style. Only asthmatic subjects with severe persistent airflow limitation may develop a poor exercise capacity due to ventilatory limitations.

PSYCHOSOCIAL COMPLICATIONS

Decreased Quality of Life

Decreased health-related quality of life and patient satisfaction are increasingly studied in chronic diseases like asthma.[54] Studies have been performed at all age groups. In 100 Canadian children with moderate severe asthma, asthma symptoms constituted the largest component of the burden of asthma.[55] Interestingly, their parents worried mostly about their child's disease, the medications, and their own inability to relieve symptoms.[55] In 1665 children (5–9 years) in Seattle, USA, the prevalence of sleep disturbances, school absences, medical service use, and parental concern was higher in asthma and asthma-like illness than in healthy children.[56] In 3109 teenagers the subjects with asthma and recent wheezing reported a lower well-being, more physical and emotional symptoms, greater limitations in activity, more comorbidities, and more negative behaviours compared with healthy teenagers.[57] In one study of adult asthmatics, women reported more daytime and nocturnal symptoms than men, despite similar levels of airway obstruction.[58] Particularly, women aged 35–55 years reported worse physical and social functioning, more bodily pain, more use of health care and medication. Investigations on quality of life in elderly patients (>40 years) with chronic nonspecific lung diseases (asthma and chronic obstructive pulmonary disease [COPD]) seen in family practices indicated that patients were more impaired in their physical and psychosocial functioning than healthy controls.[59] This was not related to the level of lung function but to respiratory symptoms like wheezing and dyspnoea. In a hospital-based control study of older (>55 years) asthmatics, subjective health status was significantly worse in asthmatics, especially for components of physical functioning, physical role limitation, energy, health change and general health perception.[60] Symptoms of depression were equally present in asthmatics and in controls.

Using the Asthma Quality of Life Questionnaire (AQLQ) of Juniper, quality of life was found to be correlated to morning peak flow[61] and severity of asthma.[62] However, there was no relationship with the level of physical activity. Patients with severe, unstable asthma appeared to have worse than expected quality of life for reasons not related to FEV_1 or to variation in peak flow.[63] Quality of life scores have shown to improve after administration of anti-inflammatory medication[64,65] and bronchodilating medication.[66-68] Thus, impaired quality of life frequently occurs in chronic asthma. The best strategies for improvement have yet to be found.

Psychological / Psychiatric Disturbances

If patients with severe asthma experience a low quality of life, one would expect that psychological and psychiatric disturbances occur rather frequently in such patients. In this respect subjects with brittle asthma are a well-known sub-group. Garden and Ayres. compared 20 asthmatic patients with a more than 40% diurnal variation in PEF and persistent respiratory symptoms despite multiple drug treatment, with 20 matched controls with less severe asthma.[69] Significantly more subjects with brittle asthma (12/20) than controls (5/20) had intercurrent or past psychiatric disorder, and 7/20 subjects with brittle asthma had a lifetime history of an anxiety disorder compared with 3/20 controls. However, there was no difference in personality profiles. Recently, the same research group demonstrated with a similar study design that subjects with brittle asthma delay

seeking medical attention more often and instead prefer self-administration with β agonists.[70] Such patients probably are at higher risk for (near) fatal asthma. Indeed, Campbell demonstrated in 77 asthmatic patients surviving a near fatal asthma attack a high level of denial towards progression of respiratory distress.[71]

Children with severe asthma may suffer from psychiatric complications like depression and anxiety disorders.[72] Because depressive illness in very severe asthmatic children is associated with greater asthma mortality, early intervention to minimize initial expression of asthmatic symptoms is advised in these patients.

Decreased Sleep Quality

Decreased sleep quality due to nocturnal airway obstruction or respiratory symptoms occurs rather frequently as shown in a large epidemiological study in England, reporting that 74% of the asthmatic population had nocturnal awakening at least once a week.[73] In the Netherlands, nocturnal awakening was reported at least once a week in 42% of 103 clinically stable asthmatic patients from a pulmonary outpatient clinic.[74] Nocturnal symptoms occur also frequently in asthmatic children: 34% of 796 asthmatic children attending the out-patient clinic of the University Hospital Groningen reported nocturnal symptoms at least once a week.[75] It is noteworthy that patients with nocturnal asthma often do not present their nocturnal symptoms spontaneously,[75-77] despite the fact that disturbed sleep interferes significantly with school and work performance,[78] and the ability to concentrate.[79] The underestimation of nocturnal asthma is the more regrettable since both bronchodilator and anti-inflammatory drugs have been shown to improve PEF variability and nocturnal symptoms as well as daytime cognitive performance in asthmatic subjects with high levels of PEF variation.[79,80] The underlying mechanisms of increased nocturnal airway obstruction are discussed in Chapter 37.

Work Disability

Asthmatic subjects are generally advised to be more selective in the jobs they undertake because they may suffer from unpredictable airway obstruction. Jobs may be lost more easily or acquired less readily because of absence or diminished work performance. Indeed, considerable influence on the choice of occupation was experienced in asthmatic subjects (aged 21) with current frequent symptoms.[81] These subjects also reported that prospective employers rather frequently had been influenced by their asthma history.[81] In another albeit uncontrolled study, significant work disability was demonstrated in 56 out-patient asthmatics with a mean age of 35 years.[82] This study reported an incidence of 19% change of job duties, 17% for reduction in wages and 20% for change in job or work status, attributed to asthma during 5 years follow-up. Interestingly, this kind of work disability was statistically correlated with the severity of asthma score, more than with the levels of airflow limitation measured at one point in time.[82] The latter is also in line with a recent study in 332 subjects with recent onset asthma.[83] Not FEV_1 but asthma severity, respiratory symptoms at the workplace and PC_{20} methacholine ≤ 4 mg ml^{-1} were significant predictors for work disability. In a large cohort of 17 319 subjects in England, Sibbald et al. investigated the relation between employment history and a history of asthma.[84] At 23 years of age the risk of unemployment was higher in subjects with a current or past history of asthma or wheeze compared with matched healthy individuals (odds ratio 1.32 and 1.54 respectively). Thus, asthma appeared to have only small adverse effects on employment in young adults.

Unfortunately, little information is available on the incidence of work disability among older asthmatics, but it is the authors' experience that many patients are unemployed.

DECLINE IN LUNG FUNCTION

After 25–35 years of age, an annual decline in FEV_1 (20 ml year^{-1}) is a normal feature in healthy subjects.[85,86] Excess annual decline is usually associated with COPD and not with asthma. However, there are by now several studies showing an excess decline in FEV_1 of approximately 20 ml year^{-1} in asthmatic subjects (Table 48.2).[86–92] This decline is larger in smoking asthmatics, but also present in non-smoking asthmatics as a group.[86,88,89] On the other hand, certainly not all asthmatics show this excess decline. Other factors associated with excess decline in FEV_1 appear to be: low baseline lung function (FEV_1% predicted),[91,92] less reversibility to β_2 agonists,[91,93] more severe bronchial hyperresponsiveness,[7,10,92,94] mucus production,[86] and male gender.[88] The association between atopic status and longitudinal changes in lung function is not clear. There are studies showing no effect,[92,95] a positive effect,[94] and a negative effect[91,96] on decline in lung function.

Childhood factors associated with a low FEV_1 (in adulthood) are: low baseline FEV_1,[6,7,97–99] more severe bronchial hyperresponsiveness,[7,94] early onset of symptoms,[100] more severe respiratory symptoms,[99,100] persistent wheezing,[101,102] female gender,[103] and smoking.[100] However, a low FEV_1 in adulthood does not necessarily imply an excess annual decline in FEV_1.

In Fig. 48.1 a model of various stages and components contributing to disease progression of asthma is shown.[104] The interplay between genetic and environmental factors probably plays an important role in the progression and outcome of asthma.[105] In this model acute inflammation is followed by chronic inflammation, which is supposed to be the key factor for tissue repair and tissue remodelling. The individual susceptibility to develop airway remodelling (the genes for irreversible airway obstruction?) has not yet been addressed.

Often the term "airway remodelling" is used to denote structural changes in the asthmatic airways. Indeed, plain radiographs frequently indicate bronchial wall thickening,[21] but more detailed information is provided by HR-CT scans.[18] CT evidence of bronchial wall thickening has been reported in up to 90% of mild to moderate severe asthmatics.[106] Morphometric studies in post-mortem or resected lung specimens have confirmed that the airways of subjects with fatal and non-fatal asthma are thicker than those of non-asthmatics.[107–109] Another study showed a direct correlation between increased airway wall thickness and irreversible airway obstruction.[110]

Microscopical studies have shown that increased airway wall thickness may be due to smooth muscle hyperplasia and hypertrophy,[111,112] mucus glands,[113,114] submucosal collagen deposition,[115,116] and increased vascularity.[117] The exact contributions of these components to irreversible airway obstruction and increased hyperresponsiveness are unclear. Subepithelial fibrosis was demonstrated to correlate with the degree of hyperresponsiveness to methacholine, and not with the FEV_1.[118] Moreover, there was a correlation with epithelial desquamation, suggesting that epithelial damage is the trigger of an airway repair process, with progressive deposition of collagen underneath the basement membrane. Submucosal fibroblasts and myofibroblasts are responsible for collagen production, a process that may be regulated by transforming growth factor-β, platelet-derived growth factor, tumour necrosis factor, interleukin-4, endothelin, histamine and tryptase.[119] The cellular and molecular mechanisms involved in the progression of

Table 48.2: Excess decline in FEV₁ in asthmatic patients.

Reference (Year)	Population	Age range (years)	Asthma (healthy)	Follow-up (years)	No[a]	(+[b]) Decline in FEV$_1$ (ml year^{-1})	Factors associated with decline	
Schachter (1984)	Rural, Conn, Lebanon	≥ 7	73 (1230)	6	2	Asthma: 24 Healthy: 6	Asthma Chronic asthma at childhood	↑ ↑
Peat (1987)	Rural, Western Australia	22–69	92 (186)	18	≥ 4	Asthma: 50 Healthy: 35 (Male non-smokers)	Asthma Smokers BHR Airway obstruction	↑ ↑? ↑ ↑
Jaakkola (1993)	Urban, Montreal	15–40	17 (374)	8	8	"New" asthma: +43 Persistent asthma: +12	Asthma Wheezing Dyspnea Atopy	↑ ↑ ↑ ↑
Ulrik (1994)	Urban, Copenhagen	20–90	177 (10556)	5	2	♂ Asthma: +39 ♀ Asthma: +11	"New" asthma Male gender Smoking Age	↑ ↑ ↑ ↑
Lange (1998)	Urban, Copenhagen	20–90	1095 (16 411)	15	3	Asthma: 38 Healthy: 22	Asthma, Smoking Mucus production	↑ ↑ ↑
Almind[c] (1992)	Out-patients, Copenhagen	18–80	214	7	2	Intr. asthma: +51 Extr. asthma: +57	Smoking Age	↑ ↑
Ulrik[d] (1992)	Out-patients, Copenhagen	28–44	143	10	2	Intr. asthma: 50 ⟨ ⟩ Extr. asthma: 23	Age Reversibility Initial FEV$_1$ Age Blood eosinophils Airway obstruction Use corticosteroids	↑ ↑ ↓ ↑ ↓ ↑ ↑

[a] Number of spirometric measurements; [b] Excess decline in FEV₁ compared with healthy individuals; [c] Excess decline in this study was estimated on basis of historical data of healthy individuals; [d] no healthy controls in this study; BHR: bronchial hyperresponsiveness; ↑: factor associated with a higher (excess) annual decline in FEV₁; ↓: factor associated with a lower (excess) annual decline in FEV₁; Intr.: intrinsic; Extr.: extrinsic.

irreversible airway obstruction are currently not clear, and specific therapeutic agents are lacking. Inflammation appears to be the initiator for tissue repair and airway remodelling. Therefore, therapy is directed at the prevention and inhibition of asthmatic airway inflammation. Until newer anti-asthma drugs are developed, we must rely on conventional anti-inflammatory drugs like corticosteroids. Inhaled corticosteroids reduce the thick-

ness of the reticular layer of the basement membrane,[120] the deposition of collagen III[121] and tenascin,[122] and the expression of insulin-like growth factor-1.[123] However, there are also two studies not showing beneficial effects on airway collagen deposition.[124,125]

Thus, it is not yet proven that (inhaled) corticosteroids are able to reduce (the development of) airway remodelling.[126] Nevertheless, several data suggest that

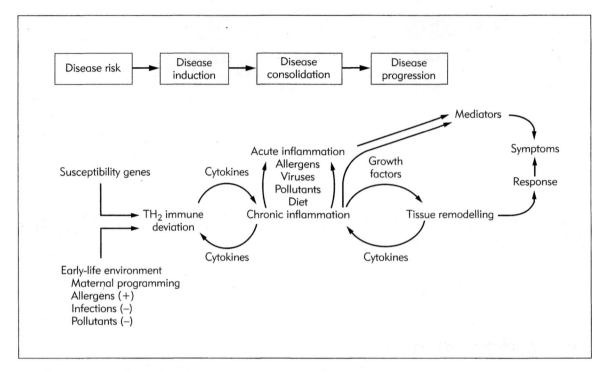

FIGURE 48.1: The evolution of asthma. (From Holgate ST. The cellular and mediator basis of asthma in relation to natural history. *Lancet* 1997; 350 (suppl. 2): 115–9, ©The Lancet Ltd. 1997.)

decline in lung function occurs more easily without anti-inflammatory therapy, and that the early institution of corticosteroids may be beneficial. Arguments favouring early institution of inhaled corticosteroids are:

- Asthma is associated with excess decline in FEV$_1$.[11,92,102,127]
- The greatest decline in lung function occurs in the early years following diagnosis.[88]
- Even in newly diagnosed asthma there is evidence for airway mucosal inflammation.[128]
- The length of the untreated period of subjects with mild asthma is reported to be associated with a lower frequency of outgrowing asthma.[10]
- The duration of pre-treatment symptoms before introducing corticosteroids has been associated retrospectively with lower PEF and FEV$_1$ values.[129]
- Asthmatic subjects not treated with inhaled corticosteroids show a loss of reversibility and a larger degree of airway obstruction in a prospective study.[130]
- A delayed introduction of inhaled corticosteroids does not lead to the expected improvement in hyperresponsiveness in adult patients with asthma.[131]

Unfortunately, we lack easy and reliable indicators both for airway inflammation and for airway remodelling in order to titrate corticosteroid therapy. Sont *et al.* showed that treatment adjustment aimed at reducing airway hyperresponsiveness on top of optimizing symptoms and lung function leads to a more effective control of asthma and to a greater reduction in thickness of the subepithelial reticular layer.[120] At this moment new methods are being explored in order to monitor airway inflammation and prevent airway remodelling. Examples are the measurement of: inflammatory cells and mediators in induced sputum;[132] nitric oxide (NO) in exhaled air;[133] eosinophil cation protein (ECP) in serum and eosinophil derived neurotoxin (EDN) in urine; glycosaminoglycans in urine.[134]

CONCLUSIONS

This chapter describes several chronic complications of asthma that require the chronic awareness of physicians. Chronic complications can be classified as pulmonary, extra-pulmonary, psychosocial, and those related to the management of asthma.

The most important pulmonary complication is the rapid decline in lung function leading to irreversible airway obstruction. Risk factors for the development of irreversible airway obstruction are, among others, more severe asthma at childhood, more severe bronchial hyperresponsiveness, lower lung function and cigarette smoking. Because specific therapeutic agents are lacking, early institution of corticosteroids is advocated in order to prevent airway remodelling. However, sufficient data to support this suggestion are currently lacking.

The extrapulmonary and psychosocial complications have been described. Particularly subjects with very severe asthma may experience a poor quality of life and tend to reduce physical activities. These patients are also prone to significant psychological and psychiatrical disturbances. Nevertheless, most asthmatic subjects are able to perform normal physical activities, experience a normal quality of life, and are normally employed.

There is a relative lack in the literature regarding the late complications of asthma in elderly patients.

KEY POINTS

1 Chronic complications can be classified as pulmonary, extra-pulmonary, psychosocial, and those related to the management of asthma.

2 Patients often adapt to their chronic impairments and disabilities. Yet some chronic complications can be reduced, cured or even prevented.

3 Persistence of asthma is asociated with early age of onset, severity of symptoms, lower lung function, atopic conditions, and female gender.

4 The most important chronic complication of asthma is the rapid decline in lung function leading to irreversible airway obstruction.

5 Risk factors for rapid decline in lung function are, among others, more severe asthma at childhood, more severe bronchial hyperresponsiveness, lower lung function and cigarette smoking.

6 Early institution of corticosteroids is advocated in order to prevent airway remodelling.

7 Subjects with very severe asthma may experience a low quality of life and tend to reduce physical activities. These patients are also prone to significant psychological and psychiatric disturbances.

8. Disappearance of symptoms does not indicate remission or cure of asthma.

9. Asthma is generally a benign disease with a good prognosis. Most asthmatic subjects are able to perform normal physical activities, experience a normal quality of life, and are normally employed.

REFERENCES

1. British Thoracic Society. Guidelines for management of asthma in adults: I–chronic persistent asthma. *BMJ* 1990; 301: 651–3.

2. Department of Health and Human Services, Public Health Service: *Report on Diagnosis and Management of Asthma*. National Institutes of Health, National Heart, Lung, and Blood Institute, Bethesda MD, USA, 1992. International Consensus.

3. Taylor WR, Newacheck PW. Impact of childhood asthma on health. *Pediatrics* 1992; 90: 657–62.

4. Lebowitz MD, Burrows B. Tucson epidemiologic study of obstructive lung diseases. II: Effects of in-migration factors on the prevalence of obstructive lung diseases. *Am J Epidemiol* 1975; 102: 153–63.

5. Martinez FD, Wright AL, Taussig LM *et al*. Asthma and wheezing in the first six years of life. *New Engl J Med* 1995; 332: 133–8.

6. Kokkonen J, Linna O. The state of childhood asthma in young adulthood. *Eur Respir J* 1993; 6: 657–61.

7. Gerritsen J, Koëter GH, Postma DS, Schouten JP, Knol K. Prognosis of asthma from childhood to adulthood. *Am Rev Respir Diseases* 1989; 140: 1325–30.

8. Roorda RJ, Gerritsen J, van Aalderen WM *et al.* Risk factors for the persistence of respiratory symptoms in childhood asthma. *Am Rev Respir Dis* 1993; 148: 1490–95.

9. Boulet LP, Turcotte H, Brochu A. Persistence of airway obstruction and hyperresponsiveness in subjects with asthma remission. *Chest* 1994; 105: 1024–31.

10. ✪ Panhuysen CI, Vonk JM, Koëter GH *et al.* Adult patients may outgrow their asthma: a 25-year follow-up study. *Am J Respir Crit Care Med* 1997; 155: 1267–72.

11. Brown PJ, Greville HW, Finucane KE. Asthma and irreversible airflow obstruction. *Thorax* 1984; 39: 131–6.

12. Connolly CK, Chan NS, Prescott RJ. The relationship between age and duration of asthma and the presence of persistent obstruction in asthma. *Postgrad Med J* 1988; 64: 422–5.

13. Braman SS, Kaemmerlen JT, Davis SM. Asthma in the elderly. A comparison between patients with recently acquired and long-standing disease. *Am Rev Respir Dis* 1991; 143: 336–40.

14. Chiang CH, Hsu K. Residual abnormalities of pulmonary function in asymptomatic young adult asthmatics with childhood-onset asthma. *J Asthma* 1997; 34: 15–21.

15. Rebuck AS. Radiological aspects of severe asthma. *Aust Radiol* 1971; 14: 264.

16. McKenzie DK, Gandevia SC. Strength and endurance of inspiratory, expiratory, and limb muscles in asthma. *Am Rev Respir Dis* 1986; 134: 999–1004.

17. Kondoh Y, Taniguchi H, Yokoyama S, Taki F, Takagi K, Satake T. Emphysematous change in chronic asthma in relation to cigarette smoking. Assessment by computed tomography. *Chest* 1990; 97: 845–9.

18. Paganin F, Seneterre E, Chanez P *et al.* Computed tomography of the lungs in asthma: influence of disease severity and etiology. *Am J Respir Crit Care Med* 1996; 153: 110–14.

19. Biernacki W, Redpath AT, Best JJK, Macnee W. Measurement of CT lung density in patients with chronic asthma. *Eur Respir J* 1997; 10: 2455–9.

20. Kraft M, Djukanovic R, Wilson S, Holgate ST, Martin RJ. Alveolar tissue inflammation in asthma. *Am J Respir Crit Care Med* 1996; 154: 1505–1510.

21. Paganin F, Trussard V, Seneterre E *et al.* Chest radiography and high resolution computed tomography of the lungs in asthma. *Am Rev Respir Dis* 1992; 146: 1084–7.

22. Martinez FD. Viral infections and the development of asthma. *Am J Respir Crit Care Med* 1995; 151: 1644–7.

23. Vaughan LM. Allergic bronchopulmonary aspergillosis. *Clin Pharmacol* 1993; 12: 24–33.

24. Patterson R, Greenberger PA, Halwig JM, Liotta JL, Roberts M. Allergic bronchopulmonary aspergillosis. Natural history and classification of early disease by serologic and roentgenographic studies. *Arch Int Med* 1986; 146: 916–18.

25. Germaud P, Tuchais E, Canfrere I, De Lajartre M, Chailléux E, Delobel M. Therapy of allergic bronchopulmonary aspergillosis with itraconazole. *Am Rev Respir Dis* 1992; 145: A736.

26. Kraft M, Cassell GH, Henson JE *et al.* Detection of *Mycoplasma pneumoniae* in the airways of adults with chronic asthma. *Am J Respir Crit Care Med* 1998; 158: 998–1001.

27. Hahn DL, Bukstein D, Luskin A, Zeitz H. Evidence for *Chlamydia pneumoniae* infection in steroid-dependent asthma. *Ann Allergy, Asthma Immunol* 1998; 80: 45–9.

28. Hamilos DL, Young RM, Peter JB, Agopian MS, Ikle DN, Barka N. Hypogammaglobulinemia in asthmatic patients. *Ann Allergy* 1992; 68: 472–81.

29. Lahood N, Emerson SS, Kumar P, Sorensen RU. Antibody levels and response to pneumococcal vaccine in steroid-dependent asthma. *Ann Allergy* 1993; 70: 289–94.

30. Kubiet M, Gonzalez-Rothi R, Cottey R, Bender B. Serum antibody response to influenza vaccine in

pulmonary patients receiving corticosteroids. *Chest* 1996; 110: 367–70.

31. Oehling AG, Akdis CA, Schapowal A, Blaser A, Schmitz M, Simon H-U. Suppression of the immune system by oral glucocorticoid therapy in bronchial asthma. *Allergy* 1997; 52: 144–54.

32. Ayres JG, Thompson RA. Low IgG subclass levels in brittle asthma and in patients with exacerbations of asthma associated with respiratory infection. *Respir Med* 1997; 91: 464–9.

33. Field SK, Underwood M, Brant R, Cowie RL. Prevalence of gastroesophageal reflux symptoms in asthma. *Chest* 1996; 109: 316–22.

34. Sontag SJ, Schnell TG, Miller TQ *et al.* Prevalence of oesophagitis in asthmatics. *Gut* 1992; 33: 872–6.

35. Peters FT, Kleibeuker JH, Postma DS. Gastric asthma: a pathophysiological entity? *Scand J Gastroenterol* 1998; 225: 19–23.

36. Martin ME, Grunstein MM, Larsen GL. The relationship of gastroesophageal reflux to nocturnal wheezing in children with asthma. *Ann Allergy* 1982; 49: 318–22.

37 Ford GA, Oliver PS, Prior JS, Butland RJ, Wilkinson SP. Omeprazole in the treatment of asthmatics with nocturnal symptoms and gastro-oesophageal reflux: a placebo-controlled cross-over study. *Postgrad Med J* 1994; 70: 350–54.

38. Boeree MJ, Peters FT, Postma DS, Kleibeuker JH. No effects of high-dose omeprazole in patients with severe airway hyperresponsiveness and (a)symptomatic gastro-oesophageal reflux. *Eur Respir J* 1998; 11: 1070–74.

39. Barish CF, Wu WC, Castell DO. Respiratory complications of gastroesophageal reflux. *Arch Int Med* 1985; 145: 1882–8.

40. Spector SL. Treatment of the unusually difficult asthmatic patient. *Allergy Asthma Proc* 1997; 18: 153–5.

41. Chappell AG. Painless myocardial infarction in asthma. *Br J Dis Chest* 1984; 78: 174–9.

42. Toren K, Lindholm NB. Do patients with severe asthma run an increased risk from ischaemic heart disease? *Int J Epidemiol* 1996; 25: 617–20.

43. Coughlin SS, Szklo M, Baughman K, Pearson TA. Idiopathic dilated cardiomyopathy and atopic disease: epidemiologic evidence for an association with asthma. *Am Heart J* 1989; 118: 768–74.

44. Coughlin SS, Metayer C, McCarthy EP *et al.* Respiratory illness, beta-agonists, and risk of idiopathic dilated cardiomyopathy. The Washington, DC, Dilated Cardiomyopathy Study. *Am J Epidemiol* 1995; 142: 395–403.

45. Martin SA, Coughlin SS, Metayer C, Rene AA, Hammond IW. Chronic respiratory illness as a predictor of survival in idiopathic dilated cardiomyopathy: the Washington, DC, Dilated Cardiomyopathy Study. *J Nat Med Ass* 1996; 88: 734–43.

46. Hart B. Replacing or reducing high dose oral corticosteroids with alternative asthma controller therapies: implications for leukotriene receptor antagonists. *Eur Respir Rev* 1998; 8: 1056–8.

47. Davison AG, Thompson PJ, Davies J, Corrin B, Turner WM. Prominent pericardial and myocardial lesions in the Churg–Strauss syndrome (allergic granulomatosis and angitis). *Thorax* 1983; 38: 793–5.

48. Calverley PM, Catterall JR, Shapiro C, Douglas NJ. Cor pulmonale in asthma. *Br J Dis Chest* 1983; 77: 303–307.

49. Kravis LP. An analysis of fifteen childhood asthma fatalities. *J Allergy Clin Immunol* 1987; 80: 467–72.

50. Malkia E, Impivaara O. Intensity of physical activity and respiratory function in subjects with and without bronchial asthma. *Scand J M Sci Sports* 1998; 8: 27–32.

51. Hubert HB, Bloch DA, Fries JF. Risk factors for physical disability in an aging cohort: the NHANES I Epidemiologic Follow up Study. *J Rheumatol* 1993; 20: 480–88.

52. Fink G, Kaye C, Blau H, Spitzer SA. Assessment of exercise capacity in asthmatic children with various degrees of activity. *Pediat Pulmonol* 1993; 15: 41–43.

53. Garfinkel SK, Kesten S, Chapman KR, Rebuck AS. Physiologic and nonphysiologic determinants of aerobic fitness in mild to moderate asthma. *Am Rev Respir Dis* 1992; 145: 741–5.

54. Blaiss MS. Outcomes analysis in asthma. *J Am Med Ass* 1997; 278: 1874–80.

55. Townsend M, Feeny DH, Guyatt GH, Furlong WJ, Seip AE, Dolovich J. Evaluation of the burden of illness for pediatric asthmatic patients and their parents. *Ann Allergy* 1991; 67: 403–408.

56. Maier WC, Arrighi HM, Morray B, Llewllyn C, Redding GJ. The impact of asthma and asthma-like illness in Seattle school children. *J Clin Epidemiol* 1998; 51: 557–68.

57. Forrest CB, Starfield B, Riley AW, Kang M. The impact of asthma on the health status of adolescents. *Pediatrics* 1997; 99: E1.

58. Osborne ML, Vollmer WM, Linton KL, Buist AS. Characteristics of patients with asthma within a large HMO: a comparison by age and gender. *Am J Respir Crit Care Med* 1998; 157: 123–8.

59. Schrier AC, Dekker FW, Kaptein AA, Dijkman JH. Quality of life in elderly patients with chronic nonspecific lung disease seen in family practice. *Chest* 1990; 98: 894–9.

60. Dyer CA, Sinclair AJ. A hospital-based case-control study of quality of life in older asthmatics. *Eur Respir J* 1997; 10: 337–41.

61. White EA, Jones PW. Morning and evening peak flow and spirometry as correlates of quality of life in asthma. *Am J Respir Crit Care Med* 1996; 153: A772.

62. Castro M, Looper L, Horrowitz MB *et al*. Correlation of physical activity with asthma severity and quality of life. *Am J Respir Crit Care Med* 1996; 153: 6.

63. Fletcher TJ, Duncanson R, Jones PW, Ayres JG. Poor quality of life in severe asthma using the AQ 20 questionnaire. *Am J Respir Crit Care Med* 1996; 153: A540.

64. Cox FM, Goodwin B, Pepsin P *et al*. Evaluation of general quality of life using the SF-36 in asthmatics receiving inhaled fluticasone propionate 500 μg/day, triamcinolone acetonide 800 μg/day or placebo. *Am J Respir Crit Care Med* 1996; 153: A801–A801.

65. Jones PW. Quality of life, symptoms and pulmonary function in asthma: long-term treatment with nedocromil sodium examined in a controlled multicentre trial. Nedocromil Sodium Quality of Life Study Group. *Eur Respir J* 1994; 7: 55–62.

66. Rutten-van Molken M, Custers F, van Doorslaer EK *et al*. Comparison of performance of four instruments in evaluating the effects of salmeterol on asthma quality of life. *Eur Respir J* 1995; 8: 888–98.

67. van der Molen T, Sears MR, de Graaf CS, Postma DS, Meyboom-de JB. Quality of life during formoterol treatment: comparison between asthma-specific and generic questionnaires. Canadian and the Dutch Formoterol Investigators. *Eur Respir J* 1998; 12: 30–34.

68. Kemp JP, Cook DA, Incaudo GA *et al*. Salmeterol improves quality of life in patients with asthma requiring inhaled corticosteroids. Salmeterol Quality of Life Study Group. *J Allergy Clin Immunol* 1998; 101: 188–95.

69. ✪ Garden GM, Ayres JG. Psychiatric and social aspects of brittle asthma. *Thorax* 1993; 48: 501–505.

70. Miles JF, Garden GM, Tunnicliffe WS, Cayton RM, Ayres JG. Psychological morbidity and coping skills in patients with brittle and non-brittle asthma: a case-control study. *Clin Exp Allergy* 1997; 27: 1151–9.

71. Campbell DA, Yellowlees PM, McLennan G *et al*. Psychiatric and medical features of near fatal asthma. *Thorax* 1995; 50: 254–9.

72. Mrazek DA. Psychiatric complications of pediatric asthma. *Ann Allergy* 1992; 69: 285–90.

73. Turner-Warwick M. Epidemiology of nocturnal asthma. *Am J Med* 1988; 85: 6–8.

74. van Keimpema AR, Ariaansz M, Tamminga JJ, Nauta JJP, Postmus PE. Nocturnal awakening and morning dip of peak expiratory flow in clinically stable asthma patients during treatment. *Respiration* 1997; 64: 29–34.

75. Meijer GG, Postma DS, Wempe JB, Gerritsen J, Knol K, van Aalderen WM. Frequency of nocturnal symptoms in asthmatic children attending a hospital outpatient clinic. *Eur Respir J* 1995; 8: 2076–80.

76. Storms WW, Bodman SF, Nathan RA, Byer P. Nocturnal asthma symptoms may be more prevalent than we think. *J Asthma* 1994; 31: 313–18.

77. Storms WW, Nathan RA, Bodman SF, Byer P. Improving the treatment of nocturnal asthma: use of an office questionnaire to identify nocturnal asthma symptoms. *J Asthma* 1996; 33: 165–8.

78. ✪ Fitzpatrick MF, Engleman H, Whyte KF, Deary IJ, Shapiro CMD. Morbidity in nocturnal asthma: sleep quality and daytime cognitive performance. *Thorax* 1991; 46: 569–73.

79. Weersink EJ, van Zomeren H, Koëter GH, Postma DS. Treatment of nocturnal airway obstruction improves daytime cognitive performance in asthmatics. *American Journal of Respir Crit Care Med* 1997; 156: 1144–50.

80. Weersink EJ, Douma RR, Postma DS, Koëter G. Fluticason propionate, salmeterol xinafoate, and their combination in the treatment of nocturnal asthma. *Am J Respir Crit Care Med* 1997; 155: 1241–6.

81. Martin AJ, Landau LI, Phelan PD. Asthma from childhood to at age 21: the patient and his disease. *BMJ* 1982; 284: 380–82.

82. Blanc PD, Jones M, Besson C, Katz P, Yelin E. Work disability among adults with asthma. *Chest* 1993; 104: 1371–7.

83. Balder B, Lindholm NB, Lowhagen O *et al*. Predictors of self-assessed work ability among subjects with recent-onset asthma. *Respir Med* 1998; 92: 729–34.

84. Sibbald B, Anderson HR, McGuigan S. Asthma and employment in young adults. *Thorax* 1992; 47: 19–24.

85. Fletcher C, Peto R. The natural history of chronic airflow obstruction. *BMJ* 1977; 1: 1645–8.

86. ✪ Lange P, Parner J, Vestbo J, Schnohr P, Jensen G. A 15-year follow-up study of ventilatory function in adults with asthma. *N Engl J Med* 1998; 339: 1194–1200.

87. ✪ Jaakkola MS, Jaakkola JJ, Ernst P, Becklake MR. Respiratory symptoms in young adults should not be overlooked. *Am Rev Respir Dis* 1993; 147: 359–66.

88. ✪ Ulrik CS, Lange P. Decline of lung function in adults with bronchial asthma. *Am J Respir Crit Care Med* 1994; 150: 629–34.

89. ✪ Almind M, Viskum K, Evald T, Dirksen A, Kok JA. A seven-year follow-up study of 343 adults with bronchial asthma. *Danish Med Bull* 1992; 39: 561–5.

90. ✪ Schachter EN, Doyle CA, Beck GJ. A prospective study of asthma in a rural community. *Chest* 1984; 85: 623–30.

91. ✪ Ulrik CS, Backer V, Dirksen A. A 10 year follow up of 180 adults with bronchial asthma: factors important for the decline in lung function. *Thorax* 1992; 47: 14–18.

92. ✪ Peat JK, Woolcock AJ, Cullen K. Rate of decline of lung function in subjects with asthma. *Eur J Respir Dis* 1987; 70: 171–9.

93. Postma DS, Lebowitz MD. Rate of decline of lung function in subjects with asthma. *Arch Int Med* 1995; 155: 1393–9.

94. van Schayck CP, Dompeling E, van Herwaarden CL, Wever AM, van Weel C. Interacting effects of atopy and bronchial hyperresponsiveness on the annual decline in lung function and the exacerbation rate in asthma. *Am Rev Respir Dis* 1991; 144: 1297–1301.

95. Gerritsen J, Koëter G, de Monchy JGR. Allergy in subjects with asthma from childhood to adulthood. *J Allergy Clin Immunol* 1990; 85: 1116–25.

96. Ostergaard PA 198 A prospective study of non-IgE-mediated asthma in children. *Acta Paediat Scand* 1988; 77: 112–17.

97. Roorda RJ, Gerritsen J, van Aalderen WM *et al*. Follow-up of asthma from childhood to adulthood: influence of potential childhood risk factors on the outcome of pulmonary function and bronchial responsiveness in adulthood. *J Allergy Clin Immunol* 1994; 93: 575–84.

98. Grol MH, Postma DS, Vonk JM *et al*. Risk factors from childhood to adulthood for bronchial responsiveness at age 32–42. *Am J Respir Crit Care Med* 1999; 160: 150–6.

99. Borsbom GJM, van Pelt W, Quanjer PH. Pubertal growth curves of ventilatory function: Relationship with childhood respiratory symptoms. *Am J Respir Crit Care Med* 147: 372–8.

100. Ulrik CS, Backer V, Dirksen A. Extrinsic and intrisic asthma from childhood to adult age: a 10 year follow-up. *Respir Med* 1995; 98: 547–54.

101. Kelly WJ, Hudson I, Phelan PD, Pain MC, Olinsky A. Childhood asthma in adult life: a further study

at 28 years of age. *Br Med J Clin Resour* 1987; 294: 1059–62.

102. Kelly WJ, Hudson I, Raven J, Phelan PD, Pain MC, Olinsky A. Childhood asthma and adult lung function. *Am Rev Respir Dis* 1988; 138: 26–30.

103. Weiss ST, Tosteson TD, Segal MR, Tager IB, Redline S, Speizer FE. Effects of asthma on pulmonary function in children. A longitudinal population-based study. *Am Rev Respir Dis* 1992; 145: 58–64.

104. ✪ Holgate ST. The cellular and mediator basis of asthma in relation to natural history. *Lancet* 1997; 350 (suppl. 2): 115–9.

105. Martinez FD. Gene by environmental interactions in the development of asthma. *Clin Exp Allergy* 1998; 28: 21–5.

106. Lynch DA, Newell JD, Tschomper BA, Cink TM, Newman LS, Bethel R. Uncomplicated asthma in adults: comparison of CT appearance of the lungs in asthmatic and healthy subjects. *Radiology* 1993; 188: 829–33.

107. James AL, Pare PD, Hogg JC. The mechanics of airway narrowing in asthma. *Am Rev Respir Dis* 1989; 139: 242–6.

108. Carroll N, Elliot J, Morton A, James A. The structure of large and small airways in nonfatal and fatal asthma. *Am Rev Respir Dis* 1993; 147: 405–410.

109. Kuwano K, Bosken CH, Pare PD, Bai TR, Wiggs BR, Hogg JC. Small airways dimensions in asthma and in chronic obstructive pulmonary disease. *Am Rev Respir Dis* 1993; 148: 1220–25.

110. Boulet L, Belanger M, Carrier G. Airway responsiveness and bronchial-wall thickness in asthma with or without fixed airflow obstruction. *Am J Respir Crit Care Med* 1995; 152: 865–71.

111. Hossain S. Quantitative measurement of bronchial muscle in men with asthma. *Am Rev Respir Dis* 1973; 107: 99–109.

112. Ebina M, Takahashi T, Chiba T, Motomiya M. Cellular hypertrophy and hyperplasia of airway smooth muscles underlying bronchial asthma. A 3-D morphometric study. *Am Rev Respir Dis* 1993; 148: 720–26.

113. Dunnill MS. The pathology of asthma, with special references to changes in the bronchial mucosa. *J Clin Pathol* 1960; 13: 27–33.

114. Takizawa T, Thurlbeck WM. Muscle and mucous gland size in the major bronchi of patients with chronic bronchitis, asthma, and asthmatic bronchitis. *Am Rev Respir Dis* 1971; 104: 331–6.

115. Roche WR, Beasley R, Williams JH, Holgate ST. Subepithelial fibrosis in the bronchi of asthmatics. *Lancet* 1989; 1: 520–24.

116. Brewster CEP, Howarth PH, Djukanovic R, Wilson J, Holgate ST, Roche WR. Myofibroblasts and subepithelial fibrosis in bronchial asthma. *Am J Respir Cell Mol Biol* 1990; 3: 507–11.

117. Li X, Wilson JW. Increased vascularity of the bronchial mucosa in mild asthma. *Am J Respir Crit Care Med* 1997; 156: 229–33.

118. Boulet LP, Laviolette M, Turcotte H *et al*. Bronchial subepithelial fibrosis correlates with airway responsiveness to methacholine. *Chest* 1997; 112: 45–52.

119. ✪ Redington AE, Howarth PH. Airway remodelling in asthma. *Thorax* 1997; 52: 310–12.

120. Sont JK, Willems LN, Krieken JHJM, Vandenbroucke JP, Sterk PJ. *A randomized trial of the clinical control and histopathological outcome of asthma when using airway hyperresponsiveness as an additional guide of long-term treatment*. Thesis Leiden University Medical Centre, 1997.

121. Trigg CJ, Manolitsas ND, Wang J *et al*. Placebo-controlled immunopathologic study of four months of inhaled corticosteroids in asthma. *Am J Respir Crit Care Med* 1994; 150: 17–22.

122. Laitinen A, Altraja A, Kampe M, Linden M, Virtanen I, Laitinen LA. Tenascin is increased in airway basement membrane of asthmatics and decreased by an inhaled steroid. *Am J Respir Crit Care Med* 1997; 156: 951–8.

123. Hoshino M, Nakamura Y, Sim JJ *et al*. Inhaled corticosteroid reduced lamina reticularis of the basement membrane by modulation of insulin-like growth factor (IGF)-I expression in bronchial asthma. *Clin Exp Allergy* 1998; 28: 568–77.

124. Djukanovic R, Wilson JW, Britten KM *et al*. Effect of an inhaled corticosteroid on airway inflammation and symptoms in asthma. *Am Rev Respir Dis* 1992; 145: 669–74.

125. Jeffery PK, Godfrey RW, Adelroth E, Nelson F, Rogers A, Johansson SA. Effects of treatment on airway inflammation and thickening of basement membrane reticular collagen in asthma. A quantitative light and electron microscopic study. *Am Rev Respir Dis* 1992; 145: 890–99.

126. Haahtela T. Airway remodelling takes place in asthma–what are the clinical implications? *Clin Exp Allergy* 1997; 27: 351–3.

127. Samet JM, Lange P. Longitudinal studies of active and passive smoking. *Am J Respir Crit Care Med* 1996; 154: S257–S265.

128. Laitinen LA, Laitinen A, Haahtela T. Airway mucosal inflammation even in patients with newly diagnosed asthma. *Am Rev Respir Dis* 1993; 147: 697–704.

129. Selroos O, Pietinalho A, Lofroos AB, Riska H. Effect of early versus late intervention with inhaled corticosteroids in asthma. *Chest* 1995; 108: 1228–34.

130. Haahtela T, Jarvinen M, Kava T *et al*. Effects of reducing or discontinuing inhaled budesonide in patients with mild asthma. *N Engl J Med* 1994; 331: 700–705.

131. Overbeek SE, Kerstjens HA, Bogaard JM, Mulder PG, Postma DS. Is delayed introduction of inhaled corticosteroids harmful in patients with obstructive airways disease (asthma and COPD)? The Dutch CNSLD Study Group. The Dutch Chronic Nonspecific Lung Disease Study Groups. *Chest* 1996; 110: 35–41.

132. Pin I, Gibson PG, Kolendowicz R *et al*. Use of induced sputum cell counts to investigate airway inflammation in asthma. *Thorax* 1992; 47: 25–9.

133. Kharitonov SA, Yates DH, Barnes PJ. Inhaled glucocorticoids decrease nitric oxide in exhaled air of asthmatic patients. *Am J Respir Crit Care Med* 1996; 153: 454–7.

134. Shute JK, Parmar J, Holgate ST, Howarth PH. Urinary glycosaminoglycan levels are increased in acute severe asthma-a role for eosinophil-derived gelatinase B? *Internat Arch Allergy and Immunol* 1997; 113: 366–7.

Part 5

Running an Asthma Service

Chapter 49

Primary Care

Mark Levy

Asthma care during the last 20 years (Table 49.1) has had a great impact on primary care, where many of these changes originated.[1] In the UK, four organizations have played a major role in this process: The National Asthma Campaign (NAC), The General Practitioners in Asthma Group (GPIAG);[2] The National Asthma and Respiratory Training Centre (NARTC) and the British Thoracic Society (BTS).

Asthma care in the community comprises three interlinked components: (1) diagnosis, i.e. the initial recognition and application of a disease label for the patient's problem; (2) organization and delivery of ongoing supervision and care – the maintenance of good health, ideally free from symptoms and attacks; and (3) acute asthma management. Our goal should be to make the transition between these areas as seamless as possible. These three facets form the focus for this chapter on primary care of patients with asthma.

Table 49.1: Major changes in management of asthma: the last 20 years

1. The development and implementation of asthma guidelines

2. The development of asthma self-management packages

3. The development of an extended role for nurses in asthma management

4. Collaboration across the interface of primary and secondary care

DIAGNOSIS

Diagnosis of asthma is the most important task for health professionals in primary care; without the label "asthma" the patient cannot be cared for properly. Diagnosis of asthma in childhood is the main topic for this section because most of the research on asthma diagnosis in primary care has focused upon children. However a few studies indicate that asthma is under-diagnosed in adults and although not discussed in depth here, this area is important for future study. Although there is no evidence of long-term positive outcome for children diagnosed and treated early, there is good evidence that undiagnosed asthmatic children are inappropriately treated[3–5] and could benefit substantially from improved management. Many children do not outgrow their asthma[6,7] – it goes into remission, hospital admissions are increasing, and there is some evidence that permanent lung damage may result from asthma. Therefore early diagnosis is a major goal for asthma care in the community. In 1978, Speight postulated unacceptable levels of under-diagnosis and under-treatment of childhood asthma;[8] and later confirmed the level of the problem[9] by showing that only a small minority of asthmatic children were actually given a diagnostic label of "asthma". Studies of general practice management of asthma continue to demonstrate that asthma is still under-diagnosed in the community.[10]

In the early 1980s, Levy and Bell identified a particular aspect of poor asthma management in children – delay in diagnosis of up to 5 years – an average of 16 respiratory consultations, to the diagnosis of childhood asthma in primary care.[11] Others verified this delay.[12,13] In the UK, the delay could possibly be explained by the nature of general practice (National Health Service) in

613

the early 1980s. Poor continuity of care resulted from mobility of patients coupled with long delays in obtaining past medical records. Doctors working in large group practices with patients consulting different doctors each time they attended and a general reluctance by doctors and patients to use the term "asthma"[14] may have contributed to delayed diagnosis. Lack of awareness of the presenting symptoms (Table 49.2) of asthma could also explain the delayed and under-diagnosis in primary care.[15]

A peer group audit of asthma diagnosis suggested that there has been a marked improvement in the speed of diagnosis of asthma in general practices in the UK. This audit[18] set out to assess the possible impact of the raised awareness of the presenting features of asthma in childhood. Two cohorts of children born in 1981 and 1986 were simultaneously audited in two self-selected groups of doctors responding to a postal invitation: (1) The General Practitioners in Asthma Group (GPIAG), a UK-based special interest group of general practitioners: 70 out of the membership (at that date) of 300 practices participated (23.3%); and (2) 63 out of a total of 225 general practices in

North West London (28%). Summary data for these 133 practices is shown in Fig. 49.1.

Firstly, the prevalence of diagnosed asthma in these practices increased from 8.7% to 10.2% in the 1981 and 1986 cohorts respectively and secondly, the average (median) age of diagnosis reduced from 5.7 to 3.2 years from 1981 to 1986 in the two cohorts respectively ($P < 0.001$). There was no difference in the ages diagnosed between the GPIAG and the North London practices and therefore this improvement in care was not limited to practices with a special interest in asthma.

Similarly a retrospective study of family doctor records in Ireland of 769 children under 5 years of age found that the mean age of diagnosis is 2.59 years.[19] In addition Barrit and Staples[20] in their second audit, 3 years after introducing the use of a specially designed asthma record card for use in their practice, found that 92% of their asthmatic children were diagnosed within one month of their first presentation with respiratory symptoms. A large prospective study of the effect of nurse education ($n = 466$ nurses caring for over 3 million people) on asthma management provided further evidence that the age of asthma diagnosis has indeed reduced. The mean age of diagnosis, in 4608 nine-year-old children studied was 4.4 years (95% CI 4.3–4.4). On average, 80.4% (95% CI 78.2–82.5) of these children were diagnosed within the practice and 62.9% (95% CI 62.4–63.3) were currently (during the previous year) prescribed inhaled steroids.[21]

Thus, there has been a reduction in the time taken to diagnose asthma signifying an improvement in asthma care by general practitioners in the UK over the last two decades. However, there are few data confirming the accuracy of this diagnosis and there are some data suggesting that general practitioners diagnose asthma and initiate treatment inappropriately.[22] This is an area for future research and improvement.

Possible Solutions: Earlier, Accurate Diagnosis of Asthma

There are many possible reasons for the demonstrated reduction in time to diagnose asthma and these deserve discussion. Increased awareness of asthma and the more unusual presenting features of this condition, following the publication of studies on the under-diagnosis and under-treatment has probably played a major role in earlier diagnosis. In the early 1980s, general practitioners were not aware that childhood

Table 49.2: Presenting symptoms of asthma in general practice[a]

Well-known
Cough
  "still coughing"
  "coughing for months"
  "no better despite antibiotics"
  "worse when laughing"
  "induced by exercise"
Wheeze
Shortness of breath
Chest tightness

Less well-knowns
Difficulty in sleeping
Spoilt holiday (spent time in hospital)
Chest pain
Vomiting
Itching[16,17] (children, usually preceding attacks, usually upper body)

[a] Any patient presenting with any of these symptoms on >3 occasions a year should be considered asthmatic until proved otherwise

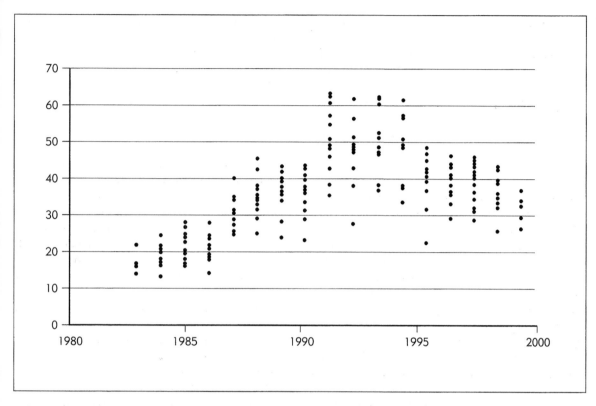

FIGURE 49.1: Data from the weekly returns service of the Royal College of General Practitioners, Birmingham, England. Each year contains 13 data points each representing the mean weekly incidence of asthma in a 4-week period (only five points in 1999). (Kindly provided by Dr D. Flemming.)

asthma presents very differently from the pattern taught and seen in hospitals (see Table 49.2). In fact, children with asthma present in a number of ways in primary care: these range from those with mild intermittent coughing to persistent coughing and wheezing; while others only present when their asthma is exacerbated by with viral infections symptoms.[15] We know that the primary care medical records often provide important clues to the diagnosis[15,23,24] and histories such as "still coughing" or "coughing for months" now alert doctors to the possibility of missed asthma. By maintaining this high level of awareness health professionals suspect asthma in any patient presenting repeatedly with respiratory symptoms, undiagnosed chest pain, disturbed sleep or more rarely, vomiting or itching.[16,17] In childhood asthma in primary care, coughing is the commonest symptom while wheezing is a relatively infrequent presenting feature of asthma; in adults asthma should be suspected if the records indicate frequent consultations for noc-

turnal respiratory symptoms, particularly following infections and in the absence of a history of smoking. Patients whose past medical records indicate a possible diagnosis of asthma could be recalled to see the doctor or nurse, for confirmation of the diagnosis by taking a detailed history and examination of the patient; which should include reversibility tests or daily peak flow diary charts. Prospectively, the diagnosis in childhood could be hastened by numbering recorded respiratory consultations from birth onwards; and because asthmatic children consult more frequently than normals,[14,25] any child consulting the doctor more than three times in any one year with respiratory symptoms has asthma until proved otherwise.[14] These principles aimed at earlier childhood diagnosis could also be applied to improve the recognition of late-onset or undiagnosed asthma in adults.

It is important to try and reduce the level of underdiagnosis of childhood asthma. However, it is vital that the accuracy of diagnosis in these children is improved.

In children mature enough to perform lung function tests such as PEF, it is possible to diagnose asthma with a great degree of confidence. However, there is considerable debate, particularly amongst paediatricians, regarding the diagnosis of asthma in children under 5 years old. This is further complicated by the complex patterns of asthma in these children. Some asthmatic children may have intermittent symptoms, only exacerbated by trigger factors such as virus infections, while others may suffer from intermittent severe attacks. Viral infections such as respiratory sincytial virus (RSV) may mimic or exacerbate asthma attacks, with the result that some of them are incorrectly diagnosed. Once a child has a medical record entry of asthma they may be "labelled as such for life". While this is entirely appropriate if correct, asthma is a dynamic condition where someone may have active uncontrolled disease at one time and in remission at others. Those of us working in primary care need to take responsibility for ensuring that our records are up to date and reflect the current status of our patients. Incorrect diagnoses may be detected through systematic follow-up of all children subsequent to the diagnosis or initiation of asthma therapy. Furthermore, a variety of diagnostic labels, used for the same patients at different times, may overcome some of these problems: for example, current asthma, asthma in remission, not asthma, wheezing episode, acute asthma, uncontrolled asthma, controlled asthma (at Step 0 through 5) and so on.

ORGANIZATION OF ASTHMA CARE IN THE COMMUNITY

Asthma accounts for a substantial proportion of the workload in primary care. The third (1990–91) Australian national survey of morbidity in general practice[26] found that respiratory consultations accounted for 23% of patient encounters ($n = 145\,799$ patient encounters with 495 doctors). Annual asthma consultations as a proportion of all encounters totalled 2.5% in all ages and 7.2% in children ($n = 42\,131$ patient encounters). The UK Morbidity Statistics from General Practice revealed a two-fold increase in patient consultations for asthma in 1991–92 compared with 10 years previously.[27] The mean weekly incidence in the UK of new episodes of asthma seem to be reducing; the explanation for this is unclear (shown in Fig. 49.1) (source: Royal College of General Practitioners, weekly returns, personal communication). Ian Gregg, one of the pioneers of primary care management of asthma asserted that, "Asthma is a disease that should be managed in the community, by primary care physicians and trained asthma nurses with access to secondary and tertiary care for emergencies and guidance on management". In support of this statement, he wrote: "(1) a general practitioner can deliver as good, if not better, care than that of an out-patient department or chest clinic where patients often see a succession of junior doctors who may have had little experience in the long-term management of asthma; and (2) the principles of treating asthma are perfectly straightforward and every aspect of its management including diagnosis, assessment and education of patients, embodies those elements of clinical practice which are the most distinctive features of primary medical care".[28] In 1983, Pereira Gray found that over 95% of asthmatic patients were being cared for exclusively by general practitioners.[29] The GPIAG National Acute Asthma Audit[30] estimated that 14.3 per 1000 patients consulted their general practitioner annually for acute asthma, and found that 86% (1546/1805) of these episodes were managed within the community. When this study was repeated in a different sample of 299 general practitioners,[31] 2031 (87%) of attacks were managed entirely by general practitioners, 251 (11%) were referred for admission to hospital, and 50 (2%) were managed by an accident and emergency department.

Guidelines assist health professionals to select appropriate asthma management and to maintain high standards of care for their patients; many of these were prepared by hospital specialists. However a survey[32] of general practitioner members of the GPIAG found a high level of agreement with the principles of management within the first set of UK guidelines.[33] Having made the diagnosis of asthma the main role of the general practitioner and asthma nurse is to enable the asthmatic patient to enjoy life without symptoms or attacks. Patients should be regularly reviewed, two or three times a year in most cases, more or less frequently in the rest depending upon the severity and timing of exacerbations and they should understand clearly how to recognize attacks and know what to do when these occur. In theory this is fine, however there is evidence of poor adherence to existing guidelines.

An Australian postal survey[34] compared selected general practitioners' self-reported asthma management practices with the Asthma Management Plan of the Thoracic Society of Australia and New Zealand.[35]

Their results suggested that most general practitioners in Australia know and practise appropriate asthma management. However, they concluded that there was room for improvement in the understanding of the use of preventive medications and use of crisis planning for severe asthma attacks and lung function measurement. Another study in Wellington, New Zealand[36] that examined general practitioners prescriptions for 228 asthmatic children, found a marked deviation from international guidelines on the management of childhood asthma. Eighty-four percent of the children were prescribed β_2-adrenoceptor agonists. Of these, 80% of those under 5 years, and 27% over 5 years of age, received these agents by the oral route. In almost half of the cases these drugs were prescribed on a regular basis, rather than intermittently as needed according to the guidelines. Fifty-two percent of patients were prescribed some form of anti-inflammatory therapy (inhaled or oral steroids, ketotifen or sodium cromoglycate); only 2% received sodium cromoglycate.

What Can be Done About Non-Adherence to Guidelines?

In 1983 Colmer and Pereira Gray[37] had the foresight to recognize the value of audit of general practice care in defining current standards of care and highlighting areas for further investigation. The department of general practice at Leicester[38] produced an extremely practical paper suggesting structured asthma audit. The idea is that practices select quality criteria for providing asthma care and divide these into three groups i.e.: "must do", "should do" and "could do" criteria (Table 49.3). Practices interested in adopting this approach may wish to amend or add to some of them. This methodology for structuring general practitioners' approach to the provision of care could be

---

Table 49.3: Three suggested levels of criteria for asthma audit. (From Ref. 39, with permission. Final draft available from the Eli Lilly National Clinical Audit Centre, Department of General Practice, University of Leicester, Gwendolien Road, Leicester LE5 4PW, UK).

"Must do" criteria
1. Diagnosed asthmatics will be recorded in the practice asthma register
2. The diagnosis has been confirmed
3. The records show that at least annually, an assessment is made of the level of control of asthma by assessment of nocturnal and day time symptoms and limitations on activities
4. The records show that at least annually the daily dose of bronchodilator has been checked and that those patients who require more than one dose daily are also receiving prophylactic medication
5. The records show that the patient's smoking habits are recorded at least annually, and for children, the smoking habits of adults in the household are recorded and advice given
6. The records show that at least annually, the inhaler technique has been checked

"Should do" criteria
7. The records show that at least annually asthmatic patients and/or their carer(s) have received education about asthma management
8. Each patient will be reviewed at regular intervals agreed with the patient, but not exceeding 12 months
9. The records show that at least annually assessment has been made about the role of precipitating factors including drugs
10. At least annually the patient's need and suitability for a peak flow meter has been assessed and a meter prescribed if required and the patient is able to use it
11. The target (ideal) peak flow should be recorded annually

"Could do" criteria
12. Information about compilations of asthma including deaths, acute admissions to hospital and severe attacks is recorded on the asthma register
13. The annual assessment of the patient has been undertaken either by a hospital physician, a general practitioner or a nurse who has received additional training about asthma

complemented by the use of asthma record cards[39] in the patient's medical notes.

Organization of Care: Asthma Clinics in General Practice

The following section contains extracts from another book,[15] with permission, and the reader is referred to this text for further information and examples of practice protocols.

Reports of nurse-run asthma clinics in the UK started appearing during the late 1980s, largely modelled upon similar care for the care of diabetic patients in the community. In 1990 National Health Service General practitioners in the UK had a new contract imposed upon them by the Government. As a result the numbers of trained asthma nurses soared, many of whom did the NARTC[40] distance learning course, pioneered by Greta Barnes, a practice nurse, and Dr Robert Pearson, a general practitioner. Unfortunately, in April 1993, the UK general practitioners' remuneration for these clinics was substantially reduced, possibly explaining why research in this field has dwindled. The relatively few published studies on the efficacy of these UK-based nurse-run clinics have shown increased patient satisfaction, reduced doctor consultations (in favour of nurse consultations) reduced episodes of acute asthma and acute home visits and reduced feelings of stigma,[41–43] which had been previously recognized.[44] Ian Charlton, who has also led the way in setting up nurse-run asthma clinics[43,45,46] found a marked drop in doctor consultations, out-of-hours visits and acute attacks of asthma during the 6 months after setting up a nurse-run asthma clinic in one practice.[45] It is unclear which aspect of these clinics brought about the changes and this is an area for further study; increased levels of education; organized follow-up and monitoring are possibilities. A controlled trial of the effect of asthma education did not improve morbidity or self-management of asthma.[47]

Usherwood and Barber's[48] doctor-run mini-clinic reduced their patients' school absence and the need for home visits for acute asthma, however their workload increased markedly. Barritt's 6-year audit of asthma care in general practice showed an initial improvement in care and outcome, however this was not enhanced significantly by the subsequent introduction of a nurse-run asthma clinic.[49]

Inappropriate self-management of acute asthma may be the reason for increased or prolonged morbidity due to asthma. A controlled study (23 active patients; 19 controls) which included monthly interviews of the effects of asthma education by a trained asthma nurse, found that self-treatment of episodes of asthma was significantly better in those patients attending the nurse-run clinic (89 out of 138, 65% episodes of uncontrolled asthma) compared with the control group (58 out of 113, 51% episodes) ($P < 0.05$). This study[50] utilized self-management plans which had been modified from Beasley et al.[51] The original plan had been modified[52] by drawing action lines on the peak flow charts thus making it easier for patients to see when their readings were dropping and approaching the zones where action was needed (Fig. 49.2).

Practicalities of Nurse-Run Asthma Clinics

Certain issues need to be addressed before a practice decides to include a nurse to care for the needs of the asthma patients in the practice. Training is essential but costly and the practice needs to be committed to fully support the nurse by assisting her to learn quickly and effectively. She will need considerable "hands-on" experience and the doctors will need to help through mentoring and by allowing her to participate in joint consultations with asthmatic patients. She will need some protected time to learn and later to run the clinic. Once she is trained, she will need to work autonomously, within the limits of her ability; however she will also need to feel reassured that an experienced doctor is available on site to assist her when she has difficulty in managing a patient. Clear guidelines need to be agreed within the practice regarding when the nurse should seek the doctor's opinion.[53] In addition, she will soon become as expert (if not more so) in the management of asthma than the doctors in the practice and she should be respected for this. The level to which the nurse is involved in the four aspects of care (Table 49.4)

Table 49.4: Tasks for the doctor or nurse running asthma clinics

Diagnosis of patients (case finding)

Monitoring and review at regular intervals
   Inhaler technique, adherence to drug regimes

Education of patients
   Self-management plans

Management of acute attacks

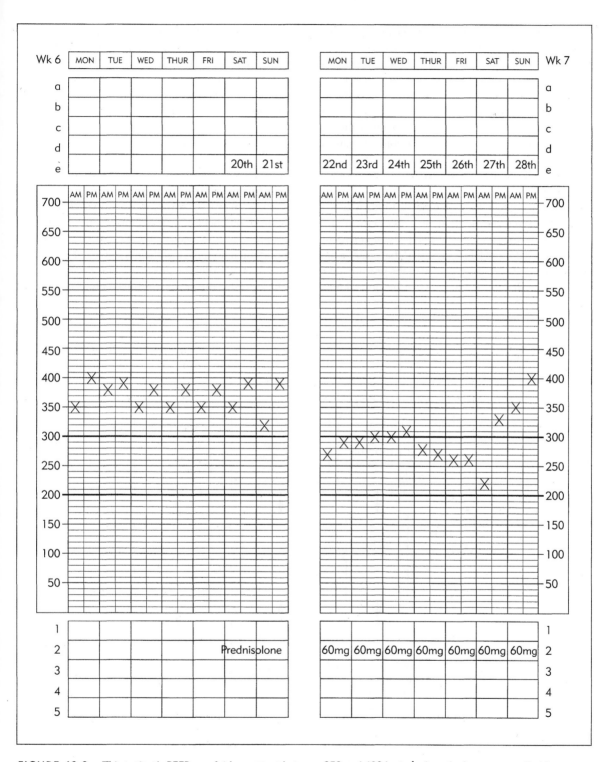

FIGURE 49.2: This patient's PEFR was fairly constant between 350 and 400 l min⁻¹ when she became unwell with influenza on the 20th of the month. Her readings soon dropped below her 75% action line, and because her asthma is usually very bad under these circumstances, she commenced a short course of oral prednisolone and managed to prevent an attack.

will obviously vary according to expertise and experience. Barnes describes three levels of nurse involvement.[40] At minimum involvement, she will record peak flows, demonstrate and check inhaler technique and set up an asthma register. At medium involvement she will carry out reversibility and exercise tests, teach home monitoring and educate patients. At maximum involvement she will have considerable autonomy in management and will quite likely be involved in treating acute episodes, particularly if the doctor is temporarily unavailable.

In an emergency the nurse needs to know how to deal with a severe attack if patients arrive at the surgery when the doctor is out on calls. This is an emergency situation and it is not being suggested that acute asthma management should be delegated to the practice nurse. The fact is that once the practice becomes known amongst its asthmatic patients as "asthma aware", they may choose to arrive at the surgery instead of emergency departments. In this event, the staff need to know what to do while contacting the doctor. It is recommended that the practice develop a protocol for the management of acute asthma perhaps modelled upon those already in existence.[15,54–60]

Asthma clinics in general practice do not necessarily mean that a specific slot of time is allocated to asthma care, although this is probably the preferred method ensuring protected time for the doctor or nurse running the clinic. In practice many asthma nurses work according to appointment systems, allowing for flexible accommodation to the needs of their patients. What is important, however, is that there is a protocol for asthma care in force within the practice. Clinic protocols need to be agreed;[61] the practice asthma register must be up

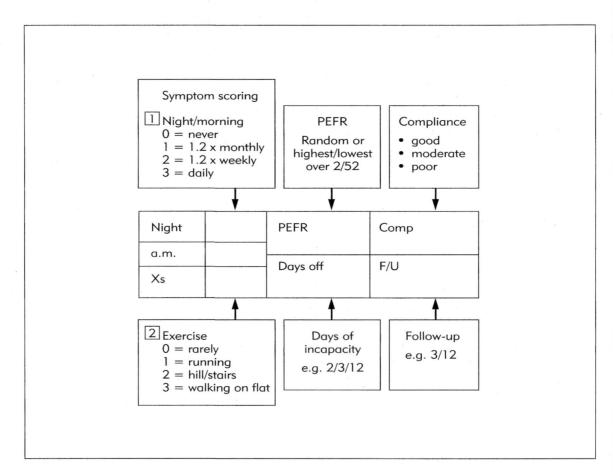

FIGURE 49.3 The Core Information Recording Stamp for use in the record when patients consult the nurse or doctor. (Source: University of Dundee Tayside Asthma Group, with permission.)

to date; systems for regular review and alert systems for identifying patients at risk should be in place. In addition, there needs to be a system for ensuring that comprehensive care is provided, thereby covering all the aspects of asthma, not necessarily at each appointment. One group[62] developed a very elegant method of educating asthma patients over a period of time by using a checklist of items (e.g. inhaler technique, self-management, effect on life-style) which were each covered in time slots of about 6 minutes on different occasions. A specially designed record card[49] helped ensure comprehensive coverage of the practice protocol and another group in Tayside developed a rubber stamp for use in the records (Fig. 49.3). Figure 49.4 is an example of a record card that could be used for asthma care in general practice.

There is opportunity for further development of a team approach to asthma care. We should not be afraid to involve our nursing colleagues in the day-to-day management and follow-up of patients with asthma.

MANAGEMENT OF ACUTE ASTHMA

Studies investigating asthma deaths clearly demonstrate a failure on the part of patients, their families and their doctors to recognize danger signs of asthma and to take early and appropriate action. Despite this well-known danger health professionals are extremely resistant to change their management of asthma from being reactive to a more proactive approach. Two recent innovations are possible means to this end: self-management plans and nurse-run asthma clinics.

ASTHMA TREATMENT (Include oral & inhaled steroid therapy)
Previous ....
....
Current ....
....

RHINITIS
Symptoms (for more than 1hr/day over 2 weeks)
Blocked nose ☐   Sneezing ☐   Runny nose ☐
Seasonal ☐   Specify ....   Perennial ☐
Allergens ....
Treatment
Previous ....
Current ....
Device technique ....
Compliance ....

OTHER MEDICAL CONDITIONS & DRUG THERAPY
....
....
....

INVESTIGATIONS
Height: cms   ☐   ft.ins.   ☐
Weight: kg.   ☐   st. lbs.   ☐
Smoking (Y/N)
If Y, how many?
If ever, when stopped
   and how many?
Blood pressure (adults only)...............................
Urine (if patient taking oral steroids): Glu ....Prot ....
CXR ....

ASTHMA CLINIC
Name ....   Sex ....
Address ....   Marital status ....
....   Dr's Name ....
Date of birth ....
INITIAL ASSESSMENT   Date ....

ASTHMATIC HISTORY
Year of onset of symptoms
Year of asthma diagnosis
Age at asthma diagnosis
Family history
Occupational history ....
Eczema (please put Y or N as approriate in all following boxes)
Hay fever/rhinitis (see back page)
Urticaria
Wheezy bronchitis
Drug allergies   Specify.........
Approx days off work/school during last year

PROVACATION		**PRESENT SYMPTOMS**	
Exercise		Respiratory infection	
Cold air		Sputum	
Respiratory infection		Cough	
Emotion		If Y, specify night or day	
Cough/sneeze		Wheezy	
Laugh		If Y, specify worse time	
Work related		**ASTHMA STATE**	
Animals		Persistent	
Seasonal element		Episodic	
Specify season			

CONTINUE ON BACK OF CARD
©National Asthma & Respiratory Training Centre

Figure 49.4   The National Asthma and Respiratory Training Centre, Asthma Clinic Record card, designed to fold into the general practitioner's records. (© The National Asthma and Respiratory Training Centre, Warwick, reproduced with permission.)

Date	Time	Height	Specify assessment, pre/post b'dilation exercise test etc	Wright PEF		Inhalation technique	Compliance	Days off school/work since last visit	SYMPTOMS (always check symptoms against the following list: cough, respiratory infection, bronchitis, sputum, exercise-induced asthma. Wheeziness worse at night and first thing in the morning?) HOME CHARTING RESULTS, EDUCATION, PLANS & THERAPY	APPT.
				Meas.	Pred or best ever					

EDUCATION
Present level of understanding   High / Med / Low   Booklet given (Y/N) ☐

COMMENT and PLANS ....
....
Re-order this card (specify 'Gold Card R') from the NARTC, The Athenaeum, 10 Church Street, Warwick CV34 4AB. Telephone (01926) 493313

Figure 49.4 *contd.*

Self-management plans are of practical help in management and education of patients and their families, and most importantly in recognizing danger signs preceding asthma attacks. Asthma clinics run by appropriately trained practice nurses offer us an opportunity to implement the use of self-management plans.

Self-Management Plans

Basic to self-management is the availability of accurate,[63,64] cheap, robust, portable peak flow meters and an individually constructed education plan.

Patients need to be taught to recognize the signs of uncontrolled or acute asthma (self-diagnosis). Asthmatics may recognize acute asthma by: increase in symptoms; decreased efficacy of their medication; or by objective measurement of their peak expiratory flow rates. Use of peak flow action levels or zones for recognizing uncontrolled asthma and subsequent adjustment of therapy[46,51,65] has become accepted by many health professionals and there is evidence of successful outcome of asthma care resulting from their use.[66]

Patients also need to understand clearly what action needs to be taken when their asthma goes out of control. The medical records should reflect that the patient has been advised how to recognize danger signs indicating asthma attacks, what to do under these circumstances and when to seek medical help (Table 49.5).

It is important to consider each patient's individual clinical history when advising on self-management plans, which should be tailored to his or her own particular circumstances. Some patients experience attacks of asthma without a corresponding drop in peak expiratory flow, and these people are best advised to adjust their medication at the onset of symptoms or during exposure to known trigger factors. For the majority of patients however, a peak flow management plan is

Table 49.5: Essential information which should be made available to all patients and parents of asthmatic children

Patients should know that their relief medication (i.e. inhaled β_2 bronchodilators) can, and indeed must, be used in high doses in emergency situations

Patients should know that their relief medication should work immediately, and this improvement should last at least 4 hours. If neither of these apply, they should seek immediate assistance from their GP and if this is not possible they should go directly to the nearest emergency treatment facility.

Patients should record their PEF in the event of symptoms of asthma and they should know what to do at various action levels of PEF, e.g. if the patients usual best PEF is 400 l min^{-1} they should increase their inhaled steroids if the readings are tending to drop towards 320 l min^{-1} (80%); they should initiate a short course of oral steroids if the readings are dropping towards 240 l min^{-1} (60%) and should seek immediate attention or call an ambulance if the readings are dropping towards 120 l min^{-1} (33%)

Relative as opposed to absolute PEF values act as clues to uncontrolled asthma. If patients' readings are tending to go down or are increasing in variation from morning to evening or from day to day, urgent action needs to be taken according to a previously agreed plan with their health professional adviser.

better because it is easier to take action based on actual figures. These plans are discussed in detail elsewhere (see Chapter 26) but are mentioned here because the primary care team has a major role to play in their implementation. There are a number of practical points to note in connection with the use of peak flow management plans:

(1) Rather than rely entirely upon single readings or predicted values, it is better to use a series of readings, when the patient is well, to determine the target "best" PEF.

(2) Different meters may give different results, even if they are of the same manufacturer type. Therefore the patient's own peak flow readings (preferably using their peak flow diary card) should always be used in making management decisions.

(3) Depending upon which scales are used on peak flow meters, there is a risk of underestimating the readings in the higher ranges (e.g. in tall people or adults) and of overestimating those in patients in the lower ranges of peak flow.[63] It is also important to realize that peak flow action levels selected at the time of diagnosing the patient's asthma, will need to be adjusted upwards as the patient improves with therapy. Once patients become familiar with the treatment protocol, they feel in control and are in a position to decide at what stage extra medication or indeed help should be sought. Figure 49.2 shows a peak flow chart with action lines drawn at 75% and 50% of the patient's best

peak flow. It was easy for her to decide to initiate a short course of oral prednisolone when she developed influenza, which resulted in a drop in her PEF.

How Are We Managing Acute Asthma Now?

A UK national asthma attack audit, which aimed to determine how acute asthma is currently managed, found that the majority of asthma attacks were managed by general practitioners in the community.[30] Asthma attacks were defined as "an episode of respiratory symptoms which prompts an urgent consultation with a doctor, is of sufficient severity to prevent the patient working or attending school or performing domestic duties or playing, and results in increased use of anti-asthma medication". This national study by the General Practitioners in Asthma Group (GPIAG) provided useful data to enable comparison of actual care of acute asthma in the community with nationally accepted guidelines available at the time in the UK.[67,68] Overall the standard of clinical care provided by the 218 participating practices was judged less than acceptable. In particular, the use of systemic steroids by general practitioners in patients who were breathless and distressed (52% patients) and those who were too breathless to talk (85% patients); and the use of nebulized bronchodilator therapy in those who were breathless and distressed (54%) and those who were too breathless to talk (82%) was unacceptably low according to the guidelines. When this audit cycle was completed in another sample of UK general practitioners,[31] some aspects of the management of asthma attacks had changed in line with guidelines; however, there is still a large gap between actual and recommended management.

Poor adherence to guidelines on asthma care is not limited to primary care: an interface audit of the provision of care in three district general hospitals outside London found that only 35% of 85 patients deemed severe enough to require nebulized bronchodilators were prescribed systemic steroids.[69]

Possible Solutions: Management of Acute Asthma

The first step is, as in the case of other chronic diseases, to reduce the possibility of our patients developing acute asthma attacks. We aim to reduce the overall levels of asthma morbidity. The scheme suggested in Fig. 49.4 may help towards this end by raising the quality of care within the practice. Next we need to assess and re-assess our management of acute asthma attacks possibly by means of ongoing audit. The national asthma attack audit data[31] have provided us with a methodology for assessing acute asthma care; this could be used to set criteria for establishing audit standards.

Systematic follow-up to the point of resolution of acute episodes needs to be improved. It is impossible for anyone to predict the duration of an episode of uncontrolled asthma and yet many doctors (often those working in accident and emergency departments) persist in advising patients prospectively of the exact duration of a course of oral steroids for these episodes. Patients are often discharged from the hospital with 5 or 6 days of prednisolone tablets: these patients complete the "course of treatment", irrespective of the resolution of their symptoms, under the false sense of security that "the doctor knows best" and assume the attack is over. Patients such as these may then be lost to follow-up – until another attack – which may even result in another preventable asthma death.

Studies on asthma death show consistently that both doctors and patients are not aware of the danger signs of asthma. Consequently help is not sought in time or medical attention is delayed, resulting in many avoidable asthma deaths. Although most asthma deaths occur in the community, a significant proportion of these had been recently treated in hospital for an acute attack.[70] It seems sensible therefore to intensify our follow-up of asthmatics, in the community, during the

few weeks following an acute attack. Without objective measurements, the timing of resolution of an attack is guess-work and it is logical to make more use of daily peak flow diary charts to help us as well as our patients decide when the danger has passed and whether or not to step down the treatment (Fig. 49.5).

Primary care physicians are in a unique position to influence outcome for patients following an acute attack, whether this has been treated in the community or hospital emergency room. An appointment with the general practitioner or nurse within 24 hours of the initial presentation with uncontrolled asthma with subsequent frequent review (daily if necessary) over the next few weeks should be included as routine in any practice protocols for acute asthma.[15] In this way patients can be monitored very closely during the vulnerable post-attack time period and are given the opportunity to learn first hand how to manage their next attack. The doctor–patient (or nurse–patient) relationship of trust and understanding is therefore enhanced and it is more likely that the patient will return for routine follow-up and review as requested.

SPECIAL INTEREST GROUPS

Groups of health professionals with a special interest in asthma exist to share experience, audit and research to improve the management of asthma in the community. In 1987, six general practitioners formed the General Practitioners in Asthma Group (GPIAG) in the UK (over 800 members, 2000). The Annual Scientific Meetings offer opportunities for peer-reviewed presentations from within the membership. The Research Unit of the GPIAG was formed in 1991 and has been invaluable in facilitating and conducting high quality research on behalf of the group. In 1999 the GPIAG established the first professorial post in the UK dedicated to primary care respiratory disease, at Aberdeen University, Scotland. In addition to its academic activities, the group has been actively represented on working parties such as those which produced national guidelines[54,71] as well as the National Asthma Campaign's Education Committee and its Task Force. It has also acted in an advisory capacity, and as a pressure group, for example to try and achieve standardization in colour coding of reliever inhalers.

Other similar groups have been formed in Australia (The General Practice Asthma Group), Canada (The Family Physician Asthma Group of Canada), and in

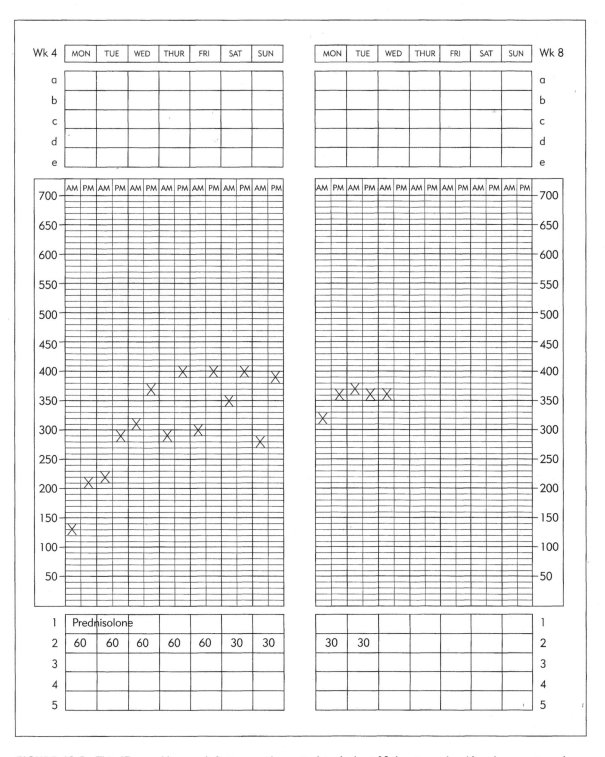

FIGURE 49.5 This 47-year-old woman's first ever asthma attack took about 10 days to resolve. After she was returned to the care of the general practitioner (a few hours after the onset of the attack) daily management decisions were assisted greatly by the PEF readings.

Ireland. The Australian Group has a membership of about 200 doctors with an expressed interest in asthma and is linked with the Australian National Asthma Campaign. At the time of writing, they are establishing their role within the infrastructure of asthma care and have applied for a government grant (part of a scheme to boost general practice) in order to finance their activities. Primary care provision of asthma care has come a long way in the last decade, and there is no doubt that special interest groups such as these will continue to play a major role in audit, research and implementation of change for the good of our patients.

The National Asthma and Respiratory Training Centre in Warwick, UK has maintained strong links with over 20 000 nurses who have attended in the past, and has established satellite training courses in other countries.

THE FUTURE

The problem of facilitating health professionals' adherence to guidelines remains a major challenge for all, right across the interface of health care. Most patients with asthma are treated in the community and it seems that most acute attacks are managed exclusively by general practitioners.[31] Hospital specialists are involved with care of those asthmatics who are either so severe that their general practitioners have sought assistance or admitted for acute episodes of asthma. This "distorted view" from the hospital perhaps leads to the erroneous, but often quoted conclusion that general practitioners cannot manage asthma. On the other hand, general practitioners see their patients discharged too early,[72] or even denied hospital admission when this is clearly in keeping with guidelines. Both parties, together with the patients want the same thing – to reduce asthma attacks and morbidity. If preventable asthma deaths are caused by problems across the interface, the way forward is to try and smooth out the transition between the hospital and community when this is required.

KEY POINTS

1 The majority of children with asthma should be diagnosed before their fourth birthday.

2 Any child consulting the doctor more than three times in any one year with respiratory symptoms has asthma until proved otherwise.

REFERENCES

1. ✪ Charlton I. The contribution primary care (general practice) has made to asthma care in the past twenty years. *Asthma Gen Pract* 1997; 5: 18–20.

2. ✪ GPIAG Website. http://www.gpiag-asthma.org

3. Hill R, Williams J, Britton J, Tattersfield A. Can morbidity associated with untreated asthma in primary schools be reduced?: a controlled intervention study. *BMJ* 1991; 303: 1169–74.

4. Anderson HR, Bailey PA, Cooper JS, Palmer JC, West S. Influence of morbidity illness label and social, family and health service factors on drug treatment of childhood asthma. *Lancet* 1981; 2: 1030–32.

5. Lee DA, Winslow NR, Speight AN, Hey EN. Prevalence and spectrum of asthma in childhood. *BMJ (Clin Res Ed)* 1983; 286: 1256–8.

6. Gerritsen J. *Prognosis of Childhood Asthma*. Assen, Netherlands: Van Gorcum, 1989.

7. Kelly WJW, Hudson I, Phelan PD, Pain MCF, Olinsky A. Childhood asthma in adult life: a further study at 28 years of life. *BMJ* 1987; 294: 1059–62.

8. Speight ANP. Is childhood asthma being underdiagnosed and undertreated? *BMJ* 1978; 2: 331–2.

9. ✪ Speight ANP, Lee DA, Hey EN. Underdiagnosis and undertreatment of asthma in childhood. *BMJ (Clin Res Ed)* 1983; 286: 1253–6.

10. Tse M, Cooper C, Bridges-Webb C, Bauman A. Asthma in general practice. Opportunities for recognition and management. *Aust Fam Physician* 1993; 22: 736–41.

11. ✪ Levy M, Bell L. General practice audit of asthma in childhood. *BMJ (Clin Res Ed)* 1984; 289: 1115–16.

12. Jones A, Sykes AP. The effect of symptom presentation on delay in asthma diagnosis in children in a general practice. *Respir Med* 1990; 84: 139–42.

13. Tudor-Hart J. Wheezing in young children: problems of measurement and management. *J R Coll Gen Pract* 1986; 36: 78–81.

14. Levy M. Delay in diagnosing asthma – is the nature of general practice to blame? [editorial]. *J R Coll Gen Pract* 1986; 36: 52–3.

15. ✪ Levy M, Hilton S. *Asthma in Practice*. London: Royal College of General Practitioners, 1999; 9–112.

16. David TJ, Wybrew M, Hennessen U. Prodromal itching in childhood asthma. *Lancet* 1984; 21: 154–5.

17. Orr AW. Prodromal itching in asthma. *J R Coll Gen Pract* 1979; 29: 287–8.

18. General Practitioners in Asthma Group (GPIAG), Levy ML. An audit of diagnosis of asthma in children. *Thorax* 1993; 48(4): 451–2 (abstract).

19. Steen HJ, Stewart MC, McAuley D, Parker S. Changing trends in approach to wheezy children by family doctors. *Ir Med J* 1993; 85: 59–60.

20. Barrit PW, Staples E. Measuring success in asthma care: a repeat audit. *Br J Gen Pract* 1991; 41: 232–6.

21. Levy ML, Barnes GR, Howe M, Neville RG. Provision of primary care asthma services in the United Kingdom. *Am Rev Resp Dis* 1998; C51, G109.

22. Dennis SM, Vickers MR, Frost CD, Price JF, Barnes PJ. The management of newly diagnosed asthma In primary care in England. *Am J Resp Crit Care Med* 1998; A634.

23. Toop LJ. Active approach to recognising asthma in general practice. *BMJ* 1985; 290: 1629–31.

24. Neville RG, Bryce FP, Robertson FM, Crombie IK, Clark RA. Diagnosis and treatment of asthma in children: usefulness of a review of medical records. *Br J Gen Pract* 1992; 42: 501–503.

25. Pietroni R, Levy M. An interdisciplinary course on asthma and diabetes in general practice. *Postgrad Educat Gen Pract* 1992; 3: 41–6.

26. Bridges-Webb C, Britt H, Miles D *et al*. Morbidity and treatment in general practice in Australia 1990–1991. *Med J Aust* 1992; 157: S1–S56.

27. Central Health Monitoring Unit. *Asthma. An Epidemiological Overview*. London: HMSO, 1995; 1–61.

28. Gregg I. The importance of asthma to the general practitioner. *Practitioner* 1987; 231: 471–7.

29. Pereira Gray D. Asthma in general practice. *Practitioner* 1983; 227: 196–201.

30. ✪ Neville RG, Clark RC, Hoskins G, Smith B. National asthma attack audit 1991–2. General Practitioners in Asthma Group. *BMJ* 1993; 306: 559–62.

31. ✪ Neville RG, Hoskins G, Smith B, Clark RA. How general practitioners manage acute asthma attacks. *Thorax* 1997; 52: 153–6.

32. Hilton SR. GPs in Asthma Group. General practice survey of acceptability and impact of the 1990 guidelines for management of adult asthma. *Thorax* 1991; 46: 741 (abstract).

33. Barnes PJ, Barnett AH, Brewis RAL *et al*. Guidelines for the management of asthma: a summary. *BMJ* 1993; 306: 776.

34. Tse M, Bridges-Webb C. Asthma mangement in general practice. *Med J Aust* 1993; 158: 766–70.

35. Woolcock A, Rubinfeld AR, Seale JP *et al*. Thoracic Society of Australia and New Zealand. Asthma management plan, 1989. *Med J Aust* 1993; 151: 650–53.

36. Thompson R, Dixon F, Watt J, Crane J, Beasley R, Burgess C. Prescribing for childhood asthma in the Wellington area: comparison with international guidelines. *NZ Med J* 1993; 106: 81–83.

37. Colmer LJ, Pereira Gray DJ. An audit of the care of asthma in a general practice. *Practitioner* 1983; 227: 271–9.

38. Eli Lilly National Clinical Audit Centre. *Monitoring Asthma*. Department of General Practitioners, University of Leicester, LE5 4PW, 1993.

39. Barritt P, Staples EB. Measuring success in asthma care: a repeat audit. *Br J Gen Pract* 1991; 41: 232–6.

40. National Asthma and Respiratory Training Centre. *NARTC Diploma in Asthma Care*. Warwick, UK: NARTC, 1988.

41. Charlton I, Charlton G, Broomfield J, Campbell M. An evaluation of a nurse-run asthma clinic in general practice using an attitudes and morbidity questionnaire. *Fam Pract* 1992; 9: 154–60.

42. ✪ Charlton I, Charlton G, Broomfield J, Mullee MA. Audit of the effect of a nurse run asthma clinic on workload and patient morbidity in a general practice. *Br J Gen Pract* 1991; 41: 227–31.

43. Charlton I. Asthma clinics: audit. *Practitioner* 1989; 233: 1522–3.

44. Sibbald B. Patient self care in acute asthma. *Thorax* 1989; 44: 97–101.

45. Charlton I. Asthma clinics: setting up. *Practitioner* 1989; 233: 1359–60.

46. Charlton I. Asthma clinics: how to run one. *Practitioner* 1989; 233: 1440–2, 1445.

47. ✪ Hilton SR, Sibbald B, Anderson HR, Freeling P. Controlled evaluation of the effects of patient education on asthma morbidity in general practice. *Lancet* 1986; 1: 26–9.

48. Usherwood TP, Barber JH. Audit of process and outcome in a mini-clinic for children with asthma. *Fam Pract* 1988; 5: 289–93.

49. Barritt PW. repeated asthma audits in family practice. *Asthma Gen Pract* 1993; 2 (1): 12 (abstract).

50. Hayward SA, Jordan M, Golden G, Levy M. A randomised controlled evaluation of asthma self management in general practice. *Asthma Gen Pract* 1996; 4: 11–13.

51. Beasley R, Cushley M, Holgate ST. A self management plan in the treatment of adult asthma. *Thorax* 1989; 44: 200–204.

52. Hayward SA, Levy M. Patient self managment of asthma [letter]. *Br J Gen Pract* 1990; 40: 166.

53. Sergeant E. Organisation of asthma care. In: Levy M, Hilton S (eds). *Asthma in Practice*. London: RCGP, 1999; 78–85.

54. The British Thoracic Society, The National Asthma Campaign, The Royal College of Physicians of London *et al.* The British Guidelines on Asthma Management: 1995 Review and Position Statement. *Thorax* 1997; 52(suppl. 1): S1–S21.

55. Beveridge RC, Grunfeld AF, Hodder RV, Verbeek PR. Guidelines for the emergency management of asthma in adults. CAEP/CTS Asthma Advisory Committee. Canadian Association of Emergency Physicians and the Canadian Thoracic Society. [Review] [167 refs]. *Can Med Ass J* 1996; 155: 25–37.

56. Ernst P, Fitzgerald JM, Spier S. Canadian Asthma Consensus Conference: Summary of reccomendations. *Can Respir J* 1996; 3: 89–100 (abstract).

57. Spelman R. *Guidelines for the diagnosis and management of asthma in general practice*. The Irish College of General Practitioners, 1996; 1–34.

58. Anon. Asthma management and prevention. *Global Initiative for Asthma* 1995; 96–3659A: 1–46 (abstract).

59. Anon. Management of childhood and adolescent asthma. 1994 consensus. South African Childhood Asthma Working Group. *SAMJ* 1994; 84: 862–6.

60. Anon. Treating infantile asthma in general practice. *Drug Therapeut Bull* 1987; 25: 61–3.

61. Levy M, Hilton S. Asthma clinic protocol – an example framework. In: *Asthma in Practice*. London: RCGP, 1999; 96–7.

62. Crosby FRG, Whyte E, Ogston S *et al.* Improving asthma control in general practice. *Thorax* 1989; 44: 344 (abstract).

63. Burge PS. Peak flow measurement. *Thorax* 1992; 47: 903.

64. Miller MR, Dickinson SA, Hitchings DR. The accuracy of portable peak flow meters. *Thorax* 1992; 47: 904–909.

65. International consensus report on diagnosis and treatment of asthma. National Heart, Lung, and Blood Institute, National Institutes of Health. Bethesda, Maryland 20892. Publication no. 92–3091, March 1992. *Eur Respir J* 1993; 5: 601–41.

66. Beasley R, D'Souza W, Te Karu H *et al.* Trial of an asthma action plan in the maori community of the wairarapa. *NZ Med J* 1993; 106: 336–8.

67. Warner JO, Gotz M, Landau LI *et al.* Management of asthma: a consensus statemtn. *Arch Dis Child* 1993; 64: 1065–79.

68. British Thoracic Society. Guidelines for management of asthma in adults: II – acute severe asthma. *BMJ* 1990; 301: 797–800.

69. Levy ML, Robb M, Bradley JL, Winter RJD. Presentation and self management in acute asthma: a prospective study in two districts. *Thorax* 1993; 48(4): 460–61 (abstract).

70. Asthma Mortality Task Force 1986. American Acadamy of Allergy and Immunology and the American Thoracic Society. *J Allergy Clin Immunol* 1987; 80: 361–514.

71. The COPD Guidelines Group of the Standards of Care Committee of the BTS. BTS Guidelines for the management of chronic obstructive pulmonary disease. *Thorax* 1997; 52: S1-S32.

72. Bucknall CE, Robertson C, Moran F, Stevenson RD. Management of asthma in hospital: a prospective audit. *BMJ* 1988; 296: 1637–9.

USEFUL ADDRESSES

General Practitioners in Asthma Group (GPIAG), Secretariat, The Medical Marketing Interface, Bath Brewery, Toll Bridge Road, Bath BA1 7DE, UK. Tel: 0225–858880; Fax: 0225 859977; http://www. gpiag-asthma.org/

National Asthma and Respiratory Training Centre, The Athenaeum, Church Street, Warwick CV34 4AB, UK. Tel: 01926 493313; Fax: 01926 493224; http:www. nartc.uk.org; E-mail: enquiries@nartc.org.uk

National Asthma Campaign, Providence House, Providence Place, London N1 ONT, UK. Tel: 020 72262260; Fax: 020 7704 0740; Helpline: 0845 01 02 03.

The General Practice Asthma Group (GPAG), Dr Ian Charlton, 7 Tilba Street, Kincumber NSW 2251, Australia. Tel: 043 692444; Fax: 043 631664.

Family Physician Asthma Group of Canada, Dr Mervyn Dean, West Coast Medical Centre, 3 Church Street, Corner Brook, NF, A2H 2Z4, Canada. Tel: 709 634 2818; Fax: 709 634 5649.

Dr R. Spellman, Health Centre, Bridgtown, Wexford, Ireland. Tel: (053) 35296.

Chapter 50

Hospital Practice

Jeff Garrett and John Kolbe

INTRODUCTION

The rationale behind a coordinated team approach to the hospital-based management of asthma is principally a philosophical one, since the approach has never been validated by way of a randomized study. Although patients who attend a specialist asthma clinic have less subsequent morbidity than those randomized to usual follow-up,[1–4] it is difficult to evaluate which aspect of care contributed most to the patients' outcome; namely education, peak flow monitoring, self-management plans, evaluation by an asthma specialist, the prescription of inhaled steroids or even that it may have been due to attendance (selection) bias.[5] On the other hand, it is beyond the scope of any hospital-based approach to medical management to substantially influence social, economic or psychological factors,[6–8] or factors which are directly under the control of the patient (illness behaviour or health-care utilization),[9] or which are dependent upon the organization and quality of medical care within the community.[6] (Fig. 50.1). Such factors are likely to have a greater influence on the patient's subsequent outcome than anything that can be achieved by way of a time-limited intervention from a team of hospital-based health-care professionals. As such, the goals of hospital-based asthma management should be realistic and communicated to those health-care professionals involved in ongoing management such that they can continue to be consistently reinforced. The aim should be to maximize the potential of the resources available to improve patients' knowledge and self-management skills[4] and to establish an individualised medical regimen after adopting a partnership approach to asthma management with the patient.[10] (Fig. 50.2)

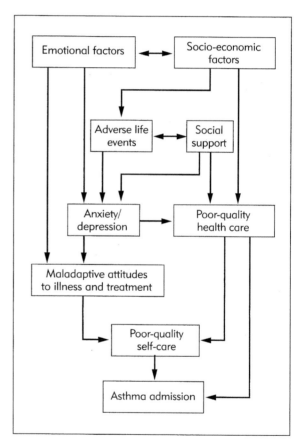

FIGURE 50.1: Interacting factors contributing to hospital admissions for asthma.

In the ideal world, the hospital team should meet with all other health-care professionals involved with managing asthma and agree on core strategies for implementing guidelines, new therapies and assessment

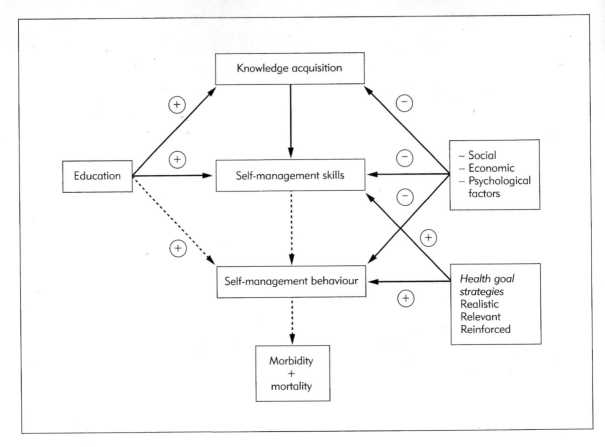

FIGURE 50.2: Strategies that reduce morbidity (premise).

tools, along with referral and follow-up procedures. Such an approach would also involve patient representatives and would involve identifying barriers to good management and where possible rectifying them. This review identifies ideals hospital medical staff should strive for in developing a system of management which should integrate where possible with primary care initiatives.

Overcoming the two key feelings (loss of control and fear) experienced by asthmatics[11] requires acquisition of knowledge, self-awareness and experience, and can be facilitated by members of the asthma management team. Adherence to management strategies can be promoted, identified and monitored by a collaborative approach to patient care.[12] Adopting a partnership approach to asthma management in a non-threatening setting (not always achievable if an in-patient) which acknowledges the problems patients may have to overcome (e.g. out of pocket expenses,

accessibility of after-hours care) is more likely to be adhered to by the patient.

The hospital-based coordinated team approach to asthma care arose out of the needs of patients and/or their caregivers and in response to either high or escalating admission rates.[13] Since a variety of personnel are available within hospitals, multidisciplinary models of health care can evolve easily. Because of the nature of hospitals, patients admitted with asthma may be managed by a variety of services, e.g. emergency department (ED), general medical team, respiratory medical team, general medical or asthma outpatient clinic, and intensive care unit (ICU). Whether to admit people with asthma to a specialist respiratory unit or to a general medical ward will usually be determined by local policy, although the outcome is superior for patients admitted to respiratory wards.[3,14,15] As a rule, patients should be admitted to the care of the same team under whom they were previously admitted or whose care they have been under in the out-patient clinic. Where general medical wards exist, it seems logical to improve levels of care by introducing guidelines[16,17] and by allowing members of the asthma management team to contribute to the management of patients admitted to a general medical ward. This approach allows medical and nursing staff working outside of specialist respiratory services to attain and then maintain expertise in asthma management. Indeed junior medical staff and nurses interact more often with the patient during an admission and it is important for both the medical team and the patient to be involved in identifying the goals of therapy so that they can be consistently reinforced. Since 70–80% of asthma admissions are preventable, junior staff providing acute medical services can develop a judgmental attitude towards patients which may be counterproductive. During the course of an asthma attack, patients commonly make self-management errors[18] related to strategies which were likely to prevent or abort the attack and which can be predicted by a variety of adverse socioeconomic and psychological factors. Taking a more detailed history about the circumstances surrounding the attack and developing an empathy with the patient is more likely to be constructive than that associated with the taking of a superficial history and adopting a judgmental attitude. Therefore the asthma management team can ensure that the philosophy of good care is endorsed, give asthma an elevated status within the hospital, ensure standards are maintained and contribute to continuity of care.

DEFINING THE ASTHMA POPULATION AND ASSESSING THEIR NEEDS

Before the final composition of the asthma management team is established and before its goals are defined, it is important to define the sociodemographic and clinical characteristics of the population of asthmatic patients who are to be targeted. For example, if the group responsible for the majority of asthma admissions are from ethnic minority groups, are socially and economically disadvantaged or disenfranchised, then attendance at a hospital-based clinic, even if it is free, is likely to be poor.[19–21] The decision to admit a patient with asthma to hospital is subject to three factors: illness behaviour, the organization of the medical care system and medical practice.[22] Whilst a common goal is to reduce the patient's severity of asthma by appropriate

use of medication and avoidance of triggers, factors outside the control of the hospital-based asthma team may influence the final results of the intervention. Poor organization of after-hours care, poor quality or absent primary health care[23–25] or financial barriers to primary health care[26] may lead to patients becoming more dependent on ED services, which tend to be used later in the course of an attack than do community-based services.[27,28] This trend is particularly strong for patients living in disadvantaged neighbourhoods, and more so if they belong to ethnic minority groups.[6] As such, and if the hospital serves a population with a high density of ethnic minority groups, then community health workers from the same ethnic background will be essential to the asthma team. If primary health care is either of poor quality or insufficient to meet the needs of the community, then the service developed within the hospital may need to formally evolve into the community.[29]

Social and economic deprivation (SED) may impact upon hospitalization for asthma and in-hospital management of asthma in a variety of ways. The relationship between SED and asthma morbidity may not be straightforward and the crucial socioeconomic predictors are likely to be cumulative measures of lifetime social circumstances, rather than those which may be currently operational. Further, certain exposures may have long-lasting effects, influences of education, welfare coverage and social infrastructure may not be reversed in the short term and may profoundly effect disease prevalence and severity, and health-care behaviour in the long term.

Across nations, higher levels of taxation, and of social expenditure, are generally associated with better health outcomes. Since large increases in income inequality tend to be related to long-term under-investment in health and human resources, it is not surprising that the strongest relationships exist between adverse health outcomes and indices of inequality of income, as opposed to the absolute level of income.[30–32] Watson et al.[33] found that the standardized asthma admission rate in Worcester (UK) was strongly associated with inequality. The relationship was strongest for admissions via the ED and was not present in those admitted via a general practitioner. Similar differences in admission rates were demonstrated in a small area analysis in Boston based on neighbourhood of domicile.[34] Carr et al.[35] have shown that hospitalization rates in New York varied 16-fold between the highest and lowest income groups. Wissow *et al.*[36] reported that the hospitalization rate for black children was three times greater than the rate for white children and we have shown the same ratio between whites and Polynesian populations in Auckland, New Zealand.[6] However, black and white children of comparable family income have nearly identical admission rates suggesting that the reported ethnic differences in asthma morbidity are likely to be due to socioeconomic differences. We have recently reconfirmed the close relationship between SED and asthma mortality, severe life-threatening asthma and asthma admissions and re-admissions.[37] Obviously, various mechanisms may be at play which increase the risk of asthma admission in communities where SED exists. These mechanisms: greater exposure to aetiologic and aggravating factors,[38,39] poor quality and/or fragmented primary health care,[40–43] reduced access to ambulatory care,[19,44] financial barriers to primary health care and asthma medications[45] and a variety of psychosocial factors[18,46–47] therefore need to be considered in all patients presenting from disadvantaged neighbourhoods.

THE ASTHMA MANAGEMENT TEAM

A variety of health professionals have skills that may be useful to an asthma management team (Table 50.1). Key people include: the physician(s), paediatrician(s) and the asthma educator. The asthma educator is often a nurse. In the hospital setting they may be closely

Table 50.1: Asthma management team personnel
Physician
Paediatrician
Asthma educator
Physiotherapist
Clinical psychologist
Dietitian
Community health worker
Pharmacist
Social worker

involved with coordination of patient care and for the reasons outlined earlier may need to also function in a patient advocacy role. There is no reason why a physiotherapist or pharmacist cannot perform the role of asthma educator. The final decision will often depend on the availability of skilled health-care workers who not only have the appropriate background of training in asthma, but also the necessary management, educational, and interpersonal skills to successfully fill the position. The final make-up of the team and its size should be influenced by the size of the hospital or by the number of people with asthma requiring hospital care and thus more comprehensive management. In small hospitals, the asthma educator's role may merge with that of a traditional nursing role, or may be combined with a nurse specialist role in managing other conditions (e.g. rehabilitation, cystic fibrosis, COPD or diabetes). Alternatively, the role may be combined with a position of responsibility in the community. In New Zealand, the asthma educator has occasionally been funded by both hospital and Asthma Society (lay) or Independant Practitioner Association (primary care-based organizations) with responsibilities to both employers. Conversely, in large hospitals or hospitals serving a large population, the asthma educator's role may evolve into that of a liaison one, providing the link between hospital-based care and community services (general practitioner, social worker, asthma society, etc). They may take a leadership role in establishing education programmes for health-care workers (either within or outside of the hospital) and in coordinating the activities of other workers involved in asthma management.

A *physician* and a *paediatrician* should be associated with the programme and should either be trained in respiratory medicine or have a subspecialty interest in the area. They should ensure that good standards of asthma care are attained and subsequently maintained. Guidelines based on a variety of consensus statements on asthma management[16,17,48,49] should be introduced to medical wards, EDs, ICUs and outpatient clinics. In association with the asthma educator, the physician/paediatrician should develop education programmes for both patients and health-care workers. A large number of education programmes are in existence[50,51] and should be adapted to meet the needs of patients using the service. In our experience, patients from disadvantaged communities with little formal education, require less emphasis on the pathophysiology of asthma, and rather more time spent on how and when to access the health-care service, on minimizing out-of-pocket costs, on accessing appropriate social welfare services and on basic survival skills. An individualized self-management plan explaining when and how to seek medical attention when confronted with worsening asthma, and how to access community support networks if social isolation exists, are needed. Physicians should develop links with the community through lay organizations such as the Asthma Society and through meetings with primary health-care physicians as well as postgraduate workshops. They should also develop a database to monitor: ICU admissions;[52] hospital admissions and re-admissions;[53] ED attendances and re-attendances including relapse rate within 1 week;[54] outpatient clinic attendances (including origin of referral);[5,19] and non-attendance rates for asthma clinic to help evaluate the overall success of the team. They should manage asthmatic patients admitted to the ward under their care, consult on asthmatic patients admitted to other wards and review their patients in specialist asthma clinics.

Asthma educators should develop asthma education programmes for both patients and health-care professionals. Ideally they should visit all patients who are admitted to hospital with an acute exacerbation of asthma. They should visit all patients on the ward who are to be referred to the asthma clinic for follow-up and all patients already under their care within the asthma clinic. They should ensure that all patients discharged from hospital have a basic understanding of asthma management, including how and when to monitor peak flows, and how to use a basic self-management plan. Such a plan should list the asthma medicines prescribed and when and how to use them, how to predict the onset of an exacerbation and what to do if confronted with an asthma attack. They should also ensure that the patient can satisfactorily use the inhaler device prescribed. They may advise the general medical team as to which patients should be followed up within the specialist asthma clinic, and they may share follow-up on some patients with the general medical team. They may seek to follow some patients in their own homes or workplace. General practitioners will often refer patients directly to the asthma educator without involvement of other members of the team.

The *physiotherapist* (physical therapist) is experienced in managing acute exacerbations of asthma, helping the patient to reduce the work of breathing by teaching relaxation techniques and breathing control and im-proving the pattern of breathing. Whilst vigorous mucociliary clearance techniques such as percussion should be discouraged during the acute phase, the physiotherapist can teach the patient self-management techniques to assist in removal of mucus plugs when they occur, particularly in conjunction with nebulization.[55] The forced expiration-technique, which uses breathing control and "huffing",[56] has been noted to be beneficial in patients with bronchopulmonary suppuration[57,58] and is helpful in reducing the tendency to bronchospasm, which can accompany coughing. For these reasons, it is beneficial to involve the physiotherapist early in the management of an acute exacerbation of asthma, both on the medical ward and in the ED. Physiotherapy can play an important role in managing patients with factitious asthma, hyperventilation syndrome[59] and in those who exhibit panic at the time of acute exacerbations of asthma. The physiotherapist visiting the medical ward can also check on inhaler technique, ensure nebulizers are being properly administered, perform spirometry and reinforce the message of good management by the asthma management team.

Psychosocial factors (recent bereavement, loss of employment, marriage break-up, psychiatric illness) have consistently been associated with an increased risk of mortality, severe life-threatening attacks and admission.[8,18,40,60–62] Psychological factors may be important in preventing patients from gaining control over their asthma. *Clinical psychologists* improve the ability of the asthma management team to evaluate the psychological dimension and, where appropriate, can apply psychological treatments. This invariably represents a very sensitive component of care. The value of working closely with a clinical psychologist with whom the asthma team develops a trust cannot be over-stated.[63] Both denial and, conversely, over-anxiety have been associated with an increased risk of morbidity and may benefit from psychological intervention.[64] The personalities of some patients are incompatible with chronic illness and its management or contribute to psychosomatic exacerbations of symptoms.[65] Some patients may not respond to education about self-management because of psychological problems, which the clinical psychologist can assess and treat or alternatively advise the asthma team regarding future management.

Whilst food allergy and chemical sensitivity contribute infrequently to poorly controlled or severe asthma in our experience, there is some evidence to suggest otherwise.[66,67] If patients are concerned about the possibility of a food allergy, it is important to take this seriously and to assess by way of a double-blind exclusion diet, which can be overseen by a *dietitian*.[68] Detailed "laboratory" assessment of possible chemical sensitivity is beyond the scope of most asthma teams,[69] but preservative-free (particularly metabisulphite-free) diets should be available to patients who have a clear history of chemical sensitivity.

Pharmacists may contribute to asthma management in a number of ways.[70,71] Their depth of knowledge of asthma medicines can be useful to the asthma team and the principles of good asthma management are more likely to be reinforced through retail pharmacies if a pharmacist in the region has taken an active interest in asthma management and involves retail pharmacies in regional initiatives. The pharmacist is an easily accessible and no-cost source of advice for the asthmatic. The retail pharmacist is likely to see the patient more often than other health-care professionals and can check on adherence and whether patients remain on medication appropriate to their needs. Whilst the role of hospital pharmacists as part of the clinical care team have been well-studied there has been no research on the effect of the extended roles of outpatient pharmacists on the process, cost and outcomes of health services delivery.

COMPONENTS OF SERVICE

Emergency Department

Patients worldwide appear to becoming more dependent on the ED for the management of acute exacerbations of asthma, particularly if they are poor.[72–74] As a result, care may become fragmented and the patient's primary physician, (if they have one), may underestimate the severity of the patient's asthma if they are not consulted at the time of an acute attack. ED physicians manage the acute attack which can be life-saving, but seldom have the opportunity to evaluate the attack in the context of the patient's overall management. Therefore, it should be the aim of the ED to maintain good communication with the patient's usual health-care provider. This can be achieved with the use of a triplicated health record of the attack within the ED; one copy is kept in the ED, one is handed to the patient and the other posted to their usual doctor. Patients ful-

filling the criteria for asthma clinic referral (Table 50.2) should be referred. Since patients referred to outpatient clinics from the ED are traditionally poor attenders[19,75] a member of the asthma management team should ideally see the patient at the time of their ED attendance or soon after discharge.

Medical Ward

Whilst assessment and comprehensive management of the acute attack remains the principal aim of the medical ward, a hospital admission provides an opportunity to improve the patient's knowledge of asthma and self-management skills. Whilst the medical ward may not be an ideal environment for health education, after a significant life event most patients are keen to learn more about their asthma and how to manage it better. Therefore, they may benefit from a referral to the asthma educator, respiratory physiotherapist or ward-based physiotherapist. Prior to discharge all patients should know how to identify early symptoms of worsening asthma, and when and how to access the medical care system if confronted with another attack. They should also be discharged with a peak flow meter and diary, a written individualized self-management plan; inhaler(s) (ensuring good technique) and should be followed up in either the asthma clinic or outpatient clinic within 2–4 weeks of discharge, since relapses occur more often within 1 month. Patients should be referred to the asthma specialist as an in-patient if their course is complicated or their response to therapy unusual. Patients from an ethnic minority group should ideally be referred to a community health worker of the same ethnicity.

Intensive Care Unit

Principal aims of therapy include assessment and comprehensive management of acute, severe, life-threatening attacks of asthma. Ideally, all patients admitted to ICU should see an asthma specialist during their hospital stay and all patients should be referred to the asthma clinic for follow-up within 2 weeks of discharge. Patients who have suffered an exacerbation of asthma sufficiently severe to warrant ICU admission are at greatest risk of either mortality[40,76–78] or further severe attacks of asthma.[5] Follow-up should be intensive until good control has been achieved, knowledge regarding appropriate self-management obtained and observed to have been put into practice, and without the need for hospital admission for 2 years (since sub-

TABLE 50.2: Guidelines for specialist consultation. (From British guidelines on the management of asthma. *Thorax* 1997; 52: 52–8.)

Adults	Children
A life-threatening asthma attack	A life-threatening asthma attack
Poor self-management ability requiring intensive education	Poor parental asthma management skills requiring intensive education
Uncertain diagnosis	Uncertain diagnosis atypical symptoms or signs
Patient not responding to therapy	Patient not responding to therapy
Unexpected side-effects from medications	Unexpected side-effects from medications
Requiring frequent courses or continuous oral corticosteroids	Requiring frequent courses or continuous oral corticosteroids
Requiring >1600 µg daily of inhaled corticosteroid	Requiring >600 µg daily in children less than 5 years and >1000 µg daily in older children or adolescents, or toddler or infant needing continuous inhaled steroid
Occupational asthma	
Abnormal lung function tests despite apparently well-controlled symptoms	
Previous admission to hospital or frequent ER attendance within the previous year	Previous admission to hospital or frequent ER attendance within the previous year

sequent ICU admissions or death are most likely to occur in this time).[5] Patients with life-threatening asthma are at higher risk of having important psychosocial problems[62,63] and may particularly benefit from a multidisciplinary approach to care.

Asthma Clinic

Patients should be followed within the outpatient clinic until satisfactory control of asthma has been obtained and self-management skills learnt. The exact timing of discharge is dependent on the quality of primary health care available to the patient and whether or not there is an ongoing need for ED attendance or hospital admission. Those patients who require continuous oral corticosteroids or an inhaled corticosteroid dose of >1600 µg BDP equivalent daily in adults or adolescents and >600 µg daily in children under 5 years should be followed in the clinic (Table 50.2). Patients and their primary care physician should be informed of

the need to refer back to the asthma clinic should good control not be maintained. Some patients may have difficulty obtaining permission from their workplace to attend an asthma clinic.[79] If they reside in areas where unemployment is high they may be afraid to admit to a medical condition that is sufficiently severe to warrant specialist medical care. If this is the case, then evening clinics may need to be introduced. Patients from lower socioeconomic group neighbourhoods or who are from an ethnic minority group have a poorer attendance rate at the asthma clinic.[19,20] Therefore, different strategies to health care delivery may need to be considered. The development of a community-based asthma education centre[29] run by an asthma educator and community health workers, in association with hospital-based and ambulatory asthma clinics, within a community of 167 000 (defined as having the highest medical and social need in New Zealand) was associated with a two-fold increase in prescription of inhaled steroids and a

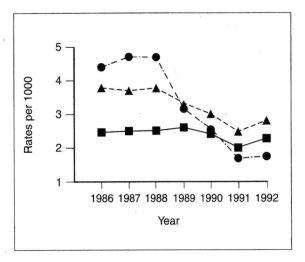

FIGURE 50.3: Asthma admission rates from the study area (●), from the rest of Auckland (■) and for New Zealand (▲) 1986–1992. (From Garrett, JE, Mercer Fenwick J, Taylor G et al. Prospective controlled evaluation of the effort of a community-based education centre in a multiracial working class neighbourhood. *Thorax* 1994; 49: 976–83, ©BMJ Publishing Group)

67% reduction in asthma admissions (to a level 30% below the national average) (Fig. 50.3). Whilst we remain unsure which component of care contributed most to the reduction in admissions, the services developed were established to best meet the needs of our patients as defined by earlier epidemiological studies.[6,19,24,54,72,79]

SUMMARY

A hospital-based approach to asthma management must be realistic in the goals it establishes for itself. For knowledge and self-management skills to be acquired during an admission to hospital or subsequent to referral to an asthma clinic, then the educational message must be realistic, relevant and consistently reinforced. Because social, economic and psychological factors have a negative impact on our ability to teach these strategies (Fig. 50.2), utilizing the expertise of a multidisciplinary team may improve the chances of success.[80] However, short-term encounters with numerous specialists and other health workers may be detrimental to the traditional doctor–patient relationship.[81] The asthma management team must aim to overcome this tendency by limiting the number of team members involved with an individual's care and by providing continuity of care by visiting and assisting with management when patients are admitted under other services.

Illness behaviour is more likely to be influenced over time. Since it is unrealistic for hospital-based asthma teams to manage patients over a prolonged period, the management goals must be pursued by primary healthcare physicians. When primary health care is deficient, then improvement in access to ambulatory care and in the quality of such care can lead to fewer hospitalizations among both medically indigent and non-indigent persons with asthma.[82] Community-based education and support centres may complement the care offered by primary health-care physicians in disadvantaged neighbourhoods and may be helpful in either establishing education to improve self-management skills or in reinforcing that which has been instituted whilst the patient was in hospital.[29,83]

ACKNOWLEDGEMENT

The authors would like to acknowledge the contributions of Kath McGregor (Asthma Nurse Educator), Pam Young (Physiotherapist), and Grant Taylor (Clinical Psychologist) to this chapter.

KEY POINTS

1 There are many potentially interacting factors which contribute to hospital admissions for asthma and include: psychosocial, quality of health care and self-care, ethnicity and economic factors.

2 To accommodate these factors the hospital approach to management must be multidisciplinary, well coordinated and of good quality and must adopt a partnership with the patient.

3 Strategies that are likely to reduce morbidity must be implemented and this includes education to improve self-management skills.

REFERENCES

1. Mayo PH, Richman J, Harris HW. Results of a program to reduce admissions for adult asthma. *Ann Intern Med* 1990; 112: 864–71.

2. ○ Zeiger RS, Heller S, Mellon MH, Wald J, Falkoff R, Schatz M. Facilitated referral to asthma specialist reduces relapse in asthma emergency room visits. *J Allergy Clin Immunol* 1991; 87: 1160–8.

3. Bucknall CE, Moran F, Robertson C, Stevenson RD. Differences in hospital asthma management. *Lancet* 1988; 1: 748–50.

4. Allen RM, Jones MP, Oldenburg B. Randomised trial of an asthma self-management plan for adults. *Thorax* 1995; 50: 731–8.

5. ○ Kolbe J, Every S, O'Hagen A, Richards G, Garrett J, Rea HH. Outcome following a severe lift threatening attack of asthma: influence of asthma clinic. *Aust N Z J Med* 1990; 20 (suppl. 1): 515.

6. Garrett JE, Mulder J, Wong-Toi H. Reasons for racial differences in A & E attendance rates for asthma. *NZ Med J* 1989; 102: 121–4.

7. Wissow LS, Gittelsohn AM, Szklo M, Starfield B, Mussman M. Poverty, race and hospitalisation for childhood asthma. *Am J Public Health* 1998; 78: 777–82.

8. Sibbald B, White P, Pharaoh C, Freeling P, Anderson HR. Relationship between psycho-social factors and asthma morbidity. *Fam Pract* 1988; 5: 12–7.

9. Maiman LA, Becker MH. The health belief: origins and correlates in psychological theory. *Health Ed Mono*; 1974; 2(4): 336–53.

10. Clark NM, Nothwehr R, Gong M. Physician–patient partnership in managing chronic illness. *Acad Med* 1995; 70(11): 957–9.

11. Snadden D, Brown JB. The experience of asthma. *Soc Sci Med* 1992; 34(12): 1351–61.

12. DiMatteo MR. Enhancing patient adherence to medical recommendations. *JAMA* 1994. 271: 1.

13. Garrett JE, Kolbe J, Richards G, Whitlock RML, Rea HH. Major reduction in asthma morbidity and continued reduction in asthma mortality in New Zealand: what lessons have been learned? *Thorax* 1995; 50: 303–11.

14. Baldwin DR, Ormerod LP, Mackay AD, Stableforth DE. Changes in hospital management of acute severe asthma by thoracic and general physicians in Birmingham and Manchester during 1978 and 1985. *Thorax* 1990; 45: 130–4.

15. Osman J, Ormerod LP, Stableforth DE. Management of acute asthma: a survey of hospital practice and comparison between thoracic and general physicians in Birmingham and Manchester. *Br J Dis Chest* 1987; 81: 232–42.

16. National Asthma Education Program. *Guidelines for the Diagnosis and Management of Asthma*. National Institutes of Health Publication No. 91–3042, 1991, (Updated 1997).

17. British Guidelines on the Management of Asthma. *Thorax* 1997; 52: S2–8.

18. ○ Kolbe J, Vamos M, Fergusson W, Elkind G, Garrett J. Differential influences on asthma self-management knowledge and self-management behaviour in acute severe asthma. *Chest* 1996; 100: 1463–8.

19. McClellan VE, Garrett JE. Attendance failure at Middlemore Hospital asthma clinic. *NZ Med J* 1989; 102: 211–3.

20. Oppenheim GL, Bergman MD, English EC. Failed appointments: a review. *J Fam Pract* 1979, 8: 789–91.

21. Deyo RA, Thomas SI. Dropouts and broken appointments. *Med Care* 1980; 18: 1146–57.

22. Anderson HR. The epidemiological value of hospital diagnostic data. In: Bennett AE (ed). *Recent Advances in Community Medicine*. Edinburgh: Churchill Livingstone, 1978; 175–94.

23. Karetsky MS. Asthma in the South Bronx: clinical and epidemiological characteristics. *J Allergy Clin Immunol* 1977; 60: 383–90.

24. Garrett JE, Mulder J, Veale A. Characteristics of asthmatics using an urban accident and emergency department. *NZ Med J* 1988; 101: 359–61.

25. Schneider KC, Dove HG. High uses of VA emergency room facilities: Are outpatients abusing the system or is the system abusing them? *Inquiry* 1983; 20: 57–64.

26. Weiss KB, Gerger PJ, Hodgson TA. An economic evaluation of asthma in the United States. *N Engl J Med* 1992; 326: 862–6.

27. Dalby BCS, Farrer JA, Harvey PW. Casualty activity analysis coding and computing. *Comput Program Biomed* 1974; 3: 254–66.

28. Torrens PR, Yedvab DG. Variations among emergency room populations: a comparison of four hospitals in New York City. *Med Care* 1970; 8: 60–75.

29. Garrett JE, Mercer Fenwick J, Taylor G, Mitchell E, Stewart J, Rea H. Prospective controlled evaluation of the effort of a community-based education centre in a multiracial working class neighbourhood. *Thorax* 1994; 49: 976–83.

30. Kaplan GA, Pamuk ER, Lynah JW, Cohen RD, Balfour JL. Inequality in income and mortality in the United States: analysis of mortality and potential pathways. *BMJ* 1996; 312: 999–1003.

31. Kennedy BP, Kawachi I, Prothro-Stith D. Income distribution and mortality: cross sectional ecological study of the Robin Hood index in the United States. *BMJ* 1996; 312: 1004–7.

32. Smith R. Gap between death rates of sick and poor widens. *BMJ* 1997; 314: 9.

33. Watson JP, Cowen P, Lewis RA. The relationship between asthma admission rates, routes of admission and socio-economic deprivation. *Eur Respir J* 1996; 9: 2087–93.

34. Gottlieb DJ, Beiser AS, O'Conner GT. Poverty, race and medication use are correlates of asthma hospitalisation rates. A small area analysis in Boston. *Chest* 1995; 108: 28–35.

35. Carr W, Zeittel L, Weiss K. Variations in asthma hospitalisations and deaths in New York City. *Am J Public Health* 1992; 82: 59–65.

36. Wissow LS, Gittelsohn AM, Szklo M, Starfield B, Mussman M. Poverty, race and hospitalisation of childhood asthma. *Am J Public Health* 1988; 78: 777–92.

37. Garrett JE, Poyser M, Kolbe J. The relationship between social and economic deprivation and asthma morbidity/mortality in New Zealand. *Eur Resp J* 1999 (in press).

38. Rosenstreich DL, Eggleston P, Kattan M *et al*. The role of cockroach allergy and exposure to cockroach allergen in causing morbidity among inner-city children with asthma. *N Engl J Med* 1997; 336: 1356–63.

39. Perry GB, Chai H, Dickey DW *et al*. Effects of particularly air pollution on asthmatics. *Am J Public Health* 1983; 73: 50–56.

40. Rea HH, Scragg R, Jackson R, Beaglehole R, Fenwick J, Sutherland PC. A case-control study of deaths from asthma. *Thorax* 1986; 41: 833–9.

41. British Thoracic Association. Death from asthma in two regions of England. *BMJ* 1982; 285: 1251–5.

42. MacDonald JB, Seaton A, Williams DA. Asthma deaths in Cardiff 1963–74: 90 deaths outside hospital. *BMJ* 1976; 1: 1493.

43. ✪ Ryan G, Stock H, Musk AW, Knight JL, Perera DM, Hobbs MST. Risk factors for death in patients admitted to hospital with asthma: a follow-up study. *Aust NZ J Med* 1991; 21: 681–5.

44. Halfon N, Newacheck PW. Childhood asthma and poverty: differential impacts and utilisation of health services. *Paediatrics* 1993; 91: 56–61.

45. Garrett J, Kolbe J, Richards G, Whitlock T, Rea H. Asthma morbidity and mortality in New Zealand. *Thorax* 1995; 50: 1020–1.

46. Kolbe J, Vamos M, Fergusson W. Socio-economic disadvantage, quality of medical care and admission for acute severe asthma. *Aust NZ J Med* 1997; 27: 294–9.

47. Campbell DA, Yellowlees PM, McLennon G, Coates JR, Frith PA, Gluyas PA *et al*. Psychiatric and medical features of near fatal asthma. *Thorax* 1995; 50: 254–9.

48. *Asthma Management Handbook*. National Asthma Campaign Limited (Australia), 1993.

49. Thoracic Society of Australia and New Zealand 1990. Consensus of Asthma: Asthma Management Plan 1989. *NZ Med J* 1990; 103: 16–8.

50. Wigal JK, Creer TL, Kutses H, Lewis P. A critique of 19 self-management programs for childhood asthma I. Development and evaluation of the programs. *Paediatr Asthma Allergy Immunol* 1990; 4: 17–39.

51. Creer TL, Wigal JK, Kutses H, Lewis P. A critique of 19 self-management programs for childhood asthma II. Comments regarding the scientific merit of the programs. *Paediatr Asthma Allergy Immunol* 1990; 4: 41–55.

52. Richards GN, Kolbe J, Fenwick J, Rea HH. Demographic characteristics of severe life threatening asthma: comparison with asthma deaths. *Thorax* 1993; 48: 1105–9.

53. Mitchell EA, Elliot RB. Hospital admissions for asthma in children: a prospective study. *NZ Med J* 1981; 94: 331–4.

54. Rea HH, Garrett JE, Mulder J, Chapman KR, White JG, Rebuck AS. Emergency room care of asthmatics: a comparison between Auckland and Toronto. *Ann Allergy* 1991; 66: 48–52.

55. Sutton PP, Gemmell HG, Innes N *et al*. Use of nebulised saline and nebulised terbutaline as an adjunct to chest physiotherapy. *Thorax* 1988; 43: 57–60.

56. Thompson BJ. The physiotherapists' role in rehabilitation of the asthmatic. *NZ J Physiotherapy* 1973; 4: 11–6.

57. Pryor JA, Webber BA. An evaluation of the forced expiration technique as an adjunct to postural drainage. *Physiotherapy* 1979; 65: 304–7.

58. Pryor JA, Webber BA, Hodson ME, Batten JC. Evaluation of the forced expiration technique as an adjunct to postural drainage in the treatment of cystic fibrosis. *BMJ* 1979; 2: 417–8.

59. Howell JBL. Behavioural breathlessness. *Thorax* 1990; 45: 287–92.

60. Cohen SI. Psychological factors. In: Clark TJH, Goodfrey S (eds). *Asthma*. London: Chapman & Hall 1977: 177–89.

61. Knapp PH, Mathe AA. Psychophysiologic aspects of bronchial asthma. In: Weiss EB, Segal MS, Stein M (eds). *Bronchial Asthma: Mechanisms and Therapeutics*, 2nd edn. Boston: Little, Brown, 1976; 914–31.

62. Gordon GMF, Ayres JG. Psychiatric and social aspects of brittle asthma. *Thorax* 1993; 48: 501–5.

63. Miklich DR. Health psychology practice with asthmatics. *Profess Psychol* 1979; 10: 580–8.

64. Yellowlees PM, Ruffin RE. Psychological defences and coping styles in patients following a life-threatening attack of asthma. *Chest* 1989; 95: 1298–303.

65. Kinsman RA, Luparello T, O'Banion K, Spector S. Multidimensional analysis of the subjective symptomotology of asthma. *Psychosom Med* 1973; 35: 250–67.

66. Taylor SL, Bush RK, Selner JC *et al*. Sensitivity to sulfited foods among sulfite-sensitive subjects with asthma. *J Allergy Clin Immunol* 1988; 81: 1159–67.

67. Stevenson DD, Simon RA, Lumry WR, Mathison DA. Adverse reactions to tartrazine. *J Allergy Clin Immunol* 1986; 78: 182–90.

68. Bernstein M, Day JH, Welsh A. Double-blind food challenge in the diagnosis of food sensitivity in the adult. *J Allergy Clin Immunol* 1980; 70: 205–10.

69. Simon RA. Sulfite challenge for the diagnosis of sensitivity. *Allergy Proc* 1989; 10: 357–62.

70. Self T. The value of demonstration and role of the pharmacist in teaching the correct use of pressurised bronchodilators. *Can Med Assoc J* 1983; 128: 129–31.

71. Smith NA. The potential for pharmacists as patient educators in asthma. *Aust J Hosp Pharm* 1988; 18: 244–8.

72. Garrett JE, Mulder J, Veale A. Trends in the use of an urban accident and emergency department by asthmatics. *NZ Med J* 1988; 101: 253–5.

73. Halfon N, Newacheek PW. Childhood asthma and poverty: differential impacts and utilization of health services. *Paediatrics* 1993; 91: 56–61.

74. Strachan DP, Anderson HR. Trends in hospital admission rates for asthma in children. *BMJ* 1992; 304: 819–20.

75. Straus JH, Tangerose S, Charney E. Referrals from an emergency room to primary care practices of an urban hospital. *Am J Public Health* 1983; 73: 57–61.

76. Sears MR, Rea HH. Patients at risk for dying of asthma: New Zealand experiences. *J Allergy Clin Immunol* 1987; 80: 477–80.

77. Strunk RC. Identification of the fatality-prone subject with asthma. *J Allergy Clin Immunol* 1989; 83: 477–85.

641

78. Garrett J, Lanes S, Kolbe J, Rea H. Risk of severe life-threatening asthma and type of prescribed B agonists: an example of confounding by severity. *Thorax* 1996; 51: 1093–9.

79. McClellan VE, Garrett JE. Asthma and the employment experience. *NZ Med J* 1990; 103: 399–401.

80. Koble J, Garrett J, Vamos M, Rea H. Influences on trends in asthma and mortality: the New Zealand experience. *Chest* 1994; 106 (suppl.): 211S–215S.

81. Korsch BM, Gozzi EK, Francis V. Gaps in doctor-patient communication. I. Doctor-patient interaction and patient satisfaction. *Pediatrics* 1968; 42: 855–71.

82. Hughes DM, McLeod M, Garner B, Goldbloom RM. Controlled trial of a home and ambulatory program for asthmatic children. *Pediatrics* 1991; 87: 54–61.

83. Clark NM, Feldman CH, Evans D, Levison MJ, Wasilewski Y, Mellins RB. The impact of health education on frequency and cost of health care use by low income children with asthma. *J Allergy Clin Immunol* 1986; 78: 108–15.

Chapter 51

Audit in Asthma

Brian Harrison

INTRODUCTION

Quality Assurance and Medical Audit

High quality in medicine, like pornography, is difficult to define but easy to recognize. It includes good professional performance, efficient use of resources, minimal risk to the patient and patient satisfaction.[1] High-quality medicine meets the users' needs effectively, efficiently and expertly and conforms to the users' requirements.[1] The most important users are the patients, but other users in this context include medical colleagues, other health care professionals and funders.

Quality is assessed under the three headings of *structure*, *process* and *outcome*. Structure comprises the basic resources of personnel, buildings and equipment. Process describes the procedures and processes involved in the use of the structure to achieve the desired outcome. Outcome is the effect of managing the condition, hopefully the restoration of the patient to as good health as possible in terms of the disease and the actual or potential side-effects and complications of the treatment.

Quality assurance is the process of recognizing and maintaining high-quality services and identifying areas of less than optimal quality and then taking steps to improve those aspects of poor quality. *Medical audit* is quality assurance applied to medicine. Both medical audit and quality assurance have four key elements that are encapsulated in the feedback loop[1] (Fig. 51.1).

Effective medical audit will reveal high-quality practices and high-quality outcomes. High quality when recognized requires praise and preservation. Most time in medical audit involves the detection, analysis and correction of deficiencies in care, but forgetting to praise and preserve the existing high-quality risks the audit process degenerating into a "witch hunt" with

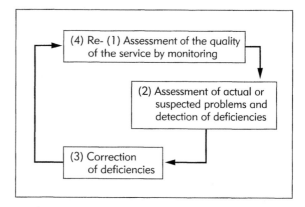

FIGURE 51.1: Medical audit: the feedback loop.

loss of the support and collaboration of those most required to correct the deficiencies and improve the service.

ASTHMA AUDIT: THE FEEDBACK LOOP

Assessing the Quality of the Service by Monitoring

There are four methods of monitoring asthma care, which are listed in Table 51.1

Sentinel-case audit and criterion-based audit require high-quality medical record systems and medical notes, though formats designed to assist the clerking of patients admitted with asthma or to provide a summary of their admission to hospital are available.[2]

Sentinal-Case Audit Sentinel-case audit involves an in-depth analysis of particularly serious departures from the norm, such as death from asthma. In the last 25 years there have been at least 13 studies of asthma deaths.[3–16] These studies have highlighted the same

Table 51.1: Methods of monitoring asthma care

Sentinel-case audit: variation from the norm in structure, process or outcome

Criterion-based audit

Departure from specified criteria (of structure, process or outcome)

Comparison of care by different groups of physicians

Patient satisfaction surveys

Peer review

potentially preventable factors (Table 51.2) that repeatedly contributed to deaths during this period of over two decades.

The two largest studies in Britain and New Zealand revealed potentially preventable factors in over 80% of the deaths. Eleven of these studies have assessed the quality of the service by monitoring and have detected deficiencies in care, but have not progressed any further around the audit loop. Studies in East Anglia in Britain have attempted to close the audit loop by reporting the results to the local medical community and then continuing the confidential enquiry into asthma deaths

Table 51.2: Potentially preventable factors contributing to asthma deaths

Underestimation of condition by patient – failure to make objective measurements; denial and/or familiarity

Underestimation of condition by doctor – failure to make objective measurements; failure of follow-up; failure to refer for specialist opinion

Under treatment with steroids

Inappropriate therapy – excessive bronchodilator therapy without adequate anti-inflammatory therapy; lack of control over repeat prescriptions

Adverse psychosocial factors – depression; denial; other psychiatric history; poverty; substance abuse; social isolation; ethnic minority; employment problems

on an annual basis.[13,16] This enquiry is analogous to the report on British Confidential Enquiry into Maternal Deaths in the UK[17] and the Confidential Enquiry into Perioperative Death.[18]

The methodology developed from the earlier British[8] and New Zealand[9] asthma death studies has several unique features[13,16] (Tables 51.3 and 51.4) and has been adopted by the UK Asthma Task Force of the National Asthma Campaign for ongoing confidential enquiries into asthma deaths in Scotland, Wales and four regions of England.

Table 51.3: Unique features of the confidential enquiries into asthma deaths

Continuing enquiry

Multidisciplinary team (Table 51.4)

Quality of care compared against recommendations in the British Thoracic Society Guidelines[19–22]

Results are fed back to the local medical community, i.e. general practitioners and hospital physicians, annually

Table 51.4: Confidential enquiry into asthma deaths: personnel and their roles

General practitioner	Reviews patient's GP notes and interviews GP
Specialist respiratory nurse	Interviews next-of-kin with agreement of GP
Public health physician	Chairs review meeting
Consultant chest physician	Coordinates enquiry, reviews hospital notes (if any)
Local chest physician	Reviews hospital notes (if any)
Research assistant	Collects names from death register, requests GP and hospital notes, administers enquiry

Criterion-Based Audit

DEPARTURE FROM SPECIFIED CRITERIA (Table 51.5) Frustration with the findings during the 1970s and 1980s that the same preventable factors were repeatedly found in surveys of asthma deaths led to the development during 1989 and 1990 of the British Guidelines on the Management of Asthma in Adults.[19,20] These have been revised and updated twice.[21,22] One of the original intentions of these guidelines was that they should be used for auditing care of patients with asthma. Subsequently a number of studies using criteria from these Guidelines have been published from primary[23–26] and secondary[27,28] care.

Lim and Harrison[2] using an earlier but similar set of local asthma management guidelines have shown that the standards recommended in such guidelines are achievable, at least on a specialist respiratory medical ward. To summarize the results: 78 patients were admitted, mainly from their general practitioner or via the accident and emergency department, with a small number admitting themselves directly to the ward. Peak expiratory flow (PEF) had been measured before admission to the ward in 76% of the patients and systemic steroids given to 74%. Full objective assessment of the severity of asthma (heart rate, systolic paradox, respiratory rate, PEF and arterial blood gases) on admission was recorded in all but one patient and all patients received systemic steroid and high-dose nebulized bronchodilator therapy. Problems with the checking of inhaler technique before discharge and of discharging patients before their PEF variability had fallen to the agreed level were identified at the first audit.

The National Asthma Attack Audit[23] used the criteria published in the British National Guidelines. Good practical assessment of the severity of the attack was reflected by the patient's state of breathlessness or distress being recorded in 97% and PEF recorded in 82%. However, the treatment of the attack was much less satisfactory, with only 56% of those having an attack severe enough to prevent normal activities being given systemic steroids and only 31% nebulized bronchodilators. Furthermore, maintenance treatment was not increased or stepped up according to the recommendations in the guidelines in over 75% of the patients already taking anti-inflammatory medication.

COMPARISON OF CARE OF PATIENTS ADMITTED TO HOSPITAL WITH ASTHMA BY DIFFERENT GROUPS OF PHYSICIANS (Fig. 51.2) Since 1987 several British studies[27–33] have shown that the processes and outcomes of care of patients with asthma are significantly better for those looked after by teams including a specialist respiratory physician than by teams containing no such specialist. In Glasgow, patients looked after by teams including a specialist respiratory physician had significantly fewer symptoms during the first 2 weeks following discharge from hospital and significantly fewer re-admissions for asthma within 1 year of discharge.[30] Repeat studies in Birmingham, Manchester and Glasgow[31,33] have shown significant improvements in management of asthma following the feedback of results from the initial surveys and further education. This improvement applies to care provided by both respiratory physicians and by general physicians, though respiratory physicians continue to provide a higher-quality service.

Table 51.5: Criterion-based audit

1. Define and agree the standard (e.g. protocols of management)

2. Measure the performance against the standard

3. Agree changes to improve the performance against the standard

4. Repeat audit to ensure the changes have had the desired and intended effect

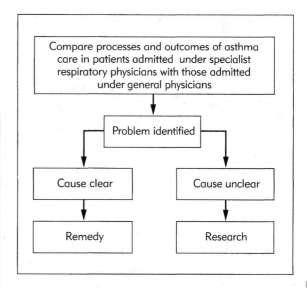

FIGURE 51.2: Comparison between groups.

A more recent multicentre audit of hospital inpatient asthma care in 36 British hospitals undertaken by the British Thoracic Society, Royal College of Physicians and National Asthma Campaign has confirmed that patients are significantly more likely to be managed in a way that matches up to the National Guidelines if they are admitted under the care of a respiratory physician[27] (Table 51.6). This assessment of asthma care of 766 patients was conducted in August and September 1990 immediately before publication of the British Guidelines. The audit was repeated in the same months a year later when the Guidelines had been widely disseminated and discussed.

The second audit, involving 900 patients, showed there had been no significant improvement in any of the variables relating to process and outcome of asthma management, but the marked differences between the management provided by specialist and non-specialist physicians persisted.[28]

These audits have highlighted differences in the quality of care received by patients admitted with asthma under the care of specialist respiratory physicians and their teams and by general physicians. They also show that when deficiencies in care and problems are demonstrated improvements can be made, but the care provided by general physicians has in no study risen to the higher quality of care provided by respiratory physicians, even when district protocols have been formulated and locally agreed.

Eight criteria or standards have evolved from these published audits (Table 51.7).[28] They can be used in any hospital. If data are submitted to the coordinating centre in Liverpool the centre provides feedback which demonstrates how their hospital performs for each item compared with the range of responses nationally over the same time period (Pearson MG, personal communication).

Patient Satisfaction Surveys Little has been published in this area in the field of asthma management. Such surveys enquire into how satisfied patients are with their out-patient or in-patient care. They can include specific

Table 51.6: Differences between respiratory and non-respiratory physicians care. (From Pearson MG, Ryland 1, Harrison BDW. A national audit of acute severe asthma in adults admitted to hospital. *Qual Health Care* 1995; 4: 24–36, with permission.)

	General physicians ($n = 340$) (%)	Respiratory physicians ($n = 426$) (%)	χ^2 (P)
Patients admitted by general practioner	40	60	$P<0.01$
Measurements of PEF on admission	83	89	$P<0.05$
Measurements of arterial blood gases on admission	58	79	$P<0.001$
No steroid therapy in first 24 hours	12	6	$P<0.01$
PEF monitored and recorded on the ward	63	83	$P<0.01$
PEF variability not measured on the ward	27	17	12.5 ($P<0.001$)
Home management plan not given	94	87	7.6 ($P<0.005$)
No steroids at all on discharge	11	4	3.98 ($P<0.05$)
No out-patient appointment made	44	9	124.0 ($P<0.001$)
Seen in out-patient department within 2 months of discharge	44	73	61.4 ($P<0.001$)

Table 51.7: Eight criteria or standards used in the ongoing British Thoracic Society audit of in-patient asthma care[28]

Peak expiratory flow on admission

Blood gases measured if oxygen saturation <92%

Systemic steroids prescribed

Peak flow variability recorded

Inhaled steroids prescribed to take home

Oral steroids prescribed to take home

Follow up out-patient appointment given

Self-management plan given

questions about, for example, the acceptability, painfulness or otherwise of arterial blood sampling, or about aspects of treatment such as waiting times or drug therapy. They can also, more importantly, question the well-being and overall function of the patient with asthma.

One survey sponsored by the National Asthma Campaign asked 1490 patients what they expected of their asthma care; 94% opted for care under a respiratory physician or asthma specialist rather than a general physician (National Asthma Campaign, Market Opinion and Research Institute Poll 1990. Information on File at NAC, Providence House, London).

Patient satisfaction surveys have tended to concentrate on the hotel aspects of care. Whilst these are clearly not unimportant, such relatively simplistic surveys must not be allowed to proliferate at the expense of surveys that are more difficult to conduct, relating to patients' medical and nursing care. A further problem with patient satisfaction surveys is that it remains difficult to ensure that enough patients complete the survey to allow the results to be representative of the whole population. Questionnaires need to be simple, specific and repeatable if the necessary compliance rates of more than 70–80% are to be obtained.

Peer Review The British Thoracic Society has established a peer review scheme in which respiratory departments in one district are visited by two consultants from separate districts in different regions of the country.[34] Consultant members of the British Thoracic Society were asked to volunteer to participate in this scheme. Volunteers agreed to be either visitors or to be visited, but could not express a preference. The pair selected to visit a particular department were provided with a demographic profile of the population served by the hospital and a statistical summary of the workload and facilities available in the department. They were also given a checklist developed specifically for the purpose of the audit or review based on published guidelines and recommendations.[35–37]

After a 2-day visit, during which the visitors were allowed unrestricted access to the department, the hospital and the staff, they gave a verbal report to the visited consultant or consultants. Errors of fact were corrected and the visitors were then asked to submit a written report, which they first showed to the visited consultant(s), to the coordinator of the review within 1 month.

Twenty-one reviews and reports were completed in the first round[34] and a further 35 reviews took place during 1997.[38] Both reviewers and reviewed have commented upon how much they learned from the visits, how they were able to exchange ideas and good practices and how problems, often recognized by the local physicians, were highlighted in a supportive way by the visitors.

It is clear that colleagues in respiratory medicine in British hospitals are generally working extremely hard and providing by and large an extremely good service. Their workload reflects the fact that respiratory diseases are responsible for 25% of acute medical admissions, 20% of new medical out-patient consultations and account for an enormous load of morbidity and mortality in society.[36]

The confidential intra-professional approach has allowed frank constructive exchanges. Inadequate staffing levels and facilities and whether or not the department uses national or local guidelines and protocols for the management of common disorders, including asthma,[19–22] can be discussed and identified. To determine whether or not the peer reviews have any impact on the provision of the service, changes that had occurred, if any, were evaluated 1 year after the visit.

Assessment and Improvement

Monitoring allows the identification and assessment of problems. Further analysis will suggest possible ways of improving and correcting the problems. When the cause of the problems is unclear this should stimulate questions and research (Fig. 51.2) with the aims of determining the cause and suggesting improvements.

Improvements can be achieved by re-education, retraining, facilitation in small groups, or by more active persuasion. Four examples that exemplify this are discussed below.

Example 1 Compared with earlier British studies[8,11] the most recent study of asthma deaths[16] has shown improved routine treatment (appropriate in 59%), improved objective monitoring with PEF measurement (adequate in 65%), but continuing deficiencies in advice, education and written management plans given to patients. Most striking was the finding that 80% of patients had psychological or social factors considered to have had an important bearing on the patient's death from asthma. This confidential enquiry has been ongoing in Norfolk since 1988. In 1989 there were ten deaths from asthma in patients aged under 65 years. In 1997 there were none. As a result of the enquiry the following changes have been introduced into the process of care:

(1) A joint clinic has been established by a chest physician and a liaison psychiatrist, to see people with asthma who have, or are suspected of having, psychological problems. The aim is to detect and hopefully help correct behaviour and attitudes that make asthma control much more difficult.

(2) When patients thought to be at risk from dying from asthma because of their psychosocial background fail to attend clinic appointments, attempts are made to contact them in their own home at a time convenient to them by a respiratory liaison nurse.

(3) We now seek to interview the next of kin of such "at-risk" patients with the patient at the clinic review in the same way as we always see the parents of children with asthma.

(4) Features found to be characteristic of patients at high risk for death from asthma and recommendations for managing such patients have been circulated to all general practitioners in the region.[16]

Example 2 In the in-patient asthma audit[2] problems were revealed with the recording of a check on inhaler technique in patients before their discharge from hospital and in patients being discharged from hospital

before their diurnal PEF variability had fallen to the recommended level.

To address the first of these, a rubber stamp was introduced for use on the patient's PEF chart. This required the signature of a trained nurse or doctor to state that they had checked the patient's inhaler technique. This, with further encouragement from senior medical and nursing staff, resulted in a significant improvement in this parameter being recorded. Adherence to the PEF variability criterion was improved by relaxing the criterion following publication of the National Guidelines,[17] by encouragement from senior medical staff, and by the requirement to specify in the notes the reason why patients were discharged before their diurnal variability had fallen to 25% or less, when this occurred.

Re-monitoring the service demonstrated marked improvement in both areas.[2] This improvement has been maintained in subsequent audits.

Example 3 The results of the multicentre audit of in-patient asthma care[27] were fed back to the coordinators in each hospital so that the results of their own hospital were identified and could be compared with the overall results. Disappointingly, the second audit one year later showed no significant improvement in any of the criteria audited.[28] This led to the following suggestions. All patients admitted with asthma should be admitted according to a protocol agreed by the local chest physicians. They should be transferred to the local chest physician's care within 24 hours of admission during the week and on Monday following the weekend. All patients requiring hospital outpatient follow-up should be seen by a respiratory physician or a member of the respiratory team. Furthermore, purchasers could help significantly in this area of quality by requiring explicitly that all patients with asthma seen in the hospital should be cared for in this way.

One result from the British Thoracic Society multicentre audit of in-patient asthma care has been the recognition that the detection of pulsus paradoxus as a sign indicative of severe asthma is of little or no value.[39] Paradox was recorded in 41% of patients and in under 5% of them was paradox of 10 mmHg or greater the only abnormal measurement. The recommendation to measure paradox and use levels of 10 mmHg or greater as an indicator of severe asthma in the original British Guidelines[20] has been dropped from the subsequent revisions.[21,22]

Example 4 The reports from the peer reviews have been sent by local physicians to their hospital management. There were numerous references to excellent services, dedicated staff and strong leadership. There were on average ten key recommendations per report. These included increased staffing, improved accommodation, new or additional equipment, service developments, improved organization, liaison and communication and improved training. A total of 52% of these recommendations required significant resources to implement. Of a further 301 "adverse" factors mentioned in the reports only 36% required significant resources to implement. One year after the 1992 reviews 38% of the key recommendations had been achieved, 15% were imminent, 38% were still thought necessary and 9% were considered unimportant or impracticable.[34]

Further Monitoring and Assessment

Clearly after the first monitoring and assessment, attempts at improvement can only be evaluated by repeated monitoring and assessment and in this way the audit loop is closed. Experience suggests that once satisfactory care is achieved further audits at regular intervals are required to maintain a high-quality service and once again recognition of high quality will be praised and rewarded.

CONCLUSIONS

Some measures of the structure, process and outcome of ambulatory and inpatient asthma care that are amenable to audit are listed in Table 51.8.

Asthma audit, like quality assurance, can be used to maintain and improve high-quality services and to assess and improve aspects of care where there are problems. To undertake such audits and to achieve the potential benefits, resources of information technology, time and money are required. In industry between 1 and 3% of turnover is spent on quality assurance.

Table 51.8: Measures in asthma care that are amenable to audit. (Modified from Harrison BDW. Audit in respiratory disease. *Respir Med* 1991; 85 (suppl. B): 47–51, with permission)

Structure of respiratory care[35-37]

Medical staff
  Senior
  Middle grade
  Pre-registration

Nursing staff
  Trained
  Untrained

Outpatient clinic facilities
Beds
Secretarial and administrative support
Pulmonary function laboratory facilities
Bronchoscopy facilities
Access to imaging facilities, ICU, pathology

Some measures of the process of outpatient asthma care[19,21,22]

Evidence of written action/management plan
Evidence of step-wise management
Recorded checks on inhaler technique
Evidence of PEF chart
Treatment
  Short-acting inhaled bronchodilator used regularly or as needed.
  Regular inhaled steroids   Y/N Dose
  Regular inhaled long-acting bronchodilator   Y/N Dose

Table 51.8: Measures in asthma care that are amenable to audit. (Modified from Harrison BDW. Audit in respiratory disease. *Respir Med* 1991; 85 (suppl. B): 47–51, with permission) (*contd.*)

Regular oral bronchodilator	Y/N Type Dose
Maintenance oral steroids	Y/N Dose
Theophylline levels monitored in patients on oral theophyllines	
Recorded evidence of spacer use if inhaled steroid dose exceeds 800 µg daily	

Smoking
   Active: current/ex/never
   Passive

Some outcome measures for outpatient asthma care[19,21,22,40]

Symptoms
   Nocturnal wakening
   Time off school/work

Pulmonary function
   PEF
     Actual value
     Best in previous 2–5 years
   FEV_1
     Actual value
     Best in previous 2–5 years
   Home PEF >80% of best
   Maximum diurnal variation in last week/month/3 months <25%

Treatment and its appropriateness to symptoms and function

Regular inhaled steroids	Y/N Daily dose
Regular bronchodilator	Y/N Daily dose
Maintenance oral steroids	Y/N Daily dose
Boosts of oral steroid/courses of oral steroids during previous month/in last year	
Number of β agonist inhalers per month	

Events
   Emergency visits to accident and emergency department in last month/year
   Urgent (unplanned) calls to, or visit to or from, GP in last month/year
   Admissions to hospital with asthma in last month/year
   Death

Some measures of the process and outcome of inpatient asthma care[19-23]

Objective assessment of severity
   PEF
   Heart rate
   Respiratory rate
   Presence/absence of cyanosis
   Oxygen saturation/blood gases

Treatment
   Systemic steroids
   High-dose β agonists inhaled/intravenous

Pre-discharge
   PEF diurnal variation <25%
   Written check on inhaler technique
   Oral steroid to take home
   Attempts to identify, and if possible correct, events preceding admission

Post-discharge
  PEF meter for home monitoring
  Treatment "stepped up" compared with maintenance therapy before admission
  Written management plan
  Follow-up appointment

Outcome
  Death
  Re-admission within 8 weeks

FEV$_1$: forced expiratory volume in 1 s; ICU: intensive care unit; PEF: peak expiratory flow.

KEY POINTS

1 Medical audit is the process of recognizing and maintaining high-quality services and identifying areas of less than optimal quality and then taking steps to improve them.

2 Sentinal case audit is best exemplified by an ongoing confidential enquiry into asthma deaths.

3 Criterion-based audit requires agreed standards with which actual practice can be compared. National guidelines and local protocols can provide these and are also of value in sentinal-case audits.

4 Repeat audits (closing the feedback loop) have demonstrated improvements in the processes of asthma care.

5 Audits of hospital in-patient practice and of asthma care in general practice have demonstrated high-quality care and also areas such as checking and recording inhaler technique, and increasing treatment during exacerbations, where improvements were necessary.

6 Audits of in-patient management of asthma have repeatedly shown significant differences between the care provided by chest physicians and that provided by general physicians.

7 Most asthmatic patients requiring hospital management and most of their general practitioners opt, wherever possible, for care under respiratory physicians.

8 High-quality *optimal* care may be expensive, but frequently low-quality care is even more expensive.

9 Asthma audit is the responsibility of the health-care professionals involved in the care of patients with asthma. It requires commitment from senior staff and will contribute to the service becoming attractive to high-quality staff.

Investment on that scale in clinical audit would transform the way our health care is delivered.

Asthma is the commonest chronic disease affecting all age groups in the developed world. Why are patients still dying unnecessarily? Why are so many patients admitted when well-established treatment strategies could have prevented those admissions? Why in survey after survey are so many patients with asthma still waking at night and still failing to lead full and unlimited lives?

High-quality excellent care is not necessarily the most expensive care. High-quality care may be expensive, but frequently low-quality care is even more expensive in terms of death, preventable morbidity and the time, hassle and litigation involved in dealing with complaints and with professional staff not performing at an acceptable level.

Asthma audit is our responsibility, the responsibility of respiratory physicians, nurses, physiotherapists, pharmacists and other health-care professionals involved in the care of patients with asthma. To be most effective professionals involved in audit need support and rewards, not sanctions. It obviously requires commitment from the senior staff, who then enable high standards and high quality to permeate throughout the system that they lead. When this happens such departments and services become "magnetic" and attract high-quality staff and provide care that is both rewarding to the patient and to those delivering and purchasing that care.

Medical audit fosters and supports the altruism of physicians wishing to provide the best possible care for their patients with asthma. It also stimulates us to maintain high-quality standards. It fosters both the effectiveness and efficiency of the service that we provide to the population of patients we serve. It helps us to ensure that patients with asthma under our care receive optimal care, that we are not denying them effective care and that we are avoiding unnecessary risks when we provide that care.

Finally, audit gives us information with which to defend ourselves against criticism and to support our claims for additional resources.

REFERENCES

1. Harrison BDW. Audit in respiratory disease. *Respir Med* 1991; 85 (suppl. B): 47–51.

2. Lim KL, Harrison BDW. A criterion based audit of inpatient asthma care. Closing the feedback loop. *J R Coll Physicians Lond* 1992; 26: 71–5.

3. Cochrane GM, Clark TJH. A survey of asthma mortality in patients between ages 35 and 64 in the Greater London hospitals. *Thorax* 1975; 30: 300–5.

4. MacDonald JB, Seaton A, Williams DA. Asthma deaths in Cardiff 1963–74: 90 deaths outside hospital. *BMJ* 1976; 1: 1493–5.

5. MacDonald JB, MacDonald ET, Seaton A, Williams DA. Asthma deaths in Cardiff 1963–74: 53 deaths in hospital. *BMJ* 1976; 2: 721–3.

6. Bateman JRM, Clarke SW. Sudden death in asthma. *Thorax* 1979; 34: 40–4.

7. Ormerod LP, Stableforth DE. Asthma mortality in Birmingham 1975–7: 53 deaths. *BMJ* 1980; 280: 687–90.

8. ○ British Thoracic Association. Death from asthma in two regions of England. *BMJ* 1982; 285: 1251–5.

9. Sears MR, Rea HH, Beaglehole RG *et al*. Asthma mortality in New Zealand: a two year national study. *NZ Med J* 1985; 98: 271–5.

10. Rea HH, Scragg R, Jackson R *et al*. A case-control study of deaths from asthma. *Thorax* 1986; 41: 833–9.

11. Eason J, Markowe HLJ. Controlled investigation of deaths from asthma in hospital in the North East Thames region. *BMJ* 1987; 294: 1255–8.

12. Robertson C, Rubinfeld AR, Bowes G. Deaths from asthma in Victoria: a 12 month survey. *Med J Aust* 1990; 152: 511–17.

13. Wareham NJ, Harrison BDW, Jenkins PF, Nicholls J, Stableforth DE. A district confidential enquiry into deaths due to asthma. *Thorax* 1993; 48: 1117–20.

14. ✪ Campbell DA, McLennan G, Coates JR *et al.* A comparison of asthma deaths and near-fatal asthma attacks in South Australia. *Eur Respir J* 1994; 7: 490–7.

15. Somerville M, Ryland I, Williams EMI, Pearson MG. Asthma deaths in Mersey in 1989–90. *J Pub Health Med* 1995; 17: 397–403.

16. ✪ Mohan G, Harrison BDW, Badminton RM *et al.* A confidential enquiry into deaths caused by asthma in an English health region: implications for general practice. *Br J Gen Pract* 1996; 46: 529–32.

17. Department of Health. *Report on British Confidential Enquiries into Maternal Deaths in the UK 1985–7.* London: Department of Health, 1991.

18. Campling EA, Devlin HB, Hoile RW, Lunn JN. *The Report of the National Confidential Enquiry into Perioperative Deaths.* London: National Confidential Enquiry into Perioperative Deaths, 1992.

19. Statement by the British Thoracic Society, Research Unit of the Royal College of Physicians of London, King's Fund Centre, National Asthma Campaign. Guidelines for management of asthma in adults: I. Chronic persistent asthma. *BMJ* 1990; 301: 651–3.

20. Statement by the British Thoracic Society, Research Unit of the Royal College of Physicians of London, King's Fund Centre, National Asthma Campaign. Guidelines for management of asthma in adults: II. Acute severe asthma. *BMJ* 1990; 301: 797–800.

21. Guidelines on the management of asthma. *BMJ* 1993; 306: 776–82 and *Thorax* 1993; 48: S1–S24.

22. ✪ The British Guidelines on Asthma Management. 1995 Review and position statement. British Thoracic Society and others. *Thorax* 1997; 52: S1–S21.

23. ✪ Neville RG, Clark RG, Hoskins G, Smith B. National asthma attack audit 1991–2. *BMJ* 1993; 306: 559–62.

24. ✪ Feder G, Griffiths C, Highton C, Eldridge S, Spence M, Southgate L. Do clinical guidelines introduced with practice based education improve care of asthma and diabetic patients: A randomised controlled trial in general practices in East London. *BMJ* 1996; 311: 1473–78.

25. Neville RG, Hoskins G, Smith B, Clark RA. Observations on the structure, process and clinical outcomes of asthma care in general practice. *Br J Gen Pract* 1996; 46: 583–7.

26. Neville RG, Hoskins G, Smith B, Clark RA. How general practitioners manage acute asthma attacks. *Thorax* 1997; 52: 152–6.

27. ✪ Pearson MG, Ryland I, Harrison BDW. A national audit of acute severe asthma in adults admitted to hospital. *Qual Health Care* 1995; 4: 24–36.

28. Pearson MG, Ryland I, Harrison BDW. Comparison of the process of care of acute severe asthma in adults admitted to hospital before and 1 year after the publication of national guidelines. *Respir Med* 1996; 90: 539–45.

29. Osman J, Ormerod LP, Stableforth DE. Management of acute asthma: a survey of hospital practice and comparison between thoracic and general physicians in Birmingham and Manchester. *Br J Dis Chest* 1987; 81: 232–41.

30. Bucknall CE, Robertson C, Moran F, Stevenson RD. Differences in hospital asthma management. *Lancet* 1988; i: 748–50.

31. Baldwin DR, Ormerod LP, Mackay AD, Stableforth DE. Changes in hospital management of acute severe asthma by thoracic and general physicians in Birmingham and Manchester during 1978 and 1985. *Thorax* 1990; 45: 130–4.

32. Bell D, Layton AJ, Gabbay J. Use of a guideline based questionnaire to audit hospital care of acute asthma. *BMJ* 1991; 302: 1440–3.

33. Bucknall CE, Robertson C, Moran F, Stevenson RD. Improving management of asthma: closing the loop or progressing along the audit spiral? *Qual Health Care* 1992; 1: 15–20.

34. ✪ Page RL, Harrison BDW. Setting up interdepartmental peer review. The British Thoracic Society scheme. *J R Coll Physicians* 1995; 29: 319–24.

35. Muers MF, Chappell AG, Farebrother M, Farrow SC, Harrison BDW, Laszlo G. Facilities for the diagnosis of respiratory disease in the UK. *J R Coll Physicians* 1988; 22: 180–4.

36. Pearson MG, Littler J, Davies PDO. Analysis of medical workload–evidence of patient to specialist mismatch. *J R Coll Physicians* 1994; 28: 230–4.

37. Corris P, Page R, Rudolf M, Wolstenholme R. *Requirements for Good Practice in Respiratory Medicine.*

London: British Thoracic Society, 1993.

38. Page RL. The BTS interdepartmental peer review scheme. Update. *BTS Newsletter* 1998; 9: 4.

39. Pearson MG, Spence DPS, Ryland I, Harrison BDW. Value of pulsus paradoxus in assessing acute severe asthma. *BMJ* 1993; 307: 659.

40. Connolly CK. Management of asthma in outpatients. *J R Coll Physicians* 1983; 17: 115–20.

Chapter 52

Economics in Asthma

Sean Sullivan, Scott Ramsey, and Kevin Weiss

INTRODUCTION

Public and private health-care systems are developing methods to minimize the cost of managing chronic diseases while maintaining high quality care for their member-populations. The goals of minimizing cost and ensuring quality often are in conflict, particularly in the era of budget constraints. The tension arises because public and private coverage of health care creates incentives for patients (and often providers) to consume care with little regard for price. Decision-makers must select disease management strategies that balance the need for fiscal responsibility with patients' desire to obtain the most technologically advanced and beneficial care. Because the process of allocating scarce resources among medical treatments can be emotional and politically charged, decision-makers would prefer to turn to rational and consistent methods of evaluation designed to maximize health for expenditure. Health economic analysis is one tool that has been developed to serve this need.

The purpose of this chapter is to briefly define the methods and uses of economic evaluation studies, to review the literature on the cost-effectiveness of asthma interventions, and to evaluate the implications of health economic studies.

BASICS OF HEALTH ECONOMIC ANALYSIS

We focus on cost-effectiveness analysis as the gold standard for economic evaluation and refer the reader to Drummond *et al.* for a detailed treatise on the methods.[1] Cost-effectiveness analysis can be defined as a set of research methods to assess and quantify the costs and clinical consequences of medical care treatments in order to estimate the "value" of an inter-

vention in relation to alternatives. Pharmacoeconomic analysis is cost-effectiveness analysis as applied to drug therapies for disease. A cost-effectiveness analysis of competing medical treatments should incorporate evidence on the clinical consequences (efficacy and safety) and total medical costs of treatment alternatives.[2]

Cost-effectiveness analysis is derived from a single equation that integrates all medical costs and outcomes into a comparative incremental ratio.

$$\text{Incremental cost-effectiveness ratio} = \frac{\text{Cost}_A - \text{Cost}_B}{\text{Effectiveness}_A - \text{Effectiveness}_B}$$

The equation shows a hypothetical cost-effectiveness comparison of two therapies, A (usually the new technology) and B (the established therapy or usual care). The incremental cost-effectiveness of A is the attributable health benefit of A relative to the incremental level of health-care expenditure for A when compared with the outcomes and costs of B. The measure of effectiveness (denominator in the equation) in a cost-effectiveness study of asthma interventions is a measure of benefit that is most suitable to the study. Here, health outcomes of treatments are expressed in "natural" units such as symptom-free days, improvement in peak expiratory flow or years of life saved. These denominators have the advantage of being readily identifiable and unambiguous aspects of a disease that are clearly affected by the treatments in question. However, important outcomes beyond the selected effectiveness measure that may also be affected by the treatment (e.g. quality of life) are ignored. A recent report by the NHLBI Workshop on Asthma Outcome Measures for Research Studies provides a useful review of the many end-points available to researchers who study asthma.[3]

As important to asthma health policy as cost-effectiveness analyses, cost-of-illness studies seek to estimate the economic burden of a disease to society. Cost-of-illness studies are not true economic evaluations, since they do not compare alternative treatments. Still, they are commonly performed as a way to raise awareness regarding the economic consequences of illnesses, particularly those where the impact on society may be undervalued by health-care policy makers and the public. For example, the often-cited study by Weiss and colleagues on the economic impact of asthma found that this "mild" chronic illness accounted for $6.2 billion in societal costs during 1990. Furthermore, more than $1 billion of these costs were as a consequence of lost days of school in children affected with the disease.[4] The literature is now replete with papers characterizing the cost-of-asthma in various countries and on select populations.[5–11]

ECONOMIC EVALUATION STUDIES OF ASTHMA INTERVENTIONS

There are a number of economic analyses of asthma interventions, but none of these meet the agreed standards for economic evaluation in health care.[12] Health economic evaluation is an evolving science. Still, there are several reasons to establish standard methods of economic evaluation. Drummond and colleagues give the following rationale for establishing standards: (1) to maintain high methodological standards; (2) to facilitate the comparison of the results of economic evaluations for different health-care interventions; and (3) to facilitate interpretation of study findings from health-care setting to setting.[13–19] The latter issue occurs both within countries with diverse health delivery systems (such as the US) and for international interpretation of studies. The National Asthma Education and Prevention Program Task Force on the Cost-effectiveness, Quality and Financing of Asthma Care has issued recommendations for cost-effectiveness evaluation of asthma interventions.[20] These recommendations include suggestions for endpoint selection, time horizon, and selection of comparators.

We now present the literature on the economics of asthma interventions by describing the studies on asthma pharmacotherapies, education programmes and other interventions.

Pharmacotherapy

Tables 52.1 and 52.2 summarize some of the important retrospective and prospective health economic evaluations of asthma pharmacotherapy.

Corticosteroids and Leukotriene Antagonists

There is substantial evidence of the positive clinical effects of combining inhaled corticosteroids with bronchodilator therapy for the management of persistent asthma.[21] This literature supports the current global recommendations for treatment. An important and as yet not fully explored research question is whether the recommendations – inhaled corticosteroids in combination with bronchodilators – are cost-effective in the treatment of mild-to-moderate or moderate-to-severe asthma.

The paper by Adelroth and Thompson examined the relationship between use of high-dose inhaled budesonide (800 μg per day) and asthma-related in-patient hospital days in 36 oral steroid-dependent patients with asthma over a 5-year period.[22] Direct medical care costs per patient declined by over 55% per year for up to 3 years after the initiation of inhaled budesonide.

Gerdtham and colleagues further investigated the benefits of inhaled steroids by associating drug consumption patterns and hospital days in 14 Swedish counties over an 11-year period.[23] The study did indicate a strong negative association between use of inhaled corticosteroids and hospital-bed-days for asthma. An approximate cost-benefit ratio was developed from the multivariate models suggestive of positive economic benefits in excess of costs on the order of between 1.5:1.0 and 2.8:1.0, depending on the analytic model.

Donahue and others, using a retrospective cohort design, evaluated 16 941 persons with asthma to determine if inhaled steroid treatment reduced the risk of asthma hospitalization.[24] The overall relative risk of hospitalization among those who received inhaled steroids was 0.5 (95% C I, 0.4–0.6) after adjusting for β-agonist use. The protective effect of inhaled steroids was most marked in persons with greatest prior β-agonist use.

Several recent studies have employed experimental research designs to investigate the cost effectiveness of inhaled corticosteroids and leukotriene antagonists.[25–33] These data are summarized in Table 52.2. While not completely comprehensive, this table provides an

Table 52.1: Non-randomized health economic studies of asthma pharmacotherapy

First author, year	Study method used	Sample size	Perspective	Treatments studied	Length of study	Costs measured	Health outcomes measured	Economic outcomes
Adelroth, 1988	Retrospective; pre/post quasi-experimental design	36 adults	Societal	Budesonide	5 years; 2 years pre, 3 years post	Direct	Reduction in need for oral steroid after introduction of inhaled budesonide	Estimated 55% reduction in direct costs
Ross, 1988	Retrospective; pre/post quasi-experimental design	53	Health system	2 groups: cromolyn users and non-users	3.2 to 3.8 years[b]	Direct	None	Estimated 92–96% reduction in health services use
Perera, 1995	Prospective pre/post quasi-experimental design	86 children	Societal	2-groups: various doses of beclomethasone and budesonide	4 years	Direct	Reduction in acute severe attacks, hospital admissions, breakthrough wheezing, missed school days, and treatment satisfaction.	Estimated 83% reduction in total costs of care; $0.04 per unit increase in patient satisfaction with treatment.
Gerdtham, 1996	Retrospective; econometric model	[a]	Societal	All inhaled corticosteroids	11 years	Direct	Reduction in hospital bed days and discharges for asthma	Estimated benefit: cost ratio of between 1.5:1 and 2.8:1
Donahue, 1997	Retrospective; cohort design	16,941	Health system	All inhaled steroids	3 years	Resource use only	Reduction in hospital admissions	Estimated 50% relative reduction in hospital admissions among persons using inhaled steroids.

[a] Unit of analysis is counties and not persons. The study represents a total of 71% of the Swedish population. [b] Cromolyn users contributed 3.2 years of data and non-users of Cromolyn contributed 3.8 years of data.

Table 52.2: Randomized health economic studies of asthma pharmacotherapy

First author, year	Study method used	Sample size	Perspective	Treatments studied	Length of study	Costs measured	Health outcomes measured	Economic outcomes
Schulpher, 1993	Randomized controlled trial	145 adults	Health system	2-groups: salmeterol and placebo	12 weeks	Direct	Episode-free days	No statistically significant difference in clinical effectiveness thus a cost-outcome was not calculated
Campbell, 1993	Randomized controlled trial	556 adults	Health system	2 groups: budesonide 400 µg compared to budesonide 800 µg	12 weeks	Direct	Lung function (FEV_1) and symptoms	Not cost-effective to increase dose of budesonide from 400 µg to 800 µg in mild to moderate patients
Connett, 1993	Randomized controlled trial	40 children	Societal	2 groups: budesonide compared to placebo	26 weeks	Direct and indirect	Lung function (FEV_1), symptoms, symptom-free days	Budesonide is dominant therapy; saved $9.43 for each symptom-free day gained
Rutten-van Molken, 1993	Randomized controlled trial	116 children	Societal	2 groups: budesonide and salbutamol, salbutamol alone	3 years[a]	Direct and indirect	Lung function (FEV_1), symptom-free days, school absences	Budesonide is cost-effective; $83 per 10% improvement in FEV_1, $4.75 per symptom-free day gained
Rutten-van Molken, 1995	Randomized controlled trial	274 adults	Societal	3 groups: beclomethasone and terbutaline, ipatropium and terbutaline, terbutaline alone	2.5 years	Direct and indirect	Lung function (FEV_1, PC_{20}), symptom-free days	Beclomethasone is cost-effective; $201 per 10% improvement in FEV_1, $5 per symptom-free day gained. Ipatropium is not cost-effective.
O'Byrne, 1996	Randomized controlled trial	57 adults	Societal	3 groups: budesonide 400 µg or 800 µg and bronchodilator compared to bronchodilator alone	16 weeks	Direct	Lung function (PEFR), symptom scores, exacerbations, emergency room visits and willingness to pay	Budesonide is cost-beneficial at 400 µg per day but not at 800 µg per day compared to bronchodilator alone
Booth, 1996	Randomized controlled trial	225 children	Societal	2 groups: sodium cromoglycate 20 mg QID compared to fluticasone 50 µg BID	8 weeks	Direct	Lung function (PEFR), symptom scores, and the probability of successful treatment	Fluticasone is cost-effective compared to sodium cromoglycate. CE ratios vary according to outcome measure selected.
Suissa, 1997	Randomized controlled trial	146 adults	Health system	2 groups: zafirlukast 20 mg BID and bronchodilator compared to bronchodilator alone	13 weeks	Resource use only	Symptom-free days, asthma episodes, health-care resource use.	Treatment with zafirlukast reduced the rate of symptom days, absence from school or work and health care contacts.
Barnes, 1999	Pooled analysis of 7 RCTs	Not stated	Health system	2 groups: budesonide, fluticasone propionate	Varied from 4 to 12 weeks	Direct	Lung function (PEFR), probability of successful treatment, symptom-free day, and episode-free day.	Fluticasone is cost-effective and may be cost saving when compared to budesonide.

[a] The study had a planned 3-year follow-up but only 39 patients reached a follow-up period of 22 months.

account of the main papers in the field. The over-arching conclusion to be derived from this literature is that treatment with inhaled corticosteroids in moderate-to-severe asthmatics is cost-effective and possibly cost-reducing when compared to β-agonist treatment alone. This result has been shown in both adults and children. There is less evidence to support any comparative economic advantage of one inhaled steroid over another. The data also suggest that the cost-effectiveness of inhaled steroids improves with increasing asthma severity. Thus, targeting effective treatments at patients with high rates of medical care service use or other markers of morbidity can reduce the costs of care, in some cases enough to offset the price of the treatments.

Long-Acting β₂ Agonists

Long-acting bronchodilators such as formoterol and salmeterol represent a relatively new approach to pro-phylactic and symptomatic treatment for asthma. Only one published study has simultaneously evaluated the impact of a long-acting agent on clinical and economic outcomes for patients with asthma.[34] In this paper, the authors reported on a retrospective cost-effectiveness analysis of a clinical trial of 145 patients diagnosed with asthma and randomized to receive 12 weeks of maintenance therapy with either long-acting formo-terol or short-acting albuterol. The primary clinical outcome measure was cumulative symptom-free days over the 12-week period. The authors concluded that there were no statistically significant differences in symptom-free days between the two treatment groups.

Inhaled Cromolyn Sodium

Ross and co-workers made use of patient and health services records in one large group practice to estimate the economic consequences of including cromolyn sodium in the treatment regimen of asthma patients.[35] A total of 53 patients were retrospectively identified from medical records and categorized into two groups: those who received cromolyn sodium for at least 1 year ($n=27$) and those who received no cromolyn sodium as part of the treatment regimen ($n=26$). Patients receiving cromolyn sodium provided an average of 3.2 years of health service utilization data, and those in the comparison group provided 3.8 years of data. Medication costs for patients on cromolyn sodium were slightly higher ($27.90 per month) than for the control group ($25.20 per month). However, emergency department and hospital costs declined significantly for cromolyn

sodium patients; after the change in medication, they experienced a 96% reduction in the rate of emergency department visits and a 92% reduction in the rate of hospital admissions. The authors made no direct mea-surement of outcomes of therapy and did not control for symptom severity or other baseline confounding that might partly explain differences in the results.

In spite of this growing literature, a number of clini-cally important questions regarding economic impact of drug therapies remain unanswered. Is early inter-vention in mild asthma cost-effective? That is, will the addition of anti-inflammatory therapy early in the course of mild asthma alter the progression of disease enough to justify the high costs of therapy? Will com-bination therapy (long-acting β agonist and inhaled steroids) be more cost-effective than less intensive treat-ment? Will treating allergy and asthma concomitantly improve the cost-effectiveness of pharmacologic inter-ventions? Will new biopharmaceuticals that show promise in asthma be priced in a way that allows access to potentially cost-effective therapies?

ASTHMA PATIENT EDUCATION PROGRAMMES

Several reports document the clinical and economic impact of patient-oriented asthma education pro-grammes. Educational interventions have included formal classroom-based medication compliance pro-grammes and asthma self-management programmes for adults and children and their parents. In general, economic evaluations of these programmes have been quite favourable, in particular when the programmes have been directed at high-risk patients or those with documented resource-intensive care needs (such as a prior hospitalization).[36–45] In a recent comprehensive (but small; $n=66$) study, Neri and colleagues conducted a prospective randomized trial comparing asthma event rates and costs before and after two education programmes: a "complete programme" that included classroom-type lessons and a "reduced programme" that included educational brochures but no formal instruction.[46] The study included cost-benefit and cost-effectiveness analyses. Compared with the year prior to the intervention, asthma-related events (attacks, medical examinations, admissions) fell significantly in the year following the evaluation for both programmes. Comparing the years pre- and post-intervention, the cost-benefit calculations revealed a cost savings of

$1181 for the complete programme and $1028 for the reduced programme. The value of asthma-related work loss was included in the calculations.

SPECIALIST CARE

Other analyses have examined the economic impact of referrals of moderate-to-severe asthmatics to specialists.[47] In retrospective chart reviews, these studies find significant reductions in sick office visits, ER visits, hospital days, and costs of care for patients. Most of these analyses, however, suffered from poor design and evaluation methods. Flaws included: failing to include the cost of the intervention; inadequate specification of the time horizon for treatment; lack of adjustment for potential confounding in patient selection; and most importantly, failure to include a control group.

CONCLUSION

Health-care decision-makers are interested in employing rational approaches to allocating scarce resources. Many embrace economic evaluations as a set of tools to improve decision-making in asthma care, given the conflicts generated by constrained health budgets and a rising demand for medical care. However, before health economic data can be integrated into the decision making process the methodologic standards of these studies must improve and common measures of outcome (such as symptom free days) must be incorporated. High standards will ensure that the internal and external validity of these studies is apparent to decision-makers and researchers and that the results

between studies are comparable. We have the tools to control asthma and most of these interventions are cost-effective. But these interventions need to be fully integrated into usual clinical practice so that the health-care system can realize the potential economic benefits.[48]

KEY POINTS

1. Treatment with inhaled corticosteroids in moderate to severe asthmatics is cost-effective and possibly cost-reducing when compared to β-agonist treatment alone.

2. Economic evaluations of asthma education programmes have been judged to be cost-beneficial, in particular when the programmes have been directed at high-risk patients or those with documented resource-intensive care needs (such as a prior hospitalization).

3. Analyses have examined the economic impact of referral of moderate-to-severe asthmatics to specialist care. These studies are inconclusive with respect to cost-effectiveness.

4. Before cost-effectiveness studies of asthma interventions can be integrated into the decision making process, the methodologic standards of these studies must improve and common measures of outcome must be incorporated.

REFERENCES

1. ✪ Drummond MF, O'Brien BJ, Stoddart GL, Torrance GW. *Methods for the Economic Evaluation of Health Care Programmes*, 2nd edn New York: Oxford University Press, 1997.

2. Banta HD, Luce BR. *Health Care Technology and its Assessment*. New York: Oxford University Press, 1993.

3. ✪ National Heart, Lung and Blood Institute: Asthma outcome measures. *Am J Respir Crit Care Med* 1994b; 149 (2): S1–S90.

4. Weiss KB, Gergen PJ, Hodgson TA. An economic evaluation of asthma in the United States. *N Engl J Med* 1992; 326: 862–6.

5. Sullivan SD. Cost and cost-effectiveness in asthma: use of pharmacoeconomics to assess the value of asthma interventions. *Immunol Allergy Clin N Am* 1996; 16 (4): 819–39.

6. Szucs TD, Anderhub H, Rutishauser M. The economic burden of asthma: direct and indirect costs in Switzerland. *Eur Respir J* 1999; 13: 281–6.

7. Graf von der Schulenburg JM, Greiner W, Molitor S, Kielhorn A. Cost of asthma therapy in relation to severity. *Med Klin* 1996; 91: 670–76.

8. Smith DH, Malone DC, Lawson KA, Okamoto LJ, Battista C, Saunders WB. A national estimate of the economic costs of asthma. *Am J Respir Crit Care Med* 1997 Sep; 156(3 Pt 1): 787–93.

9. Chew FT, Goh DY, Lee BW. The economic cost of asthma in Singapore. *Aust NZ J Med* 1999; 29(2): 228–33.

10. Lozano P, Sullivan SD, Smith DH, Weiss KB. The economic burden of asthma in U.S. children: estimates from the national medical expenditure survey. *J Allergy Clin Immunol* 1999; 104(4): 957–63.

11. Krahn MD, Berka C, Langlois P, Detsky AS. Direct and indirect costs of asthma in Canada, 1990. *CMAJ* 1996; 154(6): 821–31.

12. ❂ Gold MR, Siegel JE, Russell LB, Weinstein MC. *Cost-effectiveness in Health and Medicine*. New York, NY: Oxford University Press, 1996.

13. Drummond M, Brandt A, Luce B, Rovira J. Standardizing methodologies for economic evaluation in health care: practice, problems, and potential. *Int J Technol Assess Health Care* 1993; 9: 26–36.

14. Levenson T, Grammer LC, Yarnold PR, Patterson R. Cost-effective management of malignant potentially fatal asthma. *Allergy Asthma Proc* 1997; 18 (2): 73–8.

15. Windsor R, Bailey W, Richards J *et al.* Evaluation of the efficacy and cost-effectiveness of health education methods to increase medication adherence among adults with asthma. *Am J Public Health* 1990; 80: 1519–21.

16. Deter H. Cost-benefit analysis of psychosomatic therapy in asthma. *Psychosom Res* 1986; 30: 173–82.

17. Folgering H, Rooyakkers J, Herwaarden C. Education and cost/benefit ratios in pulmonary patients. *Monaldi Arch Chest Dis* 1994; 49 (2): 166–8.

18. Sondergaard B, Davidsen F, Kirkeby B *et al.* The economics of an intensive education programme for asthmatic patients. *Pharmacoeconomics* 1992; 1: 207–12.

19. Tougaard L, Krone T, Sorknaes A, Ellegaard H. Economic benefits of teaching patients with chronic obstructive pulmonary disease about their illness. *Lancet* 1992; 339: 1517–20.

20. ❂ Sullivan SD, Elixhauser A, Buist AS, Luce BR, Eisenberg J, Weiss KB. National Asthma Education and Prevention Program working group report on the cost effectiveness of asthma care. *Am J Respir Crit Care Med.* 1996; 154(3 Pt 2): S84–95.

21. Barnes PJ, Pedersen S. Efficacy and safety of inhaled corticosteroids in asthma. *Am Rev Resp Dis* 1993; 148(4 Pt 2): S1–S26.

22. Adelroth E, Thompson S. Advantages of high-dose inhaled budesonide. *Lancet* 1988; 1(8583): 476.

23. Gerdtham UG, Hertzman P, Boman G, Jonsson B. Impact of inhaled corticosteroids on asthma hospitalization in Sweden. *App Econ* 1996; 28: 1591–9.

24. ❂ Donahue JG, Weiss ST, Livingston JM, Goetsch MA, Greineder DK, Platt R. Inhaled steroids and the risk of hospitalization for asthma. *JAMA* 1997; 277: 887–91.

25. Campbell LM, Simpson RJ, Turbitt ML *et al.* A comparison of the cost-effectiveness of budesonide 400 μg/day and 800 μg/day in the management of mild-to-moderate asthma in general practice. *Br J Med Econ* 1993; 6: 67–74.

26. Rees TP, Lennox B, Timney AP *et al.* Comparison of increasing the dose of budesonide to 800 μg/day with a maintained dose of 400 μg/day in mild to moderate asthmatic patients. *Eur J Clin Res* 1993; 4: 67–77.

27. O'Byrne P, Cuddy L, Taylor DW, Birch S, Morris J, Syrotuik J. Efficacy and cost benefit of inhaled corticosteroids in patients considered to have mild asthma in primary care. *Can Respir J* 1996; 3 (3): 169–75.

28. Connett GJ, Lenney W, McConchie SM. The cost-effectiveness of budesonide in severe asthmatics aged one to three years. *Br J Med Econ* 1993; 6: 127–34.

29. Rutten-van Mölken MP, Van Doorslaer EK, Jansen MC, *et al.* Cost-effectiveness of inhaled corticosteroid plus bronchodilator therapy versus bronchodilator monotherapy in children with asthma. *Pharmaco Economics* 1993; 4 (4): 257–70.

30. Rutten-van Mölken MP, Van Doorslaer EK, Jansen MC, Kerstjens HA, Rutten FF. Costs and effects of inhaled corticosteroids and bronchodilators in asthma and chronic obstructive pulmonary disease. *Am J Respir Crit Care Med* 1995; 151 (4): 975–82.

31. Booth PC, Wells NEJ, Morrison AK. A comparison of the cost effectiveness of alternative prophylactic therapies in childhood asthma. *Pharmaco Economics* 1996; 10 (3): 262–8.

32. Barnes NC, Thwaites RMA, Price MJ. The cost-effectiveness of inhaled fluticasone propionate and budesonide in the treatment of asthma in adults and children. *Respir Med* 1999; 93: 402–407.

33. Suissa S, Dennis R, Ernst P, Sheehy O, Wood-Dauphinee S. Effectiveness of the leukotriene receptor antagonist zafirlukast for mild-to-moderate asthma. A randomized, double-blind, placebo-controlled trial. *Ann Intern Med.* 1997; 126 (3): 177–83.

34. Sculpher M, Buxton M. Episode-free days as endpoints in economic evaluations of asthma therapy. *Pharmaco Economics* 1993; 4 (5): 345–52.

35. Ross RN, Morris M, Sakowitz SR, Berman BA. Cost-effectiveness of including cromolyn sodium in the treatment program for asthma: a retrospective, record-based study. *Clin Ther* 1988; 10 (2): 188–203.

36. Green L. Toward cost-benefit evaluations of health education: some concepts, methods and examples. *Health Edu Monog* 1974; 2: 34–64.

37. Boulet L, Champan K, Green L, FitzGerald J. Asthma education. *Chest* 1994; 106 (4 suppl): 184S–96S.

38. Windsor R, Bailey W, Richards JJ, Manzella B, Soong S, Brooks M. Evaluation of the efficacy and cost effectiveness of health education methods to increase medication adherence among adults with asthma. *Am J Public Health* 1990; 80 (12): 1519–21.

39. Muhlhauser I, Richter B, Kraut D, Weske G, Worth H, Berger M. Evaluation of a structured treatment and teaching program on asthma. *J Intern Med* 1991; 238 (2): 157–64.

40. Trautner C, Richter B, Berger M. Cost-effectiveness of a structured treatment and teaching programme on asthma. *Eur Respir J* 1993; 6 (10): 1485–91.

41. Bolton M, Tilley B, Kuder J, Reeves T, Schultz I. The cost and effectiveness of an education program for adults who have asthma. *J Gen Intern Med* 1991; 6: 401–407.

42. Sondergaard B, Davidsen F, Kirkeby B, *et al.* The economics of an intensive education program for asthmatic patients: a prospective controlled trial. *Pharmaco Economics* 1992; 1: 207–212.

43. Fireman P, Friday G, Gira C, Vierthaler W, Michaels L. Teaching self-management skills to asthmatic children and their parents in an ambulatory care setting. *Pediatrics* 1981; 68 (3): 341–8.

44. Lewis C, Rachelefsky G, Lewis M, De la Soto A, Kaplan M. A randomized trial of ACT (asthma care training) for kids. *Pediatrics* 1984; 74 (4): 478–86.

45. Clark N, Feldman C, Evans D, Levison M, Wasilewski Y, Mellins R. The impact of health education on frequency and cost of health care use by low income children with asthma. *J Allergy Clin Immunol* 1986; 78 (1 Pt 1): 108–115.

46. ✪ Neri M, Migliori GB, Spanevello A, Berra D, Nicolini E, Landoni CV, Ballardini L, Sommaruga M, Zanon P. Economic analysis of two structured treatment and teaching programs on asthma. *Allergy* 1996; 51: 313–19.

47. Westley C, Spiecher R, Starr L, Simons P, Sanders B, Marsh W, Comer C, Harvey R. Cost effectiveness of an allergy consultation in the management of asthma. *Allergy Asthma Proc* 1997; 18 (1): 15–18.

48. ✪ Legorreta AP, Christian-Herman J, O'Connor RD, Hasan MM, Evans R, Leung KM. Compliance with national asthma management guidelines and specialty care: a health maintenance organizations experience. *Arch Intern Med* 1998; 158: 457–64.

Index

AA-2414 225

Accuhaler 264, 364

Acetaminophen (paracetamol) 422, 458

Acetylcholine 32

Acidosis, acute asthma 590–591, *591*

Activator protein-1 (AP-1) 174, 175, 176, 189, 566

Acupuncture 287, 427, 581

Acute severe asthma 4
  air flow obstruction 589–590
  air leaks/pneumothorax 590
  assisted ventilation 436
  at-risk register 436, *437*
  epidemiology 431–432
  follow-up 411, 436, 624, *625*
  haemodynamic changes 590–591
  hypoxaemic complications 590–591, *591*
  intensive care indications 436
  intrathoracic pressure elevation effects 589–590, *590*
  management
    adults 432–439
    audit 438–439, 623, 624
    children 380, 399–411
    primary care 621–624
  mucus secretion 591
  pathology 431
  peak expiratory flow (PEF) 432, 437–438
    discharge criteria 438
  pharmacotherapy
    anticholinergic bronchodilator combinations 248
    areas of uncertainty 437–438, *437*
    β-adrenergic agonists 241
    guidelines 432, *433, 434, 435*, 436–437
    systemic corticosteroids 188–189
    theophylline 248–249
  physiology 431
  pre-admission circumstances review 436
  pregnancy 501
  prevention 432
  recognition 432

respiratory muscle fatigue 589, *589*
  self-diagnosis 622

Adenosine-induced airway narrowing 224

Adhesion molecules 177

Adolescents 374–375
  functional laryngeal obstruction 378

Adrenaline (epinephrine) 237, *238*
  anaphylactic shock 399
  childhood acute asthma 399
  pregnancy 500

Aerochamber 262, 363

Age-associated mortality risk 23

Air flow obstruction 589–590
  diagnostic measurements 65

Air leaks 590

Air pollutants 11–13, 48, 150, 422
  childhood asthma 351
  childhood cough 526
  exercise-induced asthma 479
  exposure reduction 152

Airborne dusts 12–13

Airway hyperresponsiveness 27–29, *28*
  airway epithelial damage 33
  asthma diagnosis 63
  asymptomatic treatment 68
  corticosteroid effects 180
  definition 4
  diagnostic tests 67–68
  epidemiological studies 5–6
  occupational asthma 445
  questionnaire sensitivity/specificity 65
  transient asthma inflammatory response 30, *31*

Airway inflammation 27, 331
  acute severe asthma 431
  asthma diagnosis 63
  childhood asthma 339
  corticosteroid effects 179–180
  cough 527
  definition 27, 63

Airway inflammation *contd.*
  difficult (therapy-resistant) asthma   564–565
  measures   143–146, 602
  mediators   32
    blood/urine levles   70
  nocturnal asthma   565
  persisting asthma   30–32
  sputum analysis   110, *111*
  transient asthma   29–30
Airway obstruction
  chronic   595–596
  irreversible   596, 600, 601
Airway plugging   591
Airway remodelling *see* Airway structural changes
Airway resistance   81–82, 83
  increase in asthma attack   83
Airway structural changes (remodelling)   33–35, 331, 596, 600–602
  asthma treatment response   121–122
  basement membrane extracellular matrix   35
  difficult (therapy-resistant) asthma   565–566
  epithelial damage   33–34
    bronchial biopsy findings   121
  prevention   421
    inhaled corticosteroids   181–182
  smooth muscle   35
Albumin   110, 120
Albuterol *see* Salbutamol
Alcohol consumption   582
Alcohol-induced asthma   47, 553
Allergen avoidance   12, 150, 151–152, 331, 334, 422, 577
  childhood asthma   339–340, 349–353
    problems   351, 353
  pregnancy   498
  secondary measures   157–165
  see also specific allergens
Allergen-induced responses
  early (immediate)   45
  late   30, 45
  leukotriene modifier effects   223
Allergens   43–45, 68
  nomencalture   101
Allergens sensitization   9–10, 12–13, 149–150
  difficult (therapy-resistant) asthma   562
  infants   55, 149
  pre-school children   55–56
Allergic bronchopulmonary aspergillosis   71, 463–467, 509, 597
  diagnosis   463–464
  treatment   466–467
Allergic rhinitis   11, 44, 56, 112, 487
  immunotherapy   273–275, *274*

Allergy
  classification   4–5
  definition   4, 6
  diagnosis   68, 70
  investigations   101–104
    childhood asthma   344–345
    occupational asthma   445
    specific tests   102
    see also Atopy
β-adrenergic antagonists   286
β-adrenergic receptors   237
Alternaria   10, 45, 152, 163, 562
Alternative therapies   *285*, 287–288, 427–428, 581
  childhood asthma   360
American Thoracic Society   3–4
Aminophylline   248
  acute asthma   438
    children   403
  pregnancy   502
Ammonia, occupational exposure   449
Anaphylaxis   399
  food allergy   553, 554, 556
Ancillary diagnostic tests   70
Angioedema, recurrent   508–509
Angiotensin-converting enzyme (ACE) inhibitors   582
  asthma induction   47
  cough induction   509, 562
Animal allergens/pets   45, 68, 101, 102, 150, 424, 562
  cough in children   526
  environmental assay   103, 158
  exposure reduction   55, 152, 334, 351, 488
  sensitization in children   55, 56
Antacids   522
Anti-allergic drugs   197–200
Antibiotic treatment
  Chlamydia infection   562, 597
  sinusitis   542, 544–545, *545*
Anticholinergics   237, 246–248, 425, 578
  β-adrenergic agonist combined treatment   248
  childhood asthma   355
    acute   404–405
  mechanism of action   246
  nocturnal asthma   491
  pregnancy   500
Anti-fungal agents   467
Antihypertensives   582
Anti-inflammatory agents   240, 248
  childhood asthma   355–360
  pregnancy   501
  self-management plans   311, 312
Anti-inflammatory proteins, corticosteroid-induced synthesis   176
Anti-leukotrienes *see* Leukotriene antagonists

Anti-malarial drugs 213–214
Anti-tussive therapy 530–531
Anxiety 515, 517, 518, 599
  acute childhood asthma 407
Apoptosis 177
Arachidonic acid metabolism
  aspirin/NSAIDs-induced asthma 454–457, 455
  leukotriene modifiers 223–225, 224
Arterial blood gases
  acute severe asthma 431, 432, 438
    children 407
  exacerbation severity assessment 74
Asp fI 164
Aspergillus 163, 164, 463, 464, 509, 597
A. fumigatus 44, 45, 164, 463, 464, 465
A. niger 463
Aspirin challenge tests 96
Aspirin hypersensitivity 422, 543
Aspirin-sensitive asthma 46–47, 70, 453–459, 509, 562
  avoidance measures 457, 457
  clinical features 453–454
  diagnosis 454
  leukotriene antagonist effects 224, 568
  pathophysiology 454–457, 455, 456
  treatment 457–458
Assisted ventilation
  acute severe asthma 436
  childhood asthma 409–410
  complications 591–593
Asthma management team 632, 634–636, 634
Asthma Quality of Life Questionnaire 138, 599
At-risk register 436, 437
Atelectasis 591
Atmospheric temperature 48
Atopic dermatitis 55
Atopy 149, 157, 331
  childhood asthma 54–55, 56, 57, 377
  investigations 102
  occupational asthma 445
  persistent asthma risk 22
  wheezing in infancy 53, 54, 55
Attention-seeking behaviour 517
Audit 295, 643–652
  acute asthma management 438–439, 623, 624
  asthma diagnosis 614, 615
  community care
    asthma clinics 618
    quality criteria 617, 617
  criteria 646, 649, 650, 651
  criterion-based 645–647, 645
  feedback loop 643
  hospital admissions 645–646, 645, 648
  patient satisfaction surveys 646–647

peer review 647, 648
respiratory physician care 646, 646
sentinel-case 643–644
Autohaler 263, 362
Azathioprine 183, 214, 580
  clinical trials 214, 215
  side effects 214

Babyhaler 363
Bambuterol 354
Basement membrane thickening 35, 121
  asthma treatment response 121
  difficult asthma 565
Beclomethasone dipropionate (BDP) 182, 374, 426, 427, 579
  childhood asthma 356, 357, 358, 367, 368
  delivery system 263, 264
  difficult (therapy-resistant) asthma 559
  pregnancy 501
  side effects 186, 187, 188
Benzyl benzoate 159
β-adrenergic agonists 180, 181, 182, 237, 425, 426, 578
  acute severe asthma 241, 399–402, 408, 409, 436, 437
  anticholinergic combined treatments 248
  anti-inflammatory activity 240
  β_2 adrenergic receptor binding 237
  biological effects 239–240
  childhood asthma 353–355, 370, 376, 377
    acute severe attack 399–402, 408, 409
    dose 400–402, 404
    exacerbations 370
    infants 373–374, 401
    inhalation system 399–403
    systemic administration 401
  difficult (therapy-resistant) asthma 511, 559, 560, 568
  economic evaluations 656, 658, 659
  exercise-induced asthma 376, 471, 475–477, 476
  inhaled steroid combined treatment 183, 240, 245
  isomers 241–242
  long-acting 242–246, 354
    anti-leukotrienes comparison 246
    corticosteroid combinations 183
  management principles 331
  as marker of uncontrolled asthma 23, 131, 241, 310, 311, 354, 411
  mortality risk 23, 241
  nocturnal asthma 377, 489
  pregnancy 499–500, 500, 502
  self-management plans 310, 311
  short-acting 240–242
  side effects 240, 353–354, 354, 402, 592
  tolerance 241, 245–246, 354, 475, 477, 568
β-adrenergic antagonist-induced asthma 47
β-adrenergic blockers 422, 562, 582

β-adrenergic receptors   237
β₂ adrenergic receptor   237, 239
   corticosteroid-induced upregulation   176
   polymorphism   239
   signalling   237, 239
Bipolaris   164
Bisphosphonates   582
Bla g I   160
Bla g II   158, 160, 161
Blood tests   70, 145
Bone metabolism, inhaled steroid effects   186–187
Breast-feeding   11, 149, 151, 502, 557
Breath-actuated metered dose inhalers   263
Breathlessness
   acute severe asthma recognition   432
   bronchocontriction relationship (lung function tests)   85, 87
   childhood asthma diagnosis   340, 341
   clinical status assessment   127, 131
   difficult (therapy-resistant) asthma   564
   exacerbation severity assessment   72
   history-taking   64
   pulmonary mechanics   84
British Thoracic Society (BTS)   613
   audit/audit criteria   646, 647, 648, *49*
Brittle asthma   563
   associated psychiatric disorders   599
   fatal asthma risk   599
   see also Difficult (therapy-resistant) asthma; High-risk
      asthma; Unstable asthma
Bronchial aeroallergen challenge   344, 345
Bronchial biopsy   70, 120–121
Bronchial carcinoid tumour   71
Bronchial wash specimens, induced sputum comparison
      108–109
Bronchiectasis   596–597
Bronchitis
   chronic   22, 23, 85, 87
   eosinophilic   527, 530
Bronchoalveolar lavage (BAL)   70, 119–120, 121
   acute inflammatory response   30
   clinical use   122
   difficult (therapy-resistant) asthma   564
   induced sputum comparison   108–109
   nocturnal asthma   565
   persisting asthma   30, 31
   viral-associated wheeze in children   339
Bronchodilators   237–249
   acute severe asthma   436, 437
     children   407
   additional to inhaled corticosteroids   182–183
   anticholinergics   246–248
   asthma diagnosis   67

childhood asthma   353–355, 366, 367, 370, 407
   infants   373–374
glucocorticoid-resistant asthma   511
intermittent asthma   425
life-threatening asthma   436
mild persistent asthma   426
moderate persistent asthma   426
pregnancy   499–500
self-management plans   311, 312
severe asthma   427
sympathomimetics   237–246
xanthines   248–249
Bronchoscopy   119, 121–122
Bronchospasm   431
Budesonide   180, 181, 182, 190, 364, 374, 426, 579
   childhood asthma   356, 357, 358, 367, 368
   difficult (therapy-resistant) asthma   559, 566
   economic evaluations   656
   exercise-induced asthma   477, *478*
   side effects   186, 187, 188
Buteyko breathing technique   360
Butixocort   190

Calcitonin   583
Calcium channel blockers   285–286, 582
Calcium supplements   582
Can d I   104
Can f I   162
Candida   164
   oropharyngeal   185, 358
Carbon monoxide, exhaled   114
Cardiogenic pulmonary hypertension   71
Cardiovascular disorders
   asthma complications   598
   corticosteroids side effects   582
   lung function tests   85
Care delivery   295, 334
   see also Hospital practice; Primary care
Cat allergens   101, 150, 158, 161–163, 562
   exposure reduction   152, 162–163, *162*, 351
Cataracts   358
CC-10   176
Central nervous system, inhaled steroid effects   188
   children   358
Cetirizine   227
Challenge tests *see* Provocation tests
Chemical sensitizer challenge tests   95–96
Chemokines   32
   corticosteroids inhibition of transcription   176–177
Chest X-ray
   allergic bronchopulmonary aspergillosis   464–465
   childhood asthma
     acute severe   408

diagnosis 56, 57, 344
Chest wall changes in pregnancy 495
Child Health Questionnaire 137
Childhood asthma
  acute severe attack 399–411
    drugs 399–405, *404*
    follow-up 411
    general practice management 408–409
    hospital management 409–411
    at school 380
    severity assessment 405–408
    stepping down treatment 410
    treatment/monitoring 408
  adolescents 374–375
  allergens avoidance 339–340, 349–353
  allergy testing 344–345
  alternative therapies 360
  anti-inflammatory drugs 355–360
  anticholinergics 355
  bronchodilators 353–355
  chest X-ray 56, 57, 344
  chronic symptoms 596
  clinical examination 342
  compliance 347, *347*, 368, *368*, 371
  cough 525–526
  cough-variant 376
  diagnosis 53–58, 340–345, *341*
    differential diagnosis 341, 342, *342*
    infants 372, 373
    primary care 613–616, *615*
  dry powder inhalers (DPI) 265
  education 346–347, *346*
  environmental triggers 341, *341*
  exacerbations 369–370
    zone plan 369, *369*
  exercise capacity effect 598
  exercise-induced 375–386, *375*, 380
    treatment 477, *478*
  follow-up care 370–371, *371*
  food allergy-induced 553, 554, 556
  functional impairments 137, *137*
  high-risk groups 13
  holidays 380–381
  home peak flow monitoring 300
  immunotherapy 276–277, 353
  indoor environment 378–380
  infants 19, 53–54, 372–374
  inhaled steroids 355–358, 382
    clinical efficacy 181
    side effects 356–358
    systemic absorption 364, 368
  lung function tests 342–344
    peak expiratory flow (PEF) 342–343, *343*, 349

    reversibility with bronchodilator 344
    spirometry 342, 343–344
  management 339–383, *345*
    guidelines 340
    review/monitoring 348–349
    self-management plans 347, 410–411
  medication 353–368
    administration route 360–365
    drug combinations/doses 366–368
    drug selection 353–360
    mild infrequent asthma *348*, 366
    moderate asthma *348*, 366–367
    severe asthma *348*, 367–368
    step down 368
  metered dose inhaler use 262
  natural history 19–22, 53
    long-term follow-up 20
  nocturnal 376–377
  persistence 381–382, *381*
    predisposing factors 22
  prevalence 7, 339
  psychological factors 378, *379*
  quality of life assessment 137, 138
  school environment 380
  severity assessment 348–349, *348*, 405–408
  sinusitis association 538
  symptoms 340–341
    diary cards 342
    prodromal 366, *367*, 369
  systemic corticosteroids 358, 368, 370
    side effects 368
Chlamydia infection 562, 597
Chlorine, occupational exposure 449
Chlorofluorocarbon (CFC) propellants 261, 263, 264, 303, 362
Chloroquine 213, 458
  side effects 214
Chromatin, corticosteroid structural effects 175–176, *175*
Chronic difficult asthma 563
  see also Difficult (therapy-resistant) asthma
Chronic obstructive pulmonary disease (COPD) 71, 87, 189, 246, 247, 248, 487, 560, 600
Chronolog 325
Churg-Strauss syndrome 427, 509, 581, 598
Ciclesonide 190
Cladosporium 10, 45, 163
Classification 4–5
Clinical trials 332
  assessment end-points 332–333
see also specific drugs
Cockroach allergens 45, 101, 102, 150, 158, 159–161, 562
  exposure reduction 152, 161, *161*
  immunoassay 160

Cockroach allergens   *contd.*
  sensitization   22, 56
Colchicine   214–215
  clinical trials   215
  side effects   215
Cold air provocation test   94
Cold air-induced bronchoconstriction   93, 422
  leukotriene modifier effects   223
Cold freon effect   262, 263, 362
Communication
  adolescents   374, 375
  patient education   296, 301
    childhood asthma   347
Community care organization   616–621
  asthma clinics   618–621, *618*
    record cards   621, *621, 622*
Compliance   296, 300, 301, 302, 323–327, 334, 508
  adolescents   374
  assessment   324–326, *324*
    electronic recording devices   325–326
  associated factors   326
  children   347, *347*, 360, 368, *368*, 371
  difficult (therapy-resistant) asthma   560–561
  erratic   324
  improvement   326
  intentional/intelligent non-compliance   324
  patterns   326, *326*
  psychological factors   516
  unwitting non-compliance   323–324
Complications, acute   589–594
  air flow obstruction   589–590
  hypoxaemia/hypercapnia   590–591
  lobar collapse   591
  lower respiratory tract infection   591
  mechanical ventilation   591–593
  mucus secretion   591
  pharmacological treatments   591, *592*
Complications, chronic   595–603, *595*
  airway obstruction   595–596
  airway remodelling   596
  emphysema/bronchiectasis   596–597
  extrapulmonary   597–598
  lung function decline   600–602
  psychosocial   598–600
  respiratory infections   597
Congenital malformations   498, 499, 500, 501
Congestive cardiac failure   71, 560
  lung function tests   85
Connective tissue, inhaled steroid effects   187
Coping style   517
Cor pulmonale   598
Corticosteroid-dependent asthma   563
  see also Difficult (therapy-resistant) asthma

Corticosteroid-resistant asthma   189, 507–512, 522, 563
  assessment   509–510, *510*
  characteristics   507, *508*
  children   360, 368
  definition   189
  differential diagnosis   508–509
  management   510–511, *511*
  mechanisms   189, *190*
  pathophysiology   509
  see also Difficult (therapy-resistant) asthma
Corticosteroid-sparing agents   183, 203, 209, 211, 213, 579, 580
  children   355, 360
  leukotriene antagonists   225
  theophylline   355
Corticosteroids   173–192
  airway hyperresponsiveness   180
  airway inflammation   179–180
  cellular effects   177–179, *178*
  chromatin structure effects   175–176, *175*
  gene transcription regulation   173–174, *174*
    inflammatory response gene targets   176–177
  inhaled *see* Corticosteroids, inhaled
  molecular aspects   173–179
  new agents   190–191
  response prediction
    nasal eosinophilia   112
    sputum eosinophilia   110–112, *111*
  systemic *see* Corticosteroids, systemic
  topical   546
  transplacental passage   501
Corticosteroids, inhaled   424, 425, 426, 427, 579
  airway structural change
    prevention   181–182, 331
    response   601
  childhood asthma   181, 355–358, 366, 367, 368, 370, 382, 408
    delivery devices   356–357
    infants   374
    side effects   356–358, 368, 371, *372*
  clinical efficacy   180–182, *180*
  clinical use   182–183
  combination therapy   183, 190, 240, 245
    bronchodilators   182–183, 245
  comparative aspects   182
  cost-effectiveness   183, 656, *657, 658*
  difficult (therapy-resistant) asthma   560–561, 566–567
  discontinuation   181
  dose-response effects   181, 183, 356
  exercise-induced asthma   472, 477–478, *478*
  high-dose   180, 181, 182, 190
  long-acting   331
  management principles   331, 602

mortality reduction   182
mouth rinsing   364
pharmacokinetics   183–184, *184*
  new agents   190–191
pregnancy   501
self-management plans   311
side effects   184–188, *185*
  compliance issues   326
systemic absorption
  children   356–357, 364, 368
  delivery systems   185–186
therapeutic trial
  adults   68
  children   56, 57
Corticosteroids, systemic   188–189, 424, 427
  acute severe asthma   402–403, *404*, 408, 436, 437
  allergic bronchopulmonary aspergillosis   466
  alternative (steroid-sparing) treatments   577–581
  childhood asthma   358, 368, 370
    acute attack   402–403, *404*, 408
  complications   *592*
  difficult (therapy-resistant) asthma   559, 566, 567
  high-dose   312
  nocturnal asthma   490–491
  pregnancy   501, 502
  self-management plans   312
  side effects   577, *578*, 581–582
  undertreatment-associated mortality   432
Cost-effectiveness   334
  analysis   655–656
Cough   127–128, 131, 525–531, *525*
  acute complications   590, *590*
  airway inflammation   527
  assessment   527
  asthma diagnosis   340, 341, 342, 615
  children   54, 56, 340, 341, 342, 525–526
  chronic   529, *529*
  epidemiology   525
  exacerbation severity assessment   72
  history-taking   64
  management   529–531, *531*
  post-exercise   472
  recording   528–529
  virally-induced   54, 55, 56
Cough reflex   526–527
  sensitivity in asthma patients   527–528, *528*
Cough-variant asthma   5, 93, 128, 526
  children   376
Cow's milk hypersensitivity   556
CREB binding protein (CBP)   173, 175
"Credit card" self-management plan   313–314, *314*, 369
Crossed-immunoelectrophoresis   163
Current asthma   5, 6

Cushingoid appearance   581
Cyclosporin   183, 205–207, 458, 511
  children   360
  clinical trials   207, *208*
  difficult (therapy-resistant) asthma   568
  mechanism of action   205–206
  side effects   207
  steroid-sparing effect   580
Cystic fibrosis   55, 56, 57, 189, 342, 543, 544
Cytokines   32
  corticosteroids inhibition of transcription   176–177
  nitric oxide induction   113

Damp housing   10, 48, 163, 351, 379
Dapsone   183, 216
  clinical trials   216
Dartmouth COOP charts   137
Datura stramonium   246, 287
Decongestants   546
Definition of asthma   3–4, 5–6, 63, 66
Delivery systems (inhalation devices)   261–267, 423, 648
  children   360–365, *361*, 366, 367, 371
    acute severe attack   399–408
    peak expiratory flow rates needed   364, *364*
    technique   *361*, 362
  infants   374
  inhaled steroids systemic absorption   185–186
Dendritic cells   178
Denial   300, 374, 515, 518, 562
Depression   326, 515, 517, 518, 562, 599
Der f I   101, 103, 104, 158, 350
Der p I   101, 103, 104, 158, 350
Dextropropoxyphene   458
Diabetes mellitus   581, 582
Diagnosis   56, 57
  adult asthma   63–76
  airflow limitation
    measurements   65
    reversibility   67
  airway responsiveness   67–68
  algorithm   *69*
  allergy   68–70
  ancillary/confirmatory tests   66–68, 70
  children   340–345, *341*, 613–616, *615*
    infants   55
    pre-school   55–56
    school-age   56–57
  medical history   64–65, *64*
  peak expiratory flow (PEF) monitoring   66–68
  physical examination   65
  psychological factors   517
  risk factor evaluation   68–70
  spirometry   65–66

Diagnosis   contd.
   therapeutic trial   56, 57, 68
   see also Severity assessment
Diclofenac   422
Dietary risk factors   11, 149
   primary prevention   151
Dietary triggers see Food allergy
Differential diagnosis   70–71, 72
   children   55, 56, 57
   difficult (therapy-resistant) asthma   559–561, 560
Difficult (therapy-resistant) asthma   559–569
   airway inflammation mechanics   564–565
   airway responsiveness   564
   airway wall remodelling   565–566
   contributing medical factors   561–563, 561
   corticosteroid responsiveness   566
   definition   559
   differential diagnosis   559–561, 560
   economic cost   559
   epidemiology   559
   investigations   567
   management   566–568
   presentation patterns   563–564
Diisocyanates   95
Diskhaler   264, 364, 368
Diuretics   227–228, 286, 582
DLCO   87–88, 497
Dog allergens exposure reduction   152, 162
Drug-induced asthma   46–47
   agents   47
Dry powder inhalers (DPI)   261, 264–265
   children   357, 363–365, 366, 371, 400
   systemic steroid absorption   185
Dust mites   158
   see also House dust mite allergens
Dynamic hyperinflation   589
Dysphonia   184–185
Dyspnoea see Breathlessness

Early asthmatic response (EAR)   95
   allergen challenge tests   95
   chemical sensitizer challenge tests   96
Economic aspects   334, 655–660
   cost-effectiveness analysis   655–656
   difficult (therapy-resistant) asthma   559
   patient education programmes   659–660
   pharmacotherapy evaluations   656–659, 657, 658
   specialist care   660
Education, patient   295–304
   asthma management team personnel   634, 635
   childhood asthma   346–347, 346
      exacerbations management   369
   communication   296, 297, 301

   concerns of patients   301
   economic evaluations   659–660
   group education   302
   information content   299–300, 300, 302
   information-giver   296–297
   multicultural aspects   299
   potential barriers   296, 297
   pregnancy   502
   reinforcement   297, 301
   self-management   302
   sources of materials   303–304
   written information   297, 298, 299
Elastance   83–84
Electronic diaries   325
   childhood asthma   342
Electronic recording of inhalation therapy   325–326
Elimination diets   553, 553, 555–556
Emergency department services   636
Emergency self-admission service   312, 333
Emphysema   85, 87, 596–597
Endothelial cells   178–179
Endothelin-1   177
Environmental allergens   9–11, 22, 101
   control measures   101, 104, 422
      see also Allergens avoidance
   immunoassays   103, 158, 164
   indoor environment   157–158, 378–380
   sensitization   12–13
Environmental factors   48, 149–150, 331, 334
   childhood asthma   341, 341
   exposure reduction   422
Eosinophilia   71
   mortality risk   23
   sinusitis   540
Eosinophilic bronchitis   527, 530
Eosinophilic cationic protein (ECP)   30, 31, 33, 120, 564, 602
   serum level   70, 145
      induced sputum comparison   109, 109
   sputum   110
Eosinophilic pericarditis   598
Eosinophilic pneumonia   71
Eosinophils   27, 32
   activation
      asthma pathogenesis   30, 31, 32
      childhood asthma   54, 339
      epithelial damage   33
      viral infection   54
   blood counts   145
   bronchial biopsy findings   121
   bronchoalveolar lavage (BAL) studies   120
   corticosteroid effects   177
   difficult (therapy-resistant) asthma   564, 565, 566

late asthmatic response   30
  nasal   112
  sinusitis   539–540
  sputum   109, 110
  transient asthma   30
Eotaxin   32, 176, 540
Epidemiology   5–6
  allergen exposure   9–10
  childhood asthma   20–22, 55, 339
  cough   525
  dietary factors   11
  difficult (therapy-resistant) asthma   559
  gastroesophageal reflux   521
  near-fatal asthma   431
  psychological factor associations   515
Episodic asthma   5
Epithelial cells, corticosteroid effects   179
Epithelial damage   33–34
Epithelium-derived relaxing factor (EpDRF)   34
Ethane, exhaled   114
EuroQuol   138
Exacerbations   4
  childhood asthma   369–370
    bronchodilators   370
    indications for seeking medical help   370, *370*
    oral corticosteroids   370
  inhaled corticosteroids   181
  patient education   300
  peak expiratory flow (PEF) measurements   310
  pre-menstrual   502–503, 563
  self-management plans   310, 311–312
  severity assessment   72–74, *75*
  sputum eosinophilia   110
Exercise   43, 582, 598
Exercise provocation test   94, 472
Exercise-induced asthma/bronchoconstriction   43, *43*, 48,
    93, 94, 422, 471–480
  air pullutant effects   479
  children   341, 375–386, *375*, 380
  definition   471
  diagnosis   471–473, *473*
    field procedure   472–473, *474*
    hyperosmolar challenge   479, *480*
  leukotriene modifier effects   223
  management   473, 475
  mechanism   471
  non-pharmacological preventive measures   478–479
  physical training response   479
  preventive medication   475–478
  refractoriness   475
  short-acting β-adrenergic agonists   240–241
  vocal cord dysfunction   479
  warm-up   479

Exercise-induced cough   56
Exhaled gases   112–114
Expiratory reserve volume in pregnancy   496
Extracellular matrix proteins   35

Familial clustering   29
Family history   13, 22
Fatal asthma   563–564
  psychosocial factors   562
  see also Difficult (therapy-resistant) asthma; Mortality
Fatigue, respiratory muscle   589, *589*
Feeling Thermometer   138
Fel d I   101, 103, 104, 158, 161, 162, 351
Fenoterol   *238*
  delivery systems   264
  mortality risk   23, 241
Feto-placental immune response   149
Fibrinogen   110, 120
Finger clubbing   342
Fish oils   11, 149, 225–226
  clinical trials   226
Flow volume relationships   87
Flunisolide   182, 546
Flurbiprofen   46, 422
Fluticasone   181, 182, 186, 190, 579
  childhood asthma   356, 357
  delivery systems   264
  difficult (therapy-resistant) asthma   559, 566
  salmeterol combination   183, 245
Follow-up care
  acute severe asthma   436, 624, *625*
  children   370–371, *371*
    after hospital discharge   411
  outpatient clinics   637
Food additives
  allergy   422
  challenge tests   96
  childhood asthma   351
Food allergy (food-induced asthma symptoms)   47, 68, 101,
    422, 553–557
  asthma presentation   553–554
  avoidance measures   377, 378
  children   351, 377–378
    pre-school   55, 56
  diagnosis   96, 554–556
  infants   55, 149
  management   556–557
  prevalence   556
  primary preventive measures   151
Food challenge tests   96, 554–555, *555*
Forced expiratory flow (FEV$_1$)   65, 85
  acute severe asthma   431
  clinical status assessment   144

Forced expiratory flow (FEV$_1$) *contd.*
  exacerbation severity assessment   73, 74
  exercise-induced asthma   472, *473*
  long-term decline with asthma   600, *601*
Forced vital capacity (FVC)   65
Formoterol   183, 237, *238*, 354
  exercise-induced asthma   475, 477
  multi-centre studies   245
  pharmacology   242, *243*, 244, *244*
  salmeterol comparison   245
  tolerance   245–246
Functional impairments   136–137
Functional laryngeal obstruction   378
Functional residual capacity, pregnancy   496
Functional Status II (R) Scale (FSH9R)   137
Fungal allergens *see* Mould allergens
Furosemide   227

Gas exchange in pregnancy   496
Gastroesophageal reflux   49, 55, 56, 70, 488, 508,
    521–523, 530, 597–598
  diagnosis   521–522
  difficult asthma   561
  epidemiology   521
  management   522–523
  mechanisms   521
  pregnancy   499
  "silent"   521
Gastrointestinal side effects   582
Gender differences
  adult asthma persistence   23
  childhood asthma persistence   22
  wheezing in infancy   53
Gene transcription, corticosteroids-regulated   173–174
  adhesion molecules expression   177
  β$_2$ adrenoceptor expression   176
  inducible nitric oxide synthase (iNOS) inhibition   177
  inflammatory receptors   177
  mucin genes   179
  therapeutic aspects   191
General Practitioners in Asthma Group (GPIAC)   613, 614,
    616, 623, 624
Genetic aspects   29, 149
Glaucoma   583
Glucocorticoid receptors (GR)   173, *174*
  transcription factor interactions   174
Glucocorticoid response elements (GRE)   173, 176
Glucocorticoid-resistant asthma *see* Corticosteroid-resistant
    asthma
Gold therapy   183, 207–209
  clinical trials   207–209, *210*
  difficult (therapy-resistant) asthma   568
  mechanism of action   207, *209*

side effects   209, 580
  steroid-sparing effect   580
Gonadotrophin-releasing hormone agonists   563
Granulocyte macrophage-colony stimulating factor
    (GM-CSF)   32, 109, 120, 121, 149, 177, 465
Growth
  childhood asthma effects   342, 371, 382
  inhaled steroids impact   187, 357
Guaifensin   546
Guidelines   196, 295, 332
  acute severe asthma management   432, *433, 434, 435,*
    436–437, 624
  adherence in primary care   616, 617–618, 624
  audit   645, 646
  childhood asthma management   340, 346, 349
  medication in pregnancy   499, *499*

H$_1$ receptor antagonists   32, 227
  sinusitis   546
H$_2$ receptor antagonists   522, 582
Haematological effects   188
Haemodynamic changes, acute severe asthma   590–591
Health-related quality of life   135–140
  asthma-related functional impairments   136–137
  children   137, *137*
  clinical applications   139
  clinical measures correlations   135, *136*
  data interpretation   138
  definition   135
  measurement instruments   137–138
  research applications   138–139
Heating, domestic   380
Helminthosporium   163
Heparin   286
Herbal remedies   287, 427
High-risk asthma, self-management plans   316
Histamine   32, 120
Histamine/methacholine inhalation tests   67–68, 91–93
  borderline results   93
  clinical value   93
  interpretation   92–93
  methods   91–92
  sensitivity   92
History-taking   64–65, *64*
  allergy   68
  childhood asthma   340–342, *341*
    acute severe attack   406–407
  exercise-induced asthma   471–472
  gastroesophageal reflux   522
  occupational asthma   443, 445
  sinusitis   542–543
HIV infection   509

Home peak flow monitoring 300, 325
 indications *301*
Homeopathy 287, 427, 581
Hospital admission 631, *631*, 632
 acute severe asthma 432, 436, 438–439
  children 409
  follow-up 436
 as asthma status marker 73, 131
 audit 438–439, 645–646, *645*, 648
 self-management plans 312
Hospital practice 631–638
 asthma management team 632, 634–636, *634*
 childhood acute severe asthma 409–410
 emergency department 636
 intensive care 636–637
 medical ward 636
 outpatient clinics 637–638
 target populations 633–634
Hospital referral, indications in childhood asthma 346, *346*, 371
House dust mite allergens 7, 45, 68, 101, 102, 150, 158, 378, 424, 562
 avoidance measures 10, 55, 151–152, 158–159, *160*
  childhood asthma management 349–351, *350*
 environmental assay 103, 104
 mite species 158
 sensitization 9–10, 22, 56, 158
Humidity 159, 164, 349, 350, 379
 sinusitis 546
Hydrocortisone 188, 402, 458, 502
 side effects 583
Hydrofluoroalkane (HFA) propellants 261, 263, 264, 362
Hydrogen peroxide, exhaled 114
Hydroxychloroquine 183, 213, 581
Hypercapnia, acute severe asthma 590–591, *591*
Hyperinflation 589, 592
 chronic complications 596–597
Hyperosmolar challenge in exercise-induced asthma 479, *480*
Hyperosmolar dry powder provocation tests 94–95
Hypersensitivity 28
Hyperventilation 48, 517
 bronchoconstrictor response 93
Hypnosis 288
Hypogammaglobulinaemia 597
Hypokalaemia 581, 582
Hypothalamic-pituitary-adrenal axis suppression 186
 children 357
Hypoxia
 acute severe asthma 431, 432, 590–591, *591*
 exacerbations in pregnancy 502
 exercise-induced asthma 475
Hysterical conversion 509

Ibuprofen 46, 422
Idiopathic chronic persistent non-productive cough (ICPNPC) 527, 529
IgE antibodies, allergen specific
 allergy diagnosis 69
 in vitro assays 69, 103
IgG subset deficiency 55, 56, 57
Imidazole salicylate 225
Immotile cilia syndrome 543
Immune function impairment 55, 56, 543, 597
Immunoassay 69, 103
 allergic rhinitis 544
 childhood asthma diagnosis 344–345
 cockroach allergens 160
 environmental allergens 103, 157–158, 160
 food allergy-induced asthma 554
 mould allergens 163, 164
Immunoglobulin, intravenous 209–211, 286–287, 546, 581
 clinical trials 209–211
 mechanism of action 209
 side effects 211
Immunosuppressive agents 203–217, 579–580
 difficult (therapy-resistant) asthma 511, 568
Immunotherapy 273–279, *276*, 427, 578
 children 276–277, 353
 food allergy-induced asthma 557
 mechanisms 277–278, *278*
 nasal administration route 277
 pregnancy 498
 safety 277
 seasonal allergic rhinitis 273–275, *274*
 sublingual administration route 277
Inciters of asthma 43, 45
Indomethacin 46, 422, 475
Indoor environment
 aeroallergens 157–158
 childhood asthma 378–380
Inducers of asthma 43, 45
Infective complications 582
Inflammatory enzymes, corticosteroids inhibition 177
Inflammatory mediators
 antagonists 223–228
 blood/urine levles 70
 corticosteroid regulation
  gene targets 176–177
  transcription factor interactions 174
Inhaled drug-induced asthma 47
Inhaled steroids *see* Corticosteroids, inhaled
Inhalers *see* Delivery systems
Insect allergens 45
Intensive care 636–637
 indications

Intensive care *contd.*
  acute severe asthma 436
  children 409
Interleukin 1 (IL-1) receptor antagonist 176
Interleukin 1β (IL-1β) 113, 177
Interleukin 2 (IL-2) 149, 189
Interleukin 3 (IL-3) 32, 149, 177, 465
Interleukin 4 (IL-4) 32, 120, 176, 177, 178, 189, 465, 566
Interleukin 5 (IL-5) 32, 109, 120, 121, 176, 177, 178, 465, 566
Interleukin 6 (IL-6) 177, 178
Interleukin 8 (IL-8) 564
Interleukin 10 (IL-10) 32, 176, 177
Interleukin 12 (IL-12) 566
Interleukin 13 (IL-13) 189, 465
Intermittent asthma 5, 425
International asthma management plan "zone system" 314, *317, 318*
International variations in management 334
Intradermal testing 103
Intrathoracic pressure elevation effects 589–590, *590*
Intrauterine environment 149
Intrauterine growth retardation 497, 498
Ionizer therapy 288
Ipratropium bromide 32, 237
  acute severe asthma 436, 437
  childhood asthma 355, 374, 404–405, *404*
  clinical effects 246–247, *247*
  pregnancy 500
  salbutamol combination 248
  side effects 405
Irritant-induced occupational asthma (reactive airway dysfunction syndrome) 447, 449
Isocapnic hyperventilation with dry air, exercise testing 472
Isocyanates 30, 70, 95
Isoprenaline 23, *238*

Jet nebulizers 265–266

KCO 88
Ketotifen 199, 557
  children 360

Labour 502
Lansoprazole 522
Late asthmatic response (LAR) 45
  allergen challenge tests 95
  chemical sensitizer challenge tests 96
Left ventricular failure 189
Leukotriene antagonists 33, *34*, 223–225, *224*, 331, 374, 425, 426, 427, 581
  aspirin/NSAIDs-induced asthma 456, *456*, 562, 568
  childhood asthma 359–360, 361, 367, 376
  difficult (therapy-resistant) asthma 568

economic evaluations 656
exercise-induced asthma/bronchoconstriction 223, 376, 478
long-acting β-adrenergic agonists comparison 246
nocturnal asthma 491
pregnancy 501
sinusitis 546–547
Leukotrienes 32, 33, 120, 223
  aspirin/NSAIDs-induced asthma 455–456, 562
  urine levels 70
Life-threatening asthma 431
  at-risk register 436
  recognition 311, 432
  treatment 436
  see also Near-fatal asthma
Lipocortin-1 176
5–Lipoxygenase inhibitors 223
Lobar collapse 591
Local asthma task force 295, *296*
Loratidine 227
Low birthweight 13, 497, 498
Lower respiratory tract infection 591
LTC$_4$ 33
LTD$_4$ 33
LTE$_4$ 33
Lung function decline 600–602, *601*
Lung function tests 6, 57, 63, 81–88
  cardiocirculatory insufficiency 85
  childhood asthma 342–344
    acute severe asthma 407–408
    bronchial provocation tests 344
    diagnosis 57
    reversibility with bronchodilator 344
  exacerbation severity assessment 73
  flow volume relationships 87
  leukotriene modifier effects 224–225
  management aims in adults 421–422
  mortality risk 23
  nocturnal asthma assessment 487
  respiratory insufficiency 85
  ventilatory insufficiency 85
  see also Spirometry
Lung volumes in pregnancy 495–496, *496*
Lymphocytes 27, 31, 32
  bronchial biopsies 121
  bronchoalveolar lavage (BAL) 120
Lysine-aspirin inhalation test 454, 458

Macrophages, corticosteroid effects 177
Magnesium sulphate 286, 502
Major basic protein (MBP) 30, 33, 120
Management
  adults 421–428, *421*
    aims 421

childhood asthma   345–375, *345*
  principles   331–335
Mannitol challenge   94–95
Mast cells   27, 31, 32
  β-adrenergic agonist effects   240
  bronchoalveolar lavage (BAL)   120
  corticosteroid effects   177–178
  degranulation   30
  sputum   *111*, 112
Maximal breathing capacity (MBC)   85
Maximal expiratory pressure (MEP)   81
Maximal inspiratory pressure (MIP)   81
Medical history   64–65, *64*
Medical Outcomes Survey Short Form 36 (SF-36)   137
Medical ward care   636
Medroxyprogesterone acetate   563
Menfenamic acid   46
Menstrual cycle factors   49
  see also Pre-menstrual exacerbations
Metabisulphite challenge tests   96
Metabolic side effects, corticosteroids   187–188, 581
  children   358
Metaproterenol
  acute childhood asthma   401
  pregnancy   499
Metered dose inhalers (MDI)   261–264
  breath-actuated (Autohaler)   263
  children   356–357, 362, 366, 367, 400
  disadvantages   263
  method of use   261–262
  propellants   261, 263–264, 303, 362
  spacers   262–263
    indications   *262*
Methotrexate   183, 203–205, 458, 511
  children   360
  clinical trials   204–205, *206*
  difficult (therapy-resistant) asthma   568
  mechanism of action   203
  side effects   205, 580
  steroid-sparing effect   579–580
Methylergonovine   502
Methylprednisolone   188
  acute childhood asthma   402
  pregnancy   501
Mild asthma
  characteristics   425
  self-management plans   314–315
  treatment   425–426
    children   *348*, 366
Mini Asthma Quality of Life Questionnaire   138
Moderate asthma   426
  self-management plans   314–315
  treatment in children   *348*, 366–367
Mometasone   190

Monitoring treatment   93
Montelukast   223
  children   359, 376
  exercise-induced asthma   376
  pregnancy   501
  sinusitis   547
Mortality   7, 23, 73, 354, 421, 431
  acute attack follow-up in prevention   624
  confidential enquiries   *644*
  exercise-induced asthma   475
  international differences   7, 8
  pathological findings   431
  perinatal   497
  pregnancy   497
  preventable factors   432, *432*, *644*
  psychosocial factors   432, 562, 599, 647–648
  respiratory physiology   431
  risk factors   23, 73–74, 131
    children   378, *380*
    failure to recognise severity of attack   309–310
    inhaled corticosteroids in reduction   182
Mould allergens   10, 44–45, 48, 68, 101, 102, 104, 163–165, 379, 562
  antigenic determinants detection   163
  avoidance measures   152, 164–165, *165*
    childhood asthma management   351
  environmental immunoassays   164
  sensitization   56
Mouth rinsing   311, 364
  children   368
  systemic steroid absorption reduction   185
MUC2   179
MUC5AC   179
Mucolytics   286
  sinusitis   546
Mucor   163, 164
Mucus secretion   591
  corticosteroid effects   179
Multiattribute Health Utilities Index   138
Multicultural issues
  childhood asthma   347
  patient education   299
  quality of life questionnaires   139
Muscarinic agonists   422
Muscle relaxation for mechanical ventilation   593
Mycoplasma pneumoniae infection   562, 597
Myeloperoxidase   70

Naproxen   46
Nasal cytology   112
Nasal endoscopy   543–544
Nasal eosinophils   112
Nasal polyps   453, 454, 457, 543, 546, 562
Natamycin   467

National Asthma Attack Audit 645
National Asthma Campaign (NAC) 613, 624, 644, 646, 647
  self-management plan 314, *315*, *316*
National Asthma and Respiratory Training Centre (NARTC) 613, 626
Natural history 19–24, 600, *602*
  adult asthma 22–23
  childhood asthma 19–22
Near-fatal asthma 431
  psychosocial factor associations 432, 515, 517, 562
  see also Life-threatening asthma
Nebuhaler 262, 363, 364, 368, 475
Nebulizers 261, 265–266
  childhood asthma 365
    acute 399–400
  exercise-induced asthma 475
  indications for use *266*
  infants 374
Nedocromil sodium 198, 311, 425, 579
  childhood asthma 358–359, 376
  exercise-induced asthma 376, 471, 475, 477, *477*
  pregnancy 501
Neutral endopeptidase 176
Neutrophils 27, 31, 32
  corticosteroid effects 178
  difficult (therapy-resistant) asthma 565
  nasal 112
  transient asthma inflammatory response 30
Nitric oxide, exhaled 112–114, *113*, 145–146, 179
  clinical studies 113–114, *113*
  difficult (therapy-resistant) asthma 565
  inflammatory marker 70, 602
  measurement technique 114, *114*
Nitric oxide, pulmonary physiology 112
Nitric oxide synthase, inducible (iNOS) 179
  corticosteroids inhibition 177
Nitrogen dioxide 11, 48, 150, 422
NK_1 receptor 177
NK_2 receptor 177
Nocturnal asthma 48, 487–491
  airway inflammation 565
  assessment 487–488
  asthma severity marker 310
  children 376–377
  differential diagnosis 487
  inhaled corticosteroids 180–181
  interacting causative factors 488, *490*
  management 488–491
    algorithm *489*
Nocturnal waking 599
  clinical status assessment 128, 131
Non-allergic rhinitis with eosinophilia syndrome (NARES) 544

Non-compliance *see* Compliance
Non-steroidal anti-inflammatory drugs (NSAIDs) 43
Non-steroidal anti-inflammatory drugs (NSAIDs)-sensitivity 46–47, 422, 453–459, 509, 562
  avoidance measures 457, *457*
  clinical features 453–454
  diagnosis 454
    challenge tests 96
  leukotriene modifier effects 224
  pathophysiology 454–457, *455*, *456*
  treatment 457–458
Nonisotonic aerosol provocation tests 94
Noradrenaline (norepinephrine) 237
Nottingham Health Profile 137
Nuclear factor of activated T-cells (NF-AT) 176
Nuclear factor-κB (NF-κB) 174, 175, 176
Nurse-run asthma clinics 618–621, *618*, 621, *622*
  record cards 621, *621*, *622*

Occupational asthma 443–449, 562
  agents/workplaces 43, 45, *46*, *444*
  allergen avoidance 577
  chemical sensitizer challenge tests 95
  diagnosis 443, 445–446, *446*, *447*
  employer education 303
  high-risk workplace databanks 443
  high/low molecular weight agents *444*
  histamine/methacholine inhalation tests 93
  irritant-induced (reactive airway dysfunction syndrome) 447, 449
  management 446–447, *448*
  nocturnal symptoms 488
  persistence 23
  pre-employment testing 446, 449
  screening assessments 446, *448*
  specific inhalation challenges 446
  transient airway inflammatory response 30
Ocular effects, inhaled steroids 187
Oesophageal pH monitoring 521, 522
Oesophageal pressure changes 83, *84*
OKY-046 225
Omeprazole 508, 521, 522
Osteoporosis, corticosteroid side effects 567, 577, 582
  children 357–358
  preventive drug treatments 582–583, *583*
  preventive non-pharmacological treatment 582, *583*
  see also Bone metabolism
Outcomes of treatment 333
  clinical trial end-points 332–333
  perceptions of symptoms 333–334
Outpatient clinics 637–638
  see also Nurse-run asthma clinics
Oxitropium bromide 247

Oxygen administration
   acute severe asthma 431, 436
   children 409
Oxytocin 502
Ozone 11, 30, 48, 150, 422

Paediatric Asthma Caregiver Quality of Life Questionnaire
   138
Paediatric Asthma Quality of Life Questionnaire 138
Panic disorder 515, 518
Pantoprazole 522
Paracetamol (acetaminophen) 422, 458
Particulate air pollutants 11, 48
Partnership management approach 631–632, *632*
Pathophysiology 27–36, 331
   childhood asthma 339
   difficult (therapy-resistant) asthma 564–566
Patient satisfaction surveys 646–647
Peak expiratory flow rate (PEF/PEFR) 65, 87, 129–130
   acute severe asthma 431
      hospital discharge criteria 438
      recognition 432, 437–438
   asthma diagnosis 66–67
   childhood asthma 342–343, *343*, 349
      exacerbations recognition 369, 370
      inhaled device operation 364, *364*
   clinical status assessment 128–129, 131, 144, 310, 311
   compliance monitoring 325
   diary records 325, 615
      acute attack follow-up 624, *625*
   diurnal variation 130, *131*
   exacerbation severity assessment 73, 74
   exercise-induced asthma 472
   nocturnal asthma assessment 487
   occupational asthma 445–446, *445*
   self-management plans 310, 311, 618, *619*, 622–623
Peak flow meters 65, 310, 622
Peer review 647, 648
Penicillium 163
Pentamidine 47
Pentane, exhaled 114
Peptic ulceration 582
Per a I 160
Perinatal mortality 497
Persistent asthma 5
   airway inflammation 30–32
   airway structural changes 33
   children 20–22, 53, 381–382, *381*
   mild 425–426
   moderate 426
   population studies 20–23
   predisposing factors 22
   severe 427

Pets *see* Animal allergens
Pharmacological treatment 422–427, *423*
   children *see* Childhood asthma
   complications 591, *592*
   economic evaluations 656–659, *657*, *658*
   initial treatment 424
   stepwise approach 424
      maintenance therapy reduction 427
   symptom severity relationship 131
Phosphodiesterases 248
Physical examination
   asthma diagnosis 65
   childhood asthma 342
   exacerbation severity assessment 73, 74
   sinusitis 543
Placental immune response 149
Platelet activating factor 226
Platelet activating factor antagonists 226
Pleural pressure changes 83
Plicatic acid 30, 95
Pneumonitis, drug-induced 205
Pneumothorax 72, 590
Poiseuille equation 81
Pollen allergens 10–11, 44, 68, 101, 102, 104, 424
   allergic rhinitis 273
   avoidance 351
   transient asthma 29–30
Post-partum care 502
Post-traumatic stress disorder 515, 518, 562
Potential asthma 5
Practice protocols 295–296
Pranlukast 223
Pre-employment testing 446, 449
Pre-menstrual exacerbations 502–503, 563
Pre-term birth 13, 497, 498
Prednisolone 188, 189, 560, 582
   children 358, 368, 402, 408, 409, 410
   difficult (therapy-resistant) asthma 567
Prednisone 188
   difficult (therapy-resistant) asthma 567
   pregnancy 501
Pregnancy 49, 495–502
   asthma education 303
   asthma management 498–502
      medication 205, 499–501, *499*, 502
   effects of asthma 497–498
   effects on asthma 496–497, *498*
   inhaled steroids safety 188
   labour/delivery 502
   maternal exclusion diet 151
   post-partum care 502
   pulmonary function 495–496, *496*, *497*
Pressure-volume curves *84*

Prevalence   7–13
  international differences   7
  population surveys/questionnaires   6
Prevention   12–13
  acute severe asthma   432
  primary   7, 10, 149–152, *153*
  secondary   7–8, 11
  tertiary   8, 10
Primary care   613–626, *613*
  acute asthma management   621–624
  community care organization   616–621
  diagnosis   613–616
  special interest groups   624, 626
  useful addresses   629
Primary prevention   7, 10, 149–152, *153*
Propellants   261, 263, 264, 303, 362
  patient education   303
Prostaglandin D2   32–33
Prostaglandin E2   34, 502
Prostaglandin F2α   502, 503
Prostaglandins   32–33
Proton pump inhibitors   522
Provocation tests   28, *28*, 63, 91–96
  allergy diagnosis   69
  aspirin/NSAIDs-induced asthma   454
  childhood asthma diagnosis   57, 344
  epidemiological studies   6
  hyperosmolar challenge in exercise-induced asthma
    479, *480*
  occupational asthma   446
  sputum eosinophilia   110
  stimuli   *92*
    non-selective   91–95
    selective   95–96
Provocative dose (PD$_{20}$)   28
Pseudoasthma   189, 560
Psychiatric disorders   515, 562, 599
Psychological factors   48–49, 515–518
  asthma management approaches   515–518, *516*
  childhood asthma   378, *379*
  symptoms perceptions   334
Psychosocial factors
  complications   598–600
  difficult (therapy-resistant) asthma   562–563
  mortality/near-fatal asthma associations   432, 647–648
Public awareness   303
Pulmonary elastance   82–83
Pulmonary eosinophilic infiltrations   71
Pulmonary function changes, pregnancy   495–496, *497*
Pulmonary mechanics   81–83
  asthma   83–84, 564
  dyspnoea   84
  elastance   82–83, *82*

  inertance   83
  pressure measurements   83
  resistance   81–82
Pulmonary microembolism   71
Pulmonary parasitic infection   71
Pulse oximetry   74, 438
Pulsus paradoxus   407, 439

Quality Adjusted Life Years (QALYs)   138
Quality assurance   643, 649
Quality of life   598–599
  assessment *see* Health-related quality of life
Quality of Well-being Scale   138
Questionnaires   6, 64
  health-related quality of life   137–139
    cultural adaptation   139
  occupational asthma diagnosis   443
  patient satisfaction surveys   647
  sensitivity/specificity   65

RANTES   32
Reactive airway dysfunction syndrome (irritant-induced
    occupational asthma)   447, 449
Reactive oxygen species (ROS)   114
Remission   5
  population studies   23
Respiratory infections   591
  chronic   597
Respiratory insufficiency, lung function tests   85
Respiratory muscle fatigue   589, *589*
Respiratory muscle stress   83
Respiratory specialist care   646, *646*
  economic evaluations   660
Respiratory syncytial virus   54, 150, 616
Rhinoscopy   70
Rhinovirus infection   341
Rhizopus   163, 164
Risk factors   7–11, 8, *12*, 13
  chilhood asthma population studies   19, 21
  mortality *see* Mortality
  preventive approaches   9, *9*, *12*, 13
Rotadisk   264
Rotahaler/Rotacaps   264

St. George's Respiratory Questionnaire   138
Salbutamol   237, *238*, 240, 241, 324
  acute severe asthma   400, 409, 437
  childhood asthma   354, 370, 400, 409
  delivery systems   263, 264
  difficult (therapy-resistant) asthma   568
  dose dependency   240
  exercise-induced asthma   475, *476*, 477
  ipratropium bromide combination   248

isomers 241–242
Salicylic acid 422, 458
Salmeterol 183, 237, *238*, 239
  childhood asthma 354, 367, 376, 377
  economic evaluations 659
  exercise-induced asthma 376, 475, 477
  fluticasone combination 183, 245
  formoterol comparison 245
  inhaled steroid combined treatment 245
  multi-centre studies 245
  nocturnal asthma 377, 489
  pharmacology 242, *243*, 244, *244*
  pregnancy 500
  tolerance 245–246
School environment 380
School teachers 347
  education 303, 380
Secondary prevention 7–8, 11, 422
Secretory leukoprotease inhibitor 176
Sedation for mechanical ventilation 593
Self-management plans 300, 302, 309–319, 423, 618, 621,
    622–623
  acute severe asthma
    follow-up 436
    recognition 622, *623*
  childhood asthma 347, 370, 410–411
  components 309–312
  deteriorating asthma
    management 311
    recognition 309–311, *309*
  efficacy 312–313, *313*
  models 313–314, *314, 315, 316, 317, 318*
  peak expiratory flow (PEF) measurements 310, 311,
    618, *619*, 622–623
  self-referral/admission to hospital 312
  severe asthma
    management 312
    recognition 311
  stable asthma
    management 311–312
    recognition 310
  therapeutic response *311*
  unstable asthma
    management 312
    recognition 309, 310
  use in practice 314–316
    high-risk asthma 316
    mild asthma 314–315
    moderate/severe asthma 315–316
Severe asthma 427
  acute attack *see* Acute severe asthma
  children
    drug treatment *348*, 367–368

persistence in adulthood 22
  chronic symptoms 595–596
  population surveys 6
  psychosocial factors 562
  self-management plans 315–316
    management 312
    recognition 311
  sputum eosinophilia 110, *111*
Severity assessment 4, 4
  acute asthma 405–408, *406*, 432, *433, 434, 435*
  childhood asthma 348–349, *348*
    acute attack 405–408, *406*
    infants/young children 405–406
  classification 72, *73*
  exacerbations 72–74, *75*
  histamine/methacholine inhalation tests 93
  history-taking 64–65, *64*
  self-management plans *see* Self-management plans
  subjective versus objective perceptions 128–129, 144,
    300, 310, 333–334, 405, 432, 487–488
Severity classification 5, 72, *73, 424*
Sickness Impact Prolife (SIP) 137
Sinus X-ray 57, 70
Sinusitis (rhinosinusitis) 488, 509, 530, 537–548
  adjuvant medication 545–547
  antibiotic treatment 542, 544–545, *545*
  asthma association 538–541
  classification 537, *539*
  definition 537
  difficult asthma 561
  history-taking 542–543
  microbiology 541–542, *542*
  nasal ensoscopy 543–544
  physical examination 543
  predisposing conditions 537, *538*
  pregnancy 498
  surgical treatment 547
Skin tests 4, 68–69, 102–103
  allergen extracts 102
  allergic rhinitis 544
  childhood asthma diagnosis 344, 345
  epicutaneous 102–103, *102*
    wheal response 103
  food allergy-induced asthma 554
  intradermal testing 103
  occupational asthma 445
  positive/negative controls 102
Sleep apnoea 488–489
Sleep quality 599
Smoking 23, 48, 424
  adolescents 351, 374, 375
  cessation 498–499, 577–578, 582
  emphysema association 596

Smoking *contd.*
  parental/passive 11, 13, 22, 29, 150
    childhood asthma 351, *352*
    childhood cough 55, 526
    exposure reduction 152, 422
    wheezing in infancy 54
  persistent asthma risk 21, 22
  pregnancy 19, 331, 498–499
Smooth muscle changes 35
Socioeconomic status 517
Sodium cromoglycate 197–198, 287, 311, 374, 425, 426, 579
  childhood asthma 358–359, 366, 367, 376
  delivery systems 264
  economic evaluations 659
  exercise-induced asthma 376, 471, 475, 477
  food allergy-induced asthma 555, 557
  pregnancy 501
Spacer systems 185, 261, 262–263
  children 362–363, 368, 370, 400, 408
  exercise-induced asthma 475
  indications *262*
  infants 374
Special interest groups 624, 626
Spinal manipulation 288, 360
Spinhaler 264
Spirometry 85
  asthma diagnosis 65–66
  childhood asthma 342, 343–344
  exacerbation severity assessment 73
  pregnancy 496
Sputum, induced 107–112, 602
  acute inflammatory response studies 30
  asthma diagnosis 70
  bronchoscopic measures comparison 108–109
  cell counts 109, *110*, 144–145, *145*
  clinical correlates 110–112, *111*
  eosinophils 109, 110, *111*
    corticosteroid response prediction 110–112, *111*
  mast cells *111*, 112
  measurement issues 108–109, *108*
  mechanisms 107
  sample collection/analysis 107–108
Stable asthma
  management 311–312
  recognition 310
Standard Gamble 138
Stem cell factor (SCF) 178
Sulphite challenge tests 96
Sulphur dioxide 11, 48, 150, 224, 422, 479
Support groups 347
Surgical treatment 288
  sinusitis 547
Sympathomimetics 237–246
Symptom diaries, childhood asthma 342, 349

Symptoms
  childhood asthma 340–341
    acute severe attack 407
    prodromal 366, *367*, 369
  chronic 595–596
  clinical status assessment 127–128, 131, 143–144, *144*
  functional impairments 136–137
  leukotriene modifier effects 224–225
  population surveys 6
  practical assessment 131
  presenting (asthma diagnosis) 614, *614*
  progression of severity 65
  psychological factors in perception 515, 516–517
  severity-drug use relationship 131
  subjective versus objective assessment 128–129, 144, 300, 310, 333–334, 432
    children 405
    nocturnal asthma 487–488

Tachycardia 432
Tachykinins 177, 531
Tachypnoea 432
Terbutaline 237, *238*, 239, 241
  acute severe asthma 437
    children 401, 409
  delivery systems 265
  difficult (therapy-resistant) asthma 568
  exercise-induced asthma 477
  pregnancy 499, 500
Tertiary prevention 8, 10
TH$_1$ helper T cell cytokines
  asthma primary preventive approach 151
  childhood infections 150
TH$_2$ helper T cell cytokines 32
  airway inflammation 54
  allergic bronchopulmonary aspergillosis 465
  bronchoalveolar lavage (BAL) fluid 120
  nitric oxide-associated induction 113
  perpetuation in young children 150, 151
  pregnancy outcome 149
  respiratory syncytial virus response 54, 150
TH$_2$ helper T cells, corticosteroid effects 177
Theophylline 183, 237, 241, 248, 287, 426, 578
  anti-inflammatory activity 248
  childhood asthma 354–355, 367
    acute 403, *404*
  difficult (therapy-resistant) asthma 568
  exercise-induced asthma 477
  mechanism of action 248
  nocturnal asthma 489–490
  pregnancy 500–501, 502
  side effects 248, 355, 403–404, *592*
Therapeutic trial 63
  children 56, 57

diagnosis 68
  difficult asthma 560
Thromboxane A$_2$ 32–33, 225
Thromboxane B$_2$ 225
Thromboxane receptor antagonists 225
Thromboxane synthase 225
Thromboxane synthesis inhibitors 225
Thyroid disease 49
Tiffeneau index (FEV$_1$/VC) 85
Time Trade Off 138
Timolol 562
Tiotropium bromide 247–248
Tipredane 190
Toluene diisocyanate (TDI) 30, 96
Transcription factors 174, 176
Transient asthma 29–30, *31*
Transpulmonary pressure measurements 83
Triamcinolone 182
Trichophyton 163, 165, 562
Trigger factors 43, *44*
  history-taking 64, 65
  see also Environmental factors
Trivial asthma 5
Troleandomycin 183, 211–213, 581
  clinical trials 211, *213*, 214
  side effects 213
Tuberculosis 582
Tumour necrosis factor (TNFα) 113, 149, 177, 178
Turbohaler 264–265, 364, 368
Turbohaler inhalation computer (TIC) 325–326

Ultrasonic nebulizers 266
Uncontrolled asthma
  management 432
  recognition 432
Unstable asthma
  management 312
  recognition 309, 310
  see also Brittle asthma
Upper airway obstruction 71, 559
Upper respiratory tract changes in pregnancy 495
Urine tests 70, 602

Vaccination/immunization 150–151
Vasculitis 427
Ventilation in pregnancy 496
Ventilatory insufficiency, lung function tests 85
Viral live vaccines 582
Viral respiratory infection 43, 45, 150, 562
  childhood asthma
    acute severe attack 408
    management 366, 370
    trigger factor 341
  cough 54

immunostimulatory role in young children 150
  wheezing
    children 339
    infants 53, 54, 373, 374
    pathophysiology 54
Vital capacity (VC) 65, 81
Vocal cord dysfunction 508, 517, 518, 559, 560
  exercise-induced asthma 479
Volumatic 363, 368, 475
Volume replacement 591

Weakness syndromes, post-mechanical ventilation 593
Weight gain, corticosteroids-associated 581
Western red cedar 30, 95, 488
Wheal response 103
Wheezing
  children *340*
    asthma diagnosis 340, 341, 342, 615
    clinical status assessment 72, 127, 131
    history-taking 64
  infants 19, 53–54, 55, 372
    asthma diagnosis 55
    treatment 373–374, *374*
  mechanism 127
  viral-associated *see* Viral respiratory infection
Wheezy bronchitis 21, 373
Wine-induced asthma 553
Work of breathing 589
Work disability 599–600
Workplace challenge test 95
Wright peak-flow meter 129, *129*
Written information 369, 423

Xanthines 248–249
  acute asthma treatment 248–249
    children 403
  anti-inflammatory activity 248
  mechanism of action 248
  pregnancy 500–501

Yoga 287

Zafirlukast 223, 227
  children 359
  pregnancy 501
  sinusitis 546–547
Zileuton 223, 456
  pregnancy 501
  side effects 225
  sinusitis 546, 547
"Zone" self-management plans 314, *317*, *318*
  childhood asthma management 369, *369*
  peak expiratory flow (PEF) charts 618, *619*

Printed and bound by CPI Group (UK) Ltd, Croydon, CR0 4YY

08/05/2025

01864766-0001